100+ CLINICAL CASES IN PEDIATRICS

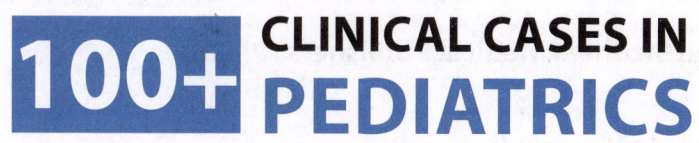

100+ CLINICAL CASES IN PEDIATRICS

Sixth Edition

R Arvind MBBS DCH DNB
Consultant Pediatrician and Neonatologist
Medical Director
Vathsalya Speciality Clinic
Bengaluru, Karnataka, India

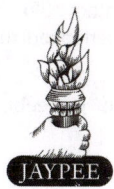

JAYPEE

JAYPEE BROTHERS MEDICAL PUBLISHERS
The Health Sciences Publisher
New Delhi | London

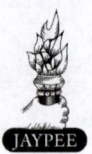

Jaypee Brothers Medical Publishers (P) Ltd.

Headquarters
Jaypee Brothers Medical Publishers (P) Ltd
EMCA House, 23/23-B
Ansari Road, Daryaganj
New Delhi 110 002, India
Landline: +91-11-23272143, +91-11-23272703
+91-11-23282021, +91-11-23245672
Email: jaypee@jaypeebrothers.com

Corporate Office
Jaypee Brothers Medical Publishers (P) Ltd
4838/24, Ansari Road, Daryaganj
New Delhi 110 002, India
Phone: +91-11-43574357
Fax: +91-11-43574314
Email: jaypee@jaypeebrothers.com

Overseas Office
JP Medical Ltd.
83, Victoria Street, London
SW1H 0HW (UK)
Phone: +44 20 3170 8910
Fax: +44 (0)20 3008 6180
Email: info@jpmedpub.com

Website: www.jaypeebrothers.com
Website: www.jaypeedigital.com

© 2025, Jaypee Brothers Medical Publishers

The views and opinions expressed in this book are solely those of the original contributor(s)/author(s) and do not necessarily represent those of editor(s) or publisher of the book.

All rights reserved. No part of this publication may be reproduced, stored or transmitted in any form or by any means, electronic, mechanical, photo copying, recording or otherwise, without the prior permission in writing of the publishers.

All brand names and product names used in this book are trade names, service marks, trademarks or registered trademarks of their respective owners. The publisher is not associated with any product or vendor mentioned in this book.

Medical knowledge and practice change constantly. This book is designed to provide accurate, authoritative information about the subject matter in question. However, readers are advised to check the most current information available on procedures included and check information from the manufacturer of each product to be administered, to verify the recommended dose, formula, method and duration of administration, adverse effects and contra indications. It is the responsibility of the practitioner to take all appropriate safety precautions. Neither the publisher nor the author(s)/editor(s) assume any liability for any injury and/or damage to persons or property arising from or related to use of material in this book.

This book is sold on the understanding that the publisher is not engaged in providing professional medical services. If such advice or services are required, the services of a competent medical professional should be sought.

Every effort has been made where necessary to contact holders of copyright to obtain permission to reproduce copyright material. If any have been inadvertently overlooked, the publisher will be pleased to make the necessary arrangements at the first opportunity.

Inquiries for bulk sales may be solicited at: jaypee@jaypeebrothers.com

100+ Clinical Cases in Pediatrics

Fourth Edition: 2016
Fifth Edition: 2021
Sixth Edition: **2025**

ISBN: 978-93-5696-572-0

Printed in India at Rajkamal Electric Press, Kundli, Haryana -131 028.

Dedicated to

My beloved father
Late Shri N Rajasekhar

Preface to the Sixth Edition

100+ Clinical Cases in Pediatrics, 6th edition is revised and updated with the recent developments in the field of pediatrics. Suggestions from the reader and students have been taken into consideration while revising the edition. All the cases have been updated including discussion, etiology, molecular and genetic science, and recent diagnostic evaluation to reach correct diagnosis and management for each case. Three new cases—adenoids, pancreatitis, and dermatomyositis—have been added in this edition.

The clinical features of the cases have been illustrated with line diagrams and photographs. The comprehensive glossary, which has been provided, has been revised and updated. This helps as ready reckoner for undergraduate and postgraduate students preparing for competitive examinations.

This book helps to improve the clinical and practical approach for undergraduate students, interns, and residents in presentation and diagnosis of clinical cases. It will be helpful for the postgraduate students and practicing pediatricians.

R Arvind

Preface to the First Edition

With the new Medical Council of India (MCI) guidelines laying more emphasis on clinical and practical skill development rather than theoretical knowledge, there is immense need for a book on common clinical cases in pediatrics. The present book attempts to fulfill this need and aims to help the undergraduate medical students, interns, and residents in diagnosis and presentation of clinical cases. It would also be helpful to the postgraduate students and the practicing pediatricians.

The most commonly encountered and typical cases have been grouped into 12 categories that include birth defects and genetic disorders, respiratory, cardiovascular, gastrointestinal, hematological, renal, central nervous system, endocrine and metabolic, nutritional, oncological disorders, disorders of connective tissue, bones and joints, and the infectious diseases. Each case has been discussed in detail under history, clinical features, differential diagnosis, complications, and treatment. At the end of each case, multiple choice questions have been added to help the student in revision. A comprehensive and exhaustive glossary has also been included. The book is well illustrated with photographs wherever required.

I thank my wife Dr Chetana, for her suggestions and professional help. I am also thankful to Rachana and Shikhar, the gems of my family, for their cooperation.

I express my deep gratitude to M/s Cyber Avenue, for typing the manuscript.

R Arvind

Acknowledgments

I thank my wife Dr Chetana for her professional help. I am thankful to my children Rachana and Shikhar for their cooperation. I express my deep gratitude to Mr Abhishek for typing the manuscript.

My special thanks are due to Shri Jitendar P Vij (Group Chairman), Mr Ankit Vij (Managing Director), Mr MS Mani (Group President), Ms Chetna Malhotra (Senior Director – Professional Publishing, Marketing and Business Development), Ms Pooja Bhandari [Director – Production (Books and Journals)], Asmi Bharati (Development Editor), and staff of M/s Jaypee Brothers Medical Publishers (P) Ltd, New Delhi, India.

Contents

Section 1	Genetics	
Case 1	Down Syndrome	3
Case 2	Klinefelter's Syndrome	14
Case 3	Turner Syndrome	18

Section 2	Respiratory System	
Case 4	Adenoids	27
Case 5	Bronchial Asthma	32
Case 6	Bronchiectasis	54
Case 7	Bronchiolitis	63
Case 8	Croup	72
Case 9	Empyema	78
Case 10	Otitis Media	85
Case 11	Pneumonia	97
Case 12	Tuberculosis	108

Section 3	Cardiovascular System	
Case 13	Atrial Septal Defect	141
Case 14	Coarctation of Aorta	148
Case 15	Infective Endocarditis	153
Case 16	Patent Ductus Arteriosus	167
Case 17	Pericarditis with Effusion	173
Case 18	Sydenham's Chorea	183
Case 19	Tetralogy of Fallot	186
Case 20	Ventricular Septal Defect	196

Section 4 Gastrointestinal System

- Case 21 Acute Gastroenteritis 207
- Case 22 Appendicitis 226
- Case 23 Congenital Hypertrophic Pyloric Stenosis 236
- Case 24 Diaphragmatic Hernia 244
- Case 25 Duodenal Atresia 253
- Case 26 Gastroesophageal Reflux 258
- Case 27 Hepatitis 270
- Case 28 Hirschsprung's Disease 278
- Case 29 Intussusception 286
- Case 30 Liver Abscess 294
- Case 31 Necrotizing Enterocolitis 301
- Case 32 Pancreatitis 310
- Case 33 Tracheoesophageal Fistula 314
- Case 34 Wilson's Disease 321

Section 5 Hematological System

- Case 35 Hemophilia 333
- Case 36 Hemorrhagic Disease of the Newborn 345
- Case 37 Henoch–Schönlein Purpura 352
- Case 38 Hereditary Spherocytosis 357
- Case 39 Idiopathic Thrombocytopenic Purpura 364
- Case 40 Iron Deficiency Anemia 374
- Case 41 Polycythemia 386
- Case 42 Sickle Cell Anemia 392
- Case 43 Thalassemia 412

Section 6 Renal System

- Case 44 Acute Poststreptococcal Glomerulonephritis 429
- Case 45 Hemolytic Uremic Syndrome 439

| Case 46 | Nephrotic Syndrome | 449 |
| Case 47 | Urinary Tract Infection | 467 |

Section 7 — Central Nervous System

Case 48	Acute Hemiplegia of Childhood	485
Case 49	Cerebral Palsy	493
Case 50	Duchenne Muscular Dystrophy	508
Case 51	Epilepsy	515
Case 52	Febrile Convulsions	526
Case 53	Guillain–Barré Syndrome	533
Case 54	Hydrocephalus	540
Case 55	Meningitis	551
Case 56	Meningomyelocele	565

Section 8 — Endocrine System

Case 57	Ambiguous Genitalia	575
Case 58	Congenital Adrenal Hyperplasia	583
Case 59	Cushing's Syndrome	594
Case 60	Diabetes Insipidus	601
Case 61	Diabetes Mellitus	610
Case 62	Hypothyroidism	617
Case 63	Precocious Puberty	627
Case 64	Undescended Testes	640

Section 9 — Infectious Diseases

Case 65	Chikungunya	649
Case 66	Congenital Rubella	653
Case 67	Congenital Syphilis	661
Case 68	Dengue Fever	670
Case 69	Herpes Zoster	679
Case 70	Human Immunodeficiency Virus	686

Case 71	Infectious Mononucleosis	696
Case 72	Malaria	704
Case 73	Measles	716
Case 74	Mumps	725
Case 75	Osteomyelitis	731
Case 76	Poliomyelitis	742
Case 77	Septic Arthritis	751
Case 78	Tetanus Neonatorum	760
Case 79	Typhoid	767
Case 80	Varicella	776
Case 81	Whooping Cough	785

Section 10 Newborn

Case 82	Birth Asphyxia	797
Case 83	Neonatal Seizures	812
Case 84	Neonatal Hypoglycemia	825
Case 85	Neonatal Pathological Jaundice	831
Case 86	Normal Newborn	850
Case 87	Premature Infant	873
Case 88	Respiratory Distress Syndrome	886

Section 11 Nutrition

Case 89	Obesity	909
Case 90	Protein–Energy Malnutrition	916
Case 91	Rickets	928
Case 92	Scurvy	939

Section 12 Neoplastic Diseases

Case 93	Ewing's Sarcoma	947
Case 94	Hodgkin's Disease	953
Case 95	Leukemia	964

Case 96	Neuroblastoma	979
Case 97	Osteosarcoma	990
Case 98	Retinoblastoma	998
Case 99	Wilms' Tumor	1006

Section 13 Rheumatic Diseases

Case 100	Acute Rheumatic Fever	1017
Case 101	Hurler's Syndrome	1031
Case 102	Dermatomyositis	1035
Case 103	Juvenile Rheumatoid Arthritis	1041

Section 14 Miscellaneous

Case 104	Congenital Dislocation of Hip	1059
Case 105	Leprosy	1067
Case 106	Marfan's Syndrome	1082
Case 107	Osteogenesis Imperfecta	1090
Case 108	Talipes	1099

Glossary 1105

Index 1129

Plate 1

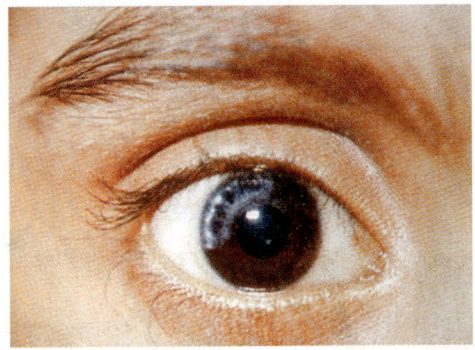

Fig. 2: Brushfield spots. *(Case 1)*

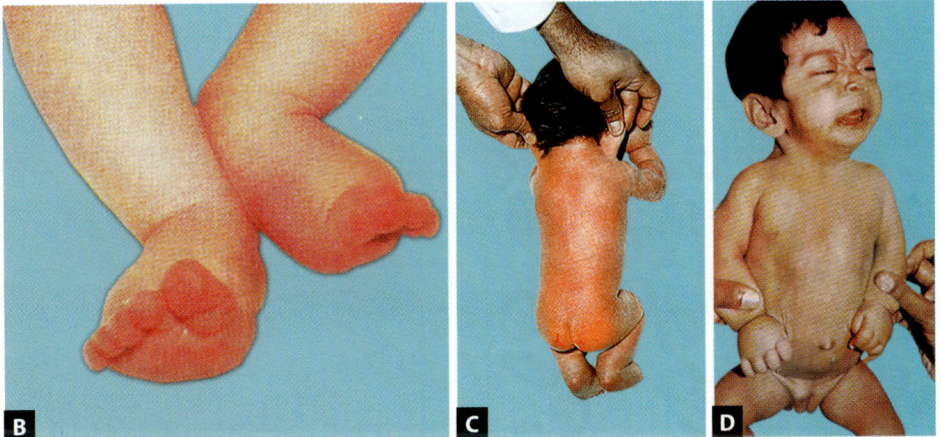

Figs. 1B to D: (B) Lymphedema of feet; (C) Low hairline; and (D) Short neck. *(Case 3)*

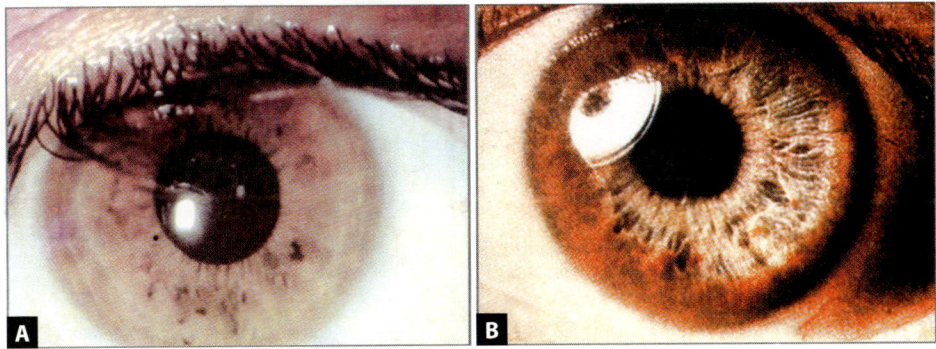

Figs. 2A and B: Kayser-Fleischer ring. *(Case 34)*

Plate 2

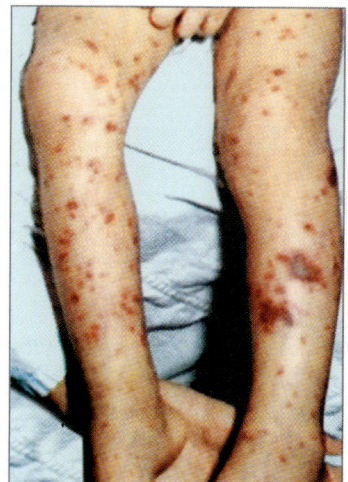

Fig. 2: Petechial rashes. *(Case 39)*

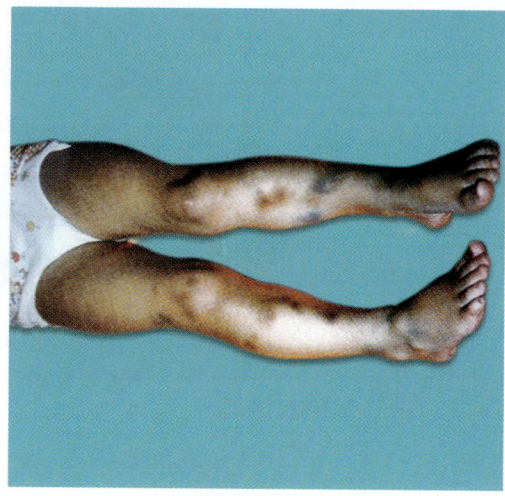

Fig. 3: Purpura. *(Case 39)*

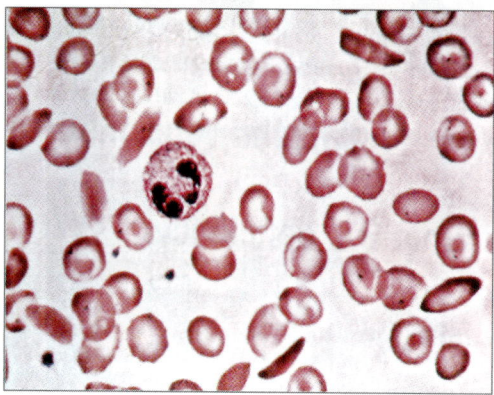

Fig. 3: Sickle cells. *(Case 42)*

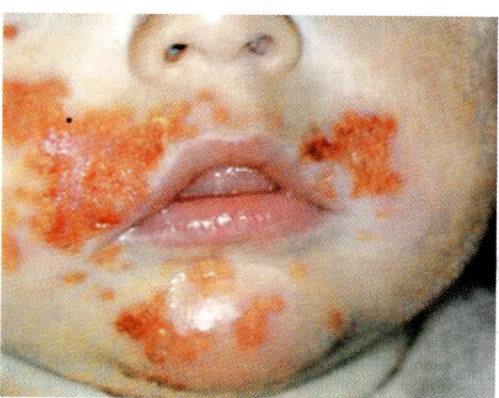

Fig. 2: Impetigo. *(Case 44)*

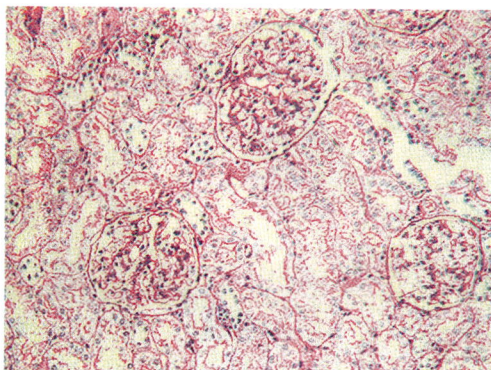

Fig. 1: Minimal change nephrotic syndrome. *(Case 46)*

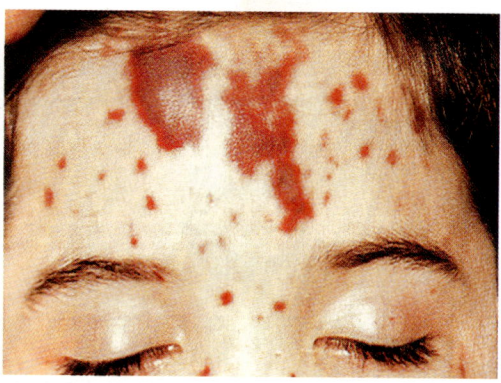

Fig. 2: Purpuric rash of meningococcus. *(Case 55)*

Plate 3

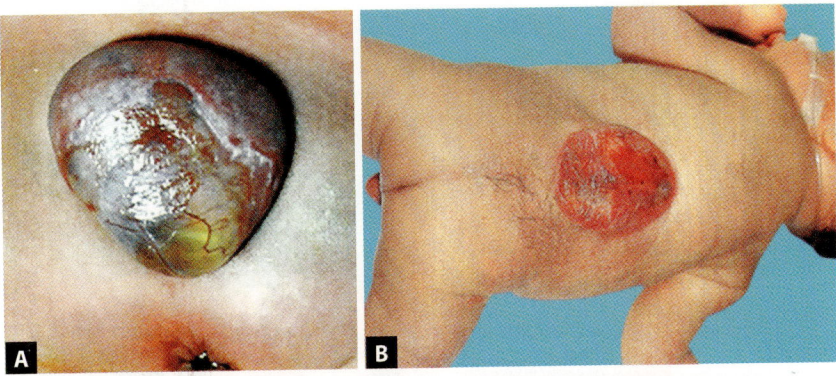

Figs. 1A and B: (A) Meningomyelocele; (B) Myelomeningocele. *(Case 56)*

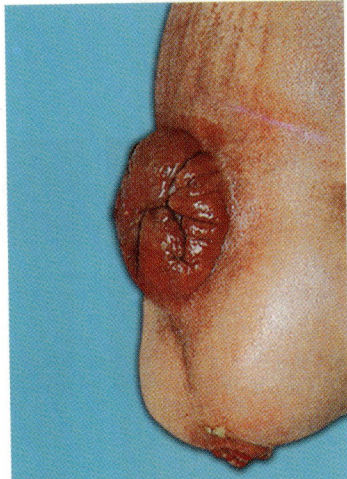

Fig. 2: Meningomyelocele. *(Case 56)*

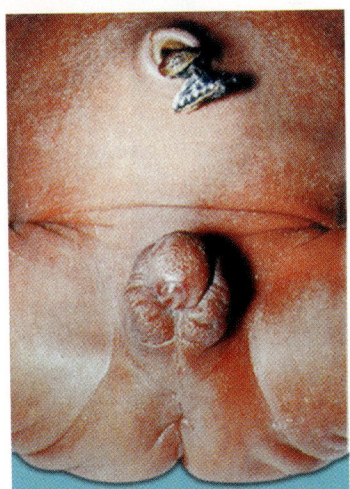

Fig. 2: Congenital adrenal hyperplasia. *(Case 58)*

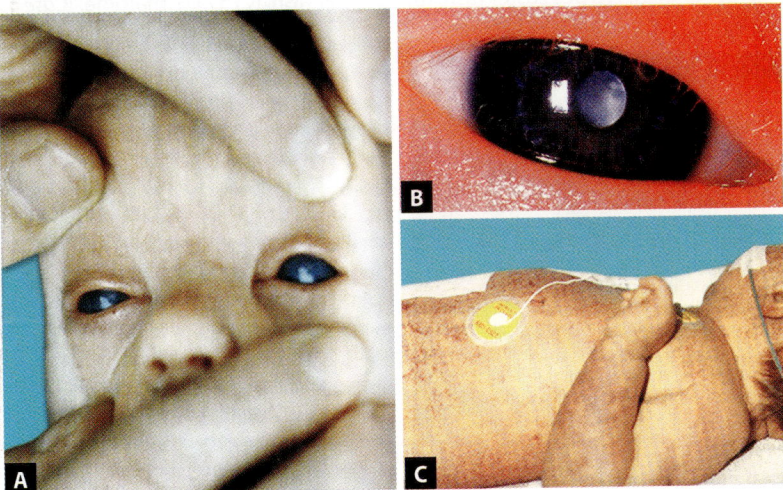

Figs. 2A to C: (A and B) Cataract and (C) Congenital rubella. *(Case 66)*

Plate 4

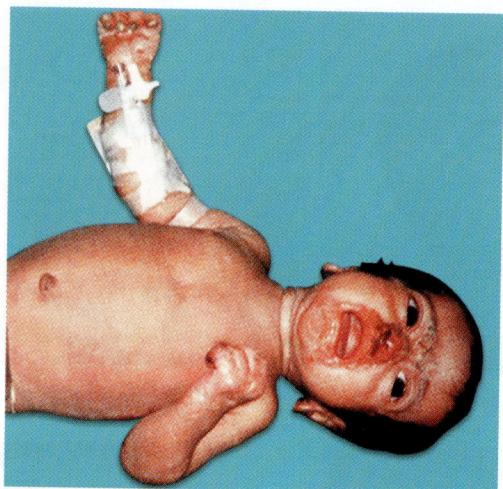

Fig. 2: Mucocutaneous manifestation of an infant. *(Case 67)*

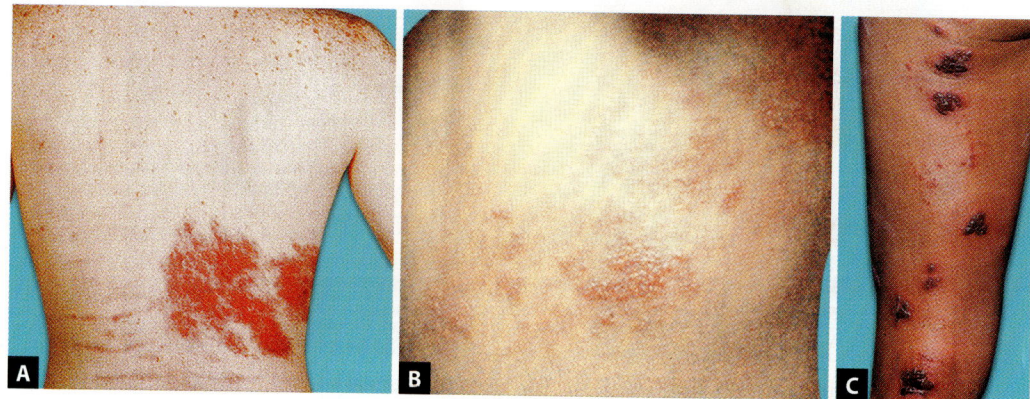

Figs. 1A to C: (A) Herpes zoster rash; (B) Vesicular rash; (C) S1 Dermatome. *(Case 69)*

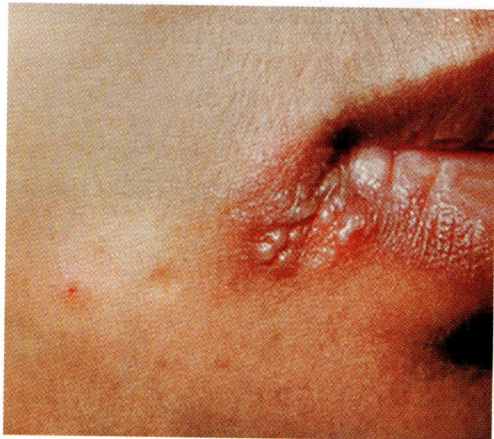

Fig. 2: Herpes simplex vesicles. *(Case 69)*

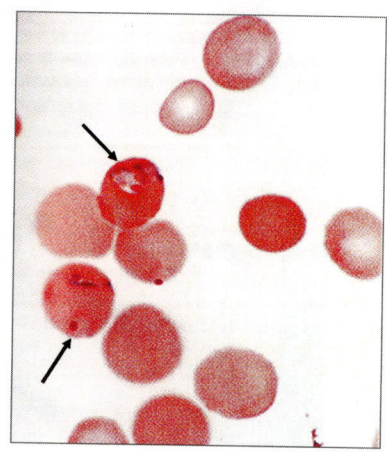

Fig. 3: Peripheral blood smear. *(Case 72)*

Plate 5

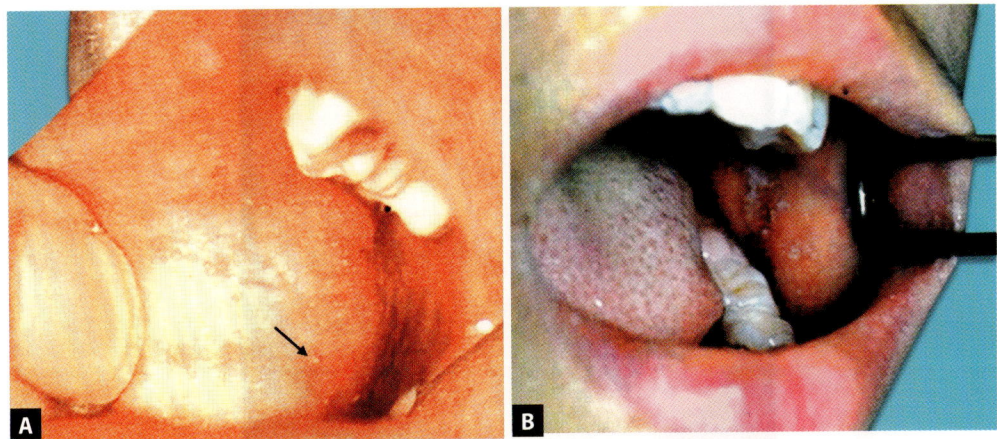

Figs. 2A and B: Koplik spots. *(Case 73)*

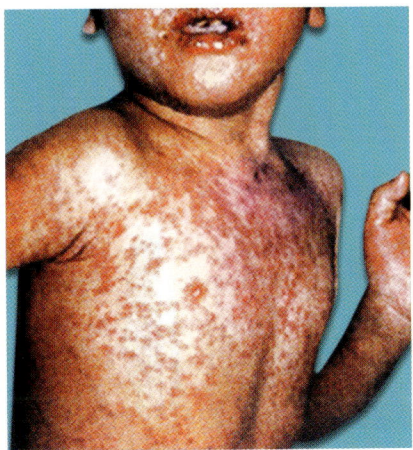

Fig. 3: Maculopapular rashes. *(Case 73)*

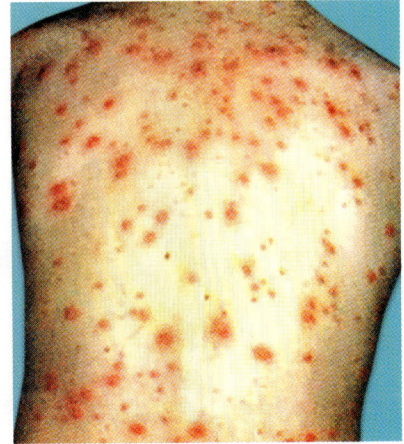

Fig. 1: Pleomorphic rashes. *(Case 80)*

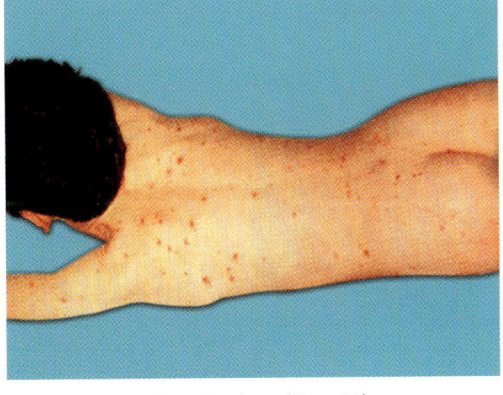

Fig. 3: Rashes. *(Case 80)*

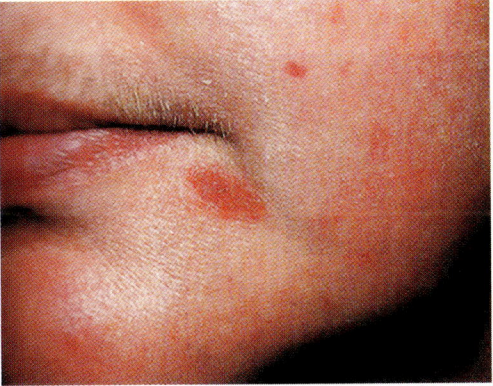

Fig. 4: Herpes simplex. *(Case 80)*

Plate 6

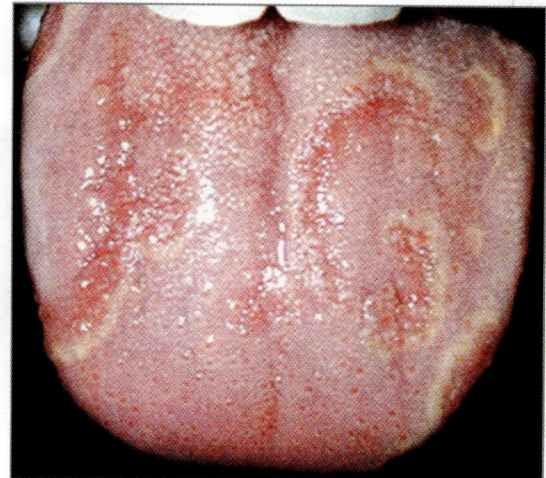

Fig. 5: Geographic tongue. *(Case 86)*

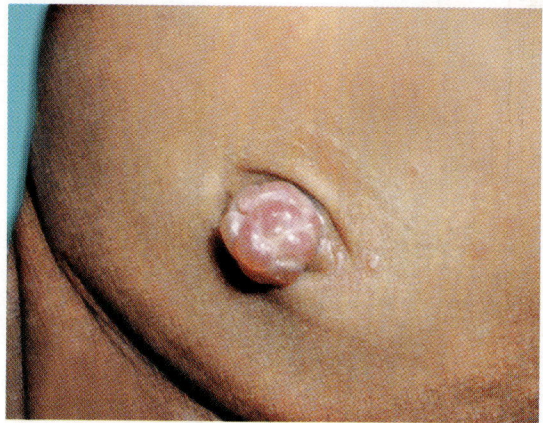

Fig. 11: Umbilical granuloma. *(Case 86)*

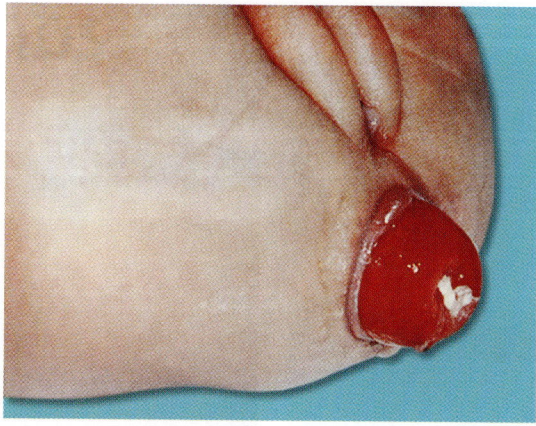

Fig. 14: Rectal prolapse. *(Case 86)*

Plate 7

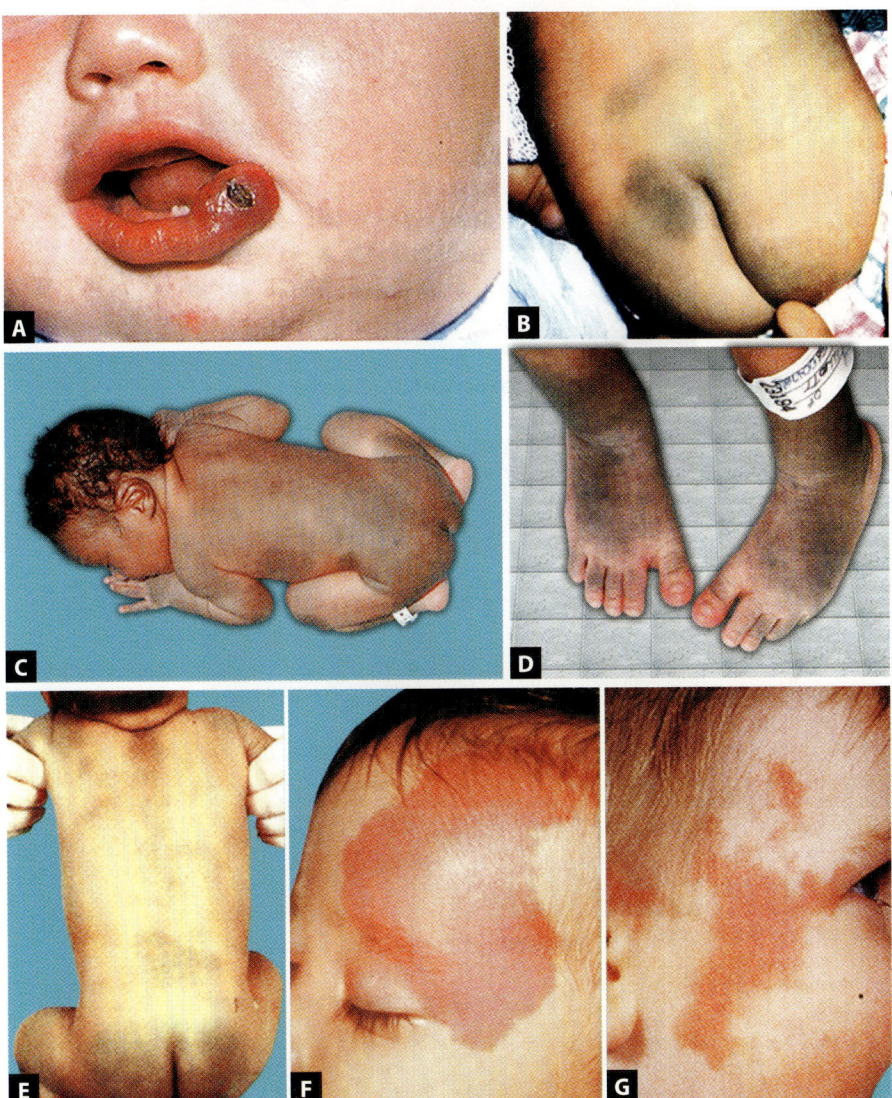

Figs. 18A to G: (A) Strawberry hemangioma; (B) Mongolian spots; (C to E) Mongolian blue spots; (F and G) Port-wine stains. *(Case 86)*

Plate 8

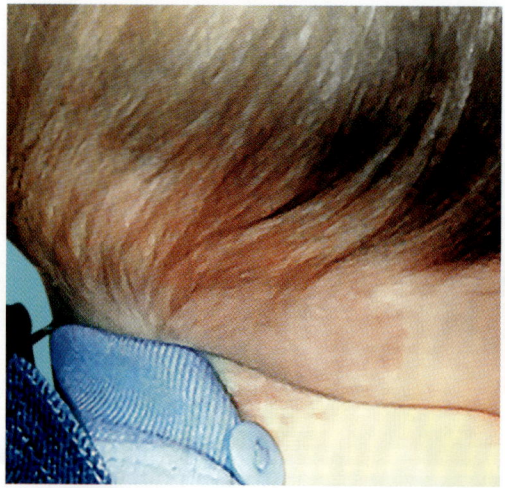

Fig. 20: Salmon patch. *(Case 86)*

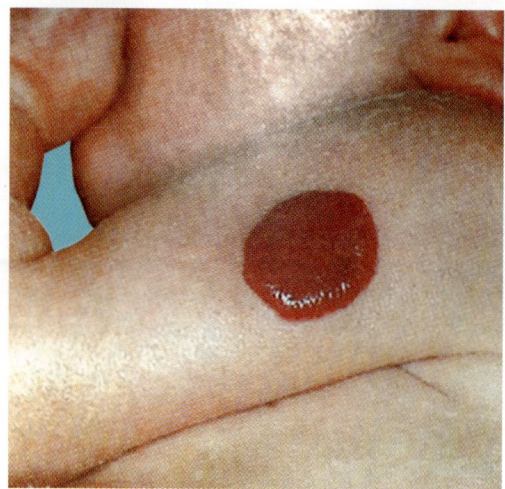

Fig. 21: Strawberry hemangioma. *(Case 86)*

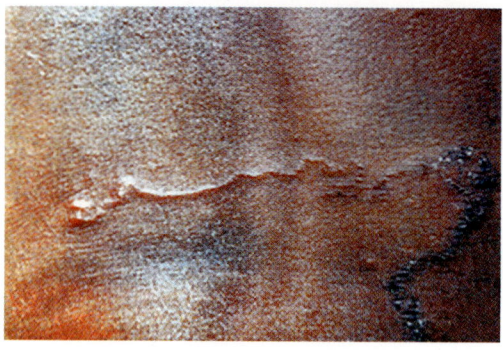

Fig. 22: Visceral larva. *(Case 86)*

Plate 9

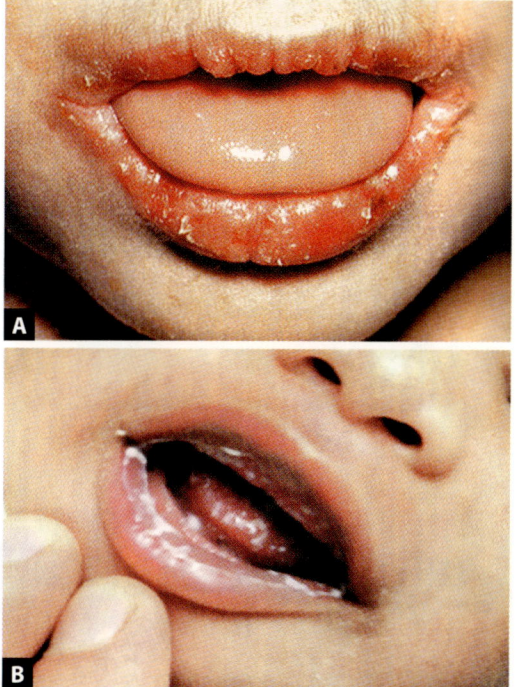

Figs. 3A and B: (A) Glossitis; (B) Oral thrush. *(Case 90)*

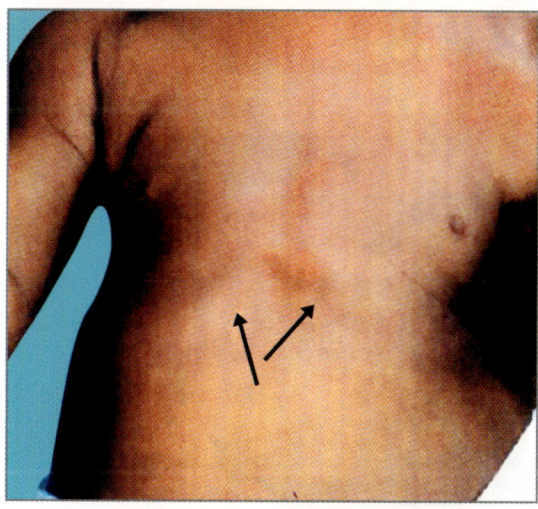

Fig. 5: Harrison sulcus. *(Case 91)*

Plate 10

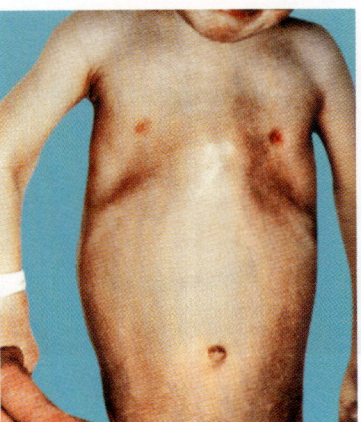

Fig. 6: Pectus carinatum. *(Case 91)*

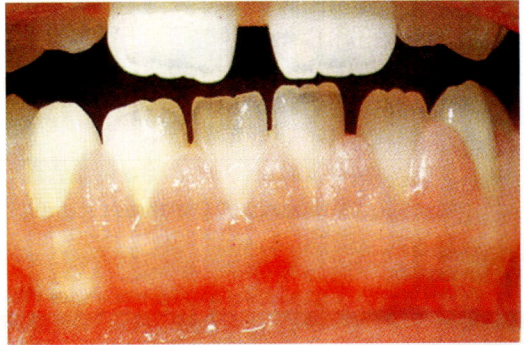

Fig. 2: Gingival hypertrophy. *(Case 92)*

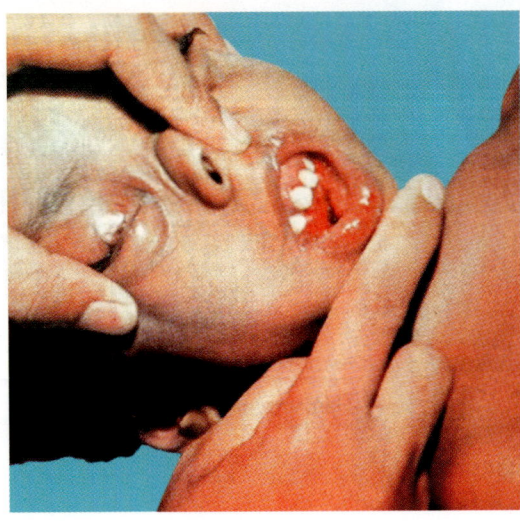

Fig. 3: Gum hypertrophy. *(Case 92)*

Plate 11

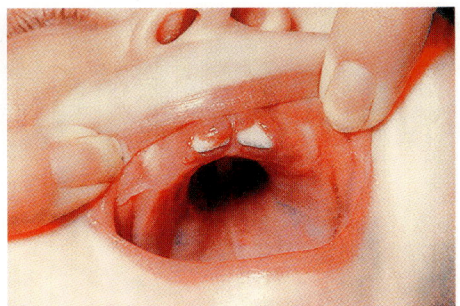

Fig. 4: Bleeding gum. *(Case 92)*

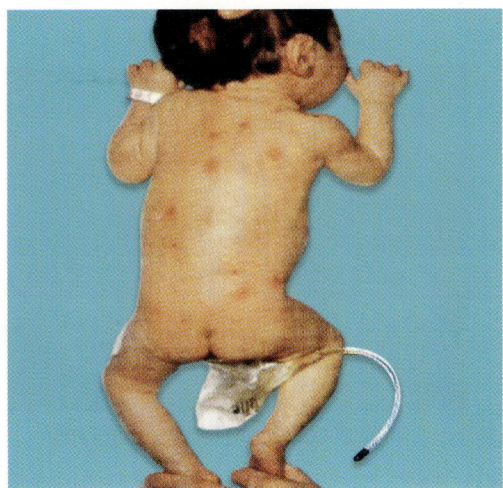

Fig. 1: Congenital leukemia. *(Case 95)*

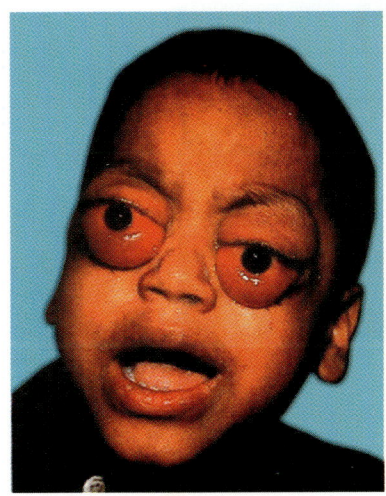

Fig. 3A: Chloroma. *(Case 95)*

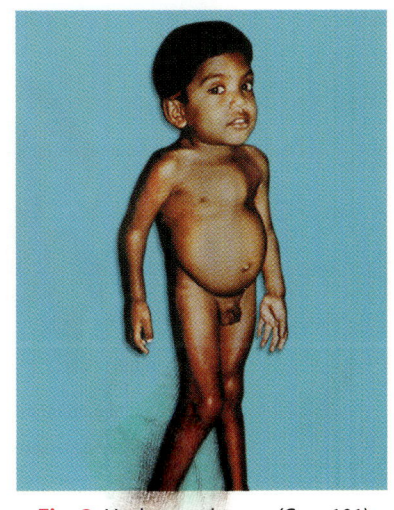

Fig. 2: Hurler syndrome. *(Case 101)*

Plate 12

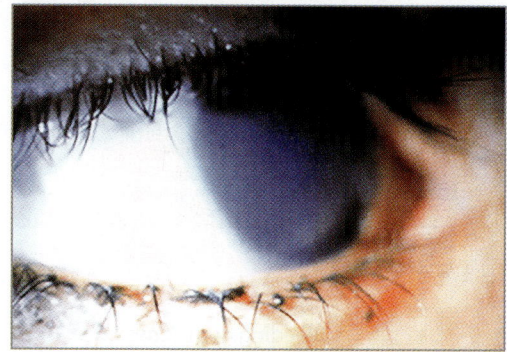

Fig. 4: Corneal clouding. *(Case 101)*

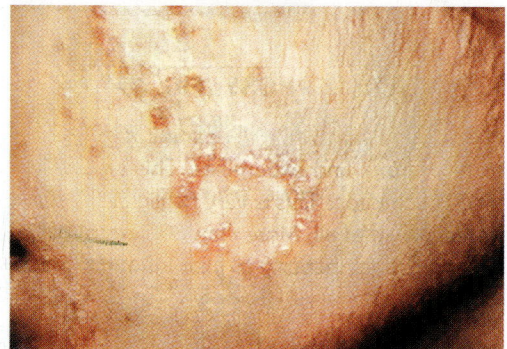

Fig. 2: Cutaneous lesions. *(Case 105)*

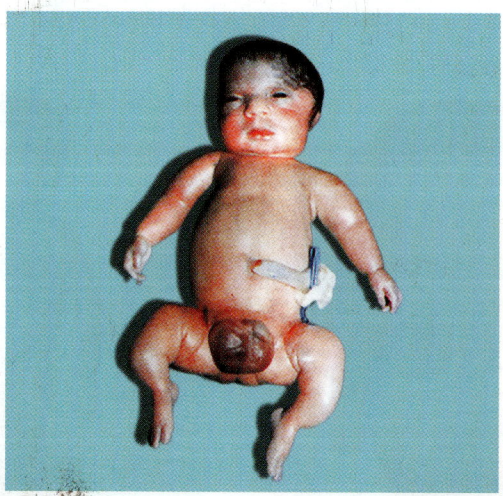

Fig. 3A: Osteogenesis imperfecta (type I). *(Case 107)*

SECTION 1

Genetics

- Case 1 **Down Syndrome**
- Case 2 **Klinefelter's Syndrome**
- Case 3 **Turner Syndrome**

CASE 1

Down Syndrome

■ PRESENTING COMPLAINTS

An 8-month-old girl was brought with the complaint of delayed developmental milestones since 6 months.

History of Presenting Complaints

An 8-month-old girl was brought to the hospital with the history of delayed developmental milestones. The mother was concerned that her child did not even develop neck control. She observed that her child was flabby and did not turn from side-to-side while lying on the bed.

Past History of the Patient

Child was born at term after a normal pregnancy. She was the first sibling of non-consanguineous marriage. Maternal age at the time of the delivery of this child was 35 years and the age of the father was 38 years. Baby cried immediately after the delivery.

The birth weight was 3.25 kg, head circumference was 35 cm, and length of the child was 49 cm. There was normal physiological jaundice after the delivery. Breast milk was given at birth and the child was exclusively on breast milk till 6 months. There were no feeding problems. The child had social smile at the age of 3 months. She did not develop neck control even at the age of 8 months for which she had been brought to the hospital. She had been completely vaccinated.

■ EXAMINATION

Child appeared small for her age. She was playing on the examination table. Her height and weight were on 3rd centile for her age and her head circumference was just below 3rd centile.

CASE AT A GLANCE	
Basic Findings	
Weight	: 6.5 kg (3rd centile)
Head circumference	: 40 cm (2nd centile)
Temperature	: 37°C
Pulse rate	: 116 beats/min
Respiratory rate	: 26 breaths/min
Blood pressure	: 60/40 mm Hg

Positive Findings

History:
- Delayed developmental milestones
- Increased maternal age
- Increased paternal age

Examination:
- Upward slanting of eyes
- Epicanthic folds
- Small nose
- Flat nasal bridge
- Broad hands
- Incurving of the little finger
- Simian crease
- Pansystolic murmur

Investigation:
- Chromosome analysis revealed three copies of chromosome 21
- Chest radiograph showed right ventricular hypertrophy

She was afebrile, pulse was 116 beats/min, respiratory rate was 26 breaths/min. Blood pressure recorded was 60/40 mm Hg. There was neither pallor, lymphadenopathy, nor edema.

Her face was round, there was upward slanting of the eyes with marked epicanthic fold. The nose was small with depressed nasal bridge. The hands were broad and small with short fingers. The little finger was incurved. There was a single palmar crease, i.e., simian crease. Neurological examination revealed the presence of generalized hypotonia. Cardiovascular system revealed the presence of the pansystolic murmur. Per abdominal examination was normal.

■ INVESTIGATION

- *Hemoglobin:* 13 g/dL
- *Total leukocyte count (TLC):* 7,800 cells/cumm
- *Differential leukocyte count (DLC):* P_{65} L_{30} E_3 M_2
- *Chromosome analysis:* Showed three copies of chromosome 21
- *X-ray chest:* Normal

■ DISCUSSION

A child with generalized hypotonia, delayed developmental milestones, upward slanting of the eyes, flat nasal bridge, and simian crease with incurving of the little finger suggests the Down syndrome. The diagnosis is supported by history advanced age of the parents.

John Langdon Down first described the phenotype of the syndrome in 1866. Hence, this was named after him as Down syndrome. It was determined that it was caused by extra chromosome 21 only in 1959.

It is the most common chromosomal disorder. The incidence (without antenatal screening) is 1 in 650 live births. It is the most common autosomal trisomy and the cause of severe learning disorder. In trisomies, there are three representatives of particular chromosome. In Down syndrome, the chromosome number 21 is represented in triplicate.

Cytogenetics

In 90% of cases, Down syndrome is associated with "regular" 21 trisomy giving a total number of 47 chromosomes. The other 10% are due to the balanced translocation involving chromosome 21. Part of an extra chromosome is attached to another. The another extra chromosome is usually 13, 14, 15, 21, or 22.

The origin of the extra chromosome is either from mother or from the father. In most cases, this is from the mother. This is common in a child of the mother conceiving at older age. This is attributed to the exposure of the maternal oocyte to the harmful environmental influences for a longer period. This is because of Graafian follicle present in the fetal life, which exists throughout the female reproductive life. Over-ripening of the ovum results from either delayed fertilization or decreased frequency of the coitus. Viral hepatitis is incorporated because of virus-induced disturbance of chromosomal segregation.

Maternal age-related chromosomal abnormalities include all trisomies and some sex chromosomal abnormalities except 45,X and 47,XYY.

The extra chromosome 21 may result from meiotic nondisjunction, translocation, and mosaicism.

- *Meiotic nondisjunction (94%):* The majority are due to errors in maternal meiosis, which increase with maternal age. Here most cases result from error at meiosis. Here the pair of chromosome 21s fails to separate. Hence one gamete has two chromosome 21s and other one has none. The fertilization of the gamete with the two chromosome 21s results with zygote trisomy 21. Meiotic nondisjunction increases with increasing maternal age. The proportion of pregnancies in elder mother is less and hence newborn affected with down syndrome is more compared with young mothers. Meiotic nondisjunction can occur in spermatogenesis, hence extra chromosome 21 can be paternal origin also. 5% are paternal-derived.

- *Translocation (5%):* Here, the chromosome 21 is translocated onto a chromosome 14 and more rarely on chromosome 13, 14, 15, 21, or 22. This is known as Robertsonian translocation. In about 95% there are three standing copies of chromosome 21 with a set of 46 chromosomes. In some cases, i.e., phenotypically normal carrier, there is balanced translocation appearing to have only 45 chromosomes, but one chromosome 21 is joined to another chromosome.
- *Mosaicism (1%):* Here some cells are normal and some have trisomy 21. This usually arises after the formation of zygote by nondisjunction mitosis. The phenotype may be milder in Down syndrome mosaicism.

CLINICAL FEATURES (FIGS. 1A TO E)

Down syndrome is usually suspected at birth because of baby's facial appearance, but is very difficult to diagnose depending on physical features. Affected infants are usually hypotonic and other clinical features are listed below. But it has to be confirmed by karyotyping. Diagnosis of Down syndrome in preterm baby is more difficult than in term baby.

GENERAL FEATURES
• Mental retardation
• Hypotonia
• Imperforate anus
• Hirschsprung's disease
• Leukemia
• High-arched palate

Diagnostic Features of Down Syndrome at Birth

- Mongoloid face
- Poor Moro reflex
- Hypotonia
- Hyper flexible joints
- Excessive skin on neck
- Slanted palpable fissure
- Pelvic dysplasia
- Anomalous auricles
- Dysplastic middle phalanx of fifth finger
- Single palmar crease
- Flat occiput
- Wide sandal gap between big and second toe

Flat facies, epicanthic fold (a fold of skin running across the inner edge of palpebral fissure), and upward slanting of the eyes are present. Nose is small with flat nasal bridge. Furrowed protruding tongue is present. The head is brachycephalic, the palpebral fissures obliqued, inward and downward toward the broad flat nose.

The eyelids show signs of chronic blepharitis, ears are large, and lips are fissured with protruded tongue. The almond-shaped eyes, presence of epicanthus, florid complexion, and absence of fatty masses help to distinguish Down syndrome from cretinism.

A variety of congenital and acquired medical problems are associated with the Down syndrome. These are best categorized

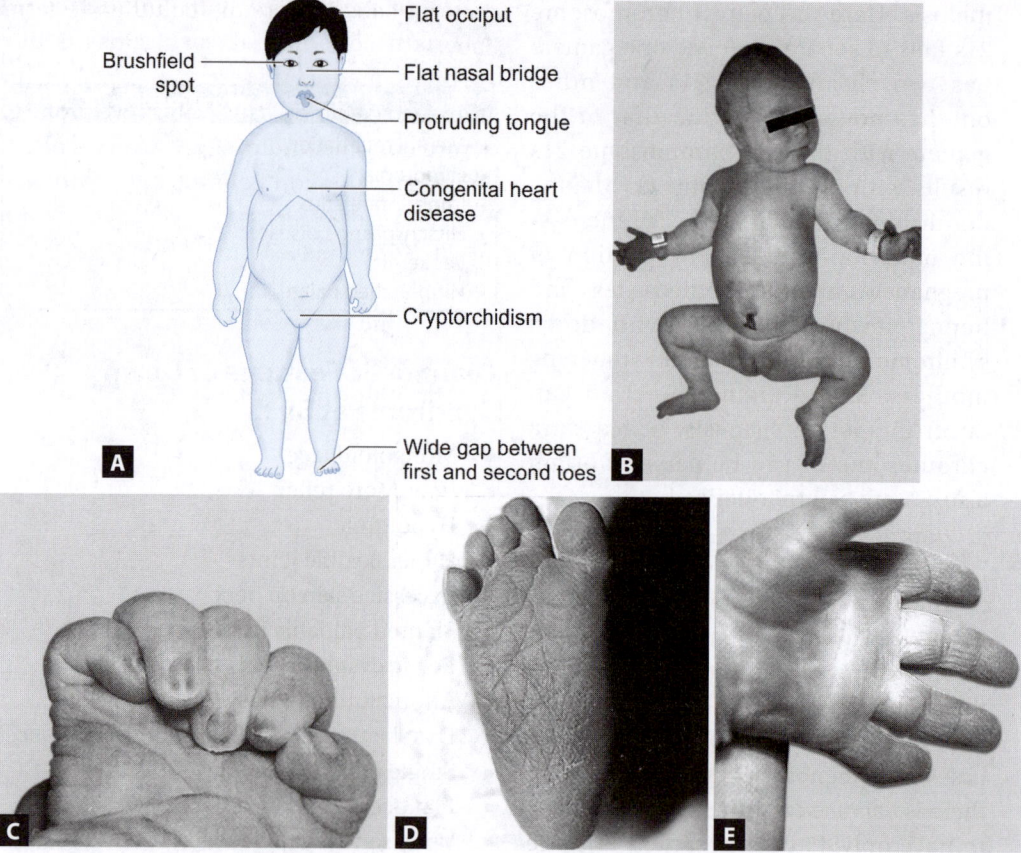

Figs. 1A to E: (A) Clinical features; (B) Down syndrome; (C) Single palmar crease; (D) Sandal gap between big and second toe; and (E) Single palmar crease.

according to the chronological age. Screening of asymptomatic individuals at regular intervals is strongly recommended.

Congenital heart disease (CHD) occurs in 40%. These are responsible for the morbidity and mortality during the first 2 years of life. All children should be evaluated before 9 months of age including echocardiography. The most common cardiac lesions are endocardial cushion defects (40%). Other lesions include atrioventricular (AV) canal, isolated ventricular septal defect (VSD), atrial septal defect (ASD), or patent ductus arteriosus (PDA), and tetralogy of Fallot.

Gastrointestinal tract anomalies are seen in 6–12% of Down syndrome patients. These include duodenal stenosis or atresia, imperforate anus, Hirschsprung's disease, tracheoesophageal fistula, esophageal atresia, bile duct atresia, malrotation, and pyloric stenosis. Physiological complications include oral motor dysfunction or gastroesophageal reflux.

Respiratory problems include recurrent otitis media, sinusitis, rhinitis, bronchiolitis, and pneumonia. These carry high mortality if associated with uncorrected heart disease. These tend to become less common with the age and growth of the craniofacial and respiratory structures.

Ophthalmic problems including Brushfield spots **(Fig. 2)** are white speckled areas

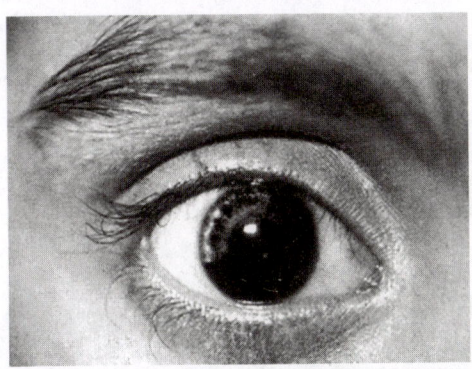

Fig. 2: Brushfield spots. *(For color version, see Plate 1)*

that occur in the periphery of iris. These are seen in 75% of patients with Down syndrome. They are also present in 7% of normal newborns. Congenital cataract is seen in about 1–2% of patients.

Thyroid problems include increased risk of congenital hypothyroidism due to the absence or aplasia of thyroid gland which occur in 1–2% of newborn. Acquired hypothyroidism is seen in 2–7% of children. The risk of Graves' disease is also increased in individuals with Down syndrome. Thyroid function tests [triiodothyronine (T3), thyroxine (T4), and thyroid-stimulating hormone (TSH)] are recommended once in neonatal period and then every year.

Transient myeloproliferative disorder (TMD) is seen in the first few months of life. There will be elevated peripheral blood leukocyte count with predominant blast forms. This will confuse the diagnosis of true congenital leukemia. Newborns with TMD are at increased risk for developing nonlymphocytic leukemia before the age of 5 years.

Patients with Down syndrome are increased risk of lymphoproliferative disorders, including acute lymphoblastic leukemia, acute myeloid leukemia, myelodysplasia, and transient lymphoproliferative syndrome.

Hearing defects with incidence of transient conductive hearing loss is due to otitis media, middle ear effusion, or impacted cerumen. These are more prone to serous otitis media during the first year of life. Routine evaluation before 6 months of age and then every year is advised. Sensorineural or mixed hearing loss may be seen.

Most males with Down syndrome are sterile, but some females have been able to reproduce, with a 50% chance of having trisomy 21 pregnancies. Two genes (*DYRK1A, DSCRI*) in the putative critical region of chromosome 21 may be targets for therapy.

Central nervous system problems include neuromotor dysfunction is characterized by generalized hypotonia with diminished primitive and deep tendon reflex. Brain size is often normal throughout gestation and during first 6 months of life. Deceleration occurs during the second half of first year. There is dysgenesis of the cerebral cortex and cerebellum. There is delay in myelination during the first year of life. This may be the primary neurological substrate of neuromuscular dysfunction.

Seizures especially infantile spasms may occur. There is delay in prelinguistic visual perception and visual motor milestones are present by the end of the first year.

Dysplasia of the brain is best reflected by changes in the brain growth and head circumference in the first few years of life. There is generalized hypocellularity of the brain and reduction in neuronal numbers and density. Decreased myelination is noted in cerebral hemisphere, basal ganglia, cerebellum, and brain stem during the first few years of life. There will be greater deficits in verbal linguistic skills relative to visual-spatial skill.

Alzheimer's disease like dementia is a known complication that occurs as early as the 4th decade and has an incidence 2–3 times higher than sporadic Alzheimer's disease.

Obstructive sleep apnea (OSA) is seen in >30%. The symptoms include snoring, restless sleep, unusual sleep position, excessive mouth breathing, daytime somnolence or behavioral changes. Predisposing factors include small oral cavity, relative macroglossia, narrowing of the upper airway, hypotonia of the pharyngeal muscles, chronic rhinitis, and enlarged tonsils or adenoids.

Intellectual disability in children with Down syndrome is variable, usually mild to moderate. Development usually progresses steadily at a slower pace, with no evidence of regression. Children learn to walk and develop communication skills and often function more effectively in social situations than would be predicted on the basis of cognitive assessment alone. Early intervention, proper medical management, and educational and vocational training can significantly affect the level of functioning in children and adolescents with Down syndrome and facilitate their transition into adulthood.

Psychiatric disorders include disruptive disorders such as attention-deficit hyperactivity disorder (ADHD), conduct/oppositional disorder, and aggression disorder. Repetitive disorders or autistic spectrum disorders are observed. Common behavioral difficulties that occur in children with Down syndrome include inattentiveness and stubbornness. The medical conditions responsible for behavioral problems include hearing loss, OSA, and side effects of medications. Stereotypic or repetitive behavior include rocking, hand flapping, staring at fingers or lights, and shaking objects.

Simian crease **(Fig. 3):** A single palmar crease is present in 45% of Down syndrome patients. Hypoplasia of the middle phalanx

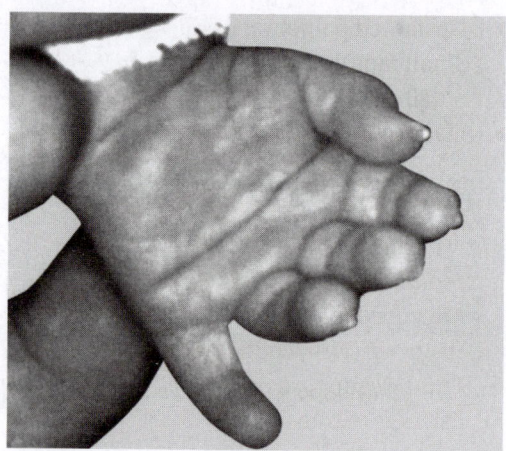

Fig. 3: Simian crease.

in the fifth finger is present. This produces clinodactyly, i.e., deflection of the finger. Hands are short and broad. Gap between first and second toe is wide, i.e., wide sandal gap.

Subluxation of joints: These children are susceptible to the subluxation of hips, patella, and cervical spine. 10–30% atlanto-occipital subluxation occurs in cervical spine. Up to 15% of children with Down syndrome have misalignment of the first cervical vertebra (C1), which places them at risk for spinal cord injury with neck hyperextension or extreme flexion.

> **ESSENTIAL DIAGNOSTIC POINTS**
> - Mental retardation
> - Small, brachycephalic head
> - *Mongoloid facies:* Upslanting, palpabral fissures; epicanthic folds; midface hypoplasia; and small, dysplastic pinnae
> - Congenital heart defects
> - Anomalies of gastrointestinal (GI) tract
> - Generalized hypotonia
> - Leukemia

Typical Craniofacial Appearance

- Round face, flat nasal bridge
- Epicanthic fold
- Brushfield spots

- Upslanted palpebral fissures
- Small mouth
- Small ears
- Flat occiput.

DIAGNOSIS

The following are the indications for the antenatal diagnosis:
- Advanced maternal age
- History of (H/o) child with Down syndrome
- Translocation carrier
- Partners of translocation carriers

The tests can be *fetal* and *maternal*.

Fetal Tests

- *Fetal umbilical blood sampling:* This is done at 18–20 weeks of gestation. Fetal blood cells are subjected to chromosomal culture. The results will be available within a week.
- *Fetal cells in the maternal circulation:* Fetal cells are found in maternal circulation in the first trimester. These cells are used for chromosomal analysis using polymerase chain reaction (PCR) technique.

Maternal Test

Maternal antenatal test can be divided into screening and diagnostic tests.

Screening Tests

All pregnant patients should undergo screening tests measuring biochemical markers in blood samples.
- *Ultrasound:* Ultrasound is the commonly used screening test to detect the structural fetal anomalies. In Down syndrome, it can be divided into first-trimester and second-trimester scanning.
  - First-trimester scanning is best done at 11 weeks of gestation. Here the nuchal soft-tissue fold is measured. It is the space between the back of the fetal neck and overlying skin. Increased thickness, i.e., >4 mm is called nuchal translucency (NT). It is associated with aneuploidy, i.e., Down syndrome.
  - Second-trimester ultrasound indicates associated markers of Down syndrome. These markers can be major or minor markers. Major markers include cardiac anomalies such as endocardial cushion defects, neural tube defects, cystic hygroma, and omphalocele. Minor markers have lower association with aneuploidy. These include NT, short femur, short middle phalanx of fifth digit, echogenic intracardiac foci, pyelectasis, hypoechogenic bowel, mild ventriculomegaly, and choroid plexus cysts.
- *Serum screening:* Here biochemical analytics are measured in maternal blood sample. Serum screening is well established in the second trimester. Here, the combination of increased human chorionic gonadotropin (hCG), decreased alpha fetoprotein, decreased unconjugated estriol, and increased inhibin are used. If three or four biochemical analytics are detected, it is called as triple/quadruple test, respectively. Quadruple test can detect up to 80% of Down syndrome pregnancies versus 70% in the triple screen. Both tests have a 5% false-positive rate. There is a method of screening during the first trimester using fetal NT thickness that can be done alone or in conjunction with maternal serum beta-hCG and pregnancy-associated plasma protein-A (PAPP-A). In the first trimester, NT alone can detect <70% of Down syndrome pregnancies, but with beta-hCG and PAPP-A.

Diagnostic Tests

There are two diagnostic tests, i.e., amniocentesis and chorionic villus sampling (CVS). Prenatal fetal karyotype with these tests is advised.

1. *Amniocentesis:* It is best done between 10 and 12 weeks by transcervical or transabdominal route, and hence diagnosis can be done in first trimester. It can be done at 16 weeks of gestation. Amniotic fluid is withdrawn with the ultrasound guidance. The amniotic fluid cells are derived from epiblast. They reflect the true constituents of embryo. These cells are cultures and cytogenetic analysis is done. The risk of miscarriage is 1:200.
2. *Chorionic villus sampling:* It is best done at or beyond 10 weeks of gestation. If it is done prior to 10 weeks, it is associated with limb anomalies. It has about 1:100 risk of miscarriage. Transabdominal CVS and cordocentesis are considered at 16–18 weeks.

With the ultrasound guidance, the chorionic villi are removed via abdominal or less commonly via vaginal route. The cells of CVS arise from trophoblast or villus core cells. These reflect more with embryonic cells. These cells are cultured and cytogenetic analysis is done. The advantages over amniocentesis are that it is done earlier in gestation and that if trisomy 21 is detected, then a surgical termination can be done.

Karyotype: It refers to the systemic arrangement of previously stained and banded chromosomes of single cells in pairs. It is performed on blood lymphocytes or skin fibroblast. The cells are cultured and arrested in mitoses during metaphase. Then they are fixed and stained.

Karyotype is mandatory to confirm the diagnosis. It is must before the diagnosis is conveyed to the parents. It is helpful for genetic counseling, as it is critical to distinguish complete trisomy 21, from trisomy 21/mosaicism or unbalanced translocation.

If there is free trisomy 21, parental chromosome need not be examined. If the baby has translocation, the parental chromosomal analysis is recommended, since one of the parents may well carry the translocation in balanced form (25% of cases). If one carries balanced translocation, other relatives should be counseled.

Detection of cell-free fetal DNA in maternal plasma is also diagnostic and replacing conventional first- and second-trimester screens. The noninvasive detection of fetal trisomy 21 by analyzing cell-free fetal DNA in maternal serum is an important advance in prenatal diagnosis of Down syndrome. Next-generation DNA sequencing has reduced the cost of this procedure, which has a high degree of accuracy (98% detection rate) and applicability.

Current tests can detect microdeletions including 22q11.2 deletion syndrome, Angelman syndrome, Prader–Willi syndrome deletion, cri du chat syndrome, Williams syndrome, and 1p36.3 deletion syndrome. Importantly, especially for microdeletions, cell-free noninvasive prenatal testing (NIPT) should be considered primarily for screening tests and follow-up invasive testing (e.g., amniocentesis) pursued for definitive diagnosis.

Radiological findings:
- 11 ribs
- Two to three ossification centers of manubrium
- Hypoplasia of the base of the skull, facial bones, and middle phalanx of fifth finger

- Accessory epiphyses at base of second metacarpal
- Coxa valga
- Bony pelvis and iliac crests are broad and flared, and acetabular and iliac angles are reduced

Dermatoglyphic findings:
- Distal palmar triradius, or large angle hypothermia pattern distal loop in third interdigital area
- Predominance of ulnar loops on the digits and radial loops or on the fourth and fifth fingers
- Hallucal area tibial pattern in the feet
- Marked crease between great and second toes

■ RECURRENT RISK

One child with trisomy 21 due to non-disjunction, the risk of recurrence 1 in 200 for mothers under age of 35 years. The risk of recurrence is 10–15% if the mother is the translocation carrier, and it is 2.5% if the father is carrier. If the parent carries rare 21:21 translocation, all the offsprings will have Down syndrome. If neither parent carries translocation (75% of the cases) risk of recurrence is <1%.

Carrier mother may produce three types of viable offspring:
1. Normal phenotype and karyotype
2. Phenotypically translocation carrier
3. Translocation carrier 21 **(Table 1)**

Carrier fathers rarely affect the offspring; they do produce both normal and carriers.

If one parent is mosaic, the risk depends upon the degree of gonadal mosaicism of the affected parent. Paternal age increases the risk of Down syndrome after the age of 55 years. For recurrence risk for families, G-banded karyotype analysis is recommended as the study of choice. The recurrence risk

TABLE 1: Recurrent risk.

Maternal age	Risk
All ages	1:650
20	1:1,530
30	1:1,000
35	1:365
40	1:100
45	1:50

for translocation carriers is higher and depends on the chromosomes involved in the translocation and the sex of the parent carrying the rearrangement.

■ TREATMENT

Medical Management

Patients are at higher risk of a number of problems and hence they should be screened for congenital heart defects, evidence of hypothyroidism and ophthalmological problems. The medical management depends upon the age of the child.

Most of the Down syndrome babies are hypotonic and many may have congenital heart defects. Feeding problems should be anticipated and managed appropriately. Breast feeding should be encouraged as the baby will have upper respiratory tract infection, atopic disease, and allergy.

Congenital cardiac defects are common and every child should have echocardiogram soon after the birth. All these heart defects should be managed in exactly the same way as any other child with congenital heart defects. In the absence of cardiac defects, many children will have long life.

Duodenal atresia is most commonly encountered gastrointestinal abnormality. There is high incidence of Hirschsprung's disease and tracheoesophageal fistula. Constipation can be a major problem and

Hirschsprung's disease should be suspected if it is severe. Celiac disease should also be kept in mind with a high index of suspicion.

These children may get recurrent upper respiratory tract infection and glue ears because of reduced cell-mediated immunity and hypertrophied tonsils and adenoids. Many of these may also develop significant hearing impairment for which they should be tested periodically.

Congenital cataracts should be detected at birth initially by routine examination for red reflex. Dense cataract should be removed as soon as possible. All children should be monitored for glaucoma periodically. Children may develop refractive errors and should be taken care.

Hypotonia may predispose to delayed motor milestones. These children may benefit from regular physiotherapy. Global developmental delay becomes evident once the child grows. Speech and language milestones may be delayed. Growth of these children should be plotted on Down syndrome growth charts rather on regular centile charts.

Developmental dysplasia of hip occurs due to hypotonia and joint laxity. This can lead to morbidity. About 15% of children with Down syndrome have radiological evidence of instability of atlantoaxial joint.

Recommended health checkup for children with Down syndrome:
- *Physical examination:* At birth, 4 weeks, 8 weeks, 6 months, and then annually
- *Eye checkup:* At birth, 6 months, 1 year, and then once in every year
- *Hearing assessment:* At birth, 6 months, and annual checkup
- *Thyroid function test:* At birth, 3 months, 6 months, and then every year.

■ COUNSELING

Antenatal Counseling

Parents should be aware of screening and definitive tests that are available. They need to understand that a screening test places them in a higher or lower risk group but does not definitely diagnose or exclude Down syndrome. When it is diagnosed by amniocentesis or CVS, the parents need to be informed of their choices. Genetic counseling about the recurrence risk should usually be delayed; this way the couple gains time to deal with the immediate issues related to the current diagnosis of Down syndrome.

The diagnosis at birth should be explained in general terms. Parents should be allowed to clear all their medical doubts. One should offer emotional support to known problems and associated disorders and importance of early intervention.

Genetic Counseling

This is done only after chromosomal analysis. The main indication is for recurrence risk and information regarding future pregnancies. The recurrence risk depends upon the mother's age. As a guide the recurrence risk for women <30 years is 0.7%. The recurrence risk for women over 30 years is same as any other women of the same age.

Health Maintenance Guidelines

- *Birth to 1 year:*
  - Karyotype confirmation and genetic counseling—newborn period
  - Cardiac evaluation and echocardiogram—newborn period
  - Confirm red reflex—newborn period
  - Check neonatal thyroid screen—newborn
  - Audiology (hearing and tympanometry)—by 6 months

- *1–12 years:*
  - Thyroid function tests—yearly
  - Vision evaluation—by 1 year
  - Audiology—yearly
  - Ear–nose–throat (ENT)
  - Cardiac
  - Gastrointestinal
  - Neurodevelopment
  - Dental evaluation at 3 years, then twice yearly
  - Cervical spine X-ray
- *12–18 years:*
  - Thyroid function tests—yearly
  - Hearing and tympanometry
  - Vision to be checked
  - Cervical spine X-ray

Developmental Intervention

This includes:
- Infant stimulation program
- Physical therapy
- Occupational therapy
- Parent support group

There will be reduction in linear growth rates, with height 2–4 standard deviation (SD) below the mean for the general population. Adolescent growth spurt usually occurs later. The final height for males ranges from 140 to 160 cm and for females between 135 and 150 cm.

The onset and progress of puberty is the same or only slightly delayed for adolescent males with Down syndrome. Males typically show decreased penile length and testicular volume, though serum testosterone levels appear normal throughout puberty. Reduced sperm count and lack of mature sperm are the causes of infertility. Females of childbearing age should be considered fertile.

Life expectancy has increased in recent decades to 50–55 years with proper health care. Neuropathologic hallmarks of Alzheimer's disease (senile plaques, neurofibrillary tangles) are present in brains of nearly all individuals with Down syndrome by age of 40 years. This is presumed to be secondary to the extra dosage of the amyloid precursor protein gene (APP) on chromosome 21. APP duplication has been reported in families with autosomal dominant Alzheimer's disease. Premature dementia is found in about one-third of the Down syndrome population by age of 60 years, with an estimated lifetime prevalence of 90% for all people with Down syndrome.

BIBLIOGRAPHY

1. Adams DJ, Clark DA. Common genetic and epigenetic syndromes. Pediatric Clin Nort Am. 2015:62(2);411-26.
2. Bull MJ; Committee on Genetics. Health supervision for children with Down Syndrome. Pediatrics. 2011;128:393-406.
3. Cassidy SB, Allanson JE. Management of Genetic Syndromes, 3rd edition. United Kingdom: Willey Blackwell; 2010.
4. Healthcare guidence, (online) available from http./www.downsyn.com/guidelines/healthcare.
5. Martin CL, Warburton D. Detection of chromosomal aberrations in clinical practice: From karyotype to genome sequence. Annu Rev Genomics Hum Genet. 2015;16:309-26.

CASE 2

Klinefelter's Syndrome

■ PRESENTING COMPLAINTS

A 13-year-old boy was brought with the complaints of:
- Bilateral enlargement of breast—6 months
- Abnormal social behavior—6 months

History of Presenting Complaints

A boy aged about 13 years was referred to the general surgeon for the management of the bilateral enlargement of the breast. According to the boy, he had noticed the enlargement of the breast for the last 6 months. But there was no discharge. He told that he had normal pubic hair development. Mother also told that his son used to be shy at the social gathering. School performance of the boy was rated as poor. School class teacher had also noticed the abnormal social behavior among his classmates. He was fighting with his peers for trivial cause.

Past History of the Patient

The boy was the third sibling of the consanguineous union. He was born at term by normal delivery. There was no significant postnatal event except for normal physiological jaundice. He was discharged on third day. He was on breast milk soon after the delivery. Weaning started by the fourth month of the child. His developmental milestones were within normal range.

CASE AT A GLANCE	
Basic Findings	
Height	: 155 cm (50th centile)
Weight	: 34 kg (20th centile)
Temperature	: 37°C
Pulse rate	: 86 beats/min, regular
Respiratory rate	: 18 breaths/min
Blood pressure	: 110/70 mm Hg

Positive Findings

History:
- Bilateral enlargement of breast
- Poor school performance
- Behavioral problems

Examination:
- Tall and poorly built
- Small testes and phallus
- Gynecomastia
- Behavioral disturbance

Investigation:
- *Karyotyping:* 47, XXY
- *Follicle-stimulating hormone (FSH):* Increased
- *Luteinizing hormone (LH):* Increased
- *Plasma testosterone:* Decreased
- *Plasma estradiol:* Increased
- *Semen analysis:* Azoospermia

These was no family history of similar problems. His two older brothers were married with two children each. Those children were doing well.

■ EXAMINATION

On examination, the child looked tall, poorly built, and undernourished. His height was on 50th centile for the age, the weight was below 20th centile. His height was 155 cm and the weight was 34 kg. His arms and legs were disproportionately long. He was sitting quietly on the examination table. There was bilateral gynecomastia. The diameter of the breast tissue was 5 cm.

The boy was afebrile, pulse was 86 beats/min, respiratory rate was 18 breaths/min, and blood pressure was 110/70 mm Hg. There was neither pallor, edema, nor lymphadenopathy. There was no icterus and clubbing.

Per abdomen examination revealed the small size of the testicle, i.e., 1.8 cm in length (normal 5.1 cm) and smaller phallic length, i.e., 5 cm (normal 6.5 cm). Pubic hair development was in feminine pattern.

Developmental assessment of the child showed retarded growth in all the parameters such as mental, social, and behavioral quadrants. His intelligence quotient was 15–20 points below the other siblings. Other systemic examinations were normal.

■ INVESTIGATION

- *Hemoglobin:* 13 g/dL
- *TLC:* 7,800 cells/cumm
- *Erythrocyte sedimentation rate (ESR):* 30 mm at the first hour
- *Chest X-ray:* Normal
- *FSH:* 5.2 U/L (normal 1.8–3.2 U/L)
- *LH:* 6 U/L (normal 0.2–4.9 U/L)
- *Plasma testosterone:* 0.5 nmol/L (normal 0.62–5.20 nmol/L)
- *Plasma estradiol:* 200 pmol/L (normal 2.9–128 pmol/L)
- *Serum prolactin:* 0.56 nmol/L (normal 0.13–0.77 nmol/L)
- *Karyotype:* 47 chromosome with sex chromosome XXY, i.e., 47,XXY
- *Semen analysis:* Revealed azoospermia
- *Testicular biopsy:* Revealed hyalinized, seminiferous, tubular membrane and adenomatous clumping of Leydig cells; there was predominance of Sertoli cells

■ DISCUSSION

This is a case of Klinefelter's syndrome. There is a failure of development of secondary sexual characters and increased gonadotropins. This was described by Klinefeter, Reifenstein, and Albright in 1942.

It is the most common sex chromosomal aneuploidy in males. The incidence is one in 1,000. It is characterized by hypogonadism, small testes, failure of development of the secondary sexual characters, and increased gonadotropins. It accounts for 10–20% of male infertility.

The classical description includes mental retardation, hypogonadism, and gynecomastia. They are on an average 10 cm taller than XY males. The altered body proportion is with low upper to lower segment ratio.

Cells deviating from the multiples of the haploid number are called aneuploid, indicating a missing or extra chromosome. This occurs most often from the meiotic nondisjunction of an X chromosome. In 54% cases, it may be maternal in origin, and in 46%, it is paternal in origin.

These individuals (80%) have a male karyotype with extra X chromosome, i.e., 47,XXY. The phenotype is male. When the number of X chromosome exceeds two, mental retardation and impairment of virilization is more. The remaining 20% have multiple sex chromosome aneuploidies (48,XXXY; 48,XXYY; 49,XXXXY), mosaicism (46,XY/47,XXY), or structurally abnormal X chromosomes; the greater the aneuploidy, the more severe the mental impairment and dysmorphism. Errors in paternal nondisjunction in meiosis I account for half the cases.

Those who have higher X chromosome counts show impaired cognition. It has been estimated that each additional X chromosome reduces the IQ by 10–15 points, when comparing these individuals with typical siblings. The main effect is seen in language skills and social domains.

■ CLINICAL FEATURES

These patients approach to the doctor with the failure of development of secondary sexual characters. These patients tend to be tall and underweight. They have relatively elongated legs. The testes tend to be small for the age and the phallus tends to be smaller than average. Cryptorchidism and hypospadias may also occur.

Development of the puberty is delayed. Feminine distribution of the pubic hair is present. 40% of the adults will have gynecomastia appearing usually soon after puberty between ages of 14 and 16 years. The most common testicular lesions are spermatogenic arrest and Sertoli cell predominance. The testes are small with the mean length of 1.8 cm as compared to 5.1 cm in normal male. The testes show normal growth early in puberty but stop in midpuberty. Testes are shrunken and hyalinized seminiferous tubules. Some are lined by Sertoli cells. Hypertrophy and clamping of Leydig cells is present. Azoospermia and infertility are encountered. Antisperm antibodies are detected.

The diagnosis is commonly made at puberty. This is because of subtleness of clinical manifestation in childhood. Other features such as behavioral or psychiatric disturbances, learning and school adjustment problems should be evaluated to rule out this syndrome. These children may be anxious, aggressive, and engage in antisocial acts. There will be verbal cognitive defects and underachievement in reading, spelling, and mathematics.

There is increased incidence of pulmonary disease, varicose veins, cancer breast, diabetes mellitus, and peptic ulcers. Lymphomas and leukemias are associated. Extragonadal germ cell tumor especially of the mediastinum and cerebral hemangiomas occur with high frequency.

> **CLINICAL FEATURES (FIG. 1)**
> - Infertility
> - Small testes with hypogonadism
> - Tall stature
> - Gynecomastia at adolescence
> - Normal pubertal development
> - Normal range intelligence
> - Educational and psychological problems

> **ESSENTIAL DIAGNOSTIC POINTS**
> - Microorchidism normal external genitalia
> - Azoospermia, sterility
> - Gynecomastia, normal-to-borderline IQ
> - Diminished fascial hair, lack of libido and potency
> - A tall eunuchoid build

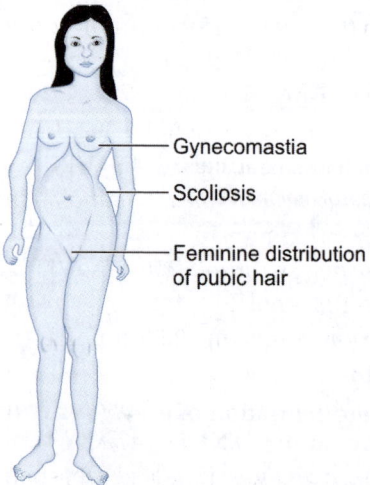

Fig. 1: Clinical features.

GENERAL FEATURES

- Behavioral problems
- Psychiatric problems
- Delayed puberty
- Mental retardation
- Tall slim
- Underweight
- Learning disabilities
- Antisocial acts

■ DIAGNOSIS

It should be suspected in prepubertal children, who have long legs, smaller than normal testes, small phallus, learning disorders, delay in language development, mental retardation, or psychosocial behavioral problems.

Gonadotropins are elevated and testosterone levels are slightly low. Estradiol levels are elevated and account for gynecomastia. Chromosome analysis reveals 47,XXY karyotype.

Testicular biopsy shows deficiency and absence of germinal cells before puberty. After puberty seminiferous tubules are hyalinized and shrunken. There is adenomatous clumping of Leydig cells. There is predominance of Sertoli cells.

LABORATORY SALIENT FINDINGS

- Gonadotropins are elevated
- Testosterone levels are slightly low
- Estradiol levels are elevated
- Chromosome analysis reveals 47, XXY karyotype
- *Testicular biopsy:* Deficiency and absence of germinal cells, seminiferous tubules are hyalinized and shrunken, adenomatous clumping of Leydig cells, predominance of Sertoli cells

The testosterone concentration is low. The concentration of estradiol is normal or increased and gonadotropin concentration is elevated. Gynecomastia occurs in 40–50% of cases as a result of increased ratio of serum estriol to testosterone. Breast cancer occurs in 4% of patients and incidence is 20 times higher than in normal males.

■ TREATMENT

Replacement therapy with long-acting testosterone preparations is recommended. It should begin at 11–12 years of age. The enanthate ester may be used. The starting dose is 25–50 mg given intramuscularly every 3–4 weeks. The increment of 50 mg is done once in every 6–9 months till the maintenance dose of adult is obtained. The maintenance dose of adult is 250–300 mg every 3 weeks. Children XXY/XY mosaicism have better prognosis. As the number of X chromosomes increases beyond two, the clinical manifestation increases correspondingly. Management includes behavioral and psychological rehabilitation.

■ BIBLIOGRAPHY

1. Adams DJ, Clark DA. Common genetic and epigenetic syndromes. Pediatric Clin North Am. 2015;62(2):411-26.
2. Carvalho CM, Lupski JR. Mechanisms underlying structural variant formation in genomic disorders. Nat Rev Genet. 2016;17(4):224-38.
3. Jones KL, Jones MC, del Campo Casanelles M. Smith's Recognizable Patterns of Human Malformation, 7th edition. United Kingdom: Elsevier Health Sciences; 2013.
4. Nevado J, Mergener R, Palomares-Bralo M, Souza KR, Vallespín E, Mena R, et al. New microdeletion and microduplication syndromes: A comprehensive review. Genet Mole Biol. 2014;37(1):210-9.

CASE 3

Turner Syndrome

■ PRESENTING COMPLAINTS

A 12-year-old girl was brought by her mother with the history of:
- Not attaining secondary sexual characters—till now
- No enlargement of breast nodule—till now

History of Presenting Complaints

A 12-year-old girl was brought by her mother with the history of not attaining the secondary sexual characters to the pediatric outpatient department. Her mother was complaining that there was not even small enlargement of the breast nodule. She told that her elder daughter had menses at this age.

Past History of the Patient

The patient was the second sibling of the non-consanguineous marriage. She was born at full term by normal delivery. Patient's mother recalled her memory and told that patient had the swelling of the lower limbs at birth. For this doctor's consultation was sought. But the doctor told that it was not the significant observation. Apart from this there was no significant postnatal event. Child was fed with the breast milk after the delivery. There was no delay in the developmental milestones. Child had been completely vaccinated.

Child used to have repeated discharge in the ears throughout her childhood. This has led to the hearing difficulty in the left ear. Her scholastic performance was rated as average. There was no family history of similar complaints.

CASE AT A GLANCE

Basic Findings
Height	: 126 cm (3rd centile)
Weight	: 36 kg (30th centile)
Temperature	: 37°C
Pulse rate	: 86 beats/min
Respiratory rate	: 16 breaths/min
Blood pressure	: 90/70 mm Hg in upper limb
	86/60 mm Hg in lower limb

Positive Findings

History:
- No secondary sexual characters
- Short stature
- Ear discharge
- No similar complaint in family

Examination:
- Short stature
- Webbing of the neck
- Broad chest
- Cubitus valgus
- No secondary sexual character
- Hearing difficulties

Investigation:
- Karyotype 45,XO
- Short metacarpal and metatarsal bone
- Ultrasound abdomen
- Follicle-stimulating hormone (FSH)—raised

■ EXAMINATION

Child was sitting shy on the examination table. She was short. Her height was 126 cm (3rd centile) and weight was 36 kg (30th centile). There was neither pallor, lymphadenopathy, clubbing, nor cyanosis.

She was afebrile. Pulse was 86 beats/min. All the peripheral pulses were felt. The respiratory rate was 16 breaths/min and was regular. The blood pressure recorded in the upper limb was 90/70 mm Hg and in the lower limb was 86/60 mm Hg. Webbing of the neck was present. Chest appeared broad with widely spaced nipple. Cubitus valgus was present. There were short fourth metacarpal and metatarsal bones. The discharge was present in the left ear. There was hearing defect. Cardiovascular system examination was normal. There was no evidence of the murmur. Abdominal examination did not reveal any mass. No secondary sexual characters were present.

■ INVESTIGATION

- *Hemoglobin:* 12 g/dL
- *TLC:* 7,500 cells/cumm
- *ESR:* 20 mm in the first hour
- *Absolute eosinophil count:* 330 cells/dL
- *Chest X-ray:* Normal
- *Skull X-ray:* Normal
- *X-ray of hand and foot:* Short metacarpal and metatarsal bone
- *Kidney–ureter–bladder (KUB):* Normal
- *Ultrasound abdomen:* Revealed streak ovaries
- *Karyotype:* 45,XO
- *FSH:* 3.6 U/L (1.8–3.2 U/L)

■ DISCUSSION

Short child with no secondary sexual characters and above clinical and laboratory finding suggests the diagnosis of Turner's syndrome. Turner syndrome was described in 1938 by Dr Henry Turner.

Half of the patients with Turner's syndrome have a 45,X chromosomal complement. The mechanism of the loss of chromosome is unknown. The genes involved in Turner phenotype are X-linked genes.

Turner's syndrome occurs in 1 in 2,500 live-born females. In the absence of the X chromosome, oocyte present in the ovary starts disappearing by the age of 2 years. The ovaries become streak ovaries in the absence of the oocytes. The majority of the 45,X chromosome fetuses are likely to be aborted. There will be considerable degree of chromosomal mosaicism, i.e., 45,X/46,XX. Formation of isochromosome of long arms of X chromosome may lead Turner phenotype with 46 chromosome because of absence of short arms. It occurs due to errors in post-zygote mitosis. The single X chromosome is often maternal.

The normal fetal ovary contains approximately 7 million oocytes, but these begin to disappear rapidly after the 5th month of gestation. At birth, there are only 2 million (1 million active follicles); by menarche, there are 400,000–500,000; and at menopause, 10,000 remain. In the absence of one X chromosome, this process is accelerated, and nearly all oocytes are gone by 2 years of age. In aborted 45,X fetuses, the number of primordial germ cells in the gonadal ridge appears to be normal suggesting that the normal process of oocyte loss is accelerated in patients with Turner syndrome. Eventually, the ovaries are described as streaks and consist only of connective tissue, with very few germ cells present.

■ CLINICAL FEATURES (FIGS. 1A TO D)

Most of them can be diagnosed at birth. These newborn will have characteristic edema of the dorsum of the hands and feet and loose skin folds are present at the nape of the neck. This is commonly seen among low-birth-weight babies.

The clinical features depend on chromosome constitution of the individuals. The patients with 45,X Turner syndrome show

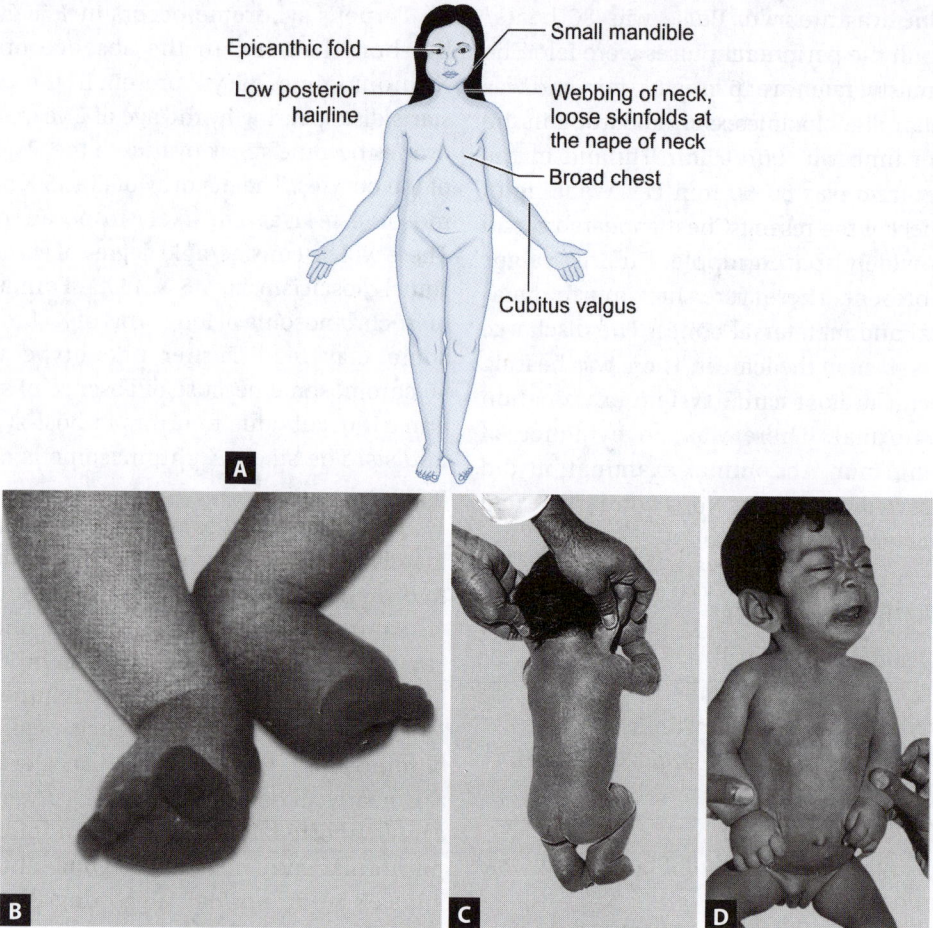

Figs. 1A to D: (A) Clinical features; (B) Lymphedema of feet; (C) Low hairline; and (D) Short neck. *(For color version, see Plate 1)*

many characteristic somatic abnormalities. Whereas those with mosaicism and structural abnormalities of X chromosome (variant Turner syndrome) show minimal somatic abnormalities. However, short stature, streak ovaries are constant findings.

In childhood, the child is of short stature. Short neck, webbing of the neck, low posterior hairline, small mandible, epicanthic fold, high-arched palate, and broad chest with widely spaced nipple are present. Cubitus valgus is also the feature. Bony anomalies include medial tibial exostosis, short fourth metacarpal and metatarsal are present. Sexual maturation fails to occur at puberty. Adult height will be <145 cm. It has been recommended to consider Turner syndrome in all girls with short stature.

ESSENTIAL DIAGNOSTIC POINTS
• Webbed neck edema of hands and feet • Coarctation of aorta • Short stature, shield chest, wide set nipples • Streak ovaries, amenorrhea • Absence of secondary sexual characters • Infertility • Malformation of urinary tract

The linear growth deceleration begins in infancy and early childhood, gets progressively more pronounced in later childhood and adolescence, and results in significant adult short stature. The height is well correlated with the midparental height (average of the parents' heights adjusted for child's sex). Specific growth curves for height have been developed for females with Turner syndrome.

Associated clinical features include the abnormalities of cardiac, renal, and of the ears. Cardiac abnormalities include mainly bicuspid aortic valve coarctation or aorta, aortic stenosis, mitral valve prolapse, and anomalous pulmonary venous drainage.

During adolescence, and certainly before pregnancy (when possible) is contemplated, repeat cardiac evaluation should be considered even in those without prior findings of cardiac abnormalities. Blood pressure should be routinely monitored even in the absence of cardiac or renal lesions and especially in those with suggestions of aortic root dilation. Cardiac magnetic resonance imaging (MRI) is a valuable tool to detect and monitor aortic root dilation.

Renal abnormalities include pelvic kidney, horseshoe kidney, double collecting system, absence of one kidney, and ureteropelvic junction obstruction. Females with Turner syndrome who had normal baseline renal ultrasound findings did not develop renal disease during a follow-up period averaging 6 years.

Inflammatory bowel disease (both Crohn disease and ulcerative colitis), gastrointestinal bleeding because of abnormal mesenteric vasculature, and delayed gastric emptying time have all been reported. Screening for celiac disease is recommended, because the risk of celiac disease is increased in Turner syndrome, with 4–6% of individuals affected. Although autoimmune diseases have been associated with Turner syndrome, the prevalence of type 1 diabetes with Turner syndrome is not very high.

Recurrent bilateral otitis media develops in approximately 75% of patients. Sensorineural hearing deficits are common, and the frequency increases with age. There will be perceptive hearing defects. This occurs as a result of the recurrent otitis media. Hypothyroidism occurs in 15–30% of adults with Turner syndrome.

In general, behavior is normal in females with Turner syndrome, but they are at an increased risk for social isolation, immaturity, and anxiety. Other conditions, such as dyslexia, nonverbal learning disability, and attention–deficit disorder, have been reported in females with Turner syndrome. In adults, deficits in perceptual spatial skills are more common than they are in the general population. Some unconfirmed data suggest the existence of an imprinted X-linked locus that affects cognitive function such as verbal and higher-order executive function skills.

Congenital lymphedema recedes in early infancy leaving only puffiness over the dorsum of the fingers and toes. Antithyroid antibodies are also present among 30–50% of patients. Crohn's disease, ulcerative colitis, gastrointestinal bleeding, scoliosis, keratoconus, pigmented nevi, and alopecia occur.

At puberty a patient may present for the first time with primary and failure of development of secondary sexual characters. Streak gonads are found with ultrasound and at laparotomy. The patients are almost invariably sterile. But menstruation and secondary sexual developmental may be induced by estrogen replacement. Girls with Turner syndrome have a normal lifespan. Hypertension and osteoporosis may be present in adult life.

Sexual maturation fails to occur. Spontaneous breast development is seen among 20%. The increased incidence of the premature menopause and increased risk of miscarriage occur.

CLINICAL FEATURES
- Persistent lymphedema of hands and feet
- Short stature—cardinal feature
- Webbing of neck or thick neck
- Cubitus valgus—wide carrying angle
- Widely spaced nipples
- CHD—coarctation of aorta
- Delayed puberty
- Ovarian dysgenesis—infertility
- Renal agenesis
- Hypothyroidism
- Recurrent otitis media
- Renal anomalies
- Normal intellectual

Primary gonadal failure is associated with early onset of adrenarche (elevation in dehydroepiandrosterone sulfate) but delayed pubarche (pubic hair development).

Antithyroid antibodies (thyroid peroxidase and/or thyroglobulin antibodies) occur in 30–50% of patients. The prevalence increases with advancing age. Cholesterol levels are elevated in adolescence, regardless of body mass index or karyotype.

GENERAL FEATURES
- High-arched palate
- Coarctation of aorta
- Horseshoe kidney
- Double collecting system
- Goiter

LABORATORY SALIENT FINDING
- Chromosomal analysis
- Ultrasonography of the heart, ovaries, and kidneys
- *Gonadotropins:* Follicle-stimulating hormone (FSH) is elevated

■ DIAGNOSIS

Chromosomal analysis should be considered. Ultrasonography of the heart, ovaries, and kidneys are indicated, skeletal abnormalities include shortening of the fourth metatarsal and metacarpal bones, epiphyseal dysgenesis, and scoliosis. Gonadotropins, especially FSH, are markedly elevated. Thyroid antibodies should be checked.

Ultrasonography of the heart, kidneys, and ovaries is indicated after the diagnosis is established. The most common skeletal abnormalities are shortening of the 4th metatarsal and metacarpal bones, epiphyseal dysgenesis in the joints of the knees and elbows, Madelung deformity, scoliosis, and, in older patients, inadequate osseous mineralization.

Plasma levels of gonadotropins, particularly FSH, are markedly elevated to greater than those of age-matched controls during infancy; at 2–3 years of age, a progressive decrease in levels occurs until they reach a nadir at 6–8 years of age, and by 10–11 years of age, they rise to adult castrate levels.

Thyroid peroxidase antibodies and thyroglobulin antibodies should be checked periodically to detect autoimmune thyroiditis, and if positive levels of T4 and TSH should be obtained.

■ DIFFERENTIAL DIAGNOSIS

This includes lymphedema, congenital syphilis, and congenital nephrotic syndrome.

■ TREATMENT

Guidelines for health supervision for children with Turner syndrome include pubertal induction as well as treatment with growth hormone and oxandrolone.

Treatment is with:
- Growth hormone therapy
- Estrogen replacement therapy for the development of secondary sexual characters at the time puberty

Growth hormone treatment should be initiated in early childhood and/or when there is evidence of height-velocity attenuation on specific Turner syndrome growth curves. Growth hormone therapy does not significantly aggravate carbohydrate tolerance and does not result in marked adverse events in patients with Turner syndrome. Serum levels of insulin-like growth factor 1 should be monitored if the patient is receiving high doses of growth hormone. If the insulin-like growth factor 1 levels are significantly elevated, the dose of growth hormone may need to be reduced.

Oxandrolone has also been used to treat the short stature associated with Turner syndrome, either alone or in combination with growth hormone. This synthetic anabolic steroid has weak androgenic effects.

Replacement therapy with estrogens is indicated, but there is little consensus about the optimal age at which to initiate treatment.

Low-dose estrogen replacement at 12 years of age permits a normal pace of puberty without interfering with the positive effect of growth hormone on the final adult height. Estrogen therapy improves verbal and nonverbal memory in females with Turner syndrome. In young women with age-appropriate pubertal development who achieve normal height, health-related quality-of-life questionnaires have yielded normal results.

Premarin is a conjugated estrogen. The dose is 0.3 mg/day or ethinyl estradiol 5–10 mg/day given daily for 3–6 months. It is effective in inducing puberty. Then the dose is increased to 0.625–1.25 mg of conjugated estrogen or 20–50 µg/day of ethinyl estradiol. Cyclical therapy with estrogen and progesterone is started after 6–12 months. Prophylactic gonadectomy is advised for Y chromosome patients due to risk of gonadoblastoma.

For oral preparations, a conjugated estrogen (Premarin), 0.15–0.625 mg daily, or micronized estradiol (Estrace), 0.5 mg given daily for 3–6 months, is usually effective in inducing puberty. The recommendations for transdermal patch therapy are 6.25 µg/100–200 µg daily that is gradually increased over 2 years to the adult dose of 100–200 µg daily. The estrogen may be cycled (taken on days 1–23) or not. A progestin (Provera) is added (taken on days 10–23) in a dose of 5–10 mg daily. In the week after the progestin, withdrawal bleeding usually occurs. Combination oral contraceptive pills may also be used for hormone replacement therapy.

Successful pregnancies have been carried to term using ovum donation and in vitro fertilization. Adolescents with few signs of spontaneous puberty may have ovaries with follicles. There remains a future possibility of using cryopreserved ovarian tissue with immature oocytes before the regression of the ovaries for the future pregnancies.

The growth hormone replacement is considered once there is evidence of growth velocity attenuation. The dosage is 0.375 mg/kg/wk. The improved growth is seen if it is started at 12–13 years. It may increase the final height of 8–10 cm.

Cyclic estrogen and progesterone therapy in phenotype female at prepubertal age, i.e., 14 years will improve physical development, induce regular menstrual cycles, and thus have great psychological benefit. An anabolic steroid-oxandrolone in very low doses of 1.25 mg daily is helpful to accelerate growth rate and increase adult height.

Cardiac evaluation is recommended periodically. Regular measurement of blood pressure at baseline and every year is advised. Renal malformations should be evaluated ultrasonographically. Regular audiometry is advised in adulthood.

■ BIBLIOGRAPHY

1. Adams DJ. Clark DA. Common genetic and epigenetic syndromes. Pediatric Clin North Am. 2015;62(2):411-26.
2. Carvallo CM, Lupski JR. Mechanisms underlying structural variant formation in genomic disorders. Nat Rev Genet. 2016;17(4):224-38.
3. Jamuar SS, Tan EC. Clinical application of next-sequencing for Mendelian diseases. Hum Genomics. 2015;9:10.
4. Levitsky LL, Luria AH, Hayes FJ, Lin AE. Turner syndrome update on biology and management across the lifespan. Curr Opin Endocrinol Diabetes Obes. 2015;22(1):65-75.

SECTION 2
Respiratory System

- Case 4 Adenoids
- Case 5 Bronchial Asthma
- Case 6 Bronchiectasis
- Case 7 Bronchiolitis
- Case 8 Croup
- Case 9 Empyema
- Case 10 Otitis Media
- Case 11 Pneumonia
- Case 12 Tuberculosis

CASE 4

Adenoids

■ PRESENTING COMPLAINTS

A 3-year-old boy was brought with the complaints of:
- Mouth breathing since 3–4 months.
- Persistent nasal discharge since 3–4 months. Snoring since 2 months.
- Cough since 15 days.

History of Presenting Complaints

A 3-year-old boy with a history of mouth breathing and persistent nasal discharge was brought to the pediatric outpatient department. The mother complained that her son had this problem since the last 3–4 months. She said that mouth breathing was more evident when the child went to sleep. Sometimes, it was associated with snoring.

There was an associated history of nasal discharge. This was associated with the nasal block. The discharge was mucopurulent in nature. There was also a history of cough. Cough used to be more during the night which disturbed his sleep. Vomiting usually occurs as a result of a cough.

Past History of the Patient

The boy was the second child of a non-consanguineous marriage. He was born at full term by normal delivery. He cried immediately after the birth. There was transient tachypnoea of newborns lasting for 24 hours.

The child was breastfed exclusively for 6 months. Weaning was started at 6 months.

CASE AT A GLANCE	
Basic Findings	
Height	: 96 cm (75th centile) 13 kg (50th centile)
Weight	: 13 kg (50th centile)
Temperature	: 37.5°C
Pulse rate	: 120 beats/min
Respiratory rate	: 24 breaths/min
Blood pressure	: 80/60 mm Hg
Positive Findings	
History:	
• Mouth breathing	
• Snoring	
• Disturbed sleep	
• Cough	
• Vomiting	
Examination:	
• Dry lips	
• Enlarged tonsils	
• Enlarged cervical lymph node	
• Nasal twang	
Investigation:	
• *TLC:* Increased	
• *DLC:* Neutrophilia	
• *Lateral chest X-ray:* Normal	
• *Neck X-ray:* Massive obstruction by hypertrophied adenoids	
(DLC: differential leukocyte count; TLC: total leukocyte count)	

The child was on family food by the age of 18 months. He had been completely immunized. His developmental milestones were normal.

■ EXAMINATION

On examination, the child was moderately built and nourished. He was active, alert, and cooperative. He was playing with dolls present on the examination table. His height was 96 cm (75th centile) and his weight was 13 kg (50th centile).

He was afebrile. The pulse rate was 120 beats/min and the respiratory rate was 24 breaths/min. The type of respiration was abdominothoracic. The blood pressure recorded was 80/60 mm Hg.

There was no pallor, icterus, or cyanosis. Enlarged cervical lymph nodes were present. His lips were dry. Nasal twang was present at the time of crying. Throat examination revealed the presence of enlarged tonsils which met each other in midline. Normal vesicular breath sounds were present. There was no respiratory distress. Other systemic examinations were normal.

■ INVESTIGATION

- *Hemoglobin:* 11 g/dL
- *Total leukocyte count (TLC):* 12,500 cells/mm^3
- *Differential leukocyte count (DLC):* $P_{75}L_{20}M_1E_3B_1$
- *Erythrocyte sedimentation rate (ESR):* 20 mm in the first hour
- *Absolute eosinophil count (AEC):* 445 cells/mm^3
- *Urine (routine):* Normal
- *X-ray neck:* Massive obstruction by the hypertrophied adenoids **(Fig. 1)**
- *X-ray chest:* Normal

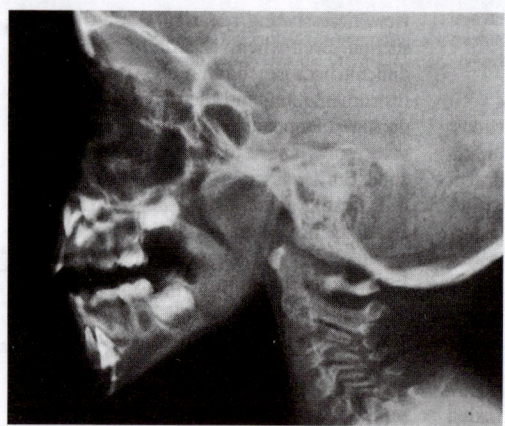

Fig. 1: X-ray of neck—massive obstruction by the hypertrophied adenoids.

■ DISCUSSION

The child presents with a history of rhinitis with mucopurulent discharge, mouth breathing, and snoring, along with a history of cough on lying down due to upper airway diseases leading to mild airway obstruction and enlarged tender cervical lymph nodes confirm the diagnosis of hypertrophied adenoids. Enlarged adenoids are invariably associated with enlarged tonsils.

Nasopharyngeal lymphoid tissue is called *adenoids*. They lie parallel to the facial tonsils. Hypertrophy and infection occur separately but often they occur together. The soft adenoid structure which is widespread in the nasopharynx, especially on the posterior wall and the roof undergoes hypertrophy. This fills up the vault of the nasopharynx and interferes with the passage of air through the nose and obstructs the Eustachian tube. Very obese children with a large and posteriorly placed tongue may develop upper airway obstruction. Other than the common cold, the next important cause of nasal obstruction is enlarged adenoids. This is more common between the ages of 4 and 8 years.

The possibility of upper airway obstruction with the increasing work of breathing may be the cause of poor appetite. Many a time it is associated with chronic pharyngitis and enlarged cervical lymph nodes. This chronic obstruction may produce hypoxia and pulmonary hypertension, hypoxia, increased work of breathing along with difficulty in swallowing resulting in failure to thrive.

The Waldeyer ring (the lymphoid tissue surrounding the opening of oral and nasal cavities into the pharynx) comprises the palatine tonsils the lingual tonsils, the pharyngeal tonsil or adenoid, lymphoid tissue surrounding the Eustachian tube orifice in the lateral wall of the nasopharynx the lingual tonsil at the base of the tongue and scattered lymphoid tissue throughout the remainder of the pharynx.

The immunologic role of the tonsils and adenoids is to induce secretory immunity and to regulate the production of immunoglobulins. Deep cervices within tonsillar tissue form tonsillar crypts that are lined with squamous epithelium and host a concentration of lymphocytes at their bases. The lymphoid of the Waldeyer ring is most immunologically active between 4 and 10 years, with a decrease after puberty. Adenotonsillar hypertrophy is greatest between 3 and 6 years, in most cases tonsils begin to involute after 8 years.

The tonsils and adenoids can be chronically infected by multiple microbes such as β-lactamase-producing organisms. Both aerobic species such as streptococci and *Haemophilus influenzae* and anaerobic species, such as *Peptostreptococcus*, *Prevotella*, and *Fusobacterium*, contribute. The tonsillar crypts can accommodate desquamated epithelial cells, lymphocytes, bacteria, and other debris, causing cryptic tonsillitis.

Airway obstruction in children is typically manifested in sleep-disordered breathing, including obstructive sleep apnea, obstructive sleep hypopnea, and upper airway resistance syndrome. Rapid enlargement of one tonsil is suggestive of a tonsillar malignancy, typically lymphoma in children.

■ CLINICAL FEATURES (FIG. 2)

Mouth breathing, persistent rhinitis, and nasal discharge are the most characteristic symptoms. Chronic mouth breathing is caused by blockage of nasal airflow. Nasal blockage is mainly because of adenoid hypertrophy.

Mouth breathing is present especially when the child lies supine. Snoring is also likely to occur. The mouth is kept open during the daytime. This indicates that the child has chronic nasopharyngitis. There will be a change in voice associated with nasal twang. Breath is offensive, and taste and smell are impaired.

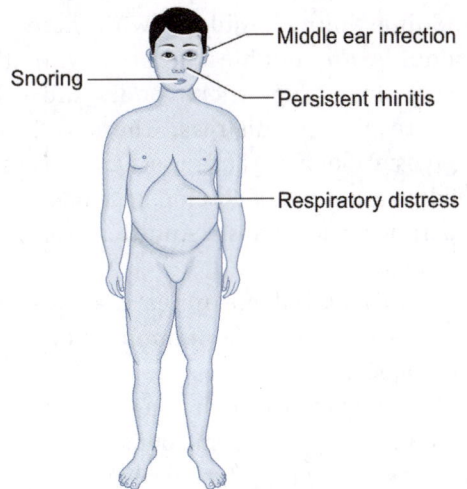

Fig. 2: Clinical features.

A harassing cough may be present, especially at night. The drainage of pus into the lower pharynx or irritation of the larynx by inspired air that has not been warmed and moistened by the passage through the nose occurs.

Symptoms of acute infection include odynophagia, dry throat, malaise fever and chills, dysphagia, referred otalgia, headache, muscle pains, and enlarged cervical nodes. Signs include a dry tongue, erythematous enlarged tonsils, tonsillar or pharyngeal exudate, palatine petechiae, and enlargement and tenderness of jugulodigastric lymph nodes.

Children with chronic tonsillitis are present with halitosis, chronic sore throat, and foreign body sensation. Signs include enlarged tonsils of different sizes often containing copious debris with crypts.

Symptoms of airway obstruction include chronic mouth breathing, nasal obstruction, hyponasal speech, hyposmia, decreased appetite, and rarely right-sided heart failure. Night symptoms include loud snoring, choking, gasping, apnea, abnormal sleep position enuresis, and sleep talking.

Some young children with marked adenoids are unable to mouth breath during sleep. They snore loudly and will have respiratory distress. There will be intercostal indrawing and nasal flaring. These children are at risk of developing hypoxemia, hyperpnea, and acidosis. Apneic spells may develop.

Obstructive sleep apnea may result. Some of them acquire pulmonary arterial hypertension.

The cough is due to drainage of pus into the lower pharynx. Chronic otitis media may be associated with infected hypertrophied adenoids. This produces blocking of the Eustachian tube orifice resulting in a middle-ear infection. Hence impaired hearing is common.

CLINICAL FEATURES
- *Mouth breathing:* Harassing cough
- *Persistent rhinitis:* Apneic speech
- *Nasal discharge:* Middle-ear infection
- *Snoring:* Nasal twang
- *Anoxic spell:* Respiratory distress

Obese children with Prader–Willi syndrome and children with large posteriorly placed tongues, i.e., with Pierre Robin syndrome, will complicate the symptoms of adenoids. Down syndrome patients will have large tongues obstructing the airway.

■ DIAGNOSIS

Adenoid enlargement is suspected in children older than 2 years who present with nasal block, mouth breathing, sleep disturbances, and chronic nasal discharge. A lateral radiograph will confirm the presence of soft tissue enlargement in the nasopharynx.

LABORATORY SALIENT FINDINGS
- Endoscopic evaluation—fiberoptic nasopharyngoscope to visualise nasopharynx.
- Lateral radiograph—adenoid hypertrophy occluding the airways

The size of the adenoids can be assessed by digital palpation during the first few years of life. A fiberoptic nasopharyngoscope can be used for visualization of the nasopharynx. Lateral pharyngeal soft tissue radiographs are helpful for detecting air column obliteration.

■ COMPLICATIONS

- Poststreptococcal glomerulonephritis
- Peritonsillar infection
- Retropharyngeal infection
- Parapharyngeal infection

TREATMENT

Tonsillectomy

Tonsillectomy alone is most commonly performed for recurrent or chronic pharyngotonsillitis. It is effective in reducing the number of infections and symptoms of chronic tonsillitis. In resistant cases of cryptic tonsillitis, tonsillectomy is curative.

Tonsillectomy should not be performed routinely for such problems unless separate indications for tonsillectomy are present. Chronic serous otitis media may improve after adenoidectomy in the patients.

Adenoidectomy

Adenoidectomy is recommended for symptomatic younger children. The pubertal growth of the midface and regression of the adenoid size tend to result in relief of adenoid-related nasal obstruction around the age of 9 years.

Adenoidectomy may be indicated for symptoms such as persistent mouth breathing, hyponasal speech, adenoid facies, and repeated, or chronic otitis media with effusion (OME).

It is indicated for the treatment of chronic nasal infection-chronic adenoiditis, chronic sinus infection with failed medical management, and recurrent bouts of acute otitis media (AOM). It may be curative in patients with nasal obstruction, chronic mouth breathing, loud snoring, and sleep-disordered breathing.

Tonsillectomy and Adenoidectomy

This is indicated in upper airway obstruction secondary to adenotonsillar hypertrophy that results in sleep disorder breathing, failure to thrive, craniofacial or occulodevelopmental abnormalities, and speech abnormalities.

Surgery of the nasal septum should be avoided in prepubertal children as it may lead to midfacial growth retardation and saddling of the nose.

BIBLIOGRAPHY

1. Baugh RF, Archer SM, Mitchell RB, Rosenfeld RM, Amin R, Burns JJ, et al. Clinical Practice guidelines: tonsillectomy in children. Surg. 2011;144(1 Suppl):S1-30.
2. Marcus CL, Brooks LJ, Draper KA, Gozal D, Halbower AC, Jones J, et al. American Academy of Pediatrics: Diagnosis and Management of childhood obstructive sleep apnea syndrome. Pediatrics. 2012;130(3): e714-55.
3. Marcus CL, Moore RH, Rosen CL, Giordani B, Garetz SL, Taylor HG, et al.; Childhood Adenotonsilectomy Trial. A randomized trial of adenotonsillectomy for childhood sleep apnea. N Engl J Med. 2013;3268(25):2366-76.

CASE 5

Bronchial Asthma

PRESENTING COMPLAINTS

A 7-year-old boy brought with the complaints of:
- Cough since 2 days
- Vomiting since 1 day
- Breathlessness since 2 hours
- Tiredness since 2 hours

History of Presenting Complaints

A 7-year-old boy was brought to the emergency room early with a history of persistent cough, breathlessness, and tiredness. According to the mother, his son went to sleep without any symptoms. She revealed later that the cough had been present since 2 days. The cough was a dry irritating type. There was a history of vomiting as a result of the cough. According to the mother, there was a disturbance of sleep, and appetite was decreased to a certain extent. The child was shown to the general practitioner.

Past History of the Patient

He was the second child of a nonconsanguineous marriage. He was born at term by normal vaginal delivery. He cried immediately after the birth. The birth weight of the child was 2.9 kg. He was on breast milk exclusively for the 4 months of age. Weaning started by the age of 4 months and was completed by 13 months. He had been vaccinated completely.

CASE AT A GLANCE	
Basic Findings	
Height	: 122 cm (50th centile)
Weight	: 24 kg (50th centile)
Temperature	: 37°C
Pulse rate	: 150 beats/min
Respiratory rate	: 60 breaths/min
Blood pressure	: 90/70 mm Hg

Positive Findings

History:
- Persistent cough
- Breathlessness
- Vomiting
- Disturbance of sleep
- Family history of bronchial asthma
- Treatment with nebulization

Examination:
- Dyspnea
- Tachycardia
- Tachypnea
- Indrawing and retraction of the chest
- Wheeze
- Hepatomegaly

Investigation:
- No abnormal findings

There was a strong family history of the father suffering from wheezing. He was on a regular inhaler for chronic management. This child had developed wheezing recently. He was symptomatic to treatment with the bronchodilator and nebulization.

■ EXAMINATION

On examination, he was moderately built and moderately nourished. Anthropometric measurements included that his height was 122 cm (50th centile), and his weight was 24 kg (50th centile).

He was afebrile, dyspneic, and was more comfortable sitting. He was sitting bending his body forward keeping his hand over the thigh. The pulse rate was 150 beats/min and the respiratory rate was 60 breaths/min. Chest retraction and indrawing of the ribs were present. The blood pressure recorded was 90/70 mm Hg. There was no pallor, no cyanosis, and no clubbing. There was no significant lymphadenopathy.

The respiratory system revealed the presence of the rhonchi, and wheeze throughout the lung fields. Per abdomen, examination showed the presence of nontender hepatomegaly. His cardiovascular system revealed tachycardia.

■ INVESTIGATION

- *Hemoglobin:* 11 g/dL
- *Total leukocyte count (TLC):* 8,800 cell/mm^3
- *Differential leukocyte count (DLC):* $P_{72}L_{18}E_8M_2$
- *Erythrocyte sedimentation rate (ESR):* 24 mm in the first hour
- *Absolute eosinophil count (AEC):* 400 cells/mm^3
- *Chest X-ray:* Normal

■ DISCUSSION

A child was brought with a history of breathlessness and tiredness. There was a strong family history of bronchial asthma. The child was having nebulization for the relief of the wheeze. On examination, there was tachypnea and hepatomegaly, and the presence of wheeze confirms bronchial asthma.

Bronchial asthma is a chronic inflammatory disease of airways affecting 15–20% of children. Diagnosing asthma in preschool children is often difficult. Nearly 50% of children will have wheeze during the first 3 years of life. In general, there are two types of wheezing:
1. Transient early wheezing
2. Persistent and recurrent wheezing

Transient Early Wheezing

This is also known as episodic viral wheeze and wheezy bronchitis. This occurs as a result of small airways being narrowed and obstructed due to inflammation and aberrant immune response to viral infection. This is more common in males and usually resolves by 5 years of age.

Persistent and Recurrent Wheezing

Preschool and school-aged children will have frequent wheezes triggered by many factors. Here immunoglobulin E (IgE) is present common to inhalant allergens. Recurrent wheezing associated with evidence allergy, i.e., skin prick test or IgE blood test is termed "atopic asthma." These have persistent symptoms and decreased lung functions. They are strongly associated with eczema, food allergy, rhinitis, and conjunctivitis.

There is increased responsiveness of the trachea and bronchi to the various stimuli. Bronchial reactivity is an essential component of bronchial asthma. There will be edema, and excessive mucus production infiltration of cells, such as eosinophils, mast cells neutrophils, and lymphocytes. There will be excessive secretion of mucus, inflammatory cells, and cellular debris. Smooth muscle spasms will also produce obstruction. This leads to the reversible widespread narrowing of airways which in turn leads to airway obstruction. Airway obstruction manifests clinically paroxysmal dyspnea, wheezing, and cough.

The various stimuli that trigger bronchial asthma may be of two types. One is extrinsic and the second is intrinsic. Extrinsic is IgE-mediated. It is mainly allergen-triggered. The intrinsic is mainly infection-triggered. It is also IgE-mediated. There is one more group. This is mixed and it is excessive and aspirin-induced.

There will be a biphasic response in the body to the allergy. This leads to bronchoconstriction. The biphasic response includes early reaction and late reaction.

Early reaction occurs within 10 minutes of exposure. Chemical mediators are released. These include histamine leukotrienes C, D, and E, prostaglandin, platelet-activating factor, and bradykinin. These are released from mast cells. The early reaction occurs due to the interaction of mast cells bounded IgE with allergen. This causes bronchoconstriction, mucosal edema, and mucosal secretion. This manifests airway obstruction. β_2 agonist drugs with inhibit this phase.

Late reaction occurs within 3–4 hours. It reaches peak reaction by 8–12 hours. This occurs due to the release of mast cell mediators. This phase cannot be inhibited by β_2 agonist drugs. This is inhibited by premedication with steroids. This suggests mucosal edema and inflammatory reaction are the cause of airway narrowing. This phase presents as clinical asthma.

There is an imbalance between excitatory and inhibitory mechanisms. Excitatory mechanisms include cholinergic, alpha-adrenergic, and noncholinergic. Inhibitory mechanisms include β-adrenergic and nonadrenergic. This increases bronchial reactiveness.

Bronchoconstriction results in increased cholinergic activity. This leads to bronchial smooth muscle spasms. Bronchodilatation occurs due to endogenous catecholamine and nonadrenergic systems. These act through β adrenergic receptors and prostaglandin E_2.

Some neuropeptides are secreted by nonadrenergic and noncholinergic nerves. These are vasoactive intestinal peptides substance P. These will relax the smooth muscles of the bronchi. These increase smooth muscle tone, mucus secretion, and microvascular leakage.

In the early phases, dyspnea, i.e., breathlessness produces hyperventilation. This causes a fall in partial pressure of arterial carbon dioxide ($PaCO_2$). Alveolar hypotension supervenes when the obstruction becomes severe. This leads to the retention of CO_2; hence, there is a rise in $PaCO_2$. With the exhaustion of the buffer mechanism, the pH of the blood falls, and respiratory acidemia occurs.

■ PATHOGENESIS

Airway inflammation is the basic pathology. It occurs due to the hyperactivity of airways to a variety of stimuli. It is initiated by the degranulation of mast cells release of mediators of inflammation. This damages the airways leading to epithelial shedding and mucus secretion. It is characterized by repeated attacks of cough with respiratory distress. The respiratory distress reverses either spontaneously or with bronchodilators. It is the result of multifactorial inheritance.

The risk factors include a family history of asthma, atopy, and bronchiolitis in infancy. Passive smoking is a predisposing factor. The triggering factors include upper respiratory tract infection (URTI), cold air, exercise, chemical irritants, and anxiety. This stimulates the release of mediators from mast cells. Exclusive breastfeeding during the first 6 months will protect against the development of asthma to a certain extent.

Viral infection triggers airway narrowing. It produces an opening up of the tight intraepithelial cell junction. The integrity of the mucosal surface is disturbed. This leads to the shelling of epithelium. Mucosal edema and mucosal secretion results in airway narrowing.

Exercise induces water loss. Water loss produces mucosal hyperosmolarity. This stimulates mediators released from mast cells. Sudden weather changes may result in the loss of heat and water from the lower airways. There will be airborne allergen in the atmosphere. This results in exacerbation of bronchial asthma. Emotional factors act through the vagus nerve. This causes the contraction of smooth muscles.

■ CLINICAL FEATURES (FIG. 1)

Symptoms vary from simple recurrent cough to severe breathlessness secondary to wheezing. Acute asthma may usually begin with a cold or bouts of spasmodic cough. Symptoms worsen during the evening or early morning or may be exaggerated by triggers, i.e., exercise and allergen exposure. A family history of asthma or allergy should be ascertained.

The cough is nonproductive in the early phase. Later the child becomes more breathless with prolonged expiration and wheezing. Accessory muscles of respiration become active. The child sweats profusely. A child looks fatigued and apprehensive. Cyanosis may appear. A child becomes restless.

In severe conditions, the child keeps his arm forward for support. Chest becomes hyperresonant because of excessive air trapping. When the obstruction becomes severe, there is decreased air entry, break sounds become feeble. Wheezing will be absent. Cyanosis appears. This is not a good sign. Wheezing reappears as the child improves clinically and airflow increases. With the remission of the attack, wheezing disappears.

Cyanosis, cardiac arrhythmias, and pulsus paradoxus indicate severe hypoxemia. The mucus plug blocks the bronchial tree and causes a collapse of small segments of the lung. Chest becomes barrel shaped in chronic intermittent cases.

The presence of a wet cough or sputum, finger clubbing, or poor growth suggests chronic infections, such as bronchiectasis and cystic fibrosis (CF).

The hallmark of bronchial asthma is wheezing. Wheezing is the whistling sound produced when the flow of air from the lung is obstructed. Obstruction may be due to the narrowing of the airway. This type of wheezing will respond positively to asthmatic therapy.

Wheezing can also be present in other diseases such as transient early wheezing, IgE-mediated atopic asthma, nonatopic asthma, CF, viral pneumonia, bronchiolitis,

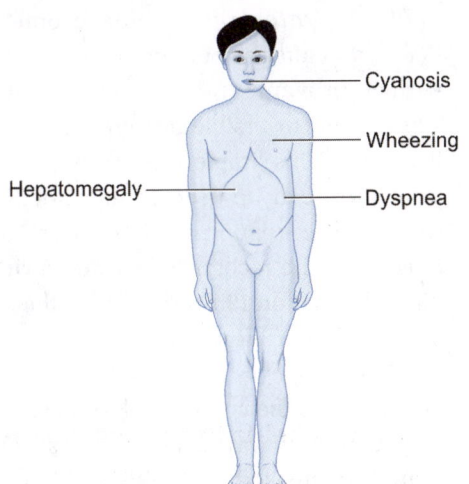

Fig. 1: Clinical features.

congestive cardiac failure, and foreign body aspiration.

> **GENERAL FEATURES**
> - Poorly built
> - Persistent coughing
> - Shortness of breath
> - Rapid breathing

> **ESSENTIAL DIAGNOSTIC POINTS**
> - Episodic symptoms of airway obstruction
> - Wheezing, cough, and breathlessness
> - Reversible airflow obstruction

DIAGNOSIS

Diagnosis of asthma is mainly by history and physical examination. The diagnosis of asthma in infants and preschoolers is often difficult due to poor cooperation in diagnostic procedures, hesitation by pediatricians, time-consuming and practicality, and ethical issues. However, early diagnosis is essential for timely treatment to improve the quality of physical and psychological development, to prevent chronic pulmonary disease due to "airway remodeling" and educate on the preventive measures, to cut health care cost, and prognosticate.

Preschoolers

The diagnosis of asthma is made based on national guidelines in UM infant who has more than three episodes of wheezing in 1 year with a family history of asthma, has atopic features, febrile episodes, and cough persisting >2 weeks with good response to bronchodilators. In some children a therapeutic trial of treatment with quick relievers and inhaled steroids for 8–12 weeks with good improvement and relapse after stopping treatment is diagnostic of asthma.

School-going Children

- *Pulmonary function tests (PFTs)*: The diagnosis of asthma is clinical in most cases; hence PFTs may not play a significant role. These investigations have an important role in the diagnosis of doubtful cases and in monitoring the response to treatment. The important parameters in spirometry include peak expiratory flow rate (PEFR), forced expiratory volume in one second (FEV_1), forced vital capacity (FVC), and FEV25–75. All parameters are decreased in asthma. FEV_1 is a commonly used parameter for documentation of the severity of asthma. FEV25–75 is effort-independent and is probably a more sensitive indicator of airway obstruction. PEFR can be measured easily with a peak expiratory flow (PEF) meter, while for other parameters a spirometer is required. PEFR may be used as a diagnostic tool in doubtful cases as well as monitoring of treatment. Abnormalities in PEFR suggestive of asthma include a diurnal variation of >20%, <80% of predicted, and improvement of >20% after bronchodilator therapy.
- *Peak expiratory flow* measurement before and after salbutamol nebulization with improvement (12–15%) is highly suggestive of reversible airway obstruction in asthma. This simple and less expensive procedure can be used to monitor the therapeutic response. Early asthma attacks can be recognized by measuring diurnal variation PEP. It measures the air coming out of larger and medium size airways.
- *Spirometry* is the central tool for defining obstructive airway disease. In asthma there is decreased FEV_1, FEV/FVC ratio, and forced expiratory flow (FEF) 25–75%.

- *Absolute eosinophil counts*: The significance of eosinophilia for distinguishing between the allergic, vasomotor, or infectious nature of chronic respiratory obstructive disease is limited. When eosinophilia is present, bronchial obstruction generally responds well to antispasmodic therapy and the condition is often reversible. The eosinophil count may be low in cases associated with infection. Steroid medication in asthma causes eosinopenia.
- *Chest X-ray* shows bilateral and symmetric air trapping in case of asthma. Patches of atelectasis of varying sizes due to mucus plugs are not unusual. The main pulmonary artery is prominent due to pulmonary hypertension. Bronchial cuffing may occur due to the presence of edema fluid in perivascular and peribronchial interstitial space. Extensive areas of collapse or consolidation should suggest an alternative diagnosis. Chest X-ray film may often be normal.
- *Allergy tests* including skin tests and radioallergosorbent allergen specific IgE (RAST) have limited usefulness. Few children need skin tests to identify sensitivity to different antigens since the role of desensitization therapy is not established.
- *Skin-prick testing:* This is often considered both as an aid to the diagnosis of atopy and to identify allergens that may be acting as triggers. *Skin testing* with allergens is the gold standard to identify the specific allergens and is used before immunotherapy for aeroallergens.
- *Total IgE level:* It is beneficial only to recognize the atopic background of asthma. It helps to predict response to steroids, the prognosis, and the possibility of development of persistent as well as strongly advocate environmental control.
- *Specific IgE level:* It is needed for specific immunotherapy and before the use of anti-IgE antibody treatment
- *Breath nitric oxide* is used in some pulmonary centers for monitoring eosinophilic airway inflammation. It is not used much in children for various reasons.

Bronchial challenge tests and other physiological tests do not have a major role in the diagnosis of asthma in children.

A prolonged whistling sound heard at the mouth during expiration is called a wheeze. Recurrent attacks of wheezing indicate bronchial asthma. Although intermittent attacks of coughing may be due to recurrent viral infections, the diagnosis of bronchial asthma should be considered. Cough, which is associated with asthma generally, worsens after exercise. Sputum is generally clear and mucoid, but expectoration of yellowish sputum (attributed to a large number of eosinophils) does not exclude the diagnosis of asthma. Chronic spasmodic cough may suggest occult asthma.

Differential Diagnosis

- *Bronchiolitis:* Bronchiolitis always occurs within the first 2 years, usually within the first 6 months of life. It is more common in winter or spring months. Generally, there is a single attack. Repeated attacks indicate viral infection associated wheeze or asthma. Hyperinflation of the chest with scattered areas of infiltration may be seen on chest X-ray. Asthma may start at any age; more than three episodes are usual, and wheezing is prominent. Infants diagnosed with bronchiolitis with a family history of allergy, having atopic eczema, or whose IgE levels are elevated are likely to develop asthma.

- *Congenital malformation* causing obstruction, e.g., vascular rings such as an aberrant right subclavian artery or double aortic arch, bronchogenic cysts, and tracheomalacia should be excluded in the differential diagnosis.
- *Aspiration of the foreign body:* Wheeze, if present is generally localized. The history of foreign body aspiration may be forgotten. An area with diminished air entry, with or without hyperresonance on percussion especially in children, may be due to obstructive emphysema because of a check-valve type of obstruction due to the foreign body. Most children develop frequent infections in the lungs around the foreign body.
- *Hypersensitivity pneumonitis:* An acute or chronic lung disease may be observed following inhalation of organic dust such as molds, wood or cotton dust, bird droppings, fur dust, grain, or following exposure to certain chemicals or drugs such as epoxy resins, para-aminosalicylic acid (PAS), and sulfonamides. In the acute form of illness, these children suffer from fever, chills, dyspnea, malaise, aches and pain, loud inspiratory vales (crackles) at the bases of the lungs, and weight loss. X-ray chest shows interstitial pneumonia. Bronchial markings are prominent. The levels of IgE antibodies to the specific antigen are increased. The skin test shows the Arthus phenomenon with local hemorrhage, edema, and local pain within 8 hours of the test. Diagnosis is established by lung biopsy.
- *Cystic fibrosis:* Children with CF may present with recurrent wheezing but over a period of time they develop clubbing. There may be clinical evidence of malabsorption. X-ray film may show evidence of hyperinflation, peribronchial cuffing, and pneumonia. Diagnosis is established by estimating sweat chloride levels.

MANAGEMENT OF ACUTE EXACERBATIONS

A stepwise approach is necessary for appropriate management. The steps in management are:
1. Assessment of severity and identification of life-threatening attack
2. Initiation of therapy
3. Assessment of response to initial therapy
4. Modification of or addition to therapy and referral

Step 1: Assessment of Severity and Identification of Life-threatening Attack

Initial assessment is necessary to rapidly determine the degree of airway obstruction and hypoxia. The features of a life-threatening attack of asthma are (1) cyanosis, silent chest, or feeble respiratory efforts; (2) fatigue or exhaustion; and (3) agitation or reduced level of consciousness.

Any child with features suggestive of a life-threatening attack should ideally be treated in a hospital where intensive care facilities are available. However, the child should receive oxygen, a bronchodilator, and a dose of steroids before making arrangements for transfer to a tertiary-level health facility. Oxygen and inhalation therapy [metered dose inhaler (MDI) with Spacer] should be continued while the child is being transferred.

Identification of life-threatening attack

The features of life-threatening asthma:
- Cyanosis
- Silent chest
- Poor respiratory effort
- Exhaustion
- Fatigue

- Altered sensorium
- PEFR <30%
- Oxygen saturation of <90%

Categorization of an acute exacerbation of asthma into mild, moderate, or severe can be done based on physical examination and objective parameters as enumerated in **Table 1**. In any child with a severe degree of respiratory distress, the presence of alteration of sensorium confusion, and cyanosis will suggest respiratory failure. Examination needs to be repeated after each step of treatment to assess the response.

An objective measurement of lung function tests becomes necessary. The two methods of objective measurements of lung function that can be used are: (1) measurements of airflow obstruction by PEFR or FEV_1 and (2) arterial blood gas (ABG) analysis or pulse oximetry.

Peak expiratory flow rate can be measured using a simple peak flow meter. A child is made to use the peak flow meter in a standing position, three times, and the best of the three values is taken as the child's PEFR during the acute attack. This is compared with the child's personal best or predicted PEFR.

It has been recommended that if pH is <7.3 or the base deficit is >5 mEq, intravenous correction with sodium bicarbonate is indicated, initially using half the calculated dose, and then repeating the ABG.

Laboratory studies are generally not indicated in a routine acute exacerbation. However, if the child is unusually ill or there is a doubt of infection, blood samples can be taken for (i) white blood cell (WBC) count for detecting polymorphonuclear leukocytosis and bacteremia which suggests bacterial infection, and (ii) serum electrolytes since

TABLE 1: Estimation of severity of acute exacerbation of asthma.

Symptom/sign	Mild	Moderate	Severe
Respiratory rate	Normal	Increased	Increased
Alertness	Normal	Normal	May be decreased
Dyspnea	Absent or mild; speaks in a complete sentence	Moderate; speaks in phrases or partial sentences	Severe; speaks only in single words or short phrases
Pulsus paradoxus	<10 mm Hg	10–20 mg Hg	20–40 mm Hg
Accessory muscle use	No or mild intercostals retractions	Moderate intercostals retractions with tracheosternal retractions, use of sternocleidomastoid muscle	Severe intercostals and tracheosternal retractions with nasal flaring
Color	Pink	Pale	Ashen gray or cyanotic
Auscultation	End expiratory wheeze only	Wheeze during the entire expiration and inspiration	Breath sounds become almost inaudible
Oxygen saturation	>95%	90–95%	<90%
$PaCO_2$	<35 mm Hg	<40 mm Hg	>40 mm Hg
PEFR	70–90% of predicted or personal best	50–70% of predicted or personal best	<50% of predicted or personal best

($PaCO_2$: partial pressure of arterial carbon dioxide; PEFR: peak expiratory flow rate)

both β-2 agonists and corticosteroids may cause hypokalemia.

A chest radiograph is indicated only when the diagnosis is doubtful or there is a suspicion of a foreign body. It is also useful in a child with high-grade fever, localized crepitations, decreased breath sounds, and other findings suggestive of infection or complications, such as pneumothorax, atelectasis, and pneumomediastinum.

Step 2: Initiation of Therapy

Principles of therapy:

The following are the broad objectives:
- The goal is to rapidly reverse the acute airflow obstruction with consequent relief of respiratory distress. This is achieved by repeated use of inhaled β-2 agonists.
- Hypoxia is treated by proper oxygenation of all acutely sick children.
- Corticosteroids are added early in an acute attack if the response to inhaled bronchodilators is not satisfactory.
- Repeated clinical and objective assessment is done to evaluate the response to the above, add other drugs if necessary, and also to detect impending respiratory failure at the earliest.

Initial therapy:
- *Oxygen:* All patients with acute severe asthma have some degree of hypoxia. Oxygen at the rate of 3–6 L/min should be started. The flow should be enough to maintain oxygen saturation above 92%.

  Table 2 discusses drug dosages in children with acute attacks of bronchial asthma.
- *β-2 agonists:* The currently recommended standard bronchodilator therapy is repeated inhalations of β-2 agonist aerosol. Salbutamol nebulizer solution (5 mg/mL) in the dose of 0.1–0.15 mg/kg diluted in 3 mL of normal saline is administered over a period of 10–15 minutes. It is preferable to use a central oxygen supply at the rate of 6–7 L/min to run the nebulizer, at least initially, to avoid hypoxia. The dose can be repeated every 20 minutes for three times and the child is reassessed after that. The rationale behind giving repeated doses of inhaled bronchodilators is that the bronchodilatation that follows the initial dose allows more distal deposition of drug particles during further dosing. This results in dilatation of smaller airways and the short dosing interval prevents any deterioration of clinical status in the intervening period. Recent studies, however, suggest that continuous nebulization may be more effective than intermittent nebulization. This method of therapy can continue for a prolonged period without having to set up nebulization at regular intervals.

  Patients are more likely to get acclimatized to continuous nebulization and therefore maintain a more constant breathing pattern. This would result in a subsequent reduction of inspiratory flow and more peripheral deposition of inhaled bronchodilator aerosol. Recommended doses are 0.1–0.5 mg/kg/h via a delivery system comprising preferably of a constant infusion pump and central oxygen supply. Higher doses of 3.4 ± 2.2 mg/kg/h have been used in ventilated patients.

  Alternatively, MDI can be used with a spacer device to give repeated inhalations of β-2 agonist. It is considered equivalent to or better than a nebulizer driven by compressed air. It does not cause oxygen desaturation unlike the former. The duration of therapy is <1 minute as compared to 15 minutes with a nebulizer. The use of MDI reduces the cost of

TABLE 2: Drug dosages in children with acute attack of bronchial asthma.

Drug	Available form	Dosage
Inhaled β-2 agonist: • Salbutamol • Metered dose inhaler • Nebulizer solution	100 µg/puff 0.5% (5 mg/mL)	• Two inhalations every 5 minutes for a total of 10–20 puffs, with 0.1–0.15 mg/kg dose up to 5 mg every 20 minutes for 1–2 hours (minimum dose 1.25 mg/dose) Or, • 0.1–0.5 mg/kg/h by continuous nebulization (maximum 15 mg/h) or 3.4 ± 2.2 mg/kg/h in ventilated patients
Terbutaline: • Metered dose inhaler • Nebulizer solution	 250 µg/puff 10 mg/mL	Two inhalations every 5 minutes for a total of 10–20 puffs • <20 kg 2.5 mg • >20 kg 5 mg
Systemic β-2 agonists: • Epinephrine HCl • Terbutaline	 1:1,000 AOL (1 mg/mL) 0.05% (0.05 mg/mL) solution for injection in 0.9% saline	• 0.01 mg/kg up to 0.3 mg subcutaneously every 20 minutes for three doses • Subcutaneous 0.005 mg/kg up to 0.3 mg every 2–6 hours as needed. An intravenous bolus of 10 µg/kg over 30 minutes followed by intravenous infusion at the rate of 0.1 µg/kg/min. Increase as necessary by 0.1 µg/kg/min every 30 minutes. The maximum dose is 4 µg/kg/min
Inhaled anticholinergics: • Ipratropium bromide • Metered dose inhaler • Nebulizer solution	 20 µg/puff 250 µg/mL	• Two inhalations every 5 minutes for a total of 10–20 puffs • 1 mL diluted in 3 mL normal saline every 20 minutes for 1–2 hours. This may be mixed with salbutamol nebulizer solution or alternated with salbutamol
Aminophylline	80% anhydrous theophylline (250 mg/10 mL injection)	Give a loading dose of 5–6 mg/kg and maintain at 0.9 mg/kg/h. If the patient is already receiving theophylline, avoid the bolus dose
Prednisolone	5, 10, and 20 mg tablets	1–2 mg/kg/dose every 6 hours for 24 hours, then 1–2 mg/kg/day in divided doses every 8–12 hours for 5–7 days
Hydrocortisone	50 mg/mL injection	10 mg/kg intravenous bolus followed by 2.5–5.0 mg/kg q6h
• Methylprednisolone • Magnesium sulfate	40 mg/mL injection 50% solution for injection (500 mg/mL)	• 4 mg/kg intravenous single dose • 30–70 mg/kg in 30 mL N/5 saline intravenous infusion over 30 minutes

therapy that is easily performed and does not require a power supply. One to two puffs every 5–10 minutes can be used for 10–20 times. One can use a commercially available large-volume (750 mL) spacer device.

In some children with severe bronchospasm, an initial dose of epinephrine may be helpful prior to initiating inhalational treatment. Oxygen desaturation seen with nebulization therapy is not seen with this form of therapy. On the contrary, a transient increase in the partial pressure of arterial oxygen (PaO$_2$) has been noticed. Injectable terbutaline may also be used in place of epinephrine. The use of epinephrine is limited by its shorter duration of action and cardiac side effects, and it cannot be repeated more than two to three times. Terbutaline has a longer duration of action, and a repeat dose may not be required for 2-6 hours.

- *Anticholinergics:* Some studies have shown that concomitant use of inhaled anticholinergics and a selective β-2 agonist produces significantly greater improvement in lung function than β-2 agonist alone. Only ipratropium bromide is used in view of negligible side effects. As it has few systemic adverse effects, its use is advocated for patients with life-threatening features or those who do not respond to initial high-dose inhaled β-2 agonists.

  Parasympathetic fibers are present in larger airways, in contrast to β-adrenergic receptors which are located in more peripheral airways. Ipratropium may also have a generalized action throughout the lung. It being an acetylcholine antagonist while salbutamol is a β-2 agonist, both acting at different sites in the lung and via different pharmacologic mechanisms, provides the basis for using these drugs together.

  An optimal dose of 250 µg contained in 1.0 mL of the respirator solution, may be mixed with salbutamol solution and both given together at an interval of 20 minutes with the nebulizer. It may also be given alternating with the dose of nebulized salbutamol. The dosing frequency may be reduced as the patient improves.

  In patients who suffer from tachycardia or marked tremors in response to a standard dose of β-2 agonists and in the younger age group (3-30 months), ipratropium may be more effective than salbutamol.

- *Corticosteroids:* Since inflammation is an important component of airway obstruction in an acute attack of asthma, there is no doubt that the use of steroids in an acute exacerbation is useful in resolving the obstruction. However, it is somewhat difficult to decide precisely when steroids should be administered.

  It is evident that the timing of the initiation of steroid therapy plays a major role in the subsequent outcome of the attack. Studies have shown that the efficacy of steroid therapy is maximal when they are started soon after the patient presents in the emergency room. In contrast, benefits were minimal when steroids were initiated 24-48 hours after observation. A single dose of intramuscular methylprednisolone in a dose of 4 mg/kg, when given as an early adjunct to the β-2 adrenergic therapy has been reported to reduce hospitalization rates. In the following situations, steroids should be started as soon as the patient presents in an emergency.
  - A child with a very severe attack of asthma.
  - Previous history of life-threatening attacks or severe attacks not responding to bronchodilators.
  - If the child is on oral steroids or high doses of inhaled steroids for prophylaxis. An oral dose of 1-2 mg/kg of prednisolone may be as effective as an equivalent dose of hydrocortisone given intravenously because the time for onset of action is the same. The total duration of therapy can be 3-7 days depending upon the response. However, children who have already been on long-term oral

steroids would require a longer course with tapering of doses over 5–10 days.

Step 3: Assessment of Response to Initial Therapy

Close monitoring for any signs of improvement or deterioration is important. The patient should be assessed after initial therapy of two to three doses of bronchodilator along with oxygen over a period of 1 hour. The plan for further management will depend on whether the response to initial therapy has been good, partial, or poor.

- *Good response:* The subject with good response to initial therapy will become free of wheezing and have no breathlessness. Heart rate and respiratory rate will decrease. Auscultation of the chest will show minimal or no rhonchi and PEFR or FEVI will improve to >70% of the predicted best. Such a child can be observed in the emergency room for 2–4 hours and if remains stable, can be discharged on bronchodilators (inhaled or oral) for the period of 5–7 days. The parents should be advised to come for follow-up and all other necessary instructions should be given for prophylaxis,
- *Partial response:* A child may show some response after bronchodilators but may still have breathlessness and wheezing. Physical examination will reveal the persistence of rhonchi. Heart rate and respiratory rate will be above the physiologic norms. Pulsus paradoxus of 10–15 mm Hg and oxygen saturation of 91–95% may be observed. Peak end expiratory reserve (PEER) will be between 40 and 70% of the predicted normal. Treatment of a child with partial response is discussed later.
- *Poor response:* If there is no subjective or objective improvement after initial therapy, it indicates a poor response. This child will continue to have severe respiratory distress and wheeze. A physical examination will reveal severe airway obstruction as indicated by significant pulsus paradoxus (≥ 15 mm Hg), use of accessory muscles, and extensive rhonchi. Oxygen saturation of $\leq 90\%$ and PEER <40% of predicted normal may be observed.

Step 4: Modification of Therapy for Patients with Partial and Poor Response to Initial Therapy

- *Continue oxygen and bronchodilator therapy:* If the response to the initial therapy is not good, oxygen and β-2 agonist inhalation should be continued. The frequency of inhalation should be decided according to the severity of respiratory distress. Children who do not have severe respiratory distress and have shown partial response may only require 2–4 hourly inhalation while children with severe distress should be given more frequent inhalations. Inhalation as frequently as every 20 minutes, or even continuous can be given without side effects for the next 2 hours and the child reassessed. If ipratropium is not used at the onset, it is added at the end of the first hour as described earlier. MDI with a spacer can also be used frequently as an effective alternate device. It should also be ascertained whether the nebulizer and MDI are being used correctly
- *Continue corticosteroids:* Corticosteroids should be continued as 1–2 mg/kg/dose of prednisolone or 2.5–5.0 mg/kg/dose of hydrocortisone every 6 hours.
- *Intravenous fluids and correction of acidosis:* Children admitted with an acute severe attack of asthma often have mild to moderate dehydration. Dehydration may

produce more viscous mucus, leading to bronchiolar plugging. Humidification of inspired air and correction of dehydration, therefore, is always indicated. However, at the same time, inappropriate hormone secretion has *been* reported in some cases of bronchial asthma. Hence fluid therapy should be individualized to keep the child in normal hydration.

Hypokalemia has been reported with frequent β adrenergic and corticosteroid therapy. It should be corrected when present. Metabolic acidosis that occurs during an acute attack may decrease the responsiveness of bronchi to bronchodilators.

- *Monitoring:* If the child is very sick and is deteriorating, he may require continuous monitoring. Repeated assessments are necessary, at least at hourly intervals, in less sick children. PEFR or FEV1 wherever possible, and ABG should be assessed for an objective evaluation, especially in very sick and young children.

ADDITION OF OTHER DRUGS

If the patient has improved with the continuation of the above therapy for about 2 hours, he can be observed for a few hours and then discharged with proper advice. In case there is no improvement, treatment is intensified with the addition of other drugs, and the child is transferred to a place where intensive care facilities are available.

Role of Aminophylline

The role of aminophylline in an acute attack of bronchial asthma is still controversial. There is no doubt that methylxanthines have bronchodilator activity, but it is uncertain whether this adds to the bronchodilator effect achieved by β-2 agonists and corticosteroids.

It is believed that aminophylline may act by mechanisms other than bronchodilation as well, such as stimulation of the respiratory drive, reduction in respiratory muscle fatiguability, and enhancement of mucociliary clearance.

A bolus dose depending upon previous treatment with methylxanthines is given followed by infusion of maintenance dose.

As soon as the patient shows a response, aminophylline infusion may be substituted by injectable deriphyllin (6 hourly bolus) or even oral theophylline if the patient is able to take it orally.

Intravenous Terbutaline

In children, with low inspiratory rates where nebulization of β-2 agonists has failed, intravenous terbutaline has been tried. Therapy is started with an initial bolus of 10 µg/kg over 30 minutes, followed by an infusion at the rate of 0.1 µg/kg/min which may be increased by 0.1 µg/kg/min every 30 minutes, up to a maximum of 4 µg/kg/min or until there is a fall in $PaCO_2$, with clinical improvement. The dose of terbutaline should be reduced by half if theophylline is used concomitantly. Significant adverse effects noted with intravenous terbutaline are tachycardia, arrhythmias, hypertension, myocardial ischemia, hyperglycemia, hypokalemia, rhabdomyolysis, lactic acidosis, and hypophosphatemia.

Magnesium Sulfate

Some patients with acute severe asthma, treated with initial nebulization therapy with β-2 agonists and corticosteroids may not improve and progress to respiratory failure. One drug which may be worth trying in these refractory patients, to avert mechanical ventilation, is magnesium sulfate. There is now evidence that magnesium sulfate can be given to children who failed to respond to initial treatment particularly if FEVI fails to rise above 60% at the end of the first hour.

It acts by counteracting calcium-mediated smooth muscle contraction, through its influence on calcium homeostasis, inhibition of acetylcholine release at the neuromuscular junction inhibition of histamine release, direct inhibition of smooth muscle contraction, and sedation. The recommended dose for infusion is 30–70 mg/kg over 20–30 minutes. It is available as a 50% solution, 0.2 mL/kg of which can be given as an infusion in 30 mL N/5 normal saline in 5% dextrose over 30 minutes. There is also evidence that nebulized salbutamol administered in isotonic magnesium sulfate provides greater benefit than if it is delivered in normal saline. Serum levels >4 mg/dL are necessary for bronchodilation.

The onset of action occurs within a few minutes of intravenous infusion and lasts for 2 hours. Side effects include a transient sensation of facial warmth, flushing, malaise, and hypotension. At serum levels >12.5 mg/dL, side effects such as areflexia, respiratory depression, and arrhythmia may be noted, but this requires administration of doses >150 mg/kg. Thus, it may be used as an adjunct to β-2 agonist therapy, though its exact place in the treatment of acute asthma remains to be determined.

■ INTENSIVE CARE MANAGEMENT

Indications for Transfer to an Intensive Care Unit

The patient is observed on the above therapy for the next few hours and is monitored frequently. The decision to transfer to the intensive care unit (ICU) will depend upon the status of the child at the time of presentation and response to therapy. Any child with signs of a life-threatening attack should be immediately transferred to ICU. If the child has been receiving therapy and has shown poor response after being observed for a few hours or develops clinical signs of impending respiratory failure such as persistent hypoxemia, exhaustion, and change in the level of the sensorium, then he should be immediately transferred to ICU. Continuous monitoring with the help of pulse oximetry or repeated ABG analysis is mandatory since most of these patients may not be in a position to perform PEFR.

Continuation of Therapy in Intensive Care Unit

The focus of care continues to be close observation and delivery of frequent nebulized β-2 agonists, combined with corticosteroids and possibly aminophylline. As mentioned earlier, a trial of intravenous terbutaline and magnesium sulfate is desirable in a child who has not responded to the above therapy due to low inspiratory flow rates.

Intubation and Controlled Ventilation

Despite maximal pharmacologic therapy, some children do not respond favorably and require intubation and mechanical ventilation. The decision to ventilate is usually reserved as a last option.

Indications for mechanical ventilation include:

- Failure of maximal pharmacologic therapy.
- Cyanosis and hypoxemia (PaO_2, <60 mm Hg).
- $PaCO_2$ >50 mm Hg and rising by >5 mm Hg/h
- Minimal chest movements
- Minimal air exchange
- Severe chest retractions
- Deterioration in mental status, lethargy, or agitation

- Recumbent and diaphoretic patient
- Pneumothorax or pneumomediastinum
- Respiratory or cardiac arrest

Arterial blood gas values alone are not indicative of the need for mechanical ventilation and should be interpreted in the context of the clinical picture. It must be stressed that in spite of being aware of the morbidity that ventilation entails, it is better to intubate a child electively rather than wait for cardiorespiratory arrest to occur.

The patient should be stabilized using 100% oxygen and administered with a bag and mask. Oral and airway secretions should be cleared, and the stomach decompressed using a nasogastric tube, to diminish the risk of aspiration. Premedication with intravenous atropine and topical anesthesia to the hypopharynx and larynx helps in decreasing bronchospasm and laryngospasm that may be produced as a result of tipper airway manipulation.

An ideal sedative that may be used for intubation is intravenous ketamine in a dose of 1–3 mg/kg. The largest recommended endotracheal tube should be used. Muscle relaxation eliminates ventilator-patient asynchrony and improves chest wall compliance. It reduces $PaCO_2$, for any given level of minute ventilation. Additionally, this gives the patient with respiratory muscle fatigue, a period of desperately needed physical rest. Vecuronium bromide, with an intermediate duration of action and without any cardiovascular or autonomic side effects, in a dose of 0.2–0.3 mg/kg may be used. Succinylcholine may be used too, but it has a short duration of action.

A volume-cycled ventilator is recommended with a low respiratory rate 8–12 breaths/min and long expiratory time [inspiratory to expiratory (I:E) ratio of 1:4 or 1:3] to prevent hyperinflation. Airway obstruction in itself causes intrinsic positive end-expiratory pressure (PEEP), therefore end-expiratory pressure PEEP should be minimal. A tidal volume of 10–12 mL/kg, and peak airway pressure of <40–50 cm of water should be maintained. High inspiratory flow rates should be kept improving gas exchange. This can usually be achieved with heavy sedation or the use of muscle relaxants. Throughout ventilation, β-2 agonists are nebulized into the inspiratory circuit of a ventilator.

In ventilated patients, a therapeutic bronchoscope with lavage after administration of saline, soda bicarbonate, and acetylcysteine has been used in very ill patients with persistent mucus plugging, to prevent atelectasis and nosocomial pneumonia.

Droperidol

Dyspnea promotes anxiety, which may impair ventilation and interfere with the efficacy of aerosol therapy. Therefore, in a pediatric ICU setup, one may use safe sedatives with bronchodilator properties. Droperidol, which has both of these properties may be used in asthmatics on assisted ventilation. It antagonizes bronchoconstriction mediated by alpha-adrenergic receptors in peripheral airways. The recommended dose is 0.22 mg/kg and its main side effect is hypotension.

Ketamine

This drug is a dissociative anesthetic with excellent sedative and analgesic properties. It relaxes smooth muscles directly, increases chest wall compliance and also decreases bronchospasm in ventilated asthmatic children. It is given in a loading dose of 0.5–1.0 mg/kg, followed by an infusion of 1.0–2.5 mg/kg/h in ventilated children. The common side effects include arrhythmias, increased secretions, and laryngospasm. It has been used in subanesthetic doses in nonventilated adults in ICU set up in the bolus dose of 0.75 mg/kg over 10 minutes, followed by an infusion at a rate of 0.15 mg/kg/h. Thus, intravenous ketamine can be used to relieve acute intractable bronchospasm, provided expert anesthetic help is available at hand.

LONG-TERM MANAGEMENT OF BRONCHIAL ASTHMA

This includes identification and elimination of exacerbating asthma or nocturnal cough, maintenance of near-normal physical activity, and parental education.

Effective long-term management includes two major areas, which are as follows:
1. Identification and elimination of precipitating factors
2. Pharmacological therapy

The goals of long-term asthma therapy include:
- To prevent chronic and troublesome symptoms, i.e., cough and breathlessness.
- To maintain normal pulmonary functions
- To maintain normal activity levels
- To prevent recurrent exacerbation of the attack

Identification and Elimination of Precipitating Factors

The common factors associated with the development and precipitation of asthma include passive smoking, associated allergic disorders, inadequate ventilation at home leading to dampness, cold air, cold food, smoke, dust, and pets in the family. Acute respiratory infection due to viruses is the most common cause of exacerbation of asthma.

Passive smoking exacerbates childhood asthma and removal from exposure leads to an improvement in symptoms. It is better that one should not have pets, especially cats and dogs. Some food and additives may trigger attacks of asthma. Cold drinks, certain preservatives, nuts, shellfish, and eggs have been associated with allergic responses.

Pharmacological Therapy

One should go in a stepwise manner. This can be achieved by following:
- Assessment of the severity of asthma
- Selection of medication
- Selection of inhalator device

Assessment of Severity

Successful management of asthma requires grading the severity of the disease according to the frequency and severity of symptoms, functional impairment, and PEFR. **Table 3** provides a guide to differentiate between mild episodic, mild persistent, moderate persistent, and severe persistent asthma. After the assessment of severity, appropriate antiasthmatic drugs are selected.

It requires the grading of the severity according to the frequency and severity of the symptoms and functional impairment. PFTs by spirometer provide objective evidence of severity. PEFR measurement is an easy alternative to spirometry. It can be performed by children older than 5–6 years of age.

Children with asthma can be classified into four groups:
1. *Mild episodic asthma* should be treated with inhaled/oral salbutamol/terbutaline, as and when required.
2. *Mild persistent asthma:* Inhaled short-acting β-agonists are given as required. Additionally, these children need daily treatment with maintenance medication, i.e., inhaled (i) cromolyn sodium (5–10 mg 6–8 hourly); or

TABLE 3: Classification of asthma for long-term management.

	Symptoms	Night-time symptoms	PEFR
Severe persistent	Continuous Limited physical activity	Frequent	≤60% predicted, variability >30%
Moderate persistent	Daily use of β-2 agonist Daily attacks affect the activity	>1 time a week	>60% <80% predicted, variability >30%
Mild persistent	>1 time a week but <1 time a week	>1 times a month	≥80% predicted, variability 20–30%
Mild intermittent	<1 time a week Asymptomatic and normal peak expiratory flow rate (PEFR) attack	≤1 times a month	≥80% predicted, variability <20%

(ii) steroids (budesonide or beclomethasone 400 µg/day or fluticasone 200 µg/day in two divided doses); or (iii) slow-release oral theophylline 5–15 mg/kg/day in two divided doses. Drug selection is based on feasibility, toxicity, compliance, and cost. The drug of choice in mild persistent asthma is a low-dose inhaled steroid.

3. *Moderate persistent asthma:* Inhaled short-acting β-agonists are given as required. Inhaled steroids (400–800 µg/day) are given in two divided doses. Long-acting β-agonists (salmeterol) 50 µg once or twice a day can be added if needed. Sustained release of theophylline is advocated in compliance with inhalation therapy is poor.

4. *Severe persistent asthma:* These children need inhalation steroids in the dose of 800–1,200 µg day in two to three divided doses for relief of symptoms long acting β-agonist and/or slow-release theophylline needs to be given regularly. Montelukast can be used at this step as an add-on treatment for better control of asthma symptoms. If there is persistence of symptoms, low dose alternate day oral prednisolone may have to be used.

5. *Bronchodilators:* This group of drugs provides immediate symptomatic relief. They may be short acting and long acting. The commonly used short-acting bronchodilators are adrenaline, terbutaline, and salbutamol. Adrenaline is given subcutaneously. The other two agents can be administered by oral, inhalation, or parenteral route. The inhalation route is preferred because of the quick onset of action and the least side effects. Long-acting β agonists include salmeterol and formoterol.

Adrenaline stimulates both α- and β-receptors. It is given subcutaneously. Terbutaline and salbutamol are specific β_2 agonists and less cardiac side effects. It can be given by inhalation. The drawback of β-agonist is the lack of anti-inflammatory effect. So, although the symptoms are received, inflammation will aggravate bronchial hyperresponsiveness.

Long-acting β-agonists include salmeterol and formoterol. Both these drugs are specific α-agonists and have a longer duration of action of 12–24 hours. The onset of action is delayed by ½–1 hours. Salmeterol offers prolonged bronchodilation and relief from the need for short-acting drugs repeatedly.

In mild-to-moderate persistent asthma, inhaled salmeterol has been found to be superior to repetitive doses of salbutamol;

however, it cannot be used as an adjunct to inhaled corticosteroids (ICSs). It appears to help in the control of exercise-induced asthma. Formoterol is a full β_2 agonist. It is as effective as salmeterol and has a more rapid acting.

Long-acting Inhaled β-Agonists

Although considered daily controller medications, long-acting inhaled β-agonists (LABAs) (salmeterol formoterol) are not intended for use as monotherapy for persistent asthma because they can increase the risk for serious asthma exacerbations (ICU admission, endotracheal intubation) and asthma-related deaths when used without an ICS. Although both salmeterol and formoterol have a prolonged duration of effect (12 hours), salmeterol has a prolonged onset of effect (60 minutes), while formoterol's onset of effect is rapid (5–10 minutes) after administration.

Corticosteroids

Asthma is a chronic inflammatory disease of the airways. Corticosteroids, being potent anti-inflammatory agents, are the cornerstone of long-term treatment of asthma. The commonly used inhaled steroid includes beclomethasone, budesonide, and fluticasone. Early interventions with ICSs after the diagnosis of asthma are made or after the initial onset of symptoms, result in a better response to treatment. This may be due to the influence of uncontrolled inflammation.

Being potent anti-inflammatory agents are the cornerstone for the long-term treatment of asthma. Steroids inhibit cytokine production, inhibit cytokine receptors, and affect various cells, such as lymphocytes, eosinophils, neutrophils, macrophagia, and mast cells.

Corticosteroids diminish the inflammation and bronchial hyperresponsiveness, and as a result airway obstruction is reduced. The advantage of inhaled administration of corticosteroids is the application of the potent medication to the sites where it is specifically needed—airways and lungs. This reduces the risk of adverse reactions.

Optimal use of inhaled steroids necessitates the use of proper techniques with the use of MDIs. Spacers result in better lung deposition. The use of spacers along with mouth rinsing after treatment reduces the amount of drug deposited in the oropharynx and swallowed. This results in lower of systemic side effects.

Prednisone, prednisolone, and methylprednisolone are rapidly and completely absorbed, with peak plasma concentrations occurring within 1–2 hours. Prednisone is an inactive prodrug that requires biotransformation via first-pass hepatic metabolism to prednisolone, its active form. Corticosteroids are metabolized in the liver into inactive compounds, with the rate of metabolism influenced by drug interactions and disease states. Anticonvulsants (phenytoin, phenobarbital, and carbamazepine) increase the metabolism of prednisolone, methylprednisolone, and dexamethasone, with methylprednisolone most significantly affected. Rifampin also enhances the clearance of corticosteroids and can result in diminished therapeutic effect. Other medications (ketoconazole and oral contraceptives) can significantly delay corticosteroid metabolism. Some macrolide antibiotics, such as erythromycin and clarithromycin, delay the clearance of only methylprednisolone.

Combination inhaled corticosteroid/long-acting β-agonist therapy: Combination ICS/LABA therapy is recommended for patients who are suboptimally controlled with ICS therapy alone and those with moderate or severe persistent asthma. In those inadequately controlled with ICS alone, combination ICS/LABA therapy is superior to add-on therapy with either an leukotriene receptor antagonist (LTRA) or theophylline or doubling the ICS dose. Benefits include improvement in baseline lung function, less need for rescue short-acting β-agonist (SABA) therapy, improved quality of life, and fewer asthma exacerbations.

Mast cell stabilizers: The drugs included in their group are cromolyn sodium, nedocromolyn sodium, and ketotifen. Cromolyn sodium reduces bronchial reactivity and symptoms induced by irritants, antigens, and exercise. It is effective as theophylline in children. If diminishes IgE antibodies, induces the release of inflammatory mediators from sensitized mast cells. It should be administered three to four times a day for good results. A recent study report suggests that it can be used in severe asthma in higher doses.

Nedocromil is another nonsteroidal drug used for the control of mild-to-moderate asthma. It is as effective as cromolyn in reducing exercise-induced symptoms and also reduces airway hyperresponsiveness to allergen challenge.

Leukotriene modifiers: Leukotriene inhibitors have an important role in the pathogenesis of asthma. They act either by decreasing the synthesis of leukotriene or antagonizing the receptors. Leukotriene inhibitors are useful in the treatment of mild-to-moderate persistent asthma and exercise-induced asthma. Their main advantages are, they are given orally once a day and they do not induce tachyphylaxis.

Leukotrienes are potent proinflammatory mediators that can induce bronchospasm, mucus secretion, and airways edema. Two classes of leukotriene modifiers have been developed: Inhibitors of leukotriene synthesis and LTRAs. Zileuton, the only synthesis inhibitor, is not approved for use in children <12 years. Because zileuton can result in elevated liver function enzyme values in 2–4% of patients and interacts with medications metabolized via the cytochrome P450 system, it is rarely prescribed for children with asthma.

Montelukast can be used in pediatric asthma patients who are >1 year of age. The pediatric dose is 5 mg once daily. Zafirlukast can be used above 12 years of age.

Theophylline: It is the oldest asthma medication. It has a concentration-dependent bronchodilator effect. Bronchodilator effect is exerted by the inhibition of phosphodiesterase. It has anti-inflammatory and immunomodulatory effects at therapeutic serum concentration. It has a role in the long-term management of asthma. It can be an alternative second-line therapy in combination with inhaled glucocorticoids in moderate persistent asthma in older children 5 years and younger. It is used as second-line therapy for mild persistent asthma in older children and adults. It is used as adjunctive therapy for the control of nocturnal symptoms in moderate severe persistent asthma.

NONSTEROIDAL ANTI-INFLAMMATORY AGENTS

Cromolyn and nedocromil are considered nonsteroidal anti-inflammatory drugs (NSAIDs), although they have little efficacy as a long-term controller for asthma. They can block exercise-induced bronchospasm (EIB) and bronchospasm caused by allergen challenge. Although both drugs are considered alternative controller agents for children with mild persistent asthma, the 2016 Global Initiative for Asthma (GINA) guidelines no longer recommend cromolyn or nedocromil. Because they inhibit EIB and allergen-triggered responses, cromolyn.

Theophylline is a phosphodiesterase inhibitor with bronchodilator and anti-inflammatory effects that can reduce asthma symptoms and rescue SABA use.

LONG-ACTING INHALED ANTICHOLINERGICS

Tiotropium is a long-acting anticholinergic agent (24-hour duration of action) that is Food and Drug Administration (FDA)-approved for use in children with asthma >12 years old.

IMMUNOTHERAPY

This consists of giving gradually increasing quantities of allergen extract to clinically sensitive subjects, so as to ameliorate the symptoms associated with subsequent exposure to allergen. This is considered in highly selected children who are sensitive to specific allergens. It is done under specialist supervision.

Allergen Immunotherapy

Allergen immunotherapy (AIT) involves administering gradually increasing doses of allergens to a person with allergic disease to reduce or eliminate the patient's allergic response to those allergens, including allergic rhinoconjunctivitis and asthma. When properly administered to an appropriate candidate, AIT is a safe, effective therapy capable not only of reducing or preventing symptoms, but also of potentially altering the natural history of the disease by minimizing disease duration and preventing disease progression. Conventional AIT is given subcutaneously [subcutaneous immunotherapy (SCIT)] under the direction of an experienced allergist. Sublingual immunotherapy (SLIT) is less potent but can still be effective and has less potential for severe allergic adverse reactions.

Inhalation Devices

Drugs used by the inhalation route are more effective and have a rapid onset of action and have fewer side effects. Also, smaller doses of the drug are needed to achieve the same pharmacological effect. Commonly available inhalation devices include MDI, MDI with spacer, MDI with spacer with face mask, dry powder inhaler (DPI), and nebulizer.

Metered Dose Inhaler

An MDI is a device, which delivers a fixed amount of medication in aerosol form each time it is activated. It can be used for exacerbation and maintenance therapy. They are effective but require considerable coordination, i.e., press and breath coordination. This may not be possible in young children.

Metered dose inhaler can be easily used for children above 10–12 years of age.

Metered Dose Inhalers with a Spacer

Use of a spacer inhalation device with an MDI should be encouraged as it results in a larger proportion of the medication being deposited in the lung, with less impact in the oropharynx. They also overcome the problems of poor technique and coordination of actuation and inspiration which occur with the use of MDIs alone. Furthermore, the use of a spacer allows MDI to be used for younger patients. MDI used with a spacer has been found to be comparable to a nebulizer in delivering salbutamol in acute exacerbation of asthma in children. Spacer has the limitation of being bulky, relatively costly, and cannot be used in young infants and toddlers. A homemade spacer prepared from a mineral water bottle has been shown to be equally effective in delivering salbutamol in acute exacerbation.

A spacer can be easily handled by children >4 years of age. Attaching a face mask to the spacer facilitates their use in very young infants and children below 4 years.

ICSs are available in MDIs using hydrofluoroalkane (HFA) as their propellant, in DPIs, or in suspension for nebulization. Fluticasone propionate, fluticasone furoate, mometasone furoate, ciclesonide, and to a lesser extent budesonide are considered second-generation ICSs, in that they have greater anti-inflammatory potency and less systemic bioavailability (and thus potential for systemic adverse effects) because of their extensive first-pass hepatic metabolism. The selection of the initial ICS dose is based on the determination of disease severity.

The risk of adverse effects from ICS therapy is related to the dose and frequency of administration. High doses (21,000 μg/day in children) and frequent administration (four times/day) are more likely to have both local and systemic adverse effects.

The most commonly encountered ICS adverse effects are local—oral candidiasis (thrush) and dysphonia (hoarse voice). Thrush results from propellant-induced mucosal irritation and local immunosuppression, and dysphonia is the result of vocal cord myopathy. These effects are dose-dependent and are most common in individuals receiving high-dose ICS or oral corticosteroid therapy. The incidence of these local effects can be greatly minimized by using a spacer with an MDI with the ICS because spacers reduce oropharyngeal deposition of the drug and propellant.

Dry Powder Inhaler

These are breath-activated devices, such as Rotahaler, Diskhaler, Spinhaler, Turbohaler, and Accuhaler. They can be used in children above 4–5 years of age. They have the advantage of being portable and eliminating the need to coordinate actuation with breathing.

Nebulizer

A nebulizer is an instrument by which the drug is delivered to the airways in form of very small drops. The required amount of drug is diluted with normal saline to make 3 mL of solution. The solution is put in the nebulizing chamber, which is run through a compressor. Alternatively, high oxygen flow (>5 L/min) through oxygen cylinders or a central supply can be used to run the nebulizer. Repeated doses of this solution are given every 20 minutes. While giving therapy through a nebulizer, it is mandatory to ensure that adequate visible vapors are being produced and the mask is held closely to the child's face with minimal leak around the mask. In case the vapor production is deficient, the tubings and the nebulizing chamber should be checked for any leakage.

■ BIBLIOGRAPHY

1. Anderson WC 3rd, Gleason MC, Miyazawa N, Szefler SJ. Approaching current and new drug therapies in for pediatric Asthma. Pediatr Clin North Am. 2017;64(6):1197-207.
2. Boulet LP, O'Byrne PM. Asthma and exercise—induced bronchoconstriction in athletsathletes. N Engl J Med. 2015;372(7): 641-8.
3. Chung KF, Wenzel SE, Brozek JL, Bush A, Castro M, Sterk PJ, et al. International ERS/ATS guidelines on definition, evaluation and treatment of severe asthma. Eur Respire J. 2014;43(2)343-73.
4. Covar RA, Strunk R, Zeiger RS, Wilson LA, Liu AH, Weiss S, et al.; Childhood Asthma Management programme and Research Group. Predictors of remitting, periodic, and persistent childhood asthma. J Allergy Clin Immunol. 2010;125(2):359-66.

5. Gilbert T, Morgan WJ, Zeiger RS, Mauger DT, Boehmer SJ, Szefler SJ, et al. Long-term inhaled corticosteroids in preschool children in at high risk for Asthma. N Engl Med. 2006; 354(19):1995-97.
6. Ginasthma.org. 2022 GINA Report, Global Strategy for Asthma Management and Prevention. [online] Available from https://ginasthma.org/gina-reports/ [Last accessed May, 2024].
7. Pike KC, Levy ML Moreiras J, Fleming L. Management of problemaetic asthma: Arch Dis Child. 2016;311-368.
8. Sears MR. Predicting asthma outcomes. J Allergy Clin Immunol. 2015;136(74):829-36;quiz 837.

CASE 6

Bronchiectasis

■ PRESENTING COMPLAINTS

An 8-year-old boy was brought with the complaints of:
- Cough since 6 months
- Bad odor since 6 months
- Fever since 1 week

History of Presenting Complaints

An 8-year-old boy with a history of prolonged cough was brought to the pediatric outpatient department (OPD). The boy gave a history of cough since the last 6 months. Cough used to be of the productive type. He was spitting out the sputum. Sputum was mucopurulent, copious, and foul smelling. Cough used to be more in the morning. The boy used to have disturbed sleep as a result of a cough. This was associated with bad odor. Along with the cough, the child used to have a fever of moderate to high degree. This fever used to be relieved after a course of antibiotics and paracetamol. There was no history of breathlessness and chest pain.

Past History of the Patient

He was the second sibling of a nonconsanguineous marriage. He was delivered at full term and delivery was uneventful. His developmental milestones were normal. He had been immunized completely. He had been treated for the primary complex at the age of 2 years. There was no family history of similar complaints. His sister was a 10-year-old and maintained good health.

■ EXAMINATION

On examination, the boy was moderately built and nourished. He was alert and comfortable. Anthropometric measurements included a height was 126 cm (70th centile) and the weight was 22 kg (50th centile).

CASE AT A GLANCE

Basic Findings
Height	: 126 cm (70th centile)
Weight	: 22 kg (50th centile)
Temperature	: 38°C
Pulse rate	: 100 beats/min
Respiratory rate	: 26 breaths/min
Blood pressure	: 90/70 mm Hg

Positive Findings

History:
- Long-duration cough
- Sputum
- Halitosis
- Bad odor
- Primary complex

Examination:
- Clubbing
- Febrile
- Coarse crepitation
- Bronchial breathing

Investigation:
- Anemia
- Total leucocyte count (TLC) increased
- *X-ray chest:* Honeycomb appearance

He was febrile, pulse rate was 100 beats/min and respiratory rate was 26 breaths/min. Blood pressure was recorded as 90/70 mm Hg.

He looked pale and clubbing was present. There was no edema and no lymphadenopathy. The respiratory system revealed the presence of coarse leathery crepitations, bronchial breathing, and percussion notes were dull at the basal region. Low-pitched rattles were felt over the affected part of the chest. Other systemic examinations were normal.

■ INVESTIGATION

- *Hemoglobin:* 8 g/dL
- *TLC:* 21,000 cells/mm^3
- *DLC:* $P_{80}L_{18}E_2$
- *ESR:* 26 mm in the first hour
- *Mantoux test:* Negative
- *Electrocardiogram (ECG):* Normal
- *X-ray chest:* Honeycomb appearance suggestive of bronchiectasis
- *Spirometry:* Normal

■ DISCUSSION

It is a chronic suppurative lung disease. It is characterized by the destruction of the bronchial and peribronchial tissues and permanent dilatation of bronchi, resulting from airway obstruction by retained mucus secretions or inflammation in response to chronic or repeated infection. It occurs either as a consequence of the preceding illness, i.e., severe pneumonia foreign body aspiration, or as a manifestation of an underlying systemic disorder, such as CF, chronic aspiration, and immunodeficiency.

Bronchiectasis may be either congenital or acquired.

Congenital bronchiectasis may be because of hypoplasia and developmental arrest of the bronchi. It occurs because of a deficiency of bronchial cartilage and due to ciliary dysfunction. It is classified into three groups:

1. *Tracheobronchial:* It occurs due to hypoplasia and/or the arrest of the developmental arrest of the bronchi. There may be tracheobronchomegaly—Mounier-Kuhn syndrome. It may be a deficiency of bronchial cartilage—Williams–Campbell syndrome. In Kartagener syndrome—congenital bronchiectasis, sinusitis, and situs inversus. This is due to ciliary dysfunction—immotile cilia syndrome. Young syndrome patients have sinusitis, bronchiectasis, and azoospermia.
2. Vascular arteriolar aneurysm and pulmonary varies lead to mucosal congestion. These predispose to infection and hence bronchiectasis.
3. Lymphatic hypoplasia leads to poor lymphatic drainage and predisposes to infection. CF is an important cause. The cause may be thick secretion, atelectasis, and infection.

Other disease entities associated with bronchiectasis are yellow nail syndrome (pleural effusion lymphedema, discolored nails) and right middle lobe syndrome. The right middle lobe syndrome is mostly associated with other generalized causes of bronchiectasis including asthma, CF, primary ciliary dyskinesia (PCD), severe pneumonia, aspiration pneumonia, foreign bodies, and immune deficient states.

■ CONDITIONS ASSOCIATED WITH BRONCHIECTASIS

- Cystic fibrosis
- Allergic bronchopulmonary aspergillosis
- Idiopathic
- Infections
- Nontuberculous mycobacteria
- Tuberculosis
- *Pasteurella multocida*

- Measles, adenovirus 21, and pertussis
- Human immunodeficiency virus (HIV)
- *Diffuse interstitial lung disease:* Rheumatoid, Sjögren, idiopathic pulmonary fibrosis, and sarcoidosis
- Primary immunodeficiency
- Postlung transplantation
- Right middle lobe syndrome
- Pulmonary ciliary dyskinesia and Kartagener syndrome
- Postinhalation injury
- Ulcerative colitis
- Asthma
- Chronic obstructive pulmonary disease
- Alpha-antitrypsin deficiency
- Diffuse panbronchiolitis–bronchiolectasis
- Yellow nail syndrome
- Young syndrome
- Swyer–James–MacLeod syndrome

Cystic fibrosis is the most common congenital cause of bronchiectasis in the developed world. In low- and middle-income settings, post-tuberculous and other postinfective causes should be considered.

Most of the cases are acquired. The basic pathology involves infection and obstruction. It is associated with the inflammatory destruction of the bronchial wall, peribronchial tissue, and accumulation of exudative material in dependent bronchi.

Aspiration of foreign bodies, food, and mucus plug in the bronchus may also produce obstruction and lead to segmental collapse. Multiple abscess may develop in the parenchymal and peribronchial tissue. Obstructive and arteritis of the small pulmonary vessels occur.

The most frequently affected lobes are the right middle lobe segments, the basal segments of the lower lobes, and the lingular segments of the left upper lobe. Aspiration of the foreign body involves the right middle lobe. Hilar adenopathy frequently affects the right middle lobe.

Due to infection, there is a loss of ciliated epithelium. Later it is regenerated as cuboidal and squamous epithelium. The elastic tissue within the bronchial wall disappears and thickening occurs because of interstitial edema, fibrosis, and round-cell infiltration. Later bronchiectasis occurs in segmental distribution.

The infection could be because of measles, pertussis, pneumonia, bronchitis, and bronchiolitis. The infection damages the bronchial wall and segmental area collapse is caused. A negative presence in the wall is exerted and dilatation occurs. The dilatation may be cylindrical, fusiform, and saccular dilatation. These result in permanent dilatation. There are four main theories.

1. *Secretion theory:* Secretion causes obstruction and mechanical distension of bronchi. Dilatation persists even after the clearance of the secretion.
2. *Traction theory:* Here infection leads to fibrosis and scarring. This exerts traction on the bronchial wall.
3. *Atelectatic theory:* Collapse leads to an increase in intrapleural pressure and hence dilatation
4. *Infection theory:* Infection damages supporting structures of the bronchial wall and subsequently leads to bronchiectasis.

Bronchiectasis can manifest in any combination of three pathologic forms, best defined by a high-resolution computed tomography (HRCT) scan. In cylindrical bronchiectasis, the bronchial outlines are regular, but there is a diffuse dilation of the bronchial unit. The bronchial lumen ends abruptly because of mucous plugging.

In varicose bronchiectasis, the degree of dilation is greater, and local constrictions cause an irregularity of outline resembling that of varicose veins. There may also be small sacculations. In saccular (cystic) bronchiectasis, bronchial dilation progresses and results in ballooning of bronchi that end in fluid- or mucus-filled sacs. This is the most severe form of bronchiectasis. Bronchiectasis lies within the disease spectrum of chronic pediatric suppurative lung disease.

The following definitions have been proposed: Prebronchiectasis (chronic or recurrent endobronchial infection with nonspecific HRCT changes; may be reversible); HRCT bronchiectasis (clinical symptoms with HRCT evidence of bronchial dilation; may persist, progress, or improve and resolve); established bronchiectasis (like the previous but with no resolution within 2 years). Early diagnosis and aggressive therapy are important to prevent the development of established bronchiectasis.

CAUSES OF ACQUIRED BRONCHIECTASIS

- Measles, whooping cough, and tuberculosis
- Pneumonia following adenovirus, herpes virus, HIV
- Immunodeficiency state, especially immunoglobulin G (IgG) and immunoglobulin A (IgA)
- Foreign body obstruction and lymph node compression producing middle lobe syndrome
- Chronic sinusitis

CLINICAL FEATURES (FIGS. 1 AND 2)

Child will typically have a chronic cough, with purulent sputum, fever, and weight loss. Sputum is copious mucopurulent. The onset of the disease is insidious. Bouts of cough are precipitated by a change in posture and waking up from a supine posture. This is because of irritation of infected secretions draining into the fresh areas of the lung. In the course of illness, the sputum may become blood-streaked, or even frank hemoptysis may occur.

Recurrent respiratory tract infection is common. Segmental wheezing is present in infants and young children. During acute exacerbation, hemoptysis may be present. This will vary in severity from blood-streaked sputum to exsanguinous hemorrhage. This follows intermittent improvement and a relapsing course. Moist and musical rales may be heard or elicited by cough. Rales, rhonchi, and decreased air entry are often heard over the bronchiectatsis area.

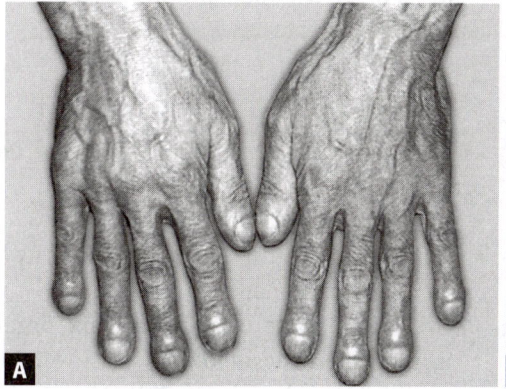 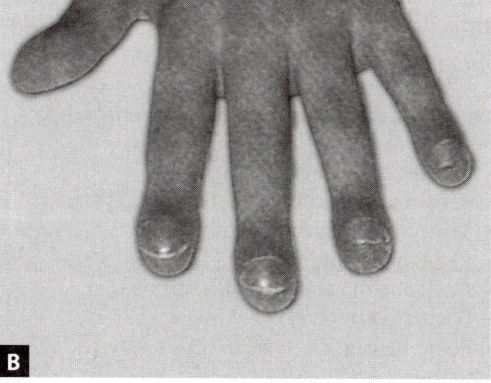

Figs. 1A and B: Clubbing of fingers.

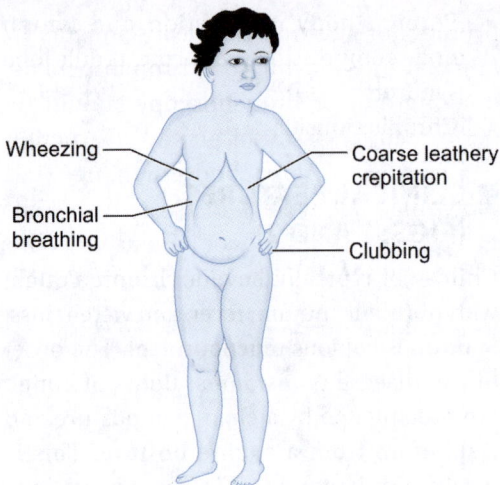

Fig. 2: Clinical features.

GENERAL FEATURES
• Cough • Foul-smelling sputum • Recurrent respiratory tract infection • Hemoptysis • Anorexia • Poor weight gain • Chest pain

In chronic cases, anorexia, irritability, and poor weight gain are common. Clubbing of the fingers may be present. Fever is less common.

Exacerbations can be defined as the presence of one major criteria (wet cough enduring longer than 72 hours, increased cough frequency over 72 hours) plus one laboratory criteria [C-reactive protein (CRP) >3 mg/L, serum interleukin-6 (IL-6) >2 ng/L, serum amyloid A >5 mg/L, elevated neutrophil percentage], two major criteria, or one major criteria plus two minor criteria (change in sputum color, breathlessness, chest pain, crackles/crepitations, and wheeze).

ESSENTIAL DIAGNOSTIC POINTS
• Chronic productive cough • Recurrent respiratory infections • Sputum is copious mucopurulent • Clubbing of fingers • Moist and musical rales may be heard • Decreased air entry • Pulmonary function tests—obstructive pattern

■ PRIMARY CILIARY DYSKINESIA

Bronchiectasis is also the end result of PCD. Also, autosomal recessive, PCD has a prevalence of 1 in 15,000–30,000, although this prevalence likely is underestimated because individuals with this disease are undiagnosed. Kartagener syndrome is the triad of bronchiectasis, sinusitis, and situs inversus. The underlying defect in PCD is an abnormal ciliary ultrastructure and function. Normally, the cilia that line the upper and lower airways have a synchronous beat that sweeps mucus from distal to proximal airways where the mucus that has foreign material can be expectorated or swallowed. In PCD, the cilia demonstrate an abnormal beating pattern or no motility at all, leading to stasis of mucus secretions. Retained mucus leads to URTIs and lower respiratory tract infections (LRTIs), and if left unchecked, these infections can cause significant damage. In the lower airways, recurrent and chronic infections can lead to bronchiectasis.

■ DIAGNOSIS

The aims of evaluating children with suspected bronchiectasis are as follows:
- To confirm the diagnosis
- The define the distribution and severity of airway involvement
- To characterize extrapulmonary organ involvement associated with bronchiectasis (e.g., cor pulmonale).

- To identify familial and treatable underlying causes of bronchiectasis.

The evaluation includes a complete medical history and physical examination, as well as laboratory testing, radiographic imaging, and PFTs.

A complete medical history, including past medical, family, travel, and environmental history, is a crucial part of the evaluation and can help identify the underlying cause of bronchiectasis. Certain features of the history should raise concern for specific underlying disorders (e.g., history of choking suggests foreign body aspiration; chronic aspiration should be considered in patients with recurrent pneumonia particularly those with neurologic dysfunction).

The general physical examination of the patient with suspected bronchiectasis may also identify the features described earlier that point to an underlying etiology, including failure to thrive, sinus and ear infections, neurologic dysfunction, and the presence of congenital anomalies. In addition, the pulmonary examination may reveal the following features: Crackles and rhonchi, which are often heard over the area of bronchiectasis; wheezing, which is less common; clubbing of the nail bed, which is a basic clinical sign of bronchiectasis; and chest wall deformity, which can be seen in obstructive lung diseases (e.g., CF), in which hyperinflation of the lungs results in increased anterior in posterior chest diameter.

On evaluation chest radiograph, findings that are suspicious for bronchiectasis include recurrent/persistent infiltrates or atelectasis in the same lobe or segment. Ciliary dyskinesia should be considered in patients with recurrent sinus and ear infections and evaluated with a nasal mucosal biopsy. Potential mechanisms of aspiration should be assessed using videofluoroscopy, esophageal pH monitoring, and/or nuclear scintigraphy. For patients with focal bronchiectasis, imaging and or bronchoscopy should be performed to assess for airway obstruction (e.g., airway foreign body or congenital pulmonary anomalies). PFTs can be helpful to evaluate the severity of lung disease and should be performed in older children. Most patients with bronchiectasis have features of obstructive lung disease, indicated by low FEV_1 and FEV/FVC ratio.

White blood cell count is often increased with polymorphonuclear leukocytosis. ESR is raised.

X-ray criteria suggesting of bronchiectasis:
- Ring-like densities with clear centers. This suggests thick-walled bronchi.
- Railroad tract
- Bronchial lumen plugged with mucopurulent material is seen as white rounded densities
- Ill-defined irregular vascular markings
- Honeycomb appearance indicating multiple small abscess cavities in later stages.

Bronchography is useful for the diagnosis. Flexible bronchoscopy combined with the installation of contrast is a safe and more convenient procedure. The findings are air-fluid levels in distended bronchi, linear array or cluster of cysts, thick bronchial walls, and dilated peripheral bronchi.

Bronchoscopy is useful in the diagnosis and management of bronchiectasis. It is used to exclude bronchial stenosis due to stricture, tumor, or foreign body in a suspected and proven case of bronchiectasis. It is useful in collecting material for staining and culture. It helps in localizing segments or lobes for contributing to massive secretion or bleeding. It helps to remove the mucus plug.

Bronchial diameter is never larger than accompanying blood vessels. If it is found, it is an early indicator of bronchiectasis—signet ring sign.

LABORATORY SALIENT FINDINGS
• Chest radiograph • Flexible bronchoscopy • CT scan helps in grading localizing and in follow-up of the progress of disease • Tuberculin test • Sputum examination

High-resolution computed tomography (CT) scan with the smaller sections is performed. It is replaced by bronchography. It is useful in detecting early disease, grading, and localizing and in follow up of the progress of disease.

Sputum should be sent for culture and sensitivity. The most common bacteria detected in cultures from the lower respiratory tract, include *Streptococcus pneumoniae*, *Staphylococcus aureus*, nontypical *H. influenzae*, and *Pseudomonas aeruginosa*. Nontuberculous mycobacterial species may also be detected. Tuberculin test (TT) is done to rule out tuberculosis.

Pilocarpine iontophoresis is done to estimate sweat chloride in patients with suspected CF.

The diagnosis of PCD can be difficult to establish. Certainly, nasal congestion is a symptom of PCD that can occur in all individuals, but in a child who has nasal congestion from birth, PCD should be considered. Most notably, patients with PCD will have a year-round, wet cough starting in infancy. Other factors that would alert the clinician to the diagnosis of PCD are neonatal respiratory distress, wheezing, bronchiectasis, recurrent sinusitis, and otitis media. Nonrespiratory issues that would raise suspicion of PCD include situs inversus or other heterotaxic syndromes, complex congenital heart disease (CHD), ectopic pregnancies, and male infertility.

The most important factor in diagnosing PCD is considering the diagnosis, after which screening and diagnostic tests help establish a diagnosis. Diagnosis requires phenotypic features of the disease and a combination of variables depending on age because not all ciliary defects result in abnormal findings on all tests. In children older than 5 years of age who are capable of performing lung function testing, nasal nitric oxide can be measured.

■ DIFFERENTIAL DIAGNOSIS

Differential diagnoses include sinusitis, tuberculosis, asthma, ciliary dyskinesia, CF, respiratory allergy, immunodeficiency status, surfactant deficiencies, and collagen vascular diseases. Foreign body aspiration and allergic bronchopulmonary aspergillosis should also be considered.

■ TREATMENT

During acute exacerbations, bacterial infections should be controlled and the airway should be kept clear of secretions. Postural drainage with a pulmonary physiotherapist may be useful.

Exacerbations can be defined as the presence of one major criteria (wet cough enduring longer than 72 hours, increased cough frequency over 72 hours) plus one laboratory criteria (CRP >3 mg/L, serum IL-6 >2 ng/L, serum amyloid A >5 mg/L, elevated neutrophil percentage), two major criteria, or one major criteria plus two minor criteria (change in sputum color, breathlessness, chest pain, crackles/crepitations, and wheeze).

There are two phases in the management of bronchiectasis, which are as follows:
1. *Immediate phase:* This includes the correction of factors damaging the lung.

Antibiotics, chest physiotherapy, and gravitational drainage are the components of this phase. Acute infection is the indication for antibiotics. Bronchoscopy is useful in this phase to remove the foreign body, to collect the material for investigation, and to remove the mucus plug. Drug treatment includes antibiotics such as penicillin, aminoglycosides, and metronidazole to be given for 3 weeks till sputum decreases and symptoms subside.
2. *Long-term or surgical plan:* In the acute phase, surgery is not indicated. It is advisable to delay surgery till the extent of the disease is defined.

Management

The management should be aggressive in localized disease to prevent the spread of the disease to other parts of normal lung tissue. Surgical removal of an area of the lung affected with severe bronchiectasis is considered when the response to medical treatment is poor. Other indications include severe localized or unilateral disease, repeated hemoptysis, and recurrent pneumonia in one area. Surgical treatment is reserved for localized. It is reserved till complications force the surgical intervention in bilateral disease. Extrinsic compression of the bronchi requires surgical intervention.

Long-term prophylactic macrolide antibiotics or nebulized antibiotics (e.g., tobramycin, colistin, and aztreonam) may be beneficial (reduced exacerbations and hospitalizations, improved lung function) but may also increase antibiotic resistance. Airway hydration (inhaled hypertonic saline or mannitol) also improves the quality of life in adults with bronchiectasis. Any underlying disorder (immunodeficiency and aspiration) that may be contributing must be addressed.

Much of the treatment of PCD has been adopted from experience with CF, enhancing mucociliary clearance with chest physiotherapy, and monitoring and treating acute exacerbations with antibiotics remain the mainstay of treatment. As with CF, individuals with PCD can become infected with organisms, such as *S. aureus*, *H. influenzae*, and *P. aeruginosa*. Intense monitoring and treatment such as identifying and treating infections are important to stabilizing lung function. Inhaled medications such as bronchodilators, hypertonic saline, and mucolytics have been used to aid in mucus clearance and are recommended on a case-by-case basis. Genetic counseling should also be offered to parents of an affected child or those who are carriers of known disease-causing mutations.

Preoperatively all children should be screened by PFT to confirm enough lung reserves so that removal of diseased lung tissue will be tolerated. Endobronchial tuberculosis is ruled out by bronchoscopy. If endobronchial tuberculosis is present, it should be treated adequately before surgery is undertaken.

Advantages of Surgical Treatment

This includes prevention of disease to nonaffected lung disease and improves the quality of work.

Contraindications of Surgery

This includes diffuse bronchitis, emphysema, or pulmonary or cardiac insufficiency.

Prevention

All lung infections should be treated adequately till the chest is clear of all signs, long after the fever has subsided. Measles and whooping cough should be prevented by specific immunization.

BIBLIOGRAPHY

1. Gupta AK, Lodha R, Kabra SK. Non cystic fibrosis bronchiectasis. Indian J Pediatr. 2015;82(10):938-44.
2. Redding GJ, Carter ER. Chronic suppurative lung disease in children: definition and spectrum of disease. Front Pediatr. 2017;5:30.
3. Salerno T, Peca D, Rossi FP, Menchini L, Danhaive O, Cutrera R. Bronchiectasis and severe respiratory insufficiency associated with a new surfactant protein C mutation. Acta Pediatr. 2013;102(1):e1-2.
4. Shapiro AJ, Zariwala MA, Ferkol T, Davis SD, Sagel SD, Dell SD, et al. Diagnosis monitoring and treatment of primary ciliary dyskinesia: PCD foundation consensus recommendations based on state of the art review. Pediatric Pulmonol. 2016;51(12): 115-32.
5. Wong C, Jayaram L, Karalus N, Eaton T, Tong C, Hockey H, Wong C, et al. Azithromycin for prevention of exacerbations in non-cystic fibrosis bronchiectasis (EMBRACE): a randomised, double-blind, placebo-controlled trial. Lancet. 21012;380(9842):660-7.

CASE 7

Bronchiolitis

PRESENTING COMPLAINTS

A 4-month-old boy was brought with complaints of:
- Cold since 3 days
- Cough since 3 days
- Fever since 2 days
- Breathlessness since 4 hours

History of Presenting Complaints

A 4-month-old boy with a history of sudden onset of breathlessness has been brought to the hospital by his mother. There was a history of fever. The child had been suffering from the cold since 3 days, but there was no history of nasal block. Later, the child developed a dry and irritating cough. This was associated with subcostal recession and intercostal indrawing. There was a history of disturbed sleep and difficulty in taking feeds.

Past History of the Patient

The child was born at full term by normal delivery. The child cried immediately after the delivery. The birth weight was 3 kg. There was no significant postnatal event except for the normal physiological jaundice. Breastfeeding was given immediately. He had attained neck control and there was a social smile. He was completely immunized.

He was the second sibling of the non-consanguineous marriage. The elder sister of the boy had a similar problem and was admitted to the hospital.

CASE AT A GLANCE

Basic Findings
Length	: 62 cm (75th centile)
Weight	: 5.5 kg (50th centile)
Temperature	: 39°C
Pulse rate	: 126 beats/min
Respiratory rate	: 56 breaths/min
Blood pressure	: 50/40 mm Hg

Positive Findings

History:
- Cold
- Cough
- Breathlessness
- Fever

Examination:
- Irritable
- Intercostal recession
- Wheezing
- Hepatomegaly

Investigation:
- Chest X-ray: Hyperinflation with patchy shadows

EXAMINATION

On examination, the child was well-built and nourished. He was crying, irritable, and dyspneic. The anthropometric measurements included. The length of the child was 62 cm (75th centile), the weight of the child was 5.5 kg (50th centile), and the head circumference was 40 cm.

The child was febrile. The pulse was 126 beats/min, the respiratory rate was 56 breaths/min, and the blood pressure recorded was 50/40 mm Hg. Subcostal recession and intercostal drawings were present.

There was no pallor, no lymphadenopathy, cyanosis, and no edema. The respiratory system revealed the presence of fine crackles audible toward the end of the inspiration, especially at the base of the lung. Per abdomen examination revealed mild distension and the presence of nontender hepatomegaly. The cardiovascular system was normal except for tachycardia.

INVESTIGATION

- *Hemoglobin:* 12 g/dL
- *TLC:* 8,600 cells/mm^3
- *DLC:* $P_{65}L_{25}E_5B_2$
- *ESR:* 20 mm in the first hour
- *X-ray chest:* Hyperinflation with small patchy shadows

DISCUSSION

A 4-month-old child was presented with a history of cough and breathlessness and it was associated with irritability and intercostal indrawing. These findings along with a hyperinflated chest radiograph led to the diagnosis of bronchiolitis. Bronchiolitis is a clinical syndrome characterized by coughing, tachypnea, labored breathing, and hypoxia.

Bronchiolitis is a common disease of the lower respiratory tract. It occurs as a result of inflammatory obstruction of bronchioles. It occurs commonly in the first 2 years of life. The peak incidence occurs approximately at 6 months of age.

Several risk factors are present. They are male infants, aged between 1 and 6 months, bottle-fed babies, in crowded places upper respiratory infections (URIs), and parental smoking.

Besides young age (<6 months) at the start of the respiratory syncytial virus (RSV) season, epidemiologic studies have identified select groups of infants at high risk for severe disease and mortality including premature birth, compromised cardiopulmonary function [chronic lung disease or CHD, trisomy 21, or immunocompromise]. Males with severe RSV LRTIs outnumber females by 1.6 to 1. Risk factors, such as low socioeconomic status, and modifiable risk factors such as exposure to second have also been associated with an increased risk for more severe RSV disease.

Bronchiolitis is more common in males, those exposed to second-hand tobacco smoke, those who have not been breastfed, and those living in crowded conditions. The risk is also higher for infants with mothers who smoked during pregnancy. Older family members, including older siblings, are a common source of infection; they might experience only minor upper respiratory symptoms (colds) given that bronchiolar edema may be less clinically apparent as airway size increases.

Humans are the only known reservoir for RSV. Studies of transmission dynamics suggest that infection of infants often follows infection of older siblings. The incubation period ranges from 2 to 8 days, most commonly 4–6 days. In infants hospitalized with primary RSV infection, continuous viral shedding for 10 or 11 days detected by polymerase chain reaction (PCR) is commonly observed; young infants and immunocompromised children may shed the virus for 3–4 weeks.

Transmission primarily occurs by inoculation of nasopharyngeal or ocular mucous membranes after direct contact with contaminated secretions or fomites. RSV can persist for 30 minutes or more on hands and for several hours on environmental surfaces. Close adherence to infection control policies is critical to limit healthcare-associated transmission.

Other viruses responsible are parainfluenza virus (type 3), rhinovirus, adenovirus, influenza type A, and *Mycoplasma pneumoniae*. Dual infection with RSV and human metapneumovirus is associated with severe bronchiolitis. The source of infection is a family member that has a respiratory disease. It is responsible for provoking wheezing at all ages.

Other agents include human metapneumovirus, rhinovirus, parainfluenza, influenza, bocavirus, and adenovirus. Viral coinfection is reported to impact severity and clinical manifestations, although its significance remains contested.

It can be classified into three types for practical purposes, i.e., (1) acute, (2) subacute, and (3) chronic type. On the pathogenetic basis, it can be classified into two types, i.e., (1) inflammatory and (2) suppurative. Bronchiolitis obliterans is a classical example of an inflammatory type of bronchiolitis.

■ PATHOGENESIS

Respiratory syncytial virus infection is first established in the upper respiratory tract by infecting the ciliated cells of the nasopharynx, paranasal sinuses, or Eustachian tubes of the inner ear. For about 1–3 days later, 30% of infants who experience their first infection will demonstrate the involvement of the lower respiratory tract. In the lower respiratory tract, RSV infects the small bronchial epithelium, spreading to the type 1 and type 2 alveolar pneumocytes. RSV infection is restricted to the respiratory epithelium and rarely spreads outside the respiratory tract. Disseminated disease has been documented in patients with T-cell deficiency. Infants are more likely to develop severe distal airway disease, because of an immature immune system, the lack of full protection from maternal antibodies, and also the smaller bronchiolar lumen of infants compared with older children and adults. In addition, in infants, collateral ventilation in alveolar regions is not well developed; thus, the impact of obstruction resulting from infection and inflammation is greater.

Bronchiolitis, which refers to inflammation of smaller intrapulmonary airways, is the single most distinctive clinical syndrome of RSV infection. The RSV is the causative agent in 50% of cases. RSV belongs to the genus *Pneumovirus* within the Paramyxoviridae family: It is an enveloped, single-stranded, negative-sense ribonucleic acid (RNA) virus with a diameter spanning 100–350 nm. The viral envelope is studded with spike-like projections that include the fusion (F) and attachment (G) surface glycoproteins, but unlike most *Paramyxoviruses*, RSV surface-proteins lack both hemagglutinin (HA) and neuraminidase (NA) activity. The G protein initiates the infection, while the F glycoprotein mediates viral penetration by fusing viral and cellular membranes, contributing to syncytia formation. These two proteins carry the antigenic determinants that elicit the production of neutralizing antibodies by the host. Human RSV exists as two antigenic subgroups, A and B, which can cocirculate during the same season and exhibit genome-wide sequence divergence.

Histopathologically

Airway plugging with mucus, necrosis of the bronchial and bronchiolar epithelium, and peribronchial inflammation with mononuclear cell predominance has been noted. The peribronchial infiltrate may extend into the adjacent pulmonary interstitium. Cytoplasmic inclusion bodies have been described, but syncytia formation is uncommon. Neutrophils are found between small airways and vascular structures and represent the predominant cell type in the bronchoalveolar lavage (BAL) of RSV-infected infants.

Bronchiolar obstruction occurs. This is because of edema and accumulation of mucus and cellular debris. This can also be because of invasion of smaller radicals of bronchial tree by the virus. This produces bronchial spasms. The bronchial lumen is reduced.

There is a marked increase in airway resistance and a reduction in airflow. Resistance to airflow is increased both during inspiration and expiration. The radius of the airway is smaller during expiration. Hence, the bronchioles have partially collapsed. The egress of the air is severely restricted during this phase. This leads to the trapping of air inside the alveoli. This produces emphysematous changes. This occurs as a result of ball valve respiratory obstruction leading to early air trapping and overinflation. When the obstruction becomes complete the trapped air in the lungs may be absorbed causing atelectasis.

This leads to ventilation-perfusion mismatch. This mismatch will lead to hypoxia. Carbon dioxide (CO_2) retention occurs leading to respiratory failure. Hyperapnea is usually not found until the respiratory rate exceeds 60 breaths/min.

Immunopathogenesis is advocated. Bronchiolitis is less severe in RSV-vaccinated babies. Protection against is mediated by antibodies to the IgG3 subclass. These antibodies have a shorter half-life and do not cross the placenta in substantial amounts so as to give protection to infants. High quantities of secretory IgA antibodies to RSV are present in the colostrum and breastfeeding reduces the likelihood of hospitalization with bronchiolitis. RSV bronchiolitis leads to the IgE synthesis. These IgE responders release chemical mediators, such as histamine, leukotriene C_4, etc. These produce smooth muscle constriction. Some may develop into asthma later in life. The presence of eosinophils in the blood and respiratory secretions suggest virus infection initiates the wheezing attack in child who is already sensitized.

■ CLINICAL FEATURES (FIG. 1)

Respiratory syncytial virus infection is heralded by initial symptoms indistinguishable from those of the common cold. The infant may show rhinitis and cough, and there may be a fever. Within 1–2 days, the cough becomes more prominent, and tachypnea may develop. At first, there will be rhinorrhea and sneezing. Rhinorrhea is a serous nasal discharge. There will be a family history of URTI in a family member. The cough may be very mild and may be associated with wheeze. These symptoms may last for several days. These may be accompanied by diminished appetite and fever. In mild cases, the symptoms disappear by 1–3 days.

With increasing respiratory effort, substernal and intercostal retractions are noted along with nasal flaring and abdominal

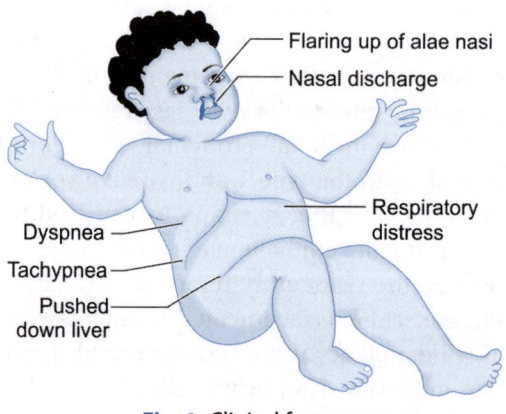

Fig. 1: Clinical features.

breathing. In more severely affected infants, symptoms may develop within several hours and the course is protracted. Respiratory distress will develop. This is characterized by paroxysmal wheeze, cough, dyspnea, and irritability. Feeding difficulty associated with increasing dyspnea will be present grunting can be present in more severe cases. The expiratory phase is prolonged, and the chest is hyperexpanded and hyperresonant, providing further evidence of generalized expiratory airflow obstruction. Those with severe disease may develop retraction in lower intercostal spaces and suprasternal notch by 3–5 days.

Apnea can be an early manifestation of RSV infection in young infants, particularly infants <8 weeks old or those with a history of premature birth or apnea of prematurity. Apnea can occur associated with respiratory tract symptoms or may be the only sign at presentation. Recurrent apnea is a serious complication. Few children will have vomiting and diarrhea.

Term infants at a postconceptual age of <44 weeks and preterm infants at a postconceptual age of <48 weeks are at the highest risk for apneic events.

Work of breathing may be markedly increased, with nasal flaring and retractions. Complete obstruction to airflow can eliminate the turbulence that causes wheezing thus the lack of audible wheezing is not reassuring in the infant shows other signs of respiratory distress. Poorly audible breath sounds suggest severe disease with nearly complete bronchiolar obstruction.

On examination, there is a varied respiratory rate. Tachypnea is usually present. There is flaring up of alae nasi, use of accessory muscles resulting in intercostal and subcostal retraction. These are shallow because of persistence distension of lungs by the trapped air. Liver and spleen are palpable, being pushed down by over or hyperinflated lungs. On auscultation, crackles or rales with or without diffuse expiratory wheezing are usually heard. Widespread crackles may be heard at the end of inspiration and in early expiration. Wheezes are audible when the expiratory phase of the breathing is prolonged. In children requiring hospitalization, hypoxemia is typical, reflecting ventilation-perfusion mismatch.

The most critical phase of the illness occurs during 48–72 hours after the onset of cough and dyspnea. Apneic spell occurs. Respiratory acidosis occurs. Periodic breathing may also occur. Hypoxic episodes will also occur. Cyanosis, apnea, and bradycardia are common.

The characteristic findings on examination are:
- Sharp dry cough
- Tachypnea
- Subcostal and intercostal recession
- Fine end-inspiratory crackles
- Hyperinflation chest
- High pitched wheezes
- Tachycardia
- Cyanosis and pallor

> **ESSENTIAL DIAGNOSTIC POINTS**
> - Acute onset of cough rhinorrhea
> - Tachypnea and expiratory wheezing
> - Nasal flaring shallow rapid respirations
> - Respiratory syncytial virus (RSV) is the most common pathogen
> - Apneic spell, respiratory acidosis, and periodic breathing

Cardiac failure is overdiagnosed. This is because of pushed-down liver secondary to overinflation of lungs. It rarely occurs in the absence of underlying cardiac disease. Over distension of one lung, i.e., MacLeod syndrome sometimes occurs.

The cause of death is prolonged apneic spells, severe uncompensated respiratory acidosis, and profound dehydration occurs due to loss of water from tachypnea, and irritability to drink water. The mortality rate is high with CHD, bronchopulmonary dysplasia, and immunodeficiency diseases.

> **CLINICAL FEATURES**
> - Mild upper respiratory tract infection
> - Sneezing
> - Cough
> - Irritability

DIFFERENTIAL DIAGNOSIS

- *Bronchial asthma:* Bronchiolitis is often confused with bronchial asthma. The latter is unusual below the age of 1 year; a family history of asthma is usually present. Several attacks occur in the same patient with or without a preceding respiratory infection. Response to bronchodilators is more consistent in children with asthma as compared to bronchiolitis.
- *Congestive heart failure:* Congestive heart failure is suggested, if there is cardiomegaly on X-ray film of the chest, tachycardia, large tender liver, raised jugular venous pressure (JVP), edema, and rales on auscultation of the lungs.
- *Foreign bodies in trachea:* These are diagnosed by the history of aspiration of the foreign body, localized wheeze, and signs of collapse or localized obstructive emphysema.
- *Bacterial pneumonia:* In bacterial pneumonia, the signs of obstruction are less pronounced, fever is high, and adventitious sounds in the lungs are prominent.

DIAGNOSIS

Bronchiolitis is a clinical diagnosis; however, other respiratory viruses also cause bronchiolitis in young children, and clinical features are insufficient to reliably distinguish RSV from these other viral infections. Specific viral diagnosis may be helpful in certain scenarios: when the diagnosis is uncertain; to reduce unnecessary use of antibiotics; or in hospitalized children at risk for severe disease or for infection control purposes. Detection of RSV from nasopharyngeal specimens may be achieved by rapid antigen tests including fluorescence-based methods such as a direct fluorescent antibody (DFA)—sensitivity 90–95%, specificity 92–97% or immunoassays such as enzyme immunoassay (EIA)—sensitivity 80%, specificity 75–100%. Detection by viral culture or by serology is not clinically practical for early diagnosis of acute RSV infection. Serology is also challenging to interpret in young infants because of the presence of maternal antibodies.

In cell culture, RSV growth is detected within 5–7 days by the typical plaque morphology with syncytium formation. Cell culture was traditionally the gold standard for diagnosis, but this technique has been replaced by the more rapid and sensitive reverse transcription–polymerase chain reaction (rt-PCR) assays. rt-PCR is the most sensitive method for RSV detection and allows the differentiation between A and B subgroups (which is useful for surveillance purposes in cases of respiratory disease outbreaks). Studies have shown that approximately 30% of children hospitalized with RSV bronchiolitis may be coinfected with another respiratory virus. Whether children with RSV bronchiolitis who are co-infected with another respiratory virus develop more severe disease is still unclear.

Respiratory viruses are now identified by PCR analysis of nasopharyngeal secretions. Nasopharyngeal secretion should be aspirated and sent for immunofluorescence, enzyme-linked immunosorbent assay (ELISA). This test will be positive for RSV in winter epidemics, occasionally adenoviral infection especially 3, 7, and 21 serotypes.

Viral testing (PCR, or rapid immuno-fluorescence) is not routinely recommended in the diagnosis of bronchiolitis but may be helpful if such testing prevents more invasive evaluations.

The chest X-ray need not be done routinely and is indicated only in children with severe respiratory distress or when there is a diagnostic dilemma. The radiographic findings of bronchiolitis include hyperinflation, patchy infiltrates that are typically migratory and attributable to postobstructive atelectasis, and peribronchial cuffing. Because bronchiolitis is not a disease of the alveolar spaces, secondary bacterial pneumonitis should be suspected if a true alveolar infiltrate is seen on a chest radiograph. The diaphragm is pushed down.

Pulse oximetry is used to measure and monitor arterial oxygen saturation (SaO_2). Blood gas analysis is usually a capillary sample performed in severe disease to identify hypercarbia when additional ventilator support is considered.

Concurrent serious bacterial infection (sepsis, pneumonia, and meningitis) is unlikely, although confirmation of viral bronchiolitis may obviate the need for a sepsis evaluation in the young febrile infant. Otitis media may complicate bronchiolitis.

> **LABORATORY SALIENT FINDINGS**
> - A radiograph of the chest shows overinflation
> - Nasopharyngeal secretion should be aspirated and sent for immunofluorescence; ELISA
> - ABG shows respiratory acidosis
> - Viral culture
> - Leukocytosis
>
> (ABG: arterial blood gas; ELISA: enzyme-linked immunosorbent assay)

■ TREATMENT

Child should be hospitalized. The child should be placed in a humid atmosphere. The child may not take feed properly because of tachypnea. Hence nasogastric tube feeding is advised. Intravenous fluid is indicated if the child is not tolerating oral feeds.

Currently, the primary treatment for RSV infection is supportive and includes nasal suctioning and hydration. In hospitalized patients close cardiorespiratory monitoring and measurement of oxygen saturation. Nasal suctioning may provide relief of upper airway obstruction, but deep suctioning of the nasopharynx is not recommended. Although infants with bronchiolitis are at risk of developing subsegmental atelectasis, chest physiotherapy has not been shown to be of clinical benefit. Humidified oxygen is frequently required when managing hospitalized infants since hypoxemia is common (oxygen saturation <90%) in more severe illnesses.

Humidified oxygen is given to relieve hypoxemia and reduce the insensible water loss due to tachypnea. This will relieve dyspnea and cyanosis. Very sick infants require a concentration of 70% through the hood. Assisted ventilation in the form of nasal or facemask CPAP or full ventilation is required in some admitted infants.

Pulse oximetry should be used to monitor oxygen saturation of >95%. The infant will be more comfortable at 30–40° angle or with the head and chest elevated.

The complications associated with hypoxemia and CO_2 retention generally begin when the respiratory rate surpasses 60 breaths/min. Admission to pediatric ICUs and use of noninvasive or invasive ventilatory support because of severe respiratory distress, hypoxemia, or apnea are required in 10–20% of children hospitalized with RSV bronchiolitis.

Indications for Hospitalization

- Moderate to severe dehydration
- Retraction apnea
- Poor feeding
- Cyanosis
- $SaO_2 < 91\%$
- Respiratory rate > 70 breaths/min
- Marked respiratory distress with retraction
- Younger than 6 months

Inhaled bronchodilators, such as albuterol or racemic epinephrine, or inhaled or systemic corticosteroids are not recommended for the management of children with RSV bronchiolitis. Nebulized hypertonic saline has been shown to increase mucociliary clearance and may be beneficial in infants who are expected to have prolonged hospitalizations (>72 hours). Last, except for AOM, bacterial infections of the lower respiratory tract are rarely associated with RSV infection; thus, antibiotic treatment is usually not indicated for LRTI.

Wheezing and rhonchi are usually present. Hence it is very difficult to differentiate from the first attack of asthma. Trial of bronchodilator salbutamol is given. A bronchodilator may be continued round the clock if there is improvement clinically.

There is improvement in lung function with the high dose 0.5 mg/kg nebulized epinephrine. This will reduce mucosal edema. This is by alpha-receptor stimulation. This produces constriction of precapillary arterioles reducing microvascular leakage.

Antibiotics are indicated in the presence of fever, clinical deterioration, high WBC count, raised CRP, and infiltration on chest X-rays.

Ribavirin is an antiviral agent. It is given by aerosol 16 hours a day for 3–5 days. It shortens the course of illness in infants with underlying CHD, chronic lung disease, and immunodeficiency.

Ribavirin is indicated:
- High risk severe or complicated RSV infection
- RSV infection with LRTI who are seriously ill.
- Mechanically ventilated infants

Ribavirin is a broad-spectrum virostatic antiviral agent with activity against RSV and other RNA viruses. Early on, small, double-blinded, placebo-controlled studies showed a beneficial effect in infants treated with aerosolized ribavirin soon after onset of disease. The required aerosol route of administration, concerns about potential toxic effects among exposed healthcare personnel, possible teratogenicity in pregnant women, conflicting results of efficacy trials, and high cost have led to infrequent use of ribavirin.

Beta-2-adrenergic drugs and ipratropium are used in infants above 6 months. If patient improvement, bronchodilators may be given every 4–6 hourly. Continuous positive airway pressure (CPAP) or assisted ventilation may be required to control respiratory failure. Extracorporeal membrane oxygenation is effective if respiratory failure is not controlled by mechanical ventilation.

■ PROGNOSIS

Most of them recover from acute infection within 2 weeks. For about 50% will have recurrent episodes of cough and wheezing. Rarely with infection adenovirus illness may result in permanent damage of airways—bronchiolitis obliterans. Bronchiolitis due to RSV infection contributes to morbidity and morbidity in children with an underlying medical disorder, including chronic disease of prematurity, CF, CHD, and immunodeficiency. Death may occur in 1% of severely ill patients due to respiratory failure.

The relationship to bronchial asthma is 25% of cases of bronchiolitis.

Children with recurrent or refractory episodes of wheezing in infancy, particularly if associated with failure to thrive, may require evaluation for chronic disorders, such as CF or immunodeficiency.

A majority of deaths due to bronchiolitis occur in children with complex medical conditions or comorbidities, such as bronchopulmonary dysplasia, CHD, and immunodeficiency.

PREVENTION

For high-risk populations, palivizumab, a monoclonal antibody to the RSV F protein, may be given monthly by intramuscular injection as a prophylactic agent. Palivizumab has been demonstrated to reduce the risk of hospitalization due to RSV bronchiolitis in certain populations, preterm infants.

BIBLIOGRAPHY

1. Colom AJ, Maffey A, Garcia Bournissen F, Teper A. Pulmonary function of a paediatric cohort of patients with postinfectious bronchiolitis obliterans. A long term follow-up. Thorax. 2015;70(2)169-74.
2. Osvald CE, Clarke JR. NICE clinical guideline: Bronchiolitis in children. Child Educ Pract Ed. 2016;101(1):46-8.
3. Teixeira MFC, Rodrigues JC, Leone C, Adde FV. Acute bronchodilator responsiveness to tiotropium in postinfectious bronchiolitis obliterans in children. Chest. 2013; 144(3):974-80.
4. Tomikawa SO, Adde FV, da Silva Filho LV, Leone C, Rodrigues JC. Follow-up on pediatric patients with bronchiolitis obliterans treated with corticosteroid pulse therapy. Orphanet J Rare Dis. 2014;9:128.
5. Walsh P, Rothenberg SJ. American Academy of Pediatrics 2014 bronchiolitis guidelines: bonfire of the evidence. West J Emerg Med. 2015;16(1):85-8.

CASE 8

Croup

PRESENTING COMPLAINTS

A 20-month-old boy was brought with the complaints of:
- Cold, cough since 2 days
- Fever since 1 day
- Noisy breathing since 4 hours
- Difficulty in breathing since 4 hours

History of Presenting Complaints

A 20-month-old boy with the sudden onset of a harsh brassy cough was brought to the hospital at about 3 AM in the morning. The cough was associated with noisy breathing. The child was irritable and uncomfortable. He was breathless. He was not able to take any feeds. He had a common cold 2 days back and had been treated with medicines. The boy had a high temperature. There was also a history of difficulty in swallowing.

Past History of the Patient

He was the only sibling of the nonconsanguineous marriage. He was born at full term with the normal delivery. His birth weight was 2.8 kg. There were no significant postnatal events. The child was breastfed for 6 months. Weaning started at the age of 4 months and the child was taking all the family food by the age of 1 year. His developmental milestones were normal. He had been completely immunized.

CASE AT A GLANCE

Basic Findings
Height	:	82 cm (75th centile)
Weight	:	11 kg (50th centile)
Temperature	:	38°C
Pulse rate	:	120 beats/min
Respiratory rate	:	64 breaths/min
Blood pressure	:	60/40 mm Hg

Positive Findings

History:
- Sudden onset of brassy cough
- Noisy breathing
- Cold 2 days back
- Breathlessness

Examination:
- Irritable
- Stridor
- Rhonchi and crepitation
- Breathlessness
- Breath sounds diminished

Investigation:
- *Chest X-ray:* Steeple sign
- *Arterial blood gas (ABG):* Features of hypoxia

EXAMINATION

The child was well built and nourished. The child was irritable and dyspneic. A noisy, brassy cough was present. Anthropometric measurements include, the height was 82 cm (75th centile), and weight was 11 kg (50th centile).

The child was febrile. Heart rate was 120 beats/min. The respiratory rate was

64 breaths/min. Intercostal indrawing was present. The subcostal recession was present. The blood pressure recorded was 60/40 mm Hg. Central cyanosis was present. There was no pallor, icterus, clubbing, and lymphadenopathy.

The respiratory system revealed the inspiratory stridor. The noisy breathing was conducted and heard all over the chest. Breath sounds were diminished. Rhonchi and aspiration are present. There was occasional expiratory stridor. Per abdomen examination revealed mild distension. No organomegaly. The cardiovascular system revealed the presence of tachycardia.

■ INVESTIGATION

- *Hemoglobin:* 14 g/dL
- *DLC:* $P_{80}L_{15}M_1E_2B_1$
- *ESR:* 20 mm in the first hour
- *Chest X-ray:* Subglottic narrowing, i.e., steeple sign
- *Serum electrolytes:*
  - Na: 130 mEq/L
  - K: 5 mEq/L
  - Cl: 90 mEq/L
- *ABG:*
  - pH < 7
  - PaO_2: 60 mm Hg
  - $PaCO_2$: 40 mm Hg
  - HCO_3: 20 mEq/L

■ DISCUSSION

The presenting symptoms and physical examination point to a diagnosis of acute laryngotracheobronchitis, i.e., croup. The croup is mainly caused by viruses. These include parainfluenza, adenovirus, RSV, influenza, and measles viruses. Sometimes bacterial infection occurs secondarily. The bacteria responsible are *Mycoplasma pneumoniae*, *H. influenzae*, group A streptococci, pneumococci, and staphylococci.

Most patients with croup are between the ages of 3 months and 5 years, with the peak in the second year of life. The incidence of croup is higher in boys. It occurs most commonly in the late fall and winter but can occur throughout the year. Approximately 15% of patients have a strong family history of croup. Recurrences are frequent from 3 to 6 years of age and decrease with growth of the airway. Recurrent croup is defined as two or more croup-like episodes. Patients with recurrent croup have a higher incidence of asthma, allergies, and gastroesophageal reflux; <9% of patients with recurrent croup demonstrate clinically significant findings on bronchoscopy (e.g., subglottic stenosis, reflux changes, and broncho/tracheomalacia).

Croup describes acute inflammatory diseases of the larynx-laryngitis, and spasmodic laryngitis, including viral croup (laryngotracheobronchitis), epiglottitis (supraglottitis), and bacterial tracheitis.

There is mucosal inflammation and increased secretions affecting the airway, but it is the edema of a subglottic area that is potentially dangerous in young children because it may result in critical narrowing of the trachea.

The airway resistance is inversely proportional to the fourth power of radius. Hence any mucosal edema in the small airways leads to a significant increase in the work of breathing, narrowing, and may lead to respiratory difficulty. Infection of these parts of the respiratory tract produces a dry, hacking cough and hoarseness of the voice giving them a common name of croup syndrome. There are four clinically distinct syndromes; these include acute laryngitis, laryngotracheobronchitis, spasmodic laryngitis, and acute epiglottis.

■ CLINICAL FEATURES (FIG. 1)

Croup is a disease of the upper airway, and alveolar gas exchange is usually normal. Hypoxia and low oxygen saturation are seen only when complete airway obstruction is imminent. The child who is hypoxic, cyanotic, pale, or obtunded needs immediate airway management.

Croup is the most common cause of acute respiratory tract infection leading to obstruction. Most of them have URIs before the cough becomes apparent. At first, there will be only a mild brassy cough with intermittent respiratory stridor. As obstruction increases, the stridor becomes obvious. It is associated with nasal flaring, suprasternal, infrasternal, and intercostal retraction.

Viral croup occurs between 6 months and 36 months of age, but the peak incidence is in the second year of life. Usually, the illness begins with rhinorrhea and within to 12–24 hours, a barking cough and stridor develop. The stridor is usually prominent during inspiration. Fever is a variable finding. The degree of airway obstruction varies from maximum to severe. The symptoms often start and are worse in the night.

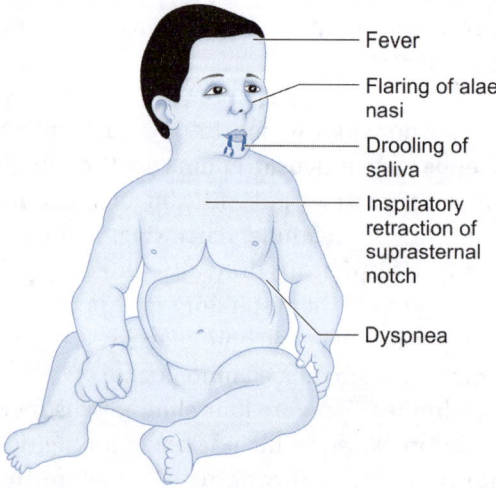

Fig. 1: Clinical features.

■ SPASMODIC CROUP

Spasmodic croup occurs most often in children 1–3 years of age and is clinically similar to acute laryngotracheobronchitis, except that the history of a viral prodrome and fever in the patient and family are often absent. The cause is viral in some cases, but allergy and other factors may also contribute.

Occurring most commonly in the evening or nighttime, spasmodic croup begins with a sudden onset that may be preceded by mild to moderate coryza and hoarseness. The child awakens with a characteristic barking, metallic cough, noisy inspiration, and respiratory distress, and appears anxious and frightened. The patient is usually afebrile. The severity of the symptoms generally diminishes within several hours and the following day, the patient often appears well except for slight hoarseness and cough. Spasmodic croup might represent more of an allergic reaction to viral antigens than direct infection, although the pathogenesis is unknown.

Sometimes there may be a fulminating course of fever, sore throat, dyspnea, rapidly progressing obstruction, and prostration. Sometimes aphonia and drooling of saliva are noted. Dysphagia is also common.

The primary findings include inflammatory edema and distribution of ciliated epithelium and exudates. As the inflammation exceeds the bronchi and bronchioles, respiratory difficulty occurs. The expiratory phase of the respiration becomes labored and prolonged. Later air hunger and restlessness occur. There will be stridor, and increasing pulse rate and deaths may occur from hypoventilation. In the hypoxic child, who may be cyanotic, pale, and obtunded, any manipulation of the pharynx may result in cardiorespiratory arrest. Subglottic edema is associated with inflammation of the trachea and bronchi (laryngotracheobronchitis) is common.

With the further compromise of the airway, air hunger, and restlessness occur. These are superseded by severe hypoxemia, hypercapnia, and weakness. These are accompanied by decreased air exchange, stridor tachycardia, and eventual death from hypoventilation.

Physical examination reveals inspiratory and expiratory stridor, flaring up of alae nasi, and inspiratory retraction of the suprasternal notch. There will be diminished breath sounds, rhonchi, and scattered crackles.

The child may assume a tripod position sitting upright and leaning forward with the chin up and mouth open while bending the arm.

ESSENTIAL DIAGNOSTIC POINTS

- Acute inflammatory disease of the larynx, including viral croup and bacterial tracheitis
- There will be stridor, and an increasing pulse rate and deaths may occur from hypoventilation
- Fulminating course of fever, sore throat, dyspnea, rapidly progressing obstruction, and prostration
- Nasal flaring, suprasternal, infrasternal, and intercostal retraction
- Subglottic edema will be associated with inflammation of the trachea and bronchi

GENERAL FEATURES

- Mild brassy cough
- Stridor
- Air hunger
- Restlessness
- Sore throat
- Aphonia
- Hypoxemia and weakness

■ DIAGNOSIS

Croup is a clinical diagnosis and does not require any investigation. Radiographs are used only if a diagnosis is uncertain. The X-ray of the neck may show the typical subglottic narrowing or steeple sign on the PA view. However, the steeple sign may be absent in patients with croup. The radiograph does not reflect the severity of airway obstruction.

Neck anteroposterior radiograph shows narrowing of the subglottic portion of the trachea producing an inverted V (steeple sign), without irregularities seen in tracheitis.

■ DIFFERENTIAL DIAGNOSIS

The differential diagnosis includes conditions that cause obstruction in the region of the larynx:

- *Laryngeal foreign body:* Sudden onset of choking and coughing without prodromal signs of infection.
- *Acute angioedema:* Usually presents with swelling of the face and neck and other manifestations of allergic reactions.
- *Retropharyngeal and peritonsillar abscess:* A peritonsillar abscess is often a clinical diagnosis whereas a radiograph or CT scan of the upper airway helps in the diagnosis of retropharyngeal abscess
- *Bacterial tracheitis:* Although, it is very rare, it is an important differential diagnosis as it may have a fulminant course and needs antibiotics.
- *Laryngeal diphtheria:* Early symptoms of diphtheria include malaise, sore throat, anorexia, and low-grade fever. Within 2–3 days a typical gray-white membrane on tonsils and/or soft palate is seen on pharyngeal examination. The fine membrane is adherent to the tissue, and forcible attempts to remove it cause bleeding.
- *Measles croup:* It always has full manifestations of systemic disease and the course may be fulminant.

- *Bronchial asthma:* A croupy cough may be an early sign of asthma.
- *Subglottic stenosis:* It presents from early infancy and is not associated with prodromal symptoms.

■ COMPLICATIONS

Complications include bronchopneumonia, cervical lymphadenitis, otitis media, meningitis, septic arthritis, tracheobronchitis, and pneumothorax.

■ TREATMENT

The mainstay of treatment for children of croup is airway management.

Indications for Hospitalization

This includes actual or suspected epiglottis, progressive stridor, severe stridor at rest, respiratory distress, hypoxemic restlessness, cyanosis, pallor, depressed sensorium, and high fever in a toxic-appearing child. Fluid should be administered for adequate hydration of the patient by intravenous route.

Basic Management

- Do not examine the throat
- Observe signs of hypoxia or deterioration
- If severe, administer nebulized adrenaline
- Urgent tracheal intubation if respiratory failure develops

Therapy includes primarily maintaining and providing adequate respiratory exchange. The use of steam often terminates laryngeal spasms and respiratory distress within minutes.

The inspired air is cooler than the body temperature and less than 100% saturated with water vapor resulting in mucosal cooling, leading to vasoconstriction and lessened edema.

Frequent continuous monitoring of the respiratory rate is essential as a rapid and rising respiratory rate may be the first sign of hypoxia and fatal respiratory obstruction.

Oxygen should be used to alleviate hypoxemia and apprehension. Persistence of the cyanosis despite giving oxygen is an indication of tracheostomy. These patients should be observed closely.

Unnecessary manipulation of the patient may induce laryngeal spasm. After the laryngeal spasm is released, its return may be prevented by the use of warm or cool humidification near the child's bed for 2–3 days. The patient should be disturbed as minimally as possible.

The use of an endotracheal or nasotracheal tube that is 0.5–1.0 mm smaller than estimated by age or height is recommended to facilitate intubation and reduce long-term sequelae. The choice of procedure should be based on the local expertise and experience with the procedure and postoperative care.

Parenteral intravenous fluid is given to make up for the insensible and respiratory water loss. This decreases the risk of vomiting if given as oral feed. Hence the risk of aspiration is taken care of. Sedatives are not indicated as the resistance by the child is the main indicator of distress.

Racemic epinephrine is given by nebulizer (0.5 mL of 2.25% solution diluted in sterile saline) and is commonly used after in doses of 2–4 mL for 15 minutes. This has a rapid onset of action within 10–30 minutes. It will give transient relief. Close observation and repeated treatment are usually necessary.

Racemic epinephrine and dexamethasone (0.5 mg/kg/dose 6–12 hours before extubation then every 6 hours for six doses with a maximum dose of 10 mg) may be useful in the treatment of upper airway edema seen postintubation.

The effectiveness of oral corticosteroids in viral croup is well established. Corticosteroids decrease the edema in the laryngeal mucosa through their anti-inflammatory action. Oral steroids are beneficial, even in mild croup, as measured by reduced hospitalization, shorter duration of hospitalization, and reduced need for subsequent interventions such as epinephrine administration.

The use of corticosteroids is indicated to reduce inflammatory edema and to prevent the obstruction of the ciliated epithelium. Dexamethasone in the dose of 0.6 mg/kg/day is used. Single intramuscular injection of dexamethasone reduces disease severity in the first 24 hours with decreased need for intubation and adrenaline nebulization. The topical nonabsorbed ICS for the treatment is budesonide. The dose is 2–4 mg. The beneficial effect of inhalation budesonide is seen. Inhalation of budesonide in doses of 2–4 mg twice a day for 2 days is useful. Oral dexamethasone (0.15 mg/kg) may be equally effective for mild to moderate croup. Heliox, a mixture of (80% helium and 20% oxygen mixture) is used to decrease respiratory difficulty.

Antibiotics such as ampicillin 100 mg/kg/day or chloramphenicol 50 mg/kg/day are used. A single daily dose of ceftriaxone may be used. Rifampicin prophylaxis for unimmunized children under 2 years should be considered.

In patients with impending respiratory failure, an airway must be established. Intubation with an endotracheal tube of slightly smaller diameter than would ordinarily be used is reasonably safe. Extubation should be accomplished within 2–3 days to minimize the risk of laryngeal injury. If a patient fails extubation, a tracheostomy may be required.

■ BIBLIOGRAPHY

1. Bjornson C, Russell KF, Vandermeer B, Durec T, Klassen TP, Jhonson DW. Nebulized epinephrine for croup in children. Database Syst Rev. 2011;2:CD006619.
2. Petrocheilou A, Tanou K, Kalampouka E, Malakasioti G, Giannios C, Kaditis AG. Viral croup: diagnosis and s treatment algorithm. Ped Pulm. 2014;49(5):421-9.
3. Russell KF, Liang Y, O'Gorman K, Johnson DW, Klassen TP. Corticosteroids for croup. Database Syst Rev. 2011;1:CD001995.
4. Tebruegge M, Pantazidou A, Thorburn K, Riordan A, Round J, De Munter C, et al. Bacterial Tracheitis: a multi-centre perspective. Scand J Infect Dis. 2009;41(8):548-57.
5. Tibballs J, Watson T. Symptoms and Signs differentiating croup and epiglottitis. Pediatr Child Health. 2011;47(3)77-82.

CASE 9

Empyema

PRESENTING COMPLAINTS

A 7-year-old boy was presented with complaints:
- Fever since 1 week
- Cough since 1 week
- Generalized weakness since 1 week
- Chest pain since 2 days
- Vomiting since 2 days

History of Presenting Complaints

A 7-year-old boy was brought to the emergency room with a high-grade fever, cough, and with generalized weakness. Fever of moderate to high degree was present since 1 week. Fever was a continuous type, sometimes associated with chill. Fever used to be relieved to some extent by antipyretics. The child had a productive cough. He was bringing out the sputum. Sputum was yellowish or white in color. The child used to have disturbed sleep because of the cough. There was an associated history of pain in the chest on the left side. The pain was increasing on taking deep inspiration. The child had been vomiting since 2 days. He was not tolerating any food.

Past History of the Patient

He was the first child of a nonconsanguineous marriage. He was born at full term by normal delivery. There was no significant postnatal event. The birth weight of the child was 3 kg. He was given breast milk. His developmental milestones were normal. His performance at school was good. There was no previous history of measles, tuberculosis, and whooping cough. There was no family history

---

CASE AT A GLANCE

Basic Findings
Height	:	120 cm (75th centile)
Weight	:	20 kg (30th centile)
Temperature	:	40°C
Pulse rate	:	120 beats/min
Respiratory rate	:	22 breaths/min
Blood pressure	:	100/70 mm Hg

Positive Findings

History:
- Cough
- Fever
- Chest pain
- Vomiting

Examination:
- Toxic
- Dehydrated
- Tenderness over the chest
- Clubbing
- Tracheal shift
- Diminished breath sounds
- Stony dullness

Investigation:
- *TLC:* Increased
- *DLC:* Neutrophilia
- *ESR:* Raised
- *X-ray chest:* Homogeneous opacity
- Thoracocentesis pus had no organism

(DLC: differential leukocyte count; ESR: erythrocyte sedimentation rate; TLC: total leukocyte count)

of similar complaints. There was no family history of tuberculosis.

■ EXAMINATION

The boy was moderately built and poorly nourished. He was looking very toxic. There were signs of moderate dehydration. His height was 120 cm (75th centile), weight was 20 kg (30th centile). He was febrile, i.e., 40°C. The pulse rate was 120 beats/min and the respiratory rate was 22 breaths/min. The blood pressure recorded was 100/70 mm Hg.

There was pallor, clubbing was present. There was no lymphadenopathy. Tenderness was present over the left inframammary region. Bony tenderness was present. The trachea was shifted to the right side. Stony dullness was present on percussion. Chest movements were diminished on the left side. Breath sounds were diminished. Other systemic examinations were normal.

■ INVESTIGATION

- *Hemoglobin:* 9.8 g/dL
- *TLC:* 22,000 cells/cumm
- *DLC:* $P_{78}L_{18}E_2M_2$
- *ESR:* 40 mm in the first hour
- *X-ray chest:* Presence of homogeneous opacity on the left side
- *Thoracocentesis:* Gram staining of the pus showed no organism
- *Pus culture and sensitivity:* Sterile

■ DISCUSSION

The child had a high-degree fever, respiratory distress, and signs of moderate dehydration. Productive cough is associated with foul-smelling sputum and the presence of clubbing are suggestive of suppurative lung disease. Tenderness at the chest, tender clubbing, and toxic look suggest empyema. Pus on thoracocentesis confirms the diagnosis.

■ PATHOPHYSIOLOGY

Empyema means a collection of thick pus in the pleural cavity. It occurs in children below 5 years. Certain organisms are common among certain age groups. The most common organism is S. pneumoniae. S. aureus is common in children <2 years of age. H. influenzae type B is common in children up to 5 years. Pneumococcus may also occur at this age. Group A streptococcus and pneumococcus are common in older children and adolescents. P. aeruginosa is suspected in immunocompromised, debilitated, hospitalized parents. It is commonly caused as a complication of staphylococcal (rarely S. pneumoniae or gram-negative bacilli) pneumonia or rupture of subdiaphragmatic or liver abscess in the pleura.

Empyema results from the rupture of lung abscess, trauma, intra-abdominal abscess, septicemia, meningitis, and malignancies. These are often loculated due to thickened pleura, fibrous septae, and inadequate drainage. They can be synpneumonic when associated with pneumonia or metapneumonic when they occur after pneumonia.

Empyema necessitans is the term used when the pus dissents through the chest wall and produces a superficial swelling in subcutaneous tissue under the skin. Empyema along with bronchopleural fistula indicates chronicity of the disease process, fibrosis. This is associated with tuberculosis empyema.

Thickening of the parietal pleura occurs if pus is not drained. It may be dissected through pleural space into the lung parenchyma. This produces broncho pleural fistula and pyopneumothorax or into the abdominal cavity. Pockets of loculated pus may eventually develop into the thick-walled abscess cavity.

Empyema has three stages: (1) Exudative, (2) fibrinopurulent, and (3) organizational. During the exudative stage, fibrinous exudate forms on the pleural surfaces.

There are three stages of development of the empyema. It is important to know the phases of development. This will help to plan the treatment and also for the prognosis.

- *Exudative phase:* It is an immediate response with the accumulation of their fluid with low cellular content. This stage lasts for a few hours to a few days. This stage responds well to the appropriate antibiotic. It requires intercostal drain placement. This may be adequate.
- *Fibrin purulent phase:* There will be a collection of pus. This contains many polymorphonuclear cells and fibrin. This lasts for about 2–10 days. It is ideally treated with decortication. In the fibrinopurulent stage, fibrinous septa form, causing loculation of the fluid and thickening of the parietal pleura. If the pus is not drained, it may dissect through the pleura into lung parenchyma, producing bronchopleural fistulas and pyopneumothorax, or into the abdominal cavity. Rarely, the pus dissects through the chest wall (i.e., empyema necessitatis).
- *Organizing phase:* There will be the formation of a "peel." This is due to the growth of fibroblast on the pleural surface. It leads to the chronic loss of lung function. With the increasing fibrous, intercostal space decreases leading to rib crowding and scoliosis. During the organizational stage, there is fibroblast proliferation; pockets of loculated pus may develop into thick-walled abscess cavities or the lung may collapse and become surrounded by a thick, inelastic envelope (peel). Open thoracotomy is the treatment of choice.

> **ESSENTIAL DIAGNOSTIC POINTS**
> - Appear toxic and have greater respiratory difficulty
> - High fever, cough, and breathlessness
> - Tenderness at the chest, tender clubbing, and toxic look
> - Pus on thoracocentesis
> - Bronchopleural fistula indicates chronicity of the disease process and fibrosis

■ CLINICAL FEATURES (FIG. 1)

The initial signs and symptoms are those of bacterial pneumonia. Most of the cases are febrile. There will be an acute history of high fever, cough, and breathlessness. They often appear toxic and have greater respiratory difficulty. In critical condition, the patient may be cyanosed. There will be a stony dull note on chest percussion, absent air entry on the affected side, and tenderness with the tracheal and mediastinal shift.

> **GENERAL FEATURES**
> - Toxic look
> - Signs of dehydration
> - Leukocytosis
> - Increased ESR

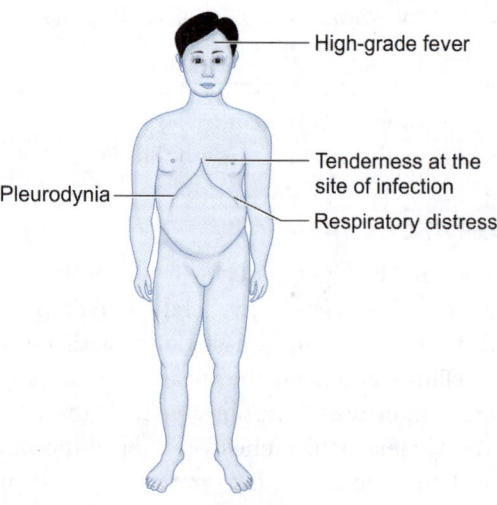

Fig. 1: Clinical features

Older children or those with chronic empyema may not look so ill. The child will show the signs of hydropneumothorax if a bronchopleural fistula develops. Clubbing may develop. Empyema necessitans should be thought about if a child develops a superficial chest wall swelling.

■ DIAGNOSIS

Increased WBC count, polymorphonuclear leukocytosis, and raised ESR support the diagnosis.

X-Ray of Chest

A standard posteroanterior (PA) view of the plain X-ray is relatively insensitive to detect pleural effusion. In general, a minimum of 400 mL of pleural fluid should be required to detect by upright chest X-ray. Decubitus films may detect as little as 50 mL of fluid. A density of >10 mm suggests sufficient volume for tapping.

In a child with worsening pneumonia, a repeat X-ray should be advised. In the presence of empyema, it will show the presence of fluid. Failure of fluid to shift on X-ray in various positions indicates loculation. They also demonstrate subpulmonic effusion.

In cases with underlying bronchopleural fistula, an air-fluid level will be present. Loculation is seen with the organization phase. Crowding of ribs with scoliosis suggests chronic empyema.

There will be the obliteration of the cardiophrenic angle, the fluid level in pyopneumothorax, and collapsed lung tracheal, and the mediastinal shift is obvious.

Significant scoliosis on the X-ray chest and evidence of parenchymal entrapment are indications for a prolonged hospital course and suggest surgical intervention.

Diagnostic Thoracocentesis

It helps in distinguishing between parapneumonic effusion and empyema. Fluid collected should be examined for gram stain in anaerobic and aerobic cultures, pH measurement, and measurement of glucose and lactate dehydrogenase (LDH).

Pus that is aspirated shows opaque fluid, polymorphs in abundance, protein content >3 g/dL, and pleural fluid. Serum protein concentration is higher, pleural LDH levels >200, and pleural LDH ratio >0.6 are diagnostic of exudates. Pus with polymorph indicates empyema. A pleural biopsy may also help in arriving at a diagnosis and etiology.

Empyema severe score includes: (1) pleural fluid pH <7.2, (2) Pleural fluid glucose level <40 mg%, and (3) Presence of anaerobic infection.

Ultrasound Chest

It is a very useful tool for diagnosis, the guidance of thoracocentesis, or pleural catheter placement. It is especially helpful when the radiograph shows a whiteout. Sonography can distinguish solid from liquid pleural abnormalities with much higher accuracy compared to skiagrams. Sonography gives valuable information regarding the size of the effusion, the presence of adhesions or loculations, and the echogenicity of the pleural fluid. The sonographic appearance of pleural fluid varies according to the stage of effusion, ranging from an anechoic completely echo-free, or sonolucent parapneumonic effusion to very echogenic fluid with septa as seen in frank empyema. Ultrasonography shows limiting membranes suggesting the presence of loculated collections even when they are not so well seen on CT scans.

Although on an ultrasound a lenticular shape may indicate the presence of loculated fluid, septa are better visualized by CT. The effusion is an empyema if bacteria are present on Gram staining at a pH is <7.20, and there are >100,000 neutrophils/mL. Cultures of the fluid must always be performed to help identify the causal organism. Using standard culture methods, the organism can be identified in up to 60% of cases. The yield improves significantly with concomitant use of nucleic acid amplification techniques. Blood cultures may be positive and have a higher yield than cultures of the pleural fluid. Leukocytosis and an elevated sedimentation rate may be found.

It may detect a smaller amount of fluid. It helps to differentiate pleural thickening from effusion. It helps in locating pleural fluid, amount of fluid, presence of loculation, and knowing about the condition of the underlying lung i.e., presence of consolidation in the underlying lobe.

It will evaluate the nature of the fluid. Pleural fluid may be transudate or exudate. Multiple echogenic foci indicate thick exudate or empyema. It differentiates lung and pleural pathology. It is useful as a prognostic indicator.

Computerized Tomography Scan

Empyema appears well-defined, smooth, round, or elliptical on CT scan. The parietal and visceral layers are separated by interposed empyema fluid, giving rise to the "split pleura sign" of empyema. CT scans should not be performed routinely as they expose the child to a very high radiation dose while most information for diagnosis and for guiding treatment decisions can be received from a good sonogram. It may have a limited role in cases that do not respond to the initial medical management or before surgery to delineate the anatomy and to rule out a lung abscess.

It helps in identifying exact anatomy, amount of pus, loculation, the thickness of "peel," and condition of underlying lung parenchyma. Margins separating the density from adjacent lung, and bone soft tissues are well defined. CT can be of value in distinguishing subpulmonic and subphrenic collections in patients with an elevated hemidiaphragm seen on X-ray.

> **LABORATORY SALIENT FINDINGS**
> - Increased white blood cell count, polymorphonuclear leukocytosis and raised erythrocyte sedimentation rate (ESR)
> - X-ray chest
> - Diagnostic thoracocentesis
> - Ultrasound chest
> - Computerized tomography (CT) scan

It is useful in differentiating pleural from parenchymal disease. This distinction is important because antibiotic therapy and postural drainage are appropriate for lung abscess, whereas thoracotomy and tube drainage are important for empyema.

■ TREATMENT

Treatment includes systemic antibiotics and thoracentesis and chest tube drainage initially with a fibrinolytic agent; if no improvement occurs, video-assisted thoracoscopic surgery (VATS) is indicated. Open decortication is indicated if fibrinolysis and VATS are ineffective. Its empyema is diagnosed early, and antibiotic treatment plus thoracentesis achieves a complete cure.

Choice of Antibiotics

It depends upon the Gram stain and culture and sensitivity. However, most of these patients are on antibiotics, so the culture may not be very useful.

When the organism is not identifiable, ampicillin with cloxacillin and cloxacillin with third-generation cephalosporin is the right combination.

Staphylococcal empyema is best treated with penicillin or vancomycin or cloxacillin. Pneumococcal infection is treated by penicillin or cefotaxime. *H. influenza* responds to cefuroxime, cefotaxime, ceftriaxone, and azithromycin.

Systemic antibiotic therapy is required for at least 2–3 weeks.

Intercostal Drainage

Pus is drained immediately and controlled by an underwater seal or continuous suction. A large bore intercostal drainage is inserted into the site where the accumulation of pus is suspected. It should achieve dependent drainage. It may achieve adequate drainage in the exudate phase, especially in the single cavity without loculation. However, it fails to achieve adequate drainage once loculation develops. Chest tubes that are no longer draining should be removed. Fibrinolytic enzymes or proteolytic enzymes are instilled into the pleural cavity. Systemic antibiotic therapy is required.

Closed-chest tube drainage is controlled by an underwater seal or continuous suction; sometimes more than one tube is required to drain loculated areas. Closed drainage is usually continued for 5–7 days. Chest tubes that are no longer draining are removed.

Instillation of fibrinolytic agents into the pleural cavity via the chest tube often promotes drainage decreases the length of time a chest tube is in place, decreases fever, lessens the need for surgical intervention, and shortens hospitalization. The optimal fibrinolytic drug and dosages have not been determined. Streptokinase 15,000 units/kg in 50 mL of 0.9% saline, urokinase 40,000 units in 40 mL saline, and alteplase (tPA) 4 mg in 40 mL of saline have been used in the pediatric population. The combination of fibrinolytic therapy with deoxyribonuclease (DNAse) is superior to the use of fibrinolytics alone to promote chest tube drainage. There is a risk of anaphylaxis with streptokinase, and all three drugs can be associated with hemorrhage and other complications.

Decortication

It is the surgical procedure. It involves the removal of fibrinous tissue from the parietal or visceral pleura to release lung entrapment.

In patients, who remain afebrile and dyspneic longer than 72 hours of initiation of therapy with intravenous antibiotics and intercostal drainage, surgical decortication is indicated. Surgical treatment is advised if pneumatoceles produce respiratory distress.

Now with a better understanding of the pathophysiology of empyema formation, once the loculi are formed, intercostal drainage will fail to resolve empyema completely. Hence on detection of empyema, if the loculation has already started developing, the patient should be subjected to primary decortication even prior to intercostal drainage.

Advantages of early decortication include the decreased length of duration of intercostal drainage and good success rate with primary treatment modality.

■ BIBLIOGRAPHY

1. Cohen E, Mahant S, Dell SD, Traubici J, Ragone A, Wadhwa A, et al. The long-term outcomes of pediatric pleural empyema: a prospective study. Arch Peditric Adoles Med. 2012;166(11)999-1004.
2. Langley JM, Kellner JD, Solomon N, Robinson JL, Le Saux N, McDonald J, et al. Empyema associated with community-

acquired pneumonia: a Pediatric Investigator's Collaborative Network on Infections in Canada (PICNIC) study. BMC Infect Dis. 2008;8:129.
3. Redden MD, Chin TY, van Driel ML. Surgical versus non-surgical management for pleural empyema. Cochrane Database Syst Rev. 2017;3(3):CD010651.
4. Walker W, Wheeler R, Legg J. Update on the causes, investigation and management of empyema in childhood. Arch Dis Child. 2011;96(5):482-8.

CASE 10

Otitis Media

■ PRESENTING COMPLAINTS
A 20-month-old boy was brought with complaints of:
- Cough and cold since 3 days
- Excessive crying since 1 day
- Discharge in right ear since 1 day

History of Presenting Complaints
A 20-month-old baby was brought to the pediatric OPD with the history of discharge in the right ear. His mother noticed the ear discharge in the morning. She gave the history of excessive crying and irritability of the child at night. She could not make out the reason for crying. She administered the paracetamol syrup and cough syrup as prescribed by a general practitioner for cough and cold, fever. She revealed that her baby had cough and cold for which she had sought the family doctor's advice.

Past History of the Patient
He was the only sibling of the nonconsanguineous marriage. He was born at full term with normal vaginal delivery. His birth weight was 3 kg. There was no significant postnatal event. The child was exclusively on breast milk for 6 months. Weaning started at the age of 4 months. Child was taking all the family food by the age of 1 year. His developmental milestones were normal. He had been completely immunized.

CASE AT A GLANCE

Basic Findings
Height	: 82 cm (75th centile)
Weight	: 11 kg (50th centile)
Temperature	: 38°C
Pulse rate	: 120 beats/min
Respiratory rate	: 26 breaths/min
Blood pressure	: 60/40 mm Hg

Positive Findings

History:
- Pain in the ear
- Discharge in the right ear
- Cough, cold, fever
- Excessive crying

Examination:
- Febrile
- Features of rhinitis
- Nasal block
- Otoscopic examination—perforation in the right ear

Investigation:
- Total leukocyte count (TLC)—increased
  – Polymorph leukocytosis

■ EXAMINATION
The child was well built and nourished. He was irritable and was not ready to lie on the examination table. Anthropometric measurements included the height 82 cm (75th centile) and weight was 11 kg (50th centile).

The child was febrile. Heart rate was 120 beats/min. The respiratory rate was

26 breaths/min. Blood pressure recorded was 60/40 mm Hg. The ear discharge was present in the right ear. Left ear was normal. There was neither pallor, icterus, clubbing, nor lymphadenopathy.

Features suggestive of rhinitis, i.e., nasal discharge and nasal block were present. Throat was congested. Otoscopic examination revealed the presence of perforation in tympanic membrane (TM). All the systemic examinations were normal.

■ INVESTIGATION

- *Hemoglobin:* 14 g/dL
- *TLC:* 12,800 cells/cumm
- *DLC:* $P_{80}L_{15}M_1E_2B_1$
- *ESR:* 20 mm in the first hour
- *Ear discharge for culture and sensitivity:* Sterile
- *Otoscopic examination:* Perforation in the TM right side

■ DISCUSSION

The child had the URI associated with cough, cold and fever. Child was irritable and was crying a lot, and later mother noticed the discharge in the ear. Along with the otoscopic findings, the diagnosis of otitis media with chronic suppurative otitis media (CSOM) was done.

Otitis media (inflammation of the middle ear) is an infection associated with middle-ear effusion (MEE) (a collection of fluid in the middle-ear space) or otorrhea (a discharge from the ear through a perforation in the TM or ventilating tube).

Otitis media can be further classified by its associated clinical symptoms, otoscopic findings, duration, frequency, and complications. The more specific classifications are AOM, OME (residual or persistent effusion), and CSOM.

Acute Otitis Media

Acute otitis media is commonly defined as inflammation of the middle ear resulting in an effusion and is associated with rapid onset of symptoms such as otalgia, fever, irritability, anorexia, or vomiting. An ear effusion is best documented by pneumatic otoscopy or tympanometry.

Otitis Media with Effusion

Otitis media with effusion is defined as an asymptomatic MEE that often follows AOM, but it may have no such antecedent history. Otoscopic findings that suggest OME include visualization of air–fluid level or bubbles, and a clear or amber-colored middle-ear fluid. Effusion is usually associated with either a mild or moderate conductive hearing impairment of 15 dB or higher. OME can also be associated with negative middle-ear pressure, which results in prominence of the malleus and a negative pressure peak on tympanometry.

To distinguish AOM from OME, signs of inflammation of the TM or symptoms of acute infection must be present. Otoscopic findings specific for AOM are a bulging TM; impaired visibility of the ossicular landmarks; a yellow, white, or bright-red color TM; opacification of the eardrum; and exudates or bullae on the eardrum.

Pathophysiology and Predisposing Factors

Eustachian tube dysfunction (ETD): The Eustachian tube regulates middle-ear pressure and allows for drainage of the middle ear. It must periodically open to prevent the development of negative pressure and effusion in the middle-ear space. If this does not occur, negative pressure leads to transudation of cellular fluid into the middle ear, as well as influx of fluids and pathogens from the nasopharynx and adenoids. Middle-ear fluid may then become infected, resulting in AOM. The Eustachian tube of infants and young children is more prone to dysfunction, because it is shorter, more compliant, and more horizontal than in adults. The Eustachian tube reaches its adult configuration by the age of 7 years. Infants with craniofacial disorders, such as Down syndrome or cleft palate, may be particularly susceptible to ETD.

Bacterial colonization: Nasopharyngeal colonization with *Streptococcus pneumoniae*, *Haemophilus influenzae*, or *Moraxella catarrhalis* increases the risk of AOM, whereas colonization with normal flora such as viridans streptococci may prevent AOM by inhibiting growth of these pathogens.

Viral URIs: URIs increase colonization of the nasopharynx with otitis pathogens. They impair Eustachian tube function by causing adenoid hypertrophy and edema of the Eustachian tube itself. It is not absolutely clear if viral pathogens are the primary cause of episodes of AOM or if they help promote bacterial infections.

Passive smoking increases the risk of persistent MEE by enhancing colonization, prolonging the inflammatory response, and impending drainage of the middle ear through the Eustachian.

Impaired host immune defenses: Immunocompromised children such as those with selective IgA deficiency usually experience recurrent AOM, rhinosinusitis, and pneumonia. However, most children who experience recurrent or persistent otitis only have selective impairments of immune defenses against specific otitis pathogens.

Bottle feeding reduces the incidence of acute respiratory infections, provides IgA antibodies that reduce colonization with otitis pathogens, and decreases the aspiration of contaminated secretions into the middle-ear space which can occur when a bottle is propped in the crib.

Season: The incidence of AOM correlates with the activity of respiratory viruses, accounting for the annual surge in otitis media cases during the winter months in temperate climates.

Genetic susceptibility: Although AOM is known to be multifactorial, and no gene for susceptibility has yet been identified, recent studies of twins and triplets suggest that as much as 70% of the risk is genetically determined.

Age: Children ages 1-3 years are at greatest risk for AOM.

Microbiology of Acute Otitis Media

Bacterial pathogens: The three most common bacterial otopathogens are *S. pneumoniae*, nontypeable *H. influenzae*, and *M. catarrhalis*. Less common bacteria include *Streptococcus pyogenes* (group A), which causes 29-10% of AOM, tends to occur in older children, and is more frequently associated with TM perforation and mastoiditis. Rare pathogens detected in the MEE include *Chlamydia*, *Mycoplasma*, *Mycobacterium tuberculosis*, and fungi.

Viral URTI is exceedingly common in infants and children and often leads to AOM. It has been suggested that certain viruses are more likely to cause AOM than others. It is likely, however, that any virus that causes URTI is able to induce AOM. A broad spectrum of respiratory viruses cause URTI; rhinoviruses and coronaviruses are the most common among them. Other common URTI viruses are adenoviruses, RSV, parainfluenza viruses, human metapneumovirus, influenza viruses, and enteroviruses.

Bacterial or viral pathogens can be detected in up to 96% of middle-ear fluid samples from patients with AOM. Polybacterial infections are seen in up to 55% of cases, with bacterial and viral coinfections occurring in up to 70%. *S. pneumoniae* and *H. influenzae* account for 35–40% and 30–35% of isolates, respectively. With widespread use of the pneumococcal conjugate vaccine starting in 2000, the incidence of AOM caused by *H. influenzae* rose while that of the *S. pneumoniae* vaccine serotypes declined. However, there has been an increase in disease caused by *S. pneumoniae* serotypes not covered by the vaccine as well as *Staphylococcus aureus*. The third most common pathogen cited is *M. catarrhalis*, which causes up to 15–25% of AOM cases. The fourth most common organism in AOM is *S. pyogenes*, which is found more frequently in school-aged children than in infants. *S. pyogenes* and *S. pneumoniae* are the predominant causes of mastoiditis. The most common viruses associated with AOM are RSV, influenza virus, adenovirus, human metapneumovirus, and enteroviruses.

Drug-resistant *S. pneumoniae* is a common pathogen in AOM and strains may be resistant to only one drug class (e.g., penicillins or macrolides) or to multiple classes. Children with resistant strains tend to be younger and to have had more unresponsive infections. Antibiotic treatment in the preceding 3 months also increases the risk of harboring resistant pathogens.

■ CLINICAL FEATURES (FIG. 1)

Symptoms of AOM are generally nonspecific, including fever, irritability, restless sleep, decreased appetite, vomiting, and diarrhea. Fever occurs in one-third to two-thirds of children with AOM, but temperatures of 40°C or more are unusual unless accompanied by invasive bacterial disease or foci elsewhere. Because AOM most often occurs during URTI, there are also symptoms such as cough, sneezing, runny nose, stuffy nose, and red/watery eyes. Purulent conjunctivitis has been associated with AOM due to nontypeable *H. influenzae*.

Ear pain may manifest as ear tugging in infants. In children 6 months to 3 years of age with URTI, ear tugging does not differentiate children with URTI and AOM from those with only URTI. Earache is not universal in AOM; about one-fifth of children older than age 2 years do not complain of ear pain. The ear pain is due to pressure of the increasing suppuration in the middle ear and is relieved when the pressure leads to ischemia of the central vessels in the capillary bed of the TM. Persistent ischemia leads to necrosis of the TM with rupture and discharge of the contents of the middle-ear abscess and virtual elimination of the otalgia. Parents often report that a child who had cried with pain was relieved and bloody pus was observed. However, the TM is so vascular that the site of perforation may not be evident even 24 hours later, and the resealed membrane may result in reaccumulation of the purulent MEE.

Hearing loss is a frequent sign in infants. It may be expressed by verbal children or detected by a parent who sees the child not responding to spoken voice.

■ DIAGNOSIS

Otologic examination should include evaluation of the position, color, and degree of translucency and mobility of the TM. The normal eardrum should be in the neutral position. Mild retraction of the TM usually indicates the presence of negative middle-ear pressure, an effusion, or both. Severe retraction of the TM identifies high negative pressure associated with MEE. Fullness or bulging of the TM is caused by increased middle-ear pressure or MEE.

The normal TM has a ground-glass appearance and is translucent. The otoscopist should be able to look through the TM and visualize the middle-ear landmarks. A blue or yellow color identifies MEE seen through a translucent TM. A red TM may indicate inflammation but may also identify engorgement of the blood vessels of the TM caused by crying, sneezing, or nose-blowing. Adequate examination of the TM to confirm the MEE is sometimes difficult, particularly in infants and small children.

The diagnosis of AOM generally requires: (1) Abrupt onset of symptoms; (2) presence of MEE (bulging of the TM, limited or absent mobility of the TM, or otorrhea); and (3) signs or symptoms of middle-ear inflammation. As AOM develops, there is a spectrum of signs seen during the progression of TM inflammation and MEE accumulation.

The guideline requires bulging TM as evidence for middle-ear inflammation. Three degrees of bulging are defined: Mild, moderate, and severe. For mild bulging of the TM, intense erythema must also be present. The American Academy of Pediatrics (AAP) guideline has tightened the AOM working definition, in order to differentiate AOM from OME, recognizing that the AOM definition likely results in high specificity but less sensitivity as it may exclude less severe presentations of AOM.

Pneumatic otoscopy is the most feasible and cost-effective method for diagnosis of AOM and OME. Mobility of the TM is identified by pressure applied to the rubber bulb attached to the pneumatic otoscope. The normal or air-filled middle ear is identified by a brisk movement inward with slight positive pressure and outward with slight negative pressure. MEE or high negative pressure within the middle ear dampens movement of the TM. Movement of the TM is best seen in the PA quadrant of the TM.

Tympanometry and acoustic reflectometry can supplement pneumatic otoscopy. Tympanometry involves varying the pressure in the external canal accompanied by a probe tone. A graphic presentation, the tympanogram provides information on middle-ear pressure and the presence of an air-filled or fluid-filled middle-ear space. Because tympanometry and pneumatic otoscopy require a seal in the external canal for a few seconds, they may be difficult to perform in the young infant who is irritable due to ear pain.

> **ESSENTIAL DIAGNOSTIC POINTS**
> - Otitis media (inflammation of the middle ear) is an infection
> - Associated with middle-ear effusion (collection of fluid in the middle-ear space)
> - Otorrhea (a discharge from the ear through a perforation in the tympanic membrane)
> - Otalgia, fever, irritability, anorexia, or vomiting
> - Otoscopic findings specific for AOM are a bulging TM; impaired visibility of the ossicular landmarks
>
> (AOM: acute otitis media; TM: tympanic membrane)

> **GENERAL FEATURES**
> - Irritability
> - Anorexia
> - Inflammation of tympanic membrane
> - Perforation of tympanic membrane

COMPLICATIONS OF OTITIS MEDIA

Untreated AOM may occasionally cause serious extracranial or intracranial complications. *Extracranial complications* include acute mastoiditis, subperiosteal and

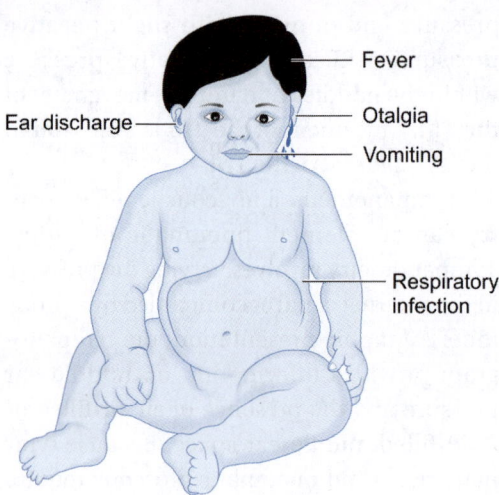

Fig. 1: Clinical features.

neck abscesses, and facial palsy. *Intracranial complications* may include meningitis or intracranial abscess. Fortunately, such complications are now less common due to increased availability of antibiotics.

Tympanosclerosis, Retraction Pockets, Adhesive Otitis

Tympanosclerosis is an acquired disorder of calcification and scarring of the TM and middle-ear structures from inflammation. If tympanosclerosis involves the ossicles, conductive hearing loss may result. The term myringosclerosis applies to calcification of the TM only and is a fairly common sequela of OME and AOM. Myringosclerosis may also develop at the site of a previous tympanostomy tube; tympanosclerosis is not a common sequela of tube placement.

Cholesteatoma

A greasy-looking mass or pearly white mass seen in a retraction pocket or perforation suggests a cholesteatoma. If infection is superimposed, serous or purulent drainage will be seen, and the middle-ear cavity may contain granulation tissue or even polyps. Persistent, recurrent, or foul-smelling otorrhea following appropriate medical management should make one suspect a cholesteatoma.

Tympanic Membrane Perforation

Occasionally, episode of AOM may result in rupture of the TM. Discharge from the ear is seen and often there is rapid relief of pain. Perforations due to AOM usually heal spontaneously within a couple of weeks. Ototopical antibiotics are recommended for a 10- to 14-day course and patients should be referred to an otolaryngologist 2–3 weeks after the rupture for examination and hearing evaluation.

When perforations fail to heal, surgical repair may be needed. TM repair is generally delayed until the child is older and Eustachian tube function has improved. Repair of the eardrum (tympanoplasty) is generally deferred until around 9 years of age, which is approximately when the Eustachian tube reaches adult orientation. In otherwise healthy children, some surgeons perform a repair earlier if the contralateral, nonperforated ear remains free of infection and effusion for 1 year.

Facial Nerve Paralysis (Fig. 2)

The facial nerve traverses the middle ear as it courses through the temporal bone to its exit at the stylomastoid foramen. Normally, the facial nerve is completely encased in bone, but occasionally bony dehiscence in the middle ear is present, exposing the nerve to infection and making it susceptible to inflammation during an episode of AOM. The acute onset of a facial nerve paralysis should not be deemed idiopathic bell palsy until all other causes have been excluded. If middle-ear fluid is present,

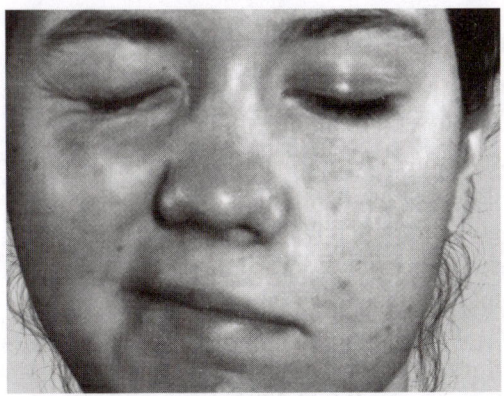

Fig. 2: Facial palsy.

prompt myringotomy and tube placement are indicated. With CT cholesteatoma or mastoiditis is suspected.

Chronic Suppurative Otitis Media

Chronic suppurative otitis media is defined as persistent otorrhea lasting longer than 6 weeks. Most often it occurs in children with tympanostomy tubes or TM perforations. Occasionally, it is an accompanying sign of cholesteatoma.

Chronic suppurative otitis media is present when persistent otorrhea occurs in a child with tympanostomy tubes or TM perforation; it starts with an acute infection that becomes chronic with mucosal edema, ulceration, granulation tissue, and eventual polyp formation. Risk factors include a history of multiple episodes of otitis media, living in crowded conditions, day care attendance, and being a member of a large family. The most common associated bacteria include *Pseudomonas aeruginosa*, *S. aureus*, proteus species, *Klebsiella pneumoniae*, and diphtheroids. Visualization of the TM, meticulous cleaning with culture of the drainage, and appropriate antimicrobial therapy, usually topical, are the keys to management.

Labyrinthitis

Suppurative infections of the middle ear can spread into the membranous labyrinth of the inner ear. Symptoms include vertigo, hearing loss, and fevers. The child often appears extremely toxic. Intravenous antibiotic therapy is used, and intravenous steroids may also be used to help decrease inflammation. Sequelae can be serious, including a condition known as labyrinthitis ossificans, or bony obliteration of the inner ear, including the cochlea, leading to profound hearing loss.

Acute Mastoiditis

The spread of infection into the mastoid bone results in acute mastoiditis. Differential diagnosis must include a severe case of otitis externa, as both processes may present with swelling and tenderness of the ear canal, periaural region, and mastoid process.

A CT scan will show clouding or coalescence of the air cells in acute mastoiditis and may be necessary to differentiate the two conditions. Untreated, this may progress to an abscess within the confines of the mastoid cells or spread externally, leading to the formation of subperiosteal or deep neck abscesses.

Acute mastoiditis should initially be treated with parenteral antibiotics directed against the aforementioned pathogens, adding coverage for gram-negative anaerobic organisms only if mastoiditis is superimposed upon a history of a chronically discharging ear, where colonization with such bacteria is common.

Surgery in the form of a cortical mastoidectomy is reserved for cases with poor response to parenteral antibiotic therapy, subperiosteal abscess, an intracranial complication or acute mastoiditis in a chronic ear.

TREATMENT OF ACUTE OTITIS MEDIA

First-line therapy
- Amoxicillin 90 mg/kg/day, up to 2 g daily; for children over 2 years or age, give for 5 days; under 2 years of age, for 10 days
- If amoxicillin has caused a rash, give cefuroxime (Ceftin) or cefdinir (Omnicef)
- If urticaria or other immunoglobulin E (IgE)-mediated events have occurred, give trimethoprim-sulfa or azithromycin (Zithromax)
- If the child is unable to take oral medication, give single intramuscular dose of ceftriaxone (Rocephin)

Second-line therapy
This is for clinical failure after 48–72 hours of treatment, or for recurrences within 4 weeks.
- Amoxicillin–clavulanate (Augmentin ES-600), given so that the patient receives amoxicillin at 90 mg/kg/day
- If amoxicillin has caused allergic symptoms, see recommendations above

Third-line therapy
- Tympanocentesis is recommended to determine the cause
- Ceftriaxone (Rocephin), two doses given intramuscularly, 48 hours apart, with the option of a third dose

Recurrences >4 weeks after the first episode
- A new pathogen is likely, so restart first-line therapy
- Be sure the diagnosis is not otitis media with effusion (OME), which may be observed for 3–6 months without treatment

The Observation Option

The choice to observe an episode of AOM and not treat with antibiotics is an option in otherwise healthy children without other underlying conditions such as cleft palate, craniofacial abnormalities, immune deficiencies, cochlear implants, or tympanostomy tubes. The decision should be made to provide antibiotic therapy if there is worsening of symptoms or lack of improvement within 48–72 hours. For infants younger than 6 months, antibiotics are always recommended on the first visit, regardless of diagnostic certainty. The clinical practice guidelines include age, presence of otorrhea, severity of symptoms, and laterality as criteria for antibiotic treatment versus observation.

Pain may be a major symptom of AOM due to pressure within the middle ear and can be substantial in the first few days of onset of illness. Antibiotic treatment does not relieve pain within the first 24 hours. Analgesics can relieve pain associated with AOM early in the course. Therefore, the child should be assessed for pain, and if pain is present, treatment for pain should be given.

Oral analgesics such as acetaminophen or ibuprofen are the mainstay of AOM pain management; they are effective for mild to moderately severe pain. Narcotic analgesics with codeine or analogs may be prescribed for severe pain; risks and benefits of using these drugs, including potential toxic effects, need to be considered. Topical agents such as benzocaine or lidocaine may offer additional brief benefit over acetaminophen in children older than 5 years.

Duration of antibiotic treatment should be 10 days for children under age 2 years, while a 7-day course should be adequate for AOM in children of age-group 2–5 years. For children of age 6 years or older with nonsevere symptoms, a 5- to 7-day course is adequate.

As it may take 1–3 days before antibiotic therapy leads to a reduction in pain, mild-to-moderate pain should be treated with ibuprofen or acetaminophen. Severe pain should be treated with narcotics, but careful and close observation is required to address possible respiratory depression, altered mental status, gastrointestinal upset, and

TABLE 1: Recommendation for initial management of uncomplicated acute otitis media (AOM).

Age	Otorrhea with AOM	Unilateral or bilateral AOM with severe symptoms	Bilateral AOM without otorrhea	Unilateral AOM without otorrhea
6 months to 2 years	Antibiotic therapy	Antibiotic therapy	Antibiotic therapy	Antibiotic therapy or additional observation
≥2 years	Antibiotic therapy	Antibiotic therapy	Antibiotic therapy or additional observation	Antibiotic therapy or additional observation

constipation. Topical analgesics have a very short duration and studies do not support efficacy in children younger than 5 years **(Table 1)**.

Antibiotic Therapy

The guideline on AOM management suggests the use of four factors in deciding whether to choose initial observation or prescribing antibiotics: Age, severity of symptoms, presence of otorrhea, and laterality of AOM. All infants and children with severe AOM, as defined by a toxic-appearing child, persistent otalgia for >48 hours, or temperature 39°C (102.2°F), should receive antibiotic therapy. AOM with otorrhea, presumably with rupture of the TM, also should receive antibiotic therapy. For those with nonsevere symptoms, initial observation is an option for children younger than 2 years of age with unilateral AOM. Children at least 2 years old with unilateral or bilateral AOM may also be observed initially. Initial observation without antibiotic prescription must be a shared decision with the child's family. If observation is offered, a mechanism must be in place to ensure follow-up and initiation of antibiotics if the child worsens or fails to improve within 72 hours of AOM onset.

High-dose amoxicillin is recommended as the first-line treatment because of its effectiveness against *S. pneumoniae* and *H. influenzae*, as well as its safety, low cost, acceptable taste, and narrow microbiologic spectrum. In children who have taken amoxicillin in the previous 30 days, those with concurrent conjunctivitis, or those for whom coverage for beta-lactamase-positive *H. influenzae* and *M. catarrhalis* is desired, therapy should be initiated with high dose of amoxicillin–clavulanate. Treatment with an effective antibiotic results in significant resolution of acute signs and symptoms within 48–72 hours. Persistent ear pain or systemic signs, including fever after 72 hours of antibiotic therapy, indicate a need for reevaluation for persistent AOM or foci elsewhere. If otologic findings support the diagnosis of persistent AOM, antibiotic treatment should be changed, depending on the initial drug.

Amoxicillin–clavulanate enhanced strength with 90 mg/kg/day of amoxicillin dosing (14:1 ratio of amoxicillin:clavulanate) is an appropriate choice when a child has had amoxicillin in the last 30 days, or is clinically failing after 48–72 hours on amoxicillin.

Alternative initial antibiotics including cefuroxime and third-generation cephalosporins are less efficacious than the first-line drugs. For penicillin-allergic children, cefdinir, cefuroxime, cefpodoxime, or ceftriaxone may be used as they are unlikely to be associated with cross-reactivity with penicillin; the exceptions are children with severe and/or recent penicillin allergy.

Three oral cephalosporins (cefuroxime, cefpodoxime, and cefdinir) are more beta-lactamase-stable and are alternative choices in children who develop a popular rash with amoxicillin. Unfortunately, coverage of highly penicillin-resistant pneumococci with these agents is poor and only the intermediate-resistance classes are covered. Of these drugs, cefdinir suspension is most palatable; the other two have a bitter aftertaste which is difficult to conceal. Flavoring agents may be helpful here.

A second-line antibiotic is indicated when a child experiences symptomatic infection within 1 month of finishing amoxicillin; however, repeated use of high-dose amoxicillin is indicated if >4 weeks have passed without symptoms. Macrolides such as azithromycin and clarithromycin are not recommended as second-line agents, because *S. pneumoniae* is resistant to macrolides in approximately 30% of respiratory isolates, and because virtually all strains of *H. influenzae* have an intrinsic macrolide efflux pump, which pumps the antibiotic out of the bacterial cell.

Reasons for failure to eradicate a sensitive pathogen include drug noncompliance, poor drug absorption, or vomiting of the drug. If a child remains symptomatic for longer than 3 days while taking a second-line agent, a tympanocentesis is useful to identify the causative pathogen. If a highly resistant pneumococcus is found or if tympanocentesis is not feasible, intramuscular ceftriaxone at 50 mg/kg/dose for 3 consecutive days is recommended. If a child has experienced a severe reaction, such as anaphylaxis, to amoxicillin, cephalosporins should not be substituted. Otherwise, the risk of cross-sensitivity is <0.1%.

Management of Otitis Media with Effusion

An audiology evaluation should be performed after approximately 3 months of continuous bilateral effusion in children younger than 3 years.

Children with hearing loss or speech delay should be referred to an otolaryngologist for possible tympanostomy tube placement. Antibiotics, antihistamines, and steroids have not been shown to be useful in the treatment of OME.

Traditionally, OME was observed for 3 months in uncomplicated cases prior to consideration for tympanostomy tube placement; longer periods of observation may be acceptable in children with normal or very mild hearing loss on audiogram, with no risk factors for speech and language issues, and no structural changes to the TM. Absolute indications for tympanostomy tubes include hearing loss >40 dB, TM retraction pockets, ossicular erosion, adhesive atelectasis, and cholesteatoma.

Penicillin resistance develops through stepwise mutations in the structure of the penicillin-binding proteins. Strains for which minimum inhibitory concentrations (MICs) of penicillin range between 0.12 and 1.0/mL are said to exhibit "intermediate" resistance. Strains for which MICs are equal to or higher than 2 mL are said to have a "high-level resistance." These strains are also resistant to other drug classes.

In patients with tympanostomy tubes with uncomplicated acute otorrhea, ototopical antibiotics (fluoroquinolone eardrops) are first-line therapy. The eardrops serve two purposes: (1) They treat the infection and (2) they physically "rinse" drainage from the tube which helps prevent plugging of the tube.

Recurrent Otitis Media

Recurrent AOM is defined as the occurrence of 2–3 separate, well-documented AOM episodes in a 6-month period, or 2–4 episodes in a 12-month period with at least 1 episode in the preceding 6 months. Antibiotic prophylaxis has been used to prevent recurrent AOM. Studies have shown that an estimated 5 children would have to be given 1 year of antibiotic prophylaxis in order to prevent 1 AOM episode. The modest benefit afforded by a prolonged course of antibiotic prophylaxis does not have longer-lasting benefit after cessation of therapy. Because of the modest benefit and the potential adverse effects associated with prolonged antibiotic use and emergence of resistance, the AAP guideline does not recommend antibiotic prophylaxis.

The use of tympanostomy tubes is recommended for recurrent AOM. Tympanostomy tubes prevent approximately 1.5 episodes of AOM in the 6 months after surgery. The disadvantages of tube placement include the cost, surgical, and anesthetic risk, and long-term sequelae such as tympanosclerosis and chronic perforation.

Tympanocentesis

If a child remains symptomatic longer than 3 days while taking a second-line agent, a tympanocentesis may be needed to identify the causative pathogen. If a highly resistant pneumococcus is found or if tympanocentesis is not feasible, intramuscular ceftriaxone in 2–3 daily doses appears to be the best third-line agent. Further studies are needed in children failing second-line therapy.

Tympanocentesis is performed by placing a needle-through the TM and aspirating the middle-ear fluid.

The fluid is sent for culture and sensitivity. Indications for tympanocentesis are: (1) AOM in an immunocompromised patient, (2) research studies, (3) evaluation for presumed sepsis or meningitis, such as in a neonate, (4) unresponsive otitis media despite courses of two appropriate antibiotics, and (5) acute mastoiditis or other suppurative complications.

Surgery

Surgical treatment, including tympanocentesis or myringotomy, results in immediate relief by draining the abscess and should be considered for the child who is toxic, who fails to improve on repeated antibiotic therapy, who has severe suppurative or nonsuppurative complications (e.g., mastoiditis or facial nerve palsy), or who has an underlying immunodeficiency. The middle-ear fluid should be cultured for bacteriologic diagnosis and susceptibility testing. Presence of multidrug-resistant (MDR) bacteria in the MEE may necessitate the use of antibiotics, such as levofloxacin or linezolid. Levofloxacin is a quinolone antibiotic that is not approved by the FDA for use in children. Linezolid is a relatively recent and expensive antibiotic that is effective against resistant gram-positive bacteria. Consultation with a pediatric infectious disease expert may help with selection of unconventional drugs.

Immunologic Evaluation and Allergy Testing

While immunoglobulin subclass deficiencies may be more common in children with recurrent AOM, there is no practical immune therapy available. More serious immunodeficiencies, such as selective IgA deficiency, should be considered in children who suffer from a combination of recurrent AOM, rhinosinusitis, and pneumonia. In the school-aged child or preschooler with an atopic background, skin testing may be beneficial in identifying allergens that can predispose to AOM.

Vaccines

The pneumococcal conjugate and influenza vaccines are recommended. The seven-valent pneumococcal conjugate vaccine (PCV7) and 13-valent pneumococcal conjugate vaccine (PCV13) are introduced. PCV7 was found to produce a 29% reduction in AOM resulting from the seven serotypes found in the vaccine, and overall, PCV7 reduced AOM by 6–7%. In recent studies, intranasal influenza vaccine reduced the number of influenza-associated cases of AOM by 30–55%.

FOLLOW-UP VISITS

The optimal timing for follow-up visits depends on the response to therapy. Children should be reassessed when symptoms of AOM continue beyond 72 hours or recur during treatment. The follow-up visit for preschool children should be 3–4 weeks after start of therapy.

PROGNOSIS

Prognosis is variable based on age of presentation. Infants who are very young at the time of first otitis media are more likely to need surgical intervention. Other factors that decrease the likelihood of resolution are onset of OME in the summer or fall, history of prior tympanostomy tubes, presence of adenoids, and hearing loss >30 dB.

BIBLIOGRAPHY

1. Lieberthal AS, Carroll AE, Chonmaitree T, Ganiats TG, Hoberman A, Jackson MA, et al. Diagnosis and management of acute otitis media. Pediatrics. 2013;131:964-99.
2. Rosenfeld RM, Shin JJ, Schwartz SR, Coggins R, Gagnon L, Hackell JM, et al. Clinical Practice Guideline: Otitis Media with Effusion (Update). Otolaryngol Head Neck Surg. 2016;154:S1-S41.
3. Siddiq S, Grainger J. The diagnosis and management of acute otitis media: American Academy of Pediatrics Guidelines 2013. Arch Dis Child Educ Pract Ed. 2015;100:193-7.
4. Stockmann C, Ampofo K, Hersh AL, Carleton ST, Korgenski K, Sheng X, et al. Role of respiratory viral activity in and acute otits media. Pediatr Infect Dis J. 2013;32:314-9.
5. Thomas NM, Brook I. Otitis media: an update on current pharmacotherapy and future perspectives. Expert Opin Pharmacother. 2014;15(8):1069-83.
6. Wald ER. Acute otitis media and acute bacterial sinusitis. Clin Infect Dis. 2011;52 Suppl 4(Suppl 4):S277-83.

CASE 11

Pneumonia

■ PRESENTING COMPLAINTS

A 6-month-old boy was brought with the complaint of:
- Cough since 3 days
- Fever since 3 days
- Noisy respiration since 2 days
- Not taking feeds since 1 day
- Breathlessness complaints since 1 day

History of the Presenting Symptom

A 6-month-old boy was brought to the pediatric emergency ward with a history of breathlessness and not taking feeds. The baby was accompanied by his mother. There was a history of fever and cough since 3 days. Fever used to be moderate to a high degree. It used to get relieved by paracetamol. Cough was associated with noisy respiration and nasal block. Cough was distressed and it was disturbing the sleep as well as intake of food. Mother has noticed mild subcostal recession and intercostals indrawing.

Past History of the Patient

The child was born at full term by normal delivery. Child cried immediately after the delivery. The birth weight was 3 kg. There was no significant postnatal event except for normal physiological jaundice. Breastfeeding was given immediately. Weaning of the food started by 4 months. At present, he is getting breast milk and cereals. He was completely immunized.

He was the second sibling of the nonconsanguineous marriage. The elder sibling is doing well with the health.

■ EXAMINATION

On examination, the child was well-built and nourished. He was crying, irritable, and

CASE AT A GLANCE

Basic Findings
Length	:	66 cm (75th centile)
Weight	:	6.3 kg (50th centile)
Temperature	:	39°C
Pulse rate	:	136 beats/min
Respiratory rate	:	56 breaths/min
Blood pressure	:	60–50 mm Hg

Positive Findings

History:
- Cold
- Cough
- Breathlessness
- Fever
- Vomiting

Examination:
- Irritable
- Dyspneic
- Crepitation
- Hepatomegaly

Investigation:
- Increased white blood cell (WBC) count
- Chest X-ray—patchy pneumonitis

dyspneic. The anthropometric measurements included the length 66 cm (75th centile), the weight was 6.3 kg (50th centile), and the head circumference was 40 cm.

The child was febrile. The pulse was 136 beats/min and respiratory rate was 56 breaths/min. The blood pressure recorded was 60–50 mm Hg. Mild subcostal recession and intercostal indrawing were present.

There was no pallor, lymphadenopathy, cyanosis, and edema. Respiratory system revealed the presence of fine crepitations at the base of the lungs. Signs of rhinitis and nasal block were present. Per abdomen examination revealed the presence of mild distension and mild nontender hepatomegaly. Cardiovascular system was normal except for tachycardia.

■ INVESTIGATION

- *Hemoglobin:* 13 g/dL
- *TLC:* 14,500 cells/mm^3
- *DLC:* $P_{68}L_{25}E_5B_2$
- *ESR:* 26 mm in the first hour
- *X-ray chest:* Increased vascular marking with bilateral patchy pneumonitis.

■ DISCUSSION

Child was having fever, cough, cold, and breathlessness. On examination, there was fever, tachycardia, and tachypnea. Respiratory system revealed the presence of crepitation at the basal of lungs. Per abdomen showed the presence of hepatomegaly. Investigation reports showed the presence of the increased WBC count suggesting pneumonia. Pneumonia is defined as inflammation of lung tissue that may result from a noninfectious or an infectious cause.

Bronchopneumonia is primarily a spreading inflammation of the terminal bronchioles and their related alveoli.

Lobar pneumonia or consolidation is a pathological state where the alveolar air has been replaced by cellular exudate and transudate.

Pneumonitis is localized inflammation of lung parenchyma due to noninfectious causes.

Interstitial pneumonia is characterized by massive proliferation and desquamation of alveolar cells and thickening of alveolar walls. Chest X-ray reveals a diffuse hazy, ground glass appearance, usually at lung bases with poorly defined hilar densities.

Persistent pneumonia is defined as the persistence of symptoms and roentgenographic abnormalities for more than 1 month.

Recurrent pneumonia is defined as two episodes of pneumonia in one year or more than three episodes at any time with radiographic clearance between two episodes of illness.

Pneumonia can be classified anatomically as lobar or lobular pneumonia, bronchopneumonia, and interstitial pneumonia. Pathologically, there is consolidation of the alveoli or infiltration of tissue with inflammatory cells.

The cause of pneumonia depends on age, immune status, and the presence of underlying chronic disease. Certain infectious agents are more common at a particular age. The causative agents of pneumonia in children according to age are given in **Table 1**.

Atypical pneumonia is caused by *Mycoplasma pneumonia* and *Chlamydia*. Atypical pneumonia is also called walking pneumonia.

Factors predisposing to bacterial pneumonia include increased number of siblings, parental smoking, preterm delivery, urban residence, poor socioeconomic status, impaired immune response, congenital and anatomic defects, lungs and tracheobronchial tree defects, CF, and congestive heart failure.

TABLE 1: Pneumonia—pathogens in various age groups.

Age	Bacteria	Viruses	Others
Neonate	• Group B Streptococci • E. coli, Klebsiella sp. Listeria monocytogenes, and S. aureus	CMV, Herpes	Chlamydia
1–3 months	• S. pneumoniae • S. aureus • H. influenzae	CMV, RSV, influenza, and parainfluenza	Chlamydia
4 months–5 years	• S. pneumoniae • S. aureus • H. influenzae • Group A Streptococcus • Klebsiella • Pseudomonas sp./M. tuberculosis	• RSV • Adenovirus • Influenza	Mycoplasma
Over 5 years	• S. pneumoniae • S. aureus • H. influenzae • M. tuberculosis	• Influenza • Varicella	• Mycoplasma • Legionella sp. • M. catarrhalis

(CMV: Cytomegalovirus; H. influenzae: Haemophilus influenzae; M. catarrhalis: Moraxella catarrhalis; M. tuberculosis: Mycobacterium tuberculosis; RSV: respiratory syncytial virus; S. aureus: Staphylococcus aureus; S. pneumoniae: Streptococcus pneumoniae)

ESSENTIAL DIAGNOSTIC POINTS

- Fever, cough, and dyspnea
- Rales or decreased breath sounds
- Wheezing
- Myalgia and malaise
- *Abnormal chest X-ray:* Infiltrates, hilar adenopathy, and pleural effusion

■ PATHOPHYSIOLOGY

Viral pneumonia usually results from the spread of infection along the airways, accompanied by direct injury of the respiratory epithelium, which results in airway obstruction from swelling, abnormal secretions, and cellular debris. The small caliber of airways in young infants makes such patients particularly susceptible to severe infection. Atelectasis, interstitial edema, and hypoxemia from ventilation–perfusion (V/Q) mismatch often accompany airway obstruction. Viral infection of the respiratory tract can also predispose to secondary bacterial infection by disturbing normal host defense mechanisms, altering secretions, and through disruptions in the respiratory microbiota.

Bacterial pneumonia most often occurs when respiratory tract organisms colonize the trachea and subsequently gain access to the lungs, but pneumonia may also result from direct seeding of lung tissue after bacteremia. When bacterial infection is established in the lung parenchyma, the pathologic process varies according to the invading organism. *M. pneumonia* attaches to the respiratory epithelium, inhibits ciliary action, and leads to cellular destruction and an inflammatory response in the submucosa. As the infection progresses, sloughed cellular debris, inflammatory cells, and mucus cause airway obstruction, with spread of infection occurring along the bronchial tree, as is seen in viral pneumonia. *Streptococcus pneumoniae* produces local edema that aids in the proliferation of organisms and their spread into adjacent portions of the lung, often resulting in the characteristic focal lobar involvement. Group A streptococcus LRTI typically results in more diffuse lung involvement with interstitial pneumonia.

The pathology includes necrosis of tracheobronchial mucosa; formation of large amounts of exudate, edema, and local hemorrhage, with extension into the interalveolar septa and involvement of lymphatic vessels with frequent pleural involvement. *Staphylococcus aureus* pneumonia manifests as confluent bronchopneumonia, which is often unilateral and characterized by the presence of extensive areas of hemorrhagic necrosis and irregular areas of cavitation of the lung parenchyma, resulting in pneumatoceles, empyema, and, at times, bronchopulmonary fistulas. Recurrent pneumonia is defined as two or more episodes in a single year or three or more episodes ever, with radiographic clearing between occurrences. An underlying disorder should be considered if a child experiences recurrent pneumonia.

Pathogens reach lungs either by hematogenous dissemination or by aspiration. Viruses are often responsible for secondary bacterial infection. Following the invasion of pulmonary tissue, an acute inflammatory response causes exudation of fluid and polymorphonuclear cells with eventual fibrin deposition and consolidation.

Consolidation of lung tissue decreases the vital capacity (VC) and compliance of lungs. Intrapulmonary right to left shunt and V/Q mismatching can cause hypoxia; even pulmonary hypertension may occur, which with added hypercapnia, can result in cardiac overload

■ CLINICAL FEATURES (FIG. 1)

Typical features of bacterial, viral, and mycoplasmal pneumonia in children are given in **Table 2**.

Cough is a common symptom. It may be absent in infants and newborn. Mere observation will provide key diagnosis. Tachypnea out of proportion to the degree of

TABLE 2: Typical features of bacterial, viral, and mycoplasmal pneumonia in children.

Items	Bacterial	Viral	Mycoplasma
Age	Any	Any	5–15 years
Season	Winter	Winter	All years
Onset	Abrupt	Variable	Insidious
Fever	High	Variable	Low grade
Tachypnea	Common	Common	Uncommon
Associated symptoms	• Mild coryza • Abdominal pain	Coryza	• Bullous myringitis • Pharyngitis
Physical findings	Evidence of consolidation	Variable	• Fine crackles • Wheezing
Leukocytosis	Common	Variable	Uncommon
Radiographic findings	Consolidation	Bilateral diffuse infiltrates	Variable
Pleural effusion	Common	Rare (adenovirus)	Small (10–20%)

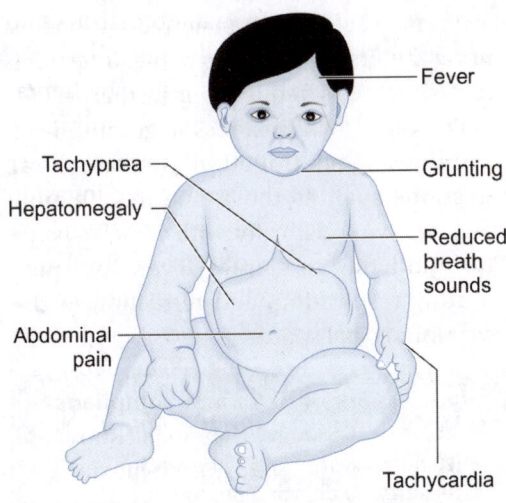

Fig. 1: Clinical features.

fever may be the only sign in infant. Grunting respiration in young children arouses a suspicion of pneumonia.

Tachypnea is the most sensitive index of disease severity. The diagnosis of pneumonia is defined as respiratory rate >60 breaths/min in children below 2 months of age, >50 breaths/min in children between 2 and 12 months of age, and >40 breaths/min in children 1–5 years of age.

Some infants with bacterial pneumonia may have associated gastrointestinal disturbances characterized by vomiting, anorexia, diarrhea, and abdominal distention secondary to a paralytic ileus. Rapid progression of symptoms is characteristic in the most severe cases of bacterial pneumonia.

GENERAL FEATURES
• Cough • Vomiting • Dehydration • Extrapulmonary infection • Congestive cardiac failure

Pneumonia may present with acute abdominal pain which is attributed to referred pain from the pleura. Apical pneumonia may be associated with meningismus and convulsions.

Localized findings include inspiratory rales, reduced breath sounds, and dullness to percussion. There may be associated abdominal pain and features of meningism depending on the localization of involved lung field.

Staphylococcus and *Klebsiella*, i.e., gram-negative organism produce pneumatocele. Pseudomonas may produce diffuse nodular pattern in lower lobes. Anaerobic infections are also associated with lung abscesses along with air/fluid levels.

Neonatal pneumonia is often difficult to recognize because of some peculiarities. These include absence of cough, fever, apneic spells, increased incidence of periodic breathing, grunting, rapid clinical deterioration, cyanosis, progressive air hunger, and septicemic features.

Pneumococcal Pneumonia

Respiratory infections due to *S pneumoniae* are transmitted by droplets and are more common in the winter months. Bacteria multiply in the alveoli and inflammatory exudate is formed. Scattered areas of consolidation occur, which coalesce around the bronchi and later become lobular or lobar in distribution. There is no tissue necrosis.

Incubation period is 1–3 days. The onset is abrupt with headache, chills, cough, and high fever. Child may develop pleuritic chest pain. In severe cases there may be grunting, chest indrawing, difficulty in feeding, and cyanosis. Bronchial breathing may be heard over areas of consolidation. Bronchophony and whispering pectoriloquy may be observed. Meningismus may be present in optical pneumonia.

X-ray findings include lobar consolidation and leukocytosis. Sputum is examined by

Gram staining and culture. Blood culture may be positive in 5–10% of cases. Demonstration of polysaccharide antigen in urine is done.

Staphylococcal Pneumonia

Staphylococcal pneumonia occurs in infancy and childhood. The pulmonary lesion may be primary infection of the parenchyma; or maybe secondary to generalized staphylococcal septicemia. It may be a complication of measles or influenza; other risk factors include CF, malnutrition, and diabetes.

The illness is characterized by the formation of multiple pneumatoceles. The pneumatoceles fluctuate in size and finally resolve and disappear within a period of a few weeks to months. Staphylococcal abscesses may erode into the pericardium causing purulent pericarditis. Empyema in a child below 2 years of age is nearly always secondary to staphylococcal infections.

The illness usually follows URTI, pyoderma, or a purulent disease

Progression of the symptoms and signs is rapid. Pulmonary infection may occasionally be complicated by disseminated disease, with metastatic abscesses in joints, bones, muscles, pericardium, liver, mastoid, or brain.

The characteristic complications of pyopneumothorax and pericarditis are highly suggestive. Pneumatoceles are present in X-ray films characteristically in pneumonia due to Staphylococci or *Klebsiella*. Staphylococci can be cultured from the blood.

Haemophilus Pneumonia

Haemophilus influenzae infections occur usually between the age of 3 months and 3 years and are nearly always associated with bacteremia. Infection usually begins in the nasopharynx and spreads locally or through the bloodstream. As the infants have transplacentally transferred antibodies during the first 3–4 months of life, infections are relatively less frequent during this period.

The onset of the illness is gradual with nasopharyngeal infection. Certain viral infections such as those due to influenza virus act synergistically with *H influenzae*. The child has moderate fever, dyspnea, grunting respiration, and retraction of the lower intercostal spaces.

> **THE WORLD HEALTH ORGANIZATION (WHO) GRADING OF PNEUMONIA**
>
> - *Pneumonia:* Fever <38.5°C, no feeding difficulties, no dehydration, cough, and tachypnea
> - *Severe pneumonia:* High-grade fever >39°C, difficulty in feeding, tachypnea, respiratory distress with intercostals retraction (ICR) or subtotal retraction (SCR), dehydration, grunt, bronchial breath sounds on auscultation with or without crackles, peripheral capillary oxygen saturation (SpO_2) ≥92 at room air, and radiological opacity on chest X-ray
> - *Very severe pneumonia:* Inability to feed, altered sensorium, intermittent apneic spells, cyanosis, excessive diaphoresis, narrow pulse pressure, academia, and SpO_2 <92 at room air.

■ DIAGNOSIS

Acute phase reactants, like complete blood count (CBC), CRP, ESR, have poor sensitivity and specificity. They neither distinguish between viral and bacterial etiology, nor help in making a decision of antibiotic choice; however, they may be useful tools for monitoring the course of the disease.

Complete blood count helps for the evidence of septicemia. WBC count >15,000 cells/mm^3, polymorphonuclear leukocytosis or count <5,000/mm^3, or febrile neutropenia are bad prognostic signs. Nasopharyngeal aspirate is investigated for viral antigens, for example, Cytomegalovirus (CMV) and adenovirus.

Radiology is not routinely required in nonsevere pneumonia to confirm the diagnosis. At times, it may correlate with the clinical signs; there is also wide variation in the interpretation by radiologists. Moreover, reliability in predicting the etiology is poor. However, Chest X-ray may be indicated in very severe disease, ambiguous picture, improvement/worsening after more than 48–72 hours of therapy, suspected complication, and known immunocompromise child. Microbiology-sputum culture or blood culture though may be more specific, but the yield is very poor (10–15%), there is also a risk of growing normal nasopharyngeal flora.

Blood culture should be obtained before initiating the antibiotic therapy. The most reliable method for the bacterial diagnosis is the culture of lung aspirate.

The definitive diagnosis of a viral infection rests on the detection of the viral genome or antigen in respiratory tract secretions. Reliable PCR assays are widely available for the rapid detection of many respiratory viruses, including RSV, parainfluenza, influenza, human metapneumovirus, adenovirus, enterovirus, and rhinovirus.

Serologic techniques can also be used to diagnose a recent respiratory viral infection but generally require testing of acute and convalescent serum samples for a rise in antibodies to a specific virus. This diagnostic technique is laborious, slow, and not generally clinically useful because the infection usually has resolved by the time it is confirmed serologically. Serologic testing may be valuable as an epidemiologic tool to define the incidence and prevalence of various respiratory viral pathogens.

Circulating antigens of streptococcal pneumonia and *H influenzae* may be detected in blood by counter immunoelectrophoresis (CIE), PCR, or latex agglutination.

Diagnostic thoracocentesis is done if there is significant pleural effusion. Gram staining and culture of pleural fluid are done. BAL should be considered in the management of severely ill children to make a prompt diagnosis.

Serology, urinary antigens, rapid antigen detection test (RADT), and cold agglutinins for mycoplasma are not easily available; they are expensive with time lagging and have poor sensitivity.

Invasive procedures, like bronchoscopy, BAL, and lung aspiration, have high sensitivity and specificity; however, they are too invasive to be advised in office practice. Pulse oximetry is a mandatory tool for monitoring the course of the disease in all hospitalized children.

> **LABORATORY SALIENT FINDINGS**
> - White blood cell (WBC) count more than 15,000 cells/mm^3, and polymorphonuclear leukocytosis
> - *Nasopharyngeal aspirate:* Viral antigens, for example, cytomegalovirus (CMV) and adenovirus
> - Blood culture
> - Counter immunoelectrophoresis (CIE), polymerase chain reaction (PCR), or latex agglutination
> - Gram staining and culture of pleural fluid

Diagnosis of pneumonia is essentially clinical and seldom requires lab support. The absence of past history of recurrent cough and presence of fever with fast breathing is a hallmark presentation in clinical diagnosis of pneumonia. It should always be remembered that there are no definite differentiating markers between viral, bacterial, and atypical pneumonia. However, there are certain clinical clues that can help to nail down an etiological diagnosis.

The definitive diagnosis of a typical bacterial infection requires isolation of an organism from the blood, pleural fluid, or lung. Culture of sputum is of little value in the diagnosis of pneumonia in young children, while percutaneous lung aspiration is invasive and not routinely performed. Blood culture is positive in only 10% of children with pneumococcal pneumonia and is not recommended for nontoxic-appearing children treated as outpatients. Blood cultures are recommended for children who fail to improve, or have clinical deterioration, have complicated pneumonia, or require hospitalization.

Urinary antigen tests should not be used to diagnose pneumonia caused by *S pneumoniae* in children because of a high rate of false positives resulting from nasopharyngeal carriage.

Pertussis infection can be diagnosed by PCR or culture of a nasopharyngeal specimen; although culture is considered the gold standard for pertussis diagnosis, it is less sensitive than the available PCR assays. Acute infection caused by *M pneumoniae* can be diagnosed on the basis of a PCR test result from a respiratory specimen or seroconversion in an IgG assay. Cold agglutinins at titers >1:64 are also found in the blood of roughly half of patients with *M pneumoniae* infections; however, cold agglutinins are nonspecific because other pathogens such as influenza viruses may also cause increase in cold agglutinin. Serologic evidence, such as anti-streptolysin O and anti-DNase B titers, may also be useful in the diagnosis of group A streptococcal pneumonia.

Clinical evidence of hyperinflation with scattered exudates on radiology is due to segmental atelectasis.

For optimum antimicrobial management of pneumonia, it is prudent to differentiate between bacterial, viral, and atypical pneumonia clinically, as it is often very difficult to isolate the offending pathogen.

Involvement of a particular lobe in the chest X-ray gives the clue to an etiological agent.
- Acute lobar pneumonia—pneumococcal pneumonia
- Right upper lobe pneumonia—aspiration pneumonia especially in neonate and infant
- Upper lobe pneumonia with cavitation-tuberculosis
- Multiple small abscess—staphylococcal/ *Klebsiella*

■ MANAGEMENT

It includes specific treatment and supportive treatment.

Specific Treatment

It includes specific antimicrobial agent. Antibiotics are selected on the basis of age of the child, epidemiology, clinical features, radiological features, and extrapulmonary manifestation.

Specific Antimicrobial Therapy in Pneumonia

- <3 months first line; cefotaxime/ceftriaxone ± aminoglycosides
- 3 months to 5 years first line; co-amoxiclav or ampicillin + chloramphenicol; second line; ceftriaxone/cefotaxime
- >5 years first line; ampicillin/penicillin G/co-amoxiclav/macrolide (if mycoplasma suspected) second line; ceftriaxone/cefotaxime and macrolide
- Suspected staphylococcal infection; cefuroxime or co-amoxiclav or IV 3rd generation cephalosporins + cloxacillin; second line; ceftriaxone/cefotaxime and vancomycin/teicoplanin/linezolid.

TABLE 3: Choice of antibiotics.

Age	First-line	Second-line
3 months–5 years	Amoxicillin	Co-amoxiclav/cefuroxime/chloramphenicol
>5 years	Amoxicillin	Macrolide/co-amoxiclav/cefuroxime

BOX 1: Indications for admission.

- Age <1 year (lobar infiltrate)
- Respiratory compromise
- Pleural effusion (always culture by thoracentesis)
- Pneumatocele
- Failure to respond to outpatient antibiotic treatment within 24–48 hours
- Dehydration

If there are indications of specific etiological agents like *Chlamydia* or *Mycoplasma*, then macrolide such as erythromycin or clarithromycin is used.

Most healthy children can be treated on outpatient setting. The most common organism responsible is *S pneumoniae*. This will respond very well to amoxicillin (500 mg/kg/day). If there is doubt on oral intake in the beginning, injectable ceftriaxone (50 mg/kg) may be given intramuscularly at the time of diagnosis and during the first 24 hours.

Alternatively, in penicillin-allergic patients, macrolide antibiotics including erythromycin (40 mg/kg in 4 divided doses) or azithromycin (10 mg/kg as a single dose) may be used.

Amoxicillin, ampicillin, amoxicillin-clavulanic acid, macrolides, and cefuroxime axetil are the orally used antibiotics **(Table 3)**.

Standard doses: 40–45 mg/kg/day in two or three divided doses;

Erythromycin: 30–40 mg/kg/day in three divided doses;

Clarithromycin: 15 mg/kg/day in two divided doses;

Azithromycin: 10 mg/kg/day in OD dose.

For the inpatients, parenteral antibiotics should be started intravenously. Indications for admission are listed in the **Box 1**. Parenteral antibiotics are continued until the patient is afebrile, has improved symptomatically, and is able to take medications by mouth. The parenteral medicine can be switched over to oral medication by that time. The total duration of treatment irrespective of route of administration is 10 days.

Patients with the pulmonary complications such a pleural effusion, empyema, abscess require 2–4 weeks of antibiotic treatment. Staphylococcal empyema requires 3–4 weeks of treatment. In these high doses, parenteral therapy is given until the complication is clear. Thereafter, oral route may be used to complete the course of treatment.

Drug Doses

- *Co-amoxiclav:* 30–40 mg/kg/day
- *Ceftriaxone:* 50–100 mg/kg/day
- *Cefotaxime:* 100–200 mg/kg/day
- *Cefuroxime:* 20–30 mg/kg/day
- *Aminoglycosides:* 15 mg/kg/day in single or two divided doses

Despite rational choice of antibiotics in right dose and for optimal duration, if there is failure in clinical improvement, one needs to check the diagnosis and rule out foreign body, aspiration pneumonia, and interstitial lung disease.

Underlying comorbidities should be looked for like lung abscess, emphysema, Bronchiectasis, left-to-right shunts, gastroesophageal reflux disease (GERD), asthma, CF, and ciliary dyskinesia.

Immunosuppression in the host like HIV and hypogammaglobulinemia should be evaluated.

The treatment of choice for pneumococcal pneumonia is penicillin (penicillin V 250 mg q 8–12 hour orally, penicillin G 0.5 MU/kg/day IV or procaine penicillin 0.6 MU IM daily for 7 days), amoxicillin (30–40 mg/kg/day for 7 days) with or without clavulanic acid is a useful alternative.

Treatment of staphylococcal pneumonia includes prompt antibiotic therapy, which should be initiated with co-amoxiclav, or a combination of cloxacillin and a third-generation cephalosporin, for example, ceftriaxone. If the patient does not show improvement in symptoms within 48 hour, therapy with vancomycin, teicoplanin, or linezolid may be necessary. Therapy should continue till all evidence of the disease disappears both clinically and radiologically, which usually takes 2 weeks in uncomplicated cases. Therapy is continued for 4–6 weeks in patients with empyema or pneumothorax. Following initial IV therapy, the remaining course may be completed with oral antibiotics.

Treatment of *Haemophilus* infection is done with ampicillin at a dose of 100 mg/kg/day or co-amoxiclav. Cefotaxime (100 mg/kg/day) or ceftriaxone (50–75 mg/kg/day) are recommended in seriously ill patients.

Supportive Treatment

Paracetamol (10–15 mg/kg/dose) every 4–6 hourly for the treatment of fever is recommended. In the presence of tachypnea, cyanosis, or chest indrawing, oxygen should be administered. IV fluid is given if the child is not tolerating the treatment orally. Oral fluids/food is encouraged as soon as tachypnea or chest retractions are under control.

Duration of Treatment

- *Pneumonia (outpatient):* 5–7 days
- *Pneumonia (inpatient):* 10–14 days
- *Atypical organism:* 10 days
- *Staphylococcus pneumonia:* 3–4 weeks

COMPLICATIONS

Complications include emphysema, pneumothorax, bronchogenic dissemination, septicemia, osteomyelitis, multiple system abscesses, septic arthritis, and meningitis.

Mortality in uncomplicated bacterial pneumonia is 1%. The most important complication is dehydration. Other complication include pleural effusion and empyema. Empyema may extend locally to involve pericardium, mediastinum, or chest wall.

Electrolytes and blood urea nitrogen (BUN) can help to assess the degree of fluid loss. Extensive involvement of lungs may lead to respiratory failure. ABGs are indicated if child has severe respiratory distress or oxygen saturation is less than 90%.

PROGNOSIS

A number of possibilities must be considered when a patient does not improve with appropriate antibiotic therapy:
- Complications such as pleural effusion or empyema
- Bacterial resistance
- Nonbacterial etiologies such as viruses or fungi and aspiration of foreign bodies or food
- Bronchial obstruction from endobronchial lesions, foreign body, or mucus plugs
- Pre-existing diseases such as immuno-deficiencies, biliary dyskinesia, CF,

pulmonary sequestration, or congenital pulmonary airway malformation
- Other noninfectious causes (including bronchiolitis obliterans, hypersensitivity pneumonitis, eosinophilic pneumonia, and granulomatosis with polyangiitis, formerly called Wegener granulomatosis)

The mortality is high in younger ages. Poor nutritional state like protein–energy malnutrition (PEM) grade III and IV, extensive bilateral bronchopneumonia, associated diseases, condition like CF, immunodeficiency state, malignancy, and associated complications like respiratory failure and congestive cardiac failure act as a poor prognostic factor.

The prognosis is usually excellent even in severe bacterial pneumonia complicated by empyema. Long-term follow-up of children with empyema has shown remarkably few, if any, residual lung function abnormalities. In contrast to adults with empyema, children seldom require surgical procedures such as decortication. Radiographic follow-up studies to document complete resolution are probably not indicated until at least 6–8 weeks have elapsed following initiation of antibiotic therapy.

BIBLIOGRAPHY

1. Das A, Patgiri SJ, Saikia L, Dowerah P, Nath R. Bacterial pathogens associated with community-acquired pneumonia in children aged below five years. Indian Pediatr. 2016;53:225-7.
2. Esposito S, Cohen R, Domingo JD, Pecurariu OF, Greenberg D, Heininger U, et al. Antibiotic therapy for pediatric community-acquired pneumonia: Do we know when, what and for how long to treat? Pediatr Infect Dis J. 2012;31(6):e78-85.
3. Iroh Tam PY. Approach to common bacterial infections: Community-acquired pneumonia. Pediatr Clin North Am. 2013; 60(2):437-53.
4. Jain S Finelli, Self WH, Wunderink RG, Fakhran S, Balk R, Bramley AM, et al. Community acquired pneumonia requiring hospitalization among U.S. Children. N Engl J Med. 2015;372(9):835-45.
5. Lodha R Kabra SK, Pandey RM. Antibiotics for community-acquired pneumonia in children. Cochrane Database Syst Rev. 2010;6:CD004874.
6. World Health Organization. (2014). Revised WHO classification and treatment of childhood pneumonia at health facilities. [online] Available from http:/apps.who.int/10665/137319-eng.pdf. [Last accessed May, 2024].

12 CASE

Tuberculosis

■ PRESENTING COMPLAINTS
A 7-year-old boy was brought with the complaint of:
- Cough since 20 days
- Fever since 20 days
- Loss of appetite since 15 days
- Loss of weight since 10 days

History of Presenting Complaints
A 7-year-old boy with a history of cough for 20 days was brought to the pediatric OPD. Cough was productive type. It used to be more in early morning. He used to bring out the white-colored mucopurulent copious sputum. Many a time the child used to have disturbed sleep because of cough. There was also a history of fever. Fever was of moderate degree, used to be more in the evening. It was not associated with chills and rigors. The boy was shown to a general practitioner and the treatment given did not relieve the fever. His appetite was decreased and mother also complained that there was a loss of weight.

Past History of the Patient
The patient was the second child of nonconsanguineous marriage. He was born at term by normal delivery. He was delivered vaginally. He cried immediately after the birth. The birth weight of the child was 2.75 kg. He was on breast milk exclusively for 4 months of age. Weaning started by the 4th month and was completed by the 13th month. He had been vaccinated completely.

There was a history of chronic cough in the father who was diagnosed to have suffered from pulmonary tuberculosis (TB) and was taking treatment.

CASE AT A GLANCE

Basic Findings
Height	: 120 cm (50th centile)
Weight	: 21 kg (50th centile)
Temperature	: 38°C
Pulse rate	: 100 beats/min
Respiratory rate	: 20 breaths/min
Blood pressure	: 80/70 mm Hg

Positive Findings

History:
- Chronic cough
- Chronic fever
- History of contact
- Decreased appetite
- Loss of weight

Examination:
- Febrile
- Pale
- Crepitations

Investigation:
- *Hemoglobin:* 9.8 g/dL
- *ESR:* 80 mm in the first hour
- *X-ray chest:* Miliary mottling
- *Mantoux test:* Positive

EXAMINATION

On examination, he was moderately built and poorly nourished. Anthropometric measurements included that his height was 120 cm (50th centile) and the weight was 21 kg (50th centile).

He was febrile, pulse rate was 100 beats/min and respiratory rate was 20 breaths/min. The blood pressure recorded was 80/70 mm Hg. There was pallor, no cyanosis, and clubbing. There was no significant lymphadenopathy.

The respiratory system revealed the presence of the occasional crepitations at the base of the lungs. Other systemic examinations were normal.

INVESTIGATION

- *Hemoglobin:* 9.8 g/dL
- *TLC:* 86,000 cells/mm^3
- *DLC:* $P_{56}L_{40}E_8M_2$
- *ESR:* 80 mm in the first hour
- X-ray chest: Suggestive of miliary mottling
- *Mantoux test:* Positive, i.e., induration >15 milliliter

DISCUSSION

Cough and fever were present for 20 days. Fever was not relieved completely by a course of antibiotics. The child had a loss of appetite and there was a history of contact with TB. Investigation report suggests the diagnosis of the primary complex. ESR was raised and Mantoux test was positive. These put the collective diagnosis of TB.

Tuberculosis is a chronic infectious disease caused by *Mycobacterium tuberculosis*. Clinical features of the disease depend on the site of the lesion, severity of infection, and host resistance. The spread of the infection to the child is by adult active TB patient. The usual mode of transmission is by inhalation of droplets of infected secretion. Measles, whooping cough, and malnutrition will flare up the TB. But childhood TB is not contagious because of low bacterial load, and no cavitating disease.

The frequency of childhood TB depends upon
- Number of infectious cases
- Closeness of contact with infectious cases
- Age of the child when exposed to TB

There are many forms of childhood TB, but common and important clinical forms are pulmonary TB, meningeal TB, miliary TB, and lymph node TB. Occasionally, mid-to-late adolescents are seen with cavities due to TB and they may be infectious.

PATHOGENESIS

Airborne transmission of *Mycobacterium bovis* and *Mycobacterium africanum* also occurs. *M. bovis* can penetrate the gastrointestinal (GI) mucosa or invade the lymphatic tissue of the oropharynx when large numbers of organisms are ingested.

Immunity

Conditions that adversely affect cell-mediated immunity predispose to progression from tuberculosis infection (TBI) to disease. Rare specific genetic defects associated with deficient cell-mediated immunity in response to mycobacteria include interleukin-12 (IL-12) receptor B1 deficiency and complete and partial interferon gamma (IFN)-γ receptor 1 chain deficiencies.

Tuberculosis infection is associated with a humoral antibody response, which plays little-known role in host defense. Shortly after infection, tubercle bacilli replicate in both free alveolar spaces and inactivated alveolar macrophages. Sulfatides in the mycobacterial cell wall inhibit fusion of the macrophage phagosomes and lysosomes, allowing the organisms to escape destruction by intracellular enzymes.

Cell-mediated immunity develops 2-12 weeks after infection, along with tissue hypersensitivity. After bacilli enter macrophages, lymphocytes that recognize mycobacterial antigens proliferate and secrete lymphokines and other mediators that attract other lymphocytes and macrophages to the area. Certain lymphokines activate macrophages, causing them to develop high concentrations of lytic enzymes that enhance their mycobactericidal capacity. A discrete subset of regulator, helper, and suppressor lymphocytes modulates the immune response. Development of specific cellular immunity prevents the progression of the initial infection in most persons.

The pathologic events in the initial TBI seem to depend on the balance among the mycobacterial antigen load; cell-mediated immunity, which enhances intracellular killing; and tissue hypersensitivity, which promotes extracellular killing. When the antigen load is small and the degree of tissue sensitivity is high, granuloma formation results from the organization of lymphocytes, macrophages, and fibroblasts. When both antigen load and degree of sensitivity are high, granuloma formation is less organized. Tissue necrosis is incomplete, resulting in the formation of caseous material. When the degree of tissue sensitivity is low, as often occurs in infants or immunocompromised persons, the reaction is diffuse and the infection is not well contained, leading to dissemination and local tissue destruction. Tumor necrosis factor (TNF) and other cytokines released by specific lymphocytes promote cellular destruction and tissue damage in susceptible persons.

Mycobacteria are nonmotile and nonspore-forming. Pleomorphic weakly gram-positive rods are typically slender and slightly bent. The cell walls contain lipids and wax that make these organisms more resistant than most others to light, alkali, acid, and the bactericidal action of antibodies. Growth is slow, with a generation time of 14-24 hours. Acid fastness, the capacity to perform stable mycolate complexes with certain arylmethane dyes, is the hallmark of mycobacteria. Cells appear red when stained with fuchsin [Ziehl-Neelsen (ZN) or Kinyoun Stain], appear purple with crystal violet, or exhibit yellow-green fluorescence under ultraviolet light. Truant stain is the most sensitive method for visualizing mycobacteria in a clinical specimen.

The infection is spread by the tuberculous patient, through inhalation, who discharges tubercle bacilli in his sputum or nasopharyngeal secretions during bouts of coughing or sneezing, etc. Such patients are open or infective cases. In the pediatric age groups, few infections may also occur by the transplacental route (congenital TB). It can spread by direct inoculation through the skin.

After the inhalation, some bacilli remain at the site of entry. Some may be carried to the lymph nodes. The inhaled tubercle bacilli may lodge in the pulmonary alveoli. It causes hyperemia and congestion. The pulmonary alveoli are filled up with exudate comprising fibrin leukocytes and tubercle bacilli. The central part of the inflamed area is necrosed. It looks like cheesy or caseous material. The epitheloid cells, fibroblasts, and giant cells with the caseous material constitute tubercular granuloma.

The inflamed area at the point of entry of the tubercle bacilli is called as primary focus. The primary focus, the draining lymphatics, and inflamed regional lymph nodes are collectively called primary complex. The areas of maximum ventilation in the lungs are usual sites of primary complex. These include right side of the lung and midzone of the lung.

During the formation of the primary complex, a few bacilli spread throughout the body by hematogenous route to form additional foci at various sites. Rich's foci are in the cortex of brain, Simon's foci in the apex of lungs, Simmonds' focus in the liver, and Weigart's focus is in the intima of blood vessels.

In most persons, the primary focus along with secondary foci heals, disappears, undergoes fibrosis, and calcifies. Uncomplicated primary complex runs a benign course. This is because the body's immune defenses can prevent them from spreading.

Further course of the infection depends on the immune response of the host. When the cell-mediated immune response is weak, the bacilli continue to multiply and the inflammatory process extends to the contiguous areas. Progressive primary disease is a serious complication of the pulmonary primary complex (PPC) in which the PPC, instead of resolving/calcifying, enlarges steadily and develops a large caseous center. The center then liquefies; this may empty into an adjacent bronchus leading to the formation of a cavity. This is associated with large numbers of tubercle bacilli. From this stage, the bacilli may spread to other parts of the lobe or the entire lung. This may lead to consolidation of the area of lung or bronchopneumonia.

A caseated lymph node may erode through the wall of the bronchus, leading to tuberculous bronchitis/endobronchial TB. Fibrosis and bronchiectatic changes may supervene. Discharge of the bacteria into the lumen may lead to its bronchial dissemination.

Hematogenous dissemination of *M. tuberculosis* occurs early in the course of the disease; this results when the bacilli find their way into bloodstream through lymph nodes. This may result in foci of infection in various organs. If the host immune system is good, then these foci are contained and disease does not occur. Seeding of apex of lungs leads to development of Simon focus. Lowering of host immunity may lead to activation of these metastatic foci and development of disease. This is especially seen in young infants, severely malnourished children, and children with immunodeficiency. Massive seeding of bloodstream with *M. tuberculosis* leads to miliary TB, where all lesions are of similar size. This usually occurs within 3–6 months after initial infection.

Extrapulmonary TB occurs when the quiescent disseminated foci of *M. tuberculosis* become active. The most common manifestation of extrapulmonary TB is peripheral lymphadenitis, especially of the cervical lymph nodes. Rarely, cutaneous TB can occur when an individual has had infectious substances such as sputum enter through a break in the skin.

Transmission of *M. tuberculosis* is virtually always by person-to-person spread via the respiratory route. Mucous droplets become airborne when the index case coughs, sneezes, laughs, or sings. Infected droplets dry and become droplet nuclei, which remain suspended in the air for hours. Environmental factors, such as poor air circulation, secondhand smoking, and indoor wood-burning stoves enhance transmission.

Two elements determine a child's risk for developing TB disease. The first is the likelihood of exposure to an individual with infectious TB, which is primarily determined by the individual's environment. The second is the ability of the person's immune system to control the initial infection and keep it clinically dormant. Without treatment, the disease develops in 5–10% of immunologically normal adults with TBI. In young children, the risk is greater; as many as 50% of those younger than 1 year with untreated TBI develop radiographic or clinical evidence of TB disease. Methods of preventing disease in infected individuals benefit children and adolescents even more than adults.

About 60% of cases of childhood TB occur in infants and children younger than 5 years. The ages of 5–14 years are often called the "favored age" because children in this range may become infected, but usually have the lowest rate of TB disease. The gender ratio for TB in children is about 1:1 in contrast to adults, in whom males predominate.

Children acquire *M. tuberculosis* from adults in their environment. Environmental risk factors include those characteristics that make it more likely that the child shares the air with an adult with infectious TB. Factors that increase the risk of a child being infected with *M. tuberculosis* include: (1) Birth or travel/residence in a country in which TB is endemic; (2) early childhood environments with exposures to multiple high-risk caregivers, for example, some orphanages; or (3) contact with high-risk adults who have had a previous residence in a jail, prison, or high-risk nursing home, and homelessness in some communities. Foreign visitors stay in the home, or locally defined risk factors contribute to TBI. Factors that increase the risk of developing disease once infected include age younger than 2 years, coinfection with HIV, other immunocompromising diseases or treatments (corticosteroids and TNF-alpha inhibitors), and malnutrition.

EVOLUTION AND TIMETABLE OF UNTREATED PRIMARY TUBERCULOSIS			
Primary infection:			
Febrile illness	Primary	Pleural effusion	Nodes
Erythema nodosum	Complex	Cavitation	(3–9 months)
Phylctenular conjunctivitis	Primary healing	Coin shadow (73% in 6 months)	
Miliary (<5 years of age)		Renal complications after 5 years	

■ CLINICAL FEATURES (FIG. 1)

The TBI may not cause any symptoms. Signs and symptoms with radiological findings appear once the disease occurs. The predisposing factors include measles, whooping cough, streptococcal infection, malnutrition, steroids, and immunosuppressive therapy.

Primary complex leads to progressive primary complex, i.e., inflammatory process extending to contagious areas. It occurs due to enlarged mediastinal lymph nodes. Sometimes cavity formation takes place. The inflamed lymph nodes may compress the neighboring bronchus, and produce obstruction. This leads to emphysema. Some bacilli may reach the bloodstream and dissemination occurs through the hematogenous route. The single massive seeding of the circulation with tubercle bacilli causes miliary TB. Miliary and meningeal TB usually occur within a year of primary lesion.

Later, the clinical features depend upon the site of infection.

Pulmonary Tuberculosis

The incubation period varies between 4 and 8 weeks. The onset of symptoms is

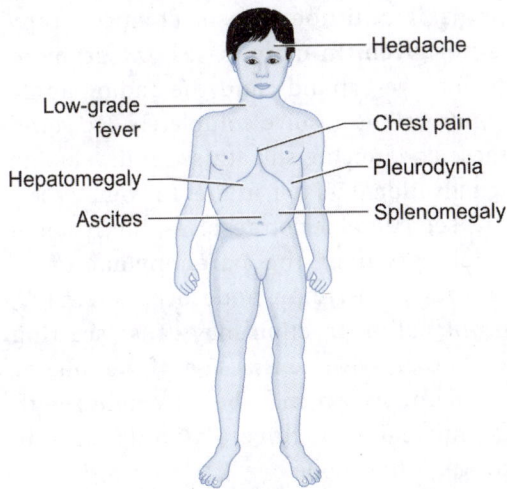

Fig. 1: Clinical features of tuberculosis (TB).

generally insidious but may be relatively acute in miliary TB. Most symptoms in children with pulmonary primary complex are constitutional in the form of mild fever, anorexia, weight loss, and decreased activity. Cough is an inconsistent symptom and may be absent even in advanced disease. Irritating dry cough can be a symptom of bronchial and tracheal compression due to enlarged lymph nodes. The PPC may be picked up accidentally during the evaluation of intercurrent infections.

Primary focus does not produce any clinical symptoms, especially in infants and young children. In older children, it may cause vague symptoms like malaise, fatigue, anorexia, weight loss, failure to thrive, and low-grade fever. This state may be sometimes flared up by the attack, whooping cough, or measles. Next step, i.e., hilar lymphadenitis may be an important feature of the primary complex. The common symptoms are cough, fever, and weight loss. This step can be diagnosed by positive TT and by radiological evidence.

Pulmonary primary complex is the result of the progression of primary disease. Children with PPC may present with high-grade fever and cough. Expectoration of sputum and hemoptysis are usually associated with advanced disease and development of cavity or ulceration of the bronchus. Abnormal chest signs consist mainly of dullness, decreased air entry, and crepitations. Cavitating pulmonary TB is uncommon in children.

Children with endobronchial TB may present with fever and troublesome cough (with or without expectoration). Dyspnea, wheezing, and cyanosis may be present.

Then the progressive primary complex produces segmental lesions. The signs and symptoms depend on extent of progressive primary lesion and type of segmental lesions produced by bronchial compression or erosion. Pleural effusion occurs as a result of discharge of caseous material of peripheral (subpleural) primary focus or enlarged regional lymph node. This occurs in the patients beyond 5 years of age.

The vast majority of children with TBI develop no signs or symptoms at any time. Occasionally, the initiation of infection is marked by several days of low-grade fever and mild cough. Rarely, the child experiences a clinically significant disease with high fever, cough, malaise, and flu-like symptoms that resolve within a week. These children have a positive test for infection, and the purpose of treating them is to prevent them from developing reactivation TB in the future.

More than 50% of infants and children with pulmonary TB have no physical findings and are discovered only via active contact tracing of an adult with TB. Infants are more likely to experience signs and symptoms because of their small airway diameters relative to the parenchymal and lymph node changes that occur. Nonproductive cough and mild dyspnea or wheezing, especially at night, are the most common symptoms. Systemic complaints such as fever, night sweats, anorexia, and decreased activity occur less often. Some infants have difficulty gaining weight or develop a true failure-to-thrive presentation that does not improve significantly until after several months of treatment.

Pulmonary signs are even less common. Some young children with bronchial obstruction have signs of air trapping, such as localized wheezing or decreased breath sounds, which may be accompanied by tachypnea or frank respiratory distress. These nonspecific symptoms and signs are sometimes alleviated by antibiotics, suggesting that bacterial superinfection distal to the focus of bronchial obstruction caused by TB has contributed to the clinical presentation of disease.

In chest radiography, the hallmark of pulmonary TB in infants and children is the relatively large size of the hilar or paratracheal lymphadenitis as compared with the less significant size of the initial parenchymal focus. Hilar lymphadenopathy is almost invariably present with childhood TB, but it may not be distinct on a plain radiograph when calcification is not present. Significant atelectasis and/or pulmonary infiltrate make it impossible to discern the lymph node enlargement. A CT scan of the chest may show the adenopathy, but this is rarely required to establish the correct diagnosis. As the hilar or mediastinal lymph nodes continue to enlarge, partial bronchial obstruction caused by external compression from the enlarged nodes causes air-trapping hyperinflation and even lobar emphysema. As the lymph nodes attach to and infiltrate the bronchial wall, reabsorption of air and atelectasis occurs.

The course of thoracic lymphadenopathy and bronchial obstruction can follow several paths if antituberculosis chemotherapy is not given. In many cases, the segment or lobe re-expands and the radiographic abnormalities resolve completely. However, these children are still at risk for developing reactivation TB later in life. In some cases, this segmental lesion resolves, but residual calcification of the parenchymal focus and regional lymph node occurs. Finally, bronchial obstruction may cause scarring and progressive contraction of the lobe or segment, which may be associated with cylindrical bronchiectasis and chronic pyogenic infection.

A rare but serious complication of TB in children occurs when the parenchymal focus enlarges and develops a large and caseous center. This progressive primary TB presents like bronchopneumonia and may be accompanied by high fever, severe cough, dullness to percussion, rales, and decreased breath sounds. Liquefaction in the center may result in the formation of a thin-walled cavity.

Adolescents with pulmonary TB may develop segmental lesions with adenopathy typical of initial infection in young children, or apical infiltrates with or without cavitation that are typical of adult reactivation TB. Regional lymphadenitis is absent in the latter type of disease. Adolescents with adult-type pulmonary TB often present with cough, fever, weight loss, fatigue, and, eventually, hemoptysis.

Tuberculous pleural effusion is uncommon in children younger than 6 years and rare in those younger than 2 years. Effusions are usually unilateral but can be bilateral. They are virtually never associated with a segmental pulmonary lesion and are rare in miliary TB.

Tuberculous pleural effusions, which can be local or general, originate from the discharge of bacilli into the pleural space from a subpleural pulmonary focus or caseated subpleural lymph node Asymptomatic local pleural effusion is so frequent in childhood pulmonary TB that it is basically a component of the primary complex. Most large and clinically significant effusions occur months to years after the initial infection.

The clinical onset of tuberculous pleurisy is usually fairly sudden. It is characterized by low-to-high fever, shortness of breath, and chest pain. On deep inspiration, there is a dullness to percussion, and diminished breath sounds on the affected side. The presentation is similar to that of pyogenic pleurisy. The fever and other symptoms may last for several weeks after the start of ultimately effective antituberculosis chemotherapy. Although corticosteroids may reduce the clinical symptoms, they have little effect on the ultimate outcome. The tuberculin skin test (TST) is positive in only 70–80% of cases. The prognosis is excellent, but radiographic resolution may take months. Scoliosis rarely complicates recovery of a long-standing effusion.

Tuberculous Lymphadenitis

It is the extension of primary lesions in the upper lung fields or abdomen. It is quite common and constitutes about 20% of TB. Cervical glands are more frequently involved. This is followed by axillary lymph nodes. Supraclavicular, tonsillar, submandibular, periauricular, axillary, and inguinal lymph nodes are commonly involved. They are less severe forms of extrapulmonary TB.

The gland may caseate and discharge its necrotic material into the skin. This results in exudative skin lesions. This is called scrofuloderma. Fine-needle aspiration cytology (FNAC) or gland biopsy is done to confirm the diagnosis.

A primary focus is visible radiologically only 30–70% of the time. TST results are usually reactive. Although spontaneous resolution may occur, untreated lymphadenitis frequently progresses to caseating necrosis, capsular rupture, and spreads to adjacent nodes and overlying skin, resulting in a draining sinus tract that may require surgical removal.

Tuberculosis of the superficial lymph nodes is the most common form of extrapulmonary TB in children. Most cases occur within 6–9 months of the initial infection, although some cases appear years later. The tonsillar, anterior cervical, and submandibular nodes become involved secondary to the extension of a primary lesion of the upper lung fields or abdomen. In areas of the world where children ingest unpasteurized products contaminated with *M. bovis*, an identical clinical entity can arise from this organism. It is important to distinguish between the two pathogens as *M. bovis* is inherently resistant to pyrazinamide (PZA), one of the first-line antituberculosis medications. Infected nodes in the inguinal, epitrochlear, or axillary regions, which are rare in children, result from regional lymphadenitis associated with TB of the skin or skeletal system.

In the early stages of infection, the lymph nodes usually enlarge gradually. The nodes are firm but not hard, discrete, and nontender. The nodes usually feel fixed to underlying or overlying tissue. Disease is most often unilateral, but bilateral involvement may occur. As the infection progresses, multiple nodes are affected, resulting in a mass of matted nodes. Systemic signs and symptoms other than low-grade fever are usually absent. The chest radiograph is usually normal, although adenopathy in the chest may be apparent.

Occasionally, the illness is more acute with rapid enlargement of cervical nodes, high fever, tenderness, and fluctuance. The infection may resolve if left untreated, but more often progresses to caseation and necrosis of the lymph node. The capsule of the node breaks down, resulting in the spread of infection to adjacent nodes. The skin overlying the massive nodes becomes thin, shiny, and erythematous. Rupture results in a draining sinus tract that may require surgical removal. However, if the correct diagnosis is made prior to rupture, the process can be cured with antituberculous therapy alone.

Abdominal Tuberculosis

It is usually secondary to the primary focus in the lungs or elsewhere in the body. It may, however, be secondary to swallowing of the infected sputum by a patient with pulmonary lesions. Patients with abdominal TB may remain asymptomatic initially.

Tuberculosis of the oral cavity or pharynx is very unusual. TB of the larynx causes chronic hoarseness and is often accompanied by upper-lobe apical pulmonary disease and sputum production in adolescents and adults. TB of the esophagus is very rare in children and may be associated with a tracheoesophageal fistula.

Tuberculous peritonitis is uncommon in adolescents and rare in young children. Whereas generalized peritonitis is caused by the dissemination of organisms, most localized disease is caused by direct extension from an abdominal lymph node, intestinal focus, or tuberculous salpingitis. Initial pain and abdominal tenderness are mild. Rarely, the lymph nodes, omentum, and peritoneum become matted in children and can be palpated as a "doughy", irregular, nontender mass. Ascites and low-grade fever are common.

Tuberculous enteritis is caused by hematogenous dissemination of organisms in most cases. However, ingestion of unpasteurized cow's milk laden with *M. bovis* causes an identical clinical picture and is still common in many areas of the world. The jejunum and ileum near Peyer's patches and the appendix are the most common sites of involvement. Mesenteric adenitis usually complicates this disease. Lymph nodes may cause intestinal obstruction or erode through the omentum to cause generalized peritonitis. This entity should be considered in any child with chronic GI complaints and a reactive TST.

Symptomatic patients show evidence of tuberculous toxemia and may present with colicky abdominal pain, vomiting, and constipation. The abdomen feels characteristically doughy. The abdominal wall is not rigid but appears tense so that the abdominal viscera cannot be palpated satisfactorily. The rolled tip omentum and enlarged lymph nodes may appear as irregular nodular masses with ascites. The liver and spleen are often enlarged. Histological examination of the liver may show granulomatous hepatitis and fatty change. There are three forms of abdominal TB.

1. *Tuberculosis mesenteric:* Glandular involvement
2. *Peritonitis:* This is of two types: (a) Ascitic and (b) plastic
   Ascitic abdominal TB is characterized by massive ascites. Plastic abdominal TB is characterized by chronic diarrhea, often alternating with constipation, chronic abdominal pain, and growth failure.
3. *Intestinal TB:* Chronic diarrhea occurs as a result of epithelial ulceration. Diagnosis is usually made by clinical findings.

Skeletal Tuberculosis

Skeletal TB results from lymphohematogenous seeding of tubercle bacilli during the initial infection. Bone infection also may originate as a result of direct extension from regional lymph node or a neighboring infected bone. The time interval between infection and clinical disease can be as short as 1 month in cases of tuberculous dactylitis, or as long as 30 months or more for TB of the hip. The infection usually begins in the metaphysis. Granulation tissue and caseation destroy bone by direct infection and by pressure necrosis. Soft-tissue abscess and extension of the infection through the epiphysis into the nearby joint often complicate the bony lesion.

Weight-bearing bones and joints are most commonly affected. A majority of cases of bone TB occur in the lower thoracic and upper lumbar vertebrae, causing TB of the spine or Pott disease. Involvement of two or more vertebrae is common; these vertebrae are usually contiguous, but there may be skip areas between lesions. Infection in the body of the vertebra leads to bony destruction and collapse. The infection may extend out from the bone, causing a paraspinal, psoas, or retropharyngeal abscess. The most frequent clinical signs and symptoms of tuberculous spondylitis in children are low-grade fever; irritability and restlessness, especially at night; back pain; and abnormal positioning in gait or refusal to walk. Spinal rigidity may be caused by profound muscle spasms.

Other sites of skeletal TB, in approximate order of frequency, are the knee, hip, elbow, and ankle. The degree of involvement can range from mild joint effusion without bone destruction to frank destruction of bone and restriction of the joint caused by chronic fibrosis. The TST is reactive in 80–90% of cases, and a culture of joint fluid or bone biopsy usually yields the organism.

Tuberculous dactylitis is a form of bone TB that is peculiar to infants and toddlers. Affected children develop distal endarteritis followed by painless swelling and cystic bone lesions in the hands.

It occurs in children if the primary TB is inadequately treated or untreated. The commonly involved bones are thoracic vertebrae. Other sites are hips, knee, and small bones of hand and feet. Kyphosis and gibbus formation leads to paraplegia. TB of bones and joints is almost always due to late hematogenesis spread from the primary complex in the lung. The common sites are spine, hip, and knee joints.

Renal Tuberculosis

It is another late manifestation of hematogenous spread. It takes around 4–5 years after the primary infection. The symptoms include frequency of micturition, dysuria, sterile pyuria, and painless hematuria. Hydronephrosis will be caused by involvement of renal pelvis and ureter.

Skin Tuberculosis

It may be in the form of erythema nodosum. Tuberculous ulcers are characterized by undermined edges. Tuberculomas are tiny papules with a concave surface. They may be multiple. Scrofuloderma is the involvement of skin overlying the caseous lymph node.

Miliary Tuberculosis

It usually occurs within the first few months. It is common below the age of 4 years. The disease is more severe in younger age. Tuberculous meningitis occurs in about 20% of miliary TB. Miliary TB occurs as a result of hematogenous dissemination. It is characterized by extensive miliary mottling of lungs and involvement of spleen, liver, and other tissues.

The lymphohematogenous spread of bacilli that accompanies the initial infection is usually asymptomatic. Patients rarely experience protracted hematogenous TB caused by the intermittent release of tubercle bacilli as a caseous focus erodes through the wall of the blood vessel in the lung. Although the clinical picture may be acute, more often, it is indolent and prolonged, with high fevers accompanying the release of organisms into the bloodstream. Early pulmonary involvement is surprisingly mild, but diffuse lung involvement becomes apparent if treatment is not given promptly.

The most common clinically significant form of disseminated TB is miliary disease, which occurs when massive numbers of bacilli are released into the bloodstream, causing disease in at least two organs. This form of disease usually occurs within 2–6 months of the primary infection. The clinical manifestations are protean, depending on the number of organisms that disseminate and the focus of infection. Lesions are usually larger and more numerous in the lungs, spleen, liver, and bone marrow than in other organs. This form of TB is most common in infants and malnourished or immunosuppressed patients.

The onset of clinical disease is sometimes explosive, with the patient becoming gravely ill in several days. More often, the onset is insidious, with the patient not being able to pinpoint the true time of initial symptoms. The most common signs include malaise, anorexia, weight loss, and low-grade fever. Within several weeks, hepatosplenomegaly and generalized lymphadenopathy develop in about 50% of cases. About this time, the fever may become higher and more sustained, but the chest radiograph is usually normal and respiratory symptoms are few. Within several more days to weeks, the lungs become filled with tubercles, causing dyspnea, cough, rales, and wheezing. As pulmonary disease progresses, alveolar air block syndrome may result in frank respiratory distress, hypoxia, and pneumothorax or pneumomediastinum. Signs or symptoms of meningitis or peritonitis are found in 20–40% of patients with advanced disease. Severe headache in a patient with miliary TB usually indicates the presence of meningitis. Abdominal pain or tenderness is usually a sign of tuberculous peritonitis. Choroid tubercles occur in patients and are highly specific for miliary TB. Unfortunately, the TST is nonreactive in as many as 50% of patients with advanced disease. X-ray chest is characteristic of demonstrating multiple minute dots. This has been described as a snowstorm appearance. Bacillus Calmette-Guérin (BCG) test is often positive.

Central Nervous System Tuberculosis

Central nervous system (CNS) disease is the most serious complication of TB in children and arises from the formation of a caseous lesion in the cerebral cortex or meninges that results from occult lymphohematogenous spread. Infants and young children are likely to experience a rapid progression to hydrocephalus, seizures, and raised intracranial pressure. In older children, signs and symptoms progress over the course of several weeks, beginning with fever, headache, irritability, and drowsiness. The disease advances with symptoms of lethargy, vomiting, nuchal rigidity, seizures, hypertonia, and focal signs. The final stage of the disease is marked by coma, hypertension, decerebrate and decorticate posturing, and death.

Central nervous system TB is the most serious complication in children and is fatal without effective treatment. This condition can arise from massive hematologic dissemination of organisms but usually arises from the formation of a caseous lesion in the cerebral cortex or meninges that develops during the occult lymphohematogenous dissemination of the initial infection. This lesion, called a Rich focus, increases in size and discharges small numbers of tubercle bacilli into the subarachnoid space. The resulting exudate may infiltrate the cortical or meningeal blood vessels, producing inflammation, obstruction, and subsequent infarction of the cerebral cortex. This exudate also interferes with the normal flow of cerebrospinal fluid (CSF) in and out of the ventricular system at the level of the basal cisterns, leading to a communicating hydrocephalus. The combination of vasculitis, infarction, cerebral edema, and hydrocephalus results in severe damage that occurs gradually or rapidly. Abnormalities in electrolyte metabolism, especially hyponatremia caused by the syndrome of inappropriate antidiuretic hormone or salt wasting, also contribute to the pathophysiology.

Tuberculous meningitis complicates about 0.3% of untreated TB infections in children. This condition is extremely rare in infants younger than 3 months because pathologic events usually need this much time to develop. It is most common in children between 6 months and 4 years of age.

The clinical progression of tuberculous meningitis may be rapid or gradual. Rapid progression occurs more frequently in infants and young children, who may experience symptoms for only several days before the onset of acute hydrocephalus, seizures, and cerebral edema. More often, the signs and symptoms progress slowly over several weeks and can be divided into three stages.

1. The first stage, which typically lasts 1-2 weeks, is characterized by nonspecific symptoms such as fever, headache, irritability, drowsiness, and malaise. Focal neurologic signs are absent, but infants may experience stagnation or loss of developmental milestones.
2. The second stage usually begins more abruptly. Lethargy, nuchal rigidity, Kernig's and Brudzinski's signs, seizures, hypertonia, vomiting, cranial nerve palsies relevant to basilar meningitis, and other focal neurologic signs are apparent. This clinical picture usually correlates with the development of hydrocephalus, increased intracranial pressure, and vasculitis.
3. The third stage is marked by coma, hemiplegia or paraplegia, hypertension, decerebrate posturing deterioration in vital signs, and eventually, death. The prognosis of tuberculous meningitis correlates closely with the clinical stage of illness at the time treatment with antituberculosis chemotherapy and corticosteroids begins.

The majority of patients in the first stage have an excellent outcome, whereas most patients diagnosed in the third stage, who survive, have permanent disabilities, including blindness, deafness, paraplegia, and mental retardation. It is imperative that antituberculosis chemotherapy be considered for any child who develops basilar meningitis and hydrocephalus or cerebral infarction with no other apparent etiology. The key to diagnosis is often identifying the adult from whom the child acquired *M. tuberculosis*.

Another manifestation of CNS TB is the tuberculoma, which presents clinically as a brain tumor. Tuberculomas account for as many as 40% of brain tumors in children in some areas of the world. These lesions, which occur most often in children younger than 10 years, are usually singular, but they may be multiple. In adults, lesions are usually supratentorial, but in children, they are often infratentorial, located at the base of the brain near the cerebellum.

The most common symptoms are headache, fever, and seizures. The paradoxical development of tuberculomas in patients with tuberculous meningitis while receiving effective chemotherapy has been recognized since the advent of CT. The cause and nature of these tuberculomas are poorly understood, but their development does not require a change in the therapeutic regimen. Whenever the condition of a child with tuberculous meningitis deteriorates or the child develops focal neurologic findings while on treatment, this phenomenon should be considered. Corticosteroids may help alleviate the occasionally severe clinical signs and symptoms. These lesions may be very slow to resolve clinically, persisting radiographically for months or years.

> **ESSENTIAL DIAGNOSTIC POINTS**
> - Tuberculosis is a chronic infectious disease caused by *Mycobacterium tuberculosis*
> - The infection is spread to the child by an adult active tuberculosis patient
> - Measles, whooping cough, and malnutrition will flare up the tuberculosis
> - The primary focus, the draining lymphatics, and inflamed regional lymph nodes are collectively called primary complex
> - Primary complex leads to progressive primary complex, i.e., inflammatory process extending to contagious areas
> - Congenital tuberculosis is suspected if the mother is known to have recently diagnosed with tuberculosis
> - Erythrocyte sedimentation rate is raised
> - Mantoux test is positive
> - Chest X-ray suggests primary complex

Cardiac Tuberculosis

Tuberculous pericarditis occurs in infected children. It arises from hematogenous dissemination or direct invasion from caseous lymph nodes in the subcarinal area. Pericardial fluid may be serofibrinous or hemorrhagic. Extensive fibrosis of the pericardial sac may lead to obliteration with development, usually years later, of constrictive pericarditis. The presenting systems are usually nonspecific: Low-grade fever, poor appetite, failure to gain weight, and chest pain. A pericardial friction rub may be heard, or, if a large effusion is already present, distant heart sounds, tachycardia, and narrow pulse pressure may suggest the diagnosis.

Congenital Tuberculosis

Congenital TB is suspected if the mother is known to have TB recently diagnosed, if the broad-spectrum antibiotics are ineffective, and if congenital infections are negative

Symptoms may be present at birth. They are also seen in the 2nd and 3rd week. Hepatosplenomegaly, respiratory distress, fever, and lymphadenopathy are present.

The fetus can be infected in utero via the umbilical cord. Placental infection results from dissemination in the mother. This results in hematogenous congenital TB. There are certain criteria that include TB lesions in the infant and one of the following:
- Lesions in the 1st week of life
- Primary hepatic complex or caseating granuloma
- Documented TB infection of the placenta or endometrium
- Exclusion of TB by a carrier in the postnatal period.

Mycobacterium tuberculosis can pass from the placenta to the fetus through the umbilical vein. The mothers of these infected infants frequently suffer from tuberculous pleural effusion, meningitis, or disseminated disease during pregnancy or soon afterward. However, the diagnosis of TB in the newborn often leads to the discovery of the mother's TB. Initial infection in the mother just before or during pregnancy is more likely to lead to congenital infection than previous infection. However, even the massive involvement of the placenta with TB does not usually give rise to congenital infection. The tubercle bacilli first reach the fetal liver, where an initial focus develops with associated involvement of regional lymph nodes. Organisms then pass through the liver into the main fetal circulation, leading to foci in the lung and other tissues. The bacilli in the lung usually remain dormant until after birth, when oxygenation and pulmonary circulation increase significantly. Congenital TB also may occur by aspiration or ingestion of infected amniotic fluid if a caseous placental lesion ruptures directly into the amniotic cavity.

Symptoms of true congenital TB may be present at birth, but more commonly begin in the 2nd or 3rd week of life. The most common signs and symptoms, in order of frequency, are respiratory distress, fever, hepatic or splenic enlargement, poor feeding, lethargy or irritability, lymphadenopathy, abdominal distention, failure to thrive, ear drainage, and skin lesions. Many infants have an abnormal chest radiograph, most often a miliary pattern. Only one-third of affected infants have meningitis. This clinical presentation in newborns is similar to that caused by bacterial sepsis and other congenital infections. The diagnosis of neonatal TB should be suspected in an infant with signs and symptoms of bacterial or congenital infection whose response to antibiotic and supportive therapy is poor and whose mother has risk factors for developing TB.

Diagnosis depends on clinical suspicion and demonstration of acid-fast bacilli (AFB) in tissue or fluids. Early morning gastric washings and open-lung biopsy are used to establish the diagnosis. Chest X-ray shows the miliary pattern.

Aspiration of infected amniotic fluid during or at the time of delivery leads to direct congenital TB.

GENERAL FEATURES
• Asymptomatic
• Poor built
• Fatigue
• Loss of appetite
• Chronic cough
• Convulsion

TUBERCULOSIS AND HUMAN IMMUNODEFICIENCY VIRUS INFECTION

In general, the clinical presentation of TB in children with HIV infection is similar to that in children without HIV infection. However, children with HIV infection more commonly have extrapulmonary TB (especially meningitis, tuberculoma, and abdominal disease). Pulmonary TB has a more aggressive picture, more often leading to substantial infiltrates or cavitation within the lung. Establishing the diagnosis of TB in an HIV-infected child can be difficult because the skin test is often negative, microbiologic confirmation of disease is difficult to achieve in many cases, and other opportunistic conditions can mimic TB. An aggressive evaluation for TB should be undertaken for any child with known HIV infection, or risk factors for HIV infection, who develops pulmonary disease or any unusual constellation of signs and symptoms.

DIFFERENTIAL DIAGNOSIS

- Typhoid
- Malaria
- Malignancy
- Urinary tract infection
- Collagen disorders
- Cirrhosis
- Rheumatic fever

DIAGNOSIS

A high index of suspicion is of considerable importance. TB should be suspected in the presence of growth failure, malnutrition, pyrexia of unknown origin (PUO), prolonged cough, recurrent chest infections, painless lymphadenopathy, asthma, pleural effusion, pneumonia not responsive to antibiotics for pyogenic infections, and unsatisfactory recovery from illnesses like typhoid, whooping cough, or measles.

Diagnosis of TB in children poses a problem due to the varied clinical presentation of TB, and since infection is paucibacillary, isolation of TB bacilli is difficult. Diagnosis is primarily passed on indirect clues such as clinical history and examination, family or contact history, radiographic abnormalities, immunization status, and FNAC/biopsy.

Bacteriological Diagnosis

Smear Examination

Demonstration of M. tuberculosis or its components: The organism can be demonstrated by (i) ZN staining, (ii) special stains, (iii) cultures, (iv) PCR, and (v) other methods.

The above methods can be used on sputum, induced sputum, gastric lavage, bronchoscopic lavage fluid, or pleural fluid. The best specimen for demonstration of *M. tuberculosis* in children is the early morning gastric aspirate (GA) obtained by using a nasogastric tube before the child arises. The yield on ZN stain is <20% and depends on the extent of pulmonary disease. For better results, at least two consecutive specimens of gastric aspiration are recommended.

Diagnosis is by clinical features, presence of contact in the family history, positive TT, and suggestive findings on chest X-ray. Demonstration of *M. tuberculosis* in a specimen from lungs is the gold standard but it is not always present.

Specimens for demonstration of M. tuberculosis: In pulmonary TB, specimens to be collected are sputum, gastric lavage, bronchoscopy lavage fluid, or pleural fluid. Recent reports suggest good results of isolation of *M. tuberculosis* from induced sputum. The latter can be safely and effectively performed in infants and young children. Induced sputum provides a satisfactory and more convenient specimen for bacteriological confirmation of pulmonary TB in both HIV-infected and uninfected children.

Method of sputum induction: Child is pretreated with 200 µg of salbutamol given via a MDI with an attached spacer or nebulizer to prevent the occurrence of bronchoconstriction. A jet nebulizer attached to oxygen at a low rate of 5 L/min or compressor can be used to deliver 5 mL of 3% sterile saline for 15 minutes. Sputum is obtained either by expectoration in children (who are able to cooperate) or by suctioning through the nasopharynx or oropharynx using a sterile, mucus extractor of catheter size six. Specimen should be transported directly to the laboratory for processing.

Gastric lavage: Early morning GA obtained by using a nasogastric tube before the child wakes up, and peristalsis empties the stomach of the respiratory secretions swallowed overnight, is the best specimen for demonstration of *M. tuberculosis*. For a higher yield, the specimen should be neutralized with sodium bicarbonate, if a delay in processing the specimen is expected.

Bronchoscopy and BAL: This has no advantage over properly done GA, bronchoscopy may be considered when there is doubt in diagnosis or a possibility of resistant TB is considered.

Young children are not able to provide sputum. In them, sputum can be induced. Following an overnight fast, the patient receives salbutamol by nebulizer followed by hypertonic saline (3% or 5%) inhalation by nebulizer. Older children may provide expectoration at the end of the procedure. In young children including infants, a nasopharyngeal aspirate is collected and processed like sputum for smear and culture to identify *M. tuberculosis*.

Smear Staining
- *ZN staining:* Yield is 20% and depends on the extent of pulmonary disease and number of specimens tested.
- *Special staining for AFB:* Fluorochrome-stained smears can be viewed more efficiently.
- Auramine O staining

Detection of AFB by ZN staining or fluorescent microscopy of sputum, gastric contents, laryngeal swabs, needle aspiration from areas of lung consolidation, lymph node, pleural, ascitic fluid, and CSF is the best way to diagnose TB.

Culture Examination

Cultures should only be obtained if the source patient is likely to have drug resistance, if bacteriological conversion or deterioration occurs during a course of supervised short-course chemotherapy, in extrapulmonary TB, and in immunocompromised children. Material can be sent for culture in Löwenstein Jenson (LJ) medium. Microscopic examination of thin-layer culture plate may lead to the detection of microcolonies of *M. tuberculosis* as early as after 7 days.

The excessively long period required for isolation of *M. tuberculosis* by conventional culture techniques has led to the development of other techniques for culture such as BACTEC radiometric assay, Septi-Chek AFB system, and mycobacterial growth indicator tube (MGIT) system. In this system, the culture is positive in majority by the end of 2 weeks though the final result is available by the end of 6 weeks.

Rapid Direct Tests

Polymerase chain reaction is the most commonly used technique of nucleic acid amplification for the diagnosis of TB. The PCR may be used to: (i) Diagnose TB rapidly by identifying deoxyribonucleic acid (DNA) from *M. tuberculosis* in clinical samples that are negative by microscopic examination; (ii) determine rapidly whether acid-fast organisms identified by microscopic examination in clinical specimens are *M. tuberculosis* or atypical mycobacteria; and (iii) identify the presence of genetic modifications known to be associated with resistance of some antimycobacterial agents. PCR is a suitable technique in childhood TB, especially when a diagnosis is difficult or needed urgently.

Serology and Antigen Testing

Enzyme-linked immunosorbent assay and radioimmunoassay (RIA) testing can be done for the detection of antibodies, IgG and IgM to mycobacterial antigens. The sensitivity and specificity depend on the type of antigen used, prevalence of TB, and recent BCG vaccination. Antigens like A60 that have less cross-reactivity have been found to have good sensitivity and specificity, particularly in TB meningitis. They may be useful in the diagnosis of extrapulmonary TB.

Radiological Diagnosis

The typical chest X-ray appearance of a pulmonary primary complex is that of an airspace consolidation of variable size, usually unifocal and homogeneous. Enlarged lymph nodes are usually seen in the hila and right paratracheal region. Adenopathy alone may be the sole manifestation of primary TB. There is no consensus regarding the most common site of involvement. Consolidation in pulmonary primary complex is usually heterogeneous and poorly marginated predilection of involvement of apical or posterior segments of upper lobe or superior segment of lower lobe.

In infected children, the chest radiographs may be normal or may demonstrate lobar, segmental involvement, multifocal involvement, hilar lymphadenopathy, pleural effusion, obstructive air trapping, miliary shadows, cavities, and pericardial effusion. Both lateral and PA views should be done since enlarged hilar nodes may be missed otherwise. In miliary TB, the chest radiograph changes may lag behind the clinical findings, so an initial negative film may bear repeating in the appropriate clinical case (cryptic miliary TB).

Occasionally, the chest radiograph may be normal and lymphadenopathy may be detected on CT. In addition, CT features such as low attenuation lymph nodes with peripheral enhancement, lymph node calcification, branching centrilobular nodules, and miliary nodules are helpful in suggesting the diagnosis in cases where the radiograph is normal or equivocal.

Other features such as segmental or lobar consolidation and atelectasis are nonspecific. Contrast-enhanced MRI is emerging as a very useful technique for diagnosing CNS TB, as it demonstrates the localized lesions, meningeal enhancement, and brainstem lesions.

X-ray skull may reveal silver beaten (also termed as copper beaten), which indicates raised intracranial tension and/or calcification when the TB is present.

Tuberculin Test

Robert Koch first proposed tuberculin, a broth culture filtrate of tubercle bacilli in 1880. In 1908, Mantoux described this intradermal test. Mantoux test can deliver tuberculin into the skin, the Heaf test or the Tine test. Reactivity to tuberculin is found if a person has been exposed to *Mycobacteria* and has intact cell-mediated immunity.

The TT is merely an index of infection, the degree of its positivity and local ulceration are no indication of an active disease or extent of disease. The degree of hypersensitivity is generally high in recently infected individuals. The reaction of TT must be considered in relation to:
- Duration of onset of hypersensitivity
- Prevalence of nonspecific tuberculous sensitivity

Mantoux test: 1TU (PPD RT23 with Tween 80) is used. It is injected intradermally on an area of healthy skin, away from obvious blood vessels on the left forearm; the site should not be swabbed with spirit or antiseptic but washed and dried at the junction of upper and middle third skin.

A tuberculin syringe with a needle 25 gauge is used intradermally, with bevel upward to produce 5–8 mm diameter wheal, which disappears within 1 hour. If no wheal is produced, the injection is too deep. It is read at 48–72 hours (any reaction observed before 48 hours may not be tuberculin hypersensitivity and should be ignored). It is read by locating the area of induration, measuring diameter not erythema with a caliper or transparent ruler.

Mountoux test is considered positive if:
- *Reaction 5 mm is positive:* Patients with HIV, patients with fibrotic lesions on chest radiograph, and close contacts of infectious TB
- *Reaction 10 mm is positive:* Recent converters >10 mm increase over 2 years in intravenous drug users known to be HIV negative, patients with predisposing medical conditions like diabetes, immunosuppressive drugs, and patients from high prevalence countries
- *Reaction >15 mm is positive:* For all others

Interpretation: Positive reaction reading, i.e., exceeding 10 mm, indicates the following:
- BCG was already given to the child
- Infection under 2 years of age, under 6 years of age provided the child is exposed to a known case of TB, and recent conversion from negative to positive.

Children with Mantoux reading of over 20 mm have high chances of a demonstrable pulmonary lesion.

False-negative reaction: Due to depressed sensitivity, an individual may show a false negative tuberculin reaction, despite the presence of TB, in the following situations:
- Poor technique
- Incubation period
- Advanced TB, for example, miliary TB, TB meningitis, etc.
- Convalescence from whooping cough or measles
- Steroid therapy
- Leukemia
- Leprosy
- Severe malnutrition

False-positive Mantoux test:
- Ruptured small venule
- Secondary infection
- Faulty interpretation (e.g., measurement of erythema)
- Recent blood transfusion

Bacillus Calmette-Guérin Diagnostic Test

There has been increasing documentation about the value of BCG vaccination as a diagnostic tool. It is believed to be far superior to TT. Its basis is hypersensitivity.

The appearance of a papule, >5 mm in diameter, during the first 24–72 hours, indicates a positive test. The grading is as follows:
- *5–10 mm diameter:* Mildly positive
- *10–20 mm diameter:* Moderately positive
- *Above 20 mm diameter:* Strongly positive

The advantages of BCG as a diagnostic measure are:
- It is a very sensitive and reliable test.
- It is generally positive even in situations like miliary TB, TB meningitis, and severe malnutrition where the Mantoux test is often false negative, despite the presence of TB.

Fine Needle Aspiration Cytology

Fine-needle aspiration cytology is a simple diagnostic technique, is now increasingly being employed and gives gratifying information.

Biopsy may show a granuloma formation with giant cells, epithelioid cells, and central caseation, which is more characteristic of TB.

Interferon Gamma Release Assay

Two blood tests, T-SPOT.TB (Oxford Immunotec; Marlborough, MA) and QuantiFERON-TB

(QFT, Qiagen; Germantown, MD) detect IFN-γ generation by the patient's T cells in response to specific *M. tuberculosis* antigens (ESAT-6, CFP-10, and TB7.7). The QFT test measures whole blood concentrations of IFN-γ and the T-SPOT.TB test measures the number of lymphocytes/monocytes producing IFN-γ. The test antigens are not present on *M. bovis*-BCG and *Mycobacterium avium* complex, the major group of environmental mycobacteria, so one would expect higher specificity compared with the TST and fewer false-positive results. Both Interferon Gamma Release Assays (IGRAs) have internal positive and negative controls. Internal positive controls allow for the detection of an anergic test response, which is useful in children who are young and immunocompromised.

Both IGRAs contain negative and positive controls in addition to the *M. tuberculosis*-specific antigens. These are used in test interpretation. A positive result is defined as when the difference in the amount of IFN-γ measured between the test antigen and the negative control is greater than a certain threshold: Over 8 spots in T-SPOT.TB and >0.35 IU/mL in QFT. Too much IFN-γ response to the negative control or too little response to the positive control yields indeterminate (QFT) or invalid (T-SPOT.TB) results. For the QFT failure to shake the sample as per manufacturer instruction increases the likelihood of an indeterminate result. Other factors associated with indeterminate results include young age and immunocompromised status.

In many clinical situations, these tests have a higher specificity than TST, better correlation with surrogate measures of recent exposure to *M. tuberculosis* in low-incidence settings, and less cross-reactivity than the TST with previous BCG vaccination. Two clear advantages of the IGRAs are the need for only one patient encounter (two with the TST) and the lack of possible boosting of the result because the patient is not exposed to any biological material. However, the sensitivity of IGRAs is similar to the TST, which ranges from 50% to 84% in studies of culture-proven TB disease in children.

Nucleic Acid Amplification Tests

The main nucleic acid amplification test (NAAT) studied in children with TB is PCR, which uses specific DNA sequences as markers for microorganisms. Compared with a clinical diagnosis of pulmonary TB in children, the sensitivity of PCR has varied from 25% to 83%, and specificity has varied from 80% to 100%. A negative PCR result never eliminates the diagnosis of TB, and the diagnosis is not confirmed by a positive PCR result.

Diagnostic Algorithm

The diagnosis of TB disease in children continues to be challenging. Even in advanced nations, the diagnosis is most often made by a combination of a positive TST, chest radiograph, physical examination, and history of contact with adult patients with TB. Newer diagnostic methods such as PCR and serodiagnosis have not given encouraging results. Newer staining and culture methods have found their place in the management of TB. There is a need to develop better techniques for the diagnosis of TB in children.

Kenneth Jones Diagnostic Criteria

In 1960, Kenneth Jones devised a scoring system for diagnosis of childhood TB **(Table 1)**. The system is helpful in arriving at an exact diagnosis.

TABLE 1: Kenneth Jones diagnostic criteria for childhood tuberculosis (TB).

Score (+3)	Score (+2)	Score (+1)	Score (−1)
• Demonstrable bacilli • Tuberculous granuloma • Positive Mantoux test	• Suggestive X-ray chest • Suggestive physical findings • Doubtful Mantoux test (5–9 mm) • Recent Mantoux conversion from negative to positive • Contact with sputum positive patient	• Nonspecific changes in X-ray chest • Compatible physical findings • History of contact • Nonspecific granuloma • Age under 2 years	Bacillus Calmette-Guérin (BCG) vaccination during the preceding 2 years

LABORATORY SAILENT FINDINGS

- Detection of acid-fast bacilli (AFB) by Ziehl–Neelson (ZN) staining
- Enzyme-linked immunosorbent assay (ELISA) and radioimmunoassay (RIA) testing for detection of antibodies IgG and IgM to mycobacterial antigens
- Polymerase chain reaction (PCR)
- Fine-needle aspiration cytology (FNAC).
- Radiological diagnosis
- Tuberculin test (TT)
- Mantoux test
- Bacillus Calmette-Guérin (BCG) test
- Computed tomography (CT) scan

The diagnosis of TB is based on clinical features, history of contact with open infective cases, demonstration of hypersensitivity to tuberculin, evidence of the radiological lesions, and laboratory investigation, i.e., TT. These are useful for diagnosis. Most frequently used tests are Mantoux test and multiple puncture test—Heaf test.

■ TREATMENT

An ideal antituberculous drug needs to possess three characteristics namely: (1) Potent bactericidal activity against metabolically active bacilli, (2) sterilizing activity against semidormant persisting bacilli, and (3) potential to prevent the emergence of resistant organisms throughout the period of chemotherapy.

Antitubercular drugs are the mainstay of treatment.

First-line drugs: Isoniazid, rifampicin, pyrazinamide (PZA), ethambutol, and streptomycin

Second-line drugs: Cycloserine, ethionamide, PAS, capreomycin, and kanamycin

Other drugs: Quinolones, rifamycin, amikacin, imipenem, and ampicillin

Mycobacteria replicate slowly and remain dormant in the body for prolonged periods. The treatment of TB is affected by the presence of naturally occurring drug-resistant organisms in large bacterial populations, even before chemotherapy is initiated. This drug resistance is caused by mutation at one of several chromosomal loci. The loci for resistance to one drug are not linked to the loci for resistance to other antituberculosis drugs.

These microbiologic characteristics of *M. tuberculosis* explain why single antimicrobial drugs cannot cure TB disease in adults. The major biologic determinant of the success of antituberculosis therapy is the size of the bacterial population within the host. For patients with a large population of bacilli, such as adults with cavities or extensive infiltrates, where many drug-resistant organisms are present initially, at least two antituberculosis drugs must be given. Conversely, for patients with infection but no disease, the bacterial population is small, drug-resistant organisms are rare or nonexistent, a single drug, such as isoniazid, can be given. Children with pulmonary TB and patients with extrapulmonary TB have medium-sized populations in which significant numbers of drug-resistant organisms may or may not be present. In general, these patients are treated with at least two, and usually three or four drugs.

Drugs for Tuberculosis

Isoniazid

Isoniazid (INH), a synthetically produced drug, is the most potent and valuable single drug in the treatment of TB. An oral dose attains a plasma concentration 20–80 times the usual level required to inhibit the growth of tubercle bacilli (0.02–0.05 ug/mL) within several hours, with high concentrations persisting for 6–8 hours in plasma and sputum. INH penetrates readily into the CSF, even in the absence of inflammation, and into caseous tissue. It is partially conjugated in the liver to an acetylated, inactive, and nontoxic form. The rate and degree of acetylation are genetically determined.

The principal side effects of INH are peripheral neuritis and hepatitis. Peripheral neuritis results from competitive inhibition of pyridoxine metabolism. This is more likely to occur at higher dosages of INH (10 mg/kg/day) in alcoholics and people who are poorly nourished. This is rarely a problem in children, although precautions must be taken during adolescence, for breastfeeding babies, during pregnancy, or when the total daily dose of INH exceeds 300 mg. Pyridoxine (10 mg for each 100 mg of isoniazid) should be given daily when indicated.

Other infrequent adverse effects of INH are convulsions (usually from a large and often intentional overdose), psychoses, loss of memory, allergic manifestations, and a lupus-like syndrome with arthritis and antinuclear antibodies.

Rifampicin

Rifampicin is a semisynthetic drug that has wide antimicrobial activity against bacteria and *mycobacteria*. It is absorbed readily from the GI tract after oral administration, with peak concentrations of 6–32 ug/mL (mean inhibitory concentration for *M. tuberculosis* is 0.5 ug/mL) occurring in 3 hours. Rifampicin readily diffuses to most tissues and body fluids; CSF levels are low but adequate for treatment. It is excreted primarily through the biliary tract and kidneys.

Rifampicin is relatively nontoxic; the principal side effect is hepatitis, which occurs with a frequency of <1%. Hepatitis seems to be more common in patients who are treated with a combination of rifampicin and isoniazid. GI disturbances, rashes, reversible leukopenia, thrombocytopenia, and elevation of BUN have been reported.

Administration of the drug may also impart an orange–red color to feces, urine, sputum, saliva, tears, and sweat. The suggested dosage is 10–20 mg/kg/day (maximum 600 mg) A liquid preparation is not commercially available but can be prepared in community pharmacies. A newer, longer-acting rifamycin called rifapentine is now available for use in combination with longer-acting for treatment of TB infection. It is not used in the treatment of TB disease in children. It has the same drug interactions and adverse effects as rifampicin.

Pyrazinamide

Pyrazinamide is a bactericidal drug that attains a therapeutic concentration in the

CSF and in macrophages. It is recommended as the third drug of a 3- or 4-drug regimen, particularly for the first 2 months of therapy. In doses of 20–40 mg/kg/day (adult dose, 2 g/day), it is well tolerated by children. Adverse reactions are rare in children but may include hepatitis, joint pain (caused by elevated levels of uric acid), and itching with or without a rash.

Ethambutol

Ethambutol is an odorless water-soluble compound rapidly absorbed from the GI tract and excreted in the urine, mainly with its form unchanged. It is bacteriostatic at the usual dose of 20 mg/kg/day. It is excreted via the kidneys and must be used with caution in patients with renal dysfunction. The only important toxic effect is retrobulbar neuritis, which infrequently results in loss of visual acuity, defects in visual fields, and inability to distinguish between red and green; the visual changes are usually reversible. This side effect should be monitored by monthly studies of visual acuity, visual fields, and tests for green color vision when possible. At doses of 20 mg/kg/day, it can be safely administered to children of all ages. Ethambutol is used as the fourth drug in a multidrug regimen, and its major purpose is to prevent the emergence of resistance to other drugs.

Corticosteroids

These drugs are controversial in the management of TB. They can be used only if effective antituberculosis therapy is in place. They are useful when the host inflammatory response to *M. tuberculosis* contributes to tissue damage. Generally accepted indications are for the management of tuberculous meningitis, tuberculous pleural effusion, pericarditis, and endobronchial disease. Prednisone at 2 mg/kg/day is used commonly for 4–6 weeks and then weaned slowly.

Second-line Drugs for Resistant Mycobacterium Tuberculosis

The emergence of MDR *M. tuberculosis* strains means that second-line drugs must be used to treat children who have acquired these strains. Second-line drugs also can be used if children are intolerant of the first-line drugs. An expert in TB should be consulted whenever a second-line drug is being considered for a child.

Second-line drugs are divided into several classes: The injectables, the fluoroquinolones, oral bacteriostatic agents, and other agents. These classes are used to determine the treatment regimens for drug-resistant TB; generally using one from each class to comprise three to four drugs active against the individual's isolate. First-line drugs with activity against the isolate are also used.

Fluoroquinolones, specifically levofloxacin and moxifloxacin, have bactericidal activity against *M. tuberculosis*. They also penetrate the tissues and CNS well. Side effects include neuropsychiatric issues, joint problems, Achilles tendon inflammation and rupture (rare in children), and prolonged QT interval. Levofloxacin is available as an oral suspension for younger children, whereas moxifloxacin must be compounded into a suspension. If an isolate is resistant to one fluoroquinolone, it is likely resistant to the other.

Streptomycin, capreomycin, amikacin, and kanamycin comprise the injectable class of second-line drugs. The injectable drugs are nephrotoxic, can cause hearing loss after prolonged use, and are quite painful when administered as intramuscular injections. The WHO recommends that children with milder forms of MDR disease can forego the injectable drugs as their risks may outweigh the benefits.

The oral bacteriostatic agent class includes cycloserine and the closely related terizidone, prothionamide and the closely related ethionamide, as well as PAS. The fifth class includes other agents such as clofazimine (used often in the treatment of *Mycobacterium leprae*, the etiologic agent responsible for leprosy, or Hansen's disease), meropenem, and linezolid. Two newly developed drugs, bedaquiline and delamanid, are being studied for their use in adult MDR-TB but can be used on a compassionate-release basis for children.

Major drugs for TB, their daily doses, route of administration, and side-effects are given in **Table 2**.

Indication for Specific Chemotherapy

The indications for specific chemotherapy are as follows:
- All children with demonstrable active tuberculous lesions, for example. Progressive primary complex, pleural effusion, miliary TB, meningitis, etc.
- All children below 5 years of age having positive tuberculin/BCG had not been already given to them
- All children whose tuberculin/BCG test has recently converted positive, provided BCG had not been given to them a few months back
- All unprotected children (BCG not given) who are exposed to open cases of TB

TABLE 2: Drugs for tuberculosis (TB).

Drug	Daily dose (mg/kg)	Route of administration	Side effects
Isoniazid	5 (preferably as a single dose)	Oral	Constipation, weight gain, euphoria, peripheral neuritis, convulsions, pellagra-like skin lesions, hepatotoxicity, very rarely bone marrow depression, and toxic encephalopathy
Streptomycin	20–50	Intramuscular	Deafness (eight cranial nerve involvement), nephrotoxicity—it may cause severe and, at times, fatal reactions in human immunodeficiency virus (HIV)-positive subjects
Thiacetazone	2–3	Oral	Hepatotoxicity, skin lesions, and agranulocytosis
Rifampicin	10–20	Oral	Rarely hepatotoxicity—intermittent administration may be accompanied by thrombocytopenia and leukopenia, an influenza-like illness and respiratory syndrome
Ethambutol	15–20	Oral	Anaphylactoid reactions, peripheral neuritis, hyperuricemia, and retrobulbar neuritis
Pyrazinamide	30	Oral	Hepatotoxicity and gout
Ethionamide	15–20	Oral	Nausea, vomiting, and pain in abdomen
Ciprofloxacin	10	Oral	Hypersensitivity and arthralgia
Amikacin	7.5	Intravenous and Intramuscular	Nephrotoxicity

Short Course Chemotherapy

Short-course chemotherapy is given in two phases.
1. *Initial intensive phase:* Here, three or four drugs are employed on a daily basis.
2. *Follow-up phase:* Here, two or three drugs are given, twice or thrice a week to reduce toxicity and improve compliance by the patient.

Indian Academy of Pediatrics Anti-Tuberculosis Treatment Regimens

The Indian Academy of Pediatrics (IAP) recommendations on anti-tuberculosis treatment (ATT) are given in **Box 1**.

Prednisolone

Role of steroids in TB: Corticosteroids, in addition to antitubercular drugs, are useful in the treatment of patients with CNS TB and occasionally pulmonary TB. These are useful in settings where the host inflammatory reaction contributes significantly to tissue damage. Short courses of corticosteroids are indicated in children with endobronchial TB that causes localized emphysema, segmental pulmonary lesions, or respiratory distress. Some children with severe miliary TB may show dramatic improvement with corticosteroids if alveolocapillary block is present. While significant improvement in symptoms can occur in children with pericardial effusion, steroids do not alter outcomes of pleural effusion. The most commonly used medication is prednisolone, at doses of 1–2 mg/kg/day for 4–6 weeks.

Prednisolone 1–2 mg/kg (double the usual dose) to take care of rifampicin steroid interaction for 4–6 weeks is used in TB meningitis (stage 2 and 3), pericardial TB, seriously ill miliary TB, and mediastinal lymph nodes causing airway compression.

> **BOX 1:** Indian Academy of Pediatrics (IAP) recommendations on treatment of childhood tuberculosis (TB).
>
> *Group 1: (Preventive therapy) 6HR*
> - Asymptomatic Mantoux positive <3 years
> - Asymptomatic Mantoux positive <5 years with grades III or IV malnutrition
> - Mantoux negative; recent converter/no signs (healed lesion—normal chest X-ray or calcification/fibrosis)
> - Children <3 years with history of positive contact
> - Children <5 years grades III or IV malnutrition with history of positive contact
>
> *Group 2: 2 HRZ/4 HR*
> - Primary complex (lungs)
> - Symptomatic Mantoux positive <3 years—without localization
> - Symptomatic Mantoux positive <5 years with grades III or IV malnutrition—without localization
> - Isolated lymphadenitis
> - Pleural effusion
>
> *Group 3: 2 HRZE/4 HR*
> - Progressive pulmonary disease
> - Tubercular lymphadenitis—multiple (in case of nonresolution of lesion, extend continuation phase by 3 months.)
>
> *Group 4: 2 HRZE/7 HR*
> - Miliary/disseminated disease
> - Cavitatory disease/bronchopneumonia
> - Osteoarticular disease
> - Abdominal, pericardial, and genitourinary disease
>
> *Group 5: 2 HRZE/10 HRE*
> - Neurotuberculosis

Steroids may also be necessary for severe hypersensitivity reactions to several anti-TB drugs. Topical steroids are used in eye, skin, and joint TB.

Indications:
- Neurotuberculosis
- Miliary TB
- TB involving serous layers
- Endobronchial TB/segmental lesions
- Genitourinary TB/sinus formation

Dose: 1–2 mg/kg/day for 4–8 weeks (for neurotuberculosis, 8–12 weeks)

Bacillus Calmette-Guérin Adenitis:
- If lymph node is small (<1.5 cm), no treatment is required.
- *Increasing size or fluctuant:* Excision or 3–6 months INH
- *Sinus formation:* Excision

MANAGEMENT OF AN INFANT BORN TO MOTHER WITH TUBERCULOSIS

It is difficult to differentiate between congenital and postnatally acquired TB. Infants born to mothers with active TB should be screened for evidence of disease by physical examination, TT, and X-ray film of chest. If physical examination and investigations are negative for disease, the infant should receive INH prophylaxis at doses of 10 mg/kg/day for 6 months.

After 3 months, the patients should be examined for evidence of infection and a repeat TT is done. If TT is negative, the infant can be immunized with BCG and INH can be stopped. If TT is positive but the infant is asymptomatic, INH prophylaxis is continued for another 3 months. Infants with congenital TB should be treated with four drugs (isoniazid, rifampicin, PZA, and ethambutol) in the intensive phase followed by two drugs (INH and rifampicin) during the maintenance phase for the next 4 months.

MANAGEMENT OF A CHILD IN CONTACT WITH AN ADULT WITH TUBERCULOSIS

Nearly one-third of children (aged <5 years) in contact with adults with active TB disease may have evidence of TB infection. The infection is more commonly associated with younger age, severe malnutrition, absence of BCG vaccination, contact with an adult who is sputum positive, and exposure to environmental tobacco smoke. Children below 5 years of age in contact with adult patients with pulmonary TB should be treated with INH prophylaxis at a dose of 10 mg/kg/day for 6 months.

MONITORING OF THERAPY

Response to treatment can be judged using the following criteria: Clinical, radiological, bacteriological, and laboratory tests.

Clinical Criteria

Clinical improvement assesses the response to therapy. The child should be seen every 2–4 weeks initially, then every 4–8 weeks. On each visit, improvement in fever, cough, appetite, and subjective well-being is assessed. The child is examined for weight gain and improvement in chest findings. Compliance is assessed by talking to parents and checking medications on each visit. A majority of children show improvement in symptoms within a few weeks.

In the presence of poor response or worsening of symptoms or signs, the initial basis of diagnosis is reviewed, especially, if there are no problems with compliance. Assessment for possibility of drug-resistant TB should be made. After the treatment is over, follow-up in every 3–6 months for the next 2 years is desirable.

Radiological Criteria

Clinical improvement precedes radiological clearance of lesions on chest X-ray films. The first chest X-ray during therapy should be done after 8 weeks, i.e., at the end of the intensive phase. In patients who show an increase or little change in radiological features coupled with delayed clinical response, prolongation of the intensive phase by 1 month is suggested. Further films are taken after 4 weeks and child, if better, should be shifted to the continuation phase; else, the child is investigated for failure of treatment and drug resistance. The degree of radiological clearance can be graded as: (i) Complete clearance, (ii) moderate-to-significant clearance (1/2–2/3 clearance), and (iii) mild clearance (decrease in size) or (iv) no clearance or appearance of a new lesion.

Microbiological Criteria

Most childhood pulmonary TB is paucibacillary. In children, where isolation of *M. tuberculosis* was possible at the time of diagnosis, every effort should be made to document the disappearance of bacilli during therapy.

TREATMENT OF EXPOSURE AND INFECTION

Children exposed to potentially infectious adults with pulmonary TB should be started on treatment with INH if the child is younger than 5 years or has other risk factors for the rapid development of TB disease. Failure to do so may result in the development of severe TB even before a test of infection becomes positive; the "incubation" of disease may be shorter than that for the test. The child should be treated for a minimum of 3 months after contact with the infectious case is broken. After 3 months, the test of infection should be repeated. If the second test is positive, infection is documented and INH should be continued for a total of 9 months; if the second test is negative, the treatment can be stopped.

Two circumstances of exposure deserve special attention. A difficult situation arises when exposed children are anergic because of HIV infection or other immunocompromise. These children are particularly vulnerable to rapid progression of TB, and it may not be possible to tell whether infection has occurred. In general, these children should be treated as if they have TB infection. The second situation is a potential exposure of a newborn to a mother or other adult with possible pulmonary TB.

In general, this exposure should be treated the same as for an older infant. The neonate should be started on INH and continued on it until TB disease in the adult can be ruled out, or for 3 months after the person with TB is no longer contagious.

Historically, treatment consisted of 9 months of INH; but in recent years, new regimens have become available. INH is usually taken everyday but can be administered twice weekly under the direct observation of a healthcare worker in cases of high-risk infection, particularly if an adult with TB disease who is also being treated twice a week is present in the home.

The summary opinion of experts is that 9 months of therapy is the optimal length of treatment for children with TB infection. The major difficulty with taking INH for 9 months is completing the regimen. Rifampicin taken daily for 4 months is effective, and completion rates with this regimen are much higher when compared to those with 9 months of INH. The rifampicin regimen causes fewer adverse events, but as children typically tolerate INH well, there is little difference between the 2 regimens in terms of safety.

The newest treatment for TB infection is a 12-dose, once-a-week regimen consisting of INH and the long-acting rifamycin–rifapentine; this regimen is referred to as 3HP. This has been studied in children from 2 to 17 years of age; it is well tolerated and at least as effective as 9 months of INH taken daily.

Adults occasionally develop a flu-like illness, joint pains, and/or skin rash caused by the rifapentine, but these are extremely rare in children. Currently, 3HP may be limited in availability and, in many locales, is available only via directly observed therapy given by the local health department.

If a child is exposed to or infected with an isoniazid-resistant but rifampicin-susceptible strain of *M tuberculosis*, rifampicin should be given for 4 months. If the infecting strain is resistant to both INH and rifampicin, a fluoroquinolone-based treatment regimen is often used, but an expert in TB should be consulted for this situation.

■ DRUG-RESISTANT TUBERCULOSIS

The incidence of *drug-resistant TB* has increased dramatically throughout the world. MDR-TB is defined as resistance to at least INH and rifampicin; *extensively drug-resistant TB* includes *MDR-TB* plus resistance to any fluoroquinolone and at least one of three injectable drugs (kanamycin, capreomycin, and amikacin).

There are two major types of drug resistance. Primary resistance occurs when a person is infected with *M. tuberculosis* that is already resistant to a particular drug. Secondary resistance occurs when drug-resistant organisms emerge as the dominant population during treatment. The major causes of secondary drug resistance are poor adherence to the medication by the patient or inadequate treatment regimens prescribed by the physician. Nonadherence to one drug is more likely to lead to secondary resistance than failure to take all drugs. Secondary resistance is rare in children because of the small size of their mycobacterial population.

The treatment of MDR-TB requires a minimum of three new drugs. Kanamycin (15 mg/kg), cycloserine (10 mg/kg), ethionamide (15 mg/kg), PAS (150–200 mg/kg) can be used. There is limited data on the use of quinolones in TB in children, but they may be used as an additional drug along with the above second-line drugs.

Treatment of drug-resistant TB is successful only when at least two bactericidal drugs are given to which the infecting strain of *M. tuberculosis* is susceptible. When a child has possible drug-resistant TB, usually at least four or five drugs should be administered initially until the susceptibility pattern is determined and a more-specific regimen can be designed. The specific treatment plan must be individualized for each patient according to the results of susceptibility testing on the isolates from the child or the adult source case. Treatment duration of 9 months with rifampicin, PZA, and ethambutol is usually adequate for isoniazid-resistant tuberculosis in children. When resistance to INH and rifampicin is present, the total duration of therapy often must be extended to 12–24 months, and intermittent regimens should not be used.

As second-line treatment options for MDR-TB in children, there is increasing use of new antituberculosis medications (bedaquiline and delamanid) and repurposed drugs (linezolid and clofazimine). Delamanid is endorsed for use in children 26 years and 220 kg in whom a four-drug regimen plus PZA cannot be used because of drug resistance, in those who experience significant drug intolerance, or in those at high risk of treatment failure. There is less evidence to support the use of bedaquiline in children. It is considered acceptable in children >12 years and >33 kg, with the same indications specified for delamanid. A baseline ECG and QTc monitoring is recommended in patients receiving bedaquiline or delamanid. Both linezolid and clofazimine are now included as core second-line agents in treatment regimens for children with MDR-TB. Both drugs require close monitoring for adverse effects and toxicity.

- Sputum examination for AFB should be done after 2 months of second-line drugs and monthly if positive till the 6th month as delayed conversion of sputum is also known. Once sputum smear and culture become negative, repeat sputum examination is advised every 3–6 months till completion of the regimen. Once it becomes negative, the injectable drugs should be omitted and at least 2 oral drugs to be continued for at least 12 months and a maximum for 18–24 months.
- Radiology does not play a significant role in the guide to the management of MDR-TB. Cough and hemoptysis are also not significant. However, fever plays a very important role in assessing the response or failure of the drug regimen.

NEWER ANTITUBERCULOUS DRUGS

In view of increasing resistance to commonly used antituberculous drugs, it is vital to discover newer agents that have antituberculous activity against resistant bacilli. Currently, some agents have emerged as promising antituberculous drugs for use in selected cases.

NEWER ANTITUBERCULOUS DRUGS

- *Quinolones:* Ciprofloxacin, ofloxacin, norfloxacin, pefloxacin, sparfloxacin, lomefloxacin, and enoxacin
- *Rifampicin derivatives:* Rifabutin and rifapentine
- *Beta-lactams with beta-lactamase inhibitors:* Amoxicillin with clavulanic acid, ticarcillin with clavulanic acid, and ampicillin with sulbactam
- *Aminoglycosides:* Kanamycin, amikacin, and capreomycin
- *Macrolides:* Clarithromycin

Steroids

In selected cases (tuberculous meningitis, severe intrathoracic TB-like pleural effusion, and extensive endobronchial disease), steroids may be given in a dose of 1–2 mg/kg/day for 2–4 weeks.

Prevention

Chemoprophylaxis in TB: It is the administration of drugs to prevent the occurrence of active disease. Usually, INH in the dose of 5 mg/kg/day is given for a duration of 6 months. This gives protection from active disease in 90% of cases.

Chemoprophylaxis is of two types:

1. *Primary chemoprophylaxis:* It is intended to prevent TB infection. It is indicated in the newborn child of a sputum-positive mother. Usually, it is given till the mother becomes sputum negative (3 months). Once the mother is sputum negative and the infant is asymptomatic but the Mantoux test is positive, chemoprophylaxis is continued for a total duration of 6 months **(Flowchart 1)**.
2. *Secondary chemoprophylaxis:* It is infact treatment of subclinical infection. It is indicated in Mantoux positive patients, asymptomatic high-risk group patients without evidence of active disease like recent converters to Mantoux positive, patients with old healed fibrotic lesions on chest radiology, HIV-positive patients, patients with chronic renal failure and hematological malignancies, and patients on corticosteroids or cytotoxic drugs.

Preventive therapy using two or more agents (for example, INH and rifampicin, or PZA and fluoroquinolone such as Ciprofloxacin) for 12 months can be considered in cases involving exposure to drug-resistant source cases.

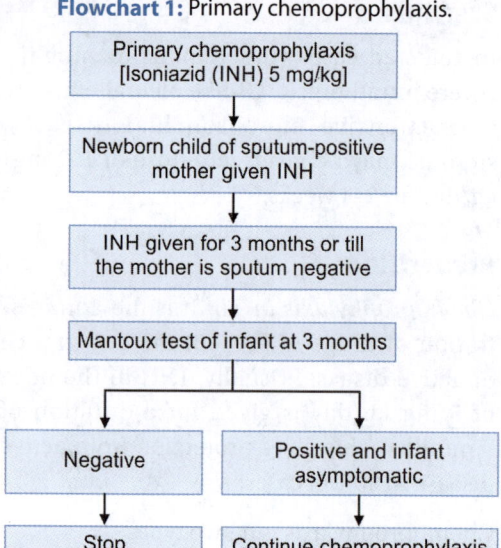

Flowchart 1: Primary chemoprophylaxis.

BOX 2: Indications for surgery in tuberculosis.
- Biopsy
- Abscess formation
- Bronchiectasis (secondary)
- Cavity formation with persistently positive sputum
- Chronic fibrosis
- Constrictive pericarditis
- Structural defects especially ureteric strictures
- Perforation of an ulcer
- Gastrointestinal hemorrhage
- Obstructive lesion
- Shunt procedure for obstructive hydrocephalus
- Pott spine with compression symptoms and signs
- Cold abscess
- Ascites
- Pleural effusion

The only available vaccine against TB is BCG, which employs live attenuated bacilli. The BCG vaccines are extremely safe in immunocompetent hosts. BCG vaccination given during infancy has little effect on the ultimate incidence of TB among adults in a population. However, many experts believe that BCG vaccines are more effective in preventing disseminated TB among infants and young children. Retrospective studies from Europe and Asia yielded estimates of the protective effect of BCG in young children of 60–80%, and the effect is particularly strong for tuberculous meningitis and severe forms of disease.

The BCG vaccines are among the safest of the childhood vaccines. Many children develop a small local ulceration, but regional suppurative lymphadenitis occurs in only 0.1–19% of vaccinees. These lesions usually resolve spontaneously, but occasionally require chemotherapy with either INH or erythromycin. Rarely, needle aspiration or surgical incision and drainage of the suppurative draining node is necessary, but this should be avoided rather than encouraged. Systemic complaints such as fever, convulsions, and irritability are extraordinarily rare after BCG vaccination. Children with undiagnosed serious immunocompromising conditions (e.g., severe combined immunodeficiency) can develop systemic and even fatal infections after neonatal BCG vaccination.

■ SURGERY

Indications of surgical intervention, greatly minimized over the years, are summarized in the **Box 2**.

■ BIBLIOGRAPHY

1. Anderson ST, Kaforou M, Brent AJ, Wright VJ, Banwell CM, Chagaluka G, et al. Diagnosis of childhood tuberculosis and host RNA expression in Africa. N Engl J Med. 2014;370(18)1712-5.
2. Chiang SS, Swanson DS, Starke JR. New diagnostics for childhood tuberculosis. Infect Dis Clin North Am. 2015;29(3);477-502.

3. Diacon AH, Pym A, Grobusch MP, de los Rios JM, Gotuzzo E, Vasilyeva I, et al. Multi drug-resistant tuberculosis and culture conversion with bedaquiline. N Engl J Med. 2014;371(8)723-32.
4. Horsburgh CR Jr, Barry CE 3rd, Lange C. Treatment of Tuberculosis. N Eng J Med. 2015;373(22);2149-60.
5. Seth V, Kabra SK, Lodha R (Eds). Essentials of Tuberculosis in Children, 3rd edition. New Delhi: Jaypee Brothers Medical Publishers (P) Ltd; 2010.
6. Starke JR. Improving tuberculosis care for children in high-burden settings. Pediatrics. 2014;134(4):655-7.

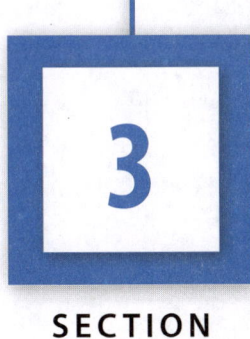

SECTION 3

Cardiovascular System

- Case 13 **Atrial Septal Defect**
- Case 14 **Coarctation of Aorta**
- Case 15 **Infective Endocarditis**
- Case 16 **Patent Ductus Arteriosus**
- Case 17 **Pericarditis with Effusion**
- Case 18 **Sydenham's Chorea**
- Case 19 **Tetralogy of Fallot**
- Case 20 **Ventricular Septal Defect**

CASE 13

Atrial Septal Defect

■ PRESENTING COMPLAINTS

A 7-year-old boy was brought with the complaint of:
- Cold since 7 days
- Cough since 7 days
- Fever since 3 days
- Tiredness since 3 days

History of Presenting Complaints

A 7-year-old boy was brought to the pediatric outpatient department with the history of repeated respiratory tract infection. He used to have respiratory illness involving cough, cold, and fever almost once in every month. Sometimes it occurs still more often. He was admitted on 3–4 occasions. Many a time he required parenteral antibiotics. His mother also told that her son would be much tired after some unaccustomed work, i.e., there was effort intolerance.

Past History of the Patient

The boy was the second sibling of non-consanguineous marriage. He was born at full term after normal delivery and cried immediately after the delivery. There was no significant postnatal event. The mother and child were sent home on third day. He was taking breast milk. Weaning was started as per the advice of the family doctor. All the developmental milestones were normal. His academic performance in school was good, but he never used to take part in sports.

■ EXAMINATION

Child was moderately built and nourished. He was attentive and was answering very promptly. Anthropometric measurements included the height 120 cm (50th centile) and the weight was 21 kg (50th centile).

The child had temperature 38°C, pulse rate was 106 beats/min, and respiratory rate was 32 breaths/min. The blood pressure recorded

---

CASE AT A GLANCE

Basic Findings
Height	: 120 cm (50th centile)
Weight	: 21 kg (50th centile)
Temperature	: 38°C
Pulse rate	: 106 beats/min
Respiratory rate	: 32 breaths/min
Blood pressure	: 70/50 mm Hg

Positive Findings

History:
- Repeated respiratory tract infection
- Effort intolerance

Examination:
- Pallor
- Parasternal heave
- Fixed split of second sound
- Ejection systolic murmur
- Crepitations at the base of lungs

Investigation:
- *Hemoglobin:* 8 g/dL
- *Electrocardiogram (ECG):* Right ventricular hypertrophy
- *X-ray chest:* Mild-to-moderate cardiomegaly

was 70/50 mm Hg. There was pallor, but there was neither icterus, cyanosis, nor edema. There was no significant lymphadenopathy.

Cardiovascular system revealed the presence of the parasternal heave. There was systolic thrill. The first heart sound was normal. There was split in second heart sound. Ejection systolic murmur was present at the left second and third intercostal spaces.

Respiratory system revealed the presence of crepitations at both the bases. Per abdomen examination was normal.

INVESTIGATION

- *Hemoglobin:* 8 g/dL
- *Total leukocyte count (TLC):* 8,500 cells/dL
- *Differential leukocyte count (DLC):* $P_{72} L_{26} M_4$
- *Erythrocyte sedimentation rate (ESR):* 22 mm in the first hour
- *Electrocardiogram (ECG):* Showed volume overload of the right ventricle, right-axis deviation, and right ventricular hypertrophy (RVH)
- *X-ray chest:* Showed mild-to-moderate cardiomegaly and pulmonary vascularity

DISCUSSION

Atrial septal defect (ASD) is an abnormal communication between two atria. There are three types: One is ostium secundum—generally located at the fossa ovalis, and second is ostium primum—located inferior to the fossa ovalis. Sinus venosus occurs in about 10% of all ASDs. Most commonly it is located at the entry of superior vena cava (SVC) into right atrium and is associated abnormal venous return as location of venosus is intimately related right upper pulmonary vein. Ostium secundum is more commonly seen, which occurs in 10% of patients with congenital heart disease (CHD).

The defect is more often sporadic but may be familial or have genetic basis (Holt-Oram syndrome). After third decade, atrial arrhythmias or pulmonary vascular disease may develop. Irreversible pulmonary hypertension results in cyanosis as atrial level shunting becomes right to left; ultimately right heart failure can occur (Eisenmenger syndrome).

In ASD secundum, a defect is seen in midatrial septum.

In ASD primum, a defect is in the lower atrial septum.

Sinus venosus defect is seen in posterosuperior atrial septum.

Interference with the development of the atrial septum at its lower margin, associated with abnormal development of the endocardial cushions produces an ostium primum ASD. This lesion is generally associated with abnormalities of the mitral and tricuspid valves (which form from the endocardial cushions) as well as defective formation of the upper portion of the interventricular septum.

A second type of ASD is the ostium secundum defect. This is a defect in the central portion of the septum in relation to the foramen ovale; it results from inadequate closure of the central hole in the septum primum by the septum secundum and is more appropriately termed a fossa ovalis defect.

A third type of ASD is the sinus venosus defect, i.e., in the superior portion of the atrial septum and generally extends into the SVC. With sinus venosus defects, there may be right-to-left shunting from the SVC into the left atrium because of deficiency in the upper part of the septum where it normally meets the SVC, and slight arterial oxygen desaturation may be found.

INCOMPETENT (PATENT) FORAMEN OVALE

With the onset of ventilation after birth, pulmonary venous return increases markedly, and left atrial pressure rises. The foramen ovale is therefore normally functionally: Closed by the membranous valve of the foramen ovale opposed to the crista dividens and the lower portion of the septum secundum. Although typically functionally closed shortly after birth, the foramen ovale remains probe-patent or larger in 30% of people. When pulmonary vascular resistance does not fall normally after birth, the resultant pulmonary hypertension and increased right ventricular (RV) end-diastolic pressure and right atrial pressure often cause right-to-left shunting across the foramen ovale and systemic hypoxemia.

In some infants, although the normal atrial pressure relationships occur after birth, the valve of the foramen ovale does not completely cover the foramen, either because the valve is too short or because the foramen ovale has become enlarged and stretched in infants in whom left atrial pressure and volume are increased, as with patent ductus arteriosus (PDA), ventricular septal defect (VSD), or left ventricular (LV) outflow obstruction secondary to aortic stenosis or coarctation. Significant left-to-right shunting may occur through an incompetent foramen ovale when left atrial pressure is high. If the cause of the increased left atrial pressure is relieved, atrial shunting generally decreases or disappears.

In some congenital heart defects, survival after birth depends on persistent patency of the foramen ovale. These defects include tricuspid, aortic, and mitral atresia and total anomalous pulmonary venous connection. In aortopulmonary transposition, a patent foramen ovale may be the only communication between the systemic and pulmonary circulations. Right-to-left shunting across the foramen ovale is also associated with RV obstructive lesions, such as pulmonic stenosis, and with pulmonary hypertension, particularly in newborns.

OSTIUM PRIMUM DEFECT

Ostium primum defect [partial atrioventricular (AV) canal defect] is the most benign form of endocardial cushion defect. The central portion of the atrial septum in the region of the mitral and tricuspid valve rings is absent, and the defect is usually large. The anterior (or septal) mitral valve leaflet is displaced and usually cleft. The tricuspid valve is generally not involved but may also have a small cleft in the septal leaflet. The magnitude of the left-to-right shunt is controlled by the same mechanisms in ostium primum as in secundum ASDs.

OSTIUM SECUNDUM DEFECT

Ostium secundum defects vary in size from a small defect to one in which only a rim of atrial tissue separates the defect from the AV valves. Usually ostium secundum defects are isolated lesions, but some may be associated with partial anomalous pulmonary venous connection (usually draining the right lung) or pulmonic stenosis.

An ostium secundum defect in the region of the fossa ovalis is the most common form of ASD and is associated with structurally normal AV valves. Secundum ASDs may be single or multiple (fenestrated atrial septum), and openings of 22 cm in diameter are common in symptomatic older children.

As the infant becomes older and pulmonary vascular resistance (PVR) drops, the RV wall becomes thinner, and the left-to-right shunt across the ASD increases. The increased blood flow through the right side of the heart results in enlargement of the right atrium and ventricle and dilation of the pulmonary artery.

Patients with the classic features of a hemodynamically significant ASD on physical examination and chest radiography, in whom echocardiographic identification of an isolated secundum ASD is made, need not undergo diagnostic catheterization before repair, with the exception of an older patient, in whom PVR may be a concern. If pulmonary vascular disease is suspected, cardiac catheterization confirms the presence of the defect and allows measurement of the shunt ratio and pulmonary pressure and resistance.

Small atrial communications are associated with small shunts. Such small defects are common at birth. Defects under 3 mm in diameter (almost all) close spontaneously, as do a high percentage of those from 5 to 6 mm diameter. Some defects become larger. Large defects are associated with large left-to-right shunts if there is low inflow resistance of the right ventricle and a low pulmonary resistance. The effect of a large shunt at the atrial level is a marked increase in flow through the right atrium and right ventricle. This extra volume load is tolerated well by the right ventricle, because it is handling the increased volume at a low pressure. Therefore, cardiac failure is unusual in infancy and when it occurs, it is generally precipitated by either a combination of defects, associated cardiomyopathy, or some other complication such as severe anemia. Persistent right-to-left shunting is unusual in ostium secundum defects, but transient right-to-left shunting is common after any Valsalva-like maneuver.

This results in the leaking of blood from left atrium to right atrium. There is not much difference in the pressure between two atria. Thus left-to-right shunt is silent. The right atrium receives the blood from left atrium also. It enlarges to accommodate the extra flow. The large volume received by the right atrium passes through the normal tricuspid valve. This produces delayed diastolic murmur. This is heard best at lower left sternal border. The right ventricle enlarges in size to accommodate the volume of blood. Because a large volume of the blood passes across the normal pulmonary valve, pulmonary ejection murmur is produced.

The shunt is variable and depends on the size of the defect, but it may be of considerable volume (as high as 20 L/min/m^2). Cineangiography, performed with the catheter through the defect and in the right upper pulmonary vein, demonstrates the defect and confirms the location of the right upper pulmonary venous drainage (normal or aberrant into SVC). Pulmonary angiography demonstrates the defect on the levophase (return of contrast to left side of heart after passing through lungs).

> **ESSENTIAL DIAGNOSTIC POINTS**
> - Right ventricular heave
> - S2 widely split and fixed
> - Grade I–III/IV ejection systolic murmur at pulmonary area
> - Diastolic flow murmur at the lower left sternal border
> - Electrocardiogram (ECG) with rsR lead VI

■ CLINICAL FEATURES (FIG. 1)

These children are generally silent, and asymptomatic. Mild effort intolerance and frequent respiratory tract infections are common. Congestive cardiac failure (CCF) is rare.

Peripheral pulses are normal and equal. Heart is hyperactive with parasternal impulse is present. Systolic thrill may be palpable along with the second left interspace. The first sound is normal and may be accentuated.

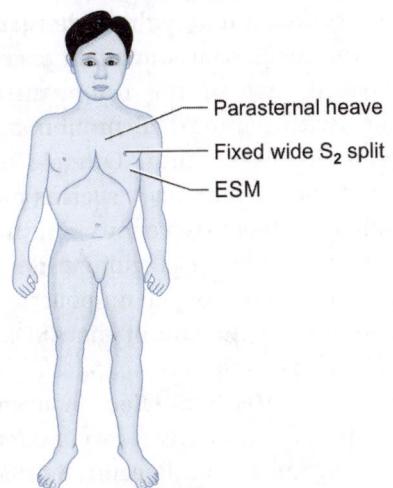

Fig. 1: Clinical features.

Second sound is widely split. The pulmonary valves close late and P2 is delayed. There will be further increase in RV volume during inspiration and hence there will be further delay in P2. Therefore second sound is widely split and fixed. The pulmonary artery and its branches enlarge to accommodate the left to right shunt. Hence, lung fields appear plethoric. The split is fixed due to RV stroke volume being equal in both inspiration and expiration.

The size of the left-to-right shunt is directly proportional to the intensity of two murmurs and heart size. Larger shunt will have more cardiomegaly and louder pulmonary and tricuspid murmurs.

The clinical features of ostium primum are similar and include RV hyperactivity, increased pulmonary flow, and a widely split second sound. In addition to the RV outflow murmur and the tricuspid mid-diastolic flow murmur, the murmurs of mitral or tricuspid regurgitation, or both, may be present.

In children with ostium secundum, large ASDs are generally asymptomatic. However, when there is pulmonary hypertension because of congenital or acquired lung disease, especially in preterm infants, the atrial septal defect may contribute to the symptoms as well as to right-to-left intracardiac shunting. The increased RV volume load causes precordial hyperactivity along the left sternal border. The first heart sound is normal, and the second heart sound is characteristically widely split, with absence of the normal respiratory variation in the width of splitting. Both components of the second sound are of normal intensity. Although fixed splitting of the second sound is characteristic in older children, this sign is occasionally absent, especially in infants or when the communication is not large.

Ejection systolic murmur is heard at second and third left intercostal spaces. There is mid-diastolic murmur in the fourth intercostal space at lower left sternal border. This is caused by increased flow across the tricuspid valve during diastole.

Flow across the ASD is not associated with a murmur. However, a long systolic ejection murmur that is crescendo–decrescendo (ejection) in type is generally heard at the upper left sternal border as a result of increased flow across the right ventricular outflow tract (RVOT) and pulmonic valve. The murmur associated with atrial septal defects can usually be differentiated from an innocent pulmonary flow murmur, which is usually shorter, by the response to the Valsalva maneuver. When intrathoracic pressure is increased, systemic venous return is immediately reduced, RV stroke volume decreases immediately, and the intensity of an innocent pulmonary flow murmur suddenly decreases.

However, with a large ASD, the left-to-right shunt across the atrial communication maintains RV stroke volume for several beats despite the decrease of systemic venous return; thus, there is little, if any, change in the intensity of the murmur in the first 3–4 beats. If the left-to-right shunt is fairly large, there is often a low-frequency, rumbling, early or mid-diastolic murmur caused by increased flow across the tricuspid valve and heard best at the lower left sternal border. A prominent third heart sound is often heard at the lowest left sternal border.

Spontaneous closure occurs in ASD <3 mm before one and a half years of age. If the defect is >8 mm, spontaneous closure is doubtful. Infective endocarditis (IE) does not occur in isolated ASDs.

Therefore, prophylaxis against IE is not required.

■ DIAGNOSIS

The ECG in ostium primum characteristically shows left-axis deviation, generally in the 20°–60° range, and RVH with an rsR pattern in right precordial leads. Chest radiographic findings depend on the magnitude of left-to-right shunting. Two-dimensional echocardiography and color Doppler flow mapping usually clearly delineate the anatomy. Congestive heart failure and arrhythmias occur, usually in late teenage or early adult life.

The chest radiograph in ostium secundum shows enlargement of the right atrium and ventricle and sometimes the outflow region of the right ventricle. The main pulmonary artery is dilated and pulmonary vascular markings are increased. However, the relationship between prominence of the pulmonary vascularity and the magnitude of the left-to-right shunt is unreliable. The ECG generally shows right-axis deviation with normal atrial complexes and normal conduction. There is RVH with a typical rsR or rSR pattern in the right precordial leads, and the S wave in the interior leads is usually notched.

Two-dimensional echocardiography in ostium secundum shows an increase in diastolic size of the right ventricle together with paradoxical motion of the interventricular septum. Other similar hemodynamic disturbances, such as partial anomalous pulmonary venous return and pulmonary or tricuspid regurgitation, may give similar findings. Septal dropout is often seen, indicating the site of the ASD, and color Doppler clearly demonstrates the flow patterns and often the defect. A negative shadow in the right atrium during contrast echocardiography can delineate the defect.

Flow velocity is increased depending upon the shunt, which brings dilatation of pulmonary artery and enlargement of right atrium and right ventricle. M-mode echo may show increased RV dimension and paradoxical motion of interventricular septum. It signifies RV volume overload; characteristic flow pattern with maximum left-to-right shunt occurs in diastole. Color flow mapping evaluates hemodynamic state of ASD. Doppler examination estimates presence in RV and pulmonary artery.

GENERAL FEATURES

- Asymptomatic
- Effort intolerance
- Repeated respiratory infection

LABORATORY SALIENT FINDINGS

- The electrocardiogram (ECG) is characterized by right-axis deviation and right ventricular hypertrophy (RVH)
- RVH and right bundle branch block (RBBB) with rSR pattern in V_1 is typical
- Radiograph of chest shows mild-to-moderate cardiomegaly, right atrial and right ventricular enlargement, and prominent main pulmonary artery segment
- Echocardiogram especially M-mode shows increased size of the right ventricle with paradoxical ventricular septal motion

COMPLICATIONS

Secundum ASD is well tolerated. Atrial arrhythmias, heart failure, and pulmonary arterial hypertension are the main complications.

TREATMENT

Medical management includes treating the chest infections. Definitive cure is by operation. The ideal age for operation is 2–5 years to prevent heart failure and arrhythmias in later life. The risk of operation is 1%. IE is very rare.

Surgical indication includes left-to-right shunt. Some consider small shunt to be an indication because of danger of paradoxical embolization and cerebrovascular accident. Another indication for surgery is left-to-right shunt with QP/QS of >1.5.

High PVR >10 units/m^2 is a contraindication to surgery.

Surgery is usually delayed till 3–4 years, because of spontaneous closure. But if CCF in infancy does not respond to medical management then surgery is indicated. The defect is repaired under cardiopulmonary bypass with either simple suture or a pericardial or a Teflon patch.

Surgical closure of the primum defect and repair of the cleft mitral valve has low risk and high effectiveness, but postoperative subaortic stenosis is common. Some patients develop severe hemolysis from red cell trauma if a small deficiency in the mitral valve leaflet directs a high-pressure jet at the atrial patch. At times, hemolysis improves, but some patients require reoperation to abolish the hemolysis.

Surgical or catheterization closure is generally recommended for symptomatic children, with large atrial level defect and associated with right heart dilatation.

Ostium primum defects are approached surgically from an incision in the right atrium. The cleft in the mitral valve is located through the atrial defect and is repaired by direct suture. The defect in the atrial septum is usually closed by insertion of a patch prosthesis. The surgical mortality rate for ostium primum defects is very low.

Transcatheter device or surgical closure is advised for all symptomatic patients, as well as for asymptomatic patients with Qp:Qs ratio of at least 2:1 and those with RV enlargement. The timing for elective closure is usually after the first year of life and before entry into school. For most patients, the procedure of choice is percutaneous catheter device closure using an atrial septal occlusion device, implanted transvenously in the cardiac catheterization laboratory.

Postoperative complications include arrhythmias and cerebrovascular accidents. The risk of operation is 1%. There is greater risk of small infants and those with high PVR.

Postoperative follow-up includes atrial and nodal arrhythmias. These occur in 7–20%. Sick sinus syndrome may supervene especially when sinus venosus defect is repaired. This eventually may require antiarrhythmic drug or pacemaker implantation.

COURSE AND PROGNOSIS

Pulmonary hypertension and reversal of shunt are rare late complications. Spontaneous closure occurs, most frequently in children with defect <4 mm in diameter.

BIBLIOGRAPHY

1. Moore J, Hegde S, El-Said H, Beekman R 3rd, Benson L, Bergersen L, et al. Transcatheter device closure of atrial septal defects: a safety review. JACC Cardiovasc Interv. 2013;6(5):433-42.

CASE 14

Coarctation of Aorta

■ PRESENTING COMPLAINTS

A 4-year-old boy was brought with the complaint of:
- Swelling of the face since 6 months
- Headache since 6 months
- Breathlessness since 3 months
- Tiredness since 2 months

History of Presenting Complaints

A 4-year-old boy was brought with history of headache and breathlessness. His mother told that his son used to have headache repeatedly and was relieved by paracetamol. She was noticing that her son used to be tired very early compared to other peers of his age. The boy used to feel pain in the legs repeatedly. He often has the swelling of the face. Then the boy visited a general practitioner for headache. The doctor recorded the blood pressure in the upper limb, which was 160/100 mm Hg. As the child had associated swelling in face, the doctor treated him as acute glomerulonephritis. He was given a course of procaine penicillin repeatedly. Later, the practitioner referred the child to the hospital for complete evaluation.

Past History of the Patient

He was the second sibling of the nonconsanguineous marriage. He was born at full term by normal delivery. He cried immediately after delivery. There was no significant postnatal development. He was discharged on third day. He was taking breast milk exclusively for 4 months. Later weaning started with cereals and fruits. He was on family food by the age of 18 months. There was no delay in developmental milestones.

CASE AT A GLANCE

Basic Findings

Height	:	105 cm (90th centile)
Weight	:	16 kg (75th centile)
Temperature	:	38°C
Pulse rate	:	110 beats/min, femoral not palpable
Respiratory rate	:	30 breaths/min
Blood pressure	:	160/100 mm Hg

Positive Findings

History:
- Headache
- Pain in legs
- Easy fatigability

Examination:
- *Hemoglobin (Hb):* 9 g/dL
- Impalpable femoral pulse
- Increased blood pressure
- Continuous murmur
- Displaced apex

Investigation:
- *X-ray chest:* Large aortic arch
- *Electrocardiogram (ECG):* Large ventricular hypertrophy
- *Echo:* Normal heart with bicuspid aortic valve
- *Barium swallow:* Characteristic E sign

Of late, he was complaining of leg pain, headache, and tiredness more frequently.

■ EXAMINATION

The boy was moderately built and nourished. He was sitting quietly and mild respiratory distress was present. The anthropometric measurements included the height 105 cm (90th centile) and the weight 16 kg (75th centile). The boy was febrile. The pulse rate was 110 beats/min and femoral pulses could not be palpated. The respiratory rate was 30 breaths/min. The blood pressure recorded in the upper limb was 160/100 mm Hg. Blood pressure could not be recorded in the lower limb.

There was pallor. There was no clubbing and no edema. Cardiovascular system revealed the apex beat was displaced in the left sixth intercostal space. Apex beat was forceful. Heart sounds were normal. Midsystolic click was heard over the aortic area. Continuous murmur was audible over the midthoracic spine. Other systemic examinations were normal.

■ INVESTIGATION

- *Hemoglobin:* 9 g/dL
- *TLC:* 9,600 cells/cumm
- *DLC:* $P_{70} L_{25} E_2 M_2 B_1$
- *ECG:* Left ventricular hypertrophy (LVH)
- *X-ray chest:* A large aortic arch that appears like figure 3 with the poststenotic dilatation of the descending aorta
- *Echo:* Normal heart with bicuspid aortic valve
- *Barium swallow:* Characteristic E sign
- *Fundoscope:* Normal

■ DISCUSSION

The child has the history of headache, leg pain, and easy fatigability. High blood pressure recording in the upper limb and absence of the femoral pulse in the lower limbs give the straight diagnosis of coarctation of aorta.

Congenital coarctation of aorta is located at the junction of the aortic arch and proximal descending aorta. It is a sharp indentation involving anterior, lateral, and posterior wall of the aorta. It may be distal or proximal to the ductus or ligamentum arteriosum and also to the left subclavian artery. Many affected females have Turner syndrome (45,XO).

Constrictions of the aorta of varying degrees may occur at any point from the transverse arch to the iliac bifurcation, but 98% occur just at the origin of the left subclavian artery at the origin of the ductus arteriosus (juxtaductal coarctation). The anomaly occurs twice as often in males as in females. Coarctation of the aorta may be a feature of *Turner syndrome* and is associated with cuspid aortic valve in >70% of patients. Mitral valve abnormalities (supravalvular mitral ring or parachute mitral valve) and subaortic stenosis are potential associated lesions. When this group of left-sided obstructive lesions occurs together, it is referred to as the *Shone complex.*

Such infants may have severe pulmonary hypertension and high pulmonary vascular resistance. Signs of heart failure are prominent. Occasionally, severely hypoplastic segments of the aortic isthmus may become completely atretic and result in an interrupted aortic arch, with the left subclavian artery arising either proximal or distal to the interruption. Coarctation associated with arch hypoplasia was once referred to as infantile type, because its severity usually led to recognition of the condition in early infancy. Adult type referred to isolated juxtaductal coarctation, which, if mild, was not usually recognized until later childhood. These terms have been replaced with the more accurate anatomic terms describing the location and severity of the defect.

Coarctation of aorta can be classified into preductal and postductal. Physiologically preductal or postductal coarctation depends upon the presence or absence of the collateral anastomosing vessels.

In preductal coarctation, if there are no collaterals, the neonate becomes symptomatic immediately, i.e., hypertension resulting in LV failure. Neonates who have postductal coarctation have some collaterals and are spared from developing reverse hypertension and congestive cardiac failure (CCF). The narrowed pulse pressure in descending aorta distal to the coarctation has been implicated in renal mechanism for the causation of hypertension.

If the postductal coarctation is present, it is operative in fetal life as it interferes with RV output reaching the descending aorta. This stimulates formation of collaterals in the fetal life.

Obstruction stimulates growth of collateral vessels between the proximal and distal segments. The intercostal vessels enlarge and become palpable at the lower border of the ribs.

Palpable collaterals are also felt at the medial and inferior angle of the scapula. Because of the decompression of the upper segment by the collateral, the resting blood pressure in the upper extremities may be normal systolic blood pressure accentuated by the exercise.

CLINICAL FEATURES (FIG.1)

Neonates or infants with more severe coarctation, usually including some degree of transverse arch hypoplasia, initially have signs of lower-body hypoperfusion, acidosis, and severe heart failure. These signs

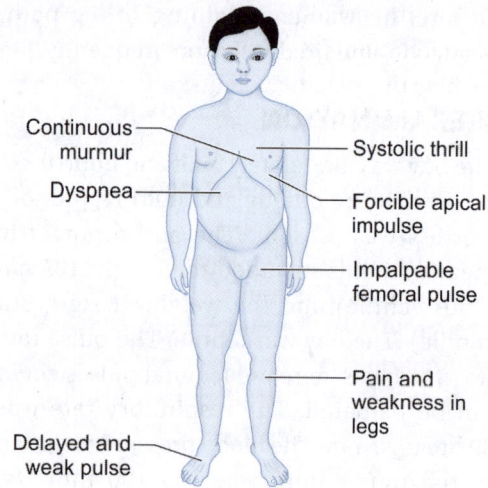

Fig. 1: Clinical features.

may be delayed days or weeks until after closure of the ductus arteriosus. If detected before ductal closure, patients may exhibit differential cyanosis, best demonstrated by simultaneous oximetry of the upper and lower extremities. On physical examination, the heart is enlarged and a systolic murmur is heard along the left sternal border with a loud S.

The symptoms may be intermittent claudication pain and weakness in the legs, and breathlessness on running. Physical examination shows delayed and weak or impalpable femorals. Infants have equal upper and lower extremity pulses from the birth until ductus arteriosus closes (ductal patency ensures flow to the descending aorta distal to the level of obstruction). It is usually diagnosed by a pulse blood pressure (>15 mm Hg) discrepancy between arms and legs on physical examination.

> **ESSENTIAL DIAGNOSTIC POINTS**
> - Pulse lag in lower extremities
> - Blowing systolic murmur in left axilla
> - Systolic blood pressure of 20 mm Hg or greater in the upper than in the lower extremity

It is important to remember that the site of coarctation does not determine whether the flow through the patent ductus arteriosus (PDA) is from left to right or from right to left. Regardless of whether the coarctation is preductal or postductal, the flow is from left to right, since the distal segment of aorta in coarctation almost never has a mean pressure below 50 mm Hg. If there is a flow through PDA, it indicates that there is severe pulmonary arterial hypertension.

It presents with heart failure in early infancy. It may be detected in evaluation of hypertension and murmur. Associated cardiac deformities may be ventricular septal defect, PDA, or aortic valve lesion.

The heart size remains normal with left ventricle forcibly heaving apical impulse. Systolic thrill may be present in the suprasternal notch. The first sound is accentuated and followed by loud constant ejection click. The second sound is normally split with loud aortic component. Ejection systolic murmur is heard maximally over back in interscapular region. The murmur starts late in systole and may appear to go through second sound suggesting continuous murmur. Continuous murmur may be heard over the collaterals in the chest wall. An aortic ejection systolic murmur and/or an aortic regurgitant murmur may also be present because of bicuspid aortic valve.

Electrocardiogram: It shows LVH. Moreover it shows RVH in infants with severe coarctation, because right ventricle serves as systemic ventricle during fetal life.

Radiograph: It shows normal-sized heart or to some degree LV enlargement. The aorta proximal to coarctation is prominent. The aortic outline may indent. The poststenotic segment is often dilated. This combination of abnormalities results in the "figure 3" on chest radiograph. Notching of ribs caused marked enlargement intercostal collaterals can be seen.

Echocardiography: Two-dimensional echo and color flow Doppler are used to visualize coarctation directly and continuous wave Doppler estimates the degree coarctation. Diastolic runoff flow is detected by continuous wave Doppler if obstruction is significant.

Barium swallow: It shows characteristic E sign and confirms the duration of coarctation. The characteristic notching of the lower ribs tends to appear beyond the age of 10 years.

GENERAL FEATURES
• Heart failure
• Hypertension
• Headache

LABORATORY SALIENT FINDINGS
• Electrocardiogram (ECG) shows left ventricular hypertrophy
• Radiograph shows normal-sized heart with prominent ascending aorta and the aortic knuckle
• Barium swallow shows characteristic E sign and confirms the duration of coarctation
• The characteristic notching of the lower ribs tends to appear beyond the age of 10 years
• *Echo:* The gradient across the narrowing is obtained with Doppler

■ COMPLICATIONS

The degree of systemic hypertension determines the severity of coarctation. Cardiac enlargement indicates LV failure and severe coarctation. Complications include severe neurological damage and even deaths because of associated cerebrovascular disease. Subarachnoid or intracerebral hemorrhage may result from the rupture of berry aneurysm. Abnormalities of the subclavian artery may occur. Other serious problems encountered are systemic hypertension, CCF, dissection of aorta, and aneurysm of aorta.

■ TREATMENT

Infants with coarctation of aorta may present in extremes secondary to LV dysfunction and low cardiac output. Resuscitative measures include prostaglandin E2 (PGE2) infusion (0.05–0.1 µg/kg/min) to reopen ductus.

Medical management includes control of CCF in infancy. The patients can be operated at any age. But the risk of operation is low if it is done between the ages of 1 and 10 years. Ideally the patients should be operated as early as possible after the age of 1 year.

Systemic hypertension may persist following operation. Coarctation is amenable to treatment by balloon angioplasty in patients with LV function. Balloon angioplasty is being increasingly utilized for the relief of recoarctation as well as primary mode of treatment in place of operative treatment.

Surgery remains the treatment of choice at most centers, Most often, the transverse aorta is splayed open and an "extended end-to-end" anastomosis performed to increase the effective cross-sectional area of the repair. The subclavian flap procedure, which involves division of the left subclavian artery and its incorporation into the wall of the repaired coarctation, has fallen out of favor because of a higher degree of residual stenosis. Some centers favor a patch aortoplasty, in which the area of coarctation is enlarged with a roof of prosthetic material.

After surgery, a striking increase in the amplitude of pulsations in the lower extremities is noted. In the immediate postoperative course, "rebound" hypertension can occur and requires medical management. This exaggerated acute hypertension gradually subsides and in most patients, antihypertensive medications can be discontinued.

■ COURSE PROGNOSIS

Children with coarctation corrected after age of 5 years are at increased risk for systemic hypertension and myocardial dysfunction.

■ BIBLIOGRAPHY

1. Allen HD, Driscoll DJ, Shaddy RE, Feltes TF. Moss and Adams' Heart Disease in Infants, Children and Adolescents, 8th edition. Philadelphia: Lippencott William and Wilkins; 2012.
2. Golden AB, Hellenbrand WE. Coarction of aorta: stenting in children and adults. Catheter Cardiovasc Interv. 2007;69:289-99.
3. Rodés-Cabau J, Miró J, Dancea A, Ibrahim R, Piette E, Lapierre C, et al. Comparison of surgical and transcatheter treatment for native coarctation of the aorta in patients >or = 1 year old. The Quebec Native Coarctation of the Aorta study. Am Heart J. 2007;154:186-92.

CASE 15: Infective Endocarditis

■ PRESENTING COMPLAINTS
A 4-year-old boy was brought with the complaint of:
- Fever since 7 days
- Pain in abdomen since 4 days
- Vomiting since 2 days
- Tiredness since 2 days

History of the Presenting Complaints
A 4-year-old boy was brought with the history of high-grade fever and tiredness. He was accompanied by his mother. She told that her son had fever since the past 1 week. To begin with it was of moderate degree. She took her son to the general practitioner. The doctor had prescribed symptomatic treatment. Later fever increased in intensity and used to be continuously associated with chills and rigors. Afterward, she also gave the history of vomiting and pain abdomen.

She revealed the history of heart murmur in her son. She showed all the reports pertaining to the cardiac problem as it was diagnosed at birth.

Past History of the Patient
The boy was the only sibling of the non-consanguineous marriage. He was born at term by normal vaginal delivery. He cried immediately after the delivery. The cry was good. The pediatrician who attended the delivery revealed the presence of congenital heart disease (CHD) and advised the parents to attend cardiac clinic later on. In the

---

CASE AT A GLANCE

Basic Findings
Height	: 99 cm (50th centile)
Weight	: 14 kg (50th centile)
Temperature	: 39°C
Pulse rate	: 120 beats/min
Respiratory rate	: 30 breaths/min
Blood pressure	: 70/50 mm Hg

Positive Findings

History:
- Fever
- Vomiting
- Murmur at birth
- Known case of VSD

Examination:
- Pallor
- Febrile
- Systolic thrill
- Systolic murmur
- Splenomegaly

Investigation:
- *Hb:* 9 g/dL
- *TLC:* Increased
- *Urine:* Microscopic hematuria
- *ECG:* Biventricular hypertrophy
- *X-ray chest:* Enlarged heart with pulmonary plethora, left atrial enlargement

(ECG: electrocardiogram; Hb: hemoglobin; TLC: total leukocyte count; VSD: ventricular septal defect)

postnatal ward, he was taking breast milk. Weaning was started as per the advice of the family doctor. All the developmental milestones were normal. His academic performance in the school was good. But he never used to take part in sports.

In the cardiac clinic, he was diagnosed with having ventricular septal defect (VSD) and was advised symptomatic treatment till the boy was 7 years old.

■ EXAMINATION

The boy was moderately built and nourished. He was looking ill and dehydrated. His anthropometric measurements included the height 99 cm (50th centile) and weight 14 kg (50th centile).

He was febrile, i.e., 39°C. His pulse rate was 120 beats/min. The respiratory rate was 30 breaths/min. The blood pressure recorded was 70/50 mm Hg. There was pallor and clubbing. There was no edema and lymphadenopathy.

Cardiovascular system examination revealed the displacement of apex beat to the anterior axillary line. Systolic thrill was felt to the left lower sternal edge. On auscultation, the pulmonary component of the second sound was loud. There was pansystolic murmur heard over the left 3rd and 4th intercostals space.

Per abdomen examination showed the presence of splenomegaly 2 mL below the costal margin. It was nontender and soft.

■ INVESTIGATION

- *Hemoglobin:* 9 g/dL
- *TLC:* 20,800 cells/cumm
- *DLC:* $P_{70} L_{28} E_2$
- *ESR:* 38 mm in the first hour
- *Urine routine:* 8-10 RBCs/HPF (red blood cells per high power field)
- *Blood culture and sensitivity:* Sterile
- *Urine culture and sensitivity:* Sterile
- *ECG:* Biventricular hypertrophy
- *X-ray chest:* Enlarged heart with pulmonary plethora and left atrial enlargement

■ DISCUSSION

A known case of rheumatic heart disease developed the high temperature associated with chills and rigors. This was associated with the clinical findings of the pallor, splenomegaly, and laboratory findings of microscopic hematuria suggests IE.

Infective endocarditis in pediatric patients is rare (5-12 per 100,000 pediatric admissions) and often associated with an underlying congenital heart defect or, increasingly, central indwelling intravascular catheters. However, structurally normal hearts may also be infected. Premature infants now account for 10% of pediatrics.

The clinical presentation of IE in children does not follow the classical presentation described in adults. Fever is the most common finding and may be associated with changing murmur and nonspecific symptoms. The primary site of infection and defense mechanisms of the host and organism determine the clinical manifestations and rate of progression. IE can involve native or prosthetic cardiac valves, septal defects, mural endocardium, patent ductus arteriosus (PDA), or intravascular devices such as catheters, occlusion devices, patches, and surgically constructed shunts. Blood cultures and echocardiography are of paramount importance to aid in the diagnosis.

Infective endocarditis is an infection of the endocardial lining of the heart and includes acute and subacute bacterial endocarditis (SBE) as well as nonbacterial endocarditis caused by viruses, fungi, and other microbiologic agents. It is a significant cause of morbidity and mortality in children and adolescents despite advances in the management and prophylaxis of the disease with antimicrobial agents. The disease represents a complex interplay between a pathogen and host factors such as endothelial disruption and immune function that is still not completely understood; the nature of the infecting organism has changed over time; diagnosis may be difficult during early stages and is thus often delayed until a more serious infection has set in.

It is often a complication of the congenital or rheumatic heart disease. It can also occur without any cardiac malformation. Rheumatic heart disease accounts for 60%. The common valves involved are mitral valve and aortic valves.

The infections which predisposes are urinary tract infection, osteomyelitis, ear infection, and tooth abscess. Important risk factors are open-heart surgery and prosthetic valves. Procedures such as tonsillectomy, rigid bronchoscopy, endoscopic biopsy, barium enema, percutaneous liver biopsy, and genitourinary procedure are predisposing factors.

Previously *Streptococcus* viridans was the agent most commonly responsible in pediatric age-groups. Now the streptococcal *aureus* leads the list. Staphylococcal endocarditis is more common in patients with no underlying heart diseases. *Streptococcus* viridans is more common after lower bowel or genitourinary disease. Fungal organisms are more common with open-heart surgery.

Congenital heart disease accounts for 25% of cases. The common CHDs are VSD, PDA, TOF, mitral valve prolapse (MVP), bicuspid aortic valve, and coarctation of aorta. Dental procedures and poor oral hygiene are important predisposing factors.

In patients with CHD, a high velocity of blood is ejected through a hole or stenotic orifice, which are more susceptible for endocarditis. Vegetations are mainly formed at the site of endocardial or frictional erosion that results from the turbulent flow.

Children with the VSD, left side valvular disease, and systemic pulmonary arterial communication including palliative shunts are at higher risk. Thus, tetralogy of Fallot (TOF), VSD, aortic stenosis, PDA, transportation of great arteries, Blalock–Taussig shunts are the most frequent structural lesions associated with endocarditis.

Surgical correction of CHD may reduce but does not eliminate the risk of endocarditis with the exception of repair of a simple ASD or PDA without prosthetic material.

■ PATHOGENESIS

Two factors are important in the pathogenesis of IE—namely, presence of structural abnormality of the heart or great arteries and bacteremia. The shear force associated with an abnormal high-velocity jet stream of blood due to a structural heart defect or trauma produced by an indwelling catheter in heart damages the endothelium.

Infective endocarditis is established by the interaction of a bloodstream pathogen with damaged endocardium. Intact endothelium is a poor stimulator of coagulation and is resistant to colonization by microorganisms; however, damaged endothelium is a potent inducer of thrombogenesis and provides a nidus to which bacteria adhere. Turbulent flow produced by certain congenital or acquired heart diseases causes sheer stress and damages the endothelium.

Thrombogenesis ensues and results in the deposition of sterile clumps of platelets, fibrin, and the formation of nonbacterial thrombotic endocarditis (NBTE). NBTE may also be produced in structurally normal hearts when indwelling intravenous (IV) catheters damage the endocardium or valvar endothelium. NBTE can then be converted to an infected vegetation in a patient with transient bacteremia or fungemia. Activities of daily living such as chewing toothbrushing, and flossing, account for most bloodstream seeding of an NBTE.

Bacteremia may also be caused by entry of organisms at the site of entry of percutaneous catheters, via the catheter lumen, or as a result of direct infection of an indwelling device at the time of placement.

Bacteremia, however, does not invariably produce IE. The propensity to adhere to an NBTE depends on the type of microorganism. Gram-positive microorganisms are most commonly responsible for IE in children, because they possess specific surface components that facilitate adherence.

Establishment of IE results from the interaction of several host and microbial factors. Following endocardial damage, bacterial access to the bloodstream from elsewhere and subsequent adherence to endocardial surfaces are required for the establishment of IE. It is now thought that the great majority of IE develops as the result of transient bacteremia related to activities of daily life, but not all bacteria are capable of initiating this process. The endocardium appears to be a preferential site of microbial adherence and may have some specificity for binding with certain bacteria. The presence of several factors, including bacterial adhesins, endothelial-binding proteins, and agglutinating antibodies that clump bacteria, promotes adherence of organisms to damaged endocardial surfaces. The Venturi effect (the reduction in fluid pressure that results when blood flows through a constricted area) deposits bacterial colonies immediately beyond the orifice that separates high- and low-pressure areas.

Classically, viridians streptococci have been the most common cause of IE, progressing along a subacute course in patients with preexisting cardiac lesions in which fever, fatigue, and immune complex-mediated clinical manifestations develop slowly over weeks or months. Enterococci behave in a fashion similar to the viridans streptococci. IE caused by *Staphylococcus aureus* has historically followed an acute course with rapid progression and poor outcome, including death, often in patients with normal hearts. Prosthetic heart valves within 2 months after implantation are prone to infection with coagulase-negative staphylococci (CONS) and *S. aureus*, as are neonates who require intensive care and intracardiac central lines.

Those organisms (*Haemophilus aphrophilus*, *Aggregatibacter actinomycetemcomitans*, *Cardiobacterium hominis*, *Eikenella corrodens*, and *Kingella kingae*) that normally inhabit the upper respiratory tract are often associated with IE when recovered from the bloodstream. Anaerobic and microaerophilic bacteria as well as polymicrobial infections are responsible for a minority of cases of IE.

The most common pathogens in neonates are *S. aureus*, CONS gram-negative bacterial species, and *Candida* species. After the first year of life, viridians group streptococci (VGS; e.g., *Streptococcus sanguis*, *Streptococcus mitis* group, *Streptococcus mutans*) and *S. aureus* are the most frequently isolated organisms in patients with underlying CHD. Importantly, *S. aureus* is the most common cause of acute (rapidly progressive) IE. CONS are also a frequent cause of IE and can cause infection in both native and prosthetic valves, indwelling vascular catheters, and prosthetic materials. Enterococcus IE occurs much less frequently in children than in adults. Gram-negative organisms cause

<109% of IE in children and include the HACEK (*Haemophilus* species, *A. actinomycetemcomitans*, *C. hominis*, *Eikenella* species, and *Kingella* species) organisms.

The prevalence of culture-negative endocarditis (CNE) is approximately 5–10%; the most common causes are recent or current antibiotic therapy or infection caused by a fastidious organism, such as *Bartonella*, *Tropheryma whipplei*, *Coxiella burnetii* (Q fever), or *Brucella*.

■ ORGANISMS

Most organisms that cause IE are gram-positive cocci including viridians group, streptococci, staphylococci, and enterococci. These organisms account for 90% cases.

- *Gram-positive cocci:*
  - Viridians group
  - Enterococci
  - Staphylococci
  - Other streptococci
  - St. *faecalis*, St. *pyogenes*, pneumococcus, anerobic and microaerophilic streptococci
- *Gram-positive bacilli:*
  - Listeria monocytogenes
  - Bacillus subitus
  - Diphtheroids
  - Nocardia israelli
- *Gram-negative organisms:*
  - Pseudomonas
  - Neisseria gonorrhoeae
  - Escherichia coli
  - Klebsiella
  - Enterobacter
- *Yeast and fungi:*
  - *Candida* species

■ CLINICAL FEATURES (FIG. 1)

Early manifestations are usually mild, especially when VGS are the infecting organisms. Prolonged fever without other

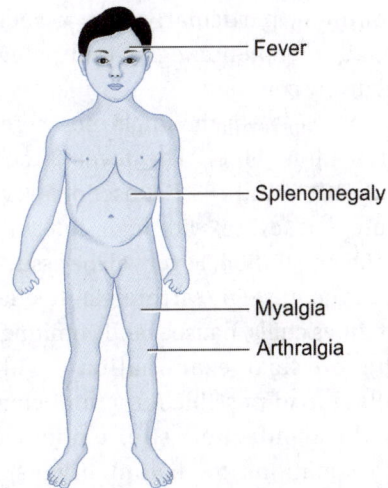

Fig. 1: Clinical features.

manifestations (except, occasionally, weight loss) persisting for several months may be the only symptom. Alternatively, the onset may be acute and severe, with high, intermittent fever and prostration.

Infective endocarditis is a multisystemic disease with various manifestations. Any fever in a patient with known cardiac disease should arouse the suspicion of IE in the presence of classical syndrome of fever, anemia, murmur, and embolic phenomenon. IE becomes a diagnostic consideration.

Clinical manifestations in newborn are nonspecific. They are indistinguishable from septicemia or CCF. These neonates have feeding difficulties, respiratory distress, and tachycardia. They have a new or changing heart murmur and hypotension. The neurological signs and symptoms such as seizures, hemiparesis, and apnea are present.

Usually, the onset and course vary between these two extremes— septicemia and CCF. The symptoms are often nonspecific and consist of low-grade fever with afternoon elevations, fatigue, myalgia, arthralgia, headache, and, at times, chills, nausea, and vomiting. New or changing heart murmurs are common, particularly with associated heart failure. Splenomegaly and petechiae are relatively common.

Prolonged fever is the single most common manifestation (90%). The fever fluctuates between 101°F and 103°F. Onset of fever may be acute and severe, with high, intermittent fever and prostration. Fever will be associated with fatigue, myalgia, arthralgia, headache, and at times chills, nausea, and vomiting.

The physical examination is highly variable due to possible structural changes at the local infection site, embolization from vegetations to distant organs, and circulating immune complexes. Serial auscultation is crucial, because it may be difficult to appreciate changes in a patient with a preexisting murmur. A new or evolving valvar lesion may cause leaflet destruction, resulting in a new or louder murmur or gallop due to congestive heart failure. Alternatively, attenuation of a continuous murmur or decrease in oxygen saturation in a cyanotic child with a prosthetic systemic to pulmonary shunt may reflect obstruction to flow due to graft infection. Heart rate and rhythm must also be closely monitored because heart block may be a sign of a life-threatening complication.

Cardiac murmur is almost universal. The appearance of the new murmur and an increase in the intensity of existing murmur are important.

Splenomegaly is seen in 25–60% of cases. It is due to reticuloendothelial proliferation caused by chronic stimulation from the bacteremia and circulating immune complexes. Splenomegaly may be absent in acute cases.

The *classical skin manifestations* develop late in the course of the disease. These manifestations include:
- *Osler node* are tender, specialized intradermal nodule in the pads of the fingers and toes.
- *Janeway lesions* are painless, small erythematous or hemorrhagic lesions on the palms and soles.
- *Splinter hemorrhages* are seen as linear lesions beneath the nails. These lesions represent vasculitis produced by circulating antigen–antibody complexes.

Embolic phenomenon: These are seen in 50% of cases. Embolization from the tricuspid valve may cause septic pulmonary emboli, resulting in breathlessness and scattered, fluffy infiltrates on chest radiographs.

Pulmonary emboli are seen in patients with VSD, PDA, and systemic pulmonary artery shunt. In 20% of cases, central nervous system (CNS) embolization is seen and results in seizure and hemiparesis. CNS complications are more common with left-sided defects such as aortic and mitral valve disease and cyanotic heart diseases. Renal embolization results in hematuria and renal failure.

Complications are often due to systemic embolization of a vegetation. Although embolic events can occur late, the majority occur in the first 2–3 weeks after diagnosis and initiation of therapy. Embolization is most commonly due to fungal or *S. aureus* infection.

Serious neurologic complications, such as embolic strokes, cerebral abscesses, mycotic aneurysms, and hemorrhage, are most often associated with staphylococcal disease and may be late manifestations. Meningismus, increased intracranial pressure, altered sensorium, and focal neurologic signs are manifestations of these complications.

Myocardial abscesses may occur with staphylococcal disease and may damage the cardiac conducting system, causing heart block, or may rupture into pericardium and produce purulent pericarditis. Pulmonary and other systemic emboli are infrequent, except with fungal disease. Many of the classic skin findings develop late in the course of the disease. They are seldom seen in appropriately treated patients. Clubbing of fingers can occur rarely in most chronic cases.

ESSENTIAL DIAGNOSTIC POINTS
- Preexisting organic heart disease
- Persistent fever
- Splenomegaly
- Leukocytosis
- Elevated erythrocyte sedimentation rate (ESR)
- Hematuria
- Positive blood culture
- Embolic phenomena

GENERAL FEATURES
- Anemia
- Hematuria
- Osler node
- Janeway lesion
- Splinter hemorrhage

■ DIAGNOSIS

Blood Culture

Blood culture is the mainstay of diagnosis of IE. It is indicated for all patients with the fever of unexplained origin and history of heart disease or previous endocarditis. Three samples of sufficient amount of blood, i.e., 1–3 mL in infants and young children and 5–7 mL in older children is optimal. It is collected with aseptic precautions every half an hour from different sites on the first day and if there is no growth by second day.

If there is no growth by second day of incubation, two more samples may be obtained. In patients, who are not acutely ill and whose blood culture is still negative, the antibiotics may be withheld for 48 hours or longer, while additional blood culture is obtained.

Of three blood cultures, one should be for anerobic culture. Three cultures can detect over 95% cases. Blood culture is negative in almost 50% cases. Most important causes for negative blood culture are prior antibiotics, anerobic organism, and fungal infection.

The critical information for appropriate treatment of IE is obtained from blood cultures. Blood specimens for culture should be obtained as promptly as possible, even if the child feels well and has no other physical findings.

In 90% of cases of endocarditis, the causative agent is recovered from the first two blood cultures. Other specimens that may be cultured include scrapings from cutaneous lesions, urine, synovial fluid, abscesses and, in the presence of manifestations of meningitis, the cerebrospinal fluid.

The microbiology laboratory and infectious disease specialist should be consulted in all suspected cases of IE. The laboratory will need to incubate cultures for at least 2 weeks if fastidious or unusual organisms are suspected, Serologies and molecular techniques, such as polymerase chain reaction (PCR), may help to identify fastidious organisms, and cell cultures may help identify intracellular organisms such as *Bartonella* or *Coxiella*. In patients who undergo surgery for IE, resected cardiac tissue is helpful as well. Several additional but nonspecific laboratory tests may help support the diagnosis. Patients often have elevated acute-phase reactants, anemia (due to hemolysis or chronic disease), and microscopic hematuria or proteinuria, leukocytosis is generally inconsistent, but patients may have a left shift. IE is diagnosed if a patient has clinical and/or echocardiographic evidence of IE but blood cultures are repeatedly negative. Conversely, positive blood culture in a child with CHD or a history of previous IE does not necessarily indicate IE.

Hematological

Anemia is seen in 50–80% cases. Usually normocytic and normochromic type of anemia is seen. It is due to hemolysis or anemia of chronic disease. Leukocytosis is present. Thrombocytopenia is unusual. It may be seen with patients with splenomegaly or disseminated intravascular coagulation (DIC). ESR is almost always elevated. It may be normal in patients with CCF.

Urine

Microscopic hematuria and proteinuria are present. They reflect immune complex injury. Renal infection may cause gross hematuria. Glomerulonephritis can cause hematuria, pyuria, and cellular casts.

There may be increase in gamma globulin, positive rheumatoid factor, presence of cryoglobulin, low complement levels, and circulatory immune complex. Antibodies against the causative organism may be increased.

According to the Duke criteria, definite IE must meet two major criteria, or 1 major and 3 minor criteria, or 5 minor criteria. Major criteria are: (1) Multiple positive blood cultures, for typical IE organisms and (2) evidence of endocardial involvement either by echocardiography or by the development of a new regurgitant murmur. Minor criteria are predisposition to IE [e.g., congenital heart disease (CHD)], fever, vascular phenomena, immunologic phenomena and microbiologic or serologic evidence that does not meet major criteria. Each of the major and minor criteria has qualifying details. Modified Duke criteria may be less specific in children than adults.

Nonspecific acute-phase reactants, such as ESR, C-reactive protein (CRP), and rheumatoid factor, are usually elevated. The tests may also be useful in following the progress of therapy.

Two-dimensional echocardiography is the principal modality for detecting vegetations. Typical echocardiographic findings include the presence of a vegetation, abscess, and new or worsening valvar insufficiency. Children have superior echocardiographic windows compared to adults, and transthoracic echocardiography (TTE) has an excellent reported sensitivity (81–97%) for detecting vegetations. Transesophageal echocardiography (EP) is more invasive, more expensive, and generally unnecessary in most pediatric cases.

LABORATORY SALIENT FINDINGS
• Blood culture • Anemia, leukocytosis, thrombocytopenia • Microscopic hematuria and proteinuria are present • Increase in gamma globulin • Positive rheumatoid factor • Presence of cryoglobulin • Low complement levels and circulatory immune complex

■ COMPLICATIONS

COMPLICATIONS OF INFECTIVE ENDOCARDITIS
• Congestive heart failure • Embolism, e.g., cerebral, pulmonary, renal, coronary • Periannular extension of abscess • Arrhythmia development, new heart block • Prosthetic device dysfunction • Valvular dehiscence • Graft or shunt occlusion • Persistent bacteremia or fungemia • Metastatic infection • Mycotic aneurysms • Glomerulonephritis/renal failure

■ TREATMENT (TABLES 1 AND 2)

It is a medical emergency, because it can damage valves, the myocardium, and other parts of the body like brain and kidney. Hence early and effective treatment will certainly prevent the morbidity and mortality of the patient.

Management requires a multidisciplinary team consisting of a pediatric cardiologist, infectious disease specialist, cardiothoracic surgeon, and general pediatrician. Empiric antibiotic treatment in a child with CHD with fever alone should be discouraged. For cases of suspected or confirmed IE, a prolonged

TABLE 1: Drug doses in endocarditis [all are given intravenously and divided into 2–4 doses/day except streptomycin given as intramuscular (IM)].

Penicillin G	10–20 million U/day	4 doses/day
Cefazolin	60 mg/kg/day	3 doses/day
Streptomycin	40 mg/kg/day (IM)	Once daily
Gentamicin	7.5 mg/kg/day	2 doses/day
Amikacin	30 mg/kg/day	3 doses/day
Ampicillin	400 mg/kg/day	4 doses/day
Cloxacillin	200 mg/kg/day	3 doses/day
Carbenicillin	400 mg/kg/day	4 doses/day
Vancomycin	60 mg/kg/day	2–3 doses/day

TABLE 2: Treatment of infective endocarditis.

Etiologic agent	Drug	Dose	Route	Duration of therapy (weeks)
Streptococcus viridans, *Streptococcus bovis* [minimal inhibitory concentration (MIC) ≤0.1 µg/mL]	1. Penicillin G Or	200,000–300,000 U/kg/24 h not to exceed 20 million U/24 h	IV	4–6
	2. Penicillin G Plus	As above no. 1	IV	2–4
	Gentamicin	3–7.5 mg/kg/h q 8 hours not to exceed 240 mg/24 h	IV	2
S. viridans, S. bovis (MIC ≥ 0.1 µg/mL)	3. Penicillin G Plus	As above no. 2	IV	4–6
	Gentamicin	As above no. 2	IV	2
S. viridans or enterococci (*S. bovis* or *Enterococcus faecalis*) (MIC > 0.5 µg/mL)	4. Penicillin G Or	As above no. 2	IV	4–6
	Ampicillin Plus	300 mg/kg/24 h q 4–6 hours not to exceed 12 g/24 h	IV	4–6
	Gentamicin	As above no. 2	IV	4–6
S. viridans, S. bovis (penicillin allergy)	5. Vancomycin Plus	40–60 mg/kg/24 h q 8–12 h not to exceed 2 g/24 h	IV	4–6
	6. Gentamicin if resistant	As above no. 2	IV	4–6
Staphylococcus aureus	7. Nafcillin Or	200 mg/kg/24 h q 4–6 hours not to exceed 12 g/24 h	IV	6–8
	Oxacillin Plus optional gentamicin	As above no. 2	IV	1–2

Contd…

Contd...

Etiologic agent	Drug	Dose	Route	Duration of therapy (weeks)
S. aureus (methicillin-resistant; penicillin allergy)	8. Vancomycin Plus optional trimethoprim sulfamethoxazole	As above no. 5 12 mg/kg/24 h trimethoprim q 8 hours not to exceed 1 g/24 h	IV IV, PO	6–8 4–8
S. aureus (with prosthetic device, methicillin-sensitive)	9. Nafcillin Plus gentamicin Plus optional rifampicin	As above no. 7 As above no. 2 10–20 mg/kg/24 h q 12 hours not to exceed 600 mg/24 h	IV IV PO	6–8 2 ≥6
S. aureus (with prosthetic device, methicillin-resistant)	10. Vancomycin Plus gentamicin Plus optional rifampicin	As above no. 5 As above no. 9 As above no. 9	IV IV PO	6–8 2 ≥6
Staphylococcus epidermidis	11. Vancomycin Plus optional rifampicin	As above no. 5 As above no. 9	IV PO	6–8 6–8
Haemophilus species	12. Ampicillin Plus optional gentamicin	As above no. 4 As above no. 2	IV IV	4–6 2–4
Unknown: Postoperative	13. Vancomycin Plus gentamicin	As above no. 5 As above no. 2	IV IV	6–8 2–4
Nonoperative	14. Nafcillin Or Vancomycin Plus gentamicin Plus optional ampicillin	As above no. 7 As above no. 5 As above no. 2 As above no. 4	IV IV IV IV	6–8 6–8 2–4 6–8

course of bactericidal IV antibiotics is given for 4–8 weeks, in patients who are not acutely ill. Antibiotics may be withheld while additional cultures are obtained. The choices of antibiotics and duration of therapy are determined by the specific pathogen, site of infection, underlying anatomy, and presence of prosthetic material. Serum concentrations of vancomycin and aminoglycosides should be monitored to achieve therapeutic levels and prevent potential side effects such as nephrotoxicity and ototoxicity.

The treatment of IE includes the treatment of the current episode and prevention of endocarditis. Antibiotics remain the mainstay of treatment. Choice of antibiotics depends on the organism isolated by blood culture. Empiric broad-spectrum antibiotics should be used when the culture is negative. Bactericidal antibiotics are used to prevent or reduce the possibility of treatment failure and relapse.

Some basic considerations apply in determining therapy for IE. High doses of parenteral antibiotics are required to exceed the bactericidal concentration for the infecting organism, and synergistic combinations are recommended in sonic situations (e.g., enterococci) to improve effectiveness or to shorten duration of treatment.

Oral antibiotics are insufficient unless bioavailability approaches 100%. Antibiotics used should be bactericidal rather than bacteriostatic, because the relatively avascular vegetations of infective endocarditis (IE) offer little access to host defenses. Pediatric and adult guidelines for therapy of specific pathogens are based on susceptibility testing and the presence or absence of prosthetic material.

Beta-lactams (including penicillins and cephalosporins) and vancomycin are used most frequently. Gentamicin is commonly added for a period of time to achieve synergy with beta-lactam or vancomycin, especially when enterococci or *S. aureus* is the causative organism. Rifampicin is useful as an adjunct when *S. aureus* infects prosthetic valves.

Antibiotic therapy should be started immediately after the diagnosis. When the virulent organism is responsible for a delay in the treatment, it may result in progressive endocardial damage. This is associated with likelihood of severe complications.

Depending upon the clinical and laboratory responses, antibiotic therapy may require modification and sometimes more prolonged treatment may be recommended. In case of non-*Staphylococcus* bacteremia usually resolves in 24 hours; the fever resolves in 5–6 days. Resolution in staphylococcal disease takes longer time.

Bacteremia generally resolves within few days after the appropriate therapy. Blood culture should be repeated to assess the adequacy of treatment and document cessation of bacteremia. Additional blood culture should be performed once or twice in 8 weeks after complication of antibiotics to ensure the complete cure.

Blood cultures should be obtained daily until bacteremia resolves; this usually occurs within several days of appropriate treatment. The efficacy of antimicrobial therapy is indicated by the disappearance of fever, sterilization of blood cultures, and normalization of inflammatory markers. Clinical and biologic surveillance (including occasional repeat blood cultures) should continue in the subsequent 6–8 weeks after completion of therapy when the risk of relapse is highest. A follow-up echocardiogram should also be performed to establish a new baseline. In most cases, this is all that is required to cure the infection and prevent life-threatening complications. However, there are cases where cardiovascular surgery may be necessary and lifesaving.

A prolonged course of therapy, i.e., at least 1 week, often 4–8 weeks is necessary, because organisms embedded within fibrin-plated matrix exist in very high concentration with relatively low rates of decrease susceptibility to beta-lactam and other cell wall active antibiotics.

Outpatient treatment can be considered in select patients; after initial inpatient management these patients must be hemodynamically stable, afebrile, have negative blood cultures, and not be at high risk for complications. There should be easy access to a hospital for prompt reevaluation should complications develop. Frequent monitoring by a home health nurse, who can assess adherence to drug therapy is also essential.

Digitalis, salt restriction, and diuretic therapy should be used for the treatment of heart failure. Surgical intervention is indicated for severe aortic or mitral valve involvement with intractable heart failure. A mycotic aneurysm, rupture of an aortic sinus, or dehiscence of an intracardiac patch requires an emergency operation.

Fungal endocarditis is difficult to manage. It has a poor prognosis regardless of treatment. It is commonly seen after the cardiac surgery especially in severely debilitated or immunosuppressed patients. The drugs of choice are amphotericin B and 5-fluorocytosine. Infected tissue is excised usually with the limited success.

ECHOCARDIOGRAPHIC FEATURES SUGGESTING FOR SURGICAL INTERVENTION

- Vegetation
- Persistent vegetation after systemic embolization
- Anterior mitral leaflet vegetation, particularly >10 mm
    - >2 embolic events during or after antimicrobial therapy
    - >1 embolic event during the first 2 weeks of antimicrobial therapy
- Increase in vegetation size despite appropriate antimicrobial therapy
- Valvar dysfunction
- Valve perforation or rupture
- Heart failure unresponsive to medical therapy
- Acute mitral or aortic regurgitation with signs of ventricular failure
- Perivalvar extension
- New heart block
- Large abscess or extension of abscess despite appropriate antimicrobial therapy
- Valvar dehiscence, rupture, or fistula

Most children with IE are cured with antibiotic therapy and occasionally surgical management. However, overall inpatient mortality remains at least 5–10%. This rate is even higher in premature infants and patients with IE caused by *S. aureus*. Specific types of CHD are also associated with poorer outcomes. Children who survive an episode of IE are at increased risk for relapse and thus must be followed closely and educated to report occurrence of fever. The pediatrician therefore plays a critical role in surveillance.

Surgical intervention, in addition to medical therapy, is generally indicated in fungal IE, when bacteremia persists despite appropriate antibiotic therapy, when congestive heart failure is uncontrolled by medical therapy, or in the presence of any of the following abscess of the valve annulus or the myocardium, systemic, embolic events, rupture of a valve leaflet or chordae, or acute valve insufficiency with cardiac failure. Prosthetic valve endocarditis per se is not an indication for surgery, but early surgical intervention may improve the outcome.

The most frequent complications of IE are congestive heart failure and arterial embolization. Intracardiac lesions that may lead to congestive heart failure include valvar insufficiency caused directly by vegetations or by chordal rupture, abscesses or the myocardium or valvar annulus, myocardial infarction, and conduction defects. Arterial emboli occur most frequently when large (<10 mm) mobile vegetations develop on valves, particularly the anterior leaflet of the mitral valve. Although vegetations slowly regress with effective therapy, sudden disappearance of vegetation should raise the possibility of embolization.

Emboli originating from left-sided vegetations can affect vascular beds in the systemic or cerebral circulation, whereas right-sided lesions produce pulmonary emboli. Cerebral emboli occur in 30% of left-sided IE and are mostly clinically silent. Magnetic resonance imaging (MRI) is often considered for detection. Mycotic aneurysms most commonly occur at vessel bifurcations and can involve any artery. Intracranial mycotic aneurysms often require surgery.

PREVENTION

Prevention of IE is more important than the diagnosis and treatment. Certain patient population with high risk is identified. Cardiac conditions have been stratified into high, moderate, and negligible risk on the basis of risk of developing endocarditis and its severity. Prophylaxis is recommended for those in high- and moderate-risk categories.

The prophylactic administration of antibiotics prior to dental procedures has been routine for over 50 years. While guidelines have continued to evolve, published data have failed to prove the effectiveness of antibiotic prophylaxis to prevent IE. There is consistent scientific evidence to suggest that dental procedures are a rare cause of IE, and prophylactic antibiotics prior to such procedures may prevent an exceedingly small number of cases. On the contrary, bacteremia from activities of daily living far exceeds that of dental procedures and is therefore much more likely to cause IE. This has resulted in a significant shift in prevention strategies toward a greater emphasis on oral hygiene and access to dental care for children with CHD. This emphasizes the necessary role of the pediatrician to lay stress on the importance of good oral hygiene, prevention of gingival and dental disease, and access to routine dental care for children at risk for IE.

Prophylaxis is now only recommended for children with a prosthetic valve or prosthetic material, certain types of CHD (unrepaired cyanotic CHD, repaired CHD with prosthetic material or device during the first 6 months after the procedure, and repaired CHD with residual defects at the site or adjacent to the site of a prosthetic patch or prosthetic device), or a previous case of IE. It is also recommended in heart transplant recipients with cardiac valvulopathy. Prophylaxis consists of a single dose of amoxicillin (50 mg/kg; maximum, 2 g) 30–60 minutes prior to all dental procedures that involve manipulation of gingival tissue, the periapical region of teeth, or perforation of the oral mucosa.

Standard Prophylaxis

Oral amoxicillin 50 mg/kg orally 1 hour before procedure and then half the dose 6 hours after the initial dose.

If allergic to penicillin, ampicillin or amoxicillin
- Erythromycin 20 mg/kg orally 2 hours before procedure and half a dose 6 hours after initial dose
- Clindamycin 10 mg/kg orally 1 hour before procedure and then half the dose 6 hours after initial dose

In Patients Unable to Take Oral Medication

Ampicillin 50 mg/kg IV/intramuscular (IM) 30 minutes before the procedure and then half the dose 6 hours after the initial dose is recommended. In patients allergic to penicillin alternatively clindamycin 10 mg IV/IM 30 minutes before the procedure and half the dose IV or oral 6 hours after the initial dose.

High-risk Patients

Ampicillin 50 mg/kg and gentamycin 2 mg/kg IV/IM 30 minutes before the procedure followed by amoxicillin 25 mg/kg orally 6 hours after the initial dose or IV/IM can be repeated 8 hours later.

In high-risk patients allergic to penicillin vancomycin 20 mg/kg IV over 1 hour started 1 hour before the procedure. No repeat dose is needed.

Antimicrobial prophylaxis prior to various procedures, including dental cleaning and other forms of dental manipulation, reduces the incidence of IE in susceptible patients.

BIBLIOGRAPHY

1. Batlimore RS, Gewitz M, Baddour LM, Beerman LB, Jackson MA, Lockhart PB, et al. Infective endocarditis in childhood: 2015 Update: A scientific statement from the American heart association. Circulation. 2015;132(15):1487-515.
2. Wilson W, Taubert KA, Gewitz M, Lockhart PB, Baddour LM, Levison M, et al.; American Heart Association Rheumatic Fever, Endocarditis, and Kawasaki Disease Committee; American Heart Association Council on Cardiovascular Disease in the Young; American Heart Association Council on Clinical Cardiology; American Heart Association Council on Cardiovascular Surgery and Anesthesia; Quality of Care and Outcomes Research Interdisciplinary Working Group. Prevention of infective endocarditis: guidelines from the American Heart Association: a guideline from the American Heart Association Rheumatic Fever, Endocarditis, and Kawasaki Disease Committee, Council on Cardiovascular Disease in the Young, and the Council on Clinical Cardiology, Council on Cardiovascular Surgery and Anesthesia, and the Quality of Care and Outcomes Research Interdisciplinary Working Group. 2007;116:1736-54.

CASE 16

Patent Ductus Arteriosus

■ PRESENTING COMPLAINTS

A 6-month-old boy was brought with the complaint of:
- Not gaining weight since 6 months
- Repeated cough and cold since 3 months

History of Presenting Complaints

A 6-month-old boy was brought to the pediatric outpatient department with history of not gaining weight. The boy used to get repeated respiratory tract infection over the last 3 months. Every time he was treated with full course of the antibiotics. His other developmental milestones were normal.

Past History of the Patient

He was the first sibling of nonconsanguineous marriage. He was delivered at full term, normally. He cried immediately after delivery. Cry of the baby was normal. The Apgar score at 1 minute was 8/10 and at 5 minutes was 10/10. The birth weight was 2.8 kg. The length was 49 cm. The head circumference was 34 cm. He started taking the breast milk regularly. He had transient tachypnea for 24 hours, and it was settled without any intervention. The child was discharged on 5th day of the delivery. The child was afebrile.

■ EXAMINATION

On examination, the baby was moderately built and poorly nourished. There was no dysmorphic features. Anthropometric measurements include the length 64 cm (50th centile) and weight 5 kg (3rd centile), and head circumference was 39 cm. The child was afebrile, the pulse rate was 126 beats/min and bounding and the respiratory rate was 26 breaths/min. The blood pressure recorded was 60/30 mm Hg. There was no cyanosis.

CASE AT A GLANCE

Basic Findings

Length	: 64 cm (50th centile)
Weight	: 5 kg (3rd centile)
Temperature	: 37°C
Pulse rate	: 126 beats/min, bounding
Respiratory rate	: 26 breaths/min
Blood pressure	: 60/30 mm Hg wide pulse pressure

Positive Findings

History:
- Failure to thrive
- Repeated respiratory infection

Examination:
- Underweight child
- Bounding pulse
- Wide pulse pressure
- Machinery murmur
- Hepatomegaly

Investigation:
- *Electrocardiogram (ECG):* Right ventricular hypertrophy
- *X-ray chest:* Cardiac enlargement and pulmonary vasculature

Cardiovascular examination revealed the presence of marked precordial impulse. The pulmonary component of the second heart sound was loud. A machinery murmur of irregular intensity and low pitch was heard. This was present both in the systole and diastole. It was audible under the left clavicle. The per abdomen examination shows the enlarged liver size of 5 cm below the costal margin. Respiratory system revealed occasional crepitation at both bases.

■ INVESTIGATION

- *Hemoglobin:* 12 g/dL
- *TLC:* 7,400 cells/cumm
- *ESR:* 26 mm in the first hour
- *ECG:* LVH
- *X-ray chest:* Cardiac enlargement, pulmonary vasculitis, and prominent pulmonary vasculature

■ DISCUSSION

A child came with the history of not gaining the weight and with repeated respiratory tract infection. On examination, the presence of the machinery murmur on auscultation, with the bounding pulse, and wide pulse pressure suggests the diagnosis of patent ductus arteriosus (PDA).

The ductus arteriosus is closed postnatally by constriction of smooth muscle in its wall. In full-term infants, this functional closure normally occurs within 10–15 hours after birth; however, complete anatomic obliteration of the ductus arteriosus is slower and it may be complete until the third postnatal month. Because PVR falls as soon as the lungs expand, in the first 10–15 hours when the ductus arteriosus is still open, a left-to-right shunt through the ductus arteriosus may occur, and a murmur may be heard.

Patent ductus arteriosus is the communication between the left pulmonary artery and descending aorta, i.e., 5 mm distal to the origin of left subclavian artery. PDA occurs in 5–10% of all CHDs. It is more common in female. Male to female ratio is 1:3. It is present in the fetal life. It closes functionally and anatomically soon after birth (1–5 days). The persistence of the ductus arteriosus is called PDA. Sometimes it may be associated with coarctation aorta.

■ CAUSES OF PERSISTENT PATENCY

A clinically apparent PDA occurs in premature infants with birth weights under 1,750 g and about 80% with birth weights under 1,000 g. The mechanisms responsible for continued patency are due to inability of the ductus arteriosus in immature infants to respond normally to an increased oxygen tension and to changes in prostaglandin concentrations.

When the term infant is found to have PDA, there is deficiency of both mucoid endothelial layer and muscular media of the ductus. Premature infants with patent ductus, however, has a normal structural anatomy. Patency is the result of immaturity. Hence PDA closes spontaneously in premature children.

The incidence of persistent patency of the ductus arteriosus in full-term infants born at high altitude is significantly higher than in those born at sea level, probably because of the lower atmospheric oxygen tension. Persistent patency of the ductus arteriosus in full term and occasional preterm infants at lower altitudes is generally related to a structural abnormality of the ductus arteriosus. Maternal rubella in the first trimester of pregnancy, however, is associated with a high incidence of persistent patency of the ductus arteriosus, and rubella virus has been cultured from ductal tissue.

It results in the left-to-right shunt, i.e., from aorta to pulmonary artery. The flow occurs both during systole and diastole. This is because pressure gradient is present throughout the cardiac cycle. The flow of the blood results in murmur. This starts in systole after the first sound. It reaches the peak at second sound. The murmur then diminishes in intensity and it is heard only in a part of diastole. This is the continuous murmur.

Patent ductus arteriosus results in the overloading of the pulmonary artery. The increased flow passing through the lungs reaches the left atrium. Left atrium enlarges to accommodate the flow. It reaches the left ventricle during diastole across the normal mitral valve.

The increased flow at the mitral valve produces the accentuation of the first heart sound and delayed diastolic murmur. The large volume of the blood in the left ventricle causes the prolongation of the LV systole. There will be increase in the size of the left ventricle to accommodate the extra volume. This produces the delayed closure of the aortic valve with large left-to-right shunt. S2 may be paradoxically split. The large LV volume is ejected into the aorta. This results in dilatation of the ascending aorta. The dilated ascending aorta results in aortic ejection click.

■ CLINICAL FEATURES (FIG. 1)

Patients are usually asymptomatic when the ductus is small. A large shunt PDA is accompanied by tachypnea, hyperdynamic circulation, and poor weight gain.

The increased volume load enlarges the left atrium and ventricle, with radiographic evidence of dilation and electrocardiographic evidence of hypertrophy. Because the ascending aorta receives the increased LV output, it is dilated. On chest radiograph, the pulmonary vascular markings indicate increased pulmonary flow. If there is

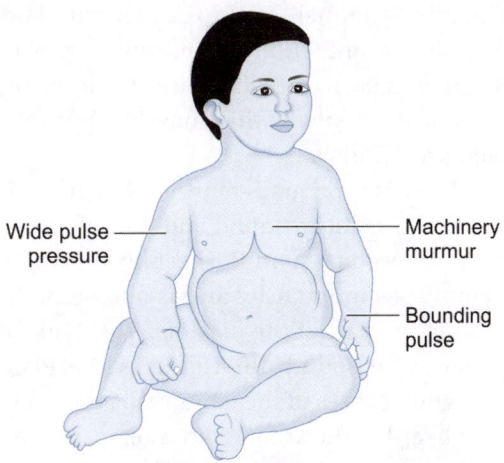

Fig. 1: Clinical features.

pulmonary hypertension, there may be signs of RV pressure overload.

These children become symptomatic in early life. They develop CCF around 6–10 weeks of age. Older children give the history of effort intolerance, palpitations, and frequent respiratory tract infections.

On examination, there is prominent bounding carotid pulsation in the neck. A leak from the systemic flow results in the flow from the aortic to pulmonary artery. This produces wide pulse pressure due to diastolic runoff through the ductus. The cardiac impulse is hyperkinetic. The systolic or continuous thrill may be palpated in the second left interspace. The first sound is accentuated. The second sound is loud, narrowly or paradoxically split with large left-to-right shunting hypertension. Paradoxical splitting is caused by volume overload of the LV and prolonged ejection of blood from this chamber.

The diagnosis of PDA is easier in full-term infants or older children than in premature infants. Because of continuous runoff of blood from the aorta to the pulmonary artery through the ductus arteriosus, the murmur in older infants and children is continuous and has a rumbling, machinery-like or "train-in-a-tunnel" quality usually with late systolic accentuation of the murmur. It is heard best below the left clavicle. If the ductus arteriosus is small, this may be the only abnormal finding.

There is continuous murmur, which starts after the first heart sound and it reaches the peak at second sound. The murmur then diminishes in intensity and is audible only during the part of the diastole. The peak at the second sound differentiates the PDA from other cases of the continuous murmur. It is heard at the second left interspace and also below the left clavicle. The other flow murmurs can be mitral delayed diastolic murmur and aortic ejection systolic murmur.

If the shunt is large, recurrent chest infection and CCF develop. Reversal of shunt takes place if a large PDA remains untreated and pulmonary hypertension develops. IE is more frequent with small PDA than large one.

ESSENTIAL DIAGNOSTIC POINTS
- Variable murmur with active precordium
- Bounding pulses
- More common in newborn premature infants
- Continuous machinery murmur

ECG: The ECG shows normal axis with LV dominance or hypertrophy. Deep "Q" waves in the left chest leads with tall "T" waves are characteristic of the volume overload in the left heart. In patients with pulmonary hypertension caused by increased blood flow, biventricular hypertrophy usually occurs.

Chest radiograph: The chest radiograph shows the cardiac enlargement. The cardiac size depends upon the size of the left-to-right shunt. The cardiac size is bigger with larger shunt. There may be left arterial enlargement. The ascending aorta and aortic knuckles are prominent. There is plethoric pulmonary vasculature.

Echocardiography: It can be imaged by 2D echo in parasternal or suprasternal notch view. The dimensions of left atrium and left ventricle provide an indirect assessment of magnitude of left-to-right shunt. It confirms the direction and degree of shunting. If suprasystemic PVR is present, flow across the ductus will be from right to left.

Cardiac catheterization: PDA closure by catheterization with a vascular plug or coils is now routine in but the smallest of neonates.

LABORATORY SALIENT FINDINGS
- Electrocardiogram (ECG) shows normal axis with left ventricular dominance or hypertrophy; deep "Q" waves in the left chest leads with tall "T" waves
- *Chest radiograph*: Cardiac enlargement, left arterial enlargement ascending aorta and aortic knuckles are prominent; plethoric pulmonary vasculature
- *Echo*: Dimension of left atrium (LA) and left ventricle (LV) provides an indirect assessment of magnitude of left-to-right shunt.

The evaluation of the size of the left-to-right shunt depends on a number of features:
- The larger the heart size, the larger the left-to-right shunt.
- The wider the pulse pressure, the larger the shunt.
- Audible delayed diastolic murmur suggests the large left-to-right shunt.

When a term infant is found to have a PDA, the wall of the ductus is deficient in both the mucoid endothelial layer and the muscular media, whereas in the premature infant the PDA usually has a normal structure. Thus a PDA persisting beyond the first few weeks of life in a term infant rarely closes spontaneously or with pharmocological intervention. If early pharmacologic or surgical intervention is not required in a premature infant, spontaneous closure occurs in most instances.

When PVR is increased, the diastolic component of the murmur may be less prominent or absent. In patients with a large left-to-right shunt, a low-pitched mitral mid-diastolic murmur may be audible at the apex as a result of the increased volume of blood flow across the mitral valve.

> **GENERAL FEATURES**
> - Failure to gain weight
> - Congestive cardiac failure
> - Repeated respiratory tract infection
> - Left ventricular hypertrophy

■ COMPLICATIONS

- Congestive cardiac failure
- Pulmonary arterial hypertension

Infective endarteritis may be seen at any age. Pulmonary or systemic emboli may occur. Rare complications include aneurysmal dilation of the pulmonary artery or the ductus, calcification of the ductus, noninfective thrombosis of the ductus with embolization, and paradoxical emboli. Pulmonary hypertension (Eisenmenger syndrome) usually develops in patients with a large PDA who do not undergo ductal closure.

■ DIFFERENTIAL DIAGNOSIS

- Coronary AV fistula
- Ruptured sinus of Valsalva
- Aortopulmonary septal defect
- Systemic AV fistula
- Pulmonary AV fistula
- Venous hum

■ TREATMENT

In the full-term infant with a PDA, spontaneous closure may occur, but much less commonly than in the premature infant. Medical management, if needed, should be instituted, and at a convenient time, surgical closure should be done.

Even if there is no heart failure, there are two reasons to close a PDA. If there is marked pulmonary hypertension as a result of a large communication, the danger of the development of pulmonary vascular disease necessitates closure, preferably before 6–8 months of age. In the older child with a small PDA, closure is often advised in view of the risk of IE, even though this risk is very low. Transcatheter closure with a coil is satisfactory if the diameter of the ductus is below 3 mm, but larger ductus can often be closed by devices such as the Amplatzer Duct Occluder.

Some ductus still need surgery, either because they are too large for a catheter-introduced device, or because an extremely premature infant has blood vessels that are too small to accept the large catheter needed to introduce coils or other devices. Surgery can be done safely by open thoracotomy or by thoracoscopy and may be a much shorter procedure than interventional catheterization. The surgical extrapleural approach to ligating the PDA has been shown to be cost-effective in developing countries.

Symptomatic PDA is common in preterm infants. Indomethacin, a prostaglandin synthesis inhibitor, is often used to close PDA in premature infants. Indomethacin does not close the PDA of full-term infants or children. The dose of indomethacin is 0.2 mg/kg/dose orally every 12–24 hours for three doses (second and third doses are 0.1 mg/kg/dose for <48-hour-old and 0.25 mg/kg/dose for <7-day-old newborn) can be used if there is adequate renal hematologic and hepatic function.

If indomethacin is not effective and ductus remains hemodynamically significant, surgical ligation should be performed. If ductus partially closes so that if shunt is no longer hemodynamically significant, a second course of indomethacin may be tried.

These patients may develop congestive cardiac failure (CCF). If the medical management cannot control the failure, then the patients may need echocardiography or cardiac catheterization for the confirmation of the diagnosis. The aortic valve around the aortic attachment of the PDA becomes more friable in adult life and increases the risk of tear during operation.

Surgical closure is indicated when the PDA and the patient is small. Patients with large left-to-right shunt require repair by 1 year to the development of progressive pulmonary vascular obstructive disease. Symptomatic PDA with normal pulmonary arterial pressure can safely coil device occluded by catheterization, ideally after the child has reached 5 kg.

Surgical indication is the anatomical existence of the lesion. Surgical procedure is performed any time between 6 months and 2 years and anytime in the older child. Procedure involves the ligation and division through left posterolateral thoracotomy, without cardiopulmonary bypass. This is safe procedure. Death occurs in <1% of patients.

Patent ductus arteriosus with pulmonary arterial hypertension need cardiac catheterization to exclude aortopulmonary defect. The patients are considered as inoperable if the right-to-left shunt has appeared because of pulmonary arterial hypertension.

Differential cyanosis occurs if the blood from the right-to-left shunt through the PDA flows down the descending aorta. Cyanosis is present in toes and not in fingers.

Infective endocarditis prophylaxis is indicated in the presence of small PDA. Catheter closure of ductus with different devices are present. These include double-umbrella device, buttoned device, and Gianturco coils.

BIBLIOGRAPHY

1. Cherif A, Jobnoun S, Khrouf N. Oral ibuprofen in early curative closure of patent ductus arteriosus in very premature infants. Am J Perinatol. 2007;24:339-45.
2. Takata H, Higaki T, Sugiyama H, Kitano M, Yamamoto E, Nakano T, et al. Long-term outcome of coil occlusion in patients with patent ductus arteriosus. Circ J. 2011; 75(2):407-12.

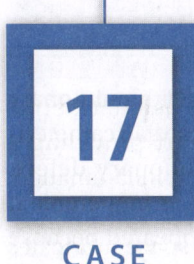

CASE 17

Pericarditis with Effusion

■ PRESENTING COMPLAINTS

An 8-year-old boy was brought with the complaint of:
- Distension of the abdomen since 6 months
- Tiredness since 2 months

History of Presenting Complaints

An 8-year-old boy was brought with the history of abdominal distension since last 6 months. His mother gave the history that her son is very weak and gets easily fatigued. She also told that the abdominal distension gradually increased in size. It was uniformly distended. There was no respiratory distress as a result of distension of the abdomen. His mother even told that he never used to play with other kids. He used to sit at one place and watched the others playing.

Past History of the Patient

He was the only sibling of the nonconsanguineous marriage. He was born at term with normal delivery. There was no significant postnatal event. The baby was discharged on fourth day. The baby was on exclusive breast milk for 6 months. Later weaning was started. He never had any problem. His developmental milestones were normal. His performance at school was good. Occasionally, he was complaining of left-sided chest pain. Recently it had increased in frequency.

CASE AT A GLANCE

Basic Findings

Height	:	125 cm (70th centile)
Weight	:	25 kg (75th centile)
Temperature	:	37°C
Pulse rate	:	100 beats/min
Respiratory rate	:	26 breaths/min
Blood pressure	:	70/50 mm Hg

Positive Findings

History:
- Abdominal distension
- Fatigability

Examination:
- Pale
- Increase in jugular venous pressure (JVP)
- Pedal pitting edema
- Muffled heart sounds
- Hepatosplenomegaly
- Shifting dullness

Investigation:
- Hypoproteinemia (4.8 g/dL)
- Hypoalbuminemia (2.4 g/dL)
- *X-ray chest:* Increase in the size of cardiac silhouette
- *Electrocardiogram (ECG):* Diffuse ST- and T-wave abnormalities; low voltage QRS complex

■ EXAMINATION

On examination, the boy was moderately built and moderately nourished. His anthropometric measurements included the height 125 cm (70th centile) and the weight 25 kg (75th centile).

He was afebrile. The pulse rate was 100 beats/min and respiratory rate was 26 breaths/min. Blood pressure recorded was 70/50 mm Hg. Jugular venous pressure (JVP) was raised especially in inspiration. There was no pallor, no lymphadenopathy, and no clubbing. Pedal pitting edema was present. Per abdomen examination revealed the presence of abdominal distension. The hepatomegaly was present about 3 cm below the costal margin. It was soft and nontender. Splenomegaly was also present. It was palpable about 2 cm below the costal margin. It was firm and nontender. Shifting dullness was present.

Cardiovascular system revealed the heart sounds are muffled and no murmur was heard. Respiratory system revealed the presence of course crepitations at the base.

■ INVESTIGATION

- *Hemoglobin:* 10 g/dL
- *TLC:* 14,000 cells/cumm
- *DLC:* $P_{72}\ L_{22}\ E_4\ M_2$
- *Platelet count:* 3,00,000/cumm
- *Total protein:* 4.8 g/dL
- *Albumin:* 2.4 g/dL
- *X-ray chest:* Increase in the size of cardiac silhouette and increase in cardio pericardial shadowing
- *ECG:* Diffuse ST- and T-wave abnormalities; low-voltage QRS complex
- *Echo:* Pericardium is closely adherent to epicardium; echo free space is present in between epicardium and pericardium.

■ DISCUSSION

Child had fluid overload, manifested by ascites, edema, and pulmonary edema. The liver is enlarged because of congestion and not of intraluminal infiltration and LV failure. Raised JVP during inspiration is Kussmaul's sign.

The pericardium serves as the external protective layer of the heart providing a barrier to trauma, malignancy, inflammation, and infection. In addition, a thin layer of fluid within the pericardial space lubricates the heart, therapy reducing the energy expenditure and shear stress encountered with cardiac motion. A basic understanding of the anatomy and physiology of the pericardium and pericardial space is necessary to recognize and properly diagnose disease processes affecting this important structure.

The pericardium is a fibrous lining surrounding the heart, consisting of two layers: The parietal (outer) layer and visceral (inner) layer. The visceral layer comes into direct contact with the epicardial surface, whereas the parietal layer contains collagenous fibers and serves as an outer protective layer. The pericardium completely envelops the atria and ventricles and terminates just superior to the semilunar valves, it also extends to surround the venae cavae and pulmonary veins near their respective entrances into the heart. Pericardial fluid is a serous, low-viscosity fluid found between the visceral pericardium and the epicardial surface of the heart. In children, approximately 10 mL of fluid is normally found within the pericardial space with larger volumes (20–30 mL) encountered in adults.

Chronic restriction to the right-side venous filling results in hepatic congestion, ascites, and pedal edema. Restriction at the left side produces pulmonary venous congestion. This manifests clinically as basal crepitation and increased frequency of chest infection. Bilateral restriction produces acute onset in cardiac tamponade. Chronic onset is seen in constructive pericarditis.

The causes of the acute pericarditis are bacterial, viral, tuberculosis, collagen, or uremic. The causes of chronic pericarditis are tuberculosis, post-pyogenic, and post-traumatic.

Pericarditis, or inflammation of the pericardium, is the most common cause of pericardial effusion in children. Pericarditis has numerous etiologies, with the most common including viral pathogens. Certain viral infections, such as enteroviruses (coxsackievirus), adenovirus, influenza, and parvovirus, have been associated. It is presumed that most cases of idiopathic pericarditis are related to viral infection, regardless of whether a prodromal illness or evidence of viral infection on laboratory testing is present. Bacterial (purulent) pericarditis is much less common and is associated with *S. aureus*, *Streptococcus pyogenes*, and *Neisseria meningitidis* organisms or mycobacterial infection (*Mycobacterium tuberculosis*). Frequently, there is a history of prior or concurrent bacterial infection by the same agent at another site, such as osteomyelitis, meningitis, or pneumonia. Unlike viral pericarditis, bacterial pericarditis does not resolve spontaneously and requires IV antibiotic therapy with pericardial drainage. The course may be fulminant, and prolonged courses of antibiotics and pericardial drainage are usually required.

Pericardial involvement occurs as a result of infective or inflammatory process. Within 48–72 hours, most cases of pericarditis will develop into the pericardial effusion. There will be accumulation of fluid within the pericardial sac. Clinical picture is determined by the degree of fluid accumulation. The normal amount of the fluid is 15–50 mL. Accumulated fluid may be serous, fibrinous, purulent, and hemorrhagic. Cardiac tamponade occurs when the amount of the pericardial fluid reaches the level that compromises cardiac functions.

Pyogenic infection will produce pyopericardium. Even a small amount may be significant clinically. There will be high fever, toxemia, and other clinical evidence of pyogenic infection such as pneumonia, empyema, and pyoderma. Tuberculosis follows the next. This is followed by viral infection.

The common causes of cardiac tamponade are tuberculosis trauma, uremia, neoplasm, and idiopathic.

In some cases pericardial disease occurs in association with a generalized process. Associations include rheumatic fever, rheumatoid arthritis, uremia, systemic lupus erythematosus (SLE), malignancy, and tuberculosis. Pericarditis after cardiac surgery (postpericardiotomy syndrome) is most commonly seen after surgical closure of an ASD.

Acute cardiac tamponade is acute heart failure due to the compression of heart by massive rapidly accumulating pericardial effusion in an otherwise nondistensible pericardial sac. There is significant rise in the intrathoracic pressure. There is rise in ventricular and diastolic atrial, systemic, and pulmonary venous pressure due to the impaired ventricular relaxation and filling, which results in poor cardiac output.

■ PATHOGENESIS

Inflammation of the pericardium may have only minor pathophysiologic consequences in the absence of significant fluid accumulation in the pericardial space. When the amount of fluid in the nondistensible pericardial space becomes excessive, pressure within the pericardium increases and is transmitted to the heart, resulting in impaired filling by compressing the chambers (atria or ventricles). Although small-to-moderate amounts of pericardial effusion can be well tolerated and clinically silent, once the noncompliant pericardium has been distended maximally, any further fluid accumulation causes abrupt impairment of cardiac filling and is termed cardiac tamponade. When untreated, tamponade can lead to shock and death. Pericardial effusions may be serous/transudative, exudative/purulent, and fibrinous and hemorrhagic.

Infectious Pericarditis

Agents identified as causing pericarditis include the enteroviruses, influenza, adenovirus, respiratory syncytial virus, and parvovirus. Because the course of this illness is usually benign, symptomatic treatment with nonsteroidal anti-inflammatory drugs (NSAIDs) is often sufficient. Persistent or early recurrence episodes may need courses of corticosteroids. Patients with large effusions and tamponade may require pericardiocentesis.

Purulent pericarditis, often caused by bacterial infections, has become much less common with the advent of new immunizations for *H. influenzae* and pneumococcal disease. Historically, purulent pericarditis was seen in association with severe pneumonias, epiglottitis meningitis, or osteomyelitis. Patients with purulent pericarditis are acutely ill. Unless the infection is recognized and treated expeditiously, the course can be fulminant, leading to tamponade and death.

Tuberculous pericarditis is rare in developed countries but can be a relatively common complication of human immunodeficiency virus (HIV) infection in regions where tuberculosis is endemic and access to antiretroviral therapy is limited. Immune complex-mediated pericarditis is a rare complication that may result in a nonpurulent (sterile) effusion following systemic bacterial infections such as meningococcus or *Haemophilus*.

Noninfectious Pericarditis

Systemic inflammatory diseases such as autoimmune, rheumatologic, and connective tissue disorders may involve the pericardium and result in serous pericardial effusions. Pericardial inflammation may be a component of the type II hypersensitivity reaction seen in patients with acute rheumatic fever. It is often associated with rheumatic valvulitis and responds quickly to anti-inflammatory agents, including corticosteroids. Tamponade is very uncommon.

Juvenile idiopathic arthritis, usually systemic-onset disease, can manifest with pericarditis. Differentiating rheumatoid pericardial inflammation from that seen with SLE is difficult and requires careful rheumatologic evaluation. Aspirin and corticosteroids can result in rapid resolution of a pericardial effusion but may be needed on a chronic basis to prevent relapse. Many of the autoinflammatory recurrent fever syndromes present with pericarditis, usually with other manifestations of those disorders.

Patients with chronic renal failure or hypothyroidism may have pericardial effusions. Clinical suspicion warrants careful screening with physical examination and, if indicated, imaging studies during the course of their illness.

The *postpericardiotomy syndrome* occurs in patients having undergone cardiac surgery and is characterized by fever, lethargy, anorexia, irritability, and chest/abdominal discomfort beginning 1–4 weeks postoperatively. There can be associated pleural effusions and serologic evidence of elevated antiheart antibodies. Postpericardiotomy syndrome is effectively treated with aspirin, NSAIDs, and in severe cases, corticosteroids. Pericardial drainage is necessary in those patients with cardiac tamponade.

Pericardial Effusion

Pericardial effusion is defined as the excess accumulation of fluid within the pericardial space. It is frequently but not universally, a manifestation of pericardial inflammation. The most common cause of pericardial effusion in children is pericarditis, which in turn has a variety of etiologies.

The causes of pericardial effusion and pericarditis can broadly be categorized into infectious, inflammatory autoimmune, traumatic, toxic, and idiopathic. Infectious etiologies are the most common, and most often in conjunction with viral infections associated with pericardial inflammation or as part of a broader cardiac inflammatory process (i.e., myocarditis).

Bacterial seeding of the pericardial space occurs less frequently; however, tuberculosis is a common cause of pericarditis and pericardial effusion in developing countries. Many autoimmune processes may have an associated pericarditis, such as SLE, in which pericardial effusion may be a presenting sign of the disease.

Trauma is a common cause of pericardial effusion via confusion of the heart or direct perforation of the pericardium by penetrating thoracic injury. Several environmental toxins and drugs can be associated with pericardial effusion; in pediatric practice, this is often associated with chemotherapeutic agents or chest irradiation in the setting of treatment for malignancy. Finally, interruption or obstruction of the lymphatic drainage in the chest, usually encountered in the postoperative setting after cardiac surgery in children, may manifest as pericardial effusion with high triglyceride content (chylopericardium).

The hemodynamic effects of pericardial effusion, as well as the presence and nature of symptoms, depend on a number of factors. The size of the fluid collection is the most important determinant of symptoms. In addition, the rate at which a pericardial effusion accumulates has an effect on symptoms. Relatively small accumulations of fluid that develop rapidly (e.g., hemopericardium occurring in the setting of trauma) may be life-threatening. In contrast, in other etiologies with a more indolent clinical course, gradual accumulation of pericardial fluid allows time for the pericardium to stretch and therefore adapt to the anatomic and physiologic changes brought about by the presence of sizeable fluid collections.

Pericardial effusions exert their adverse hemodynamic effects by impeding cardiac filling in diastole, which in turn lowers stroke volume and cardiac output. With the accumulation of sufficient pericardial fluid, intrapericardial pressure exceeds atrial pressure leading to collapse of the atrial cavity, impairment of cardiac filling, and limitation of cardiac output, a scenario known as cardiac tamponade. If unrecognized or left untreated, tamponade may quickly progress to circulatory collapse and death.

The initial physiologic response to pericardial effusion is an increase in heart rate, allowing for preservation of cardiac output in the setting of lower stroke volume. Hypotension is a late and ominous finding and may herald impending shock and circulatory collapse. In addition to tachycardia, other physical examination findings in patients with significant pericardial effusions include narrow pulse pressure, jugular venous pulsations, and tachypnea, Hepatomegaly may be present in large effusions that have enlarged gradually. Cardiac auscultation will reveal muffled or distant heart tones. A pericardial friction rub, resembling the crackling sound, created by rubbing a tuft of hair between two fingers, will often be present in small pericardial effusions but absent in large collections.

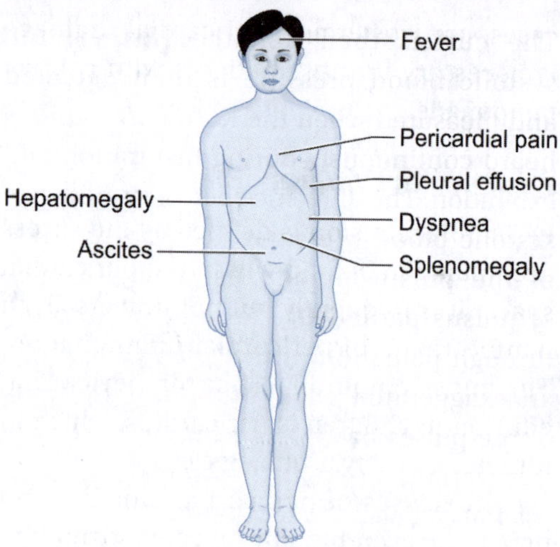

> **ESSENTIAL DIAGNOSTIC POINTS**
>
> - Retrosternal pain aggravated deep inspiration and relieved leaning forward
> - Fever
> - Pericardial friction rub
> - Tachycardia
> - Shortness of breath
> - Distention of jugular veins
> - Hepatomegaly
> - Electrocardiogram (ECG) with ST segment

Fig. 1: Clinical features.

■ CLINICAL FEATURES (FIG. 1)

The most common symptom of pericarditis is chest pain, which is usually sharp in nature and localized to the left midsternal region. Older patients may describe a sensation of heaviness in the chest, often relieved by leaning forward and exacerbated by inspiration: Frequently, there is associated fever. In younger patients, a history of irritability and feeding intolerance is common. Auscultation may reveal a pericardial friction rub, the hallmark physical examination finding in pericarditis.

The chest pain of the pericarditis is dull, sharp, and stabbing is nature. The pain radiates to epigastrium, neck, shoulder or left arm. The pain increases on lying down and on deep inspiration and decreases on sitting down and with forward bending. Child becomes dyspneic and will have cough. The type of fever depends on the etiology.

The pericardial sac is devoid of nerve supply. Hence, the pain is due to adjacent diaphragmatic or pleural irritation. The symptoms and signs in the pericardial effusion are due to the severe cardiac compression, impairment of ventricular diastolic filling, increased systemic pulmonary venous pressure, and eventually due to severely compromised cardiac output and shock.

An important physical examination finding frequently used to assess this risk is known as pulsus paradoxus. Normally, systolic blood pressure varies by a few mm Hg throughout the respiratory cycle, with the blood pressure decreasing during inspiration due to increased intrathoracic pressure. In a hemodynamically significant pericardial effusion, this normal respiratory variation in blood pressure is exaggerated, with systolic blood pressure decreasing by >10 mm Hg during inspiration. Pulsus paradoxus is caused by limitation of LV filling in the setting of a significant pericardial fluid collection. Pulsus paradoxus is demonstrated using a manual blood pressure cuff; the patient should be supine and breathing spontaneously.

The blood pressure cuff is inflated, and with deflation, auscultation is used to detect and measure the systolic blood pressure at which the Korotkoff sound is first heard.

The cuff is then deflated further; the systolic blood pressure is then detected and measured when the Korotkoff sound is heard continuously during inspiration and expiration. The difference between these two systolic blood pressures is the magnitude of the pulsus paradoxus. The presence of pulsus paradoxus can also be inferred through palpation of the pulses (in which an exaggerated change in the amplitude of the pulses can be detected with normal respiration) or in patients with invasive arterial catheters (in whom the magnitude of the blood pressure change can be observed on the cardiorespiratory monitor).

The diagnostic physical sign is pericardial friction rub. This is rough, scratchy sound. There are three components: (1) A systolic, (2) a diastolic, and (3) presystolic scratch. It can be heard anywhere over the pericardium. Pericardial friction rub is best heard with diaphragm. It is firmly pressed on the sternal border and over the base of the heart. It has to and fro components. It is always in phase with heart sounds.

Physical findings depend on the presence of fluid accumulation in the pericardial space (effusion). If the effusion is large, heart sounds are distant and muffled and a friction rub may not be present. In the absence of cardiac tamponade, the peripheral, venous, and arterial pulses are normal.

In a patient with suspected pericardial effusion, rapid clinical assessment is necessary to determine whether there is evidence of existing or impending cardiac tamponade. If the effusion develops, the cardiac silhouette increases in size. The heart sounds are muffled. These are evidences if peripheral congestion such as raised JVP, hepatomegaly, and edema. If the fluid is accumulated rapidly, then the features of cardiac tamponade such as raising JVP, paradoxical inspiratory filling of the neck veins, increasing heart rate, and pulsus paradoxus appear.

GENERAL FEATURES

- Muffled heard sound
- Low-voltage QRS complex
- Water bottle configuration

■ DIAGNOSIS

Diagnostic testing for suspected pericarditis usually involves an ECG, echocardiogram, and laboratory assessment.

Serum inflammatory markers, such as the erythrocyte sedimentation rate and CRP, are usually elevated, albeit in nonspecific fashion. Serum troponin is a sensitive marker for cardiac injury. In pericarditis, serum troponin is normal or minimally elevated; this is in contrast to myocarditis, myocardial trauma, or myocardial ischemia.

An echocardiogram is indicated to assess for pericardial effusion, AV valve regurgitation, and for determination of ventricular systolic function. In pericarditis, a pericardial effusion is usually present, and importantly, ventricular function is preserved. The presence of impaired ventricular function, significant AV or semilunar valvar regurgitation, and/or cardiac chamber dilation is suggestive of an alternative diagnosis, such as myocarditis or cardiomyopathy.

Ultrasonography: The diagnosis is easily made with ultrasonography Areas of collection whether posterior or anterior can be made. In acute cardiac tamponade, ultrasonography shows significant pericardial effusion right atrial collapse, RV diastolic collapse. There will be absent increased early diastolic filling and mitral flow velocity.

Electrocardiography: It may show sinus tachycardia with low QRS voltage amplitudes; in severe cases, electrical alternans, the presence of variation in QRS amplitude from beat to beat, can be observed. If there is associated pericarditis or myocarditis, there may be ST-segment and T-wave abnormalities. These changes are more diffusely distributed through the precordial and limb leads compared to the ST-segment and T-wave changes observed with myocardial ischemia.

Radiograph of chest: Radiograph of chest shows enlarged cardiac silhouette with water bottle configuration. It shows normal-sized heart with ragged or shaggy borders, prominent superior venal shadow margin with right atrial margin. The lungs show pleural effusion.

Echo: Normally echo shows the pericardium is closely adherent to the epicardium. The two layers can only be separated by ultrasound beam. In patients with effusion, the clear echo free space is present in between epicardium and pericardium. Serial echocardiography allows a direct, noninvasive estimate of the volume of pericardial fluid and its change over time. Cardiac tamponade is associated with compression of the atria or respiratory alteration of ventricular inflow demonstrated by Doppler imaging.

> **LABORATORY SALIENT FINDINGS**
> - *Electrocardiogram (ECG):* Diminished QRS voltages and generalized ST segment elevation, T wave flattening and inversion
> - *Ultrasonography:* Areas of collection whether posterior or anterior can be made.
> - Radiograph of chest shows enlarged cardiac silhouette with water bottle configuration, normal-sized heart with ragged or shaggy borders, lungs show pleural effusion
> - *Echo:* The echo free space between epicardium and pericardium

■ DIFFERENTIAL DIAGNOSIS

Differential diagnosis includes myocarditis, purulent pericarditis, acute rheumatic fever, juvenile rheumatoid arthritis, uremia, and neoplastic disease.

■ TREATMENT

Treatment depends on the cause of pericarditis and the size of the associated effusion. Viral pericarditis is usually self-limited and symptoms can be improved with nonsteroidal anti-inflammatory therapy. Purulent pericarditis requires immediate evacuation of the fluid and appropriate antibiotic therapy.

Idiopathic or viral-associated pericarditis is most often a self-limited process, with therapy mainly being supportive. This is in contrast to bacterial pericarditis, in which patients are systemically often bacteremic. The long-term prognosis for viral-associated pericarditis is favorable, although recurrence may occur in as much as approximately 30% of patients.

Nonsteroidal anti-inflammatory agents (ibuprofen, naproxen, and indomethacin) are often useful at alleviating symptoms Corticosteroids (prednisone, methylprednisolone) have been used in refractory cases. There has been increasing study of the mictrotubule assembly inhibitor, colchicine in the primary treatment of pericarditis, which in recent studies has been demonstrated to be superior to NSAIDs alone in effecting the resolution of symptoms. Colchicine also has value in the prevention of recurrent pericarditis. There is limited experience with the use of colchicine in infants and very young children.

Cardiac tamponade from any cause must be treated by immediate removal of the fluid, usually via pericardiocentesis.

Pericardiocentesis should also be considered if the underlying cause is unclear or identification of the pathogen is necessary for targeted therapy. In the setting of recurrent or persistent effusions, a surgical pericardiectomy or pericardial window may be necessary. Diuretics should be avoided in the patient with cardiac tamponade, because they reduce ventricular preload and can exacerbate the degree of cardiac decompensation.

Pericardiocentesis

Pericardiocentesis is done for diagnostic purpose, but if the collection is large resulting in tamponade, therapeutic removal of significant amount of fluid becomes essential.

Viral effusion needs only symptomatic treatment. It resolves spontaneously in 2–4 weeks. Other conditions such as collagen vascular disease are treated appropriately and effusion resolves slowly with steroids. Surgical drainage is rarely indicated unless the fluid is thick and fibrinous. Surgical decortication is indicated in constrictive pericarditis.

For patients with symptomatic pericardial effusion, impending cardiac tamponade, or rank tamponade, gentamicin drainage of the fluid (pericardiocentesis) by percutaneous means may be lifesaving. Surgical drainage of pericardial effusion is usually limited to patients with bacterial pericarditis or in patients with chronic, recurrent effusions (pericardial window). In the presence of tamponade, temporizing medical therapy includes oxygen, fluid resuscitation to augment preload, and avoidance of agents that decrease systemic vascular resistance (SVR). Diuretics, sometimes used in small effusions without hemodynamic compromise, should be avoided if there is concern for tamponade.

Pericardiocentesis is usually performed with real-time echocardiographic guidance. A long needle is advanced into the pericardial space from the subxiphoid region, with brisk flow of fluid from the needle confirming entry into the pericardial space. Frank blood from the needle may indicate hemopericardium or entry into heart itself. After acute drainage of fluid, a catheter is usually advanced over a wire into the pericardial space to allow for continued drainage while the inciting process for the effusion resolves. Pericardial fluid should be sent for cell count analysis, Gram stain, cytology, and culture for diagnostic purposes. Testing of pericardial fluid via PCR methods is available and can rapidly identify many viral etiologies of pericarditis.

In pyogenic pericardial effusion, the pus in the pericardial sac is surgically drained after the institution of appropriate antibiotics. Tuberculosis effusion is treated with a minimum of three antitubercular drugs and initial course of steroids. Chronic constrictive pericarditis is treated surgically. It can be prevented by early pericardiectomy.

Postpericardiotomy Syndrome

Postpericardiotomy syndrome is a distinct entity encountered in children after cardiac surgery at which the pericardium has been opened. Postpericardiotomy syndrome typically presents with fever beyond the first postoperative week (without evidence of infection elsewhere), new pericardial effusion, chest pain, friction rub, and in some cases, new pleural effusions. It is encountered in all age groups and surgeries, but for unclear reasons, it appears to be more commonly encountered in patients who have undergone atrial surgery (e.g., surgical ASD repair, AV canal defect repair). It is also common after heart transplantation.

The etiology is uncertain but is felt to have an inflammatory component. Patients may present several weeks to months after surgery, so it is important for clinicians to be aware of this diagnosis in patients with a history of cardiac surgery. Treatment includes nonsteroidal anti-inflammatory agents and pericardiocentesis for large fluid collections.

PROGNOSIS

Prognosis depends to a great extent on the cause of pericardial disease. Constrictive pericarditis can develop following infectious pericarditis (especially if bacterial or tuberculous) and can be a difficult problem to manage. Cardiac tamponade will result in death unless the fluid is evacuated.

BIBLIOGRAPHY

1. Cakir O, Gurkan F, Balci AE, Eren N, Dikici B. Purulent pericarditis in childhood: ten years of experience. J Pediatr Surg. 2002;37:1404-8.
2. Fitch MT, Nicks BA, Pariyadath M, McGinnis HD, Manthey DE. Emergency pericardiocentesis. N Engl J Med. 2012;366(12):e17.
3. LeWinter MM. Clinical practice. Acute pericarditis. N Engl J Med. 2014;371:2410-6.
4. Lilly LS. Treatment of acute and recurrent idiopathic pericarditis. Circulation. 2013;27;1723-26.
5. Ratnapalan S, Brown K, Benson L. Children presenting with acute pericarditis to the emergency room. Pediatr Emerg Care. 2011;27(7):581-5.
6. Spodick DH. Macrophysiology, microphysiology, and anatomy of the pericardium: a synopsis. Am Heart J. 1992;124:1046-51.

CASE 18

Sydenham's Chorea

■ PRESENTING COMPLAINTS

A 9-year-old boy was brought with the complaint of:
- Abnormal movement since 2 months
- Difficulty in holding the pen since 1 month.

History of Presenting Complaints

A 9-year-old girl with a history of involuntary movements came to the pediatric outpatient department. Her mother told that her daughter developed the involuntary movements two months back. In the beginning the movements were minimal which increased later on. The movements were observed to be aggravated by stress and emotional instability. The movements used to be irregular, nonrepetitive involving mainly distal parts, i.e., fingers and toes. The girl used to have difficulty in holding pen or spoon. These involuntary movements used to be absent in the night.

Past History of the Patient

She was the second sibling of the nonconsanguineous marriage. She was born at full term after normal delivery. There was no significant postnatal event. The child's developmental milestones were normal.

Her performance at school was satisfactory. There was a past history of joint pain, fever, and throat pain. For these complaints she had been treated by the general practitioner.

■ EXAMINATION

On examination, the girl appeared more clumsy with a reserved look to control her involuntary movements. She was moderately built and nourished. The anthropometric measurements included her height 128 cm (50th centile) and the weight 26 kg (75th centile). She was afebrile, her heart rate was 96 beats/min and respiratory rate was

---

CASE AT A GLANCE

Basic Findings
Height	: 128 cm (50th centile)
Weight	: 26 kg (75th centile)
Temperature	: 37°C
Pulse rate	: 96 beats/min
Respiratory rate	: 18 breaths/min
Blood pressure	: 90/60 mm Hg

Positive Findings

History:
- Girl
- Involuntary movements
- Past history of joint pain

Examination:
- Clumsy look
- Distal involuntary movements
- Pallor
- Sustained contraction at knee joint

Investigation:
- Erythrocyte sedimentation rate test (ESR): 32 mm
- Anti-streptolysin O (ASLO): 400 Todd units

18 breaths/min. The blood pressure recorded was 90/60 mm Hg.

There was neither pallor, lymphadenopathy, icterus, nor clubbing. Throat was clear. Involuntary movements were mainly found in the distal part of the extremities. The movements were nonrepetitive and quasi-purpose. Tongue used to be out of the mouth. Knee jerk showed some sustained contraction. All the systemic examinations were normal.

■ INVESTIGATION

- *Hemoglobin:* 9 g/dL
- *TLC:* 8,800 cells/cumm
- *ESR:* 32 mm in first hour
- *Anti-streptolysin O (ASLO):* 400 Todd units
- *CRP:* 1250 µg/dL (normal range: 67–1,800 µg/L)
- *X-ray chest:* Normal
- *ECG:* Normal

■ DISCUSSION

Chorea may precede or follow other manifestations of the rheumatic fever. It usually occurs in the later part of the rheumatic fever. It is one of the major criteria of the diagnosis of the rheumatic fever. One-third of these patients develop rheumatic valvular heart disease. The usual age of onset of the disease is 5–15 years.

It is an autoimmune response to CNS to group A streptococcal organism. Antineural antibodies cross-react with cytoplasm of the subthalamic and caudate nuclei. The primary pathological changes include vasculitis of the cortical arterioles and round cell infiltration of the gray and white matter.

■ CLINICAL FEATURES (FIG. 1)

Chorea is the functional overactivity of the dopaminergic system. Classically, the movements are described as irregular,

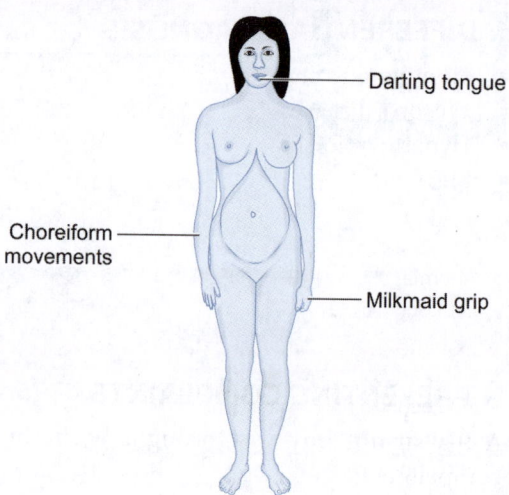

Fig. 1: Clinical features.

nonrepetitive, quasi-purpose, and involuntary. They are usually proximal but may affect fingers, hands, extremities, and face. The child may appear clumsy. Movements may be limited to one side of the body as in hemiballismus. The movements are aggravated by attention, stress, or excitement. But they disappear during sleep.

The relaxing hand grip, on and off as if she is milking the cow—milkmaid sign. The child cannot maintain the tongue in protruded position—darting tongue sign. The knee reflex may show sustained contractions resulting in a hung-up reflex. ASLO titer may not be elevated as onset of the chorea is late.

GENERAL FEATURES
• Movements aggravated by stress, attention • Absent at the time of sleep

ESSENTIAL DIAGNOSTIC POINTS
• Acute onset of choreiform movement • Associated with rheumatic endocarditis and arthritis • Autoimmune response to central nervous system (CNS) to group A streptococcal organism • Classically, the movements are described as irregular, nonrepetitive, quasi-purpose, and involuntary

DIFFERENTIAL DIAGNOSIS

- Huntington's chorea
- Wilson's disease
- Hyperthyroidism
- SLE

LABORATORY SALIENT FINDINGS

- Anemia
- Leukocytosis
- Increased ESR
- ASLO and CRP may be raised
- ECG echo to find cardiac problems
- Antineural antibodies are present
- EEG shows nonspecific seizure activity
- MRI SPECT may show basal ganglia abnormalities

(ASLO: anti-streptolysin O; CRP: C-reactive protein; ECG: electrocardiogram; EEG: electroencephalogram; ESR: erythrocyte sedimentation rate; MRI: magnetic resonance imaging; SPECT: single-photon emission computerized tomography)

TREATMENT

This disorder is usually self-limiting and may last for few weeks to few months. Child should be protected from the injury. These children may be treated with chlorpromazine, haloperidol, sodium valproate, or carbamazepine.

The dosage is determined by minimum doses for the symptom suppression. Aspirin and steroid help to limit the course of the chorea and are the important modalities of treatment in resistant cases. Antistreptococcal prophylaxis with penicillin G should be given to prevent recurrence of the rheumatic activity.

BIBLIOGRAPHY

1. Cardoso F, Seppi K, Mair KJ, Wenning GK, Poewe W. Seminar on choreas. Lancet Neurol. 2006;5(7);589-602.
2. Keller S, Dure LS. Tremor in childhood. Semin Pediatr Neurol. 2009;16(2):60-70.

CASE 19

Tetralogy of Fallot

■ PRESENTING COMPLAINTS

A 3-year-old boy was brought with the complaint of:
- Breathlessness since 1 day
- Bluish color of the lips since 2 hours
- Floppy since 1 hour.

History of Presenting Complaints

A 3-year-old boy was brought to the pediatric casualty with the history of bluish color of the lips and breathlessness. The mother of the boy told that the child was normal before going to bed last night. In the morning, he first developed difficulty in breathing and became breathless. Later, he developed the bluish color of the lips and became floppy. Then the child was brought to the hospital where he was treated with oxygen.

Past History of the Patient

The boy was born at full term with normal delivery. He cried immediately after the delivery. He was stable at birth. There was no bluish color at the time of delivery. There was no significant postnatal event except for transient tachypnea, which was settled within 24 hours.

Child was on breast milk for 6 months and weaning started later with cereals and fruits. He was on family food by the age of 15 months. His mother gave history of the dusky coloration of the lips at the age of 3 months while crying. Then he had been completely evaluated and diagnosed to have Fallot's tetralogy. Later at the age of 15 months, he became bluish even at rest. His mother had noticed that he becomes floppy having developed a bluish color.

■ EXAMINATION

The child appears moderately built and nourished. He was having breathlessness

CASE AT A GLANCE

Basic Findings

Height	: 100 cm (90th centile)
Weight	: 12 kg (80th centile)
Temperature	: 37°C
Pulse rate	: 116 beats/min
Respiratory rate	: 36 breaths/min
Blood pressure	: 90/60 mm Hg

Positive Findings

History:
- Bluish color
- Floppy
- Known tetralogy of Fallot (TOF)

Examination:
- Cyanotic spell
- Polycythemia
- Clubbing
- Ejection systolic murmur

Investigation:
- *Hemoglobin:* 18 g/dL
- *X-ray chest:* Boot-shaped heart
- *Echocardiogram (ECG):* Right-axis deviation
- *Echo:* Hypertrophied right ventricle

and was uncomfortable. He was floppy. Anthropometric measurements included his height 100 cm (above 90th centile) and the weight 12 kg (above 80th centile).

He was febrile. The pulse rate was 116 beats/min and the respiratory rate was 36 breaths/min. The blood pressure recorded was 90/60 mm Hg. There was no pallor. Clubbing was present. Cyanosis was evident.

Cardiovascular system revealed the presence of single pulmonary second sound. Ejection systolic murmur was heard over the left second intercostal space. Other systemic examination was normal.

■ INVESTIGATION

- *Hemoglobin:* 18 g/dL
- *TLC:* 12,000 cells/cumm
- *DLC:* $P_{74} L_{20} E_2 M_2$
- *ESR:* 26 mm in the first hour
- *ECG:* Right-axis deviation
- *Arterial blood gas (ABG):* pH—7; partial pressure of arterial carbon dioxide ($PaCO_2$)—55 mm Hg; partial pressure of arterial oxygen (PaO_2)—45 mm Hg; HCO_3—18 mEq/L
- *X-ray chest:* Boot-shaped heart with prominent right ventricle—pulmonary oligemia and hyperlucent lung field
- *Echo:* Hypertrophied right ventricle with a small outlet; overriding of aorta on the ventricle and VSD

■ DISCUSSION

A 3-year-old boy presented with cyanosis and breathlessness, and it was relieved after medical management. On examination, child was cyanosed and clubbing was present. Cardiovascular system revealed ejection systolic murmur. This along with chest radiograph, ECG, and echo findings, the diagnosis of Fallot's tetralogy was made. TOF occurs in 10% of all CHDs. This is the most common cyanotic CHD seen beyond infancy.

It is the most common cyanotic CHD in a child above the age of 2 years. Anatomically, it consists of VSD associated with obstruction at RV outflow. This is in the form of infundibular or infundibular plus valvular pulmonic stenosis. The right ventricle hypertrophies, not because of pulmonary stenosis (PS), but because it is pumping against systemic resistance across a (usually) large VSD. ASD occurs in 15%.

Obstruction to RV outflow with a large VSD causes a right-to-left shunt at the ventricular level with arterial desaturation. The greater the obstruction and the lower the SVR, the greater is the right-to-left shunt. TOF is associated with deletions in the long arm of chromosome 22 (22q11, DiGeorge syndrome) in as many as 15% of affected children. This is especially common in those with an associated right aortic arch.

The basic lesion is anterocephaloid malalignment of the outlet septum relative to the muscular septum. This is associated with unequal division of the truncus arteriosus into small pulmonary and large aortic components. The malalignment together with secondary hypertrophy of the muscle form the primary site of obstruction to blood flow in the infundibulum or outflow tract of the right ventricle. In addition, the pulmonary valve is often stenotic, and the pulmonary valve annulus and pulmonary arteries are often hypoplastic.

The four constituents of tetralogy includes VSD, pulmonic stenosis, overriding or dextroposed aorta and RV hypertrophy. Other associated features are right aortic arch in 25% of cases. Pulmonic annulus and main pulmonary artery are hypoplastic. Abnormal coronary artery is present.

In the most severe form of TOF with pulmonary atresia, the distal infundibular outflow tract and pulmonary valve are atretic. The pulmonary artery and main pulmonary arterial branches may be severely hypoplastic or atretic. Often, large aortopulmonary collaterals supply most of the lung. The VSD is usually large, perimembranous with outlet extension, and near the tricuspid and aortic valves. The aorta arises directly over the VSD; the degree of overriding varies greatly.

Pulmonic stenosis causes concentric RVH without cardiac enlargement and an increase in RV pressure. When the RV pressure is as high as LV or the aortic pressure, the right-to-left shunt appears to decompress the right ventricle. Increasing severity of the PS reduces flow of blood into the pulmonary artery, and increases right-to-left shunt. Because of the pulmonary outflow tract obstruction, varying amounts of systemic venous blood are shunted across the VSD into the aorta, resulting in cyanosis. Pulmonary artery pressure and pulmonary blood flow are reduced.

The flow from the right ventricle into the pulmonary artery occurs across the pulmonic stenosis and produces an ejection systolic murmur. The more severe the pulmonic stenosis, the shorter the ejection systolic murmur, and the more the cyanosis. Thus the severity of the cyanosis is directly proportional to the severity of the pulmonic stenosis. The intensity of the systolic murmur is inversely related to severity of pulmonic stenosis.

Since right ventricle is effectively decompressed by VSD, CCF never occurs. But it can occur if there are anemia, IE, systemic hypertension, myocarditis, and aortic or pulmonary wall regurgitation.

The RV outflow obstructions produce delay in P2. The ascending aorta is large and may result in aortic ejection click. Concentric RVH reduces the distensibility of the right ventricle during diastole. The right atrial contraction at the end of diastole causes a relatively large "a" waves. In acyanotic TOF, i.e., VSD with mild PS, long pansystolic murmur resulting from VSD and infundibular stenosis is audible. Ejection systolic murmur is heard in pulmonary area. Cyanosis is absent.

■ CLINICAL FEATURES (FIG. 1)

The clinical findings at birth vary with the severity of the PS, but few infants with the TOF remain asymptomatic or acyanotic. Cyanosis may not be present at birth; as long as the ductus arteriosus remains patent, there may be adequate pulmonary blood flow, or the outflow tract obstruction may not be severe at birth.

The patient may become symptomatic any time after birth. Neonates may develop anoxic spell. The most common symptoms are dyspnea on exertion and exercise intolerance. The patients assume a squatting posture as soon as they become dyspneic.

Most cases of TOF are mildly cyanosed at birth. Exertional dyspnea, squatting, and hypoxic spells develop later in life. Acyanotic

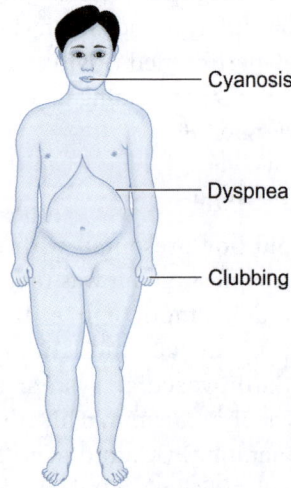

Fig. 1: Clinical features.

TOF with a large VSD will present with CCF. Presence of severe cyanosis at birth signifies atresia with VSD.

Clinical findings vary with the degree of RV outflow obstruction. Patients with mild obstruction are minimally cyanotic or acyanotic. Those with severe obstruction are deeply cyanotic from birth. Few children are asymptomatic those with significant RV outflow obstruction, many have cyanosis at birth, and nearly all have cyanosis by age of 4 months. The cyanosis usually is progressive, as subvalvular obstruction increases.

Physical examination shows a RV systolic heave along the lower left sternal border. A single loud second heart sound corresponding to aortic valve closure is generally heard best at the lower left sternal border, rather than being heard best at the upper right or both the upper right and left sternal borders. This physical sign is important, especially in a neonate when trying to differentiate an acyanotic TOF from a VSD. When closure of the pulmonary valve is audible at the upper left sternal border, it is delayed and diminished in intensity.

In patients with moderate RVOT obstruction, the mid-to-high pitch systolic murmur is loud and harsh, stenotic or pansystolic in quality, and best heard at the middle or lower left sternal border. Rarely, a continuous murmur of persistent ductus arteriosus is heard at the upper left sternal border. As there is less ejection through an increasingly stenotic pulmonary outflow tract, the murmur will shorten in duration and will increase in pitch.

Growth and development are not typically delayed, but easy fatigability and dyspnea on exertion are common. The fingers and toes show variable clubbing depending on age and severity of cyanosis. Infants who are acyanotic at birth, become cyanosed by 8–12 weeks of life. Hypoxic spell may develop depending upon the RV obstruction. Brain abscess, cerebrovascular accidents, and IE are occasional complications. Since central cyanosis predisposes to polycythemia, iron deficiency anemia, and coagulopathy are common.

Hypercyanotic episodes with paroxysmal hyperpnea may occur spontaneously or after early morning feedings or prolonged crying. The attacks may last only a few moments and have no sequelae; they may cause obtundation, limpness, deep exhaustion, or sleep; rarely, they may end in unconsciousness, convulsions, or even death.

Hypoxemic spells, also-called cyanotic or "Tet spells", are one of the hallmarks of severe TOF. These spells can occur spontaneously and at any time, but in infants occur most commonly with crying or feeding, while in older children they can occur with exercise. They are characterized by (1) sudden onset of cyanosis or deepening of cyanosis; (2) dyspnea; (3) alterations in consciousness, from irritability to syncope; and (4) decrease or disappearance of the systolic murmur (as RVOT becomes completely obstructed). These episodes most commonly start as age of 4–6 months.

Because approximately one-third of patients with the TOF begin to have hypoxic spells by 4 or 5 months of age, palliative or corrective surgery is usually done electively within a few months of birth. A few of these infants have minor spells. Their cyanosis may not increase much, but they cry inconsolably. They are often misdiagnosed as colic putting them on the abdomen with a knee–chest position aborts the crying and may make the diagnosis.

Young children with the TOF and severe cyanosis often adopt a characteristic squatting position after exertion. This maneuver increases arterial oxygen saturation (SaO_2), probably by increasing systemic arterial resistance. A final group of patients shows little or no evidence of cyanosis in infancy or early childhood (acyanotic TOF); cyanosis on exertion gradually becomes more manifest as they grow older.

In TOF, the dilated aortic root overrides a large adjacent VSD, and varying degrees of RV infundibular obstruction, pulmonary valve stenosis, and hypoplasia or narrowing of the main pulmonary artery and left pulmonary artery are revealed by echocardiogram. Doppler examination confirms the severity of the obstruction and demonstrates systolic turbulence in the main pulmonary artery.

The acute severe episodes of dyspnea and hypoxemia, termed blue spells or hypercyanotic episodes, in some infants with the TOF reflect a further acute reduction in the pulmonary blood flow. These spells may occur even if the infant is not cyanotic at rest. The precipitating mechanisms are probably multiple: Prolonged crying may decrease pulmonary blood flow because of prolonged expirations; decreases in RV preload and SVR because of sleeping, fever, or spontaneous vasomotor changes decrease pulmonary blood flow and increase the right-to-left shunt and constriction of the RV infundibulum may occur further decreasing pulmonary blood flow, although it is uncertain whether this truly occurs.

Cardiac catheterization demonstrates a systolic pressure in the right ventricle equal to the systemic pressure, since the right ventricle is connected directly to the overriding aorta. If the pulmonary artery is entered, the pressure is greatly decreased, although crossing the RVOT especially in severe cases, may precipitate a tet spell. Pulmonary artery pressure is usually lower than normal, in the range of 5–10 mm Hg. The SaO_2 level depends on the magnitude of the right-to-left shunt; in "pink tets", the systemic SaO_2 may be normal, whereas in a moderately cyanotic patient at rest, it is usually 75–85%.

Cyanotic spells are treated acutely by administration of oxygen and placing the patient in the knee–chest position (to increase SVR). IV morphine should be administered cautiously, but is helpful for its sedative effect. Propranolol produces beta blockade and may reduce the obstruction across the RVOT through its negative inotropic action. Acidosis, if present, should be corrected with IV sodium bicarbonate. Chronic oral prophylaxis of cyanotic spells with propranolol may be useful to delay surgery, but the onset of Tet spells usually prompts surgical intervention. In fact, in the current era, elective surgical repair generally occurs around the age of 3 months so as to avoid the development of Tet spells.

On examination, there is cyanosis, clubbing, and prominent "a" waves in JVP. There will be mild parasternal heave and systolic thrill is present. Ejection systolic murmur is present. Aortic ejection click may be heard. There is tachycardia. S2 is usually single in pulmonary area because aortic component is heard to dextroposed and overriding of aorta. The only indirect evidence of VSD is the presence of cyanosis. The acyanotic TOF, VSD with mild PS—long pansystolic murmur resulting in VSD and infundibular stenosis is audible. Ejection systolic murmur is heard in pulmonary area. Cyanosis is absent.

In the rare, untreated patient, major late complications include brain abscess, cerebral thrombosis with hemiplegia, and IE. Growth and development are generally delayed in proportion to the degree of cyanosis. IE is particularly common in children who have palliative systemic–pulmonary shunts rather than correction. Prophylactic antibiotic therapy is no longer routinely recommended for most of these repaired patients, although unrepaired or palliated patients still require prophylaxis.

> **GENERAL FEATURES**
> - Anoxic spell
> - Convulsions
> - Loss of consciousness

> **ESSENTIAL DIAGNOSTIC POINTS**
> - Cyanosis after neonatal period
> - Hypoxemic spells during infancy
> - Systolic ejection murmur at upper left sternal border
> - Right-sided aortic arch

■ DIAGNOSIS

Hemoglobin, hematocrit, and RBC count are usually elevated in older infants or children secondary to chronic arterial desaturation.

The radiograph of chest shows normal-sized heart with upturned apex suggestive of RVH. The absence of main pulmonary artery segment gives it the shape as coeur en sabot. The pulmonary fields are oligemic.

The heart is of normal size, and lung fields are poorly vascularized, signifying diminished pulmonary blood flow. The RVOT and main pulmonary artery segments are usually hypoplastic, resulting in a concavity of the upper left margin of the cardiac silhouette instead of the normal convexity. The right ventricle is hypertrophied, often shown by an upturning of the apex (boot-shaped heart). A characteristic "sheep's nose", coeur en sabot, or boot-shaped heart may be present, particularly with pulmonary atresia. The ascending aorta is generally large. In about 25% of the patients, a right-sided aortic arch is present and is recognized by observing a right-sided rather than left-sided indentation on the trachea. The superior vena caval shadow may be displaced to the right. When bronchial collateral circulation is well developed, diffuse fine vascular markings are noted throughout the lung.

Electrocardiogram: Right-axis deviation (+120 to +150), with RVH in cyanotic form, in acyanotic QRS axis is normal. ECG shows large overriding of the aorta, RVH, and outflow obstruction. Aortic mitral valve continuity is maintained. "T" waves are inverted in right precordial leads. "P" pulmonale may be present. There are right-axis deviation and RVH, although in the newborn infant, the diagnosis of pathologic RVH by ECG is more difficult because of the normal RV dominance at this age.

■ ECHOCARDIOGRAPHY

Two-dimensional echo and Doppler studies can make diagnosis and assess the severity of TOF. A large perimembranous infundibular VSD and overriding of aorta are visualized in long-axis parasternal view. RVOT obstruction with pulmonary valve and annulus are present. Doppler studies estimate the pressure gradient across RVOT.

Two-dimensional imaging is diagnostic, revealing thickening of the RV wall, overriding of the aorta, and a large subaortic VSD. Obstruction at the level of the infundibulum and pulmonary valve can be identified, and the size of the proximal pulmonary arteries measured. The anatomy of the coronary arteries should be visualized, as abnormal branches crossing the RVOT are at risk for transaction during surgical enlargement of the area.

Cardiac Catheterization and Angiocardiography

Pressure gradients may be noted at the pulmonary valvular level, the infundibular level, or both. RV angiography reveals RV outflow obstruction and a right-to-left shunt at the ventricular level. The major indications for cardiac catheterization are to establish coronary artery and distal pulmonary artery anatomy if not able to be clearly defined by echocardiography.

> **LABORATORY SALIENT FINDINGS**
> - The radiograph of chest shows normal-sized heart with upturned apex suggestive of right ventricular hypertrophy; the absence of main pulmonary artery segment gives it the shape as coeur en sabot; the pulmonary fields are oligemic
> - Electrocardiogram (ECG) shows large overriding of the aorta, right ventricular hypertrophy, and outflow obstruction
> - *Echo:* A large perimembranous infundibular ventricular septal defect (VSD) and overriding of aorta are visualized in long-axis parasternal view; right ventricular outflow tract obstruction with pulmonary valve and annulus
> - Doppler studies estimate the pressure gradient across right ventricular outflow tract

■ COMPLICATIONS

- Anemia
- IE
- Anoxic spell
- Hemiplegia
- Paradoxical embolism
- Brain abscess
- Right bundle branch block (RBBB)

■ TREATMENT

As with many significant congenital heart abnormalities, the treatment is ultimately surgical. For the neonate with prominent cyanosis, prompt infusion of PGE, is important. Corrective or palliative surgery is usually performed within 2–4 months of birth, but rarely in a patient who has not had surgery, medical therapy is primarily directed toward acute relief of hypercyanotic episodes and preventing the complications of right-to-left shunts.

Treatment of TOF depends on the severity of the RVOT obstruction. Infants with severe tetralogy require urgent medical treatment and surgical intervention in the neonatal period.

Neonates with marked RVOT obstruction may deteriorate rapidly because as the ductus arteriosus begins to close, pulmonary blood flow is further compromised. The IV administration of PGE (0.01–0.20 μg/kg/min), a potent and specific relaxant of ductal smooth muscle, causes dilation of the ductus arteriosus and usually provides adequate pulmonary blood flow until a surgical procedure can be performed. This agent should be administered intravenously as soon as cyanotic CHD is clinically suspected and continued through the preoperative period and during cardiac catheterization.

Infants with symptoms and severe cyanosis in the first month of life usually have marked obstruction of the RVOT. Two options are available in these infants. The first option is corrective open-heart surgery performed in early infancy and even in the newborn period in critically ill infants. This approach currently has widespread acceptance with excellent short- and long-term results and has supplanted palliative shunts for most cases. Early total repair carries the theoretical advantage that early physiologic correction allows for improved growth of the branch pulmonary arteries. In infants with less severe cyanosis, who can be maintained with good growth and absence of hypercyanotic spells, primary repair is performed electively at 4–6 months of age.

The second option, more common in previous years, is a palliative systemic-to-pulmonary artery shunt (Blalock–Taussig shunt) performed to augment pulmonary artery blood flow. The rationale for this surgery, previously, the only option for these patients, is to augment pulmonary blood flow to decrease the amount of hypoxia and improve linear growth, as well as augment growth of the branch pulmonary arteries. The modified Blalock–Taussig shunt is currently the most common aortopulmonary shunt procedure and consists of a Gore-Tex conduit anastomosed side to side from the subclavian artery to the homolateral branch of the pulmonary artery.

Hypercyanotic episodes may be treated by placing the infant on the abdomen in a knee-chest position or holding the infant with the legs flexed on the abdomen. Oxygen should be given to lessen dyspnea and cyanosis but is not very helpful because of the very low pulmonary blood flow. Morphine sulfate (0.2 mg/kg body weight subcutaneously) is especially effective in terminating a prolonged or severe attack. If the spell is protracted and severe and does not respond to the foregoing therapy, metabolic acidemia ensues, and IV fluid bolus administration and correction with IV sodium bicarbonate are essential.

Vasopressors can be given either early in the attack or if other therapies fail; phenylephrine 0.02 mg/kg intravenously or 0.1 mg/kg intramuscularly will raise systemic resistance and thus increase pulmonary blood flow. If possible, phenylephrine should be given by continuous IV infusion, generally at a dose of 2–5 mg/kg/min. Recently a nasal fentanyl spray of 2 mg/kg was reported as being effective. In infancy, these attacks may be precipitated by a relative iron-deficiency anemia (hypochromic microcytic), and such patients should have iron therapy until the hematocrit reaches levels of 50–55%.

Further increase in the hematocrit results in a marked rise in blood viscosity, with progressive impediment to blood flow, a risk of cerebral thrombosis. Any hypercyanotic episode is an absolute indication for surgery, so it is now rare to need to treat anemia except in the immediate preoperative period. If surgery is contraindicated tor some reason, oral propranolol has been given at a dosage of 0.5–1.5 mg/kg dose orally every 6 hours to prevent or reduce the frequency of paroxysmal dyspneic attacks. Some cardiologists have reported that balloon dilation and stent placement of the infundibulum and pulmonary valve may improve pulmonary blood flow enough for 6–12 months in the case that surgery needs to be delayed or is unavailable.

Medical management is limited to the management of complications and correction of anemia. Depending on the frequency and severity of hypercyanotic attacks, one or more of the following procedures should be instituted in sequence: (1) placement of the infant on the abdomen in the knee–chest position while making certain that the infant's clothing is not constrictive, (2) administration of oxygen (although increasing inspired oxygen will not reverse cyanosis caused by intracardiac shunting), and (3) injection of morphine subcutaneously in a dose not in excess of 0.2 mg/kg. Calming and holding the infant in a knee–chest position may abort progression of an early spell. Premature attempts to obtain blood samples may cause further agitation and may be counterproductive. The management of the anoxic spell includes:

- Knee–chest position
- Humidified oxygen
- Morphine 0.1–0.2 mg/kg subcutaneous injection
- Sodium bicarbonate is given to correct the acidosis
- Propranolol in the dose of 0.1 mg/kg during the anoxic spell

- Vasodilators
- Correction of anemia
- Surgery

The surgical treatment is of two types: (1) Palliative and (2) definitive.

Indications for palliative shunt procedure are as follows:
- Neonate with TOF and pulmonary atresia
- Infants with hypoplastic pulmonary annulus and hypoplastic pulmonary artery stenosis
- Severely cyanotic infants; younger than 3 months and those who have medically unmanageable hypoxic spells.

Palliative treatment consists of anastomosing a systemic artery with the pulmonary artery. This increases the pulmonary blood flow and thus increases the oxygenated blood flow reaching the systemic circulation.

Early elective surgery is indicated for infants with TOF with or without pulmonary atresia, even in the absence of symptoms. Patients with the TOF and patent RVOTs can have intracardiac surgical repair of the malformation by skilled congenital heart surgeons in the first months of life with low operative mortality. The VSD is closed, the infundibular muscle is resected, and sometimes RV outflow and main pulmonary artery patches are placed to augment the outflow tract. Pulmonary valvotomy is also performed in most patients, but enlargement of the pulmonary valve annulus with a transannular patch is avoided unless the annulus is critically small.

Balloon dilation of the pulmonary arteries can then be performed in the catheterization laboratory in anticipation of later correction.

Although repair of TOF with pulmonary atresia has in recent years become increasingly successful, the operative risk and/late complications and death are higher than for uncomplicated TOF. Unifocalization of the often discontinuous sources of pulmonary blood flow to a central system is required before the standard repair. This may be done in one or multiple stages.

Surgical correction for most patients with uncomplicated TOF results in excellent survival. Residual or recurrent small left-to-right shunts are uncommon, but residual mild or moderate RV–pulmonary outflow tract obstruction and regurgitation are common. Those who have marked pulmonary regurgitation and very dilated right ventricles may eventually develop congestive heart failure and may be at higher risk for sudden death, especially if they have very wide QRS intervals. These patients are candidates for pulmonary valve replacement, currently primarily performed surgically but increasingly being performed by catheter insertion. A few patients have surgically induced complete AV block and require an implanted pacemaker. Dysrhythmias should be suspected if these patients after surgery complain of dizzy spells, syncope, or palpitations, and appropriate diagnostic studies and therapy applied.

Balloon dilatation of RVOT and pulmonary valve has been attempted to delay surgical repair.
- *Blalock–Taussig shunt:* Subclavian artery and pulmonary artery
- *Pott's shunt:* Descending aorta to pulmonary artery
- *Waterston's shunt:* Ascending aorta and right pulmonary artery

Most preferred method is Blalock–Taussig shunt. Here, the basic heart disease remains unaltered.

Conventional (Definitive) Repair Surgery

Conventional repair surgery is indicated in symptomatic infants, who have favorable anatomy of RVOT and pulmonary artery stenosis. An early repair is advised, any time after 4 months of age. Mildly cyanotic children, who have had shunt surgery, and total repair 1–2 years after shunt operation.

The definitive operation consists of closing the VSD and resecting infundibular obstruction.

Open-heart surgery for repair of TOF is performed at ages ranging from birth to 2 years, depending on the patient's anatomy and the experience of the surgical center. The current surgical trend is toward earlier repair for symptomatic infants. The major limiting anatomic feature of total correction is the size of the pulmonary arteries. During surgery, the VSD is closed and the obstruction to RV outflow removed. Although a valve sparing procedure is preferred, in many cases a transannular patch is placed across the RVOT as the pulmonary valve is contributing to the obstruction. When a transannular patch repair is done, the patient has pulmonary insufficiency that is usually well tolerated for years. However, pulmonary valve replacement is eventually necessary once symptoms (usually exercise intolerance) and RV dilation occur. Surgical mortality is low.

This is done under cardiopulmonary bypass. The major complications include complete heart block, RBBB, residual VSD, and residual pulmonic stenosis. If the pulmonary arteries are adequate in size, and the arteries descending coronary artery is from left coronary artery, a patient with anoxic spell can be subjected to definitive repair even at the age of 3–6 months.

■ COURSE AND PROGNOSIS

Infants with severe TOF are usually deeply cyanotic at birth. These children require early surgery. Complete repair before age 2 years usually produces a good result, and patients are currently living well into adulthood. Depending on the extent of the repair required, patients frequently require additional surgery 10–15 years after their initial repair for replacement of the pulmonary valve.

Patients with TOF are at risk for sudden death due to ventricular dysrhythmias. A competent pulmonary valve without a dilated right ventricle appears to diminish arrhythmias and enhance exercise performance.

■ BIBLIOGRAPHY

1. Batra AS, McElhinney DB, Wang W, Zakheim R, Garofano RP, Daniels C, et al. Cardiopulmonary exercise function among patients undergoing transcatheter pulmonary valve implantation in the US Melody valve investigational trial. Am Heart J. 2012;163(2)280-7.
2. Valente AM, Cook S, Festa P, Ko HH, Krishnamurthy R, Taylor AM, et al. Multimodality imaging guidelines for patients with repaired tetralogy of fallot: a report from the American Society of Echocardiography: developed in collaboration with the Society for Cardiovascular Magnetic Resonance and the Society for Pediatric Radiology. J Am Soc Echocardiologr. 2014;27(2):111-41.

CASE 20

Ventricular Septal Defect

■ PRESENTING COMPLAINTS

A 4-month-old girl was brought with the complaint of:
- Not gaining weight since 2 months
- Cough and cold since 1 month
- Fever since 1 month
- Sweating since 15 days

History of Presenting Complaints

A 4-month-old girl with history of not gaining weight was brought to the pediatric outpatient department. Her mother told that her child's birth weight was 3 kg. When she was taken for immunization at 6 weeks, the weight of the child was 2.75 kg. At the time of second dose of diphtheria–pertussis–tetanus (DPT) and oral polio vaccine (OPV) at 10 weeks, the weight of the child was 3 kg. When she went to the hospital last week for the cough and cold, the weight of the child was 3.5 kg. The mother also noticed that child sweats at the time of taking feeds. She had been treated by the doctor for the lower respiratory tract infections.

Past History of the Patient

The girl was the only sibling of the nonconsanguineous marriage. She was born at full term through vaginal delivery. She cried immediately after the delivery. The birth weight was 3 kg. There was no significant postnatal event. The child was taking breast milk and was discharged on the fourth day.

The resident at the time of birth had auscultated and found the systolic murmur. It was brought to the notice of the consultant.

CASE AT A GLANCE	
Basic Findings	
Length	: 60 cm (75th centile)
Weight	: 3.5 kg (less than 3rd centile)
Temperature	: 38°C
Pulse rate	: 140 beats/min
Respiratory rate	: 46 breaths/min
Blood pressure	: 60/48 mm Hg
Positive Findings	
History:	
• Failure to thrive	
• Sweating	
• No gain in weight	
• Murmur at birth	
• Repeated infections	
Examination:	
• Underweight	
• Pallor	
• Systolic thrill	
• Hepatomegaly	
• Tachypnea	
• Febrile	
Investigation:	
• *Hemoglobin (Hb):* 9 g/dL	
• *Electrocardiogram (ECG):* Biventricular hypertrophy	
• *X-ray chest:* Enlarged heart with pulmonary plethora, left atrial enlargement	

Parents were advised to attend the cardiac clinic for assessment of murmur. According to the mother the child was getting repeated respiratory tract infections; while she was receiving the treatment, she developed the respiratory tract infection and was irritable.

■ EXAMINATION

The child was moderately built and poorly nourished. She was irritable and breathless. Subcostal recession was present. The intercostal and accessory muscle were active. Anthropometric measurements included the length 60 cm (75th centile) and weight 3.5 kg (less than 3rd centile). The head circumference was 39 cm.

She was febrile. The pulse rate was 140 beats/min, and the respiratory rate was breaths/min. Blood pressure recorded was 60/48 mm Hg. There was pallor, no lymphadenopathy, and no edema.

Sternum was prominent. Apex beat was displaced to the anterior auxiliary line. Systolic thrill was felt at the left lower sternal edge on auscultation, pulmonary component of the second sound was loud. Pansystolic murmur was present over the left 3rd and 4th intercostal spaces.

Respiratory system was normal and per abdomen examination revealed the presence of enlarged liver about 3 cm below the costal margin. It was soft and nontender.

■ INVESTIGATION

- *Hemoglobin:* 9 g/dL
- *TLC:* 9,800 cells/cumm
- *DLC:* $P_{68} L_{30} E_2$
- *ESR:* 36 mm in the first hour
- *AEC:* 346 cells/cumm
- *ECG:* Biventricular hypertrophy
- *X-ray chest:* Enlarged heart with pulmonary plethora, cardiomegaly and left atrial enlargement

■ DISCUSSION

A 4-month-old child was brought with the history of inability to gain weight and breathlessness. On examination, there was systolic thrill associated with pansystolic murmur. Radiograph of chest showed the presence of the enlarged heart with pulmonary plethora and electrocardiograph suggested biventricular hypertrophy. All these findings suggest VSD.

A VSD usually occurs as an isolated abnormality but may be associated with other congenital cardiac malformations. In view of the pattern of blood flow in the heart and great vessels of a fetus with a VSD, with diversion of blood from the aortic isthmus, narrowing the aortic isthmus or true coarctation should always be considered when an infant with a VSD has severe heart failure. VSDs are also common in corrected transposition of the great arteries. They are always present in a truncus arteriosus communis and in a double-outlet right ventricle (DORV) that, in the absence of pulmonic stenosis, has the clinical features of an isolate VSD.

Ventricular septal defect is the most common congenital heart malformation, accounting for about 30% of all CHDs. Defects in the ventricular septum occur both in the membranous portion of the septum (most common) and the muscular portion.

It is the communication between the two ventricles. It can be present in membranous or muscular part of septum. 90% of the VSDs are present in the membranous part. It can be multiple. It accounts for 20% of all CHDs.

The muscular septum has two components: (1) The inlet (trabecular) septum and (2) the outlet (infundibular) septum. The trabecular septum has three components— (1) central, (2) marginal, and (3) apical. A VSD may be classified into perimembranous outlet (infundibular), central muscular, and marginal muscular and apical muscular defects. "Bundle of His" is related to postero-inferior quadrant of perimembranous defect and superoanterior quadrant of inlet muscular defect.

The large volume of the blood passing through the lungs is seen as pulmonary plethora. The increased volume of the blood finally reaches the left atrium. This leads to left atrial enlargement. Then passing through the normal mitral valve it produces delayed diastolic murmur at the apex. It is directly related to the size of the shunt. The large flow across the mitral valve also results with accentuation of the first heart sound.

Left ventricle has two outlets: Aortic valve allowing forward flow and VSD leads to backward leak. It empties relatively early. This results in early A2 since ejection into the right ventricle and pulmonary artery is increased, and because of left-to-right shunt P2 is delayed. Therefore, second sound is widely split but varies with respiration.

Ventricular septal defects follow one of four courses. These are described in the following text.

1. *Small, hemodynamically insignificant VSDs:* Between 80% and 85% of cases, VSDs are small (<3 mm in diameter) at birth and will close spontaneously. In general, small defects in the muscular interventricular septum will close sooner than those in the membranous septum. In most cases, a small VSD never requires surgical closure. 50% of small VSDs will close by age of 2 years, and 90% by age of 6 years, with most of the remaining closing during the school years.
2. *Moderate-sized VSDs:* Asymptomatic patients with moderate-sized VSDs (3-5 mm in diameter) account for 3-5% of children with VSDs. In general, these children do not have clear indicators for surgical closure. Historically, in those who had cardiac catheterization, the ratio of pulmonary to systemic blood flow is usually <2:1, and serial cardiac catheterizations demonstrate that the shunts get progressively smaller. If the patient is asymptomatic and without evidence of pulmonary hypertension, these defects can be followed serially as some close spontaneously over time.
3. *Large VSDs with normal pulmonary vascular resistance:* These defects are usually 6-10 mm in diameter. Unless they become markedly smaller within a few months after birth, they often require surgery. The timing of surgery depends on the clinical situation. Many infants with large VSDs and normal PVR develop symptoms of failure to thrive, tachypnea, diaphoresis with feeds by age of 3-6 months, and require correction at that time. Surgery before age of 2 years in patients with large VSDs essentially eliminates the risk of pulmonary vascular disease.
4. *Large VSDs with pulmonary vascular obstructive disease:* The direction of flow across a VSD is determined by the resistance, in the systemic and pulmonary vasculature, explaining why flow is usually left to right. In large VSDs, ventricular pressures are equalized, resulting in increased pulmonary artery pressure. In addition, shear stress caused by increased volume, in the pulmonary circuit causes increased resistance over time. The vast majority of patients with inoperable pulmonary hypertension develop the condition progressively. Almost all cases of irreversible pulmonary hypertension can be prevented by surgical repair of a large VSD before age of 2 years.

The physical size of the VSD is a major (but not the only) determinant of the size of the left-to-right shunt. When the defect is large, the level of PVR in relation to SVR is the major determinant of the shunt's magnitude.

When a small communication is present (usually <5 mm), the VSD is deemed to be pressure-restrictive, meaning that RV pressure is normal or only slightly elevated. The higher pressure in the left ventricle drives the shunt left to right, and the size of the defect limits the magnitude of the shunt. In larger, nonrestrictive VSDs (usually >10 mm), RV and LV pressures are equalized. In these defects the direction of shunting and the shunt magnitude are determined by the PVR/SVR ratio.

The magnitude of intracardiac shunts is usually described by the Qp:Qs ratio. If the left-to-right shunt is small (Qp:Qs < 1.5:1), the cardiac chambers are not appreciably enlarged, and the pulmonary vascular bed is probably normal. If the shunt is large (Qp:Qs >2:1), left atrial and LV volume overload occurs, and RV and pulmonary arterial hypertension may be present if the defect is large. The main pulmonary artery, left atrium, and left ventricle are enlarged.

The hemodynamics of a VSD can also be demonstrated by cardiac catheterization, although catheterization currently is performed only when laboratory data do not fit well with the clinical findings or when pulmonary vascular disease is suspected. Oximetry demonstrates increased oxygen content in the right ventricle; because some defects eject blood almost directly into the pulmonary artery (streaming), the full magnitude of the oxygen saturation increase is occasionally apparent only when pulmonary arterial blood is sampled. Small, restrictive VSDs are associated with normal right-sided heart pressures and PVR. Large, nonrestrictive VSDs are associated with equal or near-equal pulmonary and systemic systolic pressure and variable elevations in PVR.

■ CLINICAL FEATURES (FIG. 1)

Symptoms and Signs

Patients with small or moderate left-to-right shunts usually have no cardiovascular symptoms. Patients with large left-to-right shunts are usually ill early in infancy. These infants have frequent respiratory infections and gain weight slowly. Dyspnea, diaphoresis, and fatigue are common. These symptoms can develop as early as 1–6 months of age. Older children may experience exercise intolerance. Over time, in children and adolescents with persistent large left-to-right shunt, the pulmonary vascular bed undergoes structural changes, leading to increased PVR and reversal of the shunt from left to right to right to left (Eisenmenger syndrome). Cyanosis will then be present.

- *Small left-to-right shunt:* No lifts, heaves, or thrills are present. The first sound at the apex is normal, and the second sound at the pulmonary area is split physiologically.

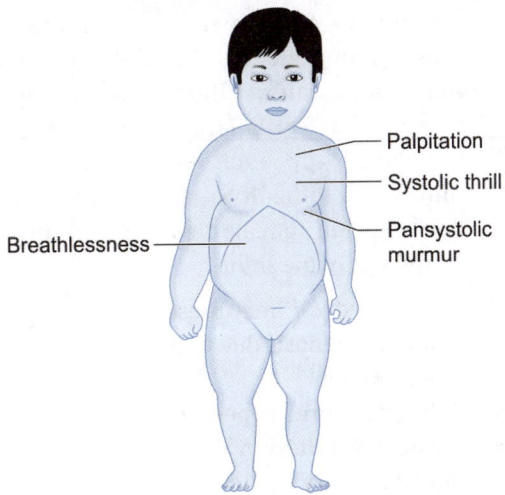

Fig. 1: Clinical features.

A grade II–IV/VI, medium-to high-pitched, harsh pansystolic murmur is heard best at the left sternal border in the third and fourth intercostal spaces. The murmur radiates over the entire precordium. No diastolic murmurs are heard.

- *Moderate left-to-right shunt:* Slight prominence of the precordium with moderate LV heave is evident. A systolic thrill may be palpable at the lower left sternal border between the third and fourth intercostal spaces. The second sound at the pulmonary area is most often split but may be single. A grade III–IV/VI, harsh pansystolic murmur is heard best at the lower left sternal border in the fourth intercostal space. A mitral diastolic flow murmur indicates that pulmonary blood flow and subsequently the pulmonary venous return are significantly increased by the large shunt.
- *Large VSDs with pulmonary hypertension:* The precordium is prominent, and the sternum bulges. Both LV and RV heaves are palpable. S2 is palpable in the pulmonary area. A thrill may be present at the lower left sternal border. S2 is usually single or narrowly split, with accentuation of the pulmonary component. The murmur ranges from grade I to IV/VI and is usually harsh and pansystolic. Occasionally, when the defect is large or ventricular pressures approach equivalency, a murmur is difficult to hear. A diastolic flow murmur may be heard, depending on the size of the shunt.

Uncomplicated VSD may present with:
- Pulmonic stenosis due to hypertrophy RV infundibulum
- Pulmonary atrial hypertension
- Aortic regurgitation due to prolapse of right coronary or noncoronary cusp of aortic valve.

■ DIAGNOSIS

Chest X-ray

In patients with small shunts, the chest radiograph may be normal. Patients with large shunts have significant cardiac enlargement involving both the left and right ventricles and the left atrium. The main pulmonary artery segment may be dilated. The pulmonary vascular markings are increased.

Electrocardiography

The ECG is normal in small left-to-right shunts. LVH usually occurs in patients with large left-to-right shunts and normal PVR. Combined ventricular enlargement occurs in patients with pulmonary hypertension caused by increased flow, increased resistance, or both. Pure RVH occurs in patients with pulmonary hypertension secondary to pulmonary vascular obstruction induced by long-standing left-to-right shunt (Eisenmenger syndrome).

Echocardiography

Two-dimensional echocardiography can reveal the size of a VSD and identify its anatomic location. Multiple defects can be detected by combining two-dimensional and color-flow imaging. Doppler can further evaluate the VSD by estimating the pressure difference between the left and right ventricles. A pressure difference greater than 50 mm Hg in the left ventricle compared to the right ventricle confirms the absence of severe pulmonary hypertension.

Cardiac Catheterization and Angiocardiography

The ability to describe the VSD anatomy and estimate the pulmonary artery pressures on the basis of the gradient across the VSD allows for the vast majority of isolated defects to be repaired without cardiac catheterization and angiocardiography. Catheterization is indicated in those patients with increased PVR. Angiocardiographic examination defines the number, size, and location of the defects.

■ TREATMENT

It is less common for moderate or large VSDs to close spontaneously, although even defects large enough to result in heart failure may occur.

In infants with a large VSD, management has two goals: Control the symptoms of heart failure and prevent the development of pulmonary vascular disease. If early treatment is successful, sometimes the shunt may diminish in size with spontaneous improvement, especially during the first year of life. The clinician must be alert not to confuse clinical improvement caused by a decrease in defect size with clinical changes caused by the development of Eisenmenger physiology. Because surgical closure can be carried out at low risk in most infants, medical management should not be pursued in symptomatic infants after an initial unsuccessful trial.

Because pulmonary vascular disease can usually be prevented when surgery is performed within the first year of life, even infants with well-controlled heart failure should not have very delayed inordinately unless there is evidence that the defect is becoming pressure-restrictive.

Isolated VSDs are the most common types of CHD, so all pediatricians need to know how they can be managed.

Spontaneous closure may eventually occur in up to 70% of patients, and many of these closures occur by 3 years of age. In a further 25%, the defect becomes smaller but may not close completely; however, the hemodynamic effects are significantly reduced. Because of these statistics, if the defect seems to be becoming smaller, surgical correction should be delayed in the hope of spontaneous closure.

Primary surgical closure of the defects can be done with very low mortality. If primary closure is not feasible because of multiple muscular defects or other complicating factors, then banding the pulmonary artery will decrease the left-to-right shunt, reduce pulmonary flow and pressure, and relieve congestive heart failure. Banding has its own complications, and removal of the band when the defect is closed later adds to the morbidity of the procedure.

Muscular defects, especially if multiple, can be difficult to close surgically. From a right ventriculotomy, the masses of hypertrophied trabeculae are daunting and make the defect(s) difficult to find. Although a left ventriculotomy simplifies surgery, a large incision in the systemic ventricle should be avoided. Some surgeons cut away all the RV trabeculae to make closing the defect easier, and others suture all the trabeculae together to close the exit holes. Because of the difficult surgery, closing the muscular defect by catheter introduction of an Amplatzer device is being used more often. Some catheterization procedures are very lengthy, and an alternative is to use a hybrid method in which a surgeon performs a small thoracotomy and the Amplatzer device is inserted more directly through a trocar. Some cardiologists have even used similar devices for nonsurgical closure of perimembranous VSDs, but this procedure has more risk of producing complete AV block and of damaging the aortic valve.

Medical Management

The medical management consists of controlling CCF, chest infections, and prevention and treatment of anemia and IE. Patients who develop symptoms can be managed with anticongestive treatment, particularly diuretics and systemic after load reduction, prior to surgery or if it is expected that the defect will close over time.

Surgical Treatment

Indications for surgical closure of a VSD include patients at any age with large defects in whom clinical symptoms and failure to thrive cannot be controlled medically; infants between 6 and 12 months of age with moderate-to-large defects associated with pulmonary hypertension, even if the symptoms are controlled by medication; and patients older than 24 months with a Qp:Qs ratio greater than 2:1. Patients with a supracristal VSD of any size are usually referred for surgery because of their higher risk for developing aortic valve regurgitation. Severe pulmonary vascular disease nonresponsive to pulmonary vasodilators is a contraindication to closure of a VSD.

Transcatheter occlusion closure has been used successfully in treating larger muscular VSDs, which may be difficult to access by surgery. Perimembranous VSD catheter closure has a high risk of postprocedural heart block and is currently not routinely performed. Hybrid methods employing a sternotomy with device placement through the anterior wall of the right ventricle under transesophageal echocardiographic and fluoroscopic visualization has been performed in difficult-to-approach muscular defects.

Surgical indication:
- Large VSDs with nonresponding CCF should be closed in the first 6 months of life.
- Significant left-to-right shunt with QP/QS of at least 2:1 indicates surgical closure.
- Older infants with large VSDs and increased pulmonary resistance.

In large VSDs, infundibular stenosis may develop which decreases the magnitude of left-to-right shunt (acyanotic TOF).

Patients with cardiomegaly, poor growth, poor exercise tolerance, or other clinical abnormalities who have a significant shunt (>2:1) typically undergo surgical repair at age of 3-6 months. The operative treatment consists of closure of the VSD with the use of Dacron patch. It can be performed through the right atrium. The operation can be done below the age of 1 year if the CCF cannot be controlled with medical management. With the evidence of pulmonary hypertension, it can be done by the age of 2 years As a result, Eisenmenger syndrome has been virtually eliminated. The surgical mortality rate for VSD closure is below 2%.

Transcatheter closure of muscular VSDs is also a possibility. Perimembranous VSDs have also been closed in children during catheterization, but a high incidence of complete heart block after placement of the occluding device has slowed the acceptance of this approach.

The complications of the surgery include complete heart block, bifascicular block, and residual ventricular defect. Postoperative follow-up includes SBE prophylaxis and pacemaker implantation in the presence of heart blocks. Surgical mortality 2-5% after the age of 6 months. It is higher in smaller infants <2 months or with associated defects.

COMPLICATIONS

In some infants with significant reductions in left-to-right shunts caused by spontaneous closing of the VSDs, mid-to-late systolic clicks have become audible. In these children, aneurysmal dilation of the thin membranous septum or tricuspid valve tissue that has grown to close the defect has occurred, with bulging of pseudoaneurysm into the right ventricle. A small opening often present at the apex of the pseudoaneurysm allows a small left-to-right shunt. Normally, the defect closes, and the pseudoaneurysm slowly shrinks, but rarely it may enlarge progressively. These pseudoaneurysms can be demonstrated by echocardiography.

A number of infants have developed progressive aortic insufficiency associated with VSD, particularly if it is subarterial. There is prolapse of an aortic valve leaflet with dilation of the aortic valve sinus, and distortion or even rupture of the aortic sinus or cusp may occur. The development of aortic insufficiency has been attributed to stress on the unsupported aortic cusp and perhaps suction on it by the jet of the shunt passing through the defect. Even with a small VSD, or one showing the evidence of closure, aortic insufficiency requires surgical closure of the defect to prevent further prolapse. It may in fact be prudent to close subarterial VSDs even before evidence of aortic valve cusp involvement is apparent.

Infective endocarditis can occur even after spontaneous closure of the defect. If IE involves the tricuspid leaflet sealing the VSD, rupture may occur and produce a direct left ventricular-to-right atrial communication. Previously, antibiotic prophylaxis for IE had been recommended for children with even small defects.

■ COURSE AND PROGNOSIS

Significant late dysrhythmias are uncommon. Functional exercise capacity and oxygen consumption are usually normal, and physical restrictions are unnecessary. Adults with corrected defects have normal quality of life.

GENERAL FEATURES
- Congestive cardiac failure
- Failure to thrive
- Frequent chest infection

ESSENTIAL DIAGNOSTIC POINTS
- Acyanotic
- Easy fatigability
- Congestive cardiac failure in infancy
- Hyperactive heart
- Biventricular enlargement
- Grade 2.3/4 pansystolic murmur maximum at lower sternal border
- P2 is usually accentuated
- Diastolic flow murmur at apex

LABORATORY SALIENT FINDINGS
- ECG shows combined ventricular hypertrophy; right ventricular hypertrophy is seen with Eisenmenger's complex
- *Chest radiograph:* Pulmonary vasculature is increased; left atrial enlargement with the large left-to-right shunt
- Echocardiogram shows increased left atrial and ventricular size and exaggerated mitral valve motion

■ BIBLIOGRAPHY

1. Butera G, Carminati M, Chessa M, Piazza L, Micheletti A, Negura DG, et al. Transcatheter closure of perimembranous ventricular septal defects: early and long-term results. J Am Coll Cardiol. 2007;50;1189-95.
2. Sondheimer HM, Rahimi-Alangi K; Current management of ventricular septal defect. Cardiol Young. 2006;16 Suppl 3:131-5.

SECTION 4
Gastrointestinal System

- Case 21 **Acute Gastroenteritis**
- Case 22 **Appendicitis**
- Case 23 **Congenital Hypertrophic Pyloric Stenosis**
- Case 24 **Diaphragmatic Hernia**
- Case 25 **Duodenal Atresia**
- Case 26 **Gastroesophageal Reflux**
- Case 27 **Hepatitis**
- Case 28 **Hirschsprung's Disease**
- Case 29 **Intussusception**
- Case 30 **Liver Abscess**
- Case 31 **Necrotizing Enterocolitis**
- Case 32 **Pancreatitis**
- Case 33 **Tracheoesophageal Fistula**
- Case 34 **Wilson's Disease**

21 CASE

Acute Gastroenteritis

■ PRESENTING COMPLAINTS

A 3-year-old girl was brought with the complaint of:
- Loose motion since 2 days
- Vomiting since 1 day
- Fever since 1 day

History of Presenting Complaints

A 3-year-old girl was brought to the pediatric outpatient department with a history of loose motion and vomiting since 2 days. According to the mother, her daughter was passing loose motion about 7–8 times/day. When a child had loose motion it was semisolid and later it became watery, not associated with blood and mucus. The mother also said that her child had vomited on the first day. The child was vomiting whatever she was taking. Vomitus is used to contain the ingested food material. The mother also revealed that she had noticed a fever since morning.

Past History of the Patient

She was the only child of a nonconsanguineous marriage. She was born at full term by normal vaginal delivery. There was no significant postnatal event. The baby was on breast milk soon after the delivery. Weaning was started in the fourth month and completed by 1 year. All the developmental milestones were normal. She was completely immunized.

CASE AT A GLANCE

Basic Findings
Height	: 100 cm (90th centile)
Weight	: 13 kg (80th centile)
Temperature	: 38°C
Pulse rate	: 120 beats/min
Respiratory rate	: 32 breaths/min
Blood pressure	: Not recordable

Positive Findings

History:
- Vomiting
- Loose motion
- Drowsy
- Fever

Examination:
- Febrile
- Signs of moderate to severe dehydration
- Sunken eyes
- Blood pressure not recordable
- Loss of skin elasticity
- Bowel sounds: Vigorous

Investigation:
- Stool examination: 8–10 pus cells

■ EXAMINATION

The girl was moderately built and nourished. She was in an altered sensorium, i.e., drowsy because of dehydration. Signs of moderate to severe dehydration were present. Her eyes were sunken, she was tired, and loss of skin elasticity was present.

Anthropometric measurements included a height of 100 cm (90th centile), a weight of

13 kg (80th centile), and a febrile child. Pulse rate was 120 beats/min and respiratory rate was 32 breaths/min and blood pressure was not recordable.

There was no pallor, lymphadenopathy, cyanosis, and clubbing. Per abdomen examination revealed mild distension, and bowel sounds were vigorous. There was no organomegaly. Respiratory and cardiovascular systems revealed no abnormalities.

■ INVESTIGATION

- *Hemoglobin:* 12 g/dL
- *Total leukocyte count (TLC):* 7,600 cells/mm^3
- *Differential leukocyte count (DLC):* $P_{80}L_{18}E_2$
- *Stool routine:*
  - 8–10 pus cells
  - Reducing substance negative
- *Electrolytes:*
  - *Na:* 110 mEq/L
  - *K:* 4 mEq/L
  - *Cl:* 8 mEq/L
- *Blood urea nitrogen (BUN):* 20 mg/dL
- *Serum creatine:* 1 mg/dL

■ DISCUSSION

Gastroenteritis is caused by an infectious agent that damages the gut mucosa and disturbs the balance between the mechanism controlling secretion and absorption within the bowel. The excessive net loss of electrolytes and water into the gut lumen results in diarrhea characterized by the passing of frequent unformed stools in the well-nourished child case. Acute diarrheal disease tends to be self-limiting with minimum mortality. Prolonged diarrhea is more common among malnourished or very young infants and is associated with an increase in mortality and morbidity.

The term diarrhea refers to the passage of three or more loose stools per day. Diarrhea is a symptom, and it is preferable to consider diarrhea if there is increased frequency, volume, and fluidity. Diarrhea is defined as an increase in the liquidity and/or frequency of the stools and can be a primary feature of both acute and chronic conditions. It reflects an increase in stool water content due to impaired water absorption and/or active water secretion by the intestine. It is also a sign when the loss of water is >15 g/kg/day in children <3 years of age and >200 g/kg/day in children >3 years of age.

Acute Diarrhea

The term acute diarrhea refers to a condition where the child passes loose stools lasting for 3–7 days.

Intermediate Diarrhea

The term intermediate diarrhea includes children with acute onset of diarrhea lasting for 8–14 days.

Dysentery

It is the term used for diarrhea with visible blood and mucus, often associated with fever and tenesmus.

Diarrheal disease is an important problem for children <5 years of age and in this age group the primary target is children between 6 months and 2 years of age. As the child grows older, the incidence decreases.

Breastfeeding has a definite impact on the occurrence of diarrheal diseases. Infants who are breastfed have a lower incidence of infective diarrhea. The protective factors in breast milk prevent diarrhea. The early introduction of cow's milk and commercial formulae increases the incidence of diarrhea.

The early introduction of weaning foods will not only be a source of infection but also result in macromolecular absorption of allergens and predispose to the onset and perpetuation of diarrhea. This is more evident if breast milk is discontinued at the time of weaning. Exclusive breastfeeding is therefore recommended till the age of 6 months.

The incidence of diarrhea is higher in bottle-fed infants than in breast-fed infants. When top milk is essential the child should be given teaspoon feeding or "palladai" feeding. This form of feeding is much superior to bottle feeding as the utensils can be cleansed properly.

Diarrhea and malnutrition form a vicious cycle and the nutritional status may worsen after an episode of diarrhea. Malnutrition is also a precipitating factor in predisposing to persistent diarrhea.

The presence of associated infections, such as urinary tract infections, acute suppurative otitis media, bronchopneumonia, and sepsis in a child with acute diarrhea are well-recognized precipitating factors for progression to persistent diarrhea if not treated promptly.

There are certain factors that are peculiar to children and infants that can aggravate the effects of diarrhea. They are as follows:

- The greater body content of water in infants.
- The larger turnover of water in the infant as compared to adults.
- The greater insensible loss of water, since the surface area is two to three times that of an adult.
- The greater metabolic requirements.
- The immaturity of the kidney in handling solutes and the poor concentration capacity.
- The inability of the infant to quench his thirst by drinking water.

Types of Acute Diarrhea

Acute diarrhea can present as:
- Acute watery diarrhea
- Acute dysentery

Etiology:

ETIOLOGY OF ACUTE WATERY DIARRHEA

- *Infections:*
  - *Viruses:* Rota, Adeno, Calici, Norwalk, and HIV
  - *Bacteria:* Vibrio cholerae, Escherichia coli, Salmonella, Shigella, staphylococci, Aeromonas hydrophila, and Plesiomonas shigelloides
  - *Protozoa:* Giardiasis, cryptosporidiosis, and Entamoeba histolytica
  - *Fungal:* Candida
  - *Systemic infections:* LRTI, UTI, and AOM
- *Diet:* Food intolerance, food allergy, and food poisoning
- *Systemic illness:* Metabolic disorders, renal disease, and endocrinopathy
- Antibiotics
- *Surgical:* Appendicitis, intussusception, short bowel syndrome
- *Miscellaneous:* Encopresis

(AOM: acute otitis media; HIV: human immunodeficiency virus; LRTI: lower respiratory tract infection; UTI: urinary tract infection)

ETIOLOGY OF ACUTE DYSENTERY

- *Infective causes:*
  - *Escherichia coli:* Enterohemorrhagic (EHEC) and enteroinvasive (EIEC)
  - *Shigella:* Shigella dysenteriae
  - *Campylobacter jejuni*
  - *Salmonella*
  - *Yersinia enterocolitica*
  - *Entamoeba histolytica*
- *Noninfective causes:*
  - Pseudomembranous colitis
  - Inflammatory bowel disease
  - Radiation-induced colitis
  - Segmental enteritis

(EHEC: enterohemorrhagic; EIEC: enteroinvasive)

The term "parenteral diarrhea" refers to a clinical state in many children who present with diarrhea where the primary disease may be outside the gastrointestinal tract (GIT), e.g., otitis media, respiratory or urinary tract infection.

Pathophysiology: Most episodes of diarrhea occur secondary to one of five types of mechanisms, including: (1) malabsorptive, (2) secretory, (3) osmotic, (4) dysmotility, and (5) inflammatory.

1. *Malabsorption diarrhea:* Malabsorption is due to a decrease in absorptive surface area, as occurs after intestinal resection (short bowel syndrome) or with intestinal villous atrophy, as seen in celiac disease. Secretory diarrhea is caused by secretagogues such as bacterial toxins (e.g., cholera), gut regulatory peptides [e.g., vasoactive intestinal polypeptide (VIP)], short-chain fatty acids, and bile salts, which can induce intestinal water secretion while inhibiting absorption.
2. *Osmotic diarrhea:* Osmotic diarrhea is a term used when the presence of unabsorbed or poorly absorbed osmotically active solutes (e.g., lactose) creates an osmotic load and inhibits water absorption, leading to a net secretion of water and consequently osmotic diarrhea. Osmotic diarrhea characteristically decreases or stops completely during fasting. The lower electrolyte concentration in osmotic diarrhea suggests that some other osmotic substance is contributing to the isotonic osmotic load in the fluid expelled from the colon.
3. *Secretory diarrhea:* This refers to diarrhea caused by abnormal ion transport in intestinal epithelial cells. A net secretory state develops in the GIT as a result of reduced absorption or increased secretion of ions and water. It can be due to the following:
   - *Abnormal mediators:* Bacterial endotoxin
   - Diffuse mucosal disease
   - Intestinal resection
   - Congenital defect of ion transport

   Secretory diarrhea characteristically persists even when the patient is in a fasting state. Osmotic diarrhea results from the intraluminal presence of malabsorbed solutes, such as lactose, which exert significant osmotic pressure that results in the secretion of water into the intestines. Secretory diarrhea does not alter with eating and the osmolality of the stool can be accounted for by normal ionic constituents. Therefore, doubling the sum of sodium and potassium concentrations in stool should equal the fecal osmolality.
4. *Inflammatory diarrhea:* Inflammation due to *Shigella* produces ulcerations in the small intestine and colon which can cause diarrhea. This results in the passage of pus, mucus, serum, and blood in addition to water and electrolytes. Inflammatory disorders cause diarrhea by several mechanisms including the release of prosecretory eicosanoids and cytokines; altered tight junction function, decreasing the mucosal absorptive capacity or the capacity to reabsorb bile acids; and/or disturbances in motility.
5. *Motility diarrhea:* Increased motility can cause diarrhea by reducing the contact time of chime with the intestinal epithelium. The reduced motility can also cause diarrhea by allowing small bowel bacterial growth, bile acid deconjugation, and malabsorption. In contrast to secretory diarrhea, dysmotility can lead to increased peristalsis, causing diarrhea due to rapid transit, or to decreased peristalsis, causing

diarrhea due to bacterial overgrowth. Motility disorders affecting the anorectum and reflexes involved in defecation may cause an increase in stool fluidity and frequency without an increase in weight.

Intestinal pathogens causing diarrhea and/or vomiting:
- *Viruses:* Rotavirus, adenovirus, and others
- *Bacteria:* Escherichia coli, Shigella, Salmonella, Campylobacter jejuni, Yersinia enterocolitica, Aeromonas, and others.
- *Parasites: Entamoeba histolytica, Giardia lamblia,* and *Cryptosporidium.*

Viral Diarrhea

Symptoms of rotavirus acute gastroenteritis (AGE) usually begin with vomiting followed by frequent passage of watery nonbloody stools, associated with fever in about half the cases. The diarrhea lacks fecal leukocytes, but stools from 20% of cases contain mucus. Recovery with complete resolution of symptoms generally occurs within 7 days. Although disaccharide malabsorption is found in 10-20% of episodes, it is rarely clinically significant.

Other viral agents elicit similar symptoms and cannot be distinguished from rotavirus based on clinical findings. In an outbreak setting, the pattern of a brief incubation period (12-48 hours), short duration of illness, and clustering of cases is shared by caliciviruses and preformed bacterial toxins. However, unlike preformed toxins, caliciviruses cause secondary infections, which confirm the contagious nature of the outbreak. Diarrheal illnesses caused by enteric adenovirus infection tend to be more prolonged than rotavirus (7-10 days), whereas astroviruses cause a shorter course (~5 days) usually without significant vomiting.

Bacterial Diarrhea

Although there is considerable overlap, fever >40°C, overt fecal blood, abdominal pain, no vomiting before diarrhea onset, and high stool frequency (>10/day) are more common with bacterial pathogens. Although high fever and overt fecal blood are often absent in bacterial enteritis, when present, there is a high probability of a bacterial etiology. The classical bacterial agents, nontyphoidal *Salmonella* (NTS), *Shigella, Campylobacter,* and *Yersinia* are present with one of five syndromes.

Acute diarrhea, the most common presentation, may be accompanied by fever and vomiting. Clinically silent bacteremia associated with uncomplicated NTS AGE can be seen among otherwise healthy children younger than 2 years living in industrialized countries.

Bloody diarrhea or *frank dysentery* is classically caused by *Shigella*. Watery diarrhea typically precedes dysentery and is often the sole clinical manifestation of mild infection.

Invasive, nonfocal disease (enteric fever) is a febrile illness associated with bacteremia without localized infection. Diarrhea may be minimal or absent. Although classically the result of *Salmonella typhi* or Paratyphi A and B, enteric fever can result from the systemic spread of the classical bacterial enteropathogens. Additional risk factors include hemolytic anemia and intravascular lesions for NTS, and iron overload, cirrhosis, and chelation therapy for *Yersinia* sepsis.

Extraintestinal invasive infections can result from either local invasion or bacteremic spread. Examples of local invasion include mesenteric adenitis, appendicitis, and rarely cholecystitis, mesenteric venous thrombosis, pancreatitis, and hepatic, or splenic abscess.

Bacteremic spread may result in pneumonia, osteomyelitis, meningitis (three conditions seen most commonly with NTS), abscesses, cellulitis, septic arthritis, and endocarditis. *Shigella* can cause noninvasive contiguous infections, such as vaginitis and urinary tract infections.

Vertical transmission of *Shigella*, NTS, and *Campylobacter* can produce perinatal infection resulting in a spectrum of illness from isolated diarrhea or hematochezia to fulminant neonatal sepsis.

Protozoal Diarrhea

Illnesses due to intestinal protozoa tend to be more prolonged, sometimes for 2 weeks or more, but usually self-limited in the otherwise healthy host. In general, the duration and severity of *Cryptosporidium* diarrhea is strongly influenced by the immune and nutritional status of the host. A protozoal etiology should be suspected when there is a prolonged diarrheal illness characterized by episodes of sometimes explosive diarrhea with nausea, abdominal cramps, and abdominal bloating.

■ CLINICAL FEATURES (FIG. 1)

Diarrhea

It is wise to ask specifically about the number and character of the stools, as the notion of what constitutes "diarrhea" varies widely. Severity is often underestimated because of the initial pooling of secretion in the gut or because watery diarrhea is easily mistaken for urine. Blood in the stools suggests an invasive organism (*Shigella*, amoebae, or necrotizing enterocolitis) or a hemorrhagic colitis induced by enema therapy with toxic substances. Blood-stained stools may also occur in *Campylobacter* infection. Frothy stools suggest carbohydrate intolerance.

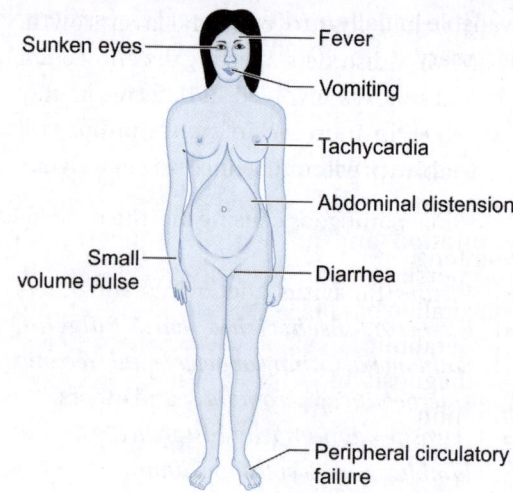

Fig. 1: Clinical features.

Pale malodorous stools suggest steatorrhoea and infection with *G. lamblia*.

Vomiting

Usually, it is present, but its severity is variable and may precede diarrhea by hours or even a day, particularly in cases of viral etiology. If bile-stained or persistent, surgical conditions must be excluded.

Constitutional Signs

Fever and toxicity are uncommon, and their presence suggests parenteral or viral etiology. An abrupt onset of diarrhea with high fever and no vomiting is characteristic of *Shigella enteritis*.

Dehydration

Dehydration occurs in a minority of cases but is the most common complication of gastroenteritis. If untreated, dehydration accounts for 60–70% of gastroenteritis deaths. Accurate and immediate assessment is critical to management. Measurement of weight changes is the most accurate method of assessment but is usually not available initially, making clinical assessment necessary.

Acidosis

Invariably present if there are signs of dehydration, characterized by deep, sighing respiration and an anxious appearance. The persistence of acidosis suggests that dehydration has not been corrected.

Metabolic alkalosis virtually excludes the diagnosis of gastroenteritis. The most common cause of protracted vomiting is pyloric stenosis or other surgical conditions.

GENERAL FEATURES
• Dehydration
• Acidotic breathing
• Seizures
• Generalized edema
• Oliguria
• Thirst
• Dry mucus membrane
• Sunken anterior fontanelle

Ileus

A distended, relatively silent abdomen suggests this diagnosis. This acute "toxic" dilatation of the gut may be caused by infection, toxemia, or hypokalemia. Potassium supplementation reduces the incidence of this complication. Necrotizing enterocolitis can occur in young malnourished infants who have had an episode of shock. It presents with signs of ileus and blood in the stools.

Seizures

These are quite common, but their cause is often obscure. Causes to be excluded are fever, hypoglycemia, electrolyte disturbances (e.g., sodium, calcium, and magnesium), cerebral vein thrombosis, and meningitis. Seizures with fever at the onset of illness suggest *Shigella entertitis*. Seizures and disturbances of central nervous function, such as coma, drowsiness, irritability, and hyperreflexia, are more common in hypernatremic dehydration.

ESSENTIAL DIAGNOSTIC POINTS
• Diarrhea
• Vomiting
• Dehydration
• Drowsiness
• Irritability
• Seizures
• Ileus
• Acidosis

■ DIAGNOSIS

Clinical examination is necessary to exclude parenteral disease and systemic infections, such as meningitis. Consider the possibility of surgical conditions, particularly if there is persistent or bile-stained vomiting, gross abdominal distension, or redness and edema of the abdominal wall.

Dehydration is the most common complication and must initially be assessed clinically. Regular weighing thereafter allows an objective measure of the process of rehydration. Many complications follow on dehydration.

Assessment of Dehydration (Table 1)

Dehydration is the single most important cause of morbidity and mortality in acute diarrhea, and the assessment of its severity is of utmost importance in the choice of fluid therapy.

Dehydration is classified as mild, moderate, or severe. In infants, fluid losses of 5% (50 mL/kg) and 10% (100 mL/kg), roughly correspond to the moderate and severe grades respectively. In older children and adults, fluid loss of 3, 5, and 7% corresponds to mild, moderate, and severe grades, respectively. Some authors use 3, 6, and 9% for older children.

TABLE 1: Features of dehydration.

	Mild	Moderate	Severe

Look at:
• Condition:
  – Eyes
  – Tears
  – Mouth and tongue
  – Thirst
	• Well, alert
	• Normal
	• Present
	• Moist
	• Drinks normally, not thirsty
		• Restless and irritable
		• Sunken
		• Absent
		• Dry
		• Thirsty, drinks eagerly
			• Lethargic or unconscious; floppy
			• Very sunken and dry
			• Absent
			• Very dry
			• Drinks poorly or not able to drink

Feel: Skin pinch	Goes back quickly	Goes back slowly	Goes back very slowly >2 seconds
Decide: Hydration status	No signs of dehydration	Has two or more signs, there is some dehydration	There is severe dehydration
Treatment plan	Treatment plan A	Treatment plan B	Treatment plan C

TABLE 2: Clinical signs of dehydration.

Body weight loss (%)	Clinical state	Signs
<5	Normal	• Thirst • Dry mucous membrane
5–10	Lethargy	• Sunken eyes or fontanelle • Reduced tissue turgor • Tachycardia • Oliguria • Lack of tears
>10	Shock	• Peripheral circulatory failure • Small pulse volume • Tachycardia • Diminished consciousness • Hypotension

Additional features (**Table 2**) such as sunken anterior fontanelle, thready pulse, shallow breathing, and decreased urine output, can also be included to grade the severity of dehydration. Treatment plan A is for those with no dehydration, plan B is for mild and moderate dehydration, and plan C is for severe dehydration.

Diagnosis

If there is no more than mild dehydration, most cases of gastroenteritis can be managed without further investigation. In severe cases, it may be useful to measure the plasma electrolytes, urea, and glucose and to determine the acid–base status, but if these results are not immediately available, do not delay the treatment of shock and dehydration.

Diagnosis of acute diarrhea is based on the clinical history of passing frequent, loose, or watery stools, with or without vomiting, fever, pain in the abdomen, or blood in the stools. Many children may have symptoms and signs of other associated illnesses, such as cough, skin rashes/measles, and urinary symptoms. The clinical triad of rotaviral diarrhea is a lever, vomiting, and profuse watery stools with a tendency for dehydration.

Dehydration is the most common and life-threatening consequence of diarrhea. Loss of water and electrolytes in diarrhea/stool results in depletion of the extracellular fluid (ECF) volume, electrolyte imbalance, and clinical manifestation of dehydration. The first symptom of dehydration appears after fluid loss of 5% of body weight. When fluid loss reaches 10%, shock often sets in, and the cascade of events that follow can culminate in death unless there is immediate intervention to rehydrate.

Routine stool examination is not recommended except in situations such as young infants with fever, suspected protozoan *Giardia* and *E. histolytica* as a cause, extragut infections or persistent colitis or disaccharide intolerance, and prolonged/persistent diarrhea with malnutrition. Stool culture is invariably noncontributory.

Diarrhea when prolonged or recurrent, then it is a major cause of malnutrition in children, owing to the use of bottle feeds, stoppage of breastfeeds, and lack of energy-dense feeds and hygiene such as hand washing, low food intake during the illness (poor appetite, vomiting, oral thrush or stomatitis, diluting/withholding of food, etc.), reduced nutrient absorption in the intestines, and increased requirements, as a result of infection. Repeated and prolonged episodes of diarrhea have even more deleterious effects and may eventually result in growth failure, intercurrent infections, and problems associated with severe malnutrition and even death.

Microbiology of stools (microscopy and culture) is necessary if a definite etiological diagnosis is required. The clinical characteristics of the illness may be helpful in identifying the probable infective agent, but in most cases, symptoms and signs are so similar as to make this impossible. Urine examination, blood culture, and cerebrospinal fluid (CSF) examination may be indicated.

In children with acute watery diarrhea without fever, and some or no signs of dehydration no investigations are required. Microscopic examination of the stool is probably the only essential investigation in these children. Children who require hospitalization (high fever, toxic appearance, and moderate to severe dehydration) require the following investigations:

> **LABORATORY SALIENT FINDINGS**
> - *Acid–base status:* Plasma electrolytes, urea, and glucose
> - *Microbiology of stools:* Microscopy and culture
> - Urine examination
> - Blood culture
> - Cerebrospinal fluid (CSF) examination

■ TREATMENT

The two main objectives in the management of acute diarrhea are as follows:
1. Prevention of dehydration and providing nutritional support
2. Treatment of dehydration if present

These objectives can be achieved by following the treatment plans as described.

The broad principles of management of acute gastroenteritis in children include oral rehydration therapy (ORT), enteral feeding and diet selection, zinc supplementation, and additional therapies, such as probiotics.

Plan A: No Dehydration

Fluids

Home-available fluids (HAFs): Children with no signs of dehydration can be managed at home with some available fluids (HAF). The HAFs are rice water, *dal* water, lassi or buttermilk, coconut water, lemon water, and plain water. The child is encouraged to take as much fluid as possible. Soft drinks, sweetened fruit drinks, and tea are unsuitable and could be potentially dangerous.

Sugar–salt solution (SSS): A homemade solution (SSS made by adding two dinger pinch of salt and one heaped teaspoon of sugar to 200 mL of water) is an effective and simple form of a replacement solution.

Limitations of SSS are the uncertain availability of sugar, lack of suitable utensils for measuring ingredients and water, and the difficulty in educating mothers to learn, retain, and use the skills required for its proper preparation and administration.

Feeding during diarrhea: Breastfeeding should always be continued during acute diarrhea. If the baby is on top milk then, animal milk need not be diluted with water during any phase of acute diarrhea. Feeding during diarrhea may increase the frequency of stool but does not worsen diarrhea nor increase the risk of dehydration. On the other hand, continued feeding during diarrhea facilitates mucosal recovery and may help in maintaining the nutritional status and preventing persistent diarrhea.

Older children who are not on breast milk should continue taking nutrient-rich food which is available at home such as cereals mixed with milk. The rationale behind continued and aggressive feeding is that the overall nutrient absorption continues to be 70% during acute diarrhea.

Feeding therefore hastens repair of the intestinal mucosa and stimulates early recovery of the pancreatic function and production of brush border enzymes. Studies have shown that the weight gain after 8 days of starting treatment was greatest in those children receiving 110 kcal/kg/day throughout their illness as compared to those who have received 55 kcal/kg/day.

Oral Rehydration Therapy

Oral rehydration solution (ORS) plus HAFs are called ORT. The HAF are *dal* water, soup, buttermilk, coconut water, and rice *kanji*. This should be encouraged as early as possible.

Children, especially infants, are more susceptible than adults to dehydration because of the greater basal fluid and electrolyte requirements per kg and because they are dependent on others to meet these demands. Dehydration must be evaluated rapidly and corrected in 4–6 hours according to the degree of dehydration and estimated daily requirements. A small minority of children, especially those in shock or unable to tolerate oral fluids, require initial intravenous (IV) rehydration, but oral rehydration is the preferred mode of rehydration and replacement of ongoing losses.

Risks associated with severe dehydration that might necessitate IV resuscitation, include age <6 months, prematurity, chronic illness, fever >38°C (100.4°F) if younger than 3 months or >39°C (102.2°F) if 3–36 months of age, bloody diarrhea, persistent emesis, poor urine output, sunken eyes, and a depressed level of consciousness.

The low-osmolality oral rehydration should be given to infants and children slowly, especially if they have emesis. It can be given initially by a dropper, teaspoon, or syringe, beginning with as little as 5 mL at a time. The volume is increased as tolerated. Oral rehydration can also be given by nasogastric (NG) tube if needed; this is not the usual route.

Limitations of ORT include shock, an ileus, intussusception, carbohydrate intolerance (rare), severe emesis, and high stool output (>10 mL/kg/h). Ondansetron (oral mucosal absorption preparation) reduces the incidence of emesis, thus permitting more effective oral rehydration, and is well established in emergency management of acute gastroenteritis in developed countries.

Composition of ORS: World Health Organization (WHO) ORS containing 75 mEq of sodium, 64 mEq of chloride, 20 mEq of potassium, and 75 mmol of glucose/L, with total osmolarity of 245 mOsm/L, is now the global standard of care and more effective than home fluids.

The high sodium content is appropriate in cholera but may not be justified in non-cholera diarrhea. This high-sodium could result in hypernatremia, especially in infants and neonates with diarrhea. Various measures to reduce the sodium load are:
- Lower sodium content in ORS
- Alternating breast milk and ORS (2:1)
- Diluting ORS in 1.5 L of water instead of 1 L. This is not scientifically approved as K^+ and HCO_3^- also get diluted.

Glucose: Optimal reabsorption of water and Na^+ occurs in the lumen when glucose and sodium are in equimolar proportion. Formulas containing more glucose become hyperosmolar and induce osmotic diarrhea, thus making ORS solution dehydrating rather than rehydrating. The standard WHO ORS recommends 20 g/L of glucose providing 111 mmol/L.

Potassium: The concentration of K^+ in ORS is 20 mEq/L. This reflects the K^+ concentration in various forms of diarrhea. This concentration cannot be decreased further.

Base: Base replacement is in the form of citrate or bicarbonate in quantity sufficient to correct mild acidosis which occurs due to dehydration or stool bicarbonate losses.

Osmolarity: The effective osmolarity should be similar to or slightly less than plasma (220–310 mOsm). The dose of ORS is 50–75 mL/kg in the first 4 hours (plan B).

Maintenance dose of ORS (Table 3): After correction of dehydration, ORS is given 50–100 mL/kg in 24 hours in between feeds. The ongoing losses can be corrected by giving 10 mL/kg for every stool. An easy formula is twice the weight of the child in teaspoons, e.g., a 5 kg child is given 10 teaspoons (50 mL).

TABLE 3: WHO guidelines for ORS in children with no dehydration (plan A).

Age	Quantity to be offered after each loose stool
• <6 months	• Quarter glass or cup (50 mL)
• 7 months to 2 years	• Quarter to half glass or cup (50–100 mL)
• 2–5 years	• Half to one glass or cup (100–200 mL)
• Older children	• As much as the child can take

(ORS: oral rehydration solution; WHO: World Health Organization)

Note: ORS in plan A is optional and can be replaced by HAF.

Guidelines for administration: ORS should be given only with a tumbler and spoon @1–2 teaspoon/min, if the child vomits, wait for 10 minutes and restart. If vomiting persists, place an NG tube and administer through the tube.

Limitations of ORS:
World Health Organization ORS:
- Does not decrease the volume of diarrhea
- Does not stop diarrhea
- Does not decrease frequency

Plan B: Some Dehydration (Mild to Moderate) (Table 4)

Moderate (5% dehydration: Vomiting not severe): It is important to restore and maintain normal hydration. Frequent reassessment is advisable. Vomiting is usually transient. Small frequent feeds or NG drips of oral rehydration fluids are usually retained.

Fluids

When there is some dehydration the fluid deficit can be calculated as per the WHO guidelines. ORS is offered at the rate of 75 mL/kg over 4 hours. In children where

TABLE 4: WHO guidelines for ORS in children with some dehydration (plan B).

Age	Weight in kg	ORS (mL)	Glass
<4 months	<5 kg	200–400	1–2
4–11 months	5–7.9 kg	400–600	2–3
12–23 months	8–10.9 kg	600–800	3–4
2–4 years	10–15.9 kg	800–1,200	4–6
5–14 years	16–29.9 kg	1,200–2,200	6–11
>15 years	30 kg or more	>2,200	12–20

the weight is not known the child's age can be used to determine the volume required although this is less precise.

Breastfeeding should be continued whatever the degree of dehydration. Infants <6 months who are not breastfed, 100–200 mL of water should be given in addition to ORS during this period. Free access to plain water for older children should be made. If the child's eyelid becomes puffy, ORS is stopped and plain water or breast milk is given instead. ORS is given according to plan A once the puffiness subsides.

After 4 hours: The child is reassessed and if there are no signs of dehydration, plan A is followed, and if signs of dehydration persist plan B is repeated. Meanwhile, food and milk are offered as mentioned in plan A. If signs of severe dehydration appear, the management is shifted to plan C.

Maintenance Dose of Oral Rehydration Solution

For about 50–100 mL/kg in 24 hours is given between feeds. For ongoing losses, ORS in the dose of 20–50 mL/kg/day or 10 mL/kg after each loose stool, should be given.

Breastfeeding should be continued, but cow milk feeds should be withheld for 6–12 hours (while rehydration is being achieved) and an electrolyte and sugar solution given by mouth or by NG tube. Avoid prolonged periods (>24 hours) of clear fluids or diluted milk feeds. Especially in malnourished children once rehydrated, milk feeds are restarted and can be given as full-strength feeds in amounts smaller than usual. Oral electrolyte and sugar solution is continued, but by 24 hours full volume (i.e., 150 mL/kg) full-strength milk feeds should begin.

For children presenting with clinical signs of dehydration, therapy should be aimed at first correcting the fluid deficit and then maintaining hydration by replacing ongoing losses while maintaining nutrition. Correction of fluid deficits can usually be accomplished via oral administration of appropriate glucose electrolyte solutions. IV fluid therapy is required in only a small number of cases in which there is an accompanying ileus, or the vomiting is of such magnitude that oral therapy fails: The fluid deficit is calculated on the basis of the clinical degree of dehydration and should provide 50 mL/kg body weight for mild dehydration (5%) and 100 mL/kg body weight for moderate dehydration (10%). The calculated deficit volume should be replaced over a period of 4–6 hours by offering frequent small volumes from a bottle, cup, or spoon, or it can be delivered as a continuous slow-rate infusion via an NG tube. Once the child is fully rehydrated, the process of providing fluids to maintain hydration should begin, and the child should be encouraged to resume regular feedings.

Plan C (Severe Dehydration) (Table 5)

Severe (5–10% dehydrated and/or serious vomiting). Requires intragastric drip of electrolyte/sugar solutions, but IV fluids are necessary if the patient suffers from shock,

TABLE 5: Intravenous fluid therapy in severe dehydration.

	First give 30 mL/kg in	Then give 70 mL/kg in
<1 year of age	1 hour*	5 hours
Older children	30 minutes	2.5 hours

*Repeat again if the radial pulse is still very weak or not detectable.

ileus, or severe vomiting. Refer the child to a hospital for treatment.

Children with moderate to severe dehydration who also have clinical findings of shock require urgent therapy to reestablish an adequate circulating blood volume. Fluid resuscitation in these cases requires IV administration of an isotonic crystalline solution, such as normal saline. An initial rapid infusion of 20 mL/kg body weight of normal saline will correct the shock in most children with dehydration due to diarrhea. In those with persistent clinical signs of shock, a second infusion of 20 mL/kg body weight can be administered. After the child's circulatory compromise has been corrected, the process of rehydration with maintenance therapy and early reintroduction of feeds as outlined previously.

Intravenous fluids are started immediately. While the drip is being set, an ORS solution is offered if the child can drink. The best IV fluid solution is Ringer's lactate solution. An ideal preparation would be Ringer's lactate with 5% dextrose. If plain Ringer's lactate is also not available, a normal saline solution (0.9% NaCl) can be used. Plain dextrose solution is not effective.

All children should be started on some ORS solution (about 5 mL/kg/h) when they can drink while on IV fluids (usually within 3–4 hours for infants or 1–2 hours for older children). If the IV line is not accessible, rehydration is done with ORS using an NG tube at 20 mL/kg/h (total of 120 mL/kg). The child is reassessed every 1–2 hours and the fluid is decreased if there is repeated vomiting or abdominal distension. If there is no improvement in hydration after 3 hours, IV fluids should be restarted, as early as possible.

General Recommendations for Intravenous Fluid Therapy

Children with diarrhea with or without vomiting would require IV fluid therapy, if there is:
- Severe dehydration with or without shock
- Persistent vomiting (>3/h)
- Failure to correct or worsening of dehydration on ORT
- High purge rate (would get reflected in persistent dehydration)
- Failure of acceptance of ORS in a dehydrated child
- Abdominal distension
- Deranged sensorium

Children presenting with shock and/or other features of severe dehydration should be given IV fluids rapidly. Ringer's lactate is preferable for initial therapy in these children as it provides extra sodium and also helps to correct acidosis, which is often present in such children.

These children should be given 20–30 mL/kg of Ringer's Lactate as a rapid infusion (within ½–1 hour). This may be repeated if the child's pulse is still feeble or the child has failed to pass urine. Thus, these children can receive 50–60 mL/kg within 2 hours of admission. If the urination is established by this time, then the remaining amount (90–100 mL/kg) of IV fluids required for correction of severe dehydration could be given over the next 6 hours as half-strength (N/2) saline.

If there is failure to pass urine even after 50–60 mL/kg of Ringer's lactate in 2 hours, then the child should be assessed for possible renal failure due to acute tubular necrosis (ATN). For this, the child's hydration status should be assessed.

If the child is still dehydrated, he should be given more fluids, but if he appears well hydrated with a good pulse, then he should be given IV furosemide (1–2 mg/kg/IV stat) to force diuresis.

If the child still fails to pass urine despite furosemide, then a diagnosis of ATN is established and the child should be managed on line of acute renal failure. It is very important that furosemide tests be given only when the child is clinically well and hydrated.

As mentioned above, IV fluids should be given for the shortest possible time. Most children can be started on ORT after correction of dehydration. Some children may still require IV fluid therapy, either because of inadequate intake of ORS or because of complications, such as abdominal distension, deranged sensorium, or convulsions.

These children should then be shifted to IV maintenance fluid therapy. Maintenance fluids are given as N/4 saline (Na^+ 37.5 mEq/L) in children <3 months of age or as N/6 saline (Na^+ 25 mEq/L) in children <3 months of age. Maintenance fluids must contain K^+ in the concentration (20 mEq/L).

Management of Electrolyte Disturbance

Hyponatremia

This is the most frequent electrolyte disturbance seen in children with diarrhea and vomiting. About 30–35% of children at the time of admission may have serum sodium <135 mEq/L. But severe hyponatremia (Na^+ <125 mEq/L) is not common.

Correction of hyponatremia: Deficit fluid therapy given with either N/2 saline or with Ringer's lactate is usually sufficient to correct mild to moderate hyponatremia (Na^+ 125–135 mEq/L) in most children. However, if the child is symptomatic (having convulsion) and his serum Na^+ is <125 mEq/L, then he or she would require more rapid correction of serum sodium. The amount of Na^+ required to correct the deficit can be calculated by the following formula:

Amount of Na^+ required = Na^+ deficit in mEq/L × 0.6 × weight in kilograms.

Hypernatremia

This is uncommon in clinical practice but does occur in Western countries where children are largely given skimmed milk feeding, containing high amounts of sodium. Inappropriate mixing of ORS or SSS is probably the only important cause of hypernatremia dehydration.

If the child arrives in shock, the initial management is still with 20–30 mL/kg of Ringer lactate till the shock is reversed. If hypernatremia is confirmed, then the child is given fluids containing 50–60 mEq/L (N/3 saline) in just maintenance amounts. This enables hypernatraemic dehydration to be corrected over 36–48 hours. More rapid correction is not desirable as it could lead to hyponatremic convulsions.

Hypokalemia

Hypokalemia is frequently seen in malnourished children with diarrhea. It may be clinically asymptomatic or the child may have hypotonia (neck flop, psedoparalysis, etc.) and abdominal distension due to paralytic ileus. Hypokalemia should be documented by measuring serum potassium.

Hypokalemia should be corrected very slowly. A mere increase in the concentration of KCl from 20 to 30–40 mEq/L in the infusion fluid is sufficient to correct hypokalemia. Potassium should never be given in higher concentrations than 40 mEq/L.

Metabolic Acidosis

This is also not uncommon. Most of the metabolic acidosis in diarrheal children occurs due to depletion of blood volume and consequent compromise of renal function. This is corrected with the correction of dehydration and restoration of blood volume as well as renal plasma flow. Severe metabolic acidosis manifests as deep and fast breathing with plasma bicarbonate levels usually below 15 mEq/L.

Symptomatic metabolic acidosis should be corrected by giving 3 mL/kg of 7.5% sodium bicarbonate solution. This should be diluted six times with 5% dextrose. Total volume (20 mL/kg) of diluted bicarbonate should be given over ½–1 hour. This would usually increase serum bicarbonate levels by 5–7 mEq/L. If plasma bicarbonate levels are available then the actual amounts of bicarbonate required can be calculated as follows:

Amount of sodium bicarbonate required (in mEq)

= Bicarbonate deficit (desired bicarbonate – actual bicarbonate) in mEq/L × 0.6
× weight in kilograms.

Correction is usually done only up to 18 mEq/L.

Once rehydration is complete, food should be reintroduced while oral rehydration is continued to replace ongoing losses from emesis or stools and for maintenance. Breastfeeding or nondiluted regular formula should be resumed as soon as possible. Foods with complex carbohydrates (rice, wheat, potatoes, bread, and cereals), lean meats, yogurt, fruits, and vegetables are also tolerated. Fatty foods or foods high in simple sugars (juices and carbonated sodas) should be avoided, the usual energy density of any diet used for the therapy of diarrhea should be around 1 kcal/g, aiming to provide an energy intake of a minimum of 100 kcal/kg/day and a protein intake of 2.3 g/kg/day. In selected circumstances when adequate intake of energy-dense food is problematic, the addition of amylase to the diet through germination techniques can also be helpful.

With the exception of acute lactose intolerance in a small subgroup, most children with diarrhea are able to tolerate milk and lactose-containing diets. Withdrawal of milk and replacement with specialized (and expensive) lactose-free formulations are unnecessary. Although children with persistent diarrhea are not lactose intolerant, administration of a lactose load exceeding 5 g/kg/day may be associated with higher purging rates and treatment failure. Alternative strategies for reducing the lactose load while feeding malnourished children who have prolonged diarrhea include the addition of milk to cereals and the replacement of milk with fermented milk products, such as yogurt.

Lactose intolerance is an important complication in some cases, but even among those children for whom lactose avoidance may be necessary, nutritionally complete diets comprised of; locally available ingredients can be used at least as effective, as commercial preparations or specialized ingredients.

Drug Therapy in Diarrhea

About >90% of cases of acute diarrheas (simple diarrheas) do not require antibiotics, however, antibiotics are frequently prescribed. Antibiotics can induce bacterial resistance and chronic carrier stage and cause disequilibrium of the intestinal ecosystem facilitating the growth of pathogenic opportunistic organisms such as the anaerobic *Clostridium difficile*.

Antibiotics are of no proven efficacy on the duration or severity of illness or the risk of complications in a wide variety of organisms ranging from viruses to some enteroinvasive bacteria, such as *Salmonella*, and parasites, such as *Cryptosporidium*.

The definite clinical indications of antibiotics are as follows:
- *Shigella* dysentery, giardiasis, infection with *E. histolytica*
- Cholera
- Septicemia/toxemia/diarrhea due to systemic illness
- Young infants with toxemia
- Moderate to severe protein-calorie malnutrition
- Immunocompromised situations

The value of antibiotics can be classified usefully as follows:
- High: *Shigella, V. cholerae, Giardia,* and *E. histolytica*
- Questionable: *Campylobacter, Yersinia, E. coli*
- No value: *Salmonella* and viruses

Antibiotics generally are not recommended for children presenting with acute bloody diarrhea unless a specific pathogen has been isolated. Antibiotics are indicated in immunocompromised children or those with septicemia due to *Salmonella, Campylobacter,* or *Yersinia*. In patients with diarrhea due to enterohemorrhagic *E. coli*, antibiotic therapy has been implicated as a risk factor for the subsequent development of hemolytic uremic syndrome (HUS). Confirmed shigellosis and cholera should be treated with an antibacterial drug. Depending on local sensitivities, trimethoprim–sulfamethoxazole (TMP-SMX) or ampicillin may be used for Shigella and azithromycin is most effective in children with cholera. Some probiotic supplements have been shown to decrease the duration of acute diarrheal illnesses. Probiotics may exert an immunomodulatory on the host and a static effect on some enteropathogens, thereby altering the intestinal microflora. *Saccharomyces boulardii*, nonpathogenic yeast has been used to treat and decrease the recurrence rate of *C. difficile* enterocolitis, and *Lactobacillus rhamnosus* GG may lessen the severity of rotaviral dehydration. Zinc is recommended as an adjunct to ORT in low-income countries. However, its efficacy in nonmalnourished children is not supported by solid evidence.

Bacterial Infections

- *Shigella dysentery:* Antibiotics shorten the duration of illness, reduce excretion of organisms, and reduce secondary attack rates in *Shigella* dysentery. However, they may increase bacterial resistance and are sometimes responsible for the HUS, such as sequelae.

    Trimethoprim–sulfamethoxazole is generally the first choice among antibiotics but has recently lost its sensitivity in most parts of our country, and hence local sensitivity patterns must be considered when choosing antibiotics. Nalidixic acid, norfloxacin, and ciprofloxacin are useful alternatives and have proven fairly safe for use in children. Course treatment with ofloxacin or cefixime has also been found to be useful both in efficacy and cost effectiveness.

- *Vibrios (cholera):* Antibiotics make a significant difference in the outcome and spread of cholera and have been listed, by WHO as "clearly indicated." The antibiotic

of choice is doxycycline (short courses do not cause major toxicity even in children <8 years of age.
- *E. coli:* These are the most commonly grown organisms in stool cultures. However, serotyping is rarely carried out in our country and therefore, the pathogenicity is always questionable.

    Enteropathogenic *E. coli* (EPEC) is commonly associated with acute watery diarrheas of infants and young children in developing countries and may be associated with significant morbidity. Antibiotics, e.g., TMP-SMX combination may be used in those with signs of toxicity. Enterotoxigenic *E. coli* (ETEC) is also a common cause of simple watery diarrhea and usually requires only supportive management. "Traveler's diarrhea" with ETEC; however, should be treated with TMP-SMX or norfloxacin, or furazolidone. Antibiotics are not useful in EIEC or EHEC types of *E. coli*.
- *Salmonella:* Diarrheas are usually mild, watery, and self-limited. Antibiotics are clearly responsible for the increased carrier stage. However, they are recommended occasionally in toxic or immunocompromised infants with septicemia.

Protozoal Infections

Drugs are clearly indicated in diarrheas due to G. lamblia. E. histolytica is not a common cause of dysentery in children. However, treatment may be necessary for diarrheas associated with trophozoite forms and for complications of amoebiasis. Although microsporidia and *Isospora* are generally amenable to antimicrobials, *Cryptosporidium* is particularly difficult to treat, and antibiotics are largely ineffective. These organisms however are usually (but not always) associated with immunocompromised states [such as human immunodeficiency virus (HIV)] and the outcome depends mainly on the management of the primary condition.

Zinc Therapy

In addition, to improving diarrhea recovery rates, the administration of zinc in community settings leads to increased use of ORS and a reduction in the inappropriate use of antimicrobials. All children older than 6 months of age with acute diarrhea in at-risk areas should receive oral zinc (20 mg/day) in some form for 10–14 days during and continued after diarrhea.

Zinc supplementation in children with diarrhea in developing countries leads to reduced duration and severity of diarrhea and could potentially prevent a large proportion of cases from recurring. Zinc administration for diarrhea management can significantly reduce all-cause mortality by 46% and hospital admission by 23%.

Probiotics

The use of probiotic nonpathogenic bacteria for the prevention and therapy of diarrhea has been successful in some settings although the evidence is inconclusive to recommend their use in all settings. In addition to restoring beneficial intestinal flora, probiotics can enhance host protective immunity, such as downregulation of pro-inflammatory cytokines and upregulation of anti-inflammatory cytokines. *S. boulardii* is effective in antibiotic-associated and in *C. difficile* diarrhea, and there is some evidence that it might prevent diarrhea in daycare centers. Lactobacillus GG (L. GG) is associated with reduced diarrheal duration and severity, which reduction is more evident in cases of childhood rotavirus diarrhea.

Saccharomyces boulardii and L. GG are the only nonbacterial biotherapeutic agents with systematic convincing data from double-blind studies against the prevention and treatment of acute diarrhea and antibiotic-associated diarrhea. The results of most prospective double-blind clinical trials with other bacterial biotherapeutic agents are disappointing, showing a lack of efficacy.

Antisecretory Drug: Racecadotril

Racecadotril is an enkephalinase inhibitor that reduces intestinal hypersecretion by inhibiting this intestinal enzyme. Racecadotril prevents the inactivation of endogenous acts as neurotransmitters in the GIT by activating opiate receptors and thus reducing the levels of cyclic adenosine monophosphate (cAMP). This results in reduced secretions of water and electrolytes without any effects on intestinal motility. Racecadotril has antisecretory effects only when hypersecretion is present and not in the basal state, unlike loperamide. It also does not produce constipation, bacterial overgrowth, or toxic megacolon so often seen with loperamide.

It is given in a dose of 1.5 mg/kg body weight every 8 hours. There are transient and mild side effects. The impact of this drug will be significant in developing countries, as it will reduce stool output during diarrhea.

Nutrition in Diarrhea

In acute diarrhea, the presence of malnutrition is an important triggering event for progression to persistent diarrhea. Diet in diarrhea, therefore, forms a crucial component in therapy and should be balanced in such a way as to supply adequate calories and nutrients and at the same time does not worsen the preexisting villous injury.

Rotavirus Immunization

Most infants acquire rotavirus diarrhea early in life; an effective rotavirus vaccine would have a major effect on reducing diarrhea mortality in developing countries.

It is now clear that the introduction of these vaccines is associated with a significant reduction in severe diarrhea and associated mortality.

Other vaccines that could potentially reduce the burden of severe diarrhea and mortality in young children are vaccines against cholera, *Shigella*, and ETEC. Preventive use of cholera vaccines in endemic countries can reduce the risk of developing cholera.

■ COMPLICATIONS OF DIARRHEA

The common complications of acute watery diarrhea are as follows:
- Dehydration
- Dyselectrolytemia
- Precipitation of malnutrition
- Secondary lactose intolerance
- Prolongation of diarrhea—persistent diarrhea
- Toxic ileus
- Hemolytic uremic syndrome
- Disseminated intravascular coagulation (DIC)
- Cortical vein thrombosis

■ FOLLOW-UP ADVICE

Children with acute diarrhea should continue the nutritional advice and utmost care should be taken to prevent another episode of diarrhea. Detailed advice regarding immunization should also be given to the parents.

BIBLIOGRAPHY

1. American Academy of Pediatrics Committee on Infectious diseases. Prevention of Rotavirus disease: Guidelines for use of rotavirus vaccine. Pediatrics. 2007;119(1): 171-82.
2. Dennehy FH. Acute diarrheal disease in children: Epidemiology, prevention, and treatment. Infect Dis Clin North Am. 2005;19(3):585-602.
3. Grimwood K, Forbes DA. Acute and persistant diarrhea. Pediatr Clin North Am. 2009; 56(6):1343-61.
4. Ryan M, Lucero Y, O'Ryan-Soriano MA, Ashkenazi S. An update on management of severe acute infectious gastroenteritis in children. Expert Rev Anti Infect Ther. 2010; 8(6):671-82.
5. Ramaswamy K, Jacobson K. Infectious diarrhea in children. Clin North Am. 2001; 30(3):611-24.
6. Thomas DW, Greer FR; American Academy of Pediatrics Committee on Nutrition; American Academy of Pediatrics Section on Gastroenterology, Hepatology, and Nutrition. Probiotics and prebiotics in pediatrics. Pediatrics. 2010;126(6):1217-31.

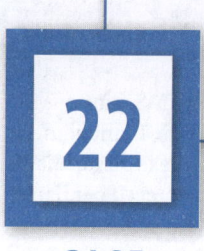

CASE 22

Appendicitis

■ PRESENTING COMPLAINTS

A 6-year-old boy was brought with the complaint of:
- Abdominal pain since 2 days
- Vomiting since 1 day
- Fever since 1 day

History of Presenting Complaints

A 6-year-old boy presented with a history of abdominal pain of sudden onset. Abdominal pain was present around the umbilicus. There was no radiation of the pain. The pain was associated with vomiting. Vomiting was of an insidious type. The child had vomited four to five times since the last 12 hours. Vomiting contains ingested food material. It was nonbilious. Abdominal pain was associated with fever. The fever was moderate to a high degree and was relieved after taking paracetamol. Fever was not associated with chills and rigors.

Past History of the Patient

The boy was the second sibling of a nonconsanguineous marriage. He was born at full term with assisted normal delivery. He cried immediately after the delivery. There was no significant postnatal event. His birth weight was 3.25 kg. He was on breast milk for the first 3 months, later weaning was started and completed by 18 months. His developmental milestones were normal. He was immunized completely. His school performance was good. He was maintaining good health except for the minor on-and-off abdominal pain.

■ EXAMINATION

On examination, the boy was moderately built and nourished. The child was in agony with the abdominal pain. The child was

---

CASE AT A GLANCE

Basic Findings
Height	: 116 cm (70th centile)
Weight	: 18 kg (50th centile)
Temperature	: 35°C
Pulse rate	: 118 beats/min
Respiratory rate	: 22 breaths/min
Blood pressure	: 100/70 mm Hg

Positive Findings

History:
- Abdominal pain
- Vomiting
- Fever
- Crying and irritability

Examination:
- Tenderness
- Guarding

Investigation:
- *TLC:* Increased
- *DLC:* Neutrophils increased
- *Urine:* Pus cells present

(DLC: differential leukocyte count; TLC: total leukocyte count)

comfortable when he was placed prone with the right lower limb flexed up at the hip. Anthropometric measurements included a height of 116 cm (70th centile), and weight was 18 kg (50th centile).

He was febrile with 38°C temperature and his pulse rate was 118 beats/min. The respiratory rate was 22 breaths/min. The blood pressure recorded was 100/70 mm Hg.

He looked pale. There was no cyanosis, no icterus, and no lymphadenopathy. Per abdomen, examination revealed the presence of diffuse periumbilical and right iliac fossa (RIF) tenderness. Mild guarding was present. There was no rebound tenderness. There was no organomegaly. Other systemic examinations were normal.

■ INVESTIGATION

- *Hemoglobin:* 7 g/dL
- *TLC:* 17,500 cells/mm^3
- *DLC:* $P_{72}L_{22}E_3M_3$
- *Erythrocyte sedimentation rate (ESR):* 20 mm in the first hour
- *Plain X-ray of abdomen:* Presence of the fecalith in the ileum
- *X-ray chest:* Normal
- *Urine microscopy:* 10–12 pus cells/high power field (HPF)

■ DISCUSSION

Appendicitis is the most common condition requiring emergency abdominal surgery in childhood. The incidence of appendicitis increases with age. It is more common among adolescents and less common among those younger than 1 year. Boys are more affected. The risk of perforation is greatest in 1–4-year-old children. Children have a higher perforation rate than adults and up to 10% of children present with complicated disease.

■ PATHOLOGY

Appendicitis is classically believed to be secondary to obstruction of the appendiceal orifice, commonly either by a fecalith or lymphoid hyperplasia after viral illness. Other causes of obstruction include parasites and tumors. It is associated with infection. One pathway to acute appendicitis begins with luminal obstruction; inspissated fecal material, lymphoid hyperplasia, ingested foreign bodies, parasites, and tumors have been implicated. Obstruction of the vermiform appendix leads to a closed loop, with mucus production, bacterial overgrowth, and resultant distension.

Luminal obstruction leads to a progressive cascade including increasing intraluminal pressures from bacterial proliferation and continued secretion of mucus, elevated intraluminal pressure, lymphatic and venous congestion and edema, impaired arterial perfusion, ischemia of the wall of the appendix, bacterial invasion of the appendiceal wall and necrosis. This occurs through all the layers of the appendiceal wall. Finally, necrosis of the wall results in perforation and contamination of the peritoneum. The perforation usually occurs at the tip of the appendix distal to obstruction to fecolith. Bacterial invasion of the mesenteric vein may result in portal vein sepsis and subsequent liver abscess. The inflammatory process associated with perforation may lead to intestinal obstructions or paralytic ileus. This progression correlates with the clinical disease progression from simple appendicitis to gangrenous appendicitis and, thereafter, appendiceal perforation. Fecaliths and appendicitis are more common in developed countries with refined, low-fiber diets than in developing countries with high-fiber diet.

Enteric infection likely plays a role in many cases in association with mucosal ulceration and invasion of the appendiceal wall by bacteria. Bacteria such as *Yersinia*, *Salmonella*, and *Shigella*, and viruses such as infectious mononucleosis, mumps, coxsackievirus B, and adenovirus are implicated. Carcinoid tumors, foreign bodies, and ascariasis have been implicated as the cause of obstruction. Abnormal mucus has been the cause of obstruction in cystic fibrosis.

As the inflammation progresses to involve serosa and overlying peritoneum, pain migrates to areas of the peritoneal irritation usually the right lower quadrant. With the perforations, pain becomes generalized. The progression from the onset of the symptoms to perforation usually occurs over 36–48 hours. Young children will have poorly developed omentum. As a consequence, of perforation, organisms may not be confined to the RIF as in adults hence it will spread throughout the peritoneal cavity.

One pathway to acute appendicitis begins with luminal obstruction; inspissated fecal material, lymphoid hyperplasia, ingested foreign bodies, parasites, and tumors have been described. Obstruction of the appendiceal lumen initiates a progressive cascade involving increasing intraluminal pressure, lymphatic and venous congestion and edema, impaired arterial perfusion, ischemia of the appendiceal wall, bacterial proliferation and invasion of the wall, and necrosis. This sequence correlates with the clinical disease progression from simple appendicitis to gangrenous appendicitis and, thereafter, appendiceal perforation.

Because the appendix has the highest concentration of gut-associated lymphoid tissue (GALT) in the intestine, some have hypothesized that the appendix may have an immune function similar to that of the thymus or bursa of Fabricius. Submucosal lymphoid follicles, which can obstruct the appendiceal lumen, are few at birth but multiply steadily during childhood, reaching a peak in number during the teen years, when acute appendicitis is most common.

Enteric infection likely plays a role in many cases of acute appendicitis in association with mucosal ulceration and invasion of the appendiceal wall by bacteria. Bacteria such as *Yersinia*, *Salmonella*, and *Shigella* spp., and viruses such as infectious mononucleosis, mumps, coxsackievirus B, and adenovirus, are implicated. In addition, case reports demonstrate the occurrence of appendicitis from ingested foreign bodies, in association with carcinoid tumors of the appendix, *Ascaris* infestation and rarely following blunt abdominal trauma.

■ CLINICAL FEATURES (FIG. 1)

Appendicitis is most common in older children, with a peak incidence between the ages of 12 and 18 years; it is rare in

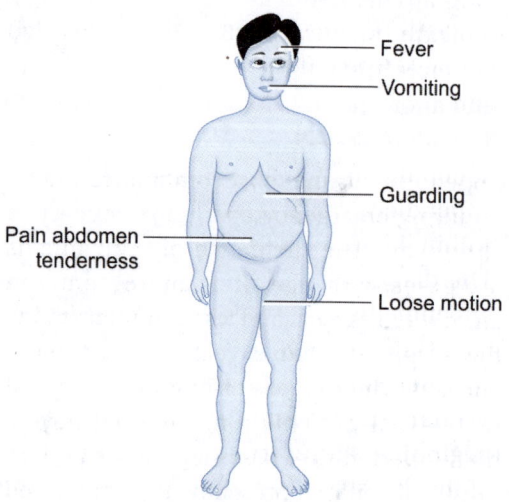

Fig. 1: Clinical features.

children younger than 5 years of age (<5% of cases) and extremely rare (<1% of cases) in children younger than 3 years of age. It affects boys slightly more often than girls. There is a seasonal peak incidence in autumn and spring. Perforation in appendicitis is more common in children compared to adults, particularly in young children; with perforation rates as high as 82% for children younger than 5 years.

History favoring a diagnosis of appendicitis includes the onset of pain before the vomiting or diarrhea, loss of appetite, and migration of pain from the periumbilical region to the RIF. Untreated appendicitis proceeds to the perforation within 48–72 hours. Therefore duration of symptoms is important in the interpretation of the signs and in determining the treatment strategy.

Clinical signs and symptoms depend upon the pathological phase of the illness. The classical triad is pain, vomiting, and fever. In the beginning, pain will be confined to the periumbilical region. Later it will be associated with nausea and vomiting.

The majority of cases of appendicitis have an "atypical" presentation. The illness typically begins insidiously with a brief (several hours) period of generalized malaise and anorexia; the child does not appear ill. The illness escalates rapidly with progressive abdominal pain followed by vomiting, and appendiceal perforation is likely to occur within 48 hours of the onset of the illness. The diagnosis before perforation in acute appendicitis in children is generally brief 36–48 hours.

Abdominal pain is consistently the primary and often the first symptom; beginning shortly (hours) after the onset of the illness. As with other visceral organs, there are no somatic pain fibers within the appendix; therefore, early appendiceal inflammation results in pain that is vague, poorly localized, unrelated to activity or position, often colicky, and periumbilical in location as a result of visceral inflammation from a distended appendix. Progression of the inflammatory process in the next 12–24 hours leads to involvement of the adjacent parietal peritoneal surfaces, resulting in somatic pain localized to the RIF. The position of the appendix is a critical factor affecting the interpretation of presenting signs and symptoms and accurate diagnosis. The pain becomes steady and more severe and is exacerbated by movement.

McBurney point is the junction of the lateral and middle third of the line joining the right iliac, suprailiac spine, and umbilicus. The most important physical finding is persistent direct tenderness to the palpation and the rigidity of the overlying rectus muscle. However, if the diagnosis is doubtful, especially in a very young child, <5 years of rectal examination, reveals important information. Localized tenderness is a later and less consistent finding when the appendix is retrocecal in position (>50% of cases). In cases of an appendix localized entirely in the pelvis, the tenderness on abdominal examination may be minimal and best appreciated on rectal examination. Later careful examination should be performed to diagnose shock as a result of sepsis and dehydration or both.

Nausea and vomiting occur in more than half the patients and usually follow the onset of abdominal pain by several hours. Anorexia is a classic and consistent finding in acute appendicitis. Fever is common and typically low-grade unless perforation has occurred. Most patients demonstrate at least mild tachycardia.

The temporal progression of symptoms from vague, mild pain, malaise, and anorexia to severe localized pain, fever, and vomiting typically occurs rapidly, in 24–48 hours in the majority of cases. If the diagnosis is delayed beyond 36–48 hours, the perforation rate exceeds. If perforation leads to diffuse peritonitis, the child generally has escalating diffuse abdominal pain and rapid development of toxicity evidenced by dehydration and signs of sepsis including hypotension, oliguria, acidosis, and high-grade fever. When several days have elapsed in the progression of appendicitis, patients often develop signs and symptoms of developing small bowel obstruction. If the appendix is retrocecal, appendicitis predictably evolves more slowly and patients are likely to relate 4–5 days of illness preceding evaluation. The pain is typically more lateral and posterior and can mimic the symptoms associated with septic arthritis of the hip or a psoas muscle abscess.

Examination findings must be interpreted relative to the temporal evolution of the illness. Abdominal tenderness may be vague or even absent early in the course of appendicitis and is often diffuse after rupture.

Rebound tenderness and referred tenderness (Rovsing sign) are also consistent findings in acute appendicitis but are not always present. Rebound tenderness is elicited by deep palpation of the abdomen followed by the sudden release of the examining hand. This is often very painful to the child and has demonstrated a poor correlation with peritonitis, so it should be avoided. Gentle finger percussion is a better test for peritoneal irritation. Similarly, digital rectal examination is uncomfortable and unlikely to contribute to the evaluation of appendicitis in most cases of appendicitis in children.

> **ESSENTIAL DIAGNOSTIC POINTS**
> - Obstruction of the lumen is the primary cause of appendicitis
> - Most common condition requiring emergency abdominal surgery
> - The obstruction is mainly caused by fecoliths
> - Infective agents may be *Yersinia*, *Salmonella* and *Shigella*
> - The classical triad is pain, vomiting, and fever
> - Rebound tenderness is tested by gentle finger percussion in all four quadrants in all the age groups

Guarding may be present, and the child may protect the area with its hand. Abdominal distension may suggest perforation or obstruction. The right lower quadrant, i.e., McBurney point should be palpated last.

Pelvic appendicitis produces rectal tenderness. Perforation leads to temporary relief of symptoms. Local muscular rigidity, psoas muscle spasms, and rebound tenderness are present. Per rectal examination is painful in pelvic appendicitis.

Psoas and obturator internus signs are pain with the passive stretch of these muscles. The psoas sign is elicited with active right thigh flexion or passive extension of the hip and is typically positive in cases of a retrocecal appendix. The obturator sign is demonstrated by adductor pain after internal rotation of the flexed thigh and is typically positive in cases of a pelvic appendix. Physical examination may demonstrate a mass in the RIF representing an inflammatory phlegmon around the appendix or a localized abscess (fluid collection).

> **GENERAL FEATURES**
> - Anorexia
> - Rebound tenderness
> - Persistent direct tenderness
> - Abdominal rigidity over the rectal muscle

DIAGNOSIS

A child with a chief complaint of migrating periumbilical to the right lower quadrant, abdominal pain, anorexia, right lower quadrant tenderness on examination, and leukocytosis is likely to have appendicitis. The differential diagnosis in a child with right lower quadrant abdominal pain includes both nonsurgical processes, such as enteritis, mesenteric adenitis, constipation, nephrolithiasis, inflammatory bowel disease, especially Crohn's disease, pneumonia, and urinary tract infections, and surgical processes, including intussusception and Meckel diverticulum.

The leukocyte count in early appendicitis may be normal and typically is only mildly elevated with a left shift ($11,000$–$16,000/mm^3$) as the illness progresses in the initial 24–48 hours. The leukocyte count may be markedly elevated ($20,000/mm^3$) in perforated appendicitis (PA) and rarely in nonperforated cases.

Urinalysis often demonstrates a few white or red blood cells, as a result of the proximity of the inflamed appendix to the ureter or bladder, but it should be free of bacteria.

C-reactive protein (CRP) increases in proportion to the degree of appendiceal inflammation but is nonspecific and not widely used. Serum amyloid A protein is consistently elevated in patients with acute appendicitis.

Plain Radiographs

Plain X-ray abdomen shows the following:
- Calcified appendicolith
- Gas fluid level in a cecum
- Small bowel dilatation without fluid level
- Amputation of the gas at the hepatic flexure due to spastic ascending colon—colon cut-off sign
- Obliteration of right psoas shadow
- Pneumoperitoneum in case of peritonitis

Barium studies show:
- Absent or incomplete filling of the appendix
- Irregularities in the appendicular lumen

Ultrasound

Ultrasonography (USG) demonstrates fecoliths, the presence of intraluminal fluid, and a thickened appendiceal wall, i.e., >2 mm in thickness when the appendix ruptures and the tip blows out the appendix becomes difficult to identify. The appendix is identified as a blind-ending, tubular, nonperistalsing segment of the bowel arising from the cecum. A noncompressible appendix, peri-appendiceal inflammation, and the presence of an appendicolith are described as reliable indicators of acute appendicitis.

The diagnosis of appendicitis relies on visualizing a noncompressible appendix that is >6 mm in diameter, lack of compressibility, has a complex mass in the RIF, or has an appendicolith. Asymmetric thickening is also an indication of inflammation. The visualized appendix usually coincides with the site of localized pain and tenderness. Findings that suggest advanced appendicitis on ultrasound (US) include asymmetric wall thickening, abscess formation, associated free intraperitoneal fluid, surrounding tissue edema, and decreased local tenderness to compression.

When the patient presents with PA, the USG can yield free fluid in the abdomen or intra-abdominal abscess and possibly a free fecalith. In large children's hospitals, USG is routinely used as a first-line diagnostic modality.

Computed Tomography Scan

In the cases, where either the appendix cannot be identified or the diagnosis is still unclear, computed tomography (CT) has been advocated. CT removes the variable of operator skill and is not affected by larger body habitus or overlying intraluminal bowel gas. However, CT introduces the risk of ionizing radiation and increased cost. Therefore, many practitioners advocate for the USG-first paradigm in the imaging for suspected appendicitis.

A CT scan may be most useful in advanced appendicitis to identify and guide percutaneous drainage of fluid collections and identification of an inflammatory mass, which might prompt a plan for initial nonoperative management.

Computed tomography scan findings include:
- Circumferential thickening of the wall of the appendix
- Phlegman—pericecal fat tissue
- Homogenous ring-like calcification—appendicolith
- Linear streaky densities in pericecal/mesenteric pelvic fascia

TABLE 1: Pediatric appendicitis scores.

Future	Score
Fever > 38°C (100.4°F)	1
Anorexia	1
Nausea/vomiting	1
Cough/percussion/hopping tenderness	2
Right lower quadrant tenderness	2
Migration of pain	1
Leukocytosis >10,000 (10^9/L)	1
Polymorphonuclear-neutrophilia >7,500 (10^9/L)	1
Total	10

LABORATORY SALIENT FINDINGS
- Leukocytosis and shift in the differential count
- Urine analysis may show the presence of pus cells as well as red blood cells
- *Plain X-ray abdomen:* Calcified appendicolith gas fluid level in the cecum
- *Barium studies:* Absent or incomplete filling of the appendix Irregularities in the appendicular lumen
- Ultrasonography demonstrates fecoliths, the presence of intra luminal fluid, and thickened appendiceal wall
- *CT scan:* Circumferential thickening of the wall of appendix phlegman—pericecal fat tissue homogenous ring-like calcification—appendicolith

■ DIFFERENTIAL DIAGNOSIS

Differential diagnosis includes Crohn's disease, Meckel's diverticulum, mesenteric adenitis, urinary tract infection, HUS, and Henoch–Schonlein purpura.

Pediatric Appendicitis Score

The pediatric appendicitis score (PAS) **(Table 1)** combines elements of history (migration of pain, anorexia, nausea, and vomiting) with physical examination findings [(right lower quadrant (RLQ) tenderness, rebound tenderness, and fever] and laboratory data [white blood cell (WBC) >10,000, polymorphonuclear neutrophils >75%] to assign a risk score in the low, intermediate, or high-risk range for acute appendicitis. Scores of S4 suggest a very low likelihood of appendicitis, whereas scores of 28 are highly sensitive and specific for appendicitis. Intermediate scores, between 4 and 7 on the PAS, are considered inconclusive and typically trigger advanced imaging studies.

■ COMPLICATIONS

Complications occur in 25–30% of children with appendicitis. The main complication is perforation. Appendicular abscess can also occur. Intra-abdominal abscess are rare. Liver abscess from the portal vein sepsis is common. Intestinal obstruction from the portal vein sepsis is common.

■ TREATMENT

Once the diagnosis of appendicitis is confirmed or highly suspected, the standard treatment for acute appendicitis is most often prompt appendectomy. Some reports suggest initial nonoperative management (antibiotics and drainage of fluid collections) as an alternative option in presentations, depending on the patient's general condition and the state of the appendix.

To be considered uncomplicated, patients had pain <48 hours, ultrasonographic or CT documentation of a nonruptured appendix, as well as an appendiceal diameter <1.1 cm without phlegmon, abscess, or fecalith. Management included a minimum of 24 hours of IV antibiotics (piperacillin-tazobactam or ciprofloxacin with metronidazole) followed by amoxicillin-clavulanate or ciprofloxacin with metronidazole to complete a 10-day total antibiotic course. The operation should proceed semielectively within 12–24 hours of diagnosis. Children with appendicitis are typically at least mildly dehydrated and require preoperative fluid resuscitation to correct hypovolemia and electrolyte abnormalities before anesthesia. Fever, if present, should be treated. Pain management begins even before a definitive diagnosis is made. In the majority of cases preoperative management can be accomplished during the period of diagnostic evaluation and prompt appendectomy can be performed.

Antibiotics

Recently the choice for antibiotic administration for appendicitis has come up for debate. Recent studies have compared the traditional triple antibiotic regimen (e.g., ampicillin, gentamicin, and clindamycin) to once-daily dosing of ceftriaxone and metronidazole and have not demonstrated a difference in the outcome. Additionally, the use of oral antibiotics prior to postoperative day 5 if the patient is able to tolerate oral medications has become more popular. Further, once the leukocytosis has resolved, patients can be safely discharged home prior to completing 5 days of IV antibiotics.

Antibiotics substantially lower the incidence of postoperative wound infections and intraperitoneal abscesses in PA, but their role is less well-defined in simple appendicitis. The antibiotic regimen should be directed against the typical bacterial flora found in the appendix, including anaerobic organisms (*Bacteroides*, *Clostridia*, and *Streptococcus* spp.) and gram-negative aerobic bacteria *E. coli*, *Pseudomonas aeruginosa*, *Enterobacter*, and *Klebsiella*.

For simple non-PA, one preoperative dose of a single broad-spectrum agent (cefoxitin) or equivalent is sufficient. The practice in perforated or gangrenous appendicitis, most surgeons prefer combination regimens, such as (piperacillin/tazobactam), ticarcillin/clavulanate, and ceftriaxone/metronidazole. The traditional triple antibiotic regimen (ampicillin, gentamicin, and clindamycin or metronidazole) is still effective but adds cost and has the concern for ototoxicity. The commonly used antibiotics are ampicillin (100 mg/kg/24 h) gentamicin (5 mg/kg/24 h), clindamycin (30 mg/kg/24 h), cefotaxime (50–100 mg/kg/24 h), and ceftriaxone (50–100 mg/kg/24 h).

Antibiotics should be given for 7–10 days and continued postoperatively for 3–5 days. Oral antibiotics are equally as effective as IV, and therefore the patient can be switched to an oral regimen and discharged once bowel function returns. This transition to oral antibiotics has significantly affected the length of stay and cost in the management of PA.

Surgery

Diagnostic laparoscopy and laparoscopic appendectomy (minimally invasive technique) for both simple and PA are the preferred approaches in most pediatric centers; open surgery is still performed in selected cases. Laparoscopic appendectomy has significant advantages in administrative factors (cost, resource utilization, and length of stay) and a slight improvement in clinical outcome measures (wound infection rate, intraabdominal abscess, analgesic requirements, and return to full activity), but has failed to establish an evidence-based preference between laparoscopic and open appendectomy in children. In non-PA, laparoscopic appendectomy appears to have lower narcotic analgesic requirements, decreased wound morbidity, and improved cosmesis, but operative times seem slightly higher, and costs are almost doubled compared to the open procedure. The length of hospitalization is similar for both approaches.

The role of laparoscopy in PA is less well-defined. There is no convincing data to recommend one approach for all patients. Most pediatric surgeons use both approaches selectively. The laparoscopic approach is used most often for obese patients, when alternative diagnoses are suspected, and in adolescent girls to better evaluate for ovarian pathology and pelvic inflammatory disease while avoiding the ionizing radiation associated with CT imaging.

Nasogastric suction should be done if there is vomiting and abdominal distension. In children with unperforated appendicitis, IV fluid and antibiotics should be started. The treatment in the perforated appendix ranges from nonsurgical to aggressive surgical resection with antibiotic irrigate, drainage of the peritoneal cavity, or even delayed wound closure. Appendiceal mass is treated with an initial conservative regimen, followed by interval appendectomy in 4–8 weeks.

Complications

The most common complications are wound infections and intra-abdominal abscesses; both are more common after perforation. Perforation and abscess formation can also lead to fistula formation in adjacent organs. Perforation rates are consistently >80% in children younger than 5 years of age. Other potential complications include postoperative ileus, diffuse peritonitis portal vein pylephlebitis (rare), and adhesive small bowel obstruction. Treatment of the wound infection is opening the wound and healing by secondary intention.

Chronic Appendicitis

The appendix may be responsible for chronic right lower quadrant pain. The literature describes two seemingly distinct pathologic entities: chronic appendicitis, where the appendix shows histologic signs of chronic inflammation, and appendiceal colic, where a nonobstructing luminal mass (e.g., fecaloma, fibrosis, kink-adhesion, foreign body, parasites, carcinoid, and lymphoid hyperplasia) is found. These diagnoses can only be definitively made following removal of the appendix. These pathologic findings can be found together or in conjunction with acute appendicitis, which further confounds the validity of this entity.

Typically, the child will complain of long-standing right lower quadrant pain and may have intermittent tenderness at Mc Burney's point. Chronic appendicitis and appendiceal colic are diseases of exclusion and will often have normal laboratory values and nondiagnostic imaging.

Perforated Appendicitis

A major area of focus and challenge in the management of acute appendicitis is the group of patients with delayed presentation (>48 hours of symptoms). In most busy centers, because acute appendicitis often has an insidious onset of generalized malaise, as many as 40–50% of patients have delayed presentation. The risk for development of postoperative complications [surgical site infection (SSI), intraabdominal abscess, small bowel obstruction] approaches 20–30% for children with PA versus an approximately 3% risk of complications in patients with simple appendicitis.

Management options for children presenting with PA include upfront appendectomy following a brief period of stabilization with IV fluids and antibiotics, antibiotics alone, and antibiotics in conjunction with percutaneous drainage of intra-abdominal fluid collections/abscesses. Antibiotics are initiated and typically continued intravenously for 1–2 days along with pain control. If the child demonstrates clinical recovery by resolution of fever and pain, and the patient can tolerate a general diet, the child ted is converted to oral antibiotics and discharged to complete an outpatient antibiotic course (typically 7–10 days of ciprofloxacin/metronidazole). A patient who fails to demonstrate clinical recovery proceeds to prompt appendectomy.

■ BIBLIOGRAPHY

1. Abbas PL, Peterson M, Stephens LJ, Rodriguez JR, Lee TC, Brandt ML, et al. Evaluating the effect of time process measures on appendectomy clinical outcomes. J Pediatr Surg. 2016;51(5):810-4.
2. Bansal S, Banever GT, Karrer FM, Partrick DA. Appendicitis in children less than 5 years old: influence of age on presentation and outcome. Am J Surg. 2012;204(6)1031-5;discussion 1035.
3. Iqbal CW, Knott EM, Mortellaro VE, Fitzgerald KM, Sharp SW, St Peter SD. Interval appendicectomy after perforated appendicitis: what are the operative risks and luminal patency rates? J Surg Res. 2012;177(1):127-30.
4. Kharbanda AB, Cosme Y, Liu K, Spitalnik SL, Dayan PS. Discriminative accuracy of novel and traditional biomarkers in children with suspected appendicitis adjusted for duration of abdominal pain. Acad Emerg Med. 2011;18(6):567-74.
5. St Peter SD, Aguayo P Fraser JD, Keckler SJ, Sharp SW, Leys CM, et al. Initial laparoscopic appendectomy versus initial nonoperative management and interval appendectomy for perforated appendicitis with abscess: a prospective, randomized trial. J Pediatr Surg. 2010;45(1):236-40.

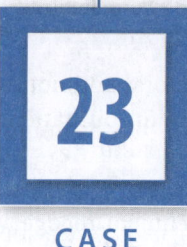

CASE 23

Congenital Hypertrophic Pyloric Stenosis

■ PRESENTING COMPLAINTS

A 10-week-old boy was brought with the complaint of:
- Persistent vomiting since 15 days
- Not gaining weight since 15 days

History of Presenting Complaints

A 10-week-old boy was brought to the pediatric outpatient department with a history of persistent vomiting since 15 days and with a history of not gaining weight. His mother said that he would vomit immediately if he completed the breastfeeds. According to the mother child used to vomit all the milk that he had taken. The milk used to come out in curdled form.

Past History of the Patient

He was the first child of a nonconsanguineous marriage. He was delivered at full term with normal delivery. He cried immediately after delivery. The birth weight was 3 kg. There was no postnatal significant event except for the prolonged physiological jaundice. The child was on breast milk from the beginning. There was no feeding problem in the beginning. He was doing well till the age of 6 weeks. His weight was 4 kg when he came for immunization. He was normal till the age of 8 weeks. Later he developed vomiting milk which he had taken. His mother had

CASE AT A GLANCE

Basic Findings
Length	:	60 cm (70th centile)
Weight	:	4.5 kg (40th centile)
Temperature	:	36.5°C
Pulse rate	:	120 beats/min
Respiratory rate	:	26 breaths/min
Blood pressure	:	60/40 mm Hg

Positive Findings

History:
- Vomiting
- Loss of weight
- Not gaining weight
- Normal at birth

Examination:
- Signs of dehydration
- Visible gastric peristalsis
- Loss of weight

Investigation:
- Electrolytes Na: 110 mEq/L
  - K: 5 mEq/L
  - Cl: 80 mEq/L
- X-ray plain:
  - Erect abdomen: Thick-walled active stomach

observed a small swelling being present in the upper part of the abdomen after the feed.

■ EXAMINATION

The boy was moderately built and nourished. Anthropometric measurements included, the weight was 4.5 kg (40th centile), and the length was 60 cm (70th centile). The head circumference was 39 cm. There were features

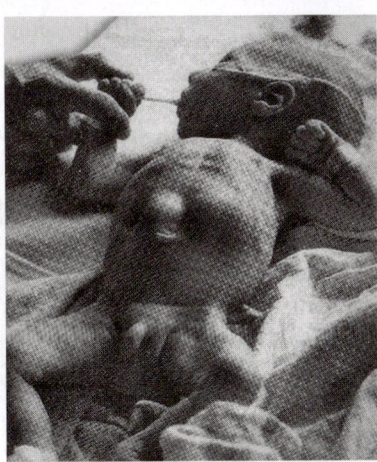

Fig. 1: Visible gastric peristalsis.

of mild dehydration. Features of a marasmic child were present.

The child was afebrile. The pulse rate was 120 beats/min, the respiratory rate was 26 breaths/min. The blood pressure recorded was 60/40 mm Hg. There was no pallor, no lymphadenopathy, and no cyanosis.

Per abdomen examination revealed the presence of a small mass **(Fig. 1)** moving from left to right. This was more evident when the child was examined after feeding. Visible gastric peristalsis was present. There was no organomegaly. Cardiovascular and respiratory systems were normal.

■ INVESTIGATION

- *Hemoglobin:* 13 g/dL
- *TLC:* 13,100 cells/cumm
- *DLC:* $P_{72}L_{26}M_2$
- *ESR:* 32 mm in the first hour
- *Absolute eosinophil count (AEC):* 360 cells/mm^3
- *Serum electrolytes:*
  - *Na:* 110 mEq/L
  - *K:* 5 mEq/L
  - *Cl:* 80 mEq/L
- *X-ray plain erect abdomen:* Thick-walled active stomach

■ DISCUSSION

The boy was normal at birth. He was doing well till the age of 6 weeks. Later he developed persistent vomiting. The presence of a visible mass moving from the left to the right side after the feeding suggests congenital hypertrophic pyloric stenosis (HPS).

It affects frequently firstborn male infants. Multifactorial inheritance is likely. Male infants are affected four times more than females. The incidence of this is more with type B and O blood groups. The cause of pyloric stenosis is unknown, but many factors have been implicated. Abnormal muscle innervation, maternal stress in the third trimester, and administration of prostaglandin E to maintain the patency of the ductus have been implicated as etiological factors.

The incidence of pyloric stenosis has increased in infants with B and O blood groups. Pyloric stenosis is occasionally associated with other congenital defects, including tracheoesophageal fistula and hypoplasia or agenesis of the inferior labial frenulum.

Pyloric stenosis has been associated with eosinophilic gastroenteritis, Apert syndrome, Zellweger syndrome, trisomy 18, Smith-Lemli-Opitz syndrome, and Cornelia de Lange syndrome. An association has been found with the use of erythromycin in neonates with the highest risk if the medication is given within the first 2 weeks of life.

Hypertrophic pyloric stenosis is a condition of infancy that occurs between 2 and 10 weeks of age, most commonly between 5 and 6 weeks of age. In premature infants, it presents at a later chronological age, but earlier postconceptional age. It is characterized by hypertrophy of the circular muscle of the pylorus causing gastric outlet obstruction.

PATHOGENESIS

Despite advances in the field, HPS is still considered idiopathic. It appears to result from the interplay of genetic predisposition with local tissue factors, as well as pre- and postnatal environmental exposures.

Hypertrophic pyloric stenosis is not congenital, as it has been shown by studying healthy newborns with US and upper gastrointestinal (UG) fluoroscopy.

All infants had normal studies after birth, but a few of them went on to develop HPS, while most did not. Pyloric stenosis does not develop without initiation of feeds, so the interaction of feeds and other pre and postnatal micro and macroenvironmental factors with the developing pyloric muscle is likely the key element to trigger the condition in genetically predisposed individuals. The majority of hypertrophy happens in the circular muscle layer, which thickens and elongates, but thickening of the mucosa is also present. The natural course of HPS is that of resolution as evidenced by the feasibility of nonoperative treatment with atropine and/or parenteral nutrition.

Diffuse hypertrophy and hyperplasia of the smooth muscle narrow the antrum of the stomach to a fine channel that easily becomes obstructed. The antral region is elongated and thickened to as much as twice its normal size. The muscular thickening is never confined to an isolated band or circular muscle fiber called the pyloric sphincter. It extends proximally well into the antrum and ends distally quite abruptly where the duodenum begins.

The appearance of the pylorus is that of an enlarged, pale muscle mass usually measuring 2–2.5 cm in length and 1–1.5 cm in diameter. Histologically the mucosa and adnexa are normal. There is marked muscle hypertrophy primarily involving the circular layer. This produces partial or complete luminal occlusion.

Milk curds produce edema of the pyloric mucosa and submucosa leading to partial luminal obstruction and hypertrophy of pyloric muscle. There is a decrease in ganglion cells in the circular muscles in the pylorus. Ganglion cells are immature.

A hereditary component of pyloric stenosis is consistent with a multifactorial, sex-modified threshold model of inheritance, in which 5.5% of sons and 2.5% of daughters of an affected father develop HPS.

There is no single gene that is responsible for HPS, but genome-wide analyses have revealed several potential contributing loci including the gene encoding the enzyme neuronal nitric oxide synthase (nNOS), a family of genes encoding transient receptor potential cation channels, and a locus adjacent to the apolipoprotein gene cluster.

Complex interactions between nerve and muscle cells and the extracellular matrix of pyloric tissue have been studied along with the influences of hormones, growth factors, and local paracrine mediators. Gastrin and prostaglandin E may be contributing factors, as well as increased levels of insulin-like growth factor-I, platelet-derived growth factor, epidermal growth factor, and transforming growth factor in pyloric muscle.

The activity of nitric oxide (NO) in hypertrophied pylorus is decreased, resulting in lower levels of NO that mediate the relaxation of smooth muscle. The distribution and interaction of extracellular matrix proteins are altered compared to the normal pylorus, and multiple abnormalities in innervation have been described. Interstitial cells of Cajal are non-neuronal cells that interact with the enteric nervous system and secrete carbon monoxide and NO, both mediators of smooth muscle relaxation. They are decreased in HPS, possibly contributing to smooth muscle spasms and hypertrophy.

Pyloric stenosis has been associated with eosinophilic gastroenteritis, Apert syndrome, Zellweger syndrome, trisomy 18, tracheoesophageal fistula, Smith–Lemli–Opitz syndrome, and Cornelia de Lange syndrome.

■ CLINICAL FEATURES (FIG. 2)

Pyloric stenosis is usually not present at birth and is more concordant in monozygotic than dizygotic twins. It has a slight association with hiatus hernia and esophageal atresia. High levels of serum gastrin may be found. Gastrin levels are elevated neurotransmitter substance that produces chronic pylorospasm leading to muscle hypertrophy. A VIP and deficiency of NO in pyloric muscle result in failed relaxation. Premature infants with HPS present 2 weeks later than term infants.

Forceful (projectile) nonbilious emesis after feeds is the hallmark of HPS. It develops progressively, increasing in frequency and force. Infants are of a typical age group (2–8 weeks) and otherwise well. They are hungry and want to eat again immediately after emesis. Weight loss and dehydration develop in more advanced cases. Hematemesis may be present if there is concomitant gastritis. Due to dehydration and loss of gastric acid, the typical metabolic finding is hypokalemic, hypochloremic metabolic alkalosis.

Initially, there is only regurgitation and occasionally nonprojectile. Vomiting becomes projectile usually within one week after the onset. It generally occurs during or shortly after the feeding but sometimes it occurs several hours later.

Nonbilious vomiting is the initial symptom of pyloric stenosis. The vomiting may or may not be projectile initially but is usually progressive, occurring immediately after a feeding. Emesis might follow each feeding, or it may be intermittent. The vomiting usually starts after 3 weeks of age, but symptoms can develop as early as the first week of life and as late as the fifth month.

In some instances, vomiting occurs after feeding. The vomiting contains only gastric content. But sometimes may be blood-stained. Approximately 20% have intermittent emesis from birth that then progresses to the classic picture. After vomiting, the infant is hungry and wants to feed again. As vomiting continues, a progressive loss of fluid, hydrogen ions, and chloride leads to critical deficits of potassium and sodium and hypochloremic metabolic alkalosis. There is a striking decrease in chloride concentration and an increase in pH and carbon dioxide content. This leads to hypochloraemic alkalosis. Correction of these chemical changes requires the replacement of sodium chloride and potassium. IV administration of 5% Dextrose in isotonic sodium chloride to which potassium chloride is added is recommended. Serum potassium levels are usually maintained, but there may be a total body potassium deficit.

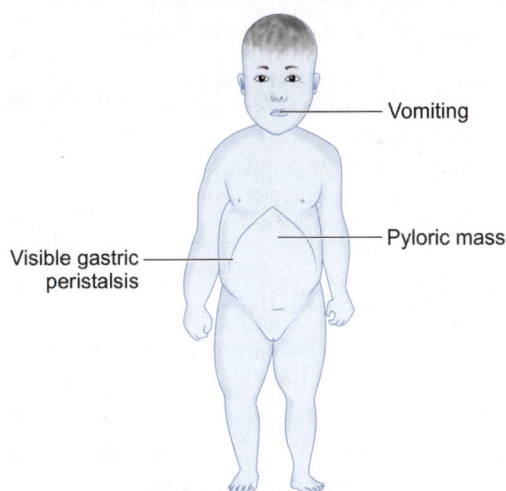

Fig. 2: Clinical features.

Hyperbilirubinemia is the most common clinical association of pyloric stenosis, also known as icteropyloric syndrome. Unconjugated hyperbilirubinemia is more common than conjugated and usually resolves with surgical correction of the pyloric stenosis. It may be associated with a decreased level of glucuronyltransferase as seen in approximately 5% of affected infants; mutations in the *UGT1A1* gene have also been implicated. If conjugated hyperbilirubinemia is a part of the presentation, other etiologies need to be investigated. Other coexistent clinical diagnoses have been described, including eosinophilic gastroenteritis, hiatal hernia, peptic ulcer, congenital nephrotic syndrome, congenital heart disease, and congenital hypothyroidism.

The diagnosis has traditionally been established by palpating the pyloric mass. The mass is firm, movable, approximately 2–2.5 cm in length, hard, best palpated from the left side, and located above and to the right of the umbilicus in the midepigastrium beneath the liver edge. The olive is easiest palpated after an episode of vomiting. After feeding, there may be a visible gastric peristaltic wave that progresses across the abdomen.

On examination, visible peristalsis preceeding from the left upper quadrant toward the pylorus in the right upper quadrant of the abdomen is more prominent after feeds, and before vomiting. Diagnosis is mainly clinical confirmation by palpating the mass. This is only feasible in a comfortable and relaxed infant with a decompressed stomach, which takes time, patience, and experience. Hyperperistaltic waves in the dilated stomach may be appreciated through the abdominal wall in the left upper quadrant.

Physical examination reveals varying degrees of dehydration and lethargy depending on the metabolic state. Weight loss may occur. Decreased elasticity of the skin and loss of subcutaneous tissue may occur. Eyes may be sunken and fat pads of cheeks may be lost giving old man's appearance.

In more advanced cases, oliguria, decreased skin turgor, lethargy, and delayed capillary refill may be present due to dehydration, and the infant may appear emaciated. Jaundice is present in up to 5% of infants presenting with HPS. This is thought to reflect a decrease in hepatic glucuronosyltransferase activity associated with starvation or may reflect an early manifestation of Gilbert syndrome.

ESSENTIAL DIAGNOSTIC POINTS

- First born male infants
- Multifactorial inheritance is likely
- A diffuse hypertrophy and hyperplasia of the smooth muscle narrows the antrum
- Abnormal muscle innervation, maternal stress in the third trimester
- Administration of prostaglandin E to maintain the patency of the ductus have been implicated as the etiological factors
- Decrease in ganglion cells in the circular muscles in pylorus
- Projectile vomiting, VGP, FTT, and jaundice

(FTT: failure o thrive; VGP: visible gastric peristalsis)

GENERAL FEATURES

- Nonbilious vomiting
- Projectile vomiting
- Prolonged physiological jaundice
- Failure to gain weight

■ INVESTIGATION

Two imaging studies are commonly used to establish the diagnosis. US examination confirms the diagnosis in the majority of cases. Criteria for diagnosis include a pyloric thickness of 3–4 mm, an overall pyloric length of 15–19 mm, and a pyloric diameter of 10-14 mm USG has a sensitivity of approximately 95%.

Ultrasonographic examination may be done in suspected patients. Serum sodium, potassium, and bicarbonate levels suggest hypokalaemic alkalosis which supports the diagnosis.

Infantile Form

A plain X-ray of the abdomen shows a dilated stomach.

Barium Study

- Elongation and narrowing of pyloric canal (2-4 cm in length)
- Double or triple track sign—crowding of mucosal folds in the pyloric channel
- String sign—passing small barium streak through a pyloric channel—double tract sign
- Twinning recess—"diamond sign"—transient triangular tent-like cleft/niche in the mid portion of the pyloric canal with the apex pointing inferiorly secondary to mucosal bulging between two separated hypertrophied muscle bundles on the greater curvature side within the pyloric canal
- Out pounding along lesser curvature due to disruption of antral peristalsis
- Mushroom sign—Kirklin sign—indentation of the base of the bulb
- Caterpillar sign—hypertrophied walls.

Ultrasonography Findings

- *Target sign:* Hypoechoic ring of hypertrophied pyloric muscle around ECHOgenic mucosa centrally on the cross section.
- *Cervic sign:* Indentation of muscle mass on fluid-filled antrum on longitudinal section
- Pyloric wall thickness >4 mm

- Pyloric muscle wall thickness >14 mm
- Elongated pyloric canal >17 mm in length
- Exaggerated peristaltic waves
- Delayed gastric emptying of fluid into duodenum

> **LABORATORY SALIENT FINDINGS**
> - Ultrasonographic examination
> - Serum sodium, potassium, and bicarbonate levels suggest hypokalemic alkalosis
> - Barium study

When contrast studies are performed, they demonstrate an elongated pyloric channel (string sign), a bulge of the pyloric muscle into the antrum (shoulder sign), and parallel streaks of barium seen in the narrowed channel, producing a "double tract sign."

■ DIFFERENTIAL DIAGNOSIS

Gastroesophageal reflux (GER), with or without a hiatal hernia, may be confused with pyloric stenosis.

Gastroesophageal reflux disease (GERD) can be differentiated from pyloric stenosis by radiographic studies.

Adrenal insufficiency from the adrenogenital syndrome can simulate pyloric stenosis, but the absence of metabolic acidosis and elevated serum potassium and urinary sodium concentrations of adrenal insufficiency aid in differentiation.

Inborn errors of metabolism can produce recurrent emesis with alkalosis (urea cycle) or acidosis (organic acidemia) and lethargy, coma, or seizures. Vomiting with diarrhea suggests gastroenteritis, but patients with pyloric stenosis occasionally have diarrhea.

- Gastroesophageal reflux
- Hiatal hernia
- Adrenal insufficiency
- Pyloric duplication
- Duodenal stenosis

TREATMENT

Hypertrophic pyloric stenosis is not a surgical emergency. Once the diagnosis of HPS is established, the priority is the restoration of intravascular volume and electrolyte and acid–base homeostasis. The infant is kept nil per os (NPO), but gastric decompression is avoided to prevent worsening fluid, acid, and electrolyte losses. Resuscitation is initiated with a normal saline bolus of 20 mL/kg, followed by one or more boluses, depending on the level of dehydration, with an end-point of establishing normal urine output. IV fluids are administered at a rate of 1.5 times maintenance, with 5% dextrose, 0.45% saline, and 20 mEq/L of potassium chloride to replace potassium lost in emesis and urine. Serum electrolytes are rechecked every 6–12 hours and IV fluids are adjusted as needed. Once serum bicarbonate and potassium are normalized, which is within 24 hours for most infants, the patient is safe to have general anesthesia. A single dose of preoperative cefazolin decreases the rate of postoperative wound infection.

Dehydration and dyselectrolytemia should be corrected rapidly. Potassium is added when renal function is restored. The stomach is washed with isotonic saline.

Extramucosal pyloromyotomy remains the standard operation. The treatment of choice is Ramstedt pyloromyotomy. At operation, or after the operation, the stomach is emptied by a catheter. The procedure is performed through a short transverse skin incision. The underlying pyloric mass is cut longitudinally to the layer of the submucosa, and the incision is closed. A Seromuscular layer of the gastric antrum and the pylorus is incised. The muscle is split with a blunt instrument allowing mucosa to bulge between split muscles laparoscopic technique is equally successful. Postoperative vomiting occurs in half the infants and is thought to be secondary to edema of the pylorus at the incision site. In most infants, however, feedings can be initiated within 12–24 hours after surgery and advanced to maintenance oral feedings within 36–48 hours after surgery. Persistent vomiting suggests an incomplete pyloromyotomy, gastritis, GERD, or another cause of the obstruction. The surgical treatment of pyloric stenosis is curative, with an operative mortality of 0–0.5%.

Oral feeding starts after 4–6 hours. 4 mL of 5% dextrose in saline solution is given hourly for 4–5 hours. Then once in 4-hour schedule is started. Persistence of vomiting beyond the fifth postoperative day suggests incomplete pyloromyotomy or associated hiatus hernia or achalasia or gastritis.

Endoscopic balloon dilation has been successful in infants with persistent vomiting secondary to incomplete pyloromyotomy.

Conservative management with nasoduodenal feedings is advisable in patients who are not good surgical candidates. Oral and IV atropine sulfate (pyloric muscle relaxant) has also been described when surgical treatment is not available. In conservative protocols, atropine is administered intravenously at a dose of 0.01 mg/kg six times a day 5 minutes before feeding. During atropine infusion, the heart rate needs to be continuously monitored by electrocardiography. Oral feeding is started at a volume of 10 mL of formula feeds six times a day. The volume is increased day by day until patients tolerate 150 mL/kg/day unless vomiting occurs more than twice a day. When patients are able to tolerate the full volume of formula without vomiting more than twice a day, 0.02 mg/kg atropine is administered orally 6 times a day before feeding.

As conservative management takes longer and oral feedings may not be tolerated at first, worsening of the nutrition status may occur and total parenteral nutrition may be required. It was also postulated that surgical management is more time and cost effective.

Fluid therapy should be continued until the infant is rehydrated and serum bicarbonate concentration is <30 mEq/L. This tells the correction of alkalosis. Correction of alkalosis is necessary to prevent postoperative apnea.

■ COMPLICATIONS

- Incomplete pyloromyotomy
- Perforation

■ BIBLIOGRAPHY

1. Leong MM, Chen SC, Hsieh CS, Chin YY, Tok TS, Wu SF, et al. Epidemiological features of infantile hypertrophic pyloric stenosis in Taiwanese children: a Nation-Wide Analysis of Cases during 1997-2007. PloS One. 2011; 6(5);e191494.
2. McAteer JP, Ledbetter DJ, Golden AB. Role of bottle feeding in the etiology of hypertrophic pyloric stenosis. JAMA Peditr. 2013;167(12):1143-9.
3. Pantelli C. New insights into the pathogenesis of infantile pyloric stenosis. Pediatr Surg Int. 2009;25(12);1043-52.
4. Rannells JD, Carver JD, Kirby RS. Infantile hypertrophic pyloric stenosis: epidemiology, genetics, and clinical update. Adv Pediatr. 2011;58(1)195-206.
5. Walker K Halliday, Holland AJ, Karskens C, Badawi N. Early developmental outcome of infants with infantile hypertrophic pyloric stenosis. J Pediatr Surg. 2010;45(12): 2369-72.

CASE 24

Diaphragmatic Hernia

■ PRESENTING COMPLAINTS

A 2-day-old male boy was brought with the complaint of:
- Excessive crying since birth
- Irritable since 6 hours
- Restless since 4 hours
- Breathlessness since 2 hours

History of Presenting Complaints

A 2-day-old male baby was brought to the hospital with severe respiratory distress. The mother was complaining that the child was irritable, restless, and crying. The child had respiratory distress. It was evident with the marked subcostal recession with the indrawing of the abdomen. The mother also complained that the child was not taking feeds and it was vomiting and not sucking at the breast. The mother said that she had noticed a bluish color on the lips and extremities.

Past History of the Patient

This boy was the second sibling of the consanguineous marriage. The child was born at term with normal vaginal delivery. He cried immediately after the delivery. He was taking feeds. There was a mild respiratory distress. The resident doctor examined and developed doubt about the position of the heart toward the right. Later he advised her to take the child to the higher institute for management.

■ EXAMINATION

On examination, the child was restless and irritable. It never used to be comfortable lying down. He was restless. Features of intrauterine growth retardation (IUGR) were present. Anthropometric measurements included a length of 51 cm (75th centile), a weight of 3 kg (50th centile), and a head circumference was 35 cm.

The child was afebrile, the heart rate was 146 beats/min. The respiratory rate was 62 breaths/min. Blood pressure was

---

CASE AT A GLANCE

Basic Findings
Length	: 51 cm (75th centile)
Weight	: 3 kg (50th centile)
Temperature	: 37°C
Pulse rate	: 146 beats/min
Respiratory rate	: 62 breaths/min
Blood pressure	: 50/40 mm Hg

Positive Findings

History:
- Respiratory distress
- Cyanosis
- Feeding difficulties

Examination:
- Tachypnea
- Scaphoid abdomen
- Shifting of the mediastinum

Investigation:
- X-ray chest—shifting of mediastinum on the right side
- Fluid and air-filled loop in the left chest

50/40 mm Hg. Cyanosis was present. There was no pallor and no icterus. There was no edema. There was a marked subcostal recession.

Per abdomen examination revealed a scaphoid abdomen. The normal physiological hepatomegaly was present on the right side below the costal margin. A cardiovascular examination revealed that heart sounds were better heard on the right side. Chest auscultation revealed the presence of bowel sounds on the left side.

■ INVESTIGATION

- *Hemoglobin:* 12 g/dL
- *Total leukocyte count (TLC):* 9,800 cells/cumm
- *Differential leukocyte count (DLC):* $P_{75}L_{20}E_3M_2$
- *C-reactive protein (CRP):* 2,000 mg/L (normal 67–1,800 mg/L)
- *X-ray chest:* Shifting of mediastinum on the right side. Free and air-filled loop in the left chest.

■ DISCUSSION

A diaphragmatic hernia is defined as communication between the abdominal and thoracic cavities with or without abdominal contents in the thorax. Etiology is usually congenital but may be traumatic. The symptoms and prognosis depend on the location of the defect and associated anomalies.

The incidence of congenital diaphragmatic hernia (CDH) is between 1/2,000 and 1/5,000 live births with females affected twice as often as males. Detects are more common on the left (85%) and are occasionally (<5%) bilateral, pulmonary hypoplasia and malrotation of the intestine are part of the lesion. Associated anomalies include central nervous system (CNS) lesions, esophageal atresia, omphalocele, and

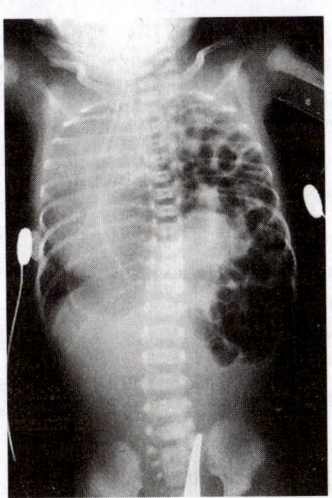

Fig. 1: Loops of bowel in left chest.

cardiovascular lesions. CDH is recognized as part of chromosomal syndromes: Trisomy 21, trisomy 13, trisomy 18, Brachmann-de Lange, Pallister–Killian, and Turner.

It is the congenital herniation of the abdominal contents into the thoracic cavity **(Fig. 1)**. Symptomatology and prognosis depend upon the location of the defect and associated anomalies. The defect may be at the esophageal hiatus (hiatal), paraesophageal (adjacent to the hiatus), retrosternal (Morgagni), or at the posterolateral (Bochdalek) portion of the diaphragm.

The term "congenital diaphragmatic hernia" typically refers to the Bochdalek form. These lesions may cause significant respiratory distress at birth, can be associated with other congenital anomalies, and have significant mortality and long-term morbidity. The size of the defect is variable ranging from a small hole to complete agenesis of this area of the diaphragm. This may be associated with anomalies in the other organ system.

■ TYPES OF DIAPHRAGMATIC HERNIA

The most common type of CDH, a Bochdalek hernia, occurs through a posterior defect in the diaphragm. Defects in the central and lateral portions of the diaphragm result in a less common anterior retrosternal hernia, a Morgagni hernia. Often, the stomach, spleen, and most of the intestines herniate into the thorax.

Herniation of the abdominal contents interferes with lung development and growth, and the resulting lung compression results in pulmonary hypoplasia that is most severe on the ipsilateral side, although both lungs may be affected. There is a marked reduction in the number of bronchi and alveoli associated with a decrease in the cross-sectional area of the pulmonary vasculature.

In addition to parenchymal maldevelopment, the intra-acinar pulmonary arteries have increased muscularization. Pulmonary capillary blood flow is decreased because of the small cross-sectional area of the pulmonary vascular bed, and flow may be further decreased by abnormal pulmonary vasoconstriction. Surfactant production may also be affected by pulmonary hypoplasia in infants with CDH.

■ PRENATAL DIAGNOSIS

Diaphragmatic hernia is often diagnosed by the fetal US, which can reveal abdominal organs and a fluid-filled bowel with peristalsis in the thorax, and a shift of the heart and mediastinum away from the side of the hernia. Polyhydramnios, pleural effusions, and ascites often are present. The differential diagnosis of these sonographic findings includes congenital cystic adenomatoid malformation, bronchogenic cysts, cystic teratoma, and neurogenic tumors. If CDH is suspected, fetal echocardiography and karyotype should be performed for potential prenatal diagnosis of commonly associated malformations. The patient should be referred to a quaternary treatment center for prenatal counseling and delivery.

■ PATHOLOGY AND ETIOLOGY

Pulmonary hypoplasia is characterized by a reduction in pulmonary mass and the number of bronchial divisions, respiratory bronchioles, and alveoli. The pathology of pulmonary hypoplasia and CDH includes abnormal septa in the terminal saccules, thickened alveoli, and thickened pulmonary arterioles. Biochemical abnormalities include relative surfactant deficiencies, increased glycogen in the alveoli, and decreased levels of phosphatidylcholine, total deoxyribonucleic acid (DNA), and total lung protein, all of which contribute to limited gas exchange.

Arriving at the diagnosis early in pregnancy allows for prenatal counseling, possible fetal interventions, and planning for postnatal care. Careful evaluation for other anomalies should include echocardiography and amniocentesis. To avoid unnecessary pregnancy termination and unrealistic expectations, an experienced multidisciplinary group must carefully counsel the parents of a child diagnosed with a diaphragmatic hernia.

A small group of infants with CDH are present beyond the neonatal period. Patients with a delayed presentation may experience vomiting as a result of intestinal obstruction or mild respiratory symptoms.

The most reliable prenatal predictor of outcome in children with CDH studied is fetal Ultrasonography (USG). A prospective study of USG at 24–26 weeks compared fetal lung-to-head ratio (LHR) with mortality. There were no survivors with LHR <1, but all babies with LHR >14 survived. A second important consideration was the presence of the liver in the thoracic cavity, which is a poor prognostic feature.

Based on the observation that hydrostatic pressure exerted by fetal lung fluid plays a critical role in lung growth and maturity, a promising experimental therapy is in utero tracheal occlusion.

Separation of developing thoracic and abdominal cavities is accompanied by closure of posterolateral pleuroperitoneal canals. This occurs in the eighth week of gestation.

Failure of this canal to close is responsible for the defect. The defect may be small and sac-like or include the entire diaphragm. Both the lungs are small but the lungs on the side of the defect may be severely affected. When little or no respiratory distress occurs, the hernia may not be detected until infancy and childhood.

There will be partial herniation of the stomach through the esophageal hiatus. Unrecognized diaphragmatic hernia has been the cause of sudden deaths in infants and toddlers. There will be phrenic nerve paralysis with displacement of abdominal contents upwards.

Failure of the development of a posterolateral portion of the diaphragm results in the persistence of the pleuroperitoneal canal or foramen of Bachdolack. This allows the viscera to occupy the chest cavity, abdomen underdeveloped, and scaphoid.

Developing lung buds project into the pericardioperitoneal cavities to form pleural cavities and the membranes fuse with dorsal mesentry of developing foregut medially and septum transversum ventrally. Closure of the pleuroperitoneal membrane is assisted by the myoblasts which ingrow.

Eventration is the upward displacement of abdominal contents into an outpouching or sac-like structure of the diaphragm.

Pulmonary hypoplasia is characterized by a reduction in pulmonary mass and the number of bronchial divisions, respiratory bronchioles, and alveoli. The pathology of pulmonary hypoplasia and CDH includes abnormal septa in the terminal saccules, thickened alveoli, and thickened pulmonary arterioles.

CLINICAL FEATURES (FIG. 2)

Clinical presentation of CDH depends on the type and size of the hernia. Infants with a large left-sided hernia may present with a scaphoid abdomen and significant respiratory symptoms in the delivery room.

The majority of the infants will have severe respiratory distress within 1 hour after the delivery. A child with delayed presentation may experience vomiting as a result of intestinal obstruction or mild respiratory symptoms. Rarely incarnation of the intestine produces ischemia with sepsis and cardiorespiratory collapse.

After delivery, a chest radiograph is needed to confirm the diagnosis. In some with an echogenic chest mass, further imaging is required. The differential diagnosis may include other diaphragm disorders, such as eventration, a cystic lung lesion (pulmonary sequestration and cystadenomatoid malformation), and others.

Respiratory distress is a cardinal sign in babies with CDH. It may occur immediately after birth or there may be a "honeymoon" period of up to 48 hours during which the baby is relatively stable. Early respiratory

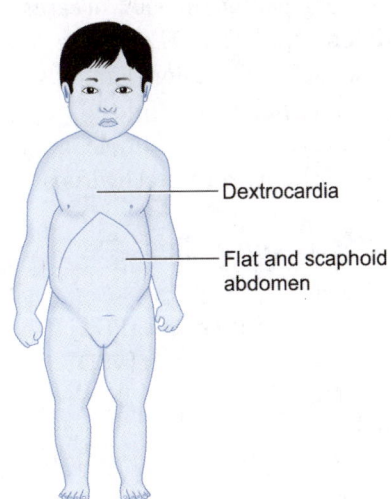

Fig. 2: Clinical features.

distress, within 6 hours after birth, is thought to be a poor prognostic sign. Respiratory distress is characterized clinically by tachypnea, grunting, use of accessory muscles, and cyanosis. Children with CDH may also have a scaphoid abdomen and increased chest wall diameter.

Bowel sounds may also be heard in the chest with decreased breath sounds bilaterally. The point of maximal cardiac impulse may be displaced away from the side of the hernia if a mediastinal shift has occurred. A chest X-ray and passage of a nasal gastric tube are all that are usually required to confirm the diagnosis.

Approximately 40% of infants with CDH have associated anomalies, most with minimal effect on survival, and others that significantly affect survival, including chromosomal and complex cardiac defects. During fetal life, the left ventricle is often small (probably as a result of increased intrathoracic pressure), and left ventricular output is reduced. Postnatally, the left ventricular size and output may improve with the correction of the hernia.

Congenital diaphragmatic hernia can be diagnosed on prenatal USG (between 16 and 24 weeks of gestation) in >50% of cases. High-speed fetal magnetic resonance imaging (MRI) can define the lesion. Findings on USG may include polyhydramnios, chest mass, mediastinal shift, gastric bubble or a liver in the thoracic cavity, and fetal hydrops.

Associated Anomalies

- Malrotation
- Patent ductus arteriosus (PDA)
- Ventricular septal defect (VSD)
- Coarctation
- Undescended testes
- Renal anomalies
- Duodenal atresia
- Meckel's diverticulum
- Hirschsprung's disease

Pulmonary hypoplasia leads to barotrauma, alveolar rupture, emphysema pneumomediastinum, and pneumothorax—surgical emphysema

Antenatal features include polyhydramnios, mediastinal displacement, and absence of intraabdominal stomach bubble.

> **ESSENTIAL DIAGNOSTIC POINTS**
> - Congenital herniation of the abdominal contents into the thoracic cavity
> - Severe respiratory distress within one hour after the delivery, including dyspnea and cyanosis
> - The lungs of the affected side are compressed and often hypoplastic
> - Abdomen is usually small and the scaphoid is contour
> - If the respiratory embarrassment is not released, shock, and hypoxia occur

In severe cases, the stomach and a large part of the intestine will displace the lungs and heart. The lungs of the affected side are compressed and often hypoplastic. There will be a decreased number of airways and blood vessels and diminished lung volume. Severe respiratory distress includes dyspnea and cyanosis since birth.

The physical finding depends upon the degree of displacement in the newborn infant. Abdomen is usually small and the scaphoid is contoured. The infant is cyanotic and has respiratory retraction. If the respiratory embarrassment is not released, shock and hypoxia occur.

Gastroesophageal reflux disease is reported in >50% of children with CDH. It is more common in those children whose diaphragmatic defect involves the esophageal hiatus. Recurrent diaphragmatic hernia is reported in 5–20% in most series. Children with patch repairs are at the highest risk.

Children with CDH typically have delayed growth in the first to second year of life. Contributing factors include poor intake and GERD energy.

GENERAL FEATURES
• Mediastinal shift • Grunting • Cyanosis • Respiratory distress

■ DIAGNOSIS

A chest radiograph is usually diagnostic. The lateral view frequently demonstrates the intestine passing through the posterior portion of the diaphragm. Chest X-ray shows gas-filled bowel loops, displacement of the lung, herniated liver, or spleen ipsilateral pneumothorax. USG and fluoroscopy are helpful in distinguishing eventration from the true hernia. CT may be necessary to exclude pneumatocele or complicated effusion.

The prenatal diagnosis of CDH can be made by using fetal sonography as early as 15 weeks of gestation. Sonographic findings include herniated abdominal viscera, abnormal anatomy of the upper abdomen, and mediastinal shift away from the herniated viscera. The high-risk fetus is identified by diagnosis early in gestation, a dilated stomach in the chest, low lung-to-thorax ratio, LHR, and polyhydramnios.

LABORATORY SALIENT FINDINGS
• *Chest radiograph:* Lateral view frequently demonstrates the intestine passing through the posterior portion of the diaphragm • Chest X-ray shows gas filled bowel loops, displacement of lung, herniated liver or spleen ipsilateral pneumothorax • Ultrasonography and fluoroscopy are helpful in distinguishing eventration from the true hernia • Computed tomography may be necessary to exclude pneumatocele or complicated effusion

■ COMPLICATIONS

Complications include abnormalities in lung function. There is a significant decrease in vital capacity and peak expiratory flow, decreased lung compliance, and tidal volume. Survivors will have restrictive lung disease and respiratory failure. Developmental delay, abnormal hearing, or vision may occur. Seizure is a neurological complication. Pectus excavatum, scoliosis, and recurrent hernia are long-term complications.

■ DIFFERENTIAL DIAGNOSIS

- Congenital pneumonia
- Aspiration pneumonitis
- Transient tachypnoea of the newborn
- Hyaline membrane disease

■ TREATMENT

Currently, the preferred management strategy for CDH is medical stabilization with appropriate cardiorespiratory support, including high-frequency oscillatory ventilation (HFOV), nitric oxide (NO), or extracorporeal membrane oxygenation (ECMO) for several days to allow for physiologic stabilization and improvement in pulmonary hypertension. The surgical approach is through a subcostal opening with primary repair if enough diaphragm tissue is available. For those with a more significant defect, closure with a patch may be required. The use of chest drains or tubes postoperatively has also decreased in the past few years, but a consensus on their use has not been reached.

Initial Management

Initial resuscitation consists of stabilization with sedation and paralysis and modest hyperventilation, i.e., the partial pressure of the carbon dioxide of 25–30 mm Hg. Volume resuscitation, dopamine, and bicarbonate are useful. If the infant stabilizes and demonstrates stable pulmonary vascular resistance without significant right to left shunt, repair of the diaphragm is performed in 24–72 hours.

Aggressive respiratory support is often needed in children with CDH. This includes rapid endotracheal intubation, sedation, and possibly paralysis. Arterial (preductal and postductal) and central venous (umbilical) lines are mandated, as are a urinary catheter and NG tube. A preductal SpO_2 value of 85% could be the minimum goal.

Gentle ventilation with permissive hypercapnia reduces lung injury, need for ECMO, and mortality. Factors that contribute to pulmonary hypertension (hypoxia, acidosis, and hypothermia) should be avoided. Echocardiography is important to guide therapeutic decisions by measuring pulmonary and system vascular pressures and defining the presence of cardiac dysfunction. Routine use of inotropes is indicated in the presence of left ventricular dysfunction. Babies with CDH may be surfactant deficient. Although surfactant is commonly used, no study has proven that it is beneficial in the treatment of CDH.

Ventilation Strategies

Conventional mechanical ventilation, HFOV, and ECMO are the three main strategies to support respiratory failure in newborns with CDH. The goal is to maintain oxygenation and carbon dioxide elimination without inducing volutrauma. The first modality to be used is conventional ventilation. Hyperventilation to induce alkalosis and decrease ductal shunting has not proved effective and should be avoided. Permissive hypercapnia has reduced lung injury and mortality rates in several studies. HFOV can be used early to prevent lung injury by using lower airway pressures.

Pulmonary hypoplasia and pulmonary hypertension are significant contributors to mortality in CDH. Pulmonary hypertension has a reactive component, due to the changing resistance of the pulmonary arterioles, and a fixed component due to the diminished cross-sectional area of the pulmonary vascular bed. Mechanical ventilation should aim to maintain appropriate lung volumes and adequate oxygenation while minimizing lung injury. Many centers prefer to use high-frequency ventilation, especially HFOV, before on and alkalosis in CDH has been replaced before and after surgery.

Extracorporeal Membrane Oxygenation

If stabilization is not possible most infants require ECMO support. ECMO with paralysis and NG suction may produce a dramatic reduction of the volume of the herniated viscera. Surfactant administration has also been shown to produce transient improvement.

The availability of ECMO and the utility of preoperative stabilization have improved the survival of babies with CDH. ECMO is the therapeutic option in children in whom conventional ventilation or conventional ventilation and HFOV fail. ECMO is most commonly used before the repair of the defect.

Birth weight and the 5-minute Apgar score may be the best predictors of outcome in patients treated with ECMO. The lower limit of weight for ECMO is 2,000 g.

The duration of ECMO for neonates with diaphragmatic hernia is longer (7–14 days) than for those with persistent fetal circulation or meconium aspiration and may last up to 2-4 weeks. The timing of repair of the diaphragm while the infant receives ECMO is controversial. The recurrence of pulmonary hypertension is associated with high mortality and weaning from ECMO support should be cautious. If the patient cannot be weaned from ECMO after repair of CDH, options include discontinuing support and, in rare cases, lung transplantation.

Surgical Repair

Prompt and aggressive, preoperative care is essential. This generally includes mechanical ventilation with 100% oxygen, sedation with narcotics, muscle paralyzes, controlled alkalosis with hyperventilation, IV sodium bicarbonate, and vasopressors.

The ideal time to repair the diaphragmatic defect is under debate. Most experts wait at least 48 hours after stabilization and resolution of the pulmonary hypertension. Good relative indicators of stability are the requirement for conventional ventilation only, a low peak inspiratory pressure, and a FiO_2 <50. If the newborn is on ECMO, the ability to be weaned from this support should be a consideration before surgical repair. In some centers, the repair is done with the cannulas in place; in other centers, the cannulas are removed.

The abdominal surgical repair approach is favored. The accompanied malrotation should be managed. The abdominal wall may be left open with the skin only closed. A subcostal approach is the most frequently used. This allows for good visualization of the defect and, if the abdominal cavity cannot accommodate the herniated contents, a polymeric silicone (silastic) patch can be placed. Both laparoscopic and thoracoscopic repairs have been reported, but these should be reserved for only the most stable infants.

Surgical repair of the diaphragmatic defect should be performed during the neonatal period. The exact timing of surgery depends on a number of variables, but over the past two decades practice has changed. In the past, surgical intervention was considered emergent, and as a consequence, postoperative management was characterized by severe pulmonary hypertension and tension pneumothoraces, resulting in poor outcomes.

Vasodilator Therapy

Nitric Oxide

Although NO is an effective treatment for infants with persistent pulmonary hypertension of the newborn (PPHN) in general, it has not had the same success for infants with CDH and may actually increase the death rate. Nonetheless, it is still widely used in the management of CDH.

Nitric oxide is a selective pulmonary vasodilator. Its use reduces ductal shunting and pulmonary pressures and results in improved oxygenation. Although it has been helpful in PPHN, randomized trials have not demonstrated improved survival or reduced need for ECMO when NO is used in newborns with CDH.

Tolazoline reduces pulmonary vascular resistance.

Thromboxane inhibitors: 5–20 mg/kg/min. *Nitroprusside/nitroglycerine/phenoxybenzamine.*

New Modalities

New modalities include surfactant replacement therapy, liquid ventilation, intratracheal pulmonary ventilation, and pulmonary lobe transplantation. Prenatal repair of the diaphragmatic hernia is abandoned as there was no improvement in survival or morbidity in randomized trials.

Current prenatal therapy of CDH is directed including the trachea, which results in enlargement of lungs with retained fluid. The baby is then delivered by a planned cesarian section, at which time the trachea is repaired or intubated, with the baby remaining in placental support.

Fetal surgery includes NO gas inhalation and intrauterine repair of diaphragmatic hernia.

■ PROGNOSIS

The incidence of spontaneous fetal demise is 7–10%. Relative predictors of a poor prognosis include an associated major anomaly, symptoms before 24 hours of age, severe pulmonary hypoplasia, herniation to the contralateral lung, and the need for ECMO. Pulmonary problems continue to be a source of morbidity for long-term survivors of CDH.

Neurocognitive defects are common and may result from disease or interventions. The abnormalities with ECMO for other diagnoses include transient and permanent developmental delay, abnormal hearing or vision, and seizures. Serious hearing loss may occur in children who are under ECMO.

Other long-term problems occurring in this population are pectus excavatum and scoliosis.

Regardless of the mode of therapy, the goal is to reverse the baby's persistent pulmonary hypertension, with right to left shunting of oxygen, and poor blood across the open foramen ovale and ductus arteriosus.

Gastroesophageal reflux disease is reported in >50% of children with CDH. GERD is more common in children whose diaphragmatic defect involves the esophageal hiatus. Intestinal obstruction is reported in up to 20% of children and may result from a midgut volvulus, adhesions, or a recurrent hernia that became incarcerated. Recurrent diaphragmatic hernia is reported in 5–20% in most series.

Children with patch repairs are at the highest risk. Children with CDH typically have delayed growth in the first 2 years of life.

Neurocognitive defects are common including transient and permanent developmental delay, abnormal hearing or vision, and seizures. Serious hearing loss may occur in up to 28% of children who underwent ECMO. The majority of neurologic abnormalities are classified as mild to moderate.

■ BIBLIOGRAPHY

1. Danzer E, Hedrick HL. Controversies in the management of severe congenital diaphragmatic hernia. Semin Fetal Neon Med. 2014;19(6):376-84.
2. Graziano JN; Congenital Diaphragmatic Hernia Study Group. Cardiac anomalies in patients with congenital diaphragmatic hernia and their prognosis: A report from the Congenital Diaphragmatic Hernia Study Group. J Peditr Surg. 2005;40(6):1045-50.
3. Kevin P Lally, William Engle; American Academy of Pediatrics Section on Surgery; American Academy of Pediatrics Committee on Fetus and Newborn. Postdischarge follow-up of infants with congenital diaphragmatic hernia. Pediatrics. 2008;121(3): 627-32.
4. van den Hout L, Schaible T, Cohen-Overbeek TE, Hop W, Siemer J, van de Ven K, et al. Actual outcome in infants with congenital diaphragmatic hernia: the role of standardized postnatal treatment protocol. Fetal Diagn Ther. 2011;29(1):55-63.

CASE 25

Duodenal Atresia

■ PRESENTING COMPLAINTS

A 2-day-old boy was brought with the complaint of:
- Persistent vomiting since birth
- Mild distension of the abdomen

History of Presenting Complaints

A 2-day-old boy was found in the postnatal ward with a history of persistent vomiting. Her mother said that in the beginning, her child was vomiting the breast milk that he was taking. Later mother noticed the greenish colored vomitus. Vomiting used to be a nonprojectile type. Mother had also noticed mild distension of the abdomen. For complaints of vomiting and mild distension, the sister in charge of the ward was given a stomach wash. The color of the stomach aspirate was greenish, and the amount was >30 mL.

Past History of the Patient

This boy was the only sibling of a consanguineous marriage. The baby was born at term with normal delivery. He cried immediately after the delivery. His birth weight was 2.8 kg. He started taking the feed immediately after delivery. The child was vomiting after taking feeds, but the resident doctor assured her considering it was normal with every newborn in the beginning. Mother gave the history of doubtful hydramnios antenatally.

■ EXAMINATION

On examination, the child was moderately built and nourished. He was just lying on the bed. The activity of the child was not satisfactory. Anthropometric measurements included a length was 50 cm (50th centile), a weight was 2.75 kg (25th centile), and a head circumference was 34 cm.

CASE AT A GLANCE

Basic Findings
Length	: 50 cm (50th centile)
Weight	: 2.75 kg (25th centile)
Temperature	: 37°C
Pulse rate	: 120 beats/min
Respiratory rate	: 38 breaths/min
Blood pressure	: 60/50 mm Hg

Positive Findings

History:
- Vomiting
- Bile-stained vomitus
- >30 mL of gastric aspirate
- Polyhydramnios

Examination:
- Mild upper abdominal distension

Investigation:
- X-ray abdomen: Double-bubble appearance

The boy was afebrile. The heart rate was 120 beats/min and the respiratory rate was 38 breaths/min. The blood pressure recorded was 60/50 mm Hg. There was no pallor, no icterus, no lymphadenopathy, and no cyanosis.

Per abdomen examination revealed mild distension in the upper abdomen. No visible gastric peristalsis. Bowel sounds were sluggish. The respiratory system revealed the presence of crepitations at the basal regions. Other systemic examinations were normal.

■ INVESTIGATION

- *Hemoglobin:* 12 g/dL
- *TLC:* 7,600 cells/mm^3
- *DLC:* $P_{80}L_{18}E_2M_0$
- *Serum electrolytes:*
  - *Na:* 110 mEq/L
  - *K:* 4 mEq/L
  - *Cl:* 98 mEq/L
- *X-ray of erect abdomen:* Double-bubble, appearance of gas and fluid-filled levels in the stomach and duodenum

■ DISCUSSION

Congenital duodenal obstruction caused by atresia is an intrinsic defect of bowel formation. Duodenal atresia is limited to the first and second parts of the duodenum. 85% of cases are distal to the entry of the bile duct into the duodenum. The most common site is at ampulla. It can also result from extrinsic compression by abnormal neighboring structures (e.g., annular pancreas and preduodenal portal vein) duplication cysts, or congenital bands associated with malrotation Although intrinsic and extrinsic causes of duodenal obstruction occur independently, they can also coexist.

Duodenal atresia complicates 1 per 10,000 live births and accounts for 25–40% of all intestinal atresias. Duodenal atresia results from failed recanalization of the intestinal lumen during gestation.

Duodenal atresia is thought to arise from delayed vacuolization of the embryonic intestinal lumen. This accounts both for the mucosal diaphragm within the duodenum and for duodenal atresia. Throughout the fourth and fifth week of normal fetal development, the duodenal mucosa exhibits rapid proliferation of epithelial cells. Persistence of these cells, which should degenerate after the seventh week of gestation leads to occlusion of the lumen (atresia) in approximately two-thirds of cases and narrowing (stenosis) in the remaining one-third.

Duodenal atresia may take several forms: The intact membrane obstructing the lumen, a short fibrous cord connecting the two blind duodenal pouches, or a gap between the nonconnecting ends of the duodenum. The membranous form of atresia is the most common. This causes the obstruction occurring distal to the ampulla of Vater.

In contrast to more distal atresias, which likely arise from prenatal vascular accidents, duodenal atresia results from failed recanalization of the intestinal lumen during gestation. Throughout the fourth and fifth week of normal fetal development, the duodenal mucosa exhibits rapid proliferation of epithelial cells. Persistence of these cells, which should degenerate after the seventh week of gestation, leads to occlusion of the lumen (atresia) in approximately two-thirds of cases and narrowing (stenosis) in the remaining one-third.

Duodenal atresia can take several forms, including a thin membrane that occludes the lumen, a short fibrous cord that connects two blind duodenal pouches, or a gap that spans two nonconnecting ends of the duodenum. The membranous form is most common, and it almost invariably occurs near the ampulla of Vater. In rare cases, the membrane is distensible and is referred to as a windsock web. This unusual form of duodenal atresia causes obstruction several centimeters distal to the origin of the membrane.

Approximately 50% of infants with duodenal atresia are premature. It is associated with Down syndrome, malrotation, esophageal atresia, congenital heart disease, and anorectal and rectal anomalies. It may occur as a result of extrinsic obstruction, such as an annular pancreas and bands of Ladd.

Tandler's Theory

Failure of recanalization of the duodenal lumen produces stenosis, atresia, and the formation of a mucosal web. The error occurs most often at the site of papilla of Vater. It is usually associated with annular pancreas, anomalies of intestinal rotation and fixation, biliary and pancreatic anomalies, duodenal obstruction, Down syndrome, malrotation, and congenital heart defects.

Duodenum gets greatly dilated with hypertrophied walls with the dilatation of pylorus and stomach. Distal duodenum becomes small and thin-walled.

■ CLINICAL FEATURES (FIG. 1)

The hallmark of the duodenal obstruction is bilious vomiting, without abdominal distension. This is usually noted on the first day of life. History of polyhydramnios may be present. This is caused by the failure of absorption of amniotic fluid in the distal intestine. This fluid may be bile stained because of intrauterine vomiting Jaundice is present in one-third of infants with prolonged vomiting, and electrolyte imbalance occurs.

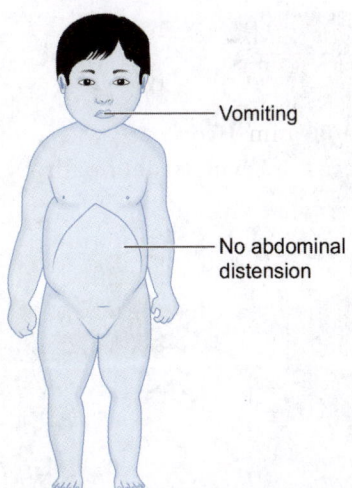

Fig. 1: Clinical features.

ESSENTIAL DIAGNOSTIC POINTS
• Bilious vomiting, without abdominal distension noted on the first day of life • History of polyhydramnios • Jaundice is present in infant with prolonged vomiting, electrolyte imbalance occurs • The most common site being at ampulla • Failure of recanalization of duodenal lumen produces stenosis, atresia, formation of a mucosal web

■ DIAGNOSIS

Prenatal USG shows a dilated, fluid-filled stomach and duodenum. Prompt amniocentesis for karyotype study is essential. Bile-stained vomiting within few hours of birth, fullness in epigastrium, rest of the abdomen is scaphoid.

LABORATORY SALIENT FINDINGS
• Prenatal USG shows dilated, fluid filled stomach and duodenum • *X-ray abdomen:* A large, air distended stomach with fluid level, markedly distended first portion of duodenum with a fluid level • Ultrasonography • CT scan • Upper GI contrast study • Fiberoptic endoscopy
(CT: computed tomography; GI: gastrointestinal; USG: ultrasonography)

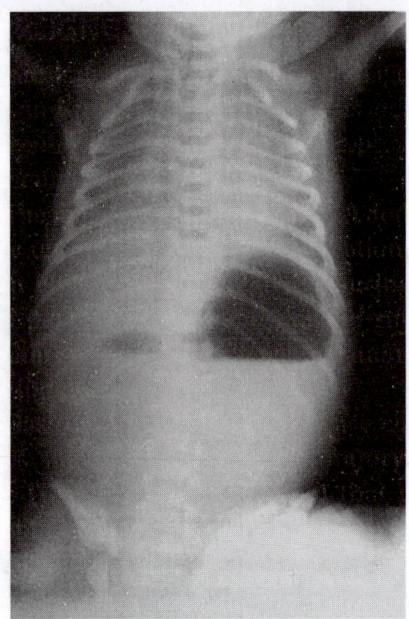

Fig. 2: Dublle bubble sign.

X-ray of Abdomen

A large, air-distended stomach with a fluid level, markedly distended the first portion of the duodenum with a fluid level. No evidence of air in the remaining GIT—double bubble sign **(Fig. 2)**. In complete atresia, a barium enema is done to determine if the malrotation is present or not.

Ultrasonography

- May show the associated annular pancreas
- May show whirlpool sign—characteristic of volvulus
- *Antenatal findings:*
  - Double bubble sign
  - Increased gastric peristalsis
  - Polyhydramnios
  - Urinary tract abnormalities

Computed Tomography Scan

- Show dilated stomach and the first part of the duodenum

- Normal caliber colon
- In case of complete obstruction, small and large bowel is collapsed.

Upper Gastrointestinal Contrast Study

It is indicated in patients who have partial obstruction to the proximal duodenum and is only modestly dilated.

Fiberoptic Endoscopy

It is indicated in older children and adults may show the presence or absence of duodenal stenosis or wet.

ECHO, a radiograph of the chest and spine is done to evaluate the associated defects.

GENERAL FEATURES
• Bilious vomiting • Icterus

Contrast studies are occasionally needed to exclude malrotation and volvulus because intestinal infarction can occur within 6–12 hours if the volvulus is not relieved. Contrast studies are generally not necessary and may be associated with aspiration. Prenatal diagnosis of duodenal atresia is readily made by fetal USG, which reveals a sonographic double-bubble. Prenatal identification of duodenal atresia is associated with decreased morbidity and fewer hospitalization days.

■ TREATMENT

The initial treatment of infants with duodenal atresia includes NG or orogastric decompression and IV fluid replacement. Echocardiography, renal US, and radiology of the chest and spine should be performed to evaluate for associated anomalies. Definitive correction of the atresia is usually postponed until life-threatening anomalies are evaluated and treated.

Treatment includes naso-orogastric decompression and IV fluid replacement. Definitive correction of atresia is usually postponed evaluating and treat the life-threatening associated anomalies.

The typical surgical repair for duodenal atresia is duodenoduodenostomy. This is done to bypass the obstruction. A distal proximal bowel is tapered in an attempt to improve peristalsis. A gastrostomy tube may be placed to drain the stomach and protect the airway. The prognosis is primarily dependent upon the presence of associated anomalies. This procedure is also preferred in cases of concomitant or isolated annular pancreas. In these instances, the duodenoduodenostorny is performed without dividing the pancreas. The dilated proximal bowel might have to be tapered to improve peristalsis.

Operative treatment includes a transverse right upper quadrant supraumbilical incision. Direst duodenostomy—standard side-to-side fusion, diamond-shaped duodenostomy. The simple duodenal web may also be excised through a longitudinal, taking care that not to damage the ampulla. If the proximal duodenum is excessively floppy or distended, antimesenteric tapering duodenoplasty is done using the autostapling device. Postoperatively, duodenal ileum may take as long as 5–12 days to settle down. Postoperatively, a gastrostomy tube can be placed to drain the stomach and protect the airway. IV nutritional support or a trans-anastomotic jejunal tube is needed until an infant starts to feed orally.

BIBLIOGRAPHY

1. Adams SD, Stanton MP. Malrotation and intestinal atresias. Early Hum Dev. 2014; 90(12);921-5.
2. Haxhija EQ, Schalamon J, Höllwarth ME. Management of isolated and associated colonic atresia. Pediatr Surg Int. 2011;27(4); 411-6.
3. Paramentier B, Peycelon M, Muller CO, El Ghoneimi A, Bonnard A. Laparoscopic management of congenital duodenal atresia or stenosis: A single-center early experience. J Pediatr Surg. 2015,50(11):1833-36.

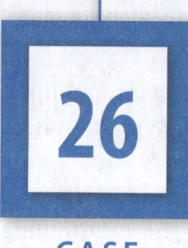

CASE 26

Gastroesophageal Reflux

■ PRESENTING COMPLAINTS

A 10-week-old baby was brought with the complaint of:
- Frequent vomiting since 15 days

History of Presenting Complaints

A 10-week-old baby was brought to the pediatric outpatient department (OPD) with a history of frequent vomiting. Her mother noticed that her daughter used to vomit as soon as she was given feeds. Later doctor explained to the mother the proper technique of feeding as well as burping. Despite proper technique, the baby used to vomit regularly about three to four times a day. Vomitus used to contain curdled milk. There was no mass or any peristaltic movements seen over the abdomen after feeding.

Past History of the Patient

The girl was the first sibling of a nonconsanguineous marriage. She was born at full term by normal delivery. She cried immediately after delivery. The birth weight of the child was 3 kg. There was no significant postnatal event. She was on breast milk on the second day itself.

■ EXAMINATION

The child was moderately built and nourished. The child was lying comfortably on an examination table. Anthropometric measurements include a length was 58 cm (97th centile), a weight was 4.5 kg (70th centile), and a head circumference was 40 cm.

She was afebrile. Anterior fontanelle was normal. Heart rate was 110 beats/min, respiratory rate was 28 breaths/min, and blood pressure recorded was 60/46 mm Hg. There was no pallor, no edema, and no lymphadenopathy. All the systemic and general examinations were normal.

■ INVESTIGATION

- *Hemoglobin:* 10 g/dL
- *TLC:* 7,000 cells/mm^3

CASE AT A GLANCE

Basic Findings

Length	: 58 cm (97th centile)
Weight	: 4.5 kg (70th centile)
Temperature	: 37°C
Pulse rate	: 110 beats/min
Respiratory rate	: 28 breaths/min
Blood pressure	: 60/46 mm Hg

Positive Findings

History:
- Vomiting

Examination:
- Normal

Investigation:
- *Barium swallow:* Shows delayed emptying of the esophagus appearance

- *DLC:* $P_{65}L_{30}M_2E_3$
- *ESR:* 20 mm at the first hour
- *Barium swallow:* Showed the delayed emptying of the esophagus

■ DISCUSSION

It is defined as an involuntary passage of gastric contents into the esophagus. The regurgitated gastric content may be saliva, ingested food, and gastric secretion. It may contain pancreatic or biliary secretion that had earlier refluxed into the stomach. This is due to duodenogastric reflux.

Gastroesophageal reflux disease (GERD) is the most common esophageal disorder in children of all ages. Gastroesophageal reflux (GER) signifies the retrograde movement of gastric contents across the lower esophageal sphincter (LES) into the esophagus, which occurs physiologically every day in all infants, older children, and adults, physiologic GER is exemplified by the effortless regurgitation of normal infants. The phenomenon becomes pathologic GERD in infants and children who manifest esophagitis-related symptoms, or extraesophageal presentations, such as respiratory symptoms and nutritional effects.

Gastroesophageal reflux is the spontaneous passage of gastric contents into the esophagus. When it reaches the mouth, it is also called regurgitation. GER is a normal physiologic process that occurs throughout the day in healthy infants, children, and adults. When GER causes bothersome symptoms, GER becomes GERD. The signs and symptoms that have been attributed to GERD range from chest pain and heartburn to cough and pneumonia.

The muscular layer distal to the midesophagus is composed of smooth muscle fibers. Hence, it is not under voluntary control. The esophagus is a hollow muscular tube. The peristaltic wave involving the external circular muscle layer is the force that propels the ingested food through the esophagus into the stomach.

The LES at the distal end of the esophageal peristalsis will transport food into the stomach. The LES is suspected to be abnormal in people who have GER. The more recent concept suggests that LES may have episodes of transient relaxation, unassociated with esophageal peristalsis. Hence it allows gastric contents to reflux into the esophagus.

The basal tone of LES at rest is independent of neurotransmitters. Relaxation of LES is mediated by inhibitory neurotransmitters. These are released from enteric neurons. A vasoactive intestinal peptide is one of the mediators. LES is tonically contracted at rest. This is abnormal in this disease. The basal tone is low. There will be episodes of transient relaxation unassociated with esophageal peristalsis, thus allowing gastric contents to reflux into the esophagus.

■ PATHOPHYSIOLOGY

The phenomenon becomes pathologic GERD in infants and children who manifest or report bothersome symptoms because of frequent or persistent GER, producing esophagitis-related symptoms, or extraesophageal presentations, such as respiratory symptoms and nutritional effects.

Factors determining the esophageal manifestations of reflux include the duration of esophageal exposure (a product of the frequency and duration of reflux episodes), the causticity of the refluxate, and the susceptibility of the esophagus to damage. The LES, defined as a high-pressure zone by manometry, is supported by the crura of the diaphragm at the gastroesophageal junction, together with valve-like functions of the esophagogastric junction anatomy, forming the antireflux barrier.

Transient lower esophageal sphincter relaxation (TLESR) is the primary mechanism allowing reflux to occur and is defined as the simultaneous relaxation of both LES and the surrounding crura. TLESRs occur independent of swallowing reduce LES pressure to 0-2 mm Hg (above gastric), and last 10-60 seconds; they appear by 26 weeks of gestation. A vagovagal reflex, composed of afferent mechanoreceptors in the proximal stomach, a brainstem pattern generator, and efferents in the LES regulate TLESRs, Gastric distention (postprandially, or from abnormal gastric emptying or air swallowing) is the main stimulus for TLESRs. Other factors influencing gastric pressure-volume dynamics, such as increased movement, straining, obesity, large-volume or hyperosmolar meals, gastroparesis, a large sliding hiatal hernia, and increased respiratory effort (coughing, wheezing) can have the same effect.

Genetic linkage is indicated by the strong evidence of GERD in studies with monozygotic twins. A pediatric autosomal dominant form with otolaryngologic and respiratory manifestations has been located on chromosome 13q14, and the locus is termed GERD1.

Gastroesophageal reflux occurs when the LES relaxes and allows tor gastric contents to enter the esophagus.

The LES, defined as a high-pressure zone by manometry, is supported by the crura of the diaphragm at the gastroesophageal junction, together with valve-like functions of the esophagogastric junction anatomy, forming the antireflux barrier. In the context of even the normal intraabdominal pressure augmentations that occur during daily life, the frequency of reflux episodes is increased by insufficient LES tone, by abnormal frequency of LES relaxations, and by hiatal herniation that prevents the LES pressure from being proportionately augmented by the crura during abdominal straining.

There are three main types of refluxes (acidic with a pH of <4, weakly acidic with a pH of 4-7, and nonacid reflux with a pH of >7). In pediatrics, the convention is to designate all reflux with a pH >4 as nonacid because it cannot be detected by pH sensors in the esophagus. The type of esophageal reflux varies depending on the timing of the reflux episode relative to a meal; reflux episodes in the 1-2 hours after a meal are typically weakly or nonacidic and those occurring 3-4 hours or more after a meal are predominately acidic, infants, who only drink formula or breast milk every 2-3 hours, are almost always refluxing nonacidic formula/breast milk, which may explain the lack of efficacy of acid suppression to improve crying and fussiness. Understanding the type of reflux present in patients is critical in order to tailor therapies appropriately.

While acidic reflux has been associated with symptoms as well as signs such as dental erosions, esophagitis, and strictures, nonacid reflux, to date, has been associated only with symptoms including extraesophageal symptoms, such as cough, wheezing, and pneumonia.

Half of all infants between 0 and 3 months of age and two-thirds of 4-6-month-old infants regurgitate at least once per day. The prevalence of regurgitation decreases dramatically after 8 months of age, which coincides with the introduction of solid food and the increase in time in the upright position. After 12 months of age, <10% of children continue to have daily regurgitation, and new onset reflux beyond this age group requires careful consideration for other diagnoses because the prevalence is low.

While regurgitation in infants is common and not typically pathologic in otherwise thriving, happy infants, the more complex problem that the clinician faces is the infant who regurgitates and has symptoms of fussiness crying, and arching.

Infant reflux becomes evident in the first few months of life, peaks at 4 months, and resolves in up to 88% by 12 months and in nearly all by 24 months. Symptoms in older children tend to be chronic, waxing and waning, but completely resolving in no more than half, which resembles adult patterns. Genetic linkage is indicated by the strong evidence of GERD in studies with monozygotic twins. A pediatric autosomal dominant form with otolaryngologic and respiratory manifestations has been located on chromosome 13q14, and the locus is termed GERD1.

Reflux may occur with increased abdominal pressure. A chronically lax sphincter is the most important mechanism. The factors contributing to the competence of the LES include the abdominal position of the sphincter, the angle of insertion of the esophagus into the stomach, and sphincter pressure. Refluxed material is returned to the stomach by the secondary peristaltic wave in the esophagus. Swallowed saliva neutralizes and washes away the last traces of acid with a primary peristaltic wave.

■ CLINICAL FEATURES (FIG. 1)

Beyond infancy, more typical symptoms of heartburn, chest pain, and epigastric pain begin to predominate. In children between 3 and 9 years of age, typical symptoms are reported in 2-7% of patients with the most common symptom being epigastric pain. In adolescents, 5% of teens report symptoms of heartburn, epigastric pain, or regurgitation.

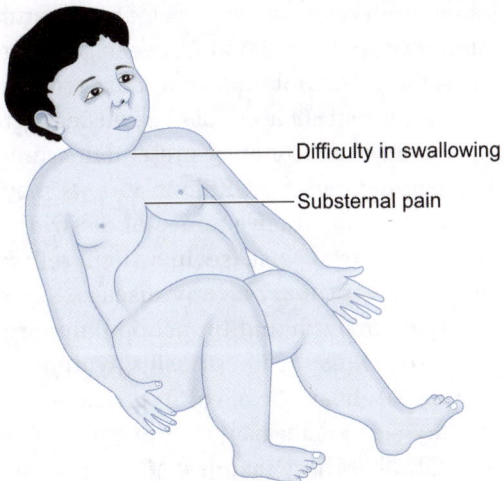

Fig. 1: Clinical features.

Clinical features are directly related to the exposure of esophageal epithelium to refluxed gastric content. Most of the infants (85%) will have vomiting during the first week of life. Some may have symptoms by 6 weeks. Patients with cerebral palsy, and Down syndrome will have an increased incidence of reflux. In 60%, symptoms disappear by 2 years. But the remainder will have symptoms till the age of 4 years.

Infantile reflux manifests more often with regurgitation (especially postprandially), signs of esophagitis (irritability, arching, choking, gagging, and feeding aversion), and resulting failure to thrive; symptoms resolve spontaneously in the majority of infants by 12-24 months. Older children can have regurgitation during the preschool years; this complaint diminishes somewhat as children age, and complaints of abdominal and chest pain supervene in later childhood and adolescence.

Older children can have regurgitation during the preschool years; this complaint diminishes somewhat as children age, and complaints of abdominal and chest pain supervene in later childhood and adolescence. Occasional children present with food refusal or neck contortions (arching, turning of head) designated Sandifer syndrome. The respiratory presentations are also age-dependent: GERD in infants may manifest as obstructive apnea or as stridor or lower airway disease in which reflux complicates primary airway disease, such as laryngomalacia and bronchopulmonary dysplasia. Otitis media, sinusitis, lymphoid hyperplasia, hoarseness, vocal cord nodules, and laryngeal edema have all been associated with GERD. Airway manifestations in older children are more commonly related to asthma or to otolaryngologic diseases, such as laryngitis and sinusitis.

The respiratory presentations are also age-dependent: GERD in infants can manifest as obstructive apnea or as stridor or lower airway disease in which reflux complicates primary airway disease, such as laryngomalacia and bronchopulmonary dysplasia. Otitis media, sinusitis, lymphoid hyperplasia, hoarseness, vocal cord nodules, and laryngeal edema have all been associated with GERD. Airway manifestations in older children are more commonly related to asthma or to otolaryngologic diseases, such as laryngitis and sinusitis.

In young infants, many episodic events such as apneic spells, "colic" crying, and sleep disturbances have been attributed to GER disease with or without esophagitis. Abnormal posturing with tilting of the head to one side and bizarre contortions of the trunk have been seen in some children with reflux. This symptom complex is referred to as "Sandifer's syndrome."

Children with pathological GER present with failure to thrive. This is because from the loss of calories, and symptoms attributable to esophagitis or with episode events like apnea in young infants. The hallmark of the severe disease is failure to thrive. This occurs as a consequence of calorie loss due to the vomited volume.

It is good to differentiate between vomiting and regurgitation. Vomiting is the forceful expulsion of the gastric contents through the mouth. It has three distinct phases, i.e., nausea, retching, and emesis. The emesis involves intense muscular activity of the respiratory and abdominal muscles. Regurgitation is an effortless passive bringing up of gastric contents that involves no muscular activity.

The aspiration of gastric content leads to inflammation and edema of the larynx and trachea. GER should be considered as a possible cause of recurrent respiratory symptoms. Recurrent bronchopulmonary infection and chronic asthma have been associated with GER.

ESSENTIAL DIAGNOSTIC POINTS

- Involuntary passage of gastric contents into the esophagus
- The lower esophageal sphincter is abnormal.
- Failure to thrive
- Recurrent respiratory symptoms
- Recurrent bronchopulmonary infection and chronic asthma.
- Aspiration pneumonia.

SYMPTOMS POSSIBLY RELATED TO REFLUX ESOPHAGITIS

- Epigastric or retrosternal pain (heartburn)
- General irritability in infants (colic)
- Weight loss and/or failure to thrive
- Hematemesis and melena
- "Noncardiac angina-like" chest pain
- Symptoms related to iron-deficiency anemia
- Dysphagia (due to esophagitis and/or structure formation)
- Belching and postprandial fullness

Aspiration pneumonia occurs in about 30% of patients. In childhood, chronic cough, wheezing, and recurrent pneumonia are common. Growth and weight gain are affected in about 60% of patients. Iron deficiency anemia is noted among 25% of the patients. About two-thirds of the patients have delayed gastric emptying and vomiting because of the pylorospasm.

The major manifestation of esophagitis is hemorrhage. Hematemesis occurs in some children. Substernal pain is less common. Dysphagia may cause irritability and anorexia in advanced cases. Reflux may rarely cause laryngospasm apnea and bradycardia.

GENERAL FEATURES
- Regurgitation of food
- Cough
- Failure to gain weight
- Esophagitis

DIFFERENTIAL DIAGNOSIS
- Hiatus hernia
- Tracheoesophageal fistula
- Esophagitis

DIAGNOSIS

Most of the esophageal tests are of some use in particular patients with suspected GERD. Contrast (usually barium) radiographic study of the esophagus and upper GIT is performed in children with vomiting and dysphagia to evaluate for achalasia, esophageal strictures and stenosis, hiatal hernia, and gastric outlet or intestinal obstruction. It has poor sensitivity and specificity in the diagnosis of GERD as a result of its limited duration and the inability to differentiate physiologic GER from GERD. Furthermore, contrast radiography neither accurately assesses mucosal inflammation nor correlates with the severity of GERD.

Upper Gastrointestinal Radiography

Barium imaging should only be used to diagnose anatomic abnormalities predisposing to reflux (e.g., hiatal hernia), to diagnose complications of reflux such as stricturing, or to look for GERD masqueraders (e.g., achalasia, pyloric stenosis, and malrotation).

Barium Swallow

Contrast (usually barium) radiographic studies of the esophagus and stomach using barium have been used to study GER. While a barium study is not specific enough in evaluating the severity of GER, it would rule out such other structural abnormalities such as a large hiatus hernia, esophageal stricture, duodenal web or an atypical pyloric stenosis, and gastric outlet or intestinal obstruction.

pH Probe Study

pH probes were considered by many to be the gold standard test to confirm a diagnosis of GERD These pf probes are inserted through the nose into the esophagus where the catheter remains with the pH sensor tip in the distal esophagus for approximately 24 hours. The catheter measures the number and duration of acid reflux episodes that have a pH of <4. Patients record symptoms during the test, and the time of these symptoms is correlated with esophageal reflux events present either before or after the symptom.

Currently, the role of pH probes are (1) to measure the total amount of acid reflux in 24 hours to clarify the role of acid in esophagitis, dental erosions, and other acid-related complications; (2) to determine how much acid reflux is still present in patients taking acid suppression medications at the time when the pH probe is performed; or (3) to correlate symptoms with acid reflux events. Because the ambient pH of the esophagus is ≥5, it is not possible for pH sensors to reliably discriminate reflux with a pH >4 from ambient esophageal pH.

Multichannel Intraluminal Impedance with pH

As with pH probes, multichannel intraluminal impedance with pH (pH-MII) catheters are also inserted through the nose into the esophagus. Unlike pH probes, there are seven impedance sensors distributed along the catheter, so bolus flow can be assessed at six different heights (between paired sensors). There is also an additional distal pH sensor on the catheter so that the pH of the refluxate can be determined.

The pH-MII test offers significant advantages over a pH probe alone, in that the catheters can (1) measure the directionality of flow, which allows for the differentiation of swallowed versus refluxed contents; (2) measure both acidic and nonacidic gastric contents; and (3) measure both distal and proximal reflux using sensors located throughout the esophagus.

The role of pH-MII in the evaluation of GERID is: (1) To determine the temporal relationship between acid and nonacid reflux events and typical and atypical symptoms; (2) to determine the relationship between full column reflux and extraesophageal symptoms; (3) to determine the efficacy of acid suppression medications when pH-MII is performed while taking medications; and (4) to diagnose the relationship between symptoms and reflux events in patients with a greater nonacidic reflux burden.

Manometry

Esophageal manometry to assess pressure profile and their dynamic changes has not been proven helpful in the practical management of GER and remains primarily a research tool today.

Scintigraphy

The goal of nuclear scintigraphy (also known as a milk scan or gastric emptying scan) is to determine the rapidity with which food or liquid empties from the stomach to determine if delays in gastric emptying may contribute to the worsening of GERD. Although the test is looking for triggers of reflux (e.g., delayed emptying), it is not used to diagnose reflux itself. This test evaluates the degree to which isotope-labeled formula or food is empty from the stomach following a 10-minute meal. Whenever possible, solid food is given during the test because delays in emptying are more often seen with solid food compared to liquid meals. Results are reported as either the percentage of meal remaining in the stomach after a fixed amount of time (usually 1 hour or hours).

Radionucleotides like 99m Tc added to the infant's feed can be monitored with a gamma counter and the time and amount of radionucleotide refluxed into the esophagus or lungs and the gastric emptying time can be studied. It has the advantage of being noninvasive and low in radiation.

Endoscopy and Biopsy

Upper Endoscopy with Biopsy of the Esophagus

The main role of endoscopy in the evaluation of patients with possible GERD is to assess for complications of GERD (e.g., erosions, Barrett esophagus, and strictures), to treat strictures with balloon dilation, and to differentiate reflux esophagitis from eosinophilic esophagitis (EoE), the latter of which can present with symptoms identical to reflux, but the therapies differ greatly, so making the correct diagnosis is critical.

Currently, the indication for endoscopy in patients with suspected GERD is (1) to evaluate for masqueraders of reflux (e.g., infectious esophagitis, EoE) in patients not responsive to acid suppression therapy; (2) to evaluate and treat complications of GERD, such as Barrett esophagus and stricturing, and (3) to assess for anatomic abnormalities (e.g., hiatal hernia, slippage of Nissen fundoplication). Definitive diagnosis of GERD by endoscopy requires the presence of erosive esophagitis with endoscopically visible breaks in the esophageal mucosa.

The flexible fiberoptic and video endoscope enable direct visualization of the esophageal mucosa as well as the study of the dynamics of the LES. Although macroscopic evidence of esophageal ulceration strongly suggests reflux esophagitis, a mucosal biopsy is required to diagnose the less severe lesions.

Endoscopy allows diagnosis of erosive esophagitis and complications such as strictures and Barrett's esophagus; esophageal biopsies can diagnose histologic reflux esophagitis in the absence of erosions while simultaneously eliminating allergic and infectious causes. Endoscopy is also used therapeutically to dilate reflux-induced strictures.

Laryngotracheobronchoscopy evaluates visible airway signs that are associated with extraesophageal GERD, such as posterior laryngeal inflammation and vocal cord nodules.

Strictures are usually demonstrated with barium esophagography. Severe esophagitis may be suspected when a ragged mucosal outline is seen on a roentgenogram. But esophagography with biopsy is the superior technique. The severity and frequency of reflux can be documented for monitoring esophageal pH with a probe in the distal esophagus.

Esophageal mucosa for microscopic study can be obtained either by endoscopic pinch biopsy or suction biopsy. Since esophagitis tends to occur in a patchy distribution, visual inspection is important before taking a biopsy even though suction biopsy is more widely used. An increased number of biopsies from different areas will significantly improve the yield for microscopic diagnosis.

Histological criteria for the diagnosis of esophagitis on endoscopic biopsies have been graded. Basal cell zone hyperplasia of the esophageal squamous epithelium and increased stromal papillary length [reflux-associated squamous hyperplasia (RASH)] are the most commonly used criteria.

> **LABORATORY SALIENT FINDINGS**
> - Barium Swallow
> - pH Probe Study
> - Esophageal manometry
> - Scintigraphy
> - Flexible fiberoptic and video endoscope enables direst visualization of the esophageal mucosa as well as study the dynamics of the LES
> - Suction biopsy
> - *Histological criteria:* Basal cell zone hyperplasia of the esophageal squamous epithelium and increased stromal papillary length (Reflux associated squamous hyperplasia – RASH)

■ TREATMENT

There are two main goals of treatment: (1) to alleviate the symptoms of GERD and/or (2) to prevent complications of GERD. The choice of therapy depends on which goal is being addressed. In the patient with esophageal atresia, the goal may be to prevent reflux esophagitis and Barrett's esophagus in adulthood. In contrast, the goal of treatment in an infant with spitting up and poor weight gain may be to reduce the regurgitation in the short term to prevent loss of calories from the regurgitation.

The main nonpharmacologic therapies in infants and children include positioning and dietary interventions. In infants, several well-designed studies have consistently shown that while right-side-down positioning may speed gastric emptying. Therefore, for infants monitored in hospital settings, left-side-down positioning is superior for reflux control. However, because of the concern that patients will roll into the prone positioning, side positioning is not recommended for infants unmonitored at home. Similarly, while prone positioning does seem to have the lowest rates of reflux of all of the positioning options, because of the risk of sudden infant death syndrome (SIDS), prone positioning cannot be recommended.

Another nonpharmacologic therapy frequently used is thickening agents added to the formula or included in the formula in the form of rice starch. While formulas with added rice starch require gastric acid to trigger the thickening in the stomach, the addition of cereal directly to the bottle thickens the formula instantly; adding thickening in this manner treats both GERD and oropharyngeal dysphagia. Typical thickening from a reflux perspective includes the addition of one teaspoon of rice cereal per ounce of formula, but the nipple should not be cut to accommodate the thickened formula, as this increases the risk of aspiration during Swallowing.

Another common cause for reflux symptoms is infant overfeeding, where patients are fed too much volume or too frequently because the symptoms of fussiness, restlessness, and discomfort are misinterpreted as hunger.

Finally, the method of administering feeds may help with reflux control. In neurologically compromised patients or in patients with significant pulmonary symptoms, transpyloric feeding has been proposed as a means to control GERD. Pediatric studies support that transpyloric feeding reduces reflux episodes to the same degree as fundoplication, and outcome studies suggest that, at least with respect to extraesophageal symptoms, transpyloric feeding has equivalent outcomes to fundoplication as well. Therefore, in patients at high risk for surgery, for patients in whom it is not clear if symptoms are reflux-related, in patients with gastric dysmotility, or as a parental preference, transpyloric feeding may serve as either a diagnostic or therapeutic intervention for GERD.

Gastroesophageal reflux is the involuntary passage of gastric contents into the esophagus. It produces esophagitis or respiratory complications. Factors such as thoracic stomach hiatal hernia, lack of intra-abdominal esophagus, and loss of cardioesophageal angle result in the incompetence of the gastroesophageal sphincter mechanism. Endoscopy with a flexible fiberoptic instrument will detect esophagitis and potential stricture formation as well as exclude other causes, such as enteropathy.

Medical therapy is better in infants than in older children. In uncomplicated cases, keeping the child prone, thickening the feeding with cereal, and careful attention at the time of burping is enough.

Conservative therapy and lifestyle modifications that form the foundation of GERD therapy can be effectively implemented through education and reassurance for parents. Dietary measures for infants include normalization of any abnormal feeding techniques, volumes, and frequencies. Thickening of feeds increases the percentage of infants with no regurgitation, decreases the frequency of daily regurgitation and emesis, and increases the infant's weight gain. However, caution should be exercised when managing preterm infants because of the possible association between xanthan gum-based thickened feeds and necrotizing enterocolitis.

Positioning measures are particularly important for infants, who cannot control their positions independently. Seated position worsens infant reflux and should be avoided in infants with GERD. Esophageal pH monitoring demonstrates more reflux episodes in infants in supine and side positions compared with the prone position.

When the infant is awake and observed, a prone position and an upright carried position can be used to minimize reflux. Lying in the flat supine position and semi-seated positions (e.g., car seats and infant carriers) in the postprandial period are considered provocative positions for GER and therefore should be avoided. The head should be elevated by elevating the head of the bed, rather than using excess pillows, to avoid abdominal flexion and compression that might worsen reflux.

A combination of modified feeding volumes, hydrolyzed infant formulas, proper positioning, and avoidance of smoke exposure satisfactorily improve GERD symptoms in infants with GERD. Older children should be counseled to avoid acidic or reflux-inducing foods. Weight reduction for obese patients and elimination of smoke exposure are other crucial measures at all ages.

Some evidence suggests a benefit to left side position and head elevation during sleep. The head should be elevated by elevating the head of the bed, rather than using excess pillows, to avoid abdominal flexion and compression that might worsen reflux.

Regurgitation is common during infancy, only in those with GER. Disease should be selected for therapy. Treatment should be in a phase schematic manner. Small frequent feeds are useful since they reduce the volume available in the stomach for reflux. Continuous NG drip feeding is an effective means of ensuring catchup growth in severe cases. However, if weight gain does not occur after a week of NG feeding, there is little benefit in continuing it.

The mainstays of therapy for GERD are acid suppression medications, either histamine (H_1) receptor antagonists (RAs) or proton pump inhibitors (PPIs).

Pharmacotherapy is directed at ameliorating the acidity of the gastric contents or at promoting their aboral movement and should be considered for those symptomatic infants and children who are either highly suspected or proven to have GERD. Antacids are the most commonly used antireflux therapy.

Histamine-2 receptor antagonists (H_2RAs) (such as cimetidine, famotidine, nizatidine, and ranitidine) are widely used antisecretory agents that act by selective inhibition of H_1 receptors on gastric parietal cells. There is a definite benefit of H_2RAs in the treatment of mild-to-moderate reflux esophagitis. H_2RAs have been recommended as first-line therapy because of their excellent overall safety profile, but they are superseded by PPIs in this role.

Ranitidine (5–10 mg/kg/day in two to three divided doses) and cimetidine have been used extensively, with the former being better tolerated and having less adverse effects. Sucralfate is comparable to H_2RAs in efficacy in adults, but its safety and usefulness in children are uproven. Omeprazole, a gastric PPI has recently been reported effective in children with severe esophagitis refractory to H_2 blockers. It may be given a trial before surgical treatment is decided.

Pantireflux effect by blocking the hydrogen-potassium adenosine triphosphatase channels of the final common pathway in gastric acid secretion. PPIs are superior to 1-12 RAs in the treatment of severe and erosive esophagitis. The use of PPIs to treat infants and children deemed to have GERD on the basis of symptoms is now the standard of care. Omeprazole (0.7–3.3 mg/kg/day, maximum 80 mg), lansoprazole-(1–3 mg/kg/day maximum 60 mg) and esomeprazole (<20 kg; 5–10 mg >20 kg; 10–20 mg OD).

Prokinetic agents have some role in treatment. Domperidone, a dopamine receptor blocker is marginally beneficial and is not widely used to treat reflux during infancy. Cisapride a 5-hydroxytryptamine receptor 4 (5-HT4) antagonist is effective without many side effects and is thought to work by enhancing neurotransmitter release that stimulates smooth muscle contraction throughout the intestinal tract. H_2 blockers do not decrease the frequency and duration of the reflux, but act by reducing the acidity of the gastric contents. Prokinetic agents available include metoclopramide (dopamine-2 and 5-HT antagonist), bethanechol (cholinergic agonist), and erythromycin (motilin receptor agonist). Most of these increase LES pressure; some improve gastric emptying or esophageal clearance.

Surgery

If the symptoms do not respond to a 6-week trial of intensive medical therapy, then surgical treatment is indicated.

The surgery done is Nissen fundoplication, which is an effective therapy for intractable GERD in children, particularly those with refractory esophagitis or strictures and those at risk for significant morbidity from chronic pulmonary disease. It may be combined with a gastrostomy for feeding or venting. Preoperative accuracy of diagnosis of GERD and the skill of the surgeon are TWO of the most important predictors of a successful outcome.

Surgical procedures aim to tighten the LES and thus prevent the reflux of gastric contents into the esophagus. Nissen fundoplication which involves a 360° wrap of the fundus around the distal 3.5 cm of the esophagus in a common procedure. It is more commonly done for neurologically impaired children with severe GERD, and the results are comparable to that in normal children.

Recent reports suggest that anterior gastric fundoplication may be equally effective. However, postoperative adhesions leading to small intestinal obstruction occur in 5–10% of cases after fundoplication.

Fundoplication procedures may be performed as open operations, by laparoscopy, or by endoluminal (gastroplication) techniques. Pediatric experience is limited with an endoscopic application of radiofrequency therapy (Stretta procedure) to a 2–3 cm area of the LES and cardia to create a high-pressure zone to reduce reflux.

Follow-up Management

The first follow-up endoscopy in those with esophagitis should be performed 4–12 weeks after instituting medical treatment. If the esophagus is normal, H_2 blockers may be discontinued. *Prokinetics* can be continued for longer periods depending on the symptomatic improvement.

Persisting esophagitis is an indication for contemplating surgery. However, since surgery is not free of complications, and GER in infants improves with age, the surgical option should be exercised only after all medical therapy has been exhausted.

Small frequent feeds are useful since they reduce the volume available in the stomach for reflux.

■ BIBLIOGRAPHY

1. Cohen S, Bueno de Mesquita M, Mimouni FB. Adverse effects reported in the use of gastroesophageal reflux disease treatments in children: a 10 years literature review. Br J Clin Pharmacol. 2015;89(2):200-8.
2. Lightdale JR, Gremse DA; Section on Gastroenterology, Hepatology, and Nutrition. Gastroesophageal reflux: management guidance for the pediatrician. Pediatrics. 2013;131(5):e1684-95.
3. Forbes D, Lim A, Ravikumara M. Gastroesophageal reflux in the 21st century. Curr Opin Pediatr. 2013;25(5):597-603.
4. Tighe M, Afzal NA, Bevan A, Hayen A, Munro A, Beattie RM. Pharmacological treatment of children with gastroesophageal reflux. Cochrane Database Syst Rev. 2014; 2014(11):CD006550.

CASE 27

Hepatitis

■ PRESENTING COMPLAINTS

A 5-year-old boy was brought with the complaint of:
- Fever since 1 week
- Vomiting since 3 days
- Abdominal pain since 3 days
- High-colored urine since 2 days

History of Presenting Complaints

A 5-year-old boy presented with the history of fever, vomiting, and abdominal pain. The boy was apparently normal till a week ago. To start with he developed the fever. Fever was moderate-to-high degree and intermittent more in the evening. There was associated history of vomiting. Vomiting was associated with nausea and was insidious. The boy was not tolerating any food and even water. Along with this, he developed pain in abdomen. The pain was present in right upper abdomen. He was not allowing anybody to touch the abdomen. There was history of passing of high-colored urine.

Past History of the Patient

He was the only child of the nonconsanguineous marriage. He was born at full term with normal delivery. He cried immediately after delivery. His birth weight was 3 kg. He was breastfed exclusively for 3 months. Weaning started later with cereals and completed by one year. His developmental milestones were normal. His performance at school was good.

■ EXAMINATION

The boy was moderately built and moderately nourished. Signs of mild dehydration were

---

CASE AT A GLANCE

Basic Findings
Height	: 108 cm (75th centile)
Weight	: 14 kg (50th centile)
Temperature	: 38°C
Pulse rate	: 110 beats/min
Respiratory rate	: 20 breaths/min
Blood pressure	: 80/60 mm Hg

Positive Findings

History:
- Fever
- Abdominal pain
- Vomiting
- High-colored urine

Examination:
- Febrile
- Jaundice
- Sign of dehydration
- Tender hepatomegaly

Investigation:
- Pallor
- Abdominal LFT
- *Alkaline phosphatase:* Increased
- *SGOT:* Increased
- *SGPT:* Increased

(LFT: liver function test; SGOT: serum glutamic oxaloacetic transaminase; SGPT: serum glutamic pyruvic transaminase)

present. This child was looking sick. His anthropometric measurements included the height 108 cm (75th centile), the weight was 14 kg (50th centile).

The child was febrile, i.e., 38°C. The heart rate was 110 beats/min. Respiratory rate was 20 breaths/min. Blood pressure recorded was 80/60 mm Hg. The child was pale and icterus was present. There was no lymphadenopathy and no edema.

Per abdomen examination revealed presence of tender hepatomegaly. Liver was palpable about 3 cm below the costal margin, soft and tender. Tenderness was present at the right upper quadrant. Cardiovascular and respiratory system was normal.

■ INVESTIGATION

- *Hemoglobin:* 12 g/dL
- *TLC:* 7,600 cells/cumm
- *DLC:* $P_{78}L_{22}E_0M_0$
- *ESR:* 22 mm at first hour
- *AEC:* 436 cells/cumm
- *Serum bilirubin:* 7 mg/dL
- *Alkaline phosphatase:* 150 U/L
- *SGOT:* 60 U/L
- *SGPT:* 150 U/L
- *X-ray chest:* Normal

■ DISCUSSION

Viral hepatitis is an important health problem in developing and developed countries of the world. Despite the availability of vaccines and prophylactic measures and improved sanitation, its incidence is almost constant. This can be explained with better understanding about epidemiological findings with changes in human ecology and behavior.

Hepatitis A virus (HAV) infection occurs throughout the world but is most prevalent in developing countries. 30–40% of the adult population has evidence of previous HAV infection. Hepatitis A is thought to account for approximately 50% of all clinically apparent acute viral hepatitis.

Hepatitis A virus infection is the most prevalent hepatotropic virus. This virus is also responsible for most forms of acute and benign hepatitis; although fulminant hepatic failure can occur.

Six major viruses are the etiologic agents responsible for most clinical cases of viral hepatitis: (1) HAV, (2) hepatitis B virus (HBV), (3) hepatitis C virus (HCV), (4) hepatitis D virus (delta agent, HDV), (5) hepatitis E virus (HEV) and (6) hepatitis G virus (HGV). Recently hepatitis F virus (HFV) has been reported as a double-stranded DNA virus. Various other causes of hepatitis are other viruses, drugs, toxins, bacteria, parasite, and other noninfectious disorders.

■ ETIOLOGY

Hepatitis A virus is a single-stranded ribonucleic acid (RNA) virus that is classified as a picornavirus. HAV causes acute hepatitis and asymptomatic infection but never chronic infection.

Infection occurs primarily via the fecal-oral route, because the virus is relatively resistant to gastric acidity, making it an extremely efficient gastrointestinal pathogen. Travel to countries where HAV is endemic is also a frequent cause of sporadic infection. In countries where it is endemic, infection is usually acquired in childhood and is most of the time asymptomatic.

These are more common in developing countries, where the prevalence rate approaches 100% in children by the age of 5 years. HAV causes only acute hepatitis and there is no complication once the acute attack subsides.

PATHOPHYSIOLOGY

Hepatitis A virus spreads by person-to-person contact and by fecal–oral route. Rarely parenteral transmission during viremia has been reported in the prodromal period. Fecal excretion of virus occurs till late in the incubation period, while, at peak just before the onset of symptoms, and at minimum a week after the onset of jaundice. HAV is highly contagious. Transmission is almost always by person-to-person contact through the fecal–oral route. Perinatal transmission occurs rarely. No other form of transmission is recognized.

The mean incubation period for HAV is approximately 15–50 days. Fecal excretion of the virus starts late in the incubation period, reaches its peak just before the onset of symptoms, and resolves by 2 weeks after the onset of jaundice in older subjects. The duration of viral excretion is prolonged in infants. Incubation period ranges from 15 to 50 days while mean period being about 4 weeks. Foodborne and waterborne outbreaks are common in crowded or unsanitary area.

Feces is infectious from 2 weeks before and one week after the onset of jaundice. Viremia is evident from the second to sixth week after the exposure. A patient is infectious in the prodromal stage, 1–2 weeks prior to illness. The risk of transmitting HAV is greatest from 2 weeks before to 1 week after the onset of jaundice. Infectivity falls rapidly with the onset of jaundice. Infective material is mainly feces, blood, and sweat.

A period of viremia precedes the presence of virus in stool and continues through the period of elevated liver enzymes. Clinical disease occurs after shedding in stool has begun. The period of peak infectivity is during the 2 weeks prior to jaundice or elevated alanine transaminase (ALT) and alkaline phosphatase, when the viral titer in the stool can be as high as 10 infectious particles per milliliter. Shedding of virus can persist for several months in young children, presumably due to physiologic immunodeficiency.

Increased risk of infection is found in contacts with infected persons, childcare centers, and household contacts. Infection is also associated with contact with contaminated food or water and after travel to endemic areas. Common source foodborne and waterborne outbreaks have occurred, including several caused by contaminated food.

The human cases are the only reservoir of the infection. The cases range from asymptomatic infection to severe form. The asymptomatic, i.e., icterus is especially common in children. There is no evidence of chronic carrier state.

PATHOLOGY

Damage to liver is by way of hepatocyte damage, cholestasis, and metabolic dysfunction. Hepatocyte damage is evidenced by release of aminotransferases into the bloodstream. Cholestasis is evident by elevation of serum alkaline phosphatase, serum nucleotidase, and urinary urobilinogen. Metabolic dysfunction results in changes in ammonia, carbohydrate, and drug metabolism.

The acute response of the liver to HAV is similar in all (A through E) hepatitis viruses. The entire liver is involved with necrosis and increased cellularity. Lobular architecture remains intact although balloon degeneration and necrosis of parenchymal cells occur initially. Diffuse Kupffer cell hyperplasia is also present along with infiltration of polymorphonuclear leukocytes and eosinophils. In neonates, giant cells are seen. During complication of fulminant hepatic failure, there is total destruction of hepatic parenchyma.

Other organ systems can be affected during acute HAV infection. Regional lymph nodes and the spleen may be enlarged. The bone marrow may be moderately hypoplastic, and aplastic anemia has been reported. Tissue in the small intestine might show changes in villous structure, and ulceration of the GIT can occur, especially in fatal cases. Acute pancreatitis and myocarditis have been reported, though rarely, and nephritis, arthritis, leukocytoclastic vasculitis, and cryoglobulinemia can result from circulating immune complexes.

Liver cell damage is most marked in the centrilobular region. Damage to hepatocytes is mediated by cell-mediated immune response. Some individual lobules are variably affected. Hepatocytes have a swollen granular appearance. Dead ones become shrunken and deeply stained. They form eosinophilic bodies by losing their nuclei. These are called Councilman bodies. These are strong indications of viral hepatitis. The portal tracts are enlarged and contain mononuclear cell infiltrate. Severe damage is accompanied by collapse of the reticulin framework, especially between central vein and portal tract. Spleen and lymph nodes may also be enlarged. During viremia myocarditis, pancreatitis and intestinal ulceration may occur.

■ CLINICAL FEATURES (FIG. 1)

The incubation period is 15–50 days with an average of 25–30 days. The onset is generally acute. During the prodromal phase, the patient has moderate fever, loss of appetite, malaise, nausea, and upper abdominal pain. After the prodromal phase, the patient passes dark-colored urine.

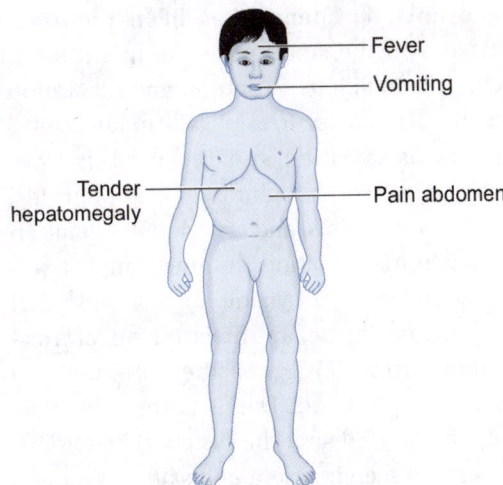

Fig. 1: Clinical features.

Fecal excretion of the virus starts late in the incubation period, reaches its peak just before the onset of symptoms, and resolves by 2 weeks after the onset of jaundice in older subjects. The duration of fecal viral excretion is prolonged in infants. The patient is, therefore, contagious before clinical symptoms are apparent and remains so until viral shedding ceases.

Hepatitis A virus is responsible for acute hepatitis only. Often, this is an anicteric illness, with clinical symptoms indistinguishable from other forms of viral gastroenteritis, particularly in young children.

The illness is much more likely to be symptomatic in older adolescents or adults, in patients with underlying liver disorders, and in those who are immunocompromised. It is characteristically an acute febrile illness with an abrupt onset of anorexia, nausea, malaise, vomiting, and jaundice. The typical duration of this illness is 7–14 days.

Other organ systems can be affected during acute HAV infection; regional lymph nodes and the spleen may be enlarged. The bone marrow may be moderately hypoplastic, and aplastic anemia has been reported. Tissues in the small intestine might show changes in villous structure, and ulceration of the GIT can occur, especially in fatal cases. Acute pancreatitis and myocarditis have been reported, though rarely, and nephritis, arthritis, vasculitis, and cryoglobulinemia can result from circulating immune complexes.

Jaundice is not visible or is so mild that it can hardly be appreciated on clinical examination and can be detected by laboratory test only. Dark-colored urine may also be noticed after the systemic symptoms. Icterus is seen in sclera and skin will remain for 1–4 weeks. Liver is enlarged and tender. Splenomegaly is present in some cases. Recovery is usual. The mortality is <1%.

ESSENTIAL DIAGNOSTIC POINTS
• Fever, chills, headache
• Fatigue, generalized weakness followed by anorexia, nausea, vomiting
• Dark-colored urine and jaundice
• Spreads by person-to-person contact and by fecal oral route
• Infective material is mainly feces, blood, and sweat
• Spleen and lymph nodes are enlarged

Thes disease is heralded by nonspecific symptoms, such as fever, chills, headache, fatigue, generalized weakness followed by anorexia, nausea, vomiting, dark-colored urine, and jaundice. The disease is benign with complete recovery in several weeks. The case fatality rate is <0.1% usually from acute liver failure.

Sometimes atypical course includes cholestatic hepatitis characterized by jaundice and severe pruritis. In most of them, symptoms resolve in 2–3 weeks after the onset and almost all patients recover completely. No chronic infection and carrier state will occur. In patients with acute hepatitis certain features may suggest fever, coryza, headache, photophobia, and cough.

Single exposure to the virus produces a humoral response and provides lifelong immunity. HAV has a single serotype.

GENERAL FEATURES
• Jaundice
• Anorexia
• Loss of weight

DIAGNOSIS

Hepatitis A virus should be suspected when there is a history of infective hepatitis in family members, school friends, or other close contacts or child has traveled to hepatitis endemic areas. Diagnosis is made by liver function tests, serologic criteria, and virus isolation.

Acute HAV infection is diagnosed by detecting antibodies to HAV, specifically, anti-HAV [immunoglobulin M (IgM)] by radioimmunoassay or, rarely, by identifying viral particles in stool.

A viral polymerase chain reaction (PCR) assay is available for research use. Anti-HAV is detectable when the symptoms are clinically apparent, and it remains positive for 4–6 months after the acute infection. A neutralizing anti-HAV (IgG) is usually detected within 8 weeks of symptom onset and is measured as part of a total anti-HAV in the serum. Anti-HAV (IgG) confers long-term protection. Rises in serum levels of ALT, AST, bilirubin, alkaline phosphatase, 5-nucleotidase, and gamma-glutamyl transpeptidase are almost universally found and do not help to differentiate the cause of hepatitis.

Basic investigations, such as urine for bile salts, bile pigments are done. Liver function tests reveal elevated ALT, AST, bilirubin, alkaline phosphatase, 5-nucleotidase and gamma-glutamyl transpeptidase. Prothrombin time may also be elevated. These tests do not help to differentiate the type of hepatitis. Serum glutamic pyruvic transaminase (SGPT) levels are very high in the first week of illness. Serum glutamic oxaloacetic transaminase (SGOT) is moderately elevated. Prothrombin time is a useful test for assessing prognosis.

Complete blood counts, blood glucose, urea, creatinine, total protein, and albumin are checked when the child is hospitalized. Hepatitis is diagnosed only if the transaminases are more than twice the upper limit of normal. In viral hepatitis, ALT is markedly increased more than 20 times the upper limit of normal and is higher than AST indicating cytoplasmic rather than mitochondrial injury.

The transaminase level remains elevated for 1–3 weeks. Serological tests for the diagnosis of hepatitis A are available. Anti-HAV is detected from onset of symptoms and persists throughout life. For initial 3–12 months anti-HAV (IgM) is detected and later on anti-HAV (IgG) is present.

Investigations for etiology are not necessary unless there are atypical manifestations or the child is hospitalized. All children should be screened for hepatitis B surface antigen (HBsAg). The presence of anti-HAV IgM or anti-HEV IgM confirms the diagnosis of acute HAV and HEV hepatitis, respectively; HBsAg positivity along with anti-HBc IgM indicates acute HBV hepatitis, whereas anti-HCV IgM positivity indicates acute HCV hepatitis.

Infection due to nonhepatotropic viruses, such as measles, paravovirus B19, herpes simplex 1 and 2, dengue virus, cytomegalovirus (CMV), Epstein–Barr virus (EBV) and HIV may present with jaundice and moderate elevation of transaminases. The associated clinical features of the underlying illness and specific serologic tests will help in diagnosis. Other causes of hepatitis such as leptospirosis, typhoid fever, Wilson disease, and autoimmune hepatitis should be excluded if there are atypical manifestations or features suggestive of nonviral hepatitis.

Ultrasound examination is done to exclude liver abscess or gallstones. Liver biopsy is not recommended in children with but is essential in those with suspected acute-on-chronic liver disease or chronic hepatitis.

- Demonstration of HAV particles or specific viral antigens in the feces
- Demonstration of rise in anti-HAV titer
- Detection of IgM antibody to HAV in patient's serum; this antibody appears early in illness persists for limited time usually for 3–4 months of life after the onset. IgG antibody indicates past infection and immunity.

Laboratory evaluation of liver function includes estimation of total and direct bilirubin, transaminases, alkaline phosphatase, prothrombin time, total protein, and albumin.

COMPLICATIONS

The complications include fulminant hepatic failure, relapse, cholestatic hepatitis, hyperbilirubinemia, aplastic anemia, renal failure, chronic hepatitis, and cirrhosis.

LABORATORY SALIENT FINDINGS

- Demonstration of HAV particles or specific viral antigens in the feces
- Demonstration of rise in anti-HAV titer
- Detection of IgM antibody to HAV in patients serum
- Serum glutamic pyruvic transaminase (SGPT) levels are very high in the first week of illness
- Serum glutamic oxaloacetic transaminase (SGOT) is moderately elevated
- Detection of IgM antibody to HAV in patients serum

(HAV: hepatitis A virus)

TREATMENT

Hepatitis A virus infection is benign in children and all recover completely. Rarely fulminant hepatic failure can occur.

There is no specific treatment for acute hepatitis. Bed rest is recommended. Good nutrition rich in carbohydrate and supplied with adequate protein should be given. There is no role of corticosteroids as it may interfere with immunologic defenses. This leads to prolongation of convalescent phase to chronic active hepatitis.

PREVENTION

Patients infected with HAV are contagious for 2 weeks before and approximately 7 days after the onset of jaundice and should be excluded from school, childcare, or work during this period. Careful handwashing is necessary, particularly after changing diapers and before preparing for serving food. In hospital settings, contact and standard precautions are recommended for 1 week after onset of symptoms.

Infection in children confers lifelong immunity. It is almost always asymptomatic or with mild symptoms and rarely culminating into fulminant hepatitis.

Indications for HAV vaccine are travelers going to areas of high prevalence, high-risk population living in crowded areas, drug users, etc., residents of communities of HAV epidemics.

Passive Immunization

Passive immunization is by immune serum globulin (IgG). It is effective in prevention of HAV infection preferably early in incubation period in the dose of 0.02 mL/kg intramuscularly. It provides protection for 3 months.

Development of an inactivated HAV vaccine, which is highly immunogenic and safe, is a major breakthrough in prevention of hepatitis A.

In addition to active immunization hepatitis A infection can be prevented by passive immunization by the administration of immune serum globulin (IgG) intramuscularly but for short period only and by enteric precautions to check the further spread of HAV.

Active Immunization

Hepatitis A Virus Vaccine

Recently, HAV vaccine is available for human use. This inactivated vaccine is prepared in cell culture and treated with formalin. Though hepatitis A infection in children confers lifelong immunity and is almost always asymptomatic or with mild symptoms and rarely culminating into fulminant hepatitis in contrast to adults in whom disease occurs in severe form, vaccination of children is useful, because these children can become carriers of the disease and could infect older siblings and adults.

Vaccination of young children in endemic areas is presently not recommended and universal childhood HAV immunization is under consideration. The dose of HAV vaccine for children aged 2–18 years is 360 U (ELISA units) intramuscular for each of the two initial injections, one month apart, followed by a booster 6–12 months after the first injection.

Immunoglobulin

Indications for intramuscular administration of Ig (0.02 mL/kg) include preexposure and postexposure prophylaxis.

Immunoglobulin is recommended for preexposure prophylaxis for susceptible travelers to countries where HAV is endemic, and it provides effective protection for up to 3 months. HAV vaccine is given any time before travel preferred for preexposure prophylaxis in healthy persons, but Ig ensures an appropriate prophylaxis in children younger than 12 months old, patients allergic to a vaccine component. If travel is planned in <2 weeks, older patients, immunocompromised hosts, and those with chronic liver disease or other medical conditions should receive both Ig and the HAV vaccine.

Immunoglobulin prophylaxis in postexposure situations should be used as soon as possible (not effective >2 weeks after exposure). It is exclusively used for children younger than 12 months old, immunocompromised hosts, those with chronic liver disease, or in whom vaccine is contraindicated.

Immunoglobulin prophylaxis in postexposure situations should be used as soon as possible (it is not effective if administered >2 weeks after exposure). It is exclusively used for children younger than 12 months old, immunocompromised hosts, those with chronic liver disease, or in whom vaccine is contraindicated. Ig is preferred in patients older than 40 years of age, with HAV vaccine preferred in healthy persons 12 months to 40 years old.

■ BIBLIOGRAPHY

1. American Academy of Pediatrics. Red Book (2012): Report of the Committee on Infectious Diseases. United States: American Academy of Pediatrics; 2012.
2. Collier MG, Tong X, Xu F. Hepatitis A hospitalizations in the United States, 2002-2011. Hepatology. 2015;61:481-5.
3. Dorell CG, Yankey D, Byrd KK, Murphy TV. Hepatitis A vaccination coverage among adolescents in the United States. Pediatrics. 2012;129:213-21.
4. Erhart LM, Ernst KC. The changing epidemiology of Hepatitis A in Arizona following intensive immunization programs (1988-2007). Vaccine. 2012;30:6103-10.
5. Satsangi S, Chawla YK Viral hepatitis: Indian scenario. Med J Armed Forces India. 2016;72:204-10.

CASE 28

Hirschsprung's Disease

PRESENTING COMPLAINTS

A 8-year-old boy was brought with the complaint of:
- Persistent soiling since 5 years
- Constipation since 5 years

History of Presenting Complaints

An 8-year-old boy came with history of persistent soiling. But on no occasion he had smeared or passed the feces. He had bowel disorder of constipation. He was responding to simple laxatives. Boy was on laxatives many a time. Bowel training later proved very difficult and approximately every 3 months he was receiving rectal washout. This was temporarily improving his incontinence. He never responded to medical management.

Past History of the Patient

He was the first child of consanguineous union. He was delivered at term by normal pregnancy. Baby cried immediately after delivery. There was no significant postnatal event. From the beginning, he had problem with bowel habits. He was having alternate loose motion and constipation. He was discharged on the 5th day. Child did not pass motion for 5 days and infant was readmitted at 10 days. No abnormalities were found. Constipation was relieved by laxatives. Other developmental milestones were normal. His school performance was good. He was not popular at school and had few friends.

EXAMINATION

Child was moderately built and moderately nourished. Anthropometric measurements included height 120 cm (50th centile) and weight 20 kg (50 centile). He was afebrile, pulse rate was 96 beats/min. The respiratory rate was 20 breaths/min. The blood pressure recorded was 90/70 mm Hg. There was

---

CASE AT A GLANCE

Basic Findings
Height	: 120 cm (50th centile)
Weight	: 20 kg (50th centile)
Temperature	: 36.8°C
Pulse rate	: 96 beats/min
Respiratory rate	: 20 breaths/min
Blood pressure	: 90/70 mm Hg

Positive Findings

History:
- Persistent soiling
- Constipation
- Used laxatives

Examination:
- Distension of abdomen

Investigation:
- *X-ray abdomen:* Narrow segment with dilated colon above
- *Barium enema:* Change with caliber between the rectum and sigmoid colon
- *Rectal biopsy:* Absence of ganglion cells in submucosa

neither pallor, lymphadenopathy, icterus, nor clubbing.

Per abdomen examination revealed presence of distension. There was no organomegaly and bowel sounds were sluggish. Other systemic examinations were normal.

■ INVESTIGATION

- *Hemoglobin:* 12 g/dL
- *TLC:* 7,600 cells/cumm
- *DLC:* $P_{68}L_{24}E_4M_2B_2$
- *Platelet count:* 3,00,000 cells/cumm
- *X-ray abdomen:* Narrow segment with dilated colon above
- *Barium enema:* Showed the evidence of a change in the caliber between rectum and sigmoid colon
- *Rectal manometry:* Absence of normal relaxation
- *Rectal biopsy:* Absence of ganglion cells in submucosa

■ DISCUSSION

Child had experienced the problem since the first week of life for passing the stools. He required laxative at that time. This suggests organic pathology. In case of long duration of soiling, the child should have either functional constipation or ultrashort segment, i.e., Hirschsprung's disease. A full-thickness biopsy of anal sphincter was performed. This confirmed the presence of aganglionic ultra-short segment leading to diagnosis of Hirschsprung's disease. Patient became continent within 3 months and remained so.

It is the most common cause of lower intestinal obstruction in neonates, with an overall incidence of 1 in 5,000 live births. The male to female ratio for Hirschsprung's disease is 4:1 for short-segment disease.

It is the most important cause of neonatal obstruction. It results in absence of ganglion cells in the bowel wall or failure of migration of embryonic neural crest cells into the bowel wall or failure of craniocaudal extension of mesenteric and submucous plexus within the wall. In the affected segment, sympathetic overactivity results in hypertension and absence of appropriate relaxation in response to absence of ganglion cells in the bowel wall or failure of migration of embryonic neural crest cells into the bowel wall or failure of craniocaudal extension of mesenteric and submucous plexus within the wall to proximal distension.

There is an increased familial incidence in long-segment disease. Hirschsprung's disease may be associated with other congenital defects, including trisomy 21, Joubert syndrome, Goldberg–Shprintzen syndrome, Smith–Lemli–Opitz syndrome, Shah–Waardenburg syndrome, cartilage-hair hypoplasia, multiple endocrine neoplasm 2 syndrome, neurofibromatosis, neuroblastoma, congenital hypoventilation (Ondine's curse), and urogenital or cardiovascular abnormalities. Hirschsprung's disease has been seen in association with microcephaly, mental retardation, abnormal facies, autism, cleft palate, hydrocephalus, and micrognathia.

Genetic defects have been identified in multiple genes that encode proteins of the RET signaling pathway (RET, GDNE, and NTN and involved in the endothelin (EDN) type B receptor pathway (EDNRB EDN3, and EVE-1). Syndromic forms of Hirschsprung's disease have been associated with the LICAM, SOX10, and ZFHXIB (formerly SIP1) genes. Observed histologically is an absence of Meissner's and Auerbach's plexuses and hypertrophied nerve bundles with high concentrations of acetylcholinesterase between the muscular layers and in the submucosa.

Hirschsprung's disease, or congenital aganglionic megacolon, is a developmental disorder (neurocristopathy) of the enteric nervous system, characterized by the absence of ganglion cells in the submucosal and myenteric plexus. It is caused by sphincter abnormal innervation of the bowel, beginning in the internal anal and extending proximally to involve variable length of the gut.

Migration of the neuroenteric cells occurs craniocaudally. Migration of cells from Auerbach's to other plexuses take place. Role of neural glycoproteins includes that of fibronectin and laminar proteins. Vagal neural crest cells are the only source of ganglion cells. There is abnormally large amount of laminin in extracellular spaces and hence there is decreased ability of ganglion cells to adhere to smooth muscle cells. There is lack of cell-to-cell adherence.

In ultrashort-segment Hirschsprung's disease, also known as anal achalasia, the aganglionic segment is limited to the internal sphincter. The clinical symptoms are similar to those of children with functional constipation. Ganglion cells are present on rectal suction biopsy, but the anorectal manometry is abnormal, with failure of relaxation of the internal anal sphincter in response to rectal distention.

■ PATHOLOGY

Hirschsprung disease is the result of an absence of ganglion cells in the bowel wall, extending proximally and continuously from the anus for variable distance. The absence of neural innervation is a consequence of arrest of neuroblast migration from the proximal to distal bowel. Without the myenteric and submucosal plexus, there is inadequate relaxation of the bowel wall and bowel wall hypertonicity, which can lead to intestinal obstruction.

Aganglionic segment is limited to rectosigmoid in 80% of patients. In 15% colon is aganglionic from anus to hepatic flexure. Incomplete parasympathetic innervation in aganglionic segment results in abnormal peristalsis, constipation, and functional intestinal obstruction. Proximal to transverse bowel, muscular hypertrophy thickens the intestinal wall. The intestine may become enormously dilated with retained feces and gas.

Histologically there is an absence of Meissner's and Auerbach's plexuses and hypertrophied nerve bundles with high concentrations of acetylcholinesterase between the muscular layers and in the submucosa.

■ PATHOPHYSIOLOGY

There is increase in adrenergic and cholinergic innervation. Adrenergic excitatory activity predominates. There is increased smooth muscle tone. There is loss of nitric oxide synthase from myenteric plexus. There is imbalance of smooth muscle contractility.

Aganglion produces colonic stasis leading to the bacterial overgrowth enteroadherent bacteria attach to unprotected intestinal epithelium. This leads to invasion of bacteria into the epithelium. Inflammatory process leads to clinical enterocolitis, systemic sepsis, and coagulopathy set in.

■ CLINICAL FEATURES (FIG. 1)

Ninety-nine percent of full-term infants pass meconium within 48 hours of birth. This disease is suspected in any full-term infant with delayed passage of stool.

Some neonates pass meconium normally but subsequently present with a history of chronic constipation. Failure to thrive with hypoproteinemia from protein-losing enteropathy is a less common presentation, because Hirschsprung's disease is usually

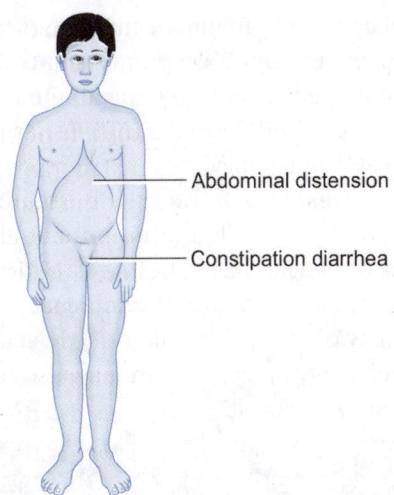

Fig. 1: Clinical features.

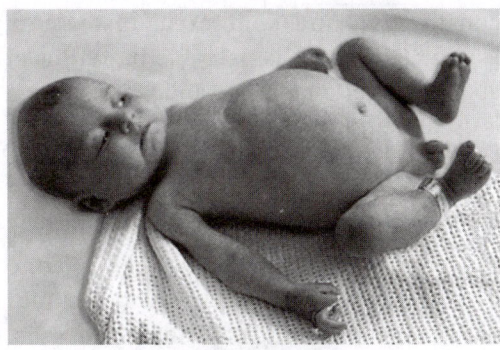

Fig. 2: Abdominal distension.

recognized early in the course of the illness but has been known to occur. Breastfed infants might not present as severely as formula-fed infants.

Stasis allows proliferation of bacteria, which can lead to enterocolitis (*Clostridium difficile*, *Staphylococcus aureus*, anaerobes, coliforms) with associated diarrhea, abdominal tenderness, sepsis, and signs of bowel obstruction. Red flags in the neonatal period then include neonatal intestinal obstruction, bowel perforation, delayed passage of meconium, abdominal distention relieved by digital rectal stimulation or enemas, chronic severe constipation, and enterocolitis.

Hirschsprung's disease is usually diagnosed in the neonatal period secondary to a distended abdomen, failure to pass meconium, and/or bilious emesis or aspirates with feeding intolerance. In 99% of healthy full-term infants, meconium is passed within 48 hours of birth, Hirschsprung's disease should be suspected in any full-term infant (the disease is unusual in preterm infants) with delayed passage of stool. Some neonates pass meconium normally but subsequently present with a history of chronic constipation.

It may manifest in first week of life as partial or complete obstruction with vomiting and abdominal distension (**Fig. 2**). This is associated with poor feeding and bilious vomiting. Temporary relief may be seen after rectal examination. Diarrhea may be prominent in neonatal period and may be associated with symptoms of intestinal obstruction. Hypoproteinemia and edema may result.

Failure to pass stool leads to dilatation of the proximal bowel and abdominal distension. Intraluminal pressure increases as bowel dilates. This leads to the decreased blood flow and deterioration of mucosal barrier. Stasis allows proliferation of bacteria, which can lead to enterocolitis (*C. difficile*, *S. aureus*, anaerobes, coliforms) with associated diarrhea, abdominal tenderness, sepsis, and signs of bowel obstruction. Early recognition of Hirschsprung's disease before the onset of enterocolitis is essential in reducing morbidity and mortality. This may be associated with septicemia and bowel obstruction.

In neonates, Hirschsprung's disease must be differentiated from meconium plug syndrome, meconium ileus, and intestinal atresia.

Episodes of constipation or diarrhea may alternate with periods of apparent normality. In older children, it may cause chronic constipation and abdominal distension. A large fecal mass is palpable in left lower abdomen. But on rectal examination rectum is usually empty.

Hirschsprung's disease in older patients must be distinguished from other causes of abdominal distention and chronic constipation. In older patients, the Currarino triad must be considered, which includes anorectal malformations (ectopic anus, anal stenosis, imperforate anus), sacral bone anomalies (hypoplasia, poor segmentation), and presacral anomaly (anterior meningoceles, teratoma, cyst).

The history often reveals constipation starting in infancy that has responded poorly to medical management. The abdomen is tympanitic and distended, with a large fecal mass palpable in the left lower abdomen. Rectal examination demonstrates a normally placed anus that easily allows entry of the finger but feels snug. The rectum is usually empty of feces, and when the finger is removed, there may be an explosive discharge of foul-smelling feces and gas. The stools, when passed, can consist of small pellets, be ribbon-like, or have a fluid consistency, unlike the large stools seen in patients with functional constipation. Intermittent attacks of intestinal obstruction from retained feces may be associated with pain and fever.

Diarrhea may fulminate into enterocolitis producing profound dehydration and shock with fluid and electrolyte loss into the lumen of the obstructed bowel. *C. difficile* has been implicated in etiology.

Features which raise the suspicion include poor growth and prominent abdominal distension with both gas and fecal retention. The abnormally increased anal tone may or may not be clinically detectable, and relatively empty rectum may also be an inconsistent feature.

GENERAL FEATURES
• Dilatation of the proximal gut • Failure to thrive • Dilated colon in radiography

■ INVESTIGATION

Full blood count may detect iron deficiency anemia. Serum protein levels reveal hypoproteinemia. Anteroposterior (AP) and lateral plain abdominal radiographs confirm stool and gas retention. The absence of gas in rectal ampulla favors Hirschsprung's disease.

Radiographic Studies

- *Plain X-ray abdomen:* Severely distended loops of intestine; relative paucity of air levels in the location of rectum force air under diaphragm (perforation of proximal intestine). Air fluid level is suggestive of obstruction.
- *Barium enema:*
  - Spastic distal segment with a dilated proximal intestine
  - Zone transition
  - Incomplete evaluation of barium—24 hours post evacuation of radiograph
  - In enterocolitis, evidence of edema, spasm, and ulceration of intestinal wall

ESSENTIAL DIAGNOSTIC POINTS
• Abnormal innervation of the bowel, beginning in the internal sphincter • There is decreased ability of ganglion cells to adhere to smooth muscle cells • Absence of ganglion cells in the bowel wall • Clinical enterocolitis, systemic sepsis, and coagulopathy set in • Failure to pass stool leads to dilatation of the proximal bowel and abdominal distension • Associated with septicemia and bowel obstruction • On rectal examination rectum is usually empty

Barium enema on unprepared colon may define the transition area between the normally innervated, dilated colon, and aganglionic narrow segment. Other diagnostic findings are:
- An abrupt change in caliber between ganglionic and aganglionic sections of the bowel
- Irregular sawtooth contraction of aganglionic segment
- Parallel transverse folds in dilated proximal colon
- A thickened nodular edematous proximal colon associated with protein losing enteropathy
- Failure to evacuate barium

Rectal examination demonstrates normal anal tone and is usually followed by explosive discharge of foul-smelling feces and gas.

Rectal suction biopsy is the gold standard for diagnosing Hirschsprung's disease. The biopsy material should contain an adequate amount of submucosa to evaluate for the presence of ganglion cells. To avoid obtaining biopsies in the normal area of hypoganglionosis, which ranges from 3 to 17 mm in length, the suction rectal biopsy should be obtained no closer than 2 cm above the dentate line. The biopsy specimen should be stained for acetylcholinesterase to facilitate interpretation. Patients with aganglionosis demonstrate a large number of hypertrophied nerve bundles that stain positively for acetylcholinesterase with an absence of ganglion cells between muscular layer and submucosa. Calretinin staining may provide a diagnosis of Hirschsprung's disease when acetylcholinesterase staining may not be sufficient.

An unprepared contrast enema is most likely to aid in the diagnosis in children older than 1 month of age, because the proximal ganglionic segment might not be significantly dilated in the first few week of life. Classic findings are based on the presence of an abrupt narrow transition zone between the normal dilated proximal colon and a smaller-caliber obstructed distal aganglionic segment. In the absence of this finding, it is imperative to compare the diameter of the rectum to that of the sigmoid colon, because a rectal diameter that is the same as or smaller than the sigmoid colon suggests Hirschsprung's disease.

Anorectal manometry evaluates the internal anal sphincter while a balloon is distended in the rectum. In healthy individuals, rectal distention initiates relaxation of the internal anal sphincter in response to rectal distention. In patients with Hirschsprung's disease, the internal anal sphincter fails to relax in response to rectal distention. Although the sensitivity and specificity can vary widely; in experienced hands, the test can be quite sensitive.

LABORATORY SALIENT FINDINGS
- Rectal examination
- Rectal suction and biopsy
- Anorectal manometry
- Barium enema
- Plain X-ray abdomen
- Iron deficiency anemia
- Hypoproteinemia

It is measured by distension of balloon placed within rectal ampulla. It shows fall of pressure in the internal anal sphincter in normal individual. But there is striking rise in pressure in patients with megacolon.

■ DIFFERENTIAL DIAGNOSIS

Differential diagnoses in newborn include meconium plug syndrome, meconium ileus, and intestinal atresia hypothyroidism, septicemia and cystic fibrosis. In older patients, the Currarino triad must be considered, which includes anorectal malformations (ectopic anus, anal stenosis, imperforate anus), sacral bone anomalies (hypoplasia, poor segmentation), and presacral anomaly (anterior meningoceles, teratoma, cyst). Other diagnoses include aerophagia, subacute intestinal obstruction-acquired megacolon, paralytic ileus, and anal fissure.

■ TREATMENT

Once the diagnosis is established it is preferable to do limited laparotomy with multiple biopsies. Colostomy is done in the most distal portion of normally ganglionated colon. Attempts to postpone surgery by repeated colonic irrigation until infant reaches satisfactory size are not justified of risk of enterocolitis.

Once the diagnosis is established, the definitive treatment is operative intervention.

There are three basic surgical options, which are described in the following text.

Summary of Surgical Procedures

- *Swenson's pull-through:* A two-layered circumferential colorectal anastomoses performed as low as possible to anocutaneous junction, thereby excising aganglionic segment nearly completely. The first successful surgical procedure, described by Swenson, was to excise the aganglionic segment and anastomose the normal proximal bowel to the rectum 1-2 cm above the dentate line. The operation is technically difficult and led to the development of two other procedures.
- *Modified Duhamell's pull-through:* Disconnections of bowel at peritoneal reflection are involved. Pull-through of the ganglionic colon through the incision made in posterior rectal wall about 1.5 cm from and margin orifice. Linear cutter stapler is used to cut and staple two opposing walls. Final outcome is creation of bowel, anterior wall made up of aganglionic rectum, and posterior wall made up of pulled-through ganglionic colon.
- *Soave's endorectal pull-through:* The endorectal pull-through procedure described by Soave involves stripping the mucosa from the aganglionic rectum and bringing normally innervated colon through the residual muscular cuff, thus bypassing the abnormal bowel from within. Advances in techniques have led to successful laparoscopic single-stage endorectal pull-through procedures, which are the treatment of choice. Removal of mucus and submucosa of rectum and pulling ganglionic intestine through the aganglionic muscular cuff and an anastomoses at anus.

In ultrashort segmental disease, aganglionic segment is limited to internal sphincter. Excision of the strip of rectal muscle, including the internal and sphincter, is diagnostic and therapeutic. When the entire colon is aganglionic ileal–anal anastomoses is the treatment of choice, preserving the part of aganglionic colon to facilitate water absorption. This helps stools to become firm.

Postoperative problems include recurrent enterocolitis, stricture, prolapse, perianal abscess, and fecal soiling.

The prognosis of surgically treated Hirschsprung's disease is generally satisfactory; the great majority of patients achieve fecal continence. Long-term postoperative problems include constipation, recurrent enterocolitis, stricture, prolapse, perianal abscesses, and fecal soiling.

BIBLIOGRAPHY

1. Frykman PK, Short SS. Hirschsprung-associated enterocolitis: prevention and therapy. Semin Pediatr Surg. 2012;21(4):328-35.
2. Parisi MA. Hirschsprung disease overview—retired chapter, for historical reference only. In: Adam MP, Feldman J, Mirzaa GM, Pagon RA, Wallace SE, Bean LJH, (Eds). In: GeneReviews [Internet]. Seattle (WA): University of Washington, Seattle; 1993.
3. Rintala RJ, Pakarinen MP. Long-term outcomes of Hirschsprung's disease. Semin Pediatr Surg. 2012;21(4):336-43.

CASE 29

Intussusception

■ PRESENTING COMPLAINTS

A 7-year-old boy was brought with the complaint of:
- Abdominal pain since 2 days
- Vomiting since 1 day
- Loose motion since 1 day

History of Presenting Complaints

A 7-year-old boy was presented with the history of abdominal pain and profuse sweating. The abdominal pain was intermittent. It was diffuse and nonlocalized. The boy developed loose motions. After sometime the loose motion was mainly mucus and blood-stained. No fecal matter was present. The child became flushed with the pain in the abdomen and lower part of the chest. Simultaneously vomiting started. It was projectile in nature and vomitus was greenish and watery in nature.

Past History of the Patient

He was the first sibling of the nonconsanguineous marriage. He was born at full term with normal delivery. He cried immediately after delivery. There was no significant postnatal event. He was discharged on the third day. He was on breast milk exclusively for 4 months. Weaning started at 4 months and completed by 18 months. There was no delay in developmental milestone. There was no previous history of attack of loose motion and vomiting.

■ EXAMINATION

The boy was moderately built and nourished. The boy looked flushed. There were signs of moderate dehydration. Anthropometric measurements included height 122 cm

---

CASE AT A GLANCE

Basic Findings
Height	: 122 (75th centile)
Weight	: 21 kg (50th centile)
Temperature	: 37.2°C
Pulse rate	: 120 beats/min
Respiratory rate	: 20 breaths/min
Blood pressure	: 100/70 mm Hg

Positive Findings

History:
- Abdominal pain, intermittent
- Vomiting
- Loose motion

Examination:
- Flushed
- Sign of dehydration
- Mass felt in epigastrium
- Skin nodule
- Subcostal tenderness

Investigation:
- *Platelets:* High
- *Erythrocyte sedimentation rate (ESR):* High
- *Barium enema:* Filling defect in the midtransverse colon

(75 centile) and the weight 21 kg (50th centile).

He was afebrile, the pulse rate was 120 beats/min and respiratory rate was 20 breaths/min. The blood pressure recorded was 100/70 mm Hg. There was neither pallor, lymphadenopathy, nor edema.

Per abdomen examination revealed presence of fullness in left upper quadrant and in left hypochondrium. There was no organomegaly. Bowel sounds were normal.

Other systemic examinations were normal. He had several birthmarks including skin nodules. There was slight subcostal tenderness.

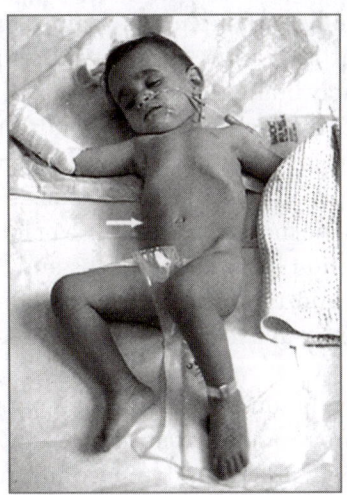

Fig. 1: Mass in upper abdomen.

■ INVESTIGATION

- *Hemoglobin:* 10 g/dL
- *TLC:* 15,000 cells/cumm
- *DLC:* $P_{78}L_{20}E_2$
- *Platelet count:* 6,00,000 cells/cumm
- *ESR:* 56 mm in the first hour
- *Blood urea:* 17 mg/dL
- *Total protein:* 4.2 g/dL
- *Total albumin:* 2.9 g/dL
- *Serum electrolytes:*
  - *Na:* 120 mEq/L
  - *K:* 4 mEq/L
  - *Cl:* 20 mEq/L
- *Barium enema:* Classical filling defect in the mid transverse colon

■ DISCUSSION

Intermittent abdominal pain associated with fullness in the abdomen **(Fig. 1)** and is associated with blood-stained mucous stools. These symptoms suggest intussusception.

Intussusception occurs when one portion of proximal intestine [intussusceptam, telescopes into a more distal portion (intussuscipiens)]. Once this prolapse has occurred, lymphatic and venous congestion develops, resulting in edema, strangulation, ischemia, and ultimately necrosis. Additionally, the lumen of the intussuscepted portion of the bowel collapses, causing intestinal obstruction. Intussusception is fatal if spontaneous reduction does not occur and it is left untreated; therefore, prompt diagnosis and treatment are critical for successful management.

Intussusception occurs when a portion of the alimentary tract is telescoped into an adjacent segment. It is the most common cause of intestinal obstruction between 5 months and 3 years of age and the most common abdominal emergency in children younger than 2 years. 60% of patients are younger than 1 year of age, and 80% of the cases occur before age 24 months; it is rare in neonates.

The incidence varies 1–4 per 1,000 live births. The male to female ratio is 4:1. If there is any underlying abnormality in GIT, this acts as a focus of the intussusception. The associated findings such as birthmarks and skin nodules are seen in neurofibroma. These are known to be associated with increased risk of developing tumor. The boy developed non-Hodgkin lymphoma. Lymphomatous infiltration can result in thickening of intestinal lining. This may act as a basis for intussusception. The condition may complicate into otitis media, gastroenteritis, and upper respiratory tract infection.

It is the most common cause of intestinal obstruction between 5 months and 3 years of age and the most common abdominal emergency in children younger than 2 years of age.

Correlation with prior or concurrent respiratory adenovirus (type C) infection has been noted, and the condition can complicate otitis media, gastroenteritis, Henoch–Schönlein purpura, or other upper respiratory tract infections.

In 2–8% of patients, recognizable lead points for the intussusception are found, such as a Meckel diverticulum, intestinal polyp, neurofibroma, intestinal duplication cysts, inverted appendix stump, leiomyomas, hamartomas, ectopic pancreatic tissue, anastomotic suture line, enterostomy tube, posttransplant lymphoproliferative disease, hemangioma, or malignant conditions such as lymphoma or Kaposi sarcoma. Intussusception can complicate mucosal hemorrhage as in Henoch–Schönlein purpura, idiopathic thrombocytopenic purpura, or hemophilia. Cystic fibrosis, celiac disease, and Crohn disease are other risk factors.

Most intussusceptions do not strangulate the bowel within the 24 hours but can eventuate in intestinal gangrene and shock.

Recurrent intussusception is noted in 5–8% and is more common after hydrostatic than surgical reduction. Chronic intussusception, in which the symptoms exist in milder form at recurrent intervals, is more likely to occur with or after acute enteritis and can arise in older children as well as in infants.

PATHOGENESIS

Intussusception is the most common cause of intestinal obstruction in children under 2 years of age. While it may occur at any age, intussusception is uncommon prior to 3 months of age, and children in the age-group 3 months to 3 years are most commonly affected. There is a peak in incidence between 5 and 7 months of age. Intussusception occurs twice as often in boys as in girls.

Pediatric intussusception is idiopathic (without an identifiable lead point) in 90% of cases. A majority of these cases are ileocolic. The mechanism is hypothesized to be an extramucosal lead point such as Peyer's patch hypertrophy or mesenteric lymphadenitis. Viral gastroenteritis (most commonly adenovirus), Henoch–Schönlein purpura, intestinal lymphoid hyperplasia, and meconium ileus have all been associated with intussusceptions.

Only 10% of pediatric intussusception can be attributed to a pathologic lead point, which includes Meckel diverticulum, intestinal polyps, intestinal duplication, hemangioma, suture line, appendix, tumors, and ectopic pancreas. Pathologic lead points should be suspected in children over 2 years of age with intussusception or in children with recurrent intussusceptions. In children with classic symptoms and normal contrast enema, small bowel to small bowel intussusceptions may be the culprit. Intussusception associated with a lead point is more likely to recur if the lead point is not excised.

Infection by concurrent respiratory adenovirus (type C) causes primary lymphoid hyperplasia or an enlarged hypertrophied ileal lymphoid patch. This then acts as leading point for intussusception.

Intussusception is noted in these conditions such as Henoch–Schönlein purpura, hemophilia, lymphoma, Peutz–Jeghers syndrome, leukemia, and cystic fibrosis. Recurrent intussusception is seen among cystic fibrosis. Seasonal peak incidence is when gastroenteritis and respiratory infection are common, i.e., during rainy and cold season.

It is postulated that gastrointestinal infection or the introduction of new food proteins results in swollen Peyer patches in the terminal ileum. Lymphoid nodular hyperplasia is another related risk factor. Prominent mounds of lymph tissue lead to mucosal prolapse of the ileum into the colon, thus causing an intussusception.

■ PATHOLOGY

Intussusceptions are most often ileocolic, less commonly cecocolic, and occasionally ileal. The upper portion of bowel, the intussusceptum, invaginates into the lower, the intussuscipiens, pulling its mesentery along with it into the enveloping loop.

Constriction of the mesentery obstructs venous return; engorgement of the intussusceptum follows, with edema, and bleeding from the mucosa leads to a bloody stool sometimes containing mucus. The apex of the intussusception can extend into the transverse, descending, or sigmoid colon, even to and through the anus in neglected cases. This presentation must be distinguished from rectal prolapse. Most intussusceptions do not strangulate the bowel within the first 24 hours but can eventuate in intestinal gangrene and shock.

Intussusception occurs when the portion of the alimentary tract is telescoped into the segment just caudal to it. The causes of this are unknown. The correlation with adenoviral infection is noted. Swollen Peyer's patches in the ileum stimulate intestinal peristalsis in an attempt to extrude the mass, thus causing intussusception.

There will be one leading point as the cause for the intussusception in 8–10% of cases. Recognizable lead points are Meckel diverticulum, intestinal polyp, neurofibroina, intestinal duplication cysts, inverted appendix stump, leiomyomas, hamartoma, ectopic pancreatic tissue, anastomotic suture line, enterostomy tube, posttransplant lymphoproliferative disease, and hemangioma malignant conditions such as lymphoma, or Kaposi sarcoma. Lead points are more common in children older than 2 years of age, the child, the higher the risk of a lead point.

At ileum and ileocecal valve, there is greater disproportion in sizes. Hence intussusception usually originates in the distal ileum and proceeds into the ascending colon. It can be either primary/secondary or simple/compound (intussusception of an intussusception).

■ CLINICAL FEATURES (FIG. 2)

Intussusception should be included in the differential diagnosis of all children with intestinal obstruction. Infants may present with the classic triad of intermittent, crampy abdominal pain, palpable abdominal mass, and "currant-jelly" stools, although the majority of children will not have all three of these symptoms at presentation. The early course is associated with sudden onset of severe paroxysms of abdominal pain.

Infants can present with diarrhea and colicky pain or restlessness alternating with listlessness without showing the pain. It may be possible to palpate typical sausage-shaped mass in the right upper abdomen. But this is often difficult in irritable child.

In typical cases, there is sudden onset, in a previously well child, of the severe paroxysmal

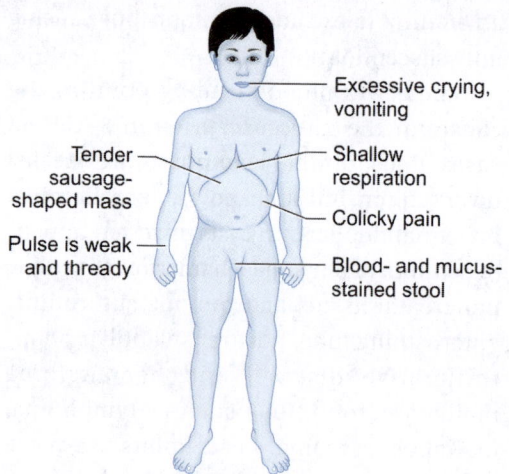

Fig. 2: Clinical features.

colicky pain that recurs at frequent intervals and is accompanied by straining efforts with legs and knees flexed and loud cries. The infant may initially be comfortable and play normally between the paroxysms of pain; but if the intussusception is not reduced, the infant becomes progressively weaker and lethargic.

At times, the lethargy is disproportionate to the abdominal signs. Eventually shock-like state may develop with the rise of body temperature, pulse becomes weak and thready, and peritonitis, can develop. The respiration is shallow and grunting. The pain may be manifested only by moaning sounds.

Vomiting occurs in most cases and is usually more frequent in the early phase. In the later phase, the vomitus becomes bile-stained.

Stools of normal appearance may be evacuated in the first few hours of symptoms. After this time, fecal excretions are small or more often do not occur, and little or no flatus is passed. Blood is generally passed in the first 12 hours, but at times not for 1–2 days, and infrequently not at all; 60% of infants pass a stool containing red blood and mucus, the currant-jelly stool. The classic triad of pain, a palpable sausage-shaped abdominal mass, and bloody or currant-jelly stool is seen in <30% of patients with intussusception.

Palpation of the abdomen usually reveals a slightly tender sausage-shaped mass, sometimes ill defined, which might increase in size and firmness during a paroxysm of pain and is most often in the right upper abdomen, with its long-axis cephalocaudal. If it is felt in the epigastrium, the long axis is transverse.

> **ESSENTIAL DIAGNOSTIC POINTS**
> - Intermittent abdominal pain with fullness in the abdomen
> - Blood-stained mucous stools
> - Associated with Meckel's diverticulum, intestinal polyp, duplication, and lymphosarcoma
> - Mostly of ileocolic and ileoileocolic type
> - Diarrhea and colicky pain or restlessness
> - Typical sausage-shaped mass in the right upper abdomen

Chronic intussusception is more likely to occur with acute enteritis. It may occur in older children and as well as in infants.

Abdominal distension and tenderness develop as intestinal obstruction becomes more acute. Recurrent intussusception is more common after hydrostatic than surgical reduction.

> **GENERAL FEATURES**
> - Severe paroxysmal colicky pain
> - Pain at frequent interval
> - Shock

DIAGNOSIS

Plain abdominal radiograph reveals the density in the area of intussusception. A barium enema will show a filling defect or a cupping in the head of the barium. A thin rim of barium may be seen trapped around the invaginating intestine in the folds of mucosa within the intussusception. Reduction of intussusception is an emergency procedure.

In children with stable vital signs erect and supine plain abdominal radiograph shows characteristic signs of absence of gas in the cecum and ascending colon, a crescentic gas shadow at the apex of the intussusception, and dilated loops of obstructed small intestine with fluid levels.

The central linear column of the barium may be visible in compressed lumen of the intussusception and a thin rim of barium may be seen trapped around the invaginating intestine in the folds of mucosa within the intussusception-coiled spring sign.

An ileoileal intussusception is best demonstrated by abdominal USG. Reduction by instillation of contrast agents, saline, or air might not be possible. Such intussusceptions can develop insidiously after bowel surgery and require reoperation if they do not spontaneously reduce. Ileoileal disease is common with Henoch–Schönlein purpura and other unidentifiable disorders and usually resolves without the need for any specific treatment. If manual operative reduction is impossible or the bowel is not viable, resection of the intussusception is necessary, with end-to-end anastomosis.

> **LABORATORY SALIENT FINDINGS**
> - Plain abdominal radiograph reveals the density in the area of intussusception
> - A barium enema will show a filling defect or a cupping in the head of the barium
> - A thin rim of barium may be seen trapped around the invaginating intestine in the folds of mucosa within the intussusception-coiled spring sign
> - Ultrasonography includes a tubular mass in longitudinal view and doughnut or target appearance in transverse images

Characteristic appearance of concentric rings or a large doughnut is observed while scanning in right lower quadrant and moving clockwise around the abdomen. Concentric rim marks the mucosal or serosal interfaces in early intussusception. When the wall of the intussusception becomes edematous, its lumen is compressed and the intussusception becomes stretched around the mass. An axial cross-section of the bowel at this stage shows a round, thick-walled doughnut. A longitudinal cross-section shows an oval, thick-walled doughnut.

Abdominal US is the standard imaging modality for intussusception, with a diagnostic accuracy of approximately 85%. Cross-sectional USG of the intussusception reveals a target sign with concentric layers of serosa and mucosa, and on longitudinal views, the tip of the intussusceptum can be seen. A target sign may also be visible on abdominal CT scan.

Saline enema under US guidance to monitor hydrostatic reduction is successful in nearly 95% cases, which acts as a part of treatment.

Contraindication of nonoperative treatment includes signs of peritonitis, signs of gangrenous bowel, free gas under the diaphragm, and multiple air fluids levels of X-ray.

Maximum permissible height of barium: It is 30 cm above the buttocks. Pressure should not exceed 120 cm H_2O. Reduction must be done by surgeon along with radiologist.

Signs of complete reduction: These include barium entering the small bowel—terminal ileum, disappearance of mass which was initially palpable, and passage of flatus and contrast through anus.

A negative filling defect and nonentrance of contrast in terminal ileum does not necessarily mean nonreduction. Edema at ileocecal valve junction leads to negative filling defect and prevents contrast of colon from entering small bowel. If the first attempt is unsuccessful, second attempt of hydrostatic reduction be done in 2-4 hours if the patient condition is stable.

The findings in USG include a tubular mass in longitudinal view and doughnut or target appearance in transverse images.

DIFFERENTIAL DIAGNOSIS

- Enterocolitis
- Meckel's diverticulum
- Anaphylactoid purpura

COMPLICATIONS

- Adhesions
- Internal herniation
- Septicemia
- Perforation
- Gangrene

TREATMENT

The first-line treatment for ileocolic intussusception in a stable child is radiographic enema reduction.

Reduction of an acute intussusception is an emergency procedure and should be performed immediately after diagnosis in preparation for possible surgery. In 75% of cases where there is no prostration, shock or peritoneal irritation, it is possible to reduce by hydrostatic pressure with the fluoroscopic guidance. The success rate of radiologic hydrostatic reduction under fluoroscopic or ultrasonic guidance is approximately 80-95% in patients with ileocolic intussusception. Spontaneous reduction of intussusception occurs in approximately 4-10% of patients.

To confirm successful reduction of the intussusception, contrast must be observed to reflux-past the ileocecal valve into the distal ileum. Following successful reduction, about 8-15% of children will have recurrence of intussusception. Most recurrences are within 6 months with one-third occurring within the first 24 hours after reduction. A second attempt at nonoperative reduction is the preferred management of recurrent ileocolic intussusception and may be safely completed within a few hours.

If there is any evidence of obstruction with abdominal distension, ileoileal-type hydrostatic reduction should not be attempted because of the risk of perforation of intussusception. In patients with prolonged intussusception and signs of shock, peritoneal irritation, intestinal perforation, or pneumatosis intestinalis, hydrostatic reduction should not be attempted.

Operative intervention is indicated if enema reduction has failed or contraindications to nonoperative reduction, such as perforation, peritonitis, or hemodynamic instability, are present. An operation is also necessary if a pathologic lead point is identified. The surgical management of intussusception begins with attempts at manual reduction. If reduction is successful and no pathologic lead points are identified, the operation is concluded. Bowel resection is required for bowel ischemic pathologic lead point, or inability to manually reduce the prolapsed segment. Resection is followed by primary bowel anastomosis or diversion, depending on the state of the child and the intestine. Traditionally, open reduction has been performed through a right-lower-quadrant abdominal incision, but the laparoscopic approach is becoming more popular.

Resection of intussusception with end-to-end anastomosis is done. Untreated intussusception in infants is almost always fatal. The chances of recovery are directly related to duration of intussusception before reduction.

Surgical treatment includes Cope's manure—gentle passing of the finger on apex of intussuscepted intestine in the descending or transverse colon, breaking down the adhesion.

■ PROGNOSIS

Untreated intussusception in infants is usually fatal; the chances of recovery are directly related to the duration of intussusception before reduction. Most infants recover if the intussusception is reduced in the first 24 hours, but the mortality rate rises rapidly after this time, especially after the second day.

The recurrence rate after reduction of intussusceptions is approximately 10%, and after surgical reduction it is 2–5%; none has recurred after surgical resection. Most recurrences occur within 72 hours of reduction. Corticosteroids may reduce the frequency of recurrent intussusception. Repeated reducible episodes caused by lymphonodular hyperplasia may respond to treatment of identifiable food allergies, if present.

■ BIBLIOGRAPHY

1. Apelt N, Featherstone N, Giuliani S. Laparoscopic treatment of intussusception in children: a systematic review. J Pediatr Surg. 2013;48(8):1789-93.
2. Fallon SC, Lopez ME, Zhang W, Brandt ML, Wesson DE, Lee TC, et al. Risk factors for surgery in pediatric intussusception. J Pediatr Surg. 2013;48(5)1032-6.
3. Fisher JG, Sparks EA, Turner CG, Klein JD, Pennington E, Khan FA, et al. Operative indications in recurrent ileocolic intussusception. J Pediatr Surg. 2015;50(1)126-30.
4. Jiang J, Jiang B, Parashar U, Nguyen T, Bines J, Patel MM. Childhood intussusception: a literature review. PLoS One. 2013; 8(7):e68482.
5. Marin JR, Alpern ER Abdominal pain in children. Emerg Med Clinic North Am. 2011;29:401-28, ix-x.
6. Niramis R, Watanatittan S, Kruatrachue A, Anuntkosol M, Buranakitjaroen V, Rattanasuwan T, et al. Management of recurrent intussusception: nonoperative or operative reduction? J Pediatr Surg. 2010; 45(11):2175-80.

CASE 30

Liver Abscess

■ PRESENTING COMPLAINTS

A 10-year-old boy was brought with the complaint of:
- Fever since 7 days
- Loss of appetite since 5 days
- Abdominal pain since 3 days

History of Presenting Complaints

A 10-year-old boy presented with a history of severe abdominal pain. The pain was present in the right upper quadrant. The pain became worse during the last 24 hours. Pain was more in the night and there was disturbed sleep because of the severe pain. Pain was not related to any food intake or to bowel habits. His mother noted that the appetite of the boy was reduced. There was no history of nausea, vomiting, or diarrhea.

He was admitted to the hospital. On admission, he was toxic and dehydrated. He was febrile, i.e., 39°C. There was moderate cervical lymphadenopathy. The hemoglobin was 12.3 g/dL and TLC was 11,700 cells/mm^3. Blood culture and sensitivity were sterile. He was observed in the hospital. The child became afebrile the next day. Later, he was discharged and advised bed rest. For about 15 days, he was on bed rest. He had a fever with night sweats but no rigors. The abdominal pain remained localized in the right upper quadrant. Pain started increasing in intensity and became almost continuous. This was producing disturbed sleep at night. There was no change in bowel and bladder habits.

Past History of the Patient

The boy was the eldest sibling of the non-consanguineous marriage. He was born at full term by normal vaginal delivery. There

---

CASE AT A GLANCE

Basic Findings
Height	: 135 cm (50th centile)
Weight	: 30 kg (50th centile)
Temperature	: 39.2°C
Pulse rate	: 126 beats/min
Respiratory rate	: 26 breaths/min
Blood pressure	: 80/60 mm Hg

Positive Findings

History:
- Fever for 3 weeks
- Chills and rigors
- Pain in the abdomen
- Decreased appetite

Examination:
- Toxic
- Guarding
- Tenderness in the right upper quadrant
- Tender hepatomegaly

Investigation:
- TLC: Increased
- ESR: Increased
- Alkaline phosphatase: Increased
- Ultrasound liver: Large liver abscess
- Platelet count decreased

was no significant postnatal event. The child had been on breast milk on the second day. He was exclusively on breast milk for 6 months. Weaning started at 6 months and he was on family food by the age of 15 months. His developmental milestones were normal. He was immunized completely. His performance at school was good.

■ EXAMINATION

The child was moderately built and moderately nourished. He was looking toxic and dehydrated. Anthropometric measurements included his height, which was 135 cm (50th centile), and weight, which was 30 kg. He was febrile. The pulse rate was 126 beats/min. The respiratory rate was 26 breaths/min. The blood pressure recorded was 80/60 mm Hg.

There was no pallor, no lymphadenopathy, and no cyanosis and clubbing. There was no icterus.

Per abdomen examination revealed an enlarged liver. Liver was palpable about 3 cm below the costal margin. It was smooth and tender. There was tenderness and guarding in the right hypochondrium. Otherwise, the abdomen was soft. Cardiovascular and respiratory system examinations were normal.

■ INVESTIGATION

- *Hemoglobin:* 11.6 g/dL
- *TLC:* 11,700 cells/mm^3
- *DLC:* $P_{72} L_{18} E_6 B_2 M_2$
- *Platelet count:* 6,00,000 cells/mm^3
- *Total protein:* 7.6 g/dL
- *Albumin:* 3.1 g/dL
- *Alkaline phosphatase:* 35.8 U/L
- *ESR:* 40 mm in the first hour
- *SGOT:* 50 U/L
- *SGPT:* 46 U/L
- *US:* Shows the large liver abscess

■ DISCUSSION

Acute illness of 3 weeks associated with the remittent onset of fever and enlarged tender hepatomegaly associated with thrombocytopenia suggests liver disorder.

Liver abscesses are usually classified as pyogenic or amebic based on etiology. The distinction is important because treatment varies substantially. Important aspects of the patient's history that suggest amebic rather than pyogenic abscess include bloody diarrhea or travel to tropical areas preceding the illness.

Hepatic abscesses are caused by bacterial infections or amebiasis. *Echinococcus granulosus* and fungal infections are other rare causes of hepatic abscesses.

The major predisposing factors for the development of liver abscess are related to immunocompromised states. These include chronic granulomatous disease (CGD), acute leukemia, steroid therapy, and a recent attack of measles.

The factors associated with the development of pyogenic liver abscess (PLA) include peritoneal abscess, prematurity, supportive umbilical vessel thrombophlebitis, skin infection, bacteremia, and surgical procedure for necrotizing enterocolitis.

Other factors that have been incriminated include malnutrition, bile duct ascariasis, trauma, aplastic anemia, and sickle cell disease.

■ PATHOGENESIS

Pyogenic liver abscesses of unknown source are classified as cryptogenic. Children with CGD, hyperimmunoglobulin E (hyper-IgE) syndrome, or malignancies are at increased risk of liver abscess.

Bacteria can reach the liver through various routes. These include contagious spread, portal vein routes, umbilical vessel, and hematogenous spread. Hepatic abscess following pancreatitis, cholangitis (subphrenic abscess), or penetrating trauma, and cryptogenic biliary tract infections are the examples of contagious spread.

Portal vein may carry the organism from the gastrointestinal tract to the liver. Hepatic abscess that occurs following pylephlebitis, intra-abdominal infection, or abscess secondary to appendicitis, inflammatory bowel disease, diverticulitis, enteritis, ulcerative colitis, and omphalitis are the example of portal vein transmission.

Hematogenous spread is the common route by which hepatic abscesses occur in children. Pyogenic hepatic abscess associated with bacteremia is an example. Umbilical vessel catheterization in the neonate can result in hepatic abscess.

Blunt trauma is known to result in liver abscesses. Cryptogenic liver, where no portal of entry can be delineated, is thought to be caused by infection of infarcted portions of liver. The biliary tract disease or gastrointestinal infection usually brings the intestinal flora to the liver. Hence, abscess associated with this condition are caused by gram-negative enteric bacilli and anaerobic organisms.

ESSENTIAL DIAGNOSTIC POINTS

- Remittent onset of fever, enlarged tender hepatomegaly and associated with thrombocytopenia
- *Immunocompromised states:* Chronic granulomatous disease, acute leukemia, steroid therapy, and measles
- Hematogenous spread is the common route
- In neonates, it is associated with fever, abdominal distension, abdominal tenderness, hepatomegaly, tachypnea, and nuchal rigidity

PATHOLOGY

The liver is enlarged. It shows solitary abscesses or multiple abscesses. Solitary abscesses are more common than multiple abscesses. Right lobe of the liver is more commonly involved. Microscopically, abscess shows disintegrating hepatocytes infiltrated by polymorphs. Areas remote from the abscess in the liver may reveal inflammation of portal tract.

Multiple abscesses are associated with ascending cholangitis giving rise to spiking temperature. Prominent symptoms include fever, nausea, vomiting, anorexia, lassitude, weakness, diarrhea, weight loss, and abdominal pain.

Pyogenic hepatic abscess is polymicrobial. *Staphylococcus aureus* is the most common organism involved. It is especially found in the solitary abscess of children with CGD. In contrast, gram-negative enteric bacilli and anaerobic organisms are frequently isolated when multiple hepatic abscesses occur. *Klebsiella, Pseudomonas, Escherichia coli,* Enterobacter, and salmonella have been isolated from these abscesses. Anaerobes such as *Streptococcus, Bacteroids fragilis,* fusobacterium, and Brucella have been identified.

CLINICAL FEATURES (FIG. 1)

Patients with infections of the liver generally present with nonspecific symptoms such as fever, fatigue, abdominal pain, or weight loss. The abdominal pain may be diffuse, and confined to the right upper quadrant, or radiate to the shoulder or back. Other symptoms may include headache, arthralgias, and adenopathy.

A history of predisposing factors and tender hepatomegaly prompt for diagnosis. Signs and symptoms are nonspecific and can include fever, night sweats, malaise, fatigue, nausea, abdominal pain with right upper quadrant tenderness, and hepatomegaly; jaundice is uncommon. Fever and pain are

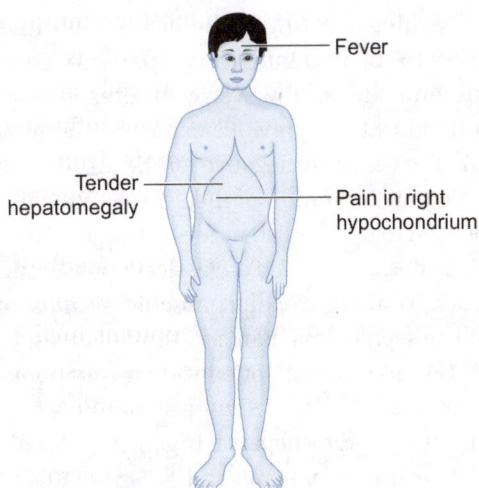

Fig. 1: Clinical features.

present in the right upper quadrant. There is tender hepatomegaly. Rapidity of onset of the symptoms with the remittent fever points toward bacterial sepsis followed by the collection of pus. Pus can be expected in the liver as there is hepatomegaly.

40% of the cases are found in CGD. The source of the infection may be pylephlebitis, generalized sepsis, cholangitis, and systemic spread from the cryptogenic biliary tract infection.

In neonates, it is associated with fever, abdominal distension, abdominal tenderness, hepatomegaly, tachypnea, and nuchal rigidity.

Amoebic Liver Abscess

Amoebic abscess presents similarly to PLA but is caused by *Entamoeba histolytica*. Jaundice is infrequently seen, and diarrhea may be seen in less than half of patients at the time of presentation; however, a history of dysentery should raise suspicion for this disease.

Amoebic liver abscesses (ALAs) may occur months to years after exposure, so obtaining a careful travel history is critical. In children, fever is the hallmark of ALA and is frequently associated with abdominal pain, distention, and enlargement and tenderness of the liver. Changes at the base of the right lung, such as elevation of the diaphragm and atelectasis or effusion, may also occur.

GENERAL FEATURES
• Nonspecific symptoms • Anorexia • Jaundice • Raised erythrocyte sedimentation rate (ESR)

■ DIAGNOSIS

Diagnosis can be challenging and is often delayed; a high index of suspicion is necessary for children with risk factors.

Routine laboratory studies may show abnormal results, but rarely are they diagnostic of PLA. Anemia and leukocytosis are common.

Liver function tests generally reflect underlying disease of the liver itself. Raised level of alkaline phosphates in serum could be indicative of underlying biliary tract obstruction or disease. Transaminase concentrations generally are normal-to-mildly elevated in a majority of the cases. A rapidly enlarging, tender liver in a patient with normal transaminase concentrations should alert the clinician to the possibility of liver abscess. Serum aminotransferase and more often the alkaline phosphatase levels are elevated. The ESR is high, and leukocytosis is common. The results of blood cultures are positive in 50% of patients.

Laboratory findings of liver infection often consist of leukocytosis, elevated ESR, and variable elevation of bilirubin, aminotransferases [alanine aminotransferase (ALT), aspartate aminotransferase (AST)], alkaline phosphatase, and gamma-glutamyl transferase (GGT). Liver US is useful in the initial evaluation of suspected liver infection because it can screen for liver abscesses or bile duct anomalies.

Chest X-rays might show elevation of the right hemidiaphragm with decreased mobility or a right pleural effusion.

Ultrasound and CT scans may be used to confirm the diagnosis of liver abscesses, to locate abscesses for performing diagnostic or therapeutic drainage procedures under the guidance of images produced by them, to study their evolution and response to therapy, and also to document healing. However, they cannot be used with certainty for differentiating a PLA from an ALA.

Radionuclide scans can be useful in the diagnosis of liver abscesses. Technetium (Tc) sulfur colloid liver scan is capable of detecting about 85% of lesions greater than 2 cm in diameter. Anterior, posterior, and lateral views reveal decreased isotope concentration in both pyogenic and amoebic abscesses. Gallium (Ga) scans can reveal areas of increased isotope concentration of pyogenic abscesses. Radionuclide scans, USG, and CT scan, are highly sensitive techniques for the detection of liver abscesses.

As with PLA, the leukocyte count and ESR are usually elevated, and ALT, AST, bilirubin, and alkaline phosphatase are normal-to-mildly elevated. Imaging studies should include US or CT of the abdomen.

Additional studies include evaluation of the stool for ova and parasites, looking for trophozoites or cysts, and testing the stool for *E. histolytica* antigen; note that stool tests may be negative in the case of extraintestinal amebiasis and that routine ova and parasite examination does not permit differentiation of *E histolytica* from nonpathogenic *Entamoeba*.

Serologic testing of the blood is positive in >90% of patients. Many patients from endemic areas, however, will already have antibodies from previous exposure; the tests can also be falsely negative for the first days of infection. Aspiration of the abscess may also be used to distinguish between pyogenic and ALA. In ALA, the fluid is classically sterile and reddish-brown in color; amebic organisms will be seen in less than one-third of cases.

Cultures of PLAs often yield mixed populations. In children, *S aureus*, *Streptococcus* sp., enteric gram-negative organisms (*E. coli*, *Klebsiella pneumoniae*, and *Serratia* in CGD patients), and anaerobic organisms are most common. Among adults, *K. pneumoniae* predominates, followed by *E. coli*, with less common aerobic gram-positive and anaerobic organisms. Blood cultures are often positive and may be helpful to determine a therapy plan.

Diagnosis of ALA is often confirmed by serum enzyme-linked immunosorbent assay (ELISA). Serology is considered reliable in nonendemic areas but can be prone to false negatives early in the infection and cannot distinguish active infection from previous exposure. Testing for *E. histolytica* presence in stool is specific but not very sensitive, and patients with ALA may not have detectable organisms in their stool.

If fluid is aspirated from the abscess cavity, it should be cultured aerobically and anaerobically. Blood culture may also show the causative organism in a great proportion or cases.

Solitary liver abscesses (70% of cases) in the right lobe of the liver (75% of cases) are more common than multiple abscesses or solitary left lobe abscesses. ELISA testing for *E. histolytica* galactose/N-acetyl-D-galactosamine (Gal/GalNAc) lectin in serum is usually positive for amebiasis.

> **LABORATORY SALIENT FINDINGS**
> - Anemia and leukocytosis are common
> - Altered liver function tests (LFT)
> - Ultrasound and computed tomography (CT) scan
> - Radionuclide scans
> - Aspirated fluid from the abscess cavity should be cultured aerobically and anaerobically
> - Blood culture

■ COMPLICATIONS

Complications include pleuropulmonary involvement, peritonitis, subphrenic or subhepatic abscess, duodenal fistula, and hemobilia.

■ DIFFERENTIAL DIAGNOSIS

- Subphrenic abscess
- Lung abscess
- Peritonitis
- Amebiasis

■ TREATMENT

The treatment modalities used in the management of PLA in children include antimicrobial therapy, needle aspiration, percutaneous catheter drainage, and open surgical drainage. Antimicrobial therapy is the mainstay of management and is instituted alone or in combination with one or more surgical techniques.

Antimicrobial Therapy

In children, a combination of penicillinase-resistant penicillin, an aminoglycosides, or a third-generation cephalosporin seems suitable. The antimicrobial agents may have to be changed depending on the clinical response and result of culture studies.

Antibiotic therapy should initially be broad spectrum but then narrowed, based on the culture results of the abscess fluid. Empirical initial antibiotic regimens include ampicillin/sulbactam, ticarcillin/clavulanic acid, or piperacillin/tazobactam. Others recommend a combination of a third-generation cephalosporin plus metronidazole. ALAs are treated with metronidazole or tinidazole plus paromomycin (oral nonabsorbable to treat the associated intestinal amebic infection). Antibiotic therapy for pyogenic abscess is IV for 2–3 weeks followed by oral therapy to complete a 4–6 weeks course.

A combination of an aminoglycoside and a third-generation cephalosporin may have to be instituted on the basis of in vitro susceptibility testing of gram-negative enteric isolates. If an anaerobic organism is isolated, the clinician may have to select from penicillin, clindamycin, metronidazole, and chloramphenicol.

Penicillin is usually adequate for gram-positive anaerobic organisms or microaerophilic streptococci while the rest are effective against gram-negative anaerobes. The duration of therapy is undecided, but most accept that it should be prolonged over at least 4 weeks.

Percutaneous Aspiration

Percutaneous aspiration and drainage of an abscess is a simple procedure that can be used to confirm the diagnosis of PLA. Pus aspirated at the procedure can be sent for microbiological testing. The results can be helpful in guiding antimicrobial therapy.

Percutaneous drainage under CT or USG guidance scores over surgical exploratory or open drainage as it decreases the morbidity associated with general anesthesia and surgical exploration. However, complications do occur. These include hemorrhage, falling off of drainage tube requiring reinsertion, and migration of the tube into the pleura giving rise to sterile pleural effusion or empyema.

Abscess fluid should be obtained by either needle aspiration or placement of a drainage catheter. Specimens should be sent for Gram stain and culture. Gram-positive bacteria are most common in children, although gram-negative bacteria and anaerobes are frequently involved, and the specimen may grow more than one pathogen. Antibiotic therapy is aimed at covering the most likely pathogens and is then refined based on culture results and susceptibilities. Treatment parenterally for 4-6 weeks is generally recommended.

Treatment of Amoebic Liver Abscess

Treatment most often begins with metronidazole (50 mg/kg/day divided into 3 doses) for 10 days, with alternatives of tinidazole, ornidazole, and nitazoxanide, which can be given for shorter periods of time. This should then be followed by a luminal amebicide such as paromomycin or iodoquinol for 10 or 20 days, respectively. This combination is effective at eradication in >90% of patients. Surgery or invasive therapy usually is not needed.

Aspiration may be indicated when fever and abdominal pain persist after 4-5 days of treatment and in large abscesses with imminent risk of rupture. In these patients, repeated aspiration may be helpful in improving symptoms and speeding symptom resolution. Complications are generally related to delay in diagnosis or rupture of the abscess, which can cause peritonitis, as well as pulmonary or even cardiac involvement. Mortality is directly related to these findings.

■ PROGNOSIS

The prognosis of PLAs depends on the rapidity with which the diagnosis is made and treatment is started. Mortality has improved over the years to about 11-16% due to a high index of suspicion that has resulted in early diagnosis and the availability of better diagnostic (especially imaging) facilities.

Following treatment, abscesses usually resolve over 6 weeks. Recurrences, though infrequent, are known to occur. Polymicrobial bacteremia, hypoalbuminemia, multiple liver abscesses, presence of complications, and an underlying immunodeficiency state are accompanied by increased mortality in patients with PLA.

■ BIBLIOGRAPHY

1. Bammigatti C, Ramasubramanian NS, Kadhiravan T, Das AK. Percutaneous needle aspiration in uncomplicated amebic liver abscess: a randomized trail. Trop Doct. 2014;43(1):19-22.
2. Mishra K, Basu S, Roychoudhury S, Kumar P. Liver abscess in children: an overview. World J Pediatr. 2010;6(3):210-6.
3. Ng KF Tan KK, Ngui R, Lim YA, Amir A, Rajoo Y, et al. Fatal case of amebic liver abscess in a child. Asian Pac J Trop Med. 2015;8(10):878-80.

CASE 31

Necrotizing Enterocolitis

■ PRESENTING COMPLAINTS

An 8-day-old boy was brought with the complaint of:
- Breathlessness since 5 days
- Distension of abdomen since 2 days
- Painful abdomen since 2 days

History of Presenting Complaints

A male baby was born preterm. He was delivered vaginally. The birth weight of the baby was 1.4 kg. Gestational age corresponds to 32 weeks. The Apgar score was 4 at 1 minute and 6 at 5 minutes. He developed respiratory distress and was shifted to neonatal intensive care unit (NICU). Child started improving without assisted ventilation. Standard low-birth-weight formula feed was given on the third day of life.

On the 8th day, distension of the abdomen was noted. Abdomen was painful on palpation. Feeding chart showed the presence of 5 mL of residual milk from the last feeding. Sister-in-charge also noticed that a higher incubator temperature was required to maintain body temperature.

■ EXAMINATION

A low-birth-weight baby was lying sick in the incubator. Features of IUGR were present. There was distension of the abdomen. Anthropometric measurements included a length of 45 cm (3rd centile), a weight of 1.3 kg, and a head circumference of 32 cm.

Activity and cry of the child were not satisfactory. He was afebrile. The heart rate was 130 beats per minute. The respiratory rate was 40 breaths per minute. The blood pressure recorded was 50/40 mm Hg.

Per abdomen examination revealed mild distension and tenderness. Bowel sounds were sluggish. No organomegaly. Other systemic examinations were normal.

CASE AT A GLANCE	
Basic Findings	
Length	: 45 cm (3rd centile)
Weight	: 1.3 kg
Temperature	: 37°C
Pulse rate	: 130 beats/min
Respiratory rate	: 40 breaths/min
Blood pressure	: 50/40 mm Hg
Positive Findings	
History:	
• Preterm baby	
• Low birth weight	
• Abdominal distension	
• Residual milk	
Examination:	
• Low birth weight	
• Features of intrauterine growth retardation (IUGR)	
• Abdominal distension, sluggish, bowel sounds not active	
Investigation:	
• Leukocytosis	
• X-ray erect abdomen—pneumatosis intestinalis	

INVESTIGATION

- *Hemoglobin:* 14 g/dL
- *TLC:* 20,000 cells/mm^3
- *DLC:* P_{88} L_{28} E_2 M_2 B_0
- *Blood culture and sensitivity (c/s):* Sterile
- *Urine c/s:* Sterile
- *Stool c/s:* Sterile
- *Bleeding time (BT):* 6 minutes (1–6 min)
- *Clotting time (CT):* 5 minutes (4–8 min)
- *Platelet count:* 4,00,000 cells/mm^3
- *Peripheral blood smear picture with leukocytosis:* Normal blood
- *Serum electrolytes:*
  - *Sodium (Na):* 120 mEq/L
  - *Potassium (K):* 4 mEq/L
  - *Chlorine (Cl):* 98 mEq/L
- *Arterial blood gases:*
  - *pH:* 7.1
  - *Partial pressure of arterial oxygen (PaO_2):* 65 mm Hg
  - *Partial pressure of arterial carbon dioxide ($PaCO_2$):* 35 mm Hg
  - *HCO_3:* 20 mEq/L
- *Erect abdomen X-ray:* Shows pneumatosis intestinalis

DISCUSSION

Necrotizing enterocolitis occurs among the premature infants who are undergoing stress in the first week of life. Clinically, it closely resembles to septicemia. This is because of associations of abdominal distension, apnea, bradycardia, instability of temperature, cyanosis, and lethargy.

Necrotizing enterocolitis is a serious gastrointestinal disease that occurs primarily in preterm infants. The disease is characterized by the rapid onset of intestinal inflammation, various degrees of mucosal or transmural necrosis of the intestine, and, in severe cases, can lead to intestinal necrosis and multiorgan dysfunctions that result in death. NEC has been reported as a complication of premature birth. It remains the most common gastrointestinal complication in preterm infants and is a major cause of morbidity and mortality in neonates.

PATHOLOGY AND PATHOGENESIS

Necrotizing enterocolitis in term infants is seen in infants with a history of birth asphyxia, Down syndrome, congenital heart disease, rotavirus infections, and Hirschsprung disease.

Necrotizing enterocolitis is a multifactorial disease primarily associated with intestinal immaturity. The triad of intestinal ischemia (injury), enteral nutrition (metabolic substrate), and bacterial translocation has classically been linked to NEC. The greatest risk factor for NEC is prematurity. The disorder probably results from an interaction between loss of mucosal integrity due to a variety of factors (ischemia, infection, and inflammation) and the host's response to that injury (circulatory, immunologic, and inflammatory), leading to necrosis of the affected area.

Clustering of cases suggests a primary role of an infectious agent. Various bacterial and viral agents, including *Escherichia coli*, *Klebsiella*, *Clostridium perfringens*, *Pseudomonas*, *Salmonella*, *Staphylococcus astrovirus*, norovirus, and rotavirus, have been recovered from cultures. Aggressive enteral feeding may predispose to the development of NEC. Stasis of the intestinal contents favors the bacterial overgrowth.

It is characterized by partial- or full-thickness intestinal ischemia usually involving the terminal ileum. The risk factors include prematurity, neonatal stress, formula feeding, surgery in newborn, umbilical artery catheterization, septicemia, and hypoalbuminemia.

Several factors have been implicated. The two main factors are mucosal injury and formula feeding.

Mucosal theory is attributed to ischemic damage to the intestinal mucosal barrier. This occurs as a result of fetal distress, perinatal asphyxia, respiratory distress syndrome, hypothermia, vascular spasm, or following exchange transfusions for hyperbilirubinemia. Mucosal injury is also attributed to diarrhea and infection. Infection produces injury to the gut.

Mucosal ischemia produces sloughing. Gas develops within the muscular layer. These may be seen as pneumocele in the X-ray. If full-thickness necrosis occurs, perforation and peritonitis develop.

Almost all patients of necrotizing enterocolitis are artificially fed prior to the onset of disease. It is assumed that there must be some substrates in formula feed that facilitate gas production in the intestinal flora. Poor systemic and gastrointestinal immunological protection against bacterial infection in preterm babies predisposes them to infection of the gut. Breast milk appears to be protective for necrotizing enterocolitis.

Many factors contribute to the development of the pathologic findings of NEC, including mucosal ischemia and subsequent necrosis, gas accumulation in the submucosa of the bowel wall (pneumatosis intestinalis), and progression of the necrosis to perforation, peritonitis, sepsis, and death. The distal part of the ileum and the proximal segment of colon are involved most frequently; in fatal cases, gangrene may extend from the stomach to the rectum (NEC totalis). The greatest risk factor for NEC is prematurity. NEC rarely occurs before the initiation of enteral feeding and is much less common in infants fed with human milk. Aggressive enteral feeding may predispose to the development of NEC.

CLINICAL FEATURES (FIG. 1)

The age at onset of NEC varies depending on the gestational age of the infant. More immature preterm infants present later in the hospital course compared to more mature preterm or term infants. NEC in term infants typically presents early, with a reported mean age of onset of 4 days.

The earliest finding often is the intolerance to feeds with vomiting. Vomitus is bile stained in 50% of cases. The first signs of impending disease may be nonspecific, including lethargy and temperature instability, or related to gastrointestinal pathology, such as abdominal distention and gastric retention. Abdominal distension is a common early finding. Abdominal wall erythema and a palpable abdominal mass are common late findings and signify more extensive disease.

The clinical findings of NEC are variable and can involve both abdominal and systemic signs and symptoms. Infants can have rapid changes in findings within a short period of time and require close monitoring for deterioration if NEC is suspected.

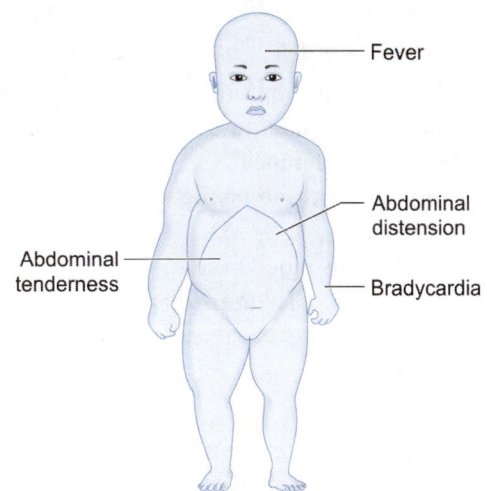

Fig. 1: Clinical features.

Nongastrointestinal signs and symptoms include temperature instability, lethargy, apnea, and bradycardia, while more severe and progressive cases demonstrate instability of vital signs, respiratory failure, and shock. Gastrointestinal signs and symptoms include poor feeding, increases in pregavage residuals, emesis, abdominal distention, and bloody stools. As NEC worsens in severity, gastrointestinal symptoms become more pronounced with marked abdominal distention, gastrointestinal hemorrhage, and abdominal wall discoloration or erythema. Abdominal wall discoloration is often an ominous sign, and a predictor of the severity of NEC.

The differential diagnosis of NEC also requires consideration of spontaneous intestinal perforation, which presents with pneumoperitoneum. This is considered to be a distinct entity from NEC and occurs earlier in the hospital course than NEC, often in the setting of no or minimal feeding; and it is more common among extremely preterm infants. (<28 weeks gestation).

Signs and Symptoms Associated with Necrotizing Enterocolitis

Gastrointestinal

- Abdominal distention
- Abdominal tenderness
- Feeding intolerance
- Delayed gastric emptying
- Vomiting
- Occult/gross blood in stool
- Change in stool pattern/diarrhea

Systemic

- Lethargy
- Apnea/respiratory distress
- Temperature instability
- Acidosis (metabolic and/or respiratory)
- Poor perfusion/shock
- DIC
- Positive results of blood cultures

Necrotizing enterocolitis may develop following a red cell transfusion. Bloody stools are seen in 25% of patients. Because of nonspecific signs, sepsis may be suspected before NEC. The spectrum of illness is broad, ranging from mild disease to severe illness with bowel perforation, peritonitis, systemic inflammatory response syndrome, shock, and death. Progression may be rapid, but it is unusual for the disease to progress from mild to severe after 72 hours.

> **ESSENTIAL DIAGNOSTIC POINTS**
> - Main factors are mucosal injury and formula feeding
> - It is characterized by partial- or full-thickness intestinal ischemia usually involving the terminal ileum
> - The risk factors include prematurity, neonatal stress, formula feedings, surgery in newborn, umbilical artery catheterization, septicemia, and hypoalbuminemia
> - The bacteria responsible for this infection include *Escherichia coli, Klebsiella, Pseudomonas, Salmonella*, and *Clostridium*
> - Stasis of the intestinal contents favors the bacterial overgrowth
> - The earliest findings often are the intolerance to feeds with vomiting
> - Vomitus is bile stained in 50% of cases
> - Abdominal distension is a common early finding
> - Abdominal wall erythema and a palpable abdominal mass are common late findings and signify more extensive disease

The illness usually develops in 1 or 2 days. The course may be fulminant with death occurring in few hours. Clinical features can be described in three stages:

- *Stage 1:*
  - *Stage IA:* Unstable temperature, apnea, bradycardia, lethargy, mild abdominal distension, and vomiting

- *Stage IB:* Blood in stools and radiograph showing mild intestinal distension
- *Stage II:* Bowel sounds are diminished with or without abdominal tenderness. There may be metabolic acidosis and mild thrombocytopenia. Pneumatosis intestinalis and dilatation of intestines are seen in abdominal radiographs.
- *Stage III:* The infant has low blood pressure, bradycardia, apnea, acidosis, DIC, and anuria. There will be frank signs of peritonitis with abdominal tenderness, distension and erythema of abdominal wall, and pneumoperitoneum is found in abdominal radiograph.

GENERAL FEATURES
• Preterm baby • Unstable temperature • Low blood pressure • Disseminated intravascular coagulation

LABORATORY SALIENT FINDINGS
• Blood in stool • Metabolic acidosis • Thrombocytopenia • Pneumatosis intestinalis and dilatation of intestines are seen in abdominal radiographs • Disseminated intravascular coagulation • Signs of peritonitis

■ DIAGNOSIS

Radiographic Findings

The primary radiographic finding in NEC is pneumatosis intestinalis, a radiographic appearance of gas within the wall of the small or large intestine. This is the hallmark of NEC and often establishes the diagnosis.

Infants with suspected NEC should have abdominal radiographs taken that include both anteroposterior views and either left-lateral decubitus or cross-table images to evaluate for free intraperitoneal air. Abdominal radiographs should be performed serially until the patient has demonstrated improvement in radiographic findings and clinical symptoms.

Other radiographic findings may include abdominal distention with evidence of ileus, portal venous gas, or pneumoperitoneum. In addition, bowel loops that remain unchanged on serial radiographic films for 24–48 hours raise the concern for ischemic bowel. Infants with evidence of pneumoperitoneum require surgery. The presence of portal venous gas may be associated with a higher eventual need for surgery, although its role as a prognostic marker for mortality is unclear.

The diagnostic evaluation of infants with suspected NEC includes evaluation for bloodstream infection, which can accompany NEC and is associated with worse outcome. Urine culture should also be obtained, as a urinary tract infection may precede the diagnosis of NEC.

Patients with NEC should have a complete blood count with differential and serum chemistry monitored. Hematologic changes that occur with NEC include thrombocytopenia, coagulopathy, anemia, neutropenia or neutrophilia, eosinophilia, and lymphopenia; further, the presence of significant hematologic abnormalities is often associated with more severe disease. In addition, infants with NEC may develop hyponatremia, hyperkalemia, and metabolic acidosis. Blood gas measurements should be performed at routine intervals to monitor for acidosis and respiratory deterioration. A lower serum pH (i.e., metabolic acidosis) is associated with advanced disease. If infants appear likely to need surgery or demonstrate worsening clinical status, coagulation studies should be obtained as DIC is often present in advanced cases of NEC.

DIFFERENTIAL DIAGNOSIS
- Septicemia
- Meconium plug syndrome
- Malrotation
- Hirschsprung disease

MANAGEMENT

Medical Management

There is no definitive treatment for established NEC, so therapy is directed at giving supportive care and preventing further injury with cessation of feeding, NG decompression, and administration of IV fluids. Careful attention to respiratory status, coagulation profile, and acid–base and electrolyte balances are important. Once blood has been drawn for culture, systemic antibiotics should be started immediately.

The treatment of NEC is based on the severity and involves bowel decompression, bowel rest, antimicrobial therapy, and monitoring of serial abdominal radiographs and laboratory parameters. Bloodstream infection develops in up to one-third of infants with NEC. Therefore, broad-spectrum antimicrobial therapy is indicated. Most bloodstream infections are caused by gram-negative bacteria, most commonly *E coli* and *Klebsiella*.

Initial management of the child with necrotizing enterocolitis without pneumoperitoneum is standardized. All oral feedings should be stopped. A NG tube is inserted to relieve distension and aspirate stomach contents. Fluid and electrolytes should be administered. Parenteral IV fluid can be used.

Careful attention to respiratory status, coagulation profile, and acid–base and electrolyte balances are important. Once blood has been drawn for culture, systemic antibiotics (with broad coverage based on the antibiotic sensitivity patterns of the gram-positive, gram-negative, and anaerobic organisms in the particular NICU) should be started immediately. Intravascular volume replacement with crystalloid or blood products, cardiovascular support with fluid boluses and/or inotropes, and correction of hematologic, metabolic, and electrolyte abnormalities are essential to stabilize the infant with NEC.

A surgeon should be consulted early in the course of treatment. The only absolute indication for surgery is evidence of perforation on the abdominal radiograph (pneumoperitoneum), present in less than half of infants with perforation or necrosis at operative exploration. Progressive clinical deterioration despite maximum medical management, a single fixed bowel loop on serial radiographs, and abdominal wall erythema are relative indications for exploratory laparotomy. Ideally, surgery should be performed after intestinal necrosis develops but before perforation and peritonitis occur.

Antibiotics must cover gram-negative and gram-positive aerobic organisms. Fungal infection is common after surgical treatment for NEC. Oral nystatin is recommended postoperation.

Antibiotic Selection and Duration

There exists wide variation in the choice of antibiotic treatment for NEC, with a combination of vancomycin and gentamicin being the two most commonly used antibiotic agents in this population. Other commonly used antibiotics include ampicillin, cephalosporins, clindamycin, metronidazole, and carbapenems. In a randomized controlled trial of 42 infants, the addition of anaerobic coverage with clindamycin to a standard regimen of ampicillin and gentamicin, compared to ampicillin and gentamicin alone, did not reduce the risk of intestinal perforation or death. However, surviving infants in the group received clindamycin, compared to ampicillin and gentamicin alone.

The best method of determining which babies require surgery consists of repeated physical examination by the same examiner, flat and left lateral decubitus abdominal radiograph every 4–6 hours for detection of pneumoperitoneum, careful monitoring of respiratory status and acid–base balance, and monitoring of leukocyte and platelet counts for the signs of sepsis.

Ventilation should be assisted in the presence of apnea or if abdominal distention is contributing to hypoxia and hypercapnia. Intravascular volume replacement with crystalloid or blood products, cardiovascular support with fluid boluses and/or inotropes, and correction of hematologic, metabolic, and electrolyte abnormalities are essential to stabilize the infant with NEC.

The patient's course should be monitored closely by means of frequent physical assessments; sequential anteroposterior and cross-lateral or lateral decubitus abdominal radiographs to detect intestinal perforation; and serial determinations of hematologic, electrolytes and acid–base status.

Shock is managed by the replacement of fluids and vasopressor agents. Plasma and platelet transfusion are used to prevent bleeding tendency. Surgical intervention is required if there is perforation.

Free intraperitoneal air is an absolute indication for surgery. However, pneumoperitoneum from the air dissecting down the chest in the ventilator-dependent child must be ruled out, so that unnecessary laparotomy is not performed.

Successful medical treatment may be followed by late-onset intestinal obstruction as a result of scarring and an intestinal long-term complication is the development of anastomotic ulcer.

Surgical Treatment

Indications for surgery include evidence of perforation on abdominal X-ray (pneumoperitoneum) or positive result of abdominal paracentesis (stool or organism on Gram stain preparation from peritoneal fluid). Failure of medical management, a single fixed bowel loop on radiographs, abdominal wall erythema, and a palpable mass are relative indications for exploratory laparotomy. Ideally, surgery should be performed after intestinal necrosis develops but before perforation and peritonitis occur.

Traditionally, management has involved an exploratory laparotomy with resection of the affected bowel. However, especially in infants with a birth weight of <1 kg, peritoneal drainage has become a more commonly used method to provide abdominal decompression until the need for a definitive laparotomy can be reassessed. However, of concern was a higher associated risk of death or neurodevelopmental impairment among infants receiving peritoneal drainage compared to initial laparotomy.

The frankly necrotic or perforated intestine should be removed and ileostomies are formed. When massive resection is necessary, the chance of the child's survival is limited. But premature infant's intestine still has potential for growth and adaption.

If ileostomy is performed, the mucous fistula should be exteriorized close to functioning ileostomy. Closure should be planned when the child is large enough, i.e., >2 kg and after a sufficient time following the event, i.e., at least 4–6 weeks to minimize the possibility of recurrence.

The children are not fed orally for at least 2–3 weeks after the onset of NEC, it frequently takes more than 1 month for those successfully treated medically to attain adequate oral caloric intake. Hyperalimentation is mandatory as soon as NEC is diagnosed. Central IV alimentation is preferred in NEC.

Gastrointestinal perforation: It is reported among 20–30% of children. It occurs within 10–48 hours after the onset of necrotizing enterocolitis. It is suspected in infants with increasing abdominal distension and abdominal mass. A serial radiograph suggests a persistent fixed loop.

- *Full-thickness necrosis of gastrointestinal tract:* These will have the sign of peritonitis. These include ascites, abdominal mass, abdominal wall erythema, and induration. Necrosed area is removed surgically.

■ MORTALITY

Cause-specific mortality from NEC is high and varies depending on the gestational age and birth weight of the infant. Factors associated with a higher risk of death included a lower gestational age, lower birth weight, treatment with assisted ventilation on the day of diagnosis, treatment with vasopressors at the time of diagnosis, and black race. The majority of deaths from NEC occur within 7 days of diagnosis.

■ LONG-TERM OUTCOMES

Neurodevelopmental impairment: It is common among preterm infants with NEC, particularly those infants that required surgery or had a comorbid bloodstream infection. If extremely low-birth-weight (ELBW) infants with NEC undergo surgery, they are at higher risk for significant long-term cognitive and motor impairment.

The ELBW infants with sepsis and NEC have a similarly high incidence of neurodevelopmental impairment of 53% compared to an incidence of 29% among ELBW infants without infection. The highest risk of adverse outcomes appears to be in infants with both surgical NEC and late bacteremia, who were found to have 8-fold higher odds of cerebral palsy compared to infants without NEC or late bacteremia.

■ PROGNOSIS

Medical management fails in approximately 20–40% of patients with pneumatosis intestinalis at diagnosis; of these, 10–30% die.

Early postoperative complications include wound infection, dehiscence, and stomal problems (prolapse and necrosis). Later complications include intestinal strictures, which develop at the site of the necrotizing lesion and appear in approximately 10% of surgically or medically managed patients. Resection of the obstructing stricture is curative.

After massive intestinal resection, complications from postoperative NEC include short bowel syndrome (malabsorption, growth failure, and malnutrition), complications related to central venous catheters (sepsis and thrombosis), and cholestatic jaundice.

Later complications include intestinal strictures, which occur in approximately 10% of surgically or medically managed patients. Preterm infants with NEC who require surgical intervention are at increased risk for adverse growth and neurodevelopmental outcomes.

■ PREVENTION

Newborns exclusively breastfed have a reduced risk of NEC. Early and aggressive increase in feeding volumes increases the risk of NEC in very low-birth-weight (VLBW) infants, although a safe feeding regimen remains unknown.

Emerging evidence indicates that the use of inhibitors of gastric acid secretion (H2-receptor blockers and proton pump inhibitors) or prolonged empirical antibiotics in early neonatal period is associated with an increased risk of NEC. Prophylactic enteral antibiotics reduced the risk of NEC.

The most effective preventive strategy for NEC is the use of *human milk*. Because early detection and treatment may prevent late deleterious consequences of NEC, considerable research is focused on the identification of biomarkers for early identification of NEC, including CRP, urinary intestinal fatty acid-binding protein (I-FABP), claudin-3 (a tight junction protein), fecal calprotectin, acylcarnitine, interleukin-6 (IL-6), IL-8, and the heart rate characteristics (HRC) index. Near-infrared spectroscopy (NIRS) may be a promising predictive diagnostic modality for NEC.

■ BIBLIOGRAPHY

1. AlFaleh K, Anabrees J. Probiotics for prevention of necrotizing enterocolitis in preterm infants. Cochrane Database Syst Rev. 2014;(4):CD005496.
2. Autmizguine J, Hornik CP, Benjamin DK Jr, Laughon MM, Clark RH, Cotten CM, et al. Anerobic antimicrobial therapy after necrotizing enterocolitis in VLBW infants. Peditrics. 2015;135(1):117-125.
3. Neu J, Walker WA. Necrotizing enterocolitis. N Engl J Med. 2011;364(3):255-64.
4. Srinivasan PS, Brandler MD, D'Souza A. Necrotising enterocolitis. Clin Perinatol. 2008;35(1):251-72.
5. Warner BB, Deych E, Zhou Y, Hall-Moore C, Weinstock GM, Sodergren E, et al. Gut bacteria dysbiosis and necrotizing enterocolitis in very low birth weight infants: A prospective case-control study. Lancet 2016;387(10031):1928-36.

CASE 32

Pancreatitis

■ PRESENTING COMPLAINTS

A 7-year-old boy was brought with the complaints of:
- Severe abdominal pain since 3 days
- Loose motion since 3 days

History of Presenting Complaints

A 7-year-old boy was admitted to the hospital with a history of severe abdominal pain. According to him, pain used to be present in the upper abdomen. There was a history of radiation of pain to the back. The pain was not related to the food intake or the bowel habits. Abdominal pain was associated with loose bulky stools. There was no history of vomiting.

Past History of the Patient

The child was the second sibling of a non-consanguineous marriage. He was born at full term by normal delivery. There was no significant postnatal event. The child was on breast milk exclusively for 3 months. Later, weaning was started. He was on family food starting from 18 months. His developmental milestones were normal. His school performance was good.

There was a history of repeated attacks of pain in the abdomen since the last 2 years. Every time it was associated with loose bulky stools. He was completely immunized.

CASE AT A GLANCE	
Basic Findings	
Height	: 116 cm (50th centile)
Weight	: 21 kg (50th centile)
Temperature	: 38°C
Pulse rate	: 120 beats/min
Respiratory rate	: 22 breaths/min
Blood pressure	: 90/70 mm Hg
Positive Findings	
History:	
• Intermittent abdominal pain	
• Bouts of loose motions	
• Back pain	
Examination:	
• Curled-up posture	
• Distended abdomen	
• Absent bowel sounds	
• Tender mass	
Investigation:	
• *Hemoglobin:* 8 g/dL	
• *TLC:* 21,000 cells/mm^3	
• *Serum amylase:* Increased	
• *X-ray abdomen:* Soft-tissue mass with calcification	

■ EXAMINATION

The boy was moderately built and nourished. He was lying in a curled-up position and crying in agony with pain. The anthropometric measurements included height that was 116 cm (50th centile) and weight that was 21 kg (50th centile).

He was afebrile. The pulse rate was 120 beats per minute and the respiratory rate was 22 breaths per minute. The blood pressure was 90/70 mm Hg. There was no pallor, lymphadenopathy, or edema.

Per abdomen examination revealed the presence of mild distension of the abdomen. A firm tender mass measuring about 4 × 6 cm was palpable in epigastrium. Bowel sounds were sluggish. No organomegaly was found. Respiratory system reveals less air entry on the left base. Other systemic examinations were normal.

■ INVESTIGATION

- *Hemoglobin:* 8 g/dL
- *TLC:* 21,000 cells/mm^3
- *DLC:* $P_{74}L_{16}M_3E_6B_1$
- *ESR:* 46 mm in the first hour
- *Random blood sugar (RBS):* 70 mg/dL
- *Serum amylase:* 200 U/L (30–100 U/L)
- *X-ray abdomen:* Soft-tissue mass with flakes of calcification in the upper abdomen (Fig. 1)

■ DISCUSSION

History of abdominal pain and ileus along with abdominal mass are signs of left-sided pleural effusion. The cause of ileus can be acute hemorrhage into existing abdominal mass. The malignant disease is ruled out as the duration of history is not favoring. Malignant disease would have produced obstruction rather than ileus. The malignant disease may be lymphoma, neuroblastoma, and nephroblastoma.

Acute pancreatitis is the most common pancreatic disorder in children. The most important causes may be blunt abdominal injuries, mumps, multisystemic disease, and congenital anomalies. Following an initial insult such as ductal obstruction, lysosomal hydrolase colocalizes with the pancreatic coenzymes within the acinar cell. The pancreatic proenzymes are then activated by cathepsin B. This leads to autodigestion and the release of active proteases. The histopathological findings of acute pancreatitis are related to the release of activated proteolytic and lipolytic enzymes. Intestinal edema appears early. As the episode of pancreatitis progresses, localized and confluent necrosis and blood vessel disruption lead to hemorrhage. This leads to an inflammatory response in the peritoneum.

There will be premature activation of trypsinogen to trypsin within the acinar cells after initial insult of ductal disruption or destruction. Trypsin then activates other pancreatic proenzymes leading to autodigestion, further enzyme activation, and release of active proteases. Lysosomal hydrolases colocalize with pancreatic proenzymes within the acinar cells.

Interstitial edema appears histopathologically in early phase. Later, there will localized and confluent necrosis and blood vessel disruption leading to hemorrhage and an inflammatory response in the peritoneum can develop.

Disorders associated with pancreatitis include acquired immunodeficiency syndrome, hemolytic uremic syndrome,

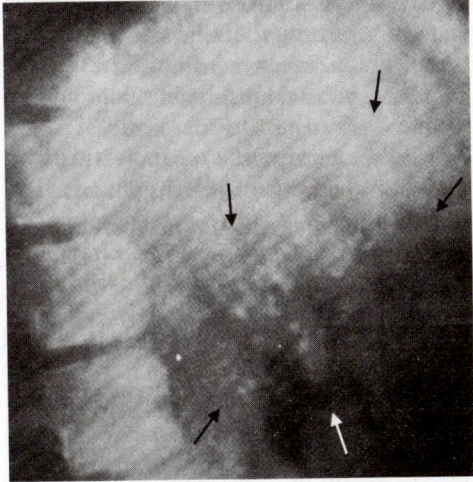

Fig. 1: X-ray abdomen showing soft-tissue mass with flakes of calcification in the upper abdomen.

Kawasaki syndrome, organic acidosis, brain tumor, and head trauma.

Morphologically, acute pancreatitis can be graded on the basis of severity as follows:
- *Mild:* Peripancreatic fat necrosis and interstitial edema
- *Moderate:* Mixed features
- *Severe:* Intrapancreatic necrosis with or without parenchymal necrosis and hemorrhage

Pancreatic inflammation can be initiated by various mechanisms. These include permeability of the pancreatic duct, overstimulation of glandular tissue, overdistension of duct, toxins, or certain metabolic abnormalities. Lecithin is activated by phospholipase A2 into the toxic lysolecithin.

CLINICAL FEATURES (FIG. 2)

Abdominal pain, persistent vomiting, and fever may develop. The abdominal pain may be present in epigastric region, and may be steady. This puts the patient in a curled-up position. The child is very uncomfortable, irritable, and appears acutely ill. The abdomen may be distended and tender. A mass may be palpable. The pain increases in intensity for 24–48 hours. The child may have persistent vomiting. This results in dehydration.

Acute hemorrhagic pancreatitis is severe form of acute pancreatitis and is very rare in children. Here, the patient is acutely ill. With severe cases, vomiting and abdominal pain, shock, high fever, jaundice, ascites, hypocalcemia, and pleural effusion can occur. A bluish discoloration may be seen around the umbilicus, i.e., Cullen sign or in the flanks, i.e., Grey Turner sign. The pancreas is necrotic and may be transformed into an inflammatory hemorrhagic mass.

In mild acute pancreatitis, there will be moderate-to-severe abdominal pain, persistent vomiting, and fever. The pain is in the epigastric region or in other upper quadrant. The steady pain makes the child to assume an antalgic position with hips and knees flexed sitting upright or lying at side. The child is uncomfortable, irritable, and acutely ill.

The abdomen may be distended and tender and a mass may be palpable. The pain can increase in intensity for 24 hours, during which vomiting may increase leading to hospitalization.

In moderately severe acute pancreatitis, there will be transient organ failure or dysfunction or development of local or systemic complications such as lung or kidney disease. Imaging may reveal sterile peripancreatic necrosis. The prognosis is good but recovery may be prolonged.

In severe acute pancreatitis, there will be persistent single or multiple organ failure. This is uncommon in children. The mortality rate is related to systemic inflammatory response syndrome, multiple organ defects, shock, renal failure, acute respiratory distress, DIC, and gastrointestinal bleeding.

Serum lipase greater than 7 times the upper limit of normal obtained within 24 hours of presentation may predict a severe course.

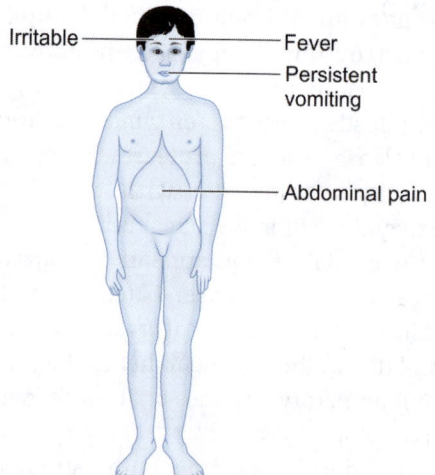

Fig. 2: Clinical features.

DIAGNOSIS

Pancreatitis is usually diagnosed by measurement of serum amylase and lipase activities. Serum amylase will be elevated for up to 4 days. Serum lipase is more specific than amylase for acute inflammatory pancreatic disease. It remains elevated for 8-14 days longer than serum amylase. Other laboratory abnormalities maybe present in acute pancreatitis include hemoconcentration, coagulopathy, leukocytosis, hyperglycemia and glycosuria, and hyperbilirubinemia.

> **LABORATORY SALIENT FINDINGS**
> - Elevated levels of amylase or lipase
> - Elevated immunoreactive trypsinogen
> - Leukocytosis and hyperglycemia
> - Hypocalcemia and falling hematocrit

Chest radiograph may show left-sided pleural effusion, pericardial effusion, and pulmonary edema. Abdominal radiograph may demonstrate a sentinel loop, dilatation of the transverse colon (cut-off sign), ileus, and pancreatic calcification.

Ultrasound and CT scan will show pancreatic enlargements, hypoechoic, sonolucent edematous pancreas, pancreatic masses, fluid collection, and abscesses. Endoscopic retrograde cholangiopancreatography (ERCP) is essential to investigate recurrent pancreatitis. Magnetic resonance cholangiopancreatography (MRCP) and endoscopic USG is required to visualize pancreatobiliary system.

DIFFERENTIAL DIAGNOSIS

Differential diagnosis includes pseudocyst, ascites, peritonitis, intestinal obstruction, appendicitis, and diabetes.

The mortality is related to systemic inflammatory response syndrome leading to multiple organ dysfunction-shock, renal failure, DIC, acute respiratory distress syndrome, intestinal bleeding, and fulminant abdominal infection.

TREATMENT

Children with uncomplicated acute pancreatitis do well and recover over a period of 2-4 days. Measurement of urinary trypsin activation peptide (TAP) is the most sensitive diagnostic test for determining severity of acute pancreatitis.

The aim is to relieve pain and restore homeostasis. Meperidine is the drug of choice for pain relief. Fluid, electrolyte, and mineral balance should be restored. NG suction is useful in patients who are vomiting. The response to treatment is usually seen within 2-4 days. Treatment of severe acute pancreatitis may involve total parenteral nutrition and surgical drainage of necrotic material or abscess. Other modalities include peritoneal lavage to reduce the risk of secondary infection and use of trypsin inhibitors. Endoscopic therapy may be beneficial in strictures.

Early refeeding decreases the complication rate and length of stay.

Antibiotics are used to treat infected necrosis. Gastric acid secretion is suppressed with proton pump inhibitors. Enteral alimentation by mouth, NG tube, or nasojejunal tube within 2-3 days of onset reduces the length of hospitalization and complication rate.

BIBLIOGRAPHY

1. Masamune A. Genetics of pancreatitis: The 2014 update. Tohoku J Exp Med. 2014: 232(2): 69-77.
2. Raizner A, Phatak UP, Baker K, Patel MG, Husain SZ, Pashankar DS. Acute necrotizing pancreatitis in children. J Pediatr. 2013; 162(4):788-92.
3. Srinath AI, Lowe ME. Pedatric pancreatitis. Pediatr Rev. 2013;34(2):79-90.

CASE 33

Tracheoesophageal Fistula

■ PRESENTING COMPLAINTS

A 6-month-old boy was brought with the complaints of:
- Cough and cold since birth
- Fever since 1 week

History of Presenting Complaints

A 6-month-old boy has been referred by a general practitioner for evaluation of repeated respiratory tract infections. His mother revealed a history of repeated attacks of cough, cold, and fever since birth. Sometimes boy used to have respiratory distress and had been hospitalized a few times. Child was given intravenous (IV) antibiotics and IV fluids.

Past History of the Patient

The boy was the only sibling of the family. Boy was born at term by normal vaginal delivery. He cried immediately after birth. Child was having bluish discoloration. Excessive froth was coming from mouth. A nasogastric (NG) tube is passed to know the patency of esophagus. But the tube could not be passed. This helps to make the diagnosis of esophageal atresia (EA). The birth weight was 2.75 kg.

Then pediatric surgeon was consulted. The tracheoesophageal fistula (TEF) was repaired with satisfactory primary repair.

CASE AT A GLANCE

Basic Findings
Length	:	70 cm (95th centile)
Weight	:	7 kg (50th centile)
Temperature	:	38°C
Pulse rate	:	128 beats/min
Respiratory rate	:	60 breaths/min
Blood pressure	:	60/50 mm Hg

Positive Findings

History:
- Repeated respiratory infections
- Bluish color at birth
- Esophageal atresia (EA)
- Surgical repair done

Examination:
- Tachypnea
- Rhonchi crepitation
- Audible wheeze

Investigation:
- X-ray chest: Air outlining the pouch

During hospital stay following the period of IV feeding, oral feeds were gradually introduced. He was given normal feeds at the time of discharge. But he had a cough and noisy breathing. His cough persisted. Despite all these, he had normal growth and development. The child was on breast milk for the first 3 months. Weaning started from the 3rd month onward. A social smile appeared at the age of 3 months. The neck control was present at the age of 3 months. The child was sitting with support at the time of admission.

EXAMINATION

On examination, the boy was moderately built and moderately nourished. The boy was alert and breathless. Anthropometric measurements included that the length was 70 cm (95th centile) and weight was 7 kg (50th centile). The head circumference was 40 cm.

He was febrile. The pulse rate was 128 beats per minute and the respiratory rate was 60 breaths per minute. Blood pressure recorded was 60/50 mm Hg. There was no pallor, no lymphadenopathy, no edema, and no cyanosis.

Respiratory system revealed the presence of rhonchi and crepitations. Wheeze was audible without a stethoscope. There was subcostal indrawing and accessory muscles were active. Cardiovascular system revealed tachycardia. Per abdomen examination was normal.

INVESTIGATION

- *Hemoglobin:* 12 g/dL
- *TLC:* 7,800 cells/mm^3
- *DLC:* $P_{55}L_{35}E_7M_3$
- *ESR:* 32 mm at first hour
- *AEC:* 660 cells/dL
- *X-ray chest:* Showed the air outlining the pouch.

DISCUSSION

Esophageal atresia is the most common congenital anomaly of the esophagus, with a prevalence of 1.7 per 10,000 live births. Of these, >90% have an associated TEF. In the most common form of EA, the upper esophagus ends in a blind pouch and the TEF is connected to the distal esophagus. The exact cause is still unknown; associated features include advanced maternal age, obesity, low socioeconomic status, and tobacco smoking.

Anatomic disorders of the esophagus in children can be congenital or acquired. The most common congenital disorder of the esophagus is EA, which can be present with or without a TEF. Other congenital esophageal disorders include esophageal webs, duplications, laryngotracheoesophageal clefts (LTEC), and esophageal stenosis from extrinsic (vascular rings) or intrinsic sources. Acquired disorders of the esophagus include strictures due to foreign body or caustic injury, Gastroesophageal reflux (GER), eosinophilic esophagitis (EoE), or diverticula.

Infants weighing <1,500 g at birth and those with severe cardiac anomalies have the highest risk for mortality. 50% of infants are nonsyndromic without other anomalies, and the rest have associated anomalies, most often associated with the VATER or VACTERL [vertebral, anorectal, (cardiac), tracheal, esophageal, renal, radial, (limb)] syndrome. Cardiac and vertebral anomalies are seen in 32% and 24%, respectively.

Around day 26 or 27 of gestation, a ventral diverticulum is formed from the caudal end of the primitive pharyngeal foregut. This laryngotracheal diverticulum undergoes elongation and differentiation and eventually forms the larynx, trachea, bronchi, and lungs. In order to separate the dorsal foregut (future esophagus) from the ventral laryngotracheal diverticulum, longitudinal tracheoesophageal folds fuse to form a septum that completely separates these structures. The traditional embryologic theory has held that failure of these folds to completely form, or improper timing of their formation, leads to the anomalies of EA and/or TEF. However, investigators have found little evidence to support that lateral folds forming a tracheoesophageal septum occur at all.

The embryogenesis of the various types of congenital esophageal stenosis is thought to be similar. An esophageal web is considered by some to represent a variant of EA. The web membrane is composed of squamous epithelium on both sides and often has a small opening which is why it often does not present on day 1 or 2 of life. Also, similar to EA-TEF, the embryology of esophageal stenosis secondary to tracheobronchial remnants is hypothesized to be due to disordered separation of the primitive foregut.

Lastly, the pathogenesis of esophageal stenosis due to fibromuscular hypertrophy is also unknown but may be similar to that of congenital pyloric stenosis.

One recent theory suggests initial normal development of the trachea and esophagus followed by fusion of the two structures to various degrees. Another theory postulates that there is an arrest of the cranial extension of the tracheoesophageal septum leading to a persistent single tube.

Esophageal atresia is more common among preterm children. Pathogenesis of this condition is defective differentiation of the primitive foregut into the trachea and esophagus. The defective growth of endodermal cells leads to atresia.

The upper part of esophagus is developed from retropharyngeal segment and lower part from pregastric segment of the first part of the primitive gut. At 4 weeks of gestation, the laryngotracheal groove is formed. Two longitudinal furrows develop. This separates the respiratory precordium from the esophagus. Altered cellular growth in this septum leads to the formation of TEF.

In more than 85% of cases, fistula between the trachea and distal esophagus accompanies atresia. Disorders in the formation and movement of the paired cranial and single caudal folds in the primitive foregut explain the variation in atresia and fistula formation.

The condition is associated with cardiovascular abnormalities, duodenal atresia, imperforate anus, urinary tract infection, and skeletal abnormalities. Antenatal maternal hydramnios is associated with this anomaly. This is associated with vertebral, anorectal, cardiac, renal, radial, and limb abnormalities.

There are five types. In the most common variety, the upper part of the esophagus ends blindly. The lower part is connected to the trachea by the fistula.

Lack of cartilage in the trachea produces variable degrees of tracheomalacia. Hence, trachea becomes floppy and vulnerable to collapse. Usually, there will be secondary problems with this surgical condition. These problems may even be present after successful correction of the condition. This is more if there is associated tracheomalacia.

■ CLINICAL FEATURES (FIG. 1)

Esophageal atresia and TEF are classified into five different types, and it is useful to use the anatomic description when referring to a specific type. By far, the most common anatomic type is EA with distal TEF, in which the fistula most frequently originates

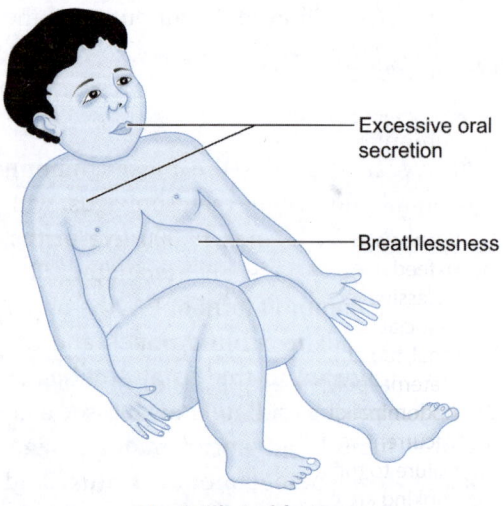

Fig. 1: Clinical features.

just proximal to the carina in the posterior trachea. The second most common type is pure EA with no TEF. The other three types are seen much less frequently and include EA with a proximal TEF, EA with a proximal and distal TEF, and finally, an H-type (or isolated) TEF without EA.

Tracheoesophageal fistula is suspected in the maternal polyhydramnios and in infants with excessive oral secretion. It sometimes presents with the cyanosis, choking, or coughing in an attempt to feed. Suction of the excessive secretion and pharynx will give temporary relief but symptoms quickly recur. Other signs may be inability to swallow or inability to pass a feeding tube. Respiratory compromise may be seen as well if there is a reflux of gastric fluid through the TEF or aspiration from the upper esophagus resulting in a chemical pneumonitis. Acute respiratory failure can be seen when inspired air goes preferentially through the fistula into the gastrointestinal tract, most commonly seen on positive pressure ventilation. In contrast, H-type TEF is often not as clinically apparent in the neonatal period and the diagnosis may be delayed. Thus, a high index of suspicion is required. Clinically, these patients often present with recurrent aspiration pneumonia, a history of coughing or choking with feeds, and cyanotic spells. Aspiration of the gastric contents produces life-threatening clinical pneumonia.

ESSENTIAL DIAGNOSTIC POINTS

- Cyanosis, choking, or coughing in an attempt to feed
- Excessive secretion and pharynx
- Associated with vertebral, anorectal, cardiac, renal, radial, and limb abnormalities
- Maternal polyhydramnios
- Abdominal distension
- Recurrent aspiration pneumonia
- Failure to thrive, slow feeding, coughing, and choking are common sequelae

The neonate typically has frothing and bubbling at the mouth and nose after birth as well as episodes of coughing, cyanosis, and respiratory distress. Feeding exacerbates these symptoms, causes regurgitation, and can precipitate aspiration.

If there is a fistula between the trachea and distal esophagus, there will be abdominal distension with tympanic note. Abdominal distension may interfere with breathing. If the fistula is in between trachea and proximal esophagus, there will be aspiration pneumonia leading to respiratory distress. If there is fistula without atresia H type, there will be recurrent aspiration pneumonia, including refractory bronchospasm and recurrent pneumonia. The diagnosis is delayed by days and months.

If the lesion occurs in extrathoracic trachea, obstruction is predominantly inspiratory. The intrathoracic lesions are more likely to collapse during expiration. These result in noisy breathing. There will be frequent episodes of bronchospasm following the surgeries. This is exaggerated by tracheomalacia.

Associated structural malformations such as tracheomalacia and esophageal stenosis should be corrected. Failure to thrive, slow feeding, coughing, and choking are common sequelae.

■ DIAGNOSIS

Prenatal diagnosis of EA–TEF is uncommon. A small gastric bubble or polyhydramnios on prenatal US can be suggestive but is not definitive. Postnatally, the diagnosis of EA with or without TEF is typically made within the 1st day of life. Failure to pass a feeding tube is often the initial step in the diagnosis. A plain chest radiograph can confirm the diagnosis by visualizing the feeding tube in the upper esophageal pouch. The image can be further enhanced by injecting a small amount of air into the feeding tube, which can help highlight the blind upper esophageal pouch consistent with EA. Injecting a very small amount of contrast while under X-ray may be helpful as well in some cases, particularly if trying to differentiate EA from traumatic misplacement of a feeding tube with a pharyngeal or esophageal injury (**Figs. 2A and B**).

The two most common types of EA–TEF can be distinguished on plain chest and abdominal X-rays. With pure EA, there will be no abdominal bowel gas visualized, while EA with distal TEF will have a normal abdominal bowel gas pattern. Rigid bronchoscopy is used to confirm the presence of a distal fistula and can also be used to assess for a rare proximal fistula.

The diagnosis of H-type TEF presents a greater challenge. Contrast esophagram, often best performed in prone position, requires a skilled radiologist, as the fistula can be quite difficult to see lower esophageal reflex (LERE). Bronchoscopy and esophagoscopy are used, to confirm the diagnosis, though the fistula can still be difficult to visualize.

Over 50% of children with EA–TEF will have other associated anomalies. All neonates with newly diagnosed EA–TEF should be evaluated for other VACTERL-related anomalies. This includes a thorough physical exam, echocardiography, renal US, spinal US, and spinal radiographs. Chromosome studies should also be sent.

GENERAL FEATURES
• Excessive oral secretion • Cyanosis • Coughing • Repeated respiratory infection • Aspiration pneumonia

LABORATORY SALIENT FINDINGS
• Inability to pass the catheter into the stomach • Plain X-ray of the chest shows the upper esophageal pouch dilated with air • Bronchoscopy detects the orifice of the fistula

■ DIFFERENTIAL DIAGNOSIS

- Traumatic postintubation
- Gastroesophageal reflux (GER)
- Hiatus hernia
- Achalasia

■ COMPLICATIONS

The main complications of the TEF include respiratory distress and ultimately congestive cardiac failure.

■ TREATMENT

Initial Management

It is a surgical emergency. Preoperatively, baby should be kept in a prone position. This is to decrease the aspiration of the gastric content. Esophageal pouch should be kept empty by content suctioning to prevent

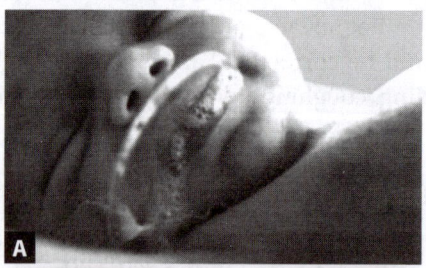
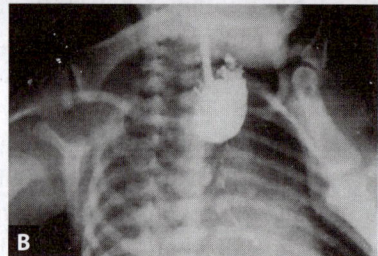

Figs. 2A and B: Tracheoesophageal fistula (TEF).

aspiration. Temperature and respiratory function are to be monitored.

Gastrostomy for feeding and surgical repair should be undertaken as early as possible. Oral feeding is started 8–10 days after the primary anastomosis. Esophagography done at 10 days will help to determine the adequacy of anastomoses. Stenosis at anastomy is common. This may require dilatation.

Initially, maintaining a patent airway, preoperative proximal pouch decompression to prevent aspiration of secretions, and use of antibiotics to prevent consequent pneumonia are paramount. Prone positioning minimizes movement of gastric secretions into a distal fistula, and esophageal suctioning minimizes aspiration from a blind pouch. Endotracheal intubation with mechanical ventilation is to be avoided if possible because it can worsen the distention of abdominal viscera.

Temporary treatments to help improve ventilation prior to urgent surgical intervention include right mainstem bronchus intubation and HFOV. However, intubation may worsen respiratory function because the positive pressure may increase airflow preferentially through the fistula. Emergent surgical management of worsening respiratory failure in these patients includes decompressive gastrostomy and ligation of the TEF. In those cases, complete repair of the EA may need to be delayed.

The timing of surgical repair depends primarily on the presence and severity of other anomalies or medical conditions.

Surgical ligation of the TEF and primary end-to-end anastomosis of the esophagus via right-sided thoracotomy constitute the current standard surgical approach. In the premature or otherwise complicated infant, a primary closure may be delayed by temporizing with fistula ligation and gastrostomy tube placement. If the gap between the atretic ends of the esophagus is >3–4 cm, primary repair cannot be done; options include using gastric, jejunal, or colonic segments interposed as a neoesophagus. These patients frequently require multiple surgical procedures to bring the two ends of the esophagus together. A gastrostomy is placed early in their management to provide access to enteral feeding and to provide access to the distal esophagus. In some cases, the two ends of the esophagus can not be surgically brought together. These patients are candidates for esophageal replacement surgery. Conduits frequently used include the stomach or colonic interposition grafts. Careful search must be undertaken for the common associated cardiac and other anomalies. Thoracoscopic surgical repair is now considered feasible and associated with favorable long-term outcomes.

Postoperative Care and Complications

Early postoperative complications following repair of EA with or without TEF include anastomotic leak, anastomotic stricture, and recurrent fistula. Often, an esophagram will be performed between postoperative days 5 and 7 to rule out a leak prior to initiating feeds. Anastomotic leaks occur in 15–20% of patients, with a majority being managed nonoperatively by providing parenteral nutrition and antibiotics until spontaneous closure is documented by a repeat esophagram. After this, oral feedings are begun. Major leaks are rare and usually present with tachypnea, sepsis, and/or tension pneumothorax on the 2nd or 3rd postoperative day. Treatment includes tube thoracostomy and possible re-exploration to control the leak and manage the sepsis.

PROGNOSIS

Prognosis depends upon the earlier diagnosis, size and maturity of the baby, associated congenital abnormalities, and the presence of pneumonitis.

The majority of children with EA and TEF grow up to lead normal complications are often challenging, particularly during the later part of life. Complications of surgery include anastomotic leak, regurgitation, and anastomotic stricture.

Gastroesophageal reflux disease contributes significantly to the respiratory disease (reactive airway disease) that often complicates EA and TEF and also worsens the frequent anastomotic strictures after repair of EA. Many patients have an associated tracheomalacia that improves as the child grows.

BIBLIOGRAPHY

1. Harmon CM, Coran AG. Congenital anomalies of the esophagus. In: Grosfeld JL, O'Neill Jr JA, Fonkalsrud EW, Coran AG (Eds). Pediatric Surgery, 5th edition. Amsterdam, Netherlands: Elsevier; 2012. pp. 893-918.
2. Kunisaki SM, Foker JE. Surgical advances in the fetus and neonate: Esophageal atresia. Clin Perinatol. 2012;39(2):349-61.
3. Provenzano MJ, Rutter MJ, von Allmen D, Manning PB, Paul Boesch R, Putnam PE, et al. Slide tracheoplasty for the treatment of tracheoesophageal fistulas. J Pediatr Surg. 2014;49(6)910-4.
4. Slater BJ, Rothenberg SS. Tracheoesophageal fistula. Semin Pediatr Surg. 2016;5(3):176-8.

CASE 34

Wilson's Disease

PRESENTING COMPLAINTS

A 10-year-old girl was brought with the complaint of:
- Yellowish color of eye since 1 month
- Altered speech since 1 month
- Altered walking since 15 days

History of Presenting Complaints

A 10-year-old girl presented with the history of deterioration of speech and gait since 1 month. Her mother noticed that there was some alteration in speech. She was able to understand all that was told. She was answering the questions after repeated hearing. Her mother had also noticed change in the walking style. She was assuming hunched posture. She was walking in short, jerky steps. Jaundice was present.

Past History of the Patient

She was the elder sibling of consanguineous marriage. She was born at term by normal vaginal delivery. She cried immediately after the delivery. She had normal physiological jaundice at birth. She was exclusively on breast milk for 6 months. Later weaning started. The child had been immunized completely. All the developmental milestones were normal. There was no significant past history apart from common cold.

CASE AT A GLANCE

Basic Findings
Height	:	132 cm (50th centile)
Weight	:	28 kg (70th centile)
Temperature	:	38°C
Pulse rate	:	96 beats/min
Respiratory rate	:	20 breaths/min
Blood pressure	:	90/70 mm Hg

Positive Findings

History:
- Speech disturbance
- Gait disturbance

Examination:
- Fine tremors
- Hunched posture
- Icterus
- KF ring
- Hepatomegaly

Investigation:
- **Hemoglobin:** 10 g/dL
- **Serum bilirubin:** Raised
- **Serum ceruloplasmin:** Decreased
- **SGOT, SGPT:** Raised
- **Serum copper:** Increased

(KF: Kayser–Fleischer; SGOT: serum glutamic oxaloacetic transaminase; SGPT: serum glutamic pyruvic transaminase)

EXAMINATION

The child was moderately built and nourished. The girl was looking pale. She was shy with hunched-up posture. Anthropometric measurements included the height

132 cm (50th centile) and the weight 28 kg (70th centile).

Child was febrile. Pulse rate was 96 beats/min and the respiratory rate was 20 breaths/min. The blood pressure recorded was 90/70 mm Hg. There was neither pallor, lymphadenopathy, nor edema. Icterus was present, and Kayser–Fleischer (KF) ring was seen.

Per abdomen examination revealed the presence of enlarged liver. Hepatomegaly was measuring about 4 cm, below the costal margin, firm and nontender. No splenomegaly and no free fluid was in the abdomen.

Higher mental function appeared normal except for speech. There was no cranial nerve involvement. The child had fine tremors when she was asked to show the hands. Deep tendon reflexes were normal. No sensory disturbances were present. Cardiovascular and respiratory systems were normal.

■ INVESTIGATION

- *Hemoglobin:* 10 g/dL
- *TLC:* 12,300 cells/cumm
- *Platelet count:* 200,000 cells/dL
- *Alkaline phosphatase:* 150 U/L (550–100 U/L)
- *Serum ceruloplasmin:* 8 mg/gL
- *Serum copper:* 1,000 µg/dL
- *Serum bilirubin:* 5 mg/dL
- *SGPT:* 1,000 U/L (normal range: 6–50 U/L)
- *SGOT:* 65 U/L (normal range: 15–55 U/L)
- *Urine 24-hour copper excretion:* 1,000 mg/dL

■ DISCUSSION

The neurological symptoms and signs are suggestive of problems associated with the basal ganglia. Hypoalbuminemia along with abnormal liver function tests suggest Wilson's disease. It is also called hepatolenticular degeneration. It is an autosomal recessive disorder characterized by degenerative changes in the brain, liver, and KF ring in cornea.

■ PATHOGENESIS

The abnormal gene for Wilson disease is found on chromosome 13 (13q14.3), and encodes ATP7B, a copper transporting P-type adenosine triphosphatase, which is mainly expressed in hepatocytes and is critical for biliary copper excretion and for copper incorporation into ceruloplasmin. Absence or malfunction of ATP7B results in decreased biliary copper excretion and diffused accumulation of copper in the cytosol of hepatocytes.

The gene locus for Wilson's disease is on the long arm of chromosome 13 and 14q21. The disease associated gene (ATP7B) encodes a copper-transporting P-type adenosine triphosphatase, the WND protein. It is likely that there are numerous mutations of the gene, and most patients have two different mutations, having acquired one from each parent. The two most frequently observed mutations are a point mutation resulting in C-to-A transversion or a frame-shift. Studies using the recently cloned ceruloplasmin gene indicate that the underlying abnormally is a defect in both translation and transcription of the ceruloplasmin mRNA.

Mutations that completely destroy gene function are associated with onset of the disease symptoms as early as 2–3 years of age.

Fetal and neonatal liver normally contains high concentration of sulfur-rich copper-binding protein, i.e., metallothionein. Serum ceruloplasmin and serum copper levels are low. Altered incorporation of copper into hepatic proteins such as ceruloplasmin is associated with diffuse accumulation of copper in cytosol of hepatocytes. Later it is deposited in other tissues, for them it is toxic.

With time, liver cells become overloaded and copper is redistributed to other tissues, including the brain and kidneys, causing toxicity, primarily as a potent inhibitor of enzymatic processes. Ionic copper inhibits pyruvate oxidase in brain and adenosine triphosphatase in membranes, leading to decreased adenosine triphosphate–phosphocreatine and potassium content of tissue.

In Wilson's disease, there is no increase in copper absorption from the GIT. The basic defect seems to be the inability of the liver to incorporate copper into apoceruloplasmin, as well as secrete copper into the bile. It has been shown that in patients with Wilson's disease, copper concentrations are very high in the lysosomes of the hepatocytes and very low in the bile.

Copper is an essential trace element and the main dietary sources include liver, shellfish, chocolate, peas, and unprocessed wheat. Normally, 50% of the ingested copper is unabsorbed, 30% is retained by the body for maintaining homeostasis.

Copper accumulated in the hepatocytes induces cell damage through reactive oxygen radicals. Release of copper from necrotic hepatocytes leads to damage of other tissues including the brain, kidneys, and red blood cells. The role of ceruloplasmin, an alpha-2 globulin produced exclusively by the liver, in the pathogenesis of Wilson's disease is unclear. In most patients with Wilson's disease, ceruloplasmin levels are low in the serum.

Altered incorporation of copper into the hepatic proteins such as ceraloplasmin is associated with diffuse accumulation in cytosol of hepatocytes. Copper inhibits pyruvate oxidase in brain, adenosine triphosphatase in the membrane. This leads to decreased ATP, phosphocreatine, and potassium content of tissue.

Characteristic histologic findings are present in the liver, but none can be considered pathognomonic. The pathologic effects on the liver are considered to be directly related to the accumulation of copper ions. Fat deposition is the earliest change seen. Fine lipid droplets of triglycerides are dispersed throughout the cytoplasma.

In the early precirrhotic stage, the changes resemble a chronic active hepatitis are focal necrosis, scattered acidophilic bodies, and moderate-to-severe steatosis. Glycogenated nuclei in periportal hepatocytes are a typical finding. Kupffer cells are hypertrophied and many contain hemosiderin.

Electron microscopy shows mitochondrial changes. As the hepatic lesion progresses collagen deposition occurs, leading on the cirrhosis. In the late cirrhotic stage, periportal fibrosis and portal inflammation are seen along with fibrous bands. The cirrhosis is often macronodular but may be of mixed type also. Cholangiolar proliferation and lymphocytic infiltration are also seen.

All grades of hepatic injury can occur. These include fatty changes, ballooned hepatocytes, glycogen granules, enlarged Kupffer cells, and minimal inflammation. These changes are similar to chronic hepatitis. There is large dense mitochondria with altered smooth endoplasmic reticulum.

PATHOPHYSIOLOGIC STAGING

A staging system explains the progression of the disease.

In stage I, there is progressive accumulation of copper in the cytosol of hepatocytes. This asymptomatic stage occurs before 5 years and continues until all hepatic binding sites for copper are saturated.

In stage II, there is redistribution of copper from the cytosol to the lysosomes of the hepatocytes and simultaneously copper is released from the liver. If the redistribution is rapid, some hepatic cell necrosis occurs and the patient develops features of liver disease. If this redistribution and release occurs slowly, the patient remains asymptomatic.

In stage III, lysosomal copper storage progresses leading to stimulation of fibrogenesis and gradual progression to cirrhosis. Copper accumulation occurs in other tissues such as brain, cornea and kidney during this stage. Rate of copper deposition determines the progression to clinical disease.

In stage IV, onset of hepatic or neurologic manifestation occurs.

In stage V, irreversible liver or brain damage takes place.

■ CLINICAL FEATURES (FIG. 1)

The clinical manifestations are related to the deposition of copper in various organs; and rarely presents before 5 years of age. Most patients present with either liver or CNS involvement, even though other organs can also be affected. About 25% of patients have multiple organs involved at presentation. In children, hepatic manifestations usually precede neurologic manifestations by many years.

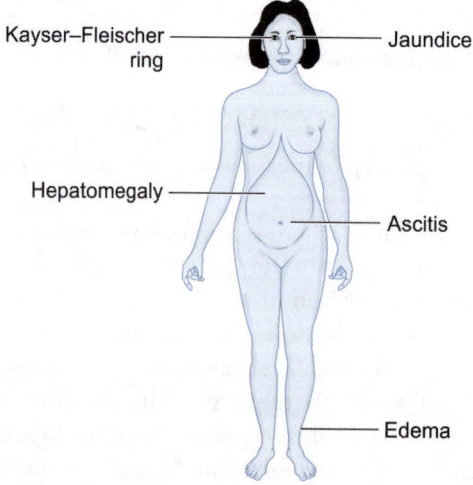

Fig. 2: Clinical features.

Wilson trait may be expressed after 2 years of age. Wilson disease is not seen before 5 years of age.

Copper enters the circulation in the non-ceruloplasmin-bound form and accumulates in various organs. The hepatic involvement is more in younger children. Neurological problems are seen in older children. Symptoms are due to copper-induced injury to various organs.

Forms of Wilsonian hepatic disease include asymptomatic hepatomegaly (with or without splenomegaly), subacute or chronic hepatitis, and acute hepatic failure (with or without hemolytic anemia). Cryptogenic cirrhosis, portal hypertension, ascites, edema, variceal bleeding, or other effects of hepatic dysfunction (delayed puberty, amenorrhea and coagulation defects) can be manifestations of Wilson disease.

Hepatic Disease

The younger is the patient, the more likely hepatic involvement will be the predominant manifestation. Girls are three times more likely than boys to present with acute hepatic failure. Clinically evident liver disease may precede neurologic manifestations by as much as 10 years. After 20 years of age, neurologic symptoms predominate.

Many young patients with Wilson's disease present as an acute self-limited hepatitis and are often thought to have viral hepatitis. Adolescents usually present with features of chronic active hepatitis. Patients with Wilson's disease may also present as fulminant hepatic failure with rapid progression and death.

Kayser–Fleischer rings are absent in young patients with hepatic Wilson disease up to 50% of the time but are present in 95% of patients with neurologic symptoms and somewhat over half of those

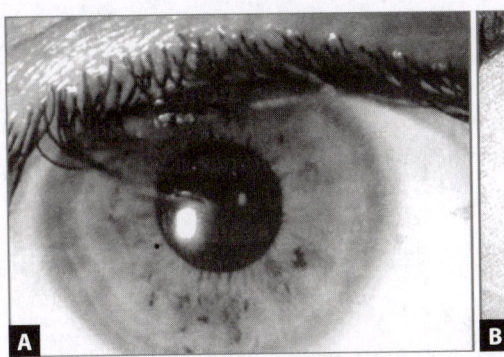 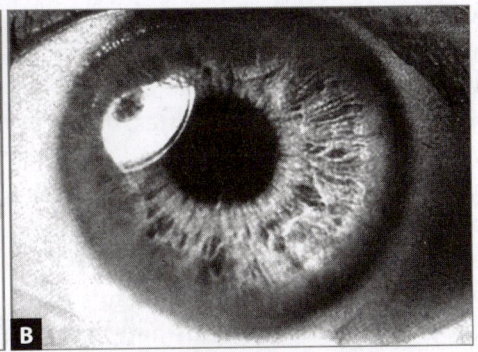

Figs. 2A and B: Kayser-Fleischer ring. (For color version, see Plate 1)

without neurologic symptoms. Psychiatric manifestations include depression, personality changes, anxiety, or psychosis.

Copper diffuses into the cornea from the aqueous humor; and this movement is inversely related to the evaporation of tears from the surface of the cornea. Since evaporation is less at the superior poles of the cornea, KF ring is first visible at the upper part of the limbus.

Sunflower cataracts are occasionally seen in association with KF rings **(Figs. 2A and B)**. They appear as a golden disc with radiating spokes, in the anterior capsule of the lens, and will resolve with therapy.

A slit-lamp examination is necessary for detection, even though it can occasionally be visible to the naked eye. The rings are first noted in the upper part, then in the lower part and finally extend laterally to complete the ring. This ring of copper granules deposited in the Descemet membrane is only a small fraction of the total corneal copper. Most of the copper is deposited in the stromal layers, which does not cause any color change and hence is not visible even under slit lamp.

Neurologic Disease

Neurologic manifestations typically begin in the second or third decade of life, even though they have been reported to occur as early as 6 years of age. Neurologic disorders can develop insidiously or precipitously, with intention tremor, dysarthria, rigid dystonia, Parkinsonism, choreiform movements, lack of motor coordination, deterioration in school performance, or behavioral changes, mask-like facies become apparent much later. Intellect is normal.

Central nervous system involvement in Wilson's disease is extensive and not limited to the basal ganglia. Studies have shown that in addition to striatal injury, there is also significant damage to the substantia nigra. However, the damage is limited exclusively to the motor system, with the sensory system being totally spared.

Neurologic disease is almost always associated with the presence of KF rings. KF rings have long been considered the hallmark of Wilson's disease. It is important to remember that they may not be seen in children with only hepatic manifestations of Wilson's disease. In addition, KF rings may also be seen in other conditions, most notably chronic active hepatitis, primary biliary cirrhosis, and intrahepatic cholestatic syndromes. KF rings appear as golden-brown or bronze or greenish-yellow discoloration (depending on the color of the iris) in the limbic region of the cornea.

Coombs-negative hemolytic anemia may be an initial manifestation, possibly related to the release of large amounts of copper from damaged hepatocytes; this form of Wilson disease is usually fatal without transplantation. During hemolytic episodes, urinary copper excretion and serum copper levels (not ceruloplasmin-bound) are markedly elevated. Hemolytic anemia may precede other manifestations and may be self-limiting or progress to persistent anemia. The hemolysis occurs due to oxidative injury to the red blood cell membranes from excess serum copper. As a consequence of hemolysis as well as cirrhosis, cholelithiasis may complicate Wilson's disease.

Electrocardiographic abnormalities have been reported in one-third of patients with Wilson's disease. Bone demineralization is the most common skeletal manifestation.

Renal defects resulting in hypercalciuria and phosphaturia with resultant hypocalcemia and hypophosphatemia are the underlying reason. Renal involvement is common and is characterized by proximal tubular dysfunction and a decrease in glomerular filtration rate.

ESSENTIAL DIAGNOSTIC POINTS

- An autosomal recessive disorder of copper metabolism
- Excessive accumulation of copper in the liver, brain, kidneys
- The basic defect is inability of the liver to incorporate copper into apo-ceruloplasmin
- *Hepatic disease:* Self-limited hepatitis; chronic active hepatitis; fulminant hepatic failure
- *Central nervous system involvement:* Basal ganglia, striatal injury substantia nigra
- Tremor, in coordination and difficulty with fine motor functions
- Dysarthria, dystonia, gait disturbances, and mask-like facies become apparent much later
- Intellect is normal
- Kayser–Fleischer rings (KF rings)

GENERAL FEATURES

- Hepatic failure
- Delayed puberty
- Amenorrhea
- Intention tremor
- Dysarthria
- Dystonia
- Behavioral changes

■ DIAGNOSIS

A high index of suspicion is the key to early diagnosis. It is a combination of clinical and family history with a few key investigations that establishes the diagnosis. The classical triad of hepatic disease, neurologic involvement, and KF rings represents a late stage in the disease process. 75% of children presenting with hepatic manifestations of Wilson's disease have decreased ceruloplasmin levels. However, a number of other conditions can also be associated with low serum ceruloplasmin levels.

Wilson disease should be considered in children and teenagers with unexplained acute or chronic liver disease, neurologic symptoms of unknown cause, acute hemolysis, psychiatric illnesses, behavioral changes, Fanconi syndrome, or unexplained bone (osteoporosis, fractures) or muscle disease (myopathy, arthralgia). The clinical suspicion is confirmed by study of indices of copper metabolism.

Most patients with Wilson disease have decreased ceruloplasmin levels (<20 mg/dL). The failure of copper to be incorporated into ceruloplasmin leads to a plasma protein with a shorter half-life and, therefore, a reduced steady-state concentration of ceruloplasmin in the circulation.

The serum "free" copper level may be elevated in early Wilson disease (>1.6 μmol/L), and urinary copper excretion (usually <40 μg/day) is increased to >100 μg/day and often up to 1,000 μg or more per day (typical findings in Wilson disease: Urine copper excretion >1.6 μmol/24 h and >0.64 μmol/24 h in children). In equivocal cases, the response of urinary copper output to chelation may be of diagnostic help. During the 24-hour urine collection patients are given two 500-mg oral doses of D-penicillamine 12 hours apart; affected patients excrete >1,600 μg/24 h.

Demonstration of KF rings, which might not be present in younger children, requires a slit-lamp examination by an ophthalmologist. After adequate treatment, KF rings resolve.

Percutaneous liver biopsy should always be performed if there are no contraindications.

Liver biopsy is of value for determining the extent and severity of liver disease and for measuring the hepatic copper content (normally <10 μg/g dry weight) but is only required if clinical signs and noninvasive tests do not allow a final diagnosis or if another liver disorder is suspected. Hepatic copper accumulation is the hallmark of Wilson disease and measurement of hepatic parenchymal copper concentration is the method of choice for diagnosis. In Wilson disease, hepatic copper content usually exceeds 250 μg/g dry weight (>4 μmol/g dry weight is the best biochemical evidence for Wilson disease but lowering the threshold to 1.2 μmol/g dry weight improves sensitivity without significantly effecting specificity).

CONDITIONS ASSOCIATED WITH LOW SERUM CERULOPLASMIN

- Malnutrition
- Protein-losing enteropathy
- Acute hepatic failure
- Nephrotic syndrome
- Hereditary hypoceruloplasminemia

Urinary copper levels may be used as a good indicator of response to therapy in Wilson's disease. 24-hour urinary copper levels greater than 1,000 μg after challenge with penicillamine in doses of 750 mg/m^2 body surface are per day in two divided doses is considered by many as diagnostic of Wilson's disease.

CONDITIONS ASSOCIATED WITH INCREASED URINARY COPPER LEVELS

- Fulminant hepatic failure
- Chronic active hepatitis
- Primary biliary cirrhosis
- Cholestatic syndrome of infancy

In those in whom liver biopsy is contraindicated, radioactive copper studies are useful. Incorporation of radiocopper into ceruloplasmin is defective in Wilson's disease. Hence the secondary rise in serum radio copper levels, which normally occurs at 24–48 hours after an oral load of the isotope is not present in patients with Wilson's disease. 65 Cu is a stable and safe copper isotope and is currently recommended for this study.

All asymptomatic relatives, especially siblings, should be screened using slit-lamp examination and measurement of serum ceruloplasmin level and 24-hour urine copper level.

Imaging studies of the brain may be helpful in diagnosis. CT scan abnormalities include ventricular dilatation, cortical atrophy, basal ganglia hypodensity, and posterior fossa atrophy.

Ophthalmic involvement results in KF ring. This is usually not seen before the age of 7 years. Screening tests for the family member includes serum ceruloplasmin level, urinary copper excretion, and sometimes liver biopsy.

Coombs-negative hemolytic anemia may be an initial manifestation, possibly related to the release of large amounts of copper from damaged hepatocytes; this form of Wilson disease is usually fatal without transplantation. During hemolytic episodes, urinary copper excretion and serum free copper levels are markedly elevated. Manifestations of renal Fanconi syndrome and progressive renal failure with alterations in tubular transport of amino acids, glucose, and uric acid may be present. Unusual manifestations include arthritis, pancreatitis, nephrolithiasis, infertility or recurrent miscarriages, cardiomyopathy, and hypoparathyroidism.

First-degree relatives of patients with Wilson disease should be screened for presymptomatic disease. This screening should include determination of the serum ceruloplasmin level and 24-hour urinary copper excretion. If these results are abnormal or equivocal, liver biopsy should be carried out to determine morphology and hepatic copper content. Genetic screening by either linkage analysis or direct DNA mutation analysis is possible, especially if the mutation for the proband case is known or the patient is from an area where a specific mutation is prevalent.

LABORATORY SALIENT FINDINGS

- Low serum ceruloplasmin levels
- 24 hour urinary copper levels greater than 1,000 μg
- Percutaneous liver biopsy
- Computed tomography (CT) scan abnormalities include ventricular dilatation, cortical atrophy, basal ganglia hypodensity, and posterior fossa atrophy

■ DIFFERENTIAL DIAGNOSIS

- Hepatitis
- Hepatic encephalopathy
- Indian childhood cirrhosis
- Hepatic copper overload syndrome
- Antitrypsin deficiency

■ COMPLICATIONS

- Copper-induced hemolysis
- Arthritis
- Renal failure
- Fanconi syndrome
- Renal tubular acidosis

■ TREATMENT

Treatment includes two aspects: (1) Induction therapy is to reduce copper to subtoxic threshold; this takes usually 4-6 months. (2) Maintenance therapy is to maintain a slightly negative copper balance so as to prevent accumulation and toxicity.

Wilson's disease is fatal if untreated, but successful outcome can be achieved with early effective therapy. Treatment is aimed at chelating excess tissue copper for urinary excretion, preventing copper absorption, and rendering tissue copper nontoxic.

Penicillamine is the drug of choice. It is a derivative of penicillin which chelates copper and enhances urinary excretion. It is administered orally in four divided doses about 30-45 minutes before food. The daily dose is 20 mg/kg body weight in young children and 750 mg/m body surface area in older children given in two divided doses.

Therapy should be initiated with small doses, and then gradually increased. Pyridoxine supplementation (25 mg thrice weekly) is recommended to offset the anti-pyridoxine effect of penicillamine. There is a dramatic increase in urinary copper excretion, about 48 hours after therapy is begun, and values up to 100 times normal may be obtained. Biochemical improvement is slow and may take many months. Improvement in clinical symptoms may, however, be seen within a few weeks of therapy.

In response to chelation, urinary copper excretion markedly increases, and with continued administration, urinary copper levels can become normal, with marked improvement in hepatic and neurologic function, and the disappearance of KF rings.

Adequacy of therapy may be assessed by serial determination of 24-hour urinary copper excretion. Calculated free serum copper has also been recommended. Values <20 indicate adequate therapy.

Approximately 20% of patients develop significant side effects with penicillamine therapy. These include fever, skin rash, granulocytopenia, or thrombocytopenia and usually occur within 3 weeks of commencing treatment. In such cases, penicillamine should be discontinued until the reactions resolve. The drug should then be reintroduced at very low doses under cover of prednisolone (0.5 mg/kg/day) and very gradually increased. Once penicillamine is tolerated, prednisolone is withdrawn.

Approximately 10–50% of patients initially treated with penicillamine for neurologic symptoms have a worsening of their condition.

Trientine (triethylene tetramine dihydrochloride) is the alternate chelating agent in patients who do not tolerate penicillamine. Triethylenetetramine dihydrochloride is a preferred alternative, and is considered first-line therapy for some patients. Trientine has few known side effects. Ammonium tetrathiomolybdate is another alternative chelating agent under investigation for patients with neurologic disease; initial results suggest that significantly fewer patients experience neurologic deterioration with this drug compared to penicillamine. It is given 1 hour before food and the dose is 20 mg/kg/day in children below 10 years of age. Older children and adults require 1.0–1.5 g daily in divided doses. Drug toxicity includes bone marrow suppression, nephrotoxicity, skin and mucosal lesions, and iron deficiency anemia. The initial dose is 120 mg/day (20 mg between meals TID and 20 mg with meals TID). Side effects include anemia, leukopenia, thrombocytopenia, and mild elevations of transaminases. Because of its extensive decoppering effect, ammonium tetrathiomolybdate also has antiangiogenic effects.

Elemental zinc (zinc acetate 50 mg thrice daily), an antagonist of copper absorption, is another alternative. Copper is absorbed in the proximal small intestine, and once it crosses the intestinal brush border, it binds to and saturates the metallothionein inside the electrolytes.

Zinc has also been used as adjuvant therapy, maintenance therapy or primary therapy in presymptomatic patients, owing to its unique ability to impair the gastrointestinal absorption of copper. Zinc acetate is given in adults at a dose of 25–50 mg of elemental zinc three times a day and 25 mg three times a day in children older than 5 years of age. Zinc induces metallothionein synthesis in the enterocytes. Metallothionein-bound copper cannot move out of the cells to reach the bloodstream. The intestinal cells therefore become loaded with this complexed copper and are then eliminated by desquamation into the intestinal lumen.

Zinc must not be given with penicillamine or trientine, since it chelates with these drugs and forms complexes that are therapeutically inactive. However, zinc acts very slowly and may take months for therapeutic benefit.

Zinc has also been used as adjuvant therapy, maintenance therapy, or primary therapy in presymptomatic patients, owing to its unique ability to impair the gastrointestinal absorption of copper. Zinc acetate can be given (adults) at a dose of 25–50 mg of elemental zinc three times a day and 25 mg three times a day in children over age of 5 years. Side effects are predominantly limited to gastric irritation but also include reduced leukocyte chemotaxis and elevations in serum lipase and/or amylase. Zinc may have a role as a first-line therapy in patients with neurologic disease, but exclusive monotherapy with zinc in symptomatic liver disease is controversial and not recommended. Antioxidants (vitamin E and curcumin) and pharmacologic chaperones (4-phenylbutyrate and curcumin) may have a role as adjunctive treatment but more research is needed.

Orthotopic liver transplantation (OLT) is indicated only in the following situations: (1) fulminant hepatic failure, (2) severe hepatic decompensation and cirrhosis, with no improvement after 2–3 months of chelation therapy, and (3) severe progressive hepatic insufficiency in a patient who discontinued treatment. OLT has also been performed for neurological manifestations of Wilson's disease, which was unresponsive to chelation therapy.

A major attempt should be made to restrict dietary copper intake to <1 mg/day. Treatment needs to be lifelong once diagnosis has been made.

PROGNOSIS

Wilson's disease is progressive and fatal if untreated. Among children who present as chronic active hepatitis, almost 50% respond to treatment. Fulminant hepatitis is frequently fatal despite chelation therapy. Patients who present with acute hepatitis or are asymptomatic do very well with treatment.

Prognosis is poor in the acute neurological form of Wilson's disease. Among patients with gradual neurological involvement, 75% respond to treatment.

BIBLIOGRAPHY

1. Arnon R, Calderon JF, Schilsky M, Emre S, Shneider BL. Wilson disease in children: serum aminotransferases and urinary copper on triethylene tetramine dihydrochloride (trientine) treatment. J Pediatr Gastroenterol Nutr. 2007;44:596-602.
2. EASL Clinical Practice Guidelines: Wilson's disease. J Hepatol. 2012;56(3):671-85.
3. Mizuochi T, Kimura A, Shimizu N, Nishiura H, Matsushita M, Yoshino M. Zinc monotherapy from the time of diagnosis for young pediatric patients with presymptomatic Wilson disease. J Pediatr Gastroenterol Nutr. 2011;53:365-7.
4. Roberts EA, Schilsky ML; American Association for Study of Liver Diseases (AASLD). Diagnosis and treatment of Wilson disease: an update. Hepatology. 2008;47:2089-111.
5. Rosencrantz R, Schilsky M. Wilson disease: pathogenesis and clinical considerations in diagnosis and treatment. Semin Liver Dis. 2011;31:245-59.

SECTION 5

Hematological System

- Case 35 **Hemophilia**
- Case 36 **Hemorrhagic Disease of the Newborn**
- Case 37 **Henoch–Schönlein Purpura**
- Case 38 **Hereditary Spherocytosis**
- Case 39 **Idiopathic Thrombocytopenic Purpura**
- Case 40 **Iron Deficiency Anemia**
- Case 41 **Polycythemia**
- Case 42 **Sickle Cell Anemia**
- Case 43 **Thalassemia**

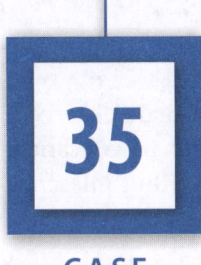

CASE 35

Hemophilia

■ PRESENTING COMPLAINTS

A 13-year-old boy was brought with the complaint of:
- Accident 3 days back
- Swelling of the joint since 2 days
- Restricted movement since 1 day

History of Presenting Complaints

A 13-year-old boy presented with history of accident in the road. There was injury to left knee. Slowly there was swelling of the joint. This led to the restricted movement of the joint at knee. His mother revealed significant past history of development of swollen tender left elbow. This had also occurred after the accidental slipping.

Past History of the Patient

He was the elder sibling of nonconsanguineous marriage. He was born at full term by normal delivery. Baby cried immediately after the delivery. The birth weight was 2.9 kg, length was 49 cm, and the head circumference was 34 cm. He was exclusively on breast milk for 4 months. His developmental milestones were normal. He was immunized completely. His performance at school was good.

■ EXAMINATION

The boy was moderately built and nourished. He was dull and anxious. He was cooperative at the time of examination. His anthropometric measurements included height 140 cm (<50th centile) and weight 38 kg (50th centile). He was short in stature.

The child was afebrile, the pulse rate was 96 beats/min and the respiratory rate was 20 breaths/min. The blood pressure recorded was 110/70 mm Hg. There was pallor, no lymphadenopathy, and no cyanosis.

Knee joint on the left side was swollen, warm, and tender. All the systemic examinations were normal.

CASE AT A GLANCE	
Basic Findings	
Height	: 140 cm (<50th centile)
Weight	: 38 kg (50th centile)
Temperature	: 37°C
Pulse rate	: 96 beats/min
Respiratory rate	: 20 breaths/min
Blood pressure	: 110/70 mm Hg
Positive Findings	
History:	
• Accident	
• Restricted movement at left knee	
• Swelling of the left knee	
Examination:	
• Swollen tender knee	
• Pallor	
Investigation:	
• Anemia	
• *Clotting factor VIII:* Decreased	
• *Active prothrombin (PT):* Prolonged	
• *von Willebrand factor:* Negative	

INVESTIGATION

- *Hemoglobin:* 9.7 g/dL
- *Total leukocyte count (TLC):* 9,900 cells/cumm
- *Platelet count:* 4,00,000 cells/cumm
- *Prothrombin time (PT):* 12 seconds
- *Active PT:* 40 seconds, i.e., prolonged (normal: 25–30 seconds)
- *Clotting factor VIII:* 5% Normal
- *Peripheral blood smear:* Normal
- *von Willebrand factor (vWF):* Normal
- *X-ray of the knee:* Joint dilated suprapatellar and popliteal bursae; epiphyseal center of the tibia and femur are enlarged

DISCUSSION

There is a history of easy bruising, joint swelling after the minor injury. This is associated with the prolonged PT and partial thromboplastin time (PTT) time and reduced level factor VII. This condition is called hemophilia A. It is a classical X-linked recessive condition. In hemophilia A, factor VIII is present, but its clotting function is defective.

The hemophilias are rare inherited bleeding disorders caused by a deficiency or an absence of coagulation factors, usually factors VIII or X. Hemophilia A or classical hemophilia is caused by mutations in the factor VIII gene (*F8*); hemophilia B, also known as Christmas disease, is caused by mutations in the factor IX gene (*F9*). The clinical hallmark of the hemophilias is soft tissue and musculoskeletal bleeding that may lead to debilitating arthropathy if untreated.

Hemophilia A and B are caused by mutations in the genes encoding for factor VIII and factor IX, respectively, which are located in the long arm of chromosome X. The genetic mutations can cause a quantitative reduction in protein expression or a qualitative decrease in protein activity, or both. Insertions, deletions, nonsense, and splice-site mutations also are observed. Patients with hemophilia B can have a variety of mutations in the F9 gene, but missense mutations are the most common.

ETIOLOGY

It is due to the congenital deficiency of the plasma coagulation factor VIII—*hemophilia A* or factor IX—*hemophilia B*.

Factors VIII and IX participate in a complex required for the activation of factor X. Together with phospholipids and calcium, they from the "tenase", or factor X-activating, complex. Factor X being activated by either the complex of factors VIII and IX or the complex of tissue factor and factor VII. In vivo, the complex of factor VIIa and tissue factor activates factor IX to initiate clotting. In the laboratory, PT measures the activation of factor X by factor VII and is therefore normal in patients with factor VIII or factor IX deficiency.

After injury, the initial hemostatic event is formation of the platelet plug, together with the generation of the fibrin clot that prevents further hemorrhage. In hemophilia A or B, clot formation is delayed and is not robust. Inadequate thrombin generation leads to failure to form a tightly cross linked fibrin clot to support the platelet plug. Patients with hemophilia slowly form a soft, friable clot. When untreated bleeding occurs in a closed space, such as a joint, cessation of bleeding may be the result of tamponade. With open wounds, in which tamponade cannot occur, profuse bleeding may result in significant blood loss. The clot that is formed may be friable, and rebleeding occurs during the physiologic lysis of clots or with minimal new trauma.

About 80% of cases of hemophilia are caused by gene carried on X-chromosome that results in a profound depression of the level of the factor VIII, i.e., antihemophilic factor in the plasma. Family history is present in 80%. Since factor VIII does not cross the placenta a bleeding may be evident in the neonatal period. A female carries hemophilia trait but only male offspring suffers from the disease.

Severity of hemophilia is dependent on the level of clotting of factor VIII or factor IX in blood. The average normal activity of clotting factor in blood is defined as 100%. The activity in an individual determines the clinical severity though the relationship is not strictly parallel. Clotting activity present in 1 mL of pooled plasma is considered as one unit.

Severely affected individuals bleed spontaneously into major joints and muscles, and usually have factor level <1% (<0.01 IU/mL). Moderately affected hemophiliacs have 1–5% (0.01–0.05 U) factor level and usually bleed only after trauma. Persons mildly affected have 6–24% (0.06–0.24 U) factor level and bleed only as a result of surgery or injury. Normal range of factor level is 50–200% (0.5–2 U).

Patients with mild hemophilia who have factor VIII or factor IX levels >5 IU/dL usually do not have spontaneous hemorrhages. These individuals may experience prolonged bleeding after dental work, surgery, or injuries from moderate trauma and may not be diagnosed until they are older.

During pregnancy higher level of factor, over 200% or 2 U, is seen. The level of activity of the clotting factor remains fairly constant throughout the life of the affected.

■ TYPES OF HEMOPHILIA

In hemophilia A, the factor VIII is deficient and in hemophilia B factor IX or Christmas factor. In addition, there are other types of hemophilia that are caused by defect in other clotting factors, such as factors II, V, VII, and X. von Willebrand's disease (vWD) is another more common hereditary disorder.

In patients with vWD, production of Willebrand factors is reduced quantitatively and qualitatively. This disorder affects both males and females equally, and is inherited in autosomal dominant way. The vWD is probably the most common inherited clotting disorder although it is generally the least severe.

■ CLINICAL FEATURES (FIG. 1)

Typically, patients with severe hemophilia can experience spontaneous musculoskeletal bleeding, while those with mild-to-moderate disease develop bleeding only after significant physical trauma or surgery. However, such spontaneous bleeding is likely induced by the routine trauma of weight-bearing on joints, as patients gain mobility and begin to ambulate late in infancy.

During the newborn period, other common presentations of hemophilia include intracranial hemorrhage (ICH) and bleeding at phlebotomy, injection, or circumcision. Therefore, infants born of known carrier mothers should not be circumcised until testing for factor VIII or factor IX has been performed. Older infants and children may experience excessive bruising, hematomas,

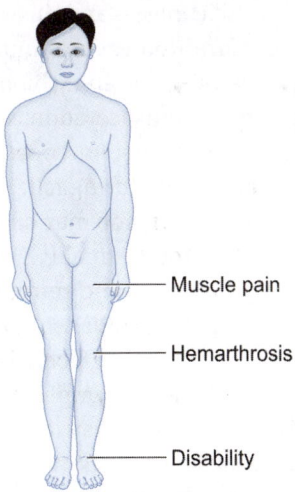

Fig. 1: Clinical features.

and intracranial, joint, muscle, or mouth bleeding after trauma. Female carriers of hemophilia can experience menorrhagia, other mucocutaneous bleeding, and surgical- and trauma-related bleeding.

Clinically, it is not possible to differentiate hemophilia A from hemophilia B. Hemophilia should be suspected in any male child with recurrent episode of prolonged bleeding, occurring spontaneously or following injury or during surgical procedures. A positive family history suggests the possibility of inherited bleeding disorder.

Patients with mild hemophilia who have factor VIII or factor IX levels >5 IU/dL usually do not have spontaneous hemorrhages. These individuals may experience prolonged bleeding after dental work, surgery, or injuries from moderate trauma and may not be diagnosed until they are older.

It usually manifests after the first year of life with unsightly bruises, prolonged bleeding after circumcision, and minor lesions from mouth. Moderate or mild hemophilia often first appears following surgery, tooth extraction, tonsillectomy, or secondary hemorrhage. Severe hemophiliacs can bleed into confined places—skull, joints, and major muscle mass—and this stops only when the pressure around surrounding tissue equals the pressure of escaping blood.

Tongue and mouth laceration is common presentation in toddlers, and occurs due to biting of tongue or lip during fall. Prolonged bleeding after circumcision may be the initial presentation. Gastrointestinal (GI) bleeding, genitourinary bleeding, and retroperitoneal bleeding are frequent in older children.

Neither factor VIII nor factor IX crosses the placenta; bleeding symptoms may be present from birth or may occur in the fetus. Obvious symptoms such as easy bruising, intramuscular hematomas, and hemarthroses begin when the child begins to cruise. Bleeding from minor traumatic lacerations of the mouth may persist for hours or days and may cause the parents to seek medical evaluation. Although bleeding may occur in any area of the body, the hallmark of hemophilic bleeding is hemarthrosis.

The hallmark of hemophilia is hemarthrosis **(Fig. 2)**. Hemorrhages in the elbow, knee and ankles cause pain and swelling. Bleeding into the joints may be induced by minor trauma; many hemarthroses are spontaneous. This will limit the movement of the joint. The earliest joint hemorrhages appear most commonly in the ankle. In the older child and adolescent, hemarthroses of the knees and elbows are also common. Recurrent bleeding may then become spontaneous because of the underlying pathologic changes in the joint. Repeated hemorrhage produces degenerative changes with osteoporosis, muscle atrophy, and ultimately fixed unstable joint. Repeated hemarthrosis develops ankylosis, synovial thickening, and atrophy of the surrounding muscles. Children with chronic arthropathy are at higher risk of developing joint bleeding.

Although most muscular hemorrhages are clinically evident owing to localized

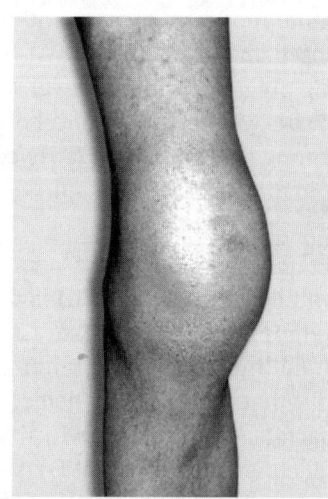

Fig. 2: Hemarthrosis.

pain or swelling, bleeding into the iliopsoas muscle requires specific mention. A patient may lose large volume of blood into the iliopsoas muscle, verging on hypovolemic shock, with only a vague area of referred pain in the groin. The hip is held in a flexed, internally rotated position owing to irritation of the iliopsoas. The diagnosis is made clinically from the inability to extend the hip but must be confirmed with ultrasonography or computed tomography (CT). Life-threatening bleeding in the patient with hemophilia is caused by bleeding into vital structures [central nervous system (CNS), upper airway] or by exsanguination (external trauma, GI or iliopsoas hemorrhage). Prompt treatment with clotting factor concentrate for these life-threatening hemorrhages is imperative. If head trauma is of sufficient concern to suggest radiologic evaluation, factor replacement should precede radiologic evaluation.

Bleeding in the muscle causes severe pain and disability. Children with retroperitoneal bleed may present with severe abdominal pain, anemia, and even shock. Intracranial bleed is uncommon. But it is major cause of death. It may be extradural, subdural, and intracerebral. CT scan is essential to confirm the bleed.

ESSENTIAL DIAGNOSTIC POINTS

- Easy bruising, joint swelling after the minor injury
- Prolonged PT and PTT time and reduced level factor VII
- Severity of hemophilia is dependent on the level of clotting of factor VIII or factor IX in blood
- Joint and muscle hemorrhages
- *Types of bleeding:* Gastrointestinal bleeding, genitourinary bleeding, and retroperitoneal bleeding, intracranial bleeding
- Computed tomography (CT) scan helps to confirm bleed

(PT: prothrombin time; PTT: partial thromboplastin time)

An individual with hemophilia B bleeds less frequently. Irritability, guarding tingling and numbness, and limitation of movement of affected joints are early symptoms. Knee and elbow joints are most frequently affected. However, any weight-bearing joint can be affected. The joints are swollen, warm, tender, and have limitation of movements.

The leading cause of mortality in hemophiliacs is intracranial bleeding. The incidence is 10–15% and risk of ICH ranges from 2% to 3.5% per year. Acute pain is one of the immediate results of untreated internal bleeding. Repeated bleeding into the same joint eventually leads to damage to joint cartilage and synovium, and results in chronic, painful, and incapacitating arthritis.

GENERAL FEATURES

- Easy bruising
- Intramuscular hematomas
- Irritability
- Intracranial bleeding
- Guarding

■ DIAGNOSIS

The laboratory screening test that is affected by a reduced level of factor VIII or factor IX is PTT. Patients with hemophilia have a normal platelet count and PT. However, the activated partial thromboplastin time (aPTT) is usually prolonged. In the event of an elevated aPTT, in a patient with bleeding symptoms, a diagnosis of hemophilia must be confirmed by specific clotting factor functional assays. In severe hemophilia, the PTT value is usually two to three times the upper limit of normal. The specific assay for factors VIII and IX will confirm the diagnosis of hemophilia. In patients with hemophilia who receive infusions of factor VIII or factor IX, a factor-specific antibody may develop. These antibodies are directed against the active clotting site and are termed inhibitors.

In such patients, the quantitative Bethesda assay for inhibitors should be performed to measure the antibody titer.

Children will have normal bleeding time (BT) with prolonged clotting and PTT. Factor VIII and factor IX deficiencies are recognized. Correction of aPTT with normal serum but not with adsorbed plasma suggests factor IX deficiency. aPTT correction with adsorbed plasma and not with normal serum suggests factor VIII deficiency. Platelet count is normal or elevated. Anemia is proportional to blood loss.

■ DIFFERENTIAL DIAGNOSIS

- Septic arthritis
- Rheumatic fever
- Idiopathic thrombocytopenic purpura (ITP)
- vWD

A reduced level of factor VIII or factor IX will result in a laboratory finding of a prolonged PTT. In 25–35% of patients with hemophilia who receive infusions of factor VII or factor IX, a factor-specific antibody may develop. These antibodies are directed against the active clotting site and are termed inhibitors. In such patients, the quantitative.

By definition, 1 IU of each factor is defined as that amount in 1 mL of normal plasma referenced against a standard established by the World Health Organization (WHO); thus, 100 mL of normal plasma has 100 IU/dL (100% activity) of each factor. Severe hemophilia is characterized as having <1% activity of the specific clotting factor, and bleeding is often spontaneous. Patients with moderate hemophilia have factor levels of 1–5% and usually require mild trauma to induce bleeding.

Through ionization of the X chromosome, some female carriers of hemophilia A or B have sufficient reduction of factor VIII or factor IX to produce mild bleeding disorders. Levels of these factors should be determined in all known or potential carriers to assess the need for treatment in the event of surgery or clinical bleeding.

Because factor VIII is carried in plasma by vWF, the ratio of factor VIII to VWF is sometimes used to diagnose carriers of hemophilia but may give false-positive or false-negative results.

> **LABORATORY SALIENT FINDINGS**
> - Normal bleeding time with prolonged clotting and partial thromboplastin time
> - Factor VIII and factor IX deficiencies
> - Platelet count is normal or elevated
> - Anemia is proportional to blood loss

■ MANAGEMENT

Management of hemophiliac children not only includes control of bleeding with replacement therapy of deficient factor, but also a comprehensive team approach. The comprehensive care of these patients involves team approach of hematologists, physiotherapists, surgeons, and orthopedic surgeons experienced in handling hemophiliac patients, dentists, psychologists, medical social workers, etc. It is essential to educate the patient and his family, and concerned people about the disease, steps to prevent bleeding, and need to seek early medical care.

The fundamental treatment of bleeding in hemophilia is replacement therapy of missing coagulation factors. Proper and prompt use of conservative and preventive measures will help in the management of bleeding, and preventing further damage to the tissues and organs. Treatment is mainly given to minimize permanent damage, for symptomatic relief of the pain, for prevention of tissue damage, to permit tissue healing, and to restore the function.

Whenever available factors like cryoprecipitate, fresh plasma, and specific factor concentrate should be administered as promptly as possible when the bleeding episode begins or is recognized. Even early minimal amount of replacement therapy in conjunction with conservative management and preventive measures helps in the management of bleeding problems in hemophiliac patients, particularly in developing countries. However, with the availability of factor concentrates, it is now possible for hemophiliacs to live a normal healthy life.

Prevention of Bleeding

Conservative management like application of ice wrapped in thick cloth applied at the local site of bleeding and pressure bandage are effective in stopping bleeding.

Local bleeding from the tooth, tongue, gingival, etc. may be stopped by applying topical thrombin preparation or gauge soaked in diluted epinephrine solution (1:10,000 aqueous epinephrine). Topical hemostatic preparation may also be applied to the skin abrasions.

Bleeding in the mouth cavity or gum may be controlled using epsilon-aminocaproic acid (EACA) (75 mg/kg/dose) or tranexamic acid (75 mg/kg/day) mixed with water and kept in mouth or gargled and then swallowed. Hematuria can be treated with watchful waiting and high fluid intake, i.e., 150–200 mL/h to prevent clot genitourinary tract.

In many cases of mild hemophilia A and most cases of vWD, desmopressin is useful as it is capable of releasing sufficient factor VIII, particularly in mild-to-moderate hemophiliac cases. This hormone desmopressin acetate (DDAVP) can be given intravenously, by subcutaneous injection, or in highly concentrated preparations by intranasal spray.

DDAVP when administered intravenously in dose of 0.3 μg/kg produces three- to fivefold increase in plasma level of factor VIII and vWF. Side effects are minimal, which include facial flushing, headache, tachycardia, abdominal cramps, nausea, hypo/hypertension.

Hemarthrosis is managed by 25 units of the factor VII per kg body weight every 12th hourly for 1 day. Aspiration of blood from the joint should not be done. Aspirin or indomethacin cannot be used to reduce the pain as these inhibit platelet functions. Hence, paracetamol, pethidine, or diazepam may be used.

Infection predisposes hemophiliacs to further bleeding and hence early antibiotic therapy is recommended during proven infection. However intramuscular injection should be avoided because of the risk of provoking hemorrhage and hematoma.

Replacement of Deficient Factor to Prevent Hemorrhage

Replacement of the deficient factor is the mainstay in management of hereditary coagulation disorder. The main aim of replacement therapy is to raise the level of deficient clotting factor to a level, which will achieve hemostasis and prompt arrest of the bleeding, and maintain it till complete healing takes place. Therefore, before giving the treatment it is essential to know the exact nature and degree of deficiency of the factor.

One unit of factor VIII or IX is the amount of factor present in 1 cc of fresh, normal citrated plasma prepared from the blood collected in 3.8% trisodium citrate solution in the proportion of 9:1.

Therapeutic materials available for the treatment of classical hemophilia are as follows:

Fresh whole blood: This is used only when there is acute blood loss or hypovolemia. However, the amount of blood and the rate of transfusion required to achieve hemostatic level of factor VIII are to be practicable. Factors VIII and V are labile, and hence they disappear from the stored blood.

Fresh frozen plasma (FFP): This became the mainstay of plasma replacement therapy. In this process, whole blood is collected in citrate–phosphate–dextrose (CPD) or in CPD adenine, and centrifuged within 4-6 hours after collection. The supernatant plasma diluted approximately 20% by anticoagulants, separated in a closed system and stored at or below –30°C.

This plasma contains essentially normal level of factors except factors V and VIII, which often lose some activities during several months of storage even at 30°C. Factor VIII level is present normally at 0.6–0.7 U/mL (60-70%). Each bag of FFP contains 180–220 mL of plasma (approximately 180–200 units of factor VIII and IX). It is readily available in the thawed material. It is useful only in the management of mild bleeding. Only 10–15 mL of plasma/kg may be given with safety in a single dose with an expected rise of 20–30% in factor VIII activity. It should be compatible with the recipient's ABO blood type to avoid transfusion reactions.

Plasma transfusion is the only known treatment for patients with rare inherited deficiency of factors V, XI, XII, and XIII. The treatment for hemorrhagic episodes in patients with Christmas disease (factor IX deficiency) is use of plasma, which need not be fresh frozen because factor IX is stable in stored plasma. However, factor concentrate may also be used. It is also useful in acquired bleeding disorders like disseminated intravascular coagulation (DIC) and hemorrhages secondary to liver disease.

Cryoprecipitate

One of the most important breakthroughs in the management of hemophilia is the development of cryoprecipitate. FFP is collected within 6 hours of procurement of blood and rapidly frozen at –70°C. It is then slowly thawed at 2°–4°C for 18-24 hours. Subsequently, plasma is separated by rapid centrifugation from the precipitate, which is refrozen and stored at temperature below –18°C for 3-12 months. The supernatant plasma is used for other purposes also as it contains all clotting factors except factor VIII and fibrinogen.

Cryoprecipitate constitutes: (1) Antihemophilic factor (factor VIII); 40–160 U/bag; (2) ristocetin factor or vWF (factor VIIIR cofactor); (3) factor VIII-related antigen (factor VIIIR Ag); (4) fibrinogen (200–250 mg of fibrinogen/bag); (5) fibronectin (cold insoluble globulin); and (6) factor XIII and trace elements of other factors.

Factor VIII Concentrate (Lyophilized Antihemophilic Factor)

Lyophilized concentrates containing 250–1,500 units of factor VIIIc in a reconstituted volume of about 25 cc and are prepared from large pools of FFP from 2,000 to 5,000 paid donors. Factor VIII is purified by combining cryoprecipitation and precipitation with glycine, polyethylene glycol, or ethanol, and further fractionated and freeze dried.

Early, appropriate therapy is the hallmark or excellent hemophilia care. When mild-to-moderate bleeding occurs, values of factor VIII or IX factor must be raised to hemostatic levels, in the 35–50% range. For life-threatening or major hemorrhages, the dose should aim to achieve 100% activity.

Dose of the factors hemostatic levels of factor VIII required may vary because of the following:
- Type of bleeding episode
- *Infection at the site of bleeding:* It increases the dose of factor VIII and the duration of therapy.
- *Interference with the wound:* It should be minimal. Handling should be appropriately timed, e.g., dressing of the wound and physiotherapy should be done after factor VIII administration.

Calculation of the dose of recombinant factor VIII (rFVIII) or recombinant factor IX (rFIX) is as follows:
- Dose of rFVIII (IU) = % Desired (rise in rFVIII) × Body weight (kg) × 0.5
- Dose of rFIX (IU) = % Desired (rise of plasma rFIX) × Body weight (kg) × 1.4

For factor VIII, the correction factor is based on the volume of distribution of factor VIII. For factor IX, the correction factor is based on the volume of distribution and the observed rise in plasma level after infusion of recombinant factor IX.

With patient severe hemophilia and hemarthrosis requires 15 U/kg of factor VII every 12–24 hours for 1–2 days. In ICH, 40–50 U/kg every 12 hours for 7–14 days is recommended.

When lyophilized products are used, dosage may be calculated to the nearest vial based on the assay amount printed on the manufacturer's label. When the bags of cryoprecipitate are used, the calculation should be to the nearest bag and should be calculated based on 100 U/bag as the average content. However, this amount varies from one blood bank to another.

Prothrombin Complex Concentrates

Lyophilized concentrates of factors II, VII, IX, X containing 500–1,000 IU of factor IX in 25 cc are marketed mainly for treatment of factor IX deficiency. However, they can be used for other rare bleeding disorders as in congenital or acquired deficiencies of factors II, VII, and X. It is also used for the patients with antibodies for factors VII and IX.

Activated Prothrombin Complex Concentrates

This product was mainly developed to bypass factor VIII or factor IX, especially for persons with a high level of inhibitors to factors VII and IX. However, high cost, high risk of transmission of hepatitis and acquired immunodeficiency syndrome (AIDS), and difficulty in laboratory monitoring for the effectiveness have limited its use.

Porcine Factor VIII Concentrate

Factor VIII concentrate made from porcine plasma has low cross-activity toward most antibodies. Use of this product was limited in the past due to severe adverse effects like anaphylaxis, thrombocytopenia, and pyrogenic reactions.

The frequency of administration of the factors mainly depends on the half-life of the involved factors. The half-life of factor VIII is 12 hours and that for factor IX 18–24 hours. Hence factor VIII needs to be infused twice a day and the second dose being at least two-thirds of the former. For Christmas disease, once a day replacement is sufficient.

Duration of treatment depends on:
- Severity of the bleeding
- Site of bleeding
- Extent of the tissue damage and how long the wound remains in fragile state
- Time required for wound healing.

For Mild Hemorrhage and Hemarthrosis

The therapy should be continued for 1–2 days or till pain in the joint subsides, for major bleeds 3–7 days, for dental extraction 7–10 days, for laparotomy 10–14 days; and for deep tissue operation 3–4 weeks. Hence, before embarking on any surgical procedure, it is necessary to ensure that sufficient material is available, patients can afford, and adequate laboratory facilities for investigations required, e.g., aPTT and factors assays, are available to monitor.

Plasma-borne Infections

Transfusion hepatitis, there are multiple causes of hepatitis A, B, non-A, non-B, hepatitis C and cytomegalovirus; chronic liver disease (CLD) retrospective reviews it has been shown that most ICH often occurs in patients with platelet counts below $20 \times 10^9/L$. When the period of thrombocytopenia is reduced, it reduces the risk of ICH.

■ TREATMENT OF HEMOPHILIA

Hemarthrosis

Hemophilia A: 50–60 IU/kg factor VIII concentrate on day 1; then 20–30 IU/kg on days 2, 3, 5 until joint function is normal or back to baseline; consider additional treatment every other day for 7–10 days. Consider prophylaxis.

Hemophilia B: 80–100 IU/kg on day 1; then 40 IU/kg on 2–4 days; consider additional treatment every other day for 7–10 days. Consider prophylaxis.

Muscular or Significant Subcutaneous Hematoma

Hemophilia A: 50 IU/kg factor VIII concentrate; 20 IU/kg every other day treatment may be needed until resolved.

Hemophilia B: 80 IU/kg factor IX concentrate; treatment every 2–3 days may be needed until resolved.

Mouth, Deciduous Tooth, or Tooth Extraction

Hemophilia A: 20 IU/kg factor VIII concentrate; antifibrinolytic therapy; remove loose deciduous tooth.

Hemophilia B: 40 IU/kg factor IX concentrate; antifibrinolytic therapy; remove loose deciduous tooth.

Epistaxis

Hemophilia A: Apply pressure for 15–20 minutes; pack with petrolatum gauze; give antifibrinolytic therapy; 20 IU/kg factor VIII concentrate if this treatment fails.

Hemophilia B: Apply pressure for 15–20 minutes; pack with petrolatum gauze; give antifibrinolytic therapy; 30 IU/kg factor IX concentrate if this treatment fails.

Major Surgery, Life-threatening Hemorrhage

Hemophilia A: 50–75 IU/kg factor VIII concentrate, then initiate 25 IU/kg q8–12 hours to maintain trough level >50 IU/dL for 5–7 days, then 50 IU/kg q 24 hours to maintain trough >25 IU/dL for 7 days.

Hemophilia B: 120 IU/kg factor IX concentrate, then 50–60 IU/kg every 12–24 hours to maintain factor IX at >40 IU/dL for 5–7 days, and then at >30 IU/dL for 7 days.

Hematuria

Hemophilia A: Bedrest; 1.5 × maintenance fluids; if not controlled in 1–2 days, 20 IU/kg factor VIII concentrate; if not controlled, give prednisone [unless patient is human immunodeficiency virus (HIV)-infected].

Hemophilia B: Bedrest; 1.5 × maintenance fluids; if not controlled in 1–2 days, 40 IU/kg factor IX concentrate; if not controlled, give prednisone (unless patient is HIV-infected).

Prophylactic Therapy

It includes 10–20 units of factor VIII twice or thrice a week to convert severe hemophilia to moderate one. Drugs such as EACA and tranexamic acid are inhibitors of fibrinolytic enzyme. These inhibit the clot lysis and promote the homeostasis. Desmopressin acetate is useful in stopping bleeding.

For minor surgery: Plasma level should be elevated to 100% 1 hour prior to procedure (50 U/kg) and maintain the plasma level above 60% for 4 days and above and 20% for subsequent 4 days.

For major surgery: Initial dose is same as above, the level is elevated to 100%, next 4 days factor level is maintained at 60% and subsequent 4 days 40% levels are maintained till all drains and sutures are removed.

For orthopedic surgery: Factor level should be maintained to 100%. After the operation plasma factor level should be maintained at 80% with 40 U/kg three times a day for 4 days. 40% level should be maintained for subsequent 4 days.

Antenatal diagnosis is possible for obtaining fetal blood at 18–20 weeks of gestation in male fetuses. Affected factors will have reduced level of procoagulant competent of factor VIII.

Hemophilia A: 20–40 IU/kg factor VIII concentrate every other day to achieve a trough level ≥1%.

Hemophilia B: 30–50 IU/kg factor IX concentrate every 2–3 days to achieve a trough level ≥1%.

■ CHRONIC COMPLICATIONS

Long-term complications of hemophilia A and B include chronic arthropathy, the development of an inhibitor to either factor VIII or factor IX, and the risk of transfusion-transmitted infectious diseases.

Historically, chronic arthropathy has been the major long-term disability associated with hemophilia. The natural history of untreated hemophilia is one of cyclic recurrent hemorrhages into specific joints, including hemorrhages into the same (target) joint. In young children, the joint distends easily, and a large volume of blood may fill the joint until tamponade ensues or therapy intervenes. After joint hemorrhage, proteolytic enzymes are released by white blood cells (WBCs) into the joint space, and heme iron induces macrophage proliferation, leading to inflammation of the synovium. The synovium thickens and develops frondlike projections into the joint that are susceptible to being pinched and may induce further hemorrhage. The cartilaginous surface becomes eroded and ultimately may even expose raw bone, leaving the joint susceptible to articular fusion. In the older patient with advanced arthropathy, bleeding into the target joint, with its thickened synovium, causes severe pain, because the joint may have little space to accommodate blood. Once a target joint is seen to be developing, the patient is usually given short- or long-term prophylaxis to prevent progression of the arthropathy and reduce inflammation.

■ INHIBITOR FORMATION

Infusion of the deficient clotting factor may initiate an immune response in patients with either factor VIII or factor IX deficiency. Inhibitors are antibodies directed against factor VII or factor IX that block the clotting activity. Failure of a bleeding episode to respond to appropriate replacement therapy is usually the first sign of an inhibitor. Many patients who have an inhibitor will lose it with continued regular infusions. Others have a higher titer of antibody with subsequent infusions and may need to go through desensitization (immune tolerance induction) programs, in which high doses of factor VIII for hemophilia A or factor IX for hemophilia B are infused in an attempt to saturate the antibody and permit the body to develop tolerance.

BIBLIOGRAPHY

1. George LA, Fogarty PF. Gene therapy for hemophilia; past present and future. Semin Hematol. 2016;53(1):46-54.
2. Kumar R, Carcao M. Inherited abnormalities of coagulation: hemophilia, von Willebrand disease, and beyond. Pediatr Clin North Am. 2013;60(6):1419-41.
3. Laffan M. New products for treatment of hemophilia. Br J Haematol. 2016;172(1):23-31.
4. Robert HR, Escobar M, White II GC. Hemophilia A and Hemophilia B. In: Lichtman MA, Beutler E (Eds). Williams Hematology, 7th edition. New York: McGraw-Hill; 2006.
5. Srivastava A, Brewer AK, Mauser-Bunschoten EP, Key NS, Kitchen S, Llinas A, et al.; Treatment Guidelines Working Group on Behalf of The World Federation of Hemophilia. Guidelines for the management of hemophilia. Haemophilia. 2013;19(1):e1-47.
6. Zimmerman B, Valentino LA. Hemophilia: in review. Pediatr Rev. 2013;34(7):289-94.

36 CASE

Hemorrhagic Disease of the Newborn

■ PRESENTING COMPLAINTS

A 3-day-old girl was brought with the complaint of:
- Blood in stool since 1 day
- Blood staining at umbilical cord since 1 day

History of Presenting Complaints

A 3-day-old girl was brought to the hospital with a history of passing the blood in motion. Her mother told that her child passed meconium for the first 2 days. Later, the child passed a yellowish-curdled type of motion two to three times. She noticed that the next motion was blood-stained and subsequent motions were bloody. Child was not irritable. The mother also complained of blood staining at the umbilical cord.

Past History of the Patient

The child was born at full term by normal vaginal delivery. The child was delivered at home. The age of the mother at the time of delivery was 17 years. There was a history of mother taking sleeping pills often. The postnatal period was normal. The birth weight of the child was 3.25 kg. The head circumference was 35 cm. The child started taking breastfeeds regularly. There was no history of cracked nipples.

■ EXAMINATION

The newborn was moderately built and nourished. There were no dysmorphic features. Features of postdated delivery were present. Anthropometric measurements include the weight of 3 kg (50th centile), the length of 50 cm (50th centile), and the head circumference of 35 cm.

The child was afebrile. Pulse rate was 116 beats per minute and respiratory rate was 34 breaths per minute. Blood pressure recorded was 56/42 mm Hg. There was no pallor, no cyanosis, and significant lymphadenopathy. Bleeding was present at the

CASE AT A GLANCE

Basic Findings
- Length : 50 cm (50th centile)
- Weight : 3 kg (50th centile)
- Temperature : 37°C
- Pulse rate : 116 beats/min
- Respiratory rate : 34 breaths/min
- Blood pressure : 56/42 mm Hg

Positive Findings

History:
- Blood in motion
- Bleeding at umbilical stump

Examination:
- Bleeding at umbilical stump
- Normal systemic examinations

Investigation:
- Prothrombin time (PT): Increased
- Partial thromboplastin time (PTT): Increased
- Decreased level of clotting factors

umbilical stump. Abdominal examination was normal. All other systemic examinations were normal.

INVESTIGATION

- *Hemoglobin:* 16.5 g/dL
- *TLC:* 10,000 cells/mm^3
- *Differential leukocyte count (DLC):* P65 L28 E6 M1 B0
- *Platelet count:* 4,00,000 cells/mm^3
- *PT:* 15 seconds
- *PTT:* 40 seconds
- Clotting factors II, VII, IX, and X are decreased

DISCUSSION

The history of ingestion of the sleeping pills could be an important factor, but the platelet count is normal, and hence it may not be thrombocytopenia. Infants with disseminated enterovirus may develop bleeding as a result of bleeding necrosis and DIC.

There is often a history of maternal peripartum illness. These babies usually present at the age of 3–5 days of life. Here, hepatosplenomegaly is present. Baby is extremely sick. Clotting factor studies would show the defects of intrinsic and extrinsic systems and thrombocytopenia. Hemorrhagic disease of newborns is usually due to vitamin K deficiency.

Vitamin K deficiency bleeding (VKDB) in the newborn, previously known as hemorrhagic disease of the newborn, is classified as early, classical, or late.

Neonates have a unique hemostatic system that places them at high risk for hemorrhagic complications, especially in the presence of illness or other stress. Plasma levels of the vitamin K-dependent coagulation factors (I, VII, IX, X, protein C and protein S) and antithrombin are low at birth and do not reach adult ranges until approximately 6 months of age. Thrombin generation and platelet function are also altered in normal newborns. Consequently, both congenital and acquired bleeding disorders that affect primary or secondary hemostasis can manifest in the newborn period. In general, hemorrhage in a healthy neonate suggests an inherited coagulation defect or immune-mediated thrombocytopenia, whereas bleeding symptoms in a sick neonate are more likely to reflect underproduction or consumption of coagulation factors and/or platelets.

Congenital hemorrhagic disorders such as hemophilia can present with bleeding in the newborn period. Common acquired hemorrhagic disorders include VKDB, disseminated intravascular coagulation, and immune-mediated thrombocytopenia.

Prodromal or warning signs (mild bleeding) may occur before serious ICH. Laboratory testing reveals that the pathophysiology of this acquired hemorrhagic disorder results because vitamin K facilitates postranscriptional carboxylation of factors I, VII, IX, and X, which is necessary for its full coagulation effects. In the absence of carboxylation, such factors form *proteins induced in vitamin K absence* (*PIVKA*), which have greatly reduced function; these can be measured and represent a sensitive marker for vitamin K status. In contrast, factors V and VIII, fibrinogen, bleeding time (BT), clot retraction, and platelet count and function are normal for maturity.

This classic form of hemorrhagic disease of the newborn, which is responsive to (and entirely prevented by) exogenous vitamin K therapy, should be distinguished from rare congenital deficiencies of clotting factors that are unresponsive to vitamin K, which can occur in otherwise well-appearing infants.

Early-onset VKDB (after birth but in first 24 hours) occurs if the mother has been treated chronically with certain drugs (e.g., anticoagulant warfarin, anticonvulsant phenytoin or phenobarbital, and cholesterol-lowering medication) that interfere with vitamin K absorption or function. These infants can have severe bleeding, which is usually corrected promptly by vitamin K administration, although some have a poor or delayed response.

Early-onset VKDB is due to the cross-placental transfer of compounds that interfere with vitamin K metabolism or function, including some anticonvulsant drugs, antibiotics, antituberculous agents, and vitamin K antagonists.

Classical VKDB occurs in the first week of life and is due to a physiological deficiency in vitamin K at birth combined with a lack of vitamin K in breast milk or inadequate feeding. Vitamin K prophylaxis has its biggest impact in preventing this type of bleeding.

Late-onset VKDB can occur at any age, although it is classically described as occurring between 2 weeks and 6 months of age. In infants, it is again due to inadequate vitamin K content in breast milk and is thus found almost universally in those exclusively breastfed.

If a mother is known to be receiving such drugs late in gestation, an infant PT should be measured using cord blood, and the infant immediately should be given 1–2 mg of vitamin K intravenously. If PT is greatly prolonged and tails to improve, or in the presence of significant hemorrhage, 10–15 mL/kg of fresh-frozen plasma should be administered. In contrast, late-onset VKDB (after 2 weeks of life) is usually associated with conditions that feature malabsorption of the fat-soluble vitamin K, such as cystic fibrosis, neonatal hepatitis, or biliary atresia, and bleeding can be severe.

Other forms of neonatal bleeding may be clinically indistinguishable from hemorrhagic disease of the newborn due to vitamin K deficiency, but they are neither prevented nor successfully treated with vitamin K. For example, an identical clinical presentation may also result from any congenital defect in blood coagulation factors. Hematomas, melena, and postcircumcision and umbilical cord bleeding may be present; up to 70% cases of hemophilia (factor VII or IX deficiency) are clinically apparent in the newborn period. Treatment of these congenital deficiencies of coagulation factors requires specific factor replacement or fresh-frozen plasma if factor concentrate is not available.

■ PATHOGENESIS

Hemorrhagic disease of the newborn resulting from severe transient deficiencies in vitamin K-dependent factors is characterized by bleeding that tends to be GI, nasal, subgaleal, intracranial, or postcircumcision. Prodromal or warning signs (mild bleeding) may occur before serious ICH. The PT, blood coagulation time, and PTT are prolonged, and levels of prothrombin (II) and factors VII, IX, and X are decreased. Vitamin K facilitates post-transcriptional carboxylation of factors II, VII, IX, and X. In the absence of carboxylation, such factors form PIVKA, which is a sensitive marker for vitamin K status. BT, fibrinogen, factors V and VIII, platelets, capillary fragility, and clot retraction are normal for maturity.

A transient deficiency of vitamin K occurs. This is probably due to the lack of free vitamin K in mother, immaturity of the liver in infants, and absence of bacterial intestinal flora, which is responsible for the synthesis of vitamin K. Severe deficiency of vitamin K-dependent factor has been reported in infants born to a mother receiving anticonvulsants during pregnancy, especially phenobarbitone and phenytoin. Transfer of vitamin K from mother to fetus is low so that newborn plasma levels are less than one-tenth of maternal levels. Hence, the concentration of vitamin-dependent factors will come down in the first few weeks of life in solely breastfed babies of inadequate intake.

A moderate decrease in factors II, VII, IX, and X normally occurs in all newborn infants by 48–72 hours after birth, with a gradual return to birth levels by 7–10 days of age. This transient deficiency of vitamin K-dependent factors is probably caused by a lack of free vitamin K from the mother and the absence of the bacterial intestinal flora responsible for the synthesis of vitamin K.

The prolongation of this deficiency is seen in premature infants between 2nd and 5th day of life. This results in a moderate decrease in vitamin K-dependent factors. These include clotting factors II, VII, IX, and X. The decrease is normally seen in all newborns by 48–72 hours after birth. They gradually return to normal by 7–10 days. This results in spontaneous and prolonged bleeding. Breast milk is a poor source of vitamin K, and hence it is more common in breastfed infants.

Breast milk is a poor source of vitamin K, therefore hemorrhagic complications are more frequent in breastfed than in formula-fed infants. This classic form of hemorrhagic disease of the newborn, which is responsive to and prevented by vitamin K therapy, must be distinguished from DIC and from the more infrequent congenital deficiencies of one or more of the other factors that are unresponsive to vitamin K. Early-onset life-threatening VKDB (onset from birth to 1–2 hours) also occurs if the mother has been treated with drugs (phenobarbital and phenytoin) that interfere with vitamin K function. Late onset (>2 weeks) is often associated with vitamin K malabsorption, as noted in neonatal hepatitis or biliary atresia.

■ CLINICAL FEATURES (FIG. 1)

The clinical features of VKDB are similar to other coagulation disorders. The typical presenting symptoms are bruising mucous membrane bleeding, excessive bleeding associated with trauma or invasive procedures, or signs of internal hemorrhage such as abdominal pain, headache, or vomiting. While so-called warning bleeds (bruising and epistaxis) may precede severe internal hemorrhage, they do not always occur. The incidence of ICH in late-onset VKDB is 30–60%. Bleeding in a newborn can be serious. A lot of blood can be lost in a few minutes from the umbilical stump and also from the ICH that may also occur.

> **ESSENTIAL DIAGNOSTIC POINTS**
> - History of maternal peripartum illness
> - Babies usually present at the age of 3–5 days of life
> - Hepatosplenomegaly is present
> - Clotting factor studies would show the defects of intrinsic and extrinsic systems
> - Thrombocytopenia
> - Usually due to vitamin K deficiency
> - Moderate decrease of clotting factors II, VII, IX, and X

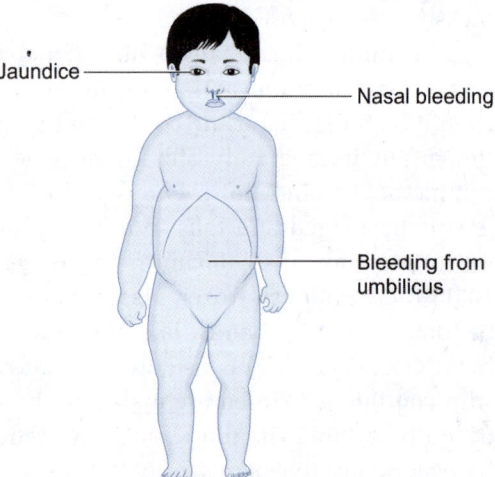

Fig. 1: Clinical features.

■ DIAGNOSIS

There will be bleeding in GI tract, nasal bleeding and ICH. BT, clotting time (CT), and PTT are prolonged. Clotting factors II, VII, IX, and X are reduced. BT, fibrinogen, factor V and factor VII, platelets, capillary fragility, and clot retraction or normal for maturity. However, severe bleeding in premature infants may require blood transfusion.

Essential investigations for all cases include hemoglobin estimation, red cell morphology, TLC, DLC, platelet count, and reticulocyte count.

Apt Test

The Apt test should be performed when there is only GI bleeding in a well neonate in the first 48 hours of life and is used to distinguish maternal from neonatal blood. One part of vomitus is mixed with five parts of distilled water and centrifuged. The pink centrifuged supernatant fluid, 1 mL of 1% sodium hydroxide is added and waited for 1–2 minutes, if the solution changes to yellow–brown color, it favors the possibility of swallowed maternal blood [hemoglobin A (HbA) gets denatured by alkali while fetal hemoglobin (HbF) stays pink].

Screening Tests

Patients suspected of having VKDB should have a complete blood count (CBC) to assess the platelet count, PT, and aPTT tests to screen for deficiencies of specific-clotting factors. The PT is always prolonged, often to a very significant degree, and the aPTT is usually increased as well. In early or mild vitamin K deficiency, it is possible that only factor VII is reduced, due to its short half-life, thus leading to a prolonged PT but normal aPTT. In the typical scenario, the PT is prolonged out of proportion to the aPTT; for example, the PT is about 4 times the mean of the normal range versus an aPTT that is approximately twice the normal.

A neonate who has a positive bleeding history or is having active bleeding should have platelet count, BT, PTT, and PT done. If the results are normal, a thrombin time and VWF testing should be considered. If the initial test results are abnormal, special tests should be planned.

Special Tests

Special tests are required to:
- Identify the deficient coagulation factor
- To determine the degree of deficiency
- To detect and quantitate immune inhibitors
- They include prothrombin consumption test, coagulation factor assays, and platelet function tests.

GENERAL FEATURES
• Gastrointestinal (GI) bleeding
• Melena
• Hematemesis
• Not taking feeds

LABORATORY SALIENT FINDINGS
• Bleeding time (BT), clotting time (CT), and partial thromboplastin time (PTT) are prolonged
• Clotting factors II, VII, IX and X are reduced

■ DIFFERENTIAL DIAGNOSIS

The differential diagnosis includes hemophilia and other congenital factor deficiencies, von Willebrand disease, platelet function abnormalities, and liver disease-associated coagulopathy. The most common disorder that can be mistaken for VKDB is liver disease-associated coagulopathy, as both result from deficiencies of some of the same clotting factors. The vitamin K-dependent factors II, VII, IX, and X are all synthesized in the liver and are deficient in both conditions. Thus, the PT, aPTT, and specific measurement of these factors will not distinguish the two conditions. Moreover, the two conditions can coexist as liver dysfunction resulting from obstructed biliary flow can lead to vitamin K deficiency. Ultimately, the lack of response to parenteral vitamin K administration may be the most important diagnostic clue.

■ TREATMENT

Intramuscular administration of 1 mg of vitamin K at the time of birth prevents the decrease in vitamin K-dependent factors in full-term infants, but it is not uniformly effective in the prophylaxis of hemorrhagic disease of the newborn, particularly in breastfed and premature infants. The disease may be effectively treated with a slow IV infusion of 1–5 mg of vitamin K, with improvement in coagulation defects and cessation of bleeding noted within a few hours. Serious bleeding, particularly in premature infants or those with liver disease, may require a transfusion of fresh-frozen plasma or whole blood. The mortality rate is low in treated patients.

A concentrated form of vitamin K-dependent coagulation factor should be avoided because of the risk of transmitting serum hepatitis.

A particularly severe form of deficiency of vitamin K-dependent coagulation factors has been reported in infants born to mothers receiving anticonvulsive medications (phenobarbital and phenytoin) during pregnancy. The infants may have severe bleeding with onset within the first 24 hours of life; the bleeding is usually corrected by vitamin K, although in some, the response is poor or delayed. PT should be measured in cord blood, and the infant should be given 1–2 mg of vitamin K intravenously. If the PT is greatly pronged and fails to improve, 10 mL/kg of fresh-frozen plasma should be administered.

The routine use of intramuscular vitamin K for prophylaxis is safe and is not associated with an increased risk of childhood cancer or leukemia. Although oral vitamin K (birth, discharge, 3–4 weeks: 1–2 mg) has been suggested as an alternative, oral vitamin K is less effective in preventing the late onset of bleeding due vitamin K deficiency, and thus cannot be recommended for routine therapy. The intramuscular route remains the method of choice.

Other forms of bleeding may be clinically indistinguishable from hemorrhagic disease of the newborn responsive to vitamin K, but they are neither prevented nor successfully treated with vitamin K. A clinical pattern identical to that of hemorrhagic disease of the newborn may also result from any of the congenital defects in blood coagulation. Hematomas, melena, and postcircumcision and umbilical cord bleeding may be present; only 5–35% of rises of factor VIII and IX deficiency become clinically apparent in the newborn period. Treatment of the rare congenital deficiencies of coagulation factors requires fresh-frozen plasma or specific factor replacement.

Once correction of vitamin K deficiency is achieved, its cause must be identified so that preventive actions can be instituted to prevent a recurrence. In early onset VKDB, this may include cessation of breastfeeding, if a mother is required to take medication that interferes with vitamin K metabolism, that may be passed to the infant via breast milk. In classical VKDB, additional vitamin K administration may be required if poor feeding is an ongoing problem or if a mother insists on exclusively breastfeeding. In late-onset VKDB, correction of the underlying disorder should be undertaken, if possible, and continued vitamin K therapy (often parentally) may be required.

■ PREVENTION

There is no question that vitamin K prophylaxis is effective at reducing the risk for VKDB in infants, but controversies exist regarding the route of administration and, to some extent, the dosing. The advantage of intramuscular prophylaxis, which is widely used, is its long duration of action, presumably from a depot effect. Newborns receiving intramuscular prophylaxis have increased levels of vitamin K for at least 4 weeks compared to those receiving no prophylaxis so far. The disadvantages are discomfort, poor acceptance by some parents, and rarely, intramuscular hematomas, local abscesses, and the potential for local nerve and vessel damage. Finally, extremely high levels of vitamin K are achieved following intramuscular injection, and it remains unknown whether this could be harmful.

Oral vitamin K prophylaxis is the preferred method. Dosing regimens vary based on local practice and guidelines. In addition to avoidance of extraordinarily high levels of vitamin K, the oral route is also more acceptable to parents. Its principal disadvantage is that administration must continue after discharge from the hospital, leading to an increased pool of at-risk infants due to poor compliance. Regardless of the chosen method, it is vital that prophylaxis must be given to all infants. In particular, babies born at home or in other nonhospital settings are at higher risk for not receiving prophylaxis, so parents should be questioned about this at first contact with the pediatrician.

■ BIBLIOGRAPHY

1. Mihatsch WA, Braegger C, Bronsky J, Campoy C, Domellöf M, Fewtrell M, et al. Prevention of vitamin K deficiency bleeding in newborn infants: a position paper by the ESPGHAN Committee on Nutrition. J Pediatr Gastroenterol Nutr. 2016;63(1);123-9.
2. Weddle M, Empey A, Crossen E, Green A, Green J, Phillipi CA. Are pediatrician complicit in vitamin K deficiency bleeding? Pediatrics. 2015;136(4)753-7.

CASE 37

Henoch–Schönlein Purpura

■ PRESENTING COMPLAINTS

A 2-year-old boy was brought with the complaint of:
- Rashes since 1 day
- Uneasiness since 1 day

History of Presenting Complaints

A 2-year-old boy was brought to the casualty with a history of florid rash over the forearm, hands, trunk, buttocks, and lower limbs. All these developed spontaneously within the last 24 hours. Mother described rashes as circular, red in color with increased redness in center. There was a flushed area surrounding the rash. In spite of these rashes, he was playful. In between, he used to have brief episodes of uneasiness. There was no history of itching.

Past History of the Patient

He was the only sibling of a nonconsanguineous marriage. He was born at full term by normal delivery. Baby cried immediately after the delivery. The birth weight of the baby was 3 kg. Child was given breastfeed immediately. He was on exclusive breast milk for 4 months. Later weaning was started at 4 months, and he was on family food by 18 months. There was no postnatal significant event except for the normal physiological jaundice. Developmental milestones were normal. Child had been completely immunized.

CASE AT A GLANCE

Basic Findings
Height	: 88 cm (90th centile)
Weight	: 13 kg (70th centile)
Temperature	: 37°C
Pulse rate	: 120 beats/min
Respiratory rate	: 32 breaths/min
Blood pressure	: 60/40 mm Hg

Positive Findings

History:
- Rashes
- Sudden onset
- No itching

Examination:
- Rashes over the lower limbs and buttocks

Investigation:
- *Urine:* Red blood cells (RBCs)++, Protein+
- *Immunoglobulin A (IgA) level:* Increased
- *Stool:* RBCs present

■ EXAMINATION

The boy was moderately built and nourished. He was playful and was playing with the toys on the examination table. Anthropometric measurements included height of 88 cm (90th centile) and weight of 13 kg (70th centile).

The child was afebrile. The pulse rate was 120 beats per minute, the respiratory rate was 32 breaths per minute. The blood pressure recorded was 60/40 mm Hg. The rashes were present over the forearms, hands, trunk, buttocks, and lower limbs. These rashes are used to blanch on pressure.

There was no pallor, no lymphadenopathy, and no cyanosis. All the systemic examinations were normal.

■ INVESTIGATION

- *Hemoglobin:* 10 g/dL
- *TLC:* 11,000 cells/mm^3
- *Platelets:* 4,50,000 cells/mm^3
- *PT:* 18 seconds
- *IgA level:* 5 g/dL (increased)
- *C3 complement:* Normal
- *Urine:* RBCs++
  Protein++
- *Stools:* RBCs+

■ DISCUSSION

Henoch–Schönlein Purpura (HSP) is also known as anaphylactoid purpura. It is the vasculitis of small vessels. This illness is more frequent in children than adults. Most cases occur between 2–8 years of age. It is more common in males and in the winter season.

The specific pathogenesis of HSP is not known. The cytokine tumor necrosis factor-alpha (TNF-α) and interleukin 6 (IL-6) have been implicated in active disease. It is an IgA-mediated vasculitis. Perivascular accumulation of white cells is present.

Henoch–Schönlein purpura, recently renamed IgA vasculitis, is an acute leukocytoclastic vasculitis, affecting mainly the small vessels of the skin, joints, GI tract, and kidneys. HSP is the most common form of systemic vasculitis in childhood.

The main features of the disease include nonthrombocytopenic palpable purpura (present in 100% of affected children), arthritis or arthralgias (75–85%), colicky abdominal pain with or without GI hemorrhage (60–85%), and renal involvement (10–50%). Although it can occur at any age, HSP is overwhelmingly a disease of childhood.

The mean age of patients is 6 years. The clinical features of HSP may be atypical at the extremes of age, typically presenting with milder manifestations in infants younger than 2 years of age and a more severe course in adults.

The disease occurs more frequently in males, although sex differences are not seen in patients older than age 16 years. HSP has a seasonal pattern, with peaks in winter and spring. It is an IgA-mediated, leukocytoclastic vasculitis characterized by neutrophil infiltration and fibrinoid necrosis in the walls of arterioles, capillaries, and postcapillary venules, with deposition of IgG, IgA, and C3.

The etiology of the disease is unknown. HSP often follows a respiratory infection. A wide variety of pathogens and other environmental exposures that have been associated with HSP include bacterial infections (group A beta-hemolytic streptococci, *Legionella*, *Yersinia*, *Mycoplasma*), viral infections [Epstein–Barr virus (EBV), varicella-zoster virus, cytomegalovirus, parvovirus, hepatitis B virus], drugs (penicillin and other B-lactam antibiotics, chlorpromazine, quinidine, thiazide diuretics), vaccines (measles, yellow fever, and cholera), food additives, and insect bites. Of all the pathogens linked to HSP, group A beta-hemolytic *Streptococcus* has been studied the most.

GENERAL FEATURES
• Acute onset
• Fatigue
• Rash—maculopapular, petechiae, and purpura
• Renal involvement

■ CLINICAL FEATURES (FIG. 1)

The onset of the disease may be acute or insidious. There will be low-grade fever and fatigue. Headache, loss of appetite and

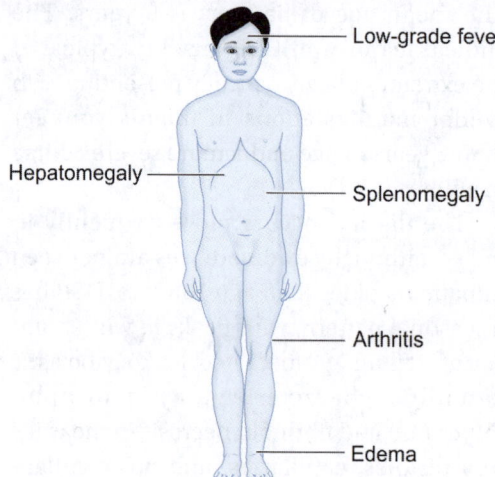

Fig. 1: Clinical features.

abdominal pain are early symptoms. It is a benign self-limiting disease, which resolves after fluctuating course. It involves GI tract, renal system, and joints.

The hallmark of the disease is rash. Initially, they begin as pinkish maculopapules that blanch on pressure. These may progress to petechiae or purpura. These are palpable purpura that evolve from red to purple to rusty brown. These tend to occur in crops. These last from 3–10 days. These appear on legs and feet above the knees and buttocks. This condition can easily be distinguished from other causes because platelet count is in a normal range. Damage to the cutaneous vessels results in local angioedema. Edema occurs primarily in dependent areas—waist, eyes, and buttocks.

Skin lesions, present in all patients because the diagnosis depends on a recognizable rash, are the initial manifestation in about 50% of patients. The typical rashes begin as small wheals or erythematous maculopapules that evolve into petechial or purpuric lesions, more prominent on dependent and pressure-bearing areas. Although usually located over the lower extremities or buttocks, the rashes may involve the upper extremities, trunk, and face. In young children, HSP might present as edema and purpura involving the face and ears. Skin lesions tend to occur in crops and last from 5 days to 4 weeks. Angioedema of the scalp perineal area and extremities may precede the onset of the rash.

Arthritis is the second most common feature of HSP, occurring in roughly 75% of patients and most often affecting knees and ankles. In about 25% of patients, arthritis/arthralgias of large joints is the initial symptom of HSP, often preceding the appearance of a skin rash by 24–48 hours. Because joint swelling is often periarticular, there may be no true joint effusion despite significant pain in motion. Joint symptoms typically resolve spontaneously after a few days without residual deformity but may recur with exacerbations or recurrences of HSP.

Gastrointestinal involvement occurs in 50–75% of patients. The most common complaint is colicky abdominal pain, frequently associated with vomiting. Pain may be severe enough to mimic an acute abdomen and may precede the onset of rash in as many as 10–15% of patients, again confusing the clinical picture. GI bleeding is usually occult, but 30% of patients have grossly bloody or melanotic stools. Upper GI series show nonspecific changes such as thickening of the bowel wall, "thumb printing", and filling defects. Ultrasound studies are abnormal in as many as 80% of patients with GI involvement and reveal increased echogenicity and thickening of the wall of the second portion of the duodenum and/or hydrops of the gallbladder. Endoscopy may reveal lesions with a similar appearance to the palpate purpura seen in the skin. These findings are not present in patients with HSP without GI complaints. Intussusception has been reported in 1–5% of patients; other uncommon complications may include perforation or bowel infarct.

Edema and damage to GI tract may lead to intermittent abdominal pain. This is often colicky in nature. Some may have hematemesis, melena, and diarrhea. There will be associated intussusception, perforation, and bowel obstruction.

Renal involvement occurs in 40– 50% of patients with HSP and is most commonly limited to transient urinary abnormalities such as microscopic hematuria or hematuria plus mild proteinuria leading to chronic renal failure, nephritis, and nephrotic syndrome. Unlike arthritis and GI involvement, nephritis rarely, if ever, precedes the onset of purpura. Patients with nephritis develop urinary abnormalities within 4 weeks, but they may occur up to 3 months after the onset of symptoms. Urinalysis should be done each week while the disease is active, then monthly for the next 3 months: If all analyses are normal, nephritis is unlikely to occur. If at any time there is evidence of nephritis, long-term monitoring of urinalyses, protein excretion, renal function, and blood pressure is warranted until the urinary abnormalities resolve. There will be a focal segmental increase in mesangial cells and matrix. Renal histopathology shows lesions indistinguishable from those of IgA nephropathy (Berger's disease).

Central nervous system involvement leads to the development of seizures, paresis, and coma. Other rare complications include rheumatoid-like nodules, cardiac and eye involvement, mononeuropathies, pancreatitis, and pulmonary and intramuscular damage.

CLINICAL FEATURES
- Acute onset
- Low-grade fever
- Fatigue
- Rash—maculopapular, petechiae, and purpura
- Arthritis
- Edema
- Hepatosplenomegaly
- Renal involvement

■ DIAGNOSIS

Diagnostic criteria include purpura or petechiae (mandatory), more extensive in the lower extremities, and one of the following four criteria:

1. Abdominal pain
2. Histopathology (IgA deposition on biopsy)
3. Arthritis or arthralgia
4. Renal involvement

Routine laboratory tests are neither specific nor diagnostic. There will be moderate thrombocytosis and leukocytosis. Erythrocyte sedimentation rate (ESR) may be raised. Anemia may be present. Immunofluorescent microscopy reveals mesangial deposits of IgA, frequently in association with IgG, C3, and fibrin. The predominant deposits of IgA suggest IgA nephropathy. Definitive diagnosis is confirmed by biopsy of the involved cutaneous sites. Elevated levels of antistreptolysin O (ASLO) titer are noted.

■ DIFFERENTIAL DIAGNOSIS

Differential diagnosis includes:
- Meningococcemia
- Systemic lupus erythematosus (SLE)
- Polyarteritis nodosa
- Goodpasture syndrome
- Kawasaki disease

■ COMPLICATIONS

- Nephrotic syndrome
- Bowel perforation

- Scrotal swelling
- Chronic renal disease

TREATMENT

Treatment is largely supportive. Most children may be managed as outpatients with appropriate analgesia and hydration. Development of GI and renal complications may be monitored by assessing stool guaiac tests, blood pressure, and urine dipsticks as outpatient unless severe intestinal or renal involvement necessitates hospital admission.

Antibiotics are given for streptococcal infection. Steroids are helpful in arthralgia and abdominal pain. Hydration of the patient should be corrected by IV fluid and/or by plenty of oral fluid. Diet should be easily digestible to the gut of the patient. Acetaminophen is used to control pain, edema, fever, and malaise. Other associated systemic diseases are managed accordingly.

Intestinal complications (e.g., hemorrhage, obstruction, and intussusception) may be life threatening and managed with corticosteroids, barium enema reduction, surgical reduction, or resection of intussusception. Oral or IV corticosteroids (1-2 mg/kg/24 hours) are often associated with the dramatic improvement of both GI and CNS complications.

Nonsteroidal anti-inflammatory drugs (NSAIDs) may be used to manage severe joint pain, although they should be avoided in the setting of significant renal disease. Prednisone in a dosage of 1-2 mg/kg/day is helpful in the management of painful edema, scrotal swelling, and severe disabling arthritis. Steroids also may be used in children with severe abdominal pain, although their efficacy has not been proven. Treatment of HSP nephritis remains controversial. Therapies of severe renal disease, particularly chronic changes such as crescent formation, include IV pulses of methylprednisolone, cyclophosphamide, and azathioprine, alone or in different combinations.

BIBLIOGRAPHY

1. Barut K, Sahin S, Kasapcopur O. Peditric vasculitis. Curr Opin Rheumatol. 2016;28(1): 29-38.
2. McCarthy HJ, Tizard EJ. Clinical practice: diagnosis and management of Henoch-Schönlein purpura. Eur J Pediatr. 2010;169(6); 643-50.
3. Ting TV. Diagnosis and management of cutaneous vasculitis in children. Pediatr Clin North Am. 2014;61(2):321-46.

CASE 38

Hereditary Spherocytosis

PRESENTING COMPLAINTS

A 10-year-old boy was brought with the complaint of:
- Cough and cold since 1 week
- Throat pain since 3 days
- Decreased appetite since 3 days
- Abdominal pain since 1 day

History of Presenting Complaints

A 10-year-old boy presented to the casualty with a history of abdominal pain. Pain was present on the left upper part of the abdomen. It was severe colicky pain. It was present since day 1. It was not related to bowel and bladder disturbances. It was not related to food intake. One week back, the child had received treatment for cough, cold, and throat pain. There was no history of vomiting and disturbed sleep. According to the mother, the child's appetite has come down.

Past History of the Patient

The boy was the eldest sibling of non-consanguineous marriage. He was born at full term by normal delivery. There was no significant postnatal event. His developmental milestones were normal. His performance at school was normal.

■ EXAMINATION

On examination, the patient was moderately built and nourished. He was looking sick because of the abdominal pain. The anthropometric measurements included the height of 132 cm (50th centile) and the weight of 28 kg (50th centile).

He was febrile. The pulse rate was 106 beats per minute, the respiratory rate was 26 breaths per minute. The blood pressure recorded was 110/80 mm Hg. Pallor and icterus were present. There was neither lymphadenopathy nor clubbing.

CASE AT A GLANCE

Basic Findings
Height	: 132 cm (50th centile)
Weight	: 28 kg (50th centile)
Temperature	: 38°C
Pulse rate	: 106 beats per minute
Respiratory rate	: 26 breaths per minute
Blood pressure	: 100/80 mm Hg

Positive Findings

History:
- Upper respiratory tract infections (URTI)
- Abdominal pain

Examination:
- Pallor
- Icterus
- Splenomegaly

Investigation:
- *Bilirubin:* Raised
- *Peripheral blood smear:* Small round red cells
- *Coombs test:* Negative

Throat examination revealed the presence of enlarged congested tonsils. Per abdomen examination revealed splenomegaly about 4 cm below the left costal margin. It was tender and soft on palpation. Cardiovascular system examination revealed presence of ejection systolic murmur at the base. There was no radiation of the murmur. Other systemic examinations were normal.

INVESTIGATION

- *Hemoglobin:* 9 g/dL
- *TLC:* 38,600 cells/mm^3
- *Serum bilirubin:* 4.9 g/dL unconjugated bilirubin is raised
- *Mean corpuscular volume (MCV):* 60 fL
- *Mean corpuscular hemoglobin concentration (MCHC):* >36%
- *Platelet count:* 2,50,000 cells/mm^3
- *Reticulocyte count:* 2%
- *Osmotic fragility test:* Increased
- *Peripheral blood smear:* Small red round cells
- *X-ray skull:* Showed widening of diploic space in the frontal and parietal bones
- *Coombs test:* Negative
- *Urine:* Normal

DISCUSSION

The child is anemic and icteric. Raised serum bilirubin is unconjugated type and is the indicator of hemolysis. Pancytopenia is present. Reticulocyte count was low as a result of hemolysis. A negative Coombs test indicates bone marrow hypoplasia.

Hereditary spherocytosis (HS) usually is transmitted as an autosomal dominant or, less commonly, as an autosomal recessive disorder. 25% of patients have no previous family history. The pathophysiology underlying HS involves five proteins that are key components of the cytoskeleton responsible for RBC's shape.

Abnormalities of *ankyrin or spectrin* are the most common molecular defects. Defects in these membrane proteins result in uncoupling of the vertical interactions of the lipid bilayer with the underlying membrane skeleton, with subsequent release of membrane microvesicles. The loss of membrane surface area without a proportional loss of cell volume causes decreased erythrocyte deformability. This impairs cell passage from the splenic cords to the splenic sinuses, leading to the trapping and premature destruction of HS erythrocytes by the spleen.

The need for transfusions in infancy is not indicative of more severe disease later in life because they are typically slow to mount an adequate reticulocyte response to last a few months after birth.

HS patients are susceptible to aplastic crises primarily as a result of *parvovirus B19* infection, *hypoplastic crises* associated with other infections, and *megaloblastic crises* caused by folate deficiency. During these crises, high RBC turnover in the setting of erythroid marrow failure can result in profound anemia (hematocrit <10%), high-output heart failure, cardiovascular collapse, and death. Leukocyte and platelet counts may also fall.

PATHOGENESIS

Abnormalities of spectrin or ankyrin are the most common molecular defects. Dominant defects have been described in β-spectrin and band 3. Recessive defects have been described in α-spectrin and protein 4.2. Both dominant and recessive defects have been described in ankyrin.

A deficiency in spectrin, band 3, ankyrin, or protein 4.2 results in uncoupling in the "vertical" interactions of the lipid bilayer skeleton and subsequent release of membrane microvesicles. The most common molecular defects are abnormalities of the spectrin or ankyrin. The loss of membrane surface area without a proportional loss of cell volume causes sphering of the RBCs. There is associated increase in cation permeability, cation transport, adenosine triphosphate use, and glycolysis. The decreased deformability of the spherocytic RBCs impairs cell passage from the splenic cords to the splenic sinuses, and the spherocytes are destroyed prematurely in the spleen. The decreased abnormality of the spherocytic RBCs impairs cell passage from the splenic cords to splenic sinuses. The spherocytic RBCs are destroyed prematurely in the spleen. Splenectomy improves the RBCs lifespan and cures anemia.

Defects in the erythrocyte membrane lead to loss of membrane surface area and eventual morphologic change. Spherocytes have a decreased ability to deform and quickly become trapped in the sinusoids of the spleen; the majority of hemolysis in spherocytosis, thus, occurs in the extravascular compartment.

The characteristic spherocytic red cell is smaller than the normal erythrocyte and lacks the central pallor of the biconcave disc when the red cells are placed in a hypotonic saline solution. Water and sodium enter the cell causing them to swell.

Hereditary spherocytosis and beta-thalassemia should be considered as the spleen was palpable and red cells were microcytic. Coombs test will be positive if there is an autoimmune process. Acute leukemia with pancytopenia is ruled out because of the presence of unconjugated bilirubin.

Children with congenital hemolytic disease may develop an acute hemolytic crisis or an aplastic crisis. Acute hemolytic crisis is caused by hemolytic episodes provoked by antimalarials. Reticulocyte count remains increased in glucose-6-phosphate dehydrogenase (G6PD). However, the test should be repeated once the acute episode is resolved, and the reticulocyte count have returned to normal.

Other possible diagnoses include:
- Paroxysmal cold hemoglobinuria, which is usually precipitated by viral infection
- Autoimmune hemolytic anemia in which Coombs test is negative
- *Cold agglutinin disease:* This follows a viral infection, especially by *mycoplasma*.
- *Congenital hemolytic anemia*: X-linked inheritance should be explained to the parents. They should be alarmed of the provoking factors such as infections and drugs.

Hereditary spherocytosis is associated with splenomegaly with the red cells that are spherical in shape. Affected cells are unduly permeable to sodium and acquire the spherocytic shape because of the loss of membrane function and increase in volume.

The spleen is intimately involved in the hemolytic process. Splenic circulation imposes a metabolic environment that is characterized by stressful spherocytic cells. Repeated passage through the splenic circulation produces sequestration and destruction. The spherocyte is relatively rigid and passes with difficulty through the minute apertures between splenic cord and sinuses.

In neonates, it may manifest with anemia and hyperbilirubinemia, and slight jaundice may be present after infancy. This may be enough to require phototherapy and exchange transfusion. Spleen is almost always palpable. Pigmentary gallstones have been reported as early as 4–5 years of age.

Evidence of hemolysis includes reticulocytosis, anemia, and hyperbilirubinemia.

Abnormality of the red cell membrane can be demonstrated by osmotic fragility studies. Because of the high RBC turnover and high-tuned erythroid marrow activity, children are prone to aplastic crisis. This occurs as a result of parvovirus.

The diagnosis can be made on the triad of spherocytosis, increased osmotic fragility, and dominant inheritance.

■ CLINICAL FEATURES (FIG. 1)

In the neonatal period, HS is a significant cause of hemolytic disease and can manifest as anemia and hyperbilirubinemia, sufficiently severe to require phototherapy or exchange transfusions. Hemolysis may be more prominent in the newborn because hemoglobin F binds 2,3-DPG poorly, and the increased level of free 2,3-DPG destabilizes interactions among spectrin, actin, and protein 4.1 in the RBC membrane.

Some patients remain asymptomatic into adulthood, but others have severe anemia with pallor, jaundice, fatigue, and exercise intolerance. Severe cases may be marked by expansion of the diploë of the skull as a result of marrow hyperplasia (frontal bossing), but to a lesser extent than in thalassemia major. Depending on the severity of the anemia and the comorbidities associated with severe anemia, some patients benefit from a splenectomy.

After infancy, splenomegaly is common; there is no correlation between spleen size and disease severity. Bilirubin gallstone formation is a function of age; they can form as early as age 4–5 years and are present in the majority of adult patients.

Children with HS are also susceptible to aplastic crises, primarily as a result of parvovirus B19 infection, and to hypoplastic crises associated with various other infections. Turnover in the setting of erythroid marrow failure can result in profound anemia (hematocrit <10%), high-output heart failure, cardiovascular collapse, and death. WBC and platelet counts can also fall. Rare complications associated with HS include splenic sequestration crisis, gout, cardiomyopathy, priapism, leg ulcers, and spinocerebellar degeneration.

Typical manifestations of spherocytosis include partially compensated hemolysis with variable anemia and substantial reticulocytosis. Affected children have intermittent jaundice and palpable splenomegaly, and are at risk for developing pigmented (bilirubin) gallstones due to chronic hemolysis. Because of the dependence on an active marrow output of reticulocytes, severe anemia requiring erythrocyte transfusion (aplastic crisis) can occur in association with acute parvovirus B19 infection and may be the initial clinical presentation. In the newborn period, spherocytosis is often associated with nonphysiologic jaundice in the first 24 hours of life; anemia may be exaggerated during the 1st year of life requiring periodic RBC transfusions.

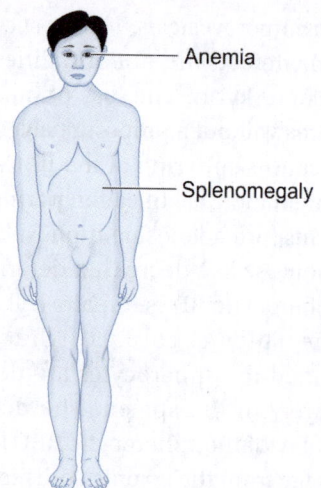

Fig. 1: Clinical features.

Spherocytosis should be considered in any child with anemia, especially if there is a positive family history and splenomegaly. The CBC shows mild-to-moderate anemia with an increased reticulocyte but normal leukocyte and platelet counts. The MCHC is often increased and virtually pathognomonic for spherocytosis when greater than 36 g/dL. Small, dense spherocytes without central pallor can be identified on the peripheral smear, along with larger reticulocytes. A negative direct antiglobulin test [(DAT), formerly known as the direct Coombs test] excludes an autoimmune hemolytic process. The gold standard to establish the diagnosis of spherocytosis is to demonstrate an increased osmotic fragility; this testing may not be required if clinical presentation and family history are consistent with spherocytosis.

> **FEATURES OF HEMOLYTIC ANEMIA**
> - Dark colored urine; dark brown and red
> - Jaundice
> - Pallor
> - Tachycardia
> - Spleen and/liver enlargement

■ LABORATORY FINDINGS

The diagnosis of HS can be established from a positive family history and the presence of typical clinical and laboratory features of the disease: splenomegaly, spherocytes on the blood smear, reticulocytosis, and an elevated MCHC. If these are present, no additional testing is necessary to confirm the diagnosis.

The classic incubated osmotic fragility test can detect the presence of spherocytes in the blood; however, it is not specific to HS and may be abnormal in other hemolytic anemias. The RBCs are incubated in progressive dilutions of sodium chloride causing the RBCs to swell and eventually lyse. Spherocytes lose at a higher sodium chloride concentration than biconcave cells in hypotonic solutions because they have a lower surface area to volume ratio. Unfortunately, this test has poor sensitivity relative to other screening assays and can miss up to 20% of mild HS cases.

Evidence of hemolysis includes and indirect hyperbilirubinemia. The hemoglobin level usually is 6–10 g/dL, but it can be in the normal range. The reticulocyte percentage is often increased to 6–20%, with a mean of approximately 10%. The MCV is normal, although the MCHC is often increased (36–38 g/dL, RBCs). The RBCs on the blood smear vary in size and include polychromatophilic reticulocytes and spherocytes. X-ray shows erythroid hyperplasia. The spherocytes are smaller in diameter and appear hyperchromic as a result of the high hemoglobin concentration. The central pallor is less conspicuous than in normal cells. Spherocytes may be the predominant cells or may be relatively sparse, depending on the severity of the disease. Other evidence of hemolysis includes decreased haptoglobin and the presence of gallstones on ultrasonography.

The presence of spherocytes can be confirmed by osmatic fragility test. The rare causes of spherocytes include thermal injury, Clostridia septicemia, and Wilson's disease.

Diagnosis in the neonatal period requires a high index of suspicion because the disease presents differently than in older children, particularly in de novo and recessively inherited cases where family history is not available for guidance. Jaundice is frequently observed and kernicterus can occur. Hemolytic anemia may be severe enough to require blood transfusion. In fact, HS is the leading cause of Coombs-negative hemolytic anemia requiring transfusion in the 1st month of life. Splenomegaly is uncommon in neonates.

Clinically, HS should be differentiated from other inherited disorders presenting with episodic anemia, jaundice, and splenomegaly, such as other red cell membranopathies, enzymopathies, unstable hemoglobin, and autoimmune hemolytic anemia.

> **LABORATORY SALIENT FINDINGS**
> - Spherocytosis
> - Reticulocytosis
> - Negative Coombs test
> - Elevated indirect bilirubin
> - Increased osmatic fragility
> - Erythroid hyperplasia
> - Splenomegaly and gallstones
> - Elevated mean corpuscular hemoglobin concentration (MCHC)

> **GENERAL FEATURES**
> - Hyperbilirubinemia
> - Fatigue
> - Exercise intolerance
> - Pigmentary gallstones

DIFFERENTIAL DIAGNOSIS

- ABO incompatibility
- Isoimmune hemolytic anemia
- Thermal injury
- Clostridia septicemia
- Wilson's disease

> **ESSENTIAL DIAGNOSTIC POINTS**
> - Anemia and jaundice
> - Family history of jaundice gallstones
> - Splenomegaly
> - Spherocytosis with reticulosis
> - Increased osmotic fragility
> - Negative Coombs test

TREATMENT

General Supportive Care

Parents should be advised of the risk of newborn jaundice and the potential need for phototherapy and exchange transfusion after birth to decrease bilirubin levels. Infants born to parents with known HS should be monitored carefully as hyperbilirubinemia may peak several days after birth. A minority of infants will be transfusion-dependent until the development of adequate erythropoiesis to compensate for the ongoing hemolysis. Continued transfusion-dependence is not common after 6–12 months of age.

Once the baseline level of disease severity is reached, an annual visit to the hematologist usually is sufficient. Growth should be monitored, exercise tolerance and spleen size should be documented, and parents should receive anticipatory guidance regarding the risk of aplastic crisis secondary to parvovirus, and hypoplastic crises with other infections. Parents and patients should be informed of an increased risk for gallstone development. The degree of splenomegaly does not correlate with disease severity. Folic acid supplementation is recommended in moderate and severe HS because of an enhanced requirement with increased erythropoiesis.

Treatment is splenectomy. It should be delayed until the patient is 5–6 years old. If anemia is severe enough to impair growth or if aplastic crisis is frequent, the operation may be considered earlier.

Red blood cell transfusion can be given during an aplastic crisis. Splenectomy prevents gallstones and eliminates the throat of aplastic crisis. After splenectomy, jaundice and reticulocytosis disappear. Immunization against *Haemophilus influenzae* type b, *Streptococcus pneumoniae*, and *Neisseria meningitidis* should be done. Post splenectomy, patients should receive penicillin to prevent sepsis. Patients should receive folic acid supplementation to prevent deficiency due high turnover of red cells and accelerated erythropoiesis throughout life.

Indications for Splenectomy

- Severe anemia
- Reticulocytosis
- Aplastic crisis
- Poor growth
- Cardiomegaly

Guidelines for Splenectomy

In children undergoing splenectomy, a concomitant cholecystectomy should be performed if there are gallstones. It is controversial whether to perform a concomitant splenectomy in less severely ill patients who are undergoing cholecystectomy for gallstone disease. Postsplenectomy thrombocytosis is frequently observed, but requires no treatment and usually resolves spontaneously. The patient, household contacts, and other frequent contacts should be current with their vaccinations. Prophylactic antibiotics are typically prescribed at least until the patient is 5 years old or at least 2 years after splenectomy. Folate supplementation should be continued if the hemoglobin level and reticulocyte count do not normalize.

Because the spherocytes are destroyed almost exclusively in the spleen, splenectomy eliminates most of the hemolysis. After splenectomy, the anemia, hyperbilirubinemia, and incidence of gallstones are significantly lessened, if not completely eradicated. However, splenectomy is associated with immediate surgical morbidities in addition to a lifelong increased risk for sepsis, particularly that caused by pneumococcal species. This risk is not completely eliminated with the requisite preoperative and postoperative vaccination against pneumococcus, meningococcus, and *H. influenzae* type b.

Splenectomy is recommended for patients with severe HS. It should be considered for patients with moderate HS and frequent hypoplastic or aplastic crises, poor growth, or cardiomegaly. It is generally not recommended for patients with mild HS. When splenectomy is indicated, it should be performed after the age of 6 years, if possible, to avoid the heightened risk of postsplenectomy sepsis in younger children.

The laparoscopic approach has less surgical morbidity and is recommended if the surgeon is adequately trained in this approach. Partial splenectomy may be beneficial but needs further study.

■ BIBLIOGRAPHY

1. Bolton-Maggs PH, Langer JC, Iolascon A, Tittensor P, King MJ; General Haematology Task Force of the British Committee for Standards in Haematology. Guidelines for the diagnosis and management of hereditary spherocytosis-2011 update. Br J Haematol. 2012;156(1)37-49.
2. Da Costa L, Galimand J, Fenneteau O, Mohandas N. Hereditory spherocytosis, elliptocytosis, and other red cell membrane disorders. Blood Rev. 2013;27(4);167-78.
3. Gallagher PG. Abnormalities of erythrocyte membrane. Pediatr Clin North Am. 2013; 60(6):1349-62.
4. Gupta N, Sharma S, Seth T, Mishra P, Mahapatra M, Kumar S, et al. Rituximab in steriod refractory autoimmune hemolytic anemia. Indian J Pediatr. 2012;79(6):803-5.

CASE 39

Idiopathic Thrombocytopenic Purpura

■ PRESENTING COMPLAINTS

A 3-year-old girl was brought with the complaint of:
- Cough and cold since 2 weeks
- Fever since 3 days
- Rashes since 1 day
- Bleeding in the mucous membrane of the mouth

History of Presenting Complaints

A 3-year-old girl presented with a history of sudden onset of bruising and generalized rashes all over the body. There was a history of bleeding in the mucous membrane of the mouth in the gum and lips. There was bleeding in the nose also. There was no itching. There was a past history of cough and cold which had been treated by a family doctor about 2 weeks before.

Past History of the Patient

She was the eldest sibling of a nonconsanguineous marriage. She was born at full term after normal delivery. She cried immediately after the delivery. There was no significant postnatal event. The child's developmental milestones were normal. Her performance at school was good.

■ EXAMINATION

The girl was moderately built and moderately nourished. She was sitting quietly on the examination table. Anthropometric measurements included height was 95 cm (50th centile) and weight was 13 kg (50th centile).

The child was afebrile. The pulse rate was 120 beats/min. The respiratory rate was 20 breaths/min. The blood pressure recorded was 60/44 mm Hg. There was no pallor, no lymphadenopathy, no icterus, and no edema.

There was a hematoma on the upper lip. Bleeding from the gingiva was present.

CASE AT A GLANCE

Basic Findings
Height	: 95 cm (50th centile)
Weight	: 13 kg (50th centile)
Temperature	: 37°C
Pulse rate	: 120 beats/min
Respiratory rate	: 20 breaths/min
Blood pressure	: 60/44 mm Hg

Positive Findings

History:
- Rashes
- Cough and cold 15 days back
- Bleeding in gum

Examination:
- Hematoma
- Bleeding in the gingival region
- Macular nonblanching erythematous rashes

Investigation:
- Bleeding time (BT) prolonged
- Platelet decreased
- Peripheral blood smear shows large platelets
- Bone marrow examination reveals increased megakaryocytes

There were multiple bruises of varying size and color. Superficial macular nonblanching erythematous rashes were present over the eyelids and cheeks. There was a fresh gaze over the skin with marked bruising and hematoma over the left side of the forehead as well as over the right flank and left knee.

■ INVESTIGATION

- *Hemoglobin:* 12 g/dL
- *Total leukocyte count (TLC):* 7,800 cells/mm^3
- *Platelet count:* 40,000/mm^3
- *Bleeding time (BT):* 6 minutes (1–5 minutes)
- *Clotting time (CT):* 7 minutes (4–8 minutes)
- *Erythrocyte sedimentation rate (ESR):* 12 mm in the first hour
- *Peripheral blood smear:* Megathrombocytes, i.e., large platelets are seen
- *Bone marrow:* Normal granulocytes examination and erythrocytic series, increased number of eosinophils and megakaryocytes.

■ DISCUSSION

The child had a preceding viral infection. This is followed by the acute onset of bruises and petechiae. Generalized petechiae are suggestive of thrombocytopenia. Leukemia is ruled out as there is absence of pallor and lymphadenopathy, and the features are suggestive of bone marrow failure. It is the most commonly acquired bleeding disorder. It is a benign disorder.

About 70% of idiopathic thrombocytopenic purpura (ITP) follow lower respiratory tract infection (LRTI). This may act as a trigger factor, where an immune process results in the development of platelet antibodies. Bone marrow aspirate shows a normal or increased number of megakaryocytes. Every common infectious virus has been described in association with ITP including EBV and HIV.

In a small number of children, after 1-4 weeks of exposure to a common viral infection, an autoantibody directed against the platelet surface develops with a resultant sudden onset of thrombocytopenia. A recent history of viral illness is described in 50–65% of cases of childhood ITP. The peak age is 1–4 years, although the age ranges from early in infancy to the elderly. In childhood, males and females are equally affected. ITP seems to occur more often in late winter and spring after the peak season of viral respiratory illness. The most common cause of acute onset of thrombocytopenia in an otherwise well child is (autoimmune) idiopathic thrombocytopenic purpura (ITP).

■ PATHOGENESIS

Idiopathic thrombocytopenic purpura (ITP) is an acquired disorder that has a multifactorial etiology including the generation of antiplatelet autoantibodies and subsequent reticuloendothelial (RE) clearance, direct T-cell cytotoxicity, and abnormal platelet production in the bone marrow.

Some children develop an acute presentation of an autoimmune disease that is unknown. The extract antigenic target for most such antibodies in most cases of childhood acute ITP remains undetermined. However, in chronic ITP, many patients demonstrate antibodies against the platelet glycoprotein complex. After binding the antibody to the platelet surface, circulating antibody-coated platelets are recognized by the fragment crystallizable (Fc) receptor on splenic macrophages, ingested, and destroyed. Most common viruses have been described in association with ITP, including EBV and HIV. EBV-related ITP is usually of short duration and follows the course of infectious mononucleosis. HIV-associated ITP is usually chronic. In some patients, ITP appears to arise in children infected with *Helicobacter pylori* or rarely following vaccines.

Platelet-associated immunoglobulin can be demonstrated in the plasma of patients. It is attributed to the interaction of the platelets and immune complexes formed during antibody response to viral infection. The platelets are sequestrated in the spleen and survival time is diminished.

It is associated with petechial and mucocutaneous bleeding and occasionally it hemorrhages into the tissue. There is a profound deficiency of circulating platelets despite an adequate number of megakaryocytes in the bone marrow. An increased amount of immunoglobulin G (IgG) has been found bound to platelets and may represent immune complexes absorbed on the platelet surface.

■ CLINICAL FEATURES (FIG. 1)

The classical presentation is a sudden onset of generalized petechiae **(Fig. 2)** and purpura **(Fig. 3)**. This occurs in healthy children between 1 and 4 years of age. There will be a history of preceding viral infection for 1–4 weeks with an average of 2 weeks. Hemorrhage in the mucous membrane may be prominent with hemorrhagic bullae on the gums and lips. Nasal bleeds may be severe. Findings on physical examination are normal, other than the finding of petechiae and purpura. Splenomegaly, lymphadenopathy, bone pain, and pallor are rare.

Immune thrombocytopenia diagnosis is classified as either primary or secondary ITP. Primary ITP, or ITP not triggered by another disorder, occurs in up to 75% of children. Secondary ITP is triggered by another

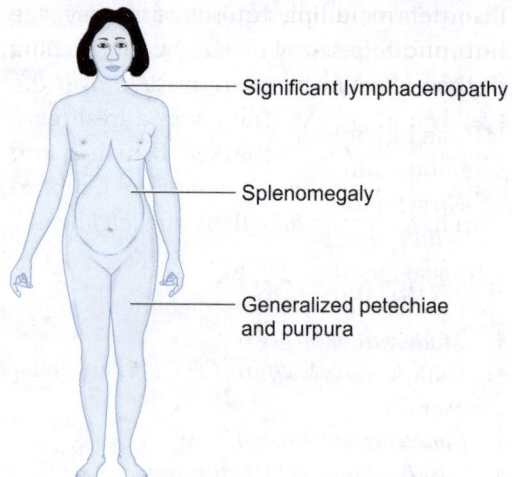

Fig. 1: Clinical features.

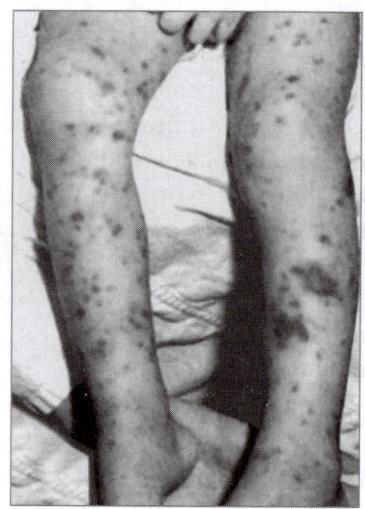

Fig. 2: Petechial rashes. *(For color version, see Plate 2)*

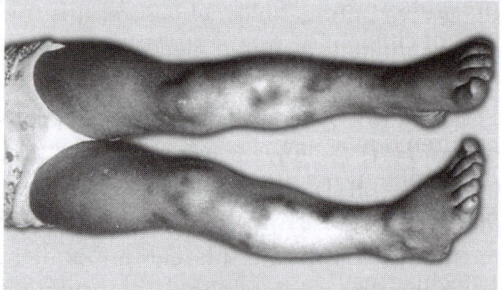

Fig. 3: Purpura. *(For color version, see Plate 2)*

disorder, including autoimmune diseases, immunodeficiency syndromes, thyroid disease, infection, or pregnancy.

ITP can be clinically classified on the basis of symptoms and signs as:
- No symptoms
- *Mild symptoms:* Bruising and petechiae, occasional minor epistaxis, very little interference with daily living.
- *Moderate:* More severe skin and mucosal lesions, more troublesome epistaxis and menorrhagia
- *Severe:* Bleeding episodes—menorrhagia, epistaxis, melena requiring transfusion or hospitalization, symptoms interfering seriously with the quality of life.

The presence of abnormal findings, such as hepatosplenomegaly, bone or joint pain, remarkable lymphadenopathy other cytopenias, and congenital anomalies suggests other diagnoses (leukemia, syndromes). The possibility of systemic illness is considered in chronic ITP. The onset is insidious and occurs in adolescents.

The course of illness is benign and self-limiting spontaneous remissions occur within a few weeks. Severe bleeding is rare in 70–80% of children who present with acute ITP, spontaneous resolution occurs within 6 months. Therapy does not appear to affect the natural history of the illness. 1% of patients develop an intracranial hemorrhage (ICH). There is no evidence that therapy prevents serious bleeding. Approximately 20% of children who present with acute ITP go on to have chronic ITP. The prognosis may be related more to age, as ITP in younger children is more likely to resolve whereas the development of chronic ITP in adolescents approaches 50%.

The serious complication is ICH. Petechiae may be seen all over the body, over the bony prominence and anterior surface of the leg. The spleen is often not palpable, but the tip of the spleen is just palpable. The presence of splenomegaly with thrombocytopenia requires aggressive evaluation of associated problems, such as collagen vascular disorders and hypersplenism.

The chronic idiopathic thrombocytopenic purpura persists for >6 months. Some children are steroid-responsive and dependent. Splenectomy may be eventually indicated but a late spontaneous remission may be the possibility. They also interfere with the sequestration of platelets by the spleen as they prevent the interaction of sensitized lymphocytes in the spleen with homologous platelets.

GENERAL FEATURES
• Sudden onset of generalized petechiae and purpura • Bleeding from the gums and mucous membrane • Intracranial hemorrhage

◼ DIAGNOSIS

Diagnosis is chiefly based on the clinical history, physical examination, and evidence of thrombocytopenia in the peripheral smear.

Severe thrombocytopenia (platelet count $<20 \times 10/L$) is common, and platelet size is normal or increased, reflective of increased platelet turnover. In acute ITP, the hemoglobin value, WBC count, and differential count should be normal. Hemoglobin may be decreased if there have been profuse nosebleeds or menorrhagia. Laboratory evidence reveals isolated thrombocytopenia with a normal coagulation profile (PT and PTT). Platelet-associated IgG antibodies have been demonstrated in patients with idiopathic thrombocytopenic purpura.

Bone marrow examination is recommended only in circumstances where the diagnosis is not clear due to the presence of atypical features. Indications for bone marrow aspiration/biopsy include an abnormal WBC count or differential or unexplained anemia as well as findings on history and physical examination suggestive of a bone marrow failure syndrome or malignancy. Current recommendations do not include routine bone marrow studies before initiating steroid treatment or in the case of a patient who fails intravenous immunoglobulin (IVIG) therapy. Bone marrow examination is essential to exclude acute leukemia. Bone marrow examination shows normal granulocytic and erythrocytic series, with characteristically normal or increased numbers of megakaryocytes. Some of the megakaryocytes may appear to be immature and are reflective of increased platelet turnover.

Thrombopoietin levels are not recommended, as they are often not increased despite increased peripheral destruction. This observation led to the development of new therapies with recombinant thrombopoietin agonists.

Other laboratory tests should be performed as indicated by the history and physical examination. Studies on HIV should be done in at-risk populations, especially sexually active teens. Platelet antibody testing is seldom useful in acute ITP. A direct antiglobulin test (DAT) (Coomb's test) should be done if there is unexplained anemia to rule out Evans syndrome (autoimmune hemolytic anemia and thrombocytopenia) or before instituting therapy with IV anti-D.

Direct antiglobulin test, formerly known as direct Coombs test) and serum immunoglobulins are recommended in all newly diagnosed ITP patients, as these markers may be associated with an underlying tendency toward autoimmunity. Antinuclear antibody (ANA) testing can be obtained in patients with high suspicion of autoimmune disease.

> **LABORATORY SALIENT FINDINGS**
> - Thrombocytopenia
> - Immunoglobulin G (IgG) antibodies
> - Normal coagulation profile
> - *Bone marrow:* Increased number of megakaryocytes

■ DIFFERENTIAL DIAGNOSIS

Differential diagnosis includes congenital syndrome, such as megakaryocytic cytopenia, DIC, hemolytic uremic syndrome (HUS), HIV, and lymphoma.

■ CLINICAL COURSE

In approximately 75% of children, ITP is a self-limited condition with spontaneous resolution regardless of interventions and treatments during the course of the disease. After remission, the chance of having another episode of ITP is small (<5%), and following recovery, children are not at increased risk for other blood disorders or cancers. The most feared outcome, ICH, is fortunately rare, occurring in <1% of affected children.

The International Working Group Consensus Report recommends the following categories to stratify ITP cases according to the duration of the disease in order to facilitate guidance and treatment decisions.

A simple classification system has been proposed to characterize the severity of bleeding in ITP on the basis of symptoms and signs rather than platelet count, as follows:
- No symptoms
- *Mild symptoms:* Bruising and petechiae, occasional minor epistaxis, very little interference with daily living
- *Moderate symptoms:* More severe skin and mucosal lesions, more troublesome epistaxis, and menorrhagia

- *Severe symptoms:* Bleeding episodes-menorrhagia, epistaxis, melena requiring transfusion or hospitalization, symptoms interfering seriously with the quality of life
- *Newly diagnosed:* 0–3 months from diagnosis
- *Persistent:* 3–12 months from diagnosis
- *Chronic:* >12 months from diagnosis.

This categorization was changed from the former terminology (acute, <6 months, and chronic, >6 months, from diagnosis) due to the large number of children entering spontaneous remission beyond 12 months from diagnosis.

■ COMPLICATIONS

Severe hemorrhage and bleeding into the vital organs, ICH are more serious. The biggest risk factor for hemorrhage is a platelet count of <10,000/dL.

ESSENTIAL DIAGNOSTIC POINTS
- Decreased platelet count
- Petechiae
- Ecchymosis
- Normal coagulation profile
- Bone marrow: Normal or increased megakaryocyte

■ TREATMENT

Acute ITP has a self-limiting and benign course. By 1 year only 10% of children with ITP remain thrombocytopenic. The chronic ITP still improves as long as 5–10 years after the diagnosis. About 5% of patients have recurrent ITP. Recovery occurs in 50–60% of the children within 4–6 weeks and remaining within 6 months. The mortality rate in the majority varies between 0.5 and 1%. It is mainly due to ICH and severe GI hemorrhage.

Indications for the treatment:
- Platelet count below $20 \times 10^9/L$
- Presence of severe mucosal bleeds
- Presence of menorrhagia
- Chronic ITP
- Symptonic with atypical presentation.

There are no data showing that treatment affects either short- or long-term clinical outcomes of ITP. Many patients with new-onset ITP have mild symptoms, with findings limited to petechiae and purpura on the skin, despite severe thrombocytopenia. Compared with untreated control subjects, treatment appears to be capable of inducing a more rapid rise in platelet count to the theoretically safe level of $>20 \times 10/L$.

Acute Immune Thrombocytopenia

Given the typically mild clinical symptoms and expectation of resolution in childhood ITP, most experts recommend observation without treatment regardless of the platelet count in children with no symptoms or with only mild cutaneous findings. However, for children with wet bleeding symptoms, including wet purpura, epistaxis, or menorrhagia, treatment is recommended to elevate the platelet count to a hemostatic range, facilitating cessation of bleeding and decreasing the risk of ICH and other forms of life-threatening bleeding. Treatment to raise the platelet count and lessen bleeding symptoms includes corticosteroids, IVIG, and anti-D immunoglobulin. These front-line therapies function at least in part by interfering with the immune destruction of antibody-coated platelets. Initial approaches to the management of ITP include the following:

- No therapy other than education and counseling of the family and patient for patients with minimal, mild, and moderate symptoms, as defined earlier. This approach emphasizes the usually benign nature of ITP and avoids the therapeutic roller coaster that ensues once interventional therapy is begun. This approach is far less costly, and side effects are minimal.

- Disorders that cause increased platelet destruction on a nonimmune basis are usually serious systemic illnesses with obvious clinical findings, such as HUS and DIC.
- A single dose of IVIG (0.8–1.0 g/kg) or a short course of corticosteroids should be used as first-line treatment. IVIG at a dose of 0.8–1.0 g/kg/day for 1–2 days induces a rapid rise in platelet count (usually >20 × 10/L) in 95% of patients within 48 hours. IVIG appears to induce a response by downregulating Fe-mediated phagocytosis of antibody-coated platelets. Side effects include fever and chills during the infusion, headache, and rarely, aseptic meningitis. IVIG therapy is both expensive and time-consuming to administer. Additionally, after infusion, there is a high frequency of headaches and vomiting, suggestive of IVIG-induced aseptic meningitis.
- *Prednisone:* Corticosteroid therapy has been used for many years to treat acute and chronic ITP in adults and children. Prednisolone is given in doses of 1–4 mg/kg/day for 2–4 weeks and then tapered. Platelets usually rise about 3–5 days after steroid initiation, but it can take up to 2 weeks for an effect to be seen. Side effects of steroids include weight gain, irritability, hypertension, and hyperglycemia. Dexamethasone is also given at a dose of 20 mg/m^2 over 4 days every four to six courses. Prednisolone appears to induce a more rapid rise in platelet count than in untreated patients with ITP. Corticosteroid therapy is usually continued for a short course until a rise in platelet count to >20 × 10^9/L. has been achieved to avoid the long-term side effects of corticosteroid therapy, especially growth failure, diabetes mellitus, and osteoporosis.

The other important modes of steroid action include decreased clearance of opsonized platelets and decreased production of antiplatelet antibodies. Platelet count was observed to recover more rapidly with corticosteroids than with no therapy. Similarly, a short course of oral prednisolone therapy (4 mg/kg/day × 4 days without tapering) was safe, inexpensive, and effective. The efficacy of corticosteroids has been demonstrated in terms of platelet recovery time and not in terms of morbidity or mortality.

Several studies have shown that IV pulse methylprednisolone (30 mg/kg/day for 3 days) is more effective in increasing the platelet count to a safer level.

- *Intravenous (IV) anti-D therapy:* For rhesus (Rh)-positive patients, IV anti-D at a dose of 50–75 µg/kg causes a rise in platelet counts to >20 × 10^9/L in 80–90% of patients within 48–72 hours. When given to Rh-positive individuals, IV anti-D induces mild hemolytic anemia. Red blood cell (RBC)-antibody complexes bind to macrophage Fe receptors and interfere with platelet destruction, thereby causing a rise in platelet count. IV anti-D is ineffective in Rh-negative patients.

Anti-Rd (D) acts by a mechanism similar to that of IV-IgG. IV (or intramuscular) anti-Rh (D) has been advocated as a cheaper alternative to IV-IgG in Rh-(positive) nonsplenectomized patients. It is more effective in acute ITP than in chronic ITP.

Each of these medications may be used to treat ITP exacerbations, which commonly occur several weeks after an initial course of therapy. In the special case of ICH, multiple modalities should be used, including platelet transfusion, IVIG, high-dose corticosteroids, and prompt consultation by neurosurgery and surgery.

The choice of therapy depends on a variety of factors, including the side effect profile of each agent and the indication for treatment, as well as patient-related factors. Platelet transfusion is generally avoided due to the expected rapid antibody-mediated clearance of transfused platelets and a theoretical risk of increased antibody development but can be used in the management of serious or life-threatening bleeding.

Antifibrinolytic agents (aminocaproic acid and tranexamic acid) can be helpful adjuncts to therapy for mucosal bleeding symptoms. Medications that affect platelet number or function (aspirin, NSAIDs) should be avoided. Activity restrictions may be required depending on the platelet count and bleeding symptoms.

In the case of severe or life-threatening hemorrhage, an aggressive approach with a combination of therapies is warranted. IVIG and high-dose IV steroids should be given, with consideration of platelet transfusion/drip to facilitate hemostasis acutely. If the patient has signs and symptoms worrisome for ICH, expeditious imaging should be obtained with surgical and neurosurgical consultations as needed. Urgent/emergent splenectomy can be lifesaving in the setting of uncontrolled bleeding or neurologic compromise.

Splenectomy

The role of splenectomy should be reserved on two occasions, i.e., in older children ≥4 years with severe idiopathic thrombocytopenic purpura that has lasted longer than 1 year (chronic idiopathic thrombocytopenic purpura) and whose symptoms are not relieved by medical therapy. It is also considered in severe complications, such as ICH.

Results are immediate as platelet antibodies are developed in the spleen. Titers of antibodies decrease rapidly after splenectomy. Platelet concentration should be readily available to control excessive bleeding during surgery.

The majority of patients (65–88%) achieve remission immediately after splenectomy. The results of splenectomy are immediate as the antiplatelet antibodies are synthesized in the spleen.

Splenectomy is associated with a lifelong risk of overwhelming postsplenectomy infection caused by encapsulated organisms, increased risk of thrombosis, and the potential development of pulmonary hypertension in adulthood. As an alternative to splenectomy, rituximab has been used off-label in children to treat chronic ITP. In 30–40% of children, rituximab has induced a partial or complete remission.

Intracranial Hemorrhage

Intracranial hemorrhage is a life-threatening complication of ITP. Its incidence has been reported to vary from 0.1 to 1%. It was believed that ICH occurs during the first few days of onset of ITP and when the platelet count is $<20 \times 10^9$/L.

The current principle of therapy for ICH is to rapidly increase the platelet count either by splenectomy, platelet transfusions, or by IV-IgG. Splenectomy reduces the destruction of both autologous and transfused platelets. 60–70% of patients sustain permanent remission following splenectomy. Emergency craniotomy is indicated in patients with posterior fossa hemorrhage and progressive neurologic deterioration.

Chronic Immune Thrombocytopenia

Management of patients with chronic ITP is based on the evaluation of the patient's bleeding symptoms, platelet count, overall quality of life, and ability to perform daily activities. Because approximately one-third of patients will have spontaneous remission of their chronic ITP even years after diagnosis, management often consists of observation alone, with pharmacologic intervention reserved for severe thrombocytopenia or bleeding episodes, or before anticipated hemostatic challenges (invasive procedures or high-risk physical activities). However, some children with chronic ITP have more severe thrombocytopenia or significant and frequent bleeding episodes, or quality-of-life impairments that necessitate more definitive and durable treatment. Options include rituximab, thrombopoietin receptor agonists, alternative immunosuppressive regimens, and splenectomy. Splenectomy is successful in approximately 70% of the children but concerns over the risk of thrombosis and long-term risk of severe infection, as well as favorable side effect profiles of nonsurgical options, limit its use.

The monoclonal CD20 antibody rituximab has been reported to elicit a complete platelet response for up to a year in 30% of patients with chronic ITP. Infusion reactions, risk of hypogammaglobulinemia and/or infections, and very rare risk of progressive multifocal leukomalacia can occur. The thrombopoietin agonists romiplostim and eltrombopag are efficacious in approximately 70% of children and are increasingly used due to their favorable side effect profiles to and potential for long-term use. These agents work by increasing in platelet production, to compensate for peripheral loss and increase circulating platelet count. Short-term side effects are generally mild and improve with duration of use. Serious side effects are rare and include the risk of thrombosis and the potential for bone marrow fibrosis. Eltrombopag is an oral agent taken once daily. The dose is weight-based with a maximum dose of 75 mg. Liver function abnormalities are possible and generally reversible on drug discontinuation. Romiplostim is administered subcutaneously once weekly. The manufacturer recommends weight-based dosing and escalating to a maximum of 10 µg/kg.

THERAPY FOR CHRONIC ITP

Blockade of reticuloendothelial system:
- Corticosteroids:
  - Standard of high dose
  - Low dose on alternate days
  - Pulse steroids
- IV-IgG
- Anti-Rh (D) globulin:
  - Vince alkaloids (Vincristine and vinblastine)
  - Splenectomy
  - Anti-Fc receptor antibody
- *Immunosuppression:*
  - Cyclophosphamide
  - Cyclosporine
  - Azathioprine
  - Interferons
  - Danazol
  - Splenectomy
- *Removal of antiplatelet antibodies:*
  - Plasmapheresis
  - Exchange transfusion
  - Immunoadsorption

Refractory ITP: It is not benign. The mortality rate is 5.1%. Drugs used are Vinca alkaloids, cyclophosphamide, azathioprine, cycloserine, and danazol.

■ BIBLIOGRAPHY

1. Arnold DM, Kukaswadia S, Nazi I, Esmail A, Dewar L, Smith JW, et al. A systematic evaluation of laboratory testing for

drug-induced immune thrombocytopenia. J Thromb Haemost. 2013;11(1):169-79.
2. Bolton-Maggs PH, Chalmers EA, Collins PW, Harrison P, Kitchen S, Liesner RJ, et al. A review of platelet disorders with guidelines for their management on behalf of the UKHCDO.
3. George JN. Clinical practice. Thrombotic thrombocytopenic purpura N Engl Med. 2006;354(18)1927-35.
4. Nurden AT. Qualitative disorders of platelets and megakaryocytes. J Thromb Haemost. 2005;3(8)1773-82.
5. Rodeghiero F, Stasi R, Gernsheimer T, Michel M, Provan D, Arnold DM, et al. Standardization of terminology, definitions and outcome criteria in immune thrombocytopenic purpura of adults and children: report from an international working group. Blood. 2009;113(11)2386-93.

CASE 40

Iron Deficiency Anemia

■ PRESENTING COMPLAINTS

A 3-year-old boy was brought with the complaint of:
- Repeated attack of cough and cold since 6 months
- Tiredness since 6 months
- On and off pain in the abdomen since 6 months
- Not taking feeds regularly since 1 month

History of Presenting Complaints

A 3-year-old boy came to the pediatric outpatient department with a history of fatigue and repeated attacks of cough and cold since 6 months. According to the mother her son was getting repeated chest infections. She also complained that every time he was getting relief only after the administration of antibiotics. She has also noted that her son was becoming pale day by day. Later she also noticed that he was not playing with the friends. He was just sitting in one place. He was quite irritable. He was not taking food regularly.

Past History of the Patient

He was the only child of a nonconsanguineous marriage. He was born at term with normal delivery. His birth weight was 3 kg. He cried immediately after the delivery. There was no significant postnatal event. He was discharged on the fifth day. He was on breastfeeding exclusively for 4 months. Weaning started at 4 months, and he was on family food for 15 months. His developmental milestones

CASE AT A GLANCE

Basic Findings
Height	: 90 cm (50th centile)
Weight	: 13 kg (50th centile)
Temperature	: 37°C
Pulse rate	: 110 beats/min
Respiratory rate	: 26 breaths/min
Blood pressure	: 60/40 mm Hg

Positive Findings

History:
- Fatigue
- Repeated respiratory infection
- Pain in abdomen

Examination:
- Pallor
- Koilonychia
- Bald tongue
- Ejection systolic murmur

Investigation:
- *Hb:* Decreased
- *ESR:* Raised
- *MCH:* Decreased
- *MCV:* Decreased
- *MCHC:* Decreased
- *Reticulocytes:* Increased
- *Serum iron level:* Decreased

(ESR: erythrocyte sedimentation rate; Hb: hemoglobin; MCH: mean corpuscular hemoglobin; MCHC: mean corpuscular hemoglobin concentration; MCV: mean corpuscular volume)

were normal. The boy had been completely immunized.

EXAMINATION

The boy was moderately built and poorly nourished. He was sitting quietly on the examination table. He was not interested in his surroundings. Anthropometric measurements included height was 90 cm (50th centile), and weight was 13 kg (50th centile).

The boy was afebrile. The heart rate was 110 beats/min, the respiratory rate was 26 breaths/min. The blood pressure recorded was 60/40 mm Hg. There was gross pallor, koilonychia was present. There was no lymphadenopathy and no icterus. There was no cyanosis.

The tongue was bald. The cardiovascular system revealed the presence of an ejection systolic murmur heard at the base. The respiratory system revealed the presence of crepitations at the base of the lungs. The per abdomen examination was normal.

INVESTIGATION

- *Hemoglobin:* 6 g/dL
- *TLC:* 7,900 cells/mm^3
- *ESR:* 40 mm in the first hour
- *Absolute eosinophil count (AEC):* 650 cells/mm^3
- *MCV:* 65 pg
- *Mean corpuscular hemoglobin (MCH):* 25 pg
- *MCHC:* 24%
- *Reticulocyte count:* 3%
- *Serum iron levels:* 28 μg/dL
- *Total iron-binding capacity (TIBC):* 360 μg/dL

DISCUSSION

Iron deficiency is the most common cause of nutritional anemia. Children during the phase of rapid growth such as preschool age and adolescence are at higher risk for the development of iron deficiency anemia (IDA).

Iron is important in several iron-dependent enzymes including catalase, peroxidase, cytochromes, and ribonucleotide reductase. It is a major constituent of hemoglobin which is important for oxygen carriage in multicellular organisms.

The term, newborns possess about 75 mg of elemental iron/kg (0.25–0.5 g of total body iron), largely acquired during the transfer of maternal iron stores during the third trimester of pregnancy. They must then gain 4.5 g of iron throughout their childhood (1 mg/day) to achieve nearly 5.0 g of body iron in the average adult. An additional 0.2–0.5 mg/day of absorbed iron is required to balance normal physiologic iron losses.

Most iron in neonates is in circulating hemoglobin. The relatively high hemoglobin concentration of the newborn infant falls during the first 2–3 months of life, considerable iron is recycled. These iron stores are usually sufficient for blood formation in the first 6–9 months of life in term infants. Stores are depleted sooner in low-birth-weight infants or infants with perinatal blood loss because their iron stores are smaller. Delayed (1–3 minutes) clamping of the umbilical cord can improve iron status and reduce the risk of iron deficiency, whereas early clamping (<30 seconds) puts infants at risk for iron deficiency.

Blood loss must be considered as a possible cause in every case of IDA, particularly in older children and adolescents. Chronic IDA from adult bleeding may be caused by a lesion of the gastrointestinal tract (GIT), such as peptic ulcer, Meckel diverticulum, polyp, hemangioma, and inflammatory bowel disease.

In developing countries, infections with hookworm, *Trichuris trichiura*, *Plasmodium*, and *Helicobacter pylori* often contribute to iron deficiency. Celiac disease and giardiasis may interfere with iron absorption.

■ PREDISPOSING FACTORS

They are low socioeconomic status with poor hygiene and nutrition, worm infestation; high socioeconomic group with only bottle feeding and improper weaning and poor breastfeeding; adolescent girls on slimming diet; preterm babies; low birth weight babies born to anemic mother, and rapid growth in children.

■ IRON SOURCES

It can be divided into dietary hem iron, and nonhem dietary iron. Hem iron is available in meat, fish, and blood products. It is of high bioavailability with 20–30% absorbed from these foods.

■ ETIOLOGY

Iron adequacy is the balance between the iron required on one hand, and the iron available and absorbed on the other hand. This can be disturbed leading to the deficiency by increased requirements.

Increased Requirement

The iron requirement is more in infancy, during the period of rapid growth. This makes the full-term prone to deficiency by 4–6 months. In preterm the deficiency may be seen by 6–8 weeks.

Healthy-term infants who are on exclusively breastfeeds are at risk for iron deficiency after they are 6 months old. The lower iron stores of premature infants are more rapidly depleted as compared with term infant.

Breastfed infants require less iron from other food. During the first year of life, because of relatively small quantities of iron, it is often difficult to attain sufficient.

Infants who are breastfed exclusively should require iron supplements after 4 months. Increased requirements of iron are more during the infancy period of rapid growth. This makes full-term newborns prone to deficiency by 4–6 weeks.

Iron is more required during adolescence, menstruation, pregnancy, and lactation. If the diet is poor or iron is not supplemented, iron deficiency will occur. Low birth weight babies are prone to develop iron deficiency.

Decreased Availability

Iron availability depends on the iron content of the diet, the type of iron, and the absorptive capacity of the GI tract.

In infancy, breast milk is the main source of iron. Though the iron content of breast milk is less, it has high bioavailability. Hence exclusive breastfeeding protects the baby from iron deficiency in the first 4–6 months of life. After this, the baby needs a generous iron supply from proper weaning food. At this stage, bottle feeding only a milk-based diet and improper food habits lead to iron deficiency. Hence proper weaning, breastfeeding, and iron supplementation will prevent iron deficiency in infancy.

Only one-tenth of the dietary iron is absorbed by the GI mucosa. Most of the iron is in ferric form. This is converted into the ferrous form. This is easily absorbed. This conversion is facilitated by hydrochloric acid in the gastric juices. Absorption of iron takes place in the first and second parts of the duodenum and at times in the jejunum.

The intestinal mucosa controls it. In the normal state, when the iron in the food is in excess, the mucosa holds the iron in the apoferritin in the mucosal cell. This desquamates in 2–3 days hence getting rid of excess iron.

In the deficiency state, the mucosal cell transports the iron rapidly through the blood circulation. Here it combines with transferrin. It is transported to the site of utilization and storage.

Absorption of iron is decreased by GI tract diseases, such as diarrhea, celiac disease, hypoproteinemia, GI surgery, worm infestations, and cow's milk allergy. Recurrent infections lead to reduced intake, poor absorption, and increased losses due to bleeding.

Increased Blood Losses

Each milliliter of packed red blood cell (PRBC) has 1 mg of iron. Hence bleeding can lead to loss of iron from the body. Excessive loss of iron can occur due to GI bleeding due to polyps, piles, fissures, Meckel's diverticulum, and worms, such as hookworms, *T. trichiura*, schistosomiasis, and varices.

There could be other forms of chronic blood loss in patients with bleeding disorders. Bleeding as a case of iron deficiency is less common in infancy. It should be thought of in an older child or adult male with unexplained iron deficiency.

Once the iron is assimilated into the body, it is not easily excreted. An average loss of iron per day in children is 0.9 mg/day. 0.6 mg/day is lost in the GIT in the form of RBCs, bile, or exfoliated mucosal cells. The rest is lost from the desquamated cells of the skin and urinary tract.

■ PATHOGENESIS

Body iron is predominantly incorporated into the hemoglobin of circulating erythrocytes and their marrow precursors. Phagocytosis of senescent erythrocytes by RE macrophages and degradation of hemoglobin allows for recovery and recycling of heme iron that provides the majority of the daily iron requirement to the bone marrow. Only a small fraction of the average daily iron requirement is obtained from dietary iron.

In iron-sufficient states, an estimated 10% of dietary iron is absorbed. Therefore, children's diets must contain 10–15 mg of iron to maintain a positive iron balance. During periods of maximal growth-infancy and adolescence-iron requirements for the expanding blood volume and muscle mass may exceed dietary iron accrual, placing those individuals at risk for iron deficiency. In infancy, particularly when exclusively breastfed, an adequate level of iron intake is difficult to achieve if iron supplementation, iron-fortified formula, or iron-rich foods are not provided.

Some disorders disrupt the integrity of the enteric mucosa and hinder iron absorption. Inflammatory bowel diseases, particularly Crohn's disease and celiac disease, can damage the duodenum, where most iron absorption occurs, and GI bleeding may exacerbate the problem. Children who undergo GI surgery and/or reconstruction may also be at risk for poor iron absorption.

An oral iron challenge can be used to assess iron absorption. This involves obtaining a tasting serum iron level followed by a level 1–2 hours after an oral dose of 1–2 mg/kg of elemental iron, preferably with ferrous sulfate. Failure to observe a marked increase over the baseline level is concerning for iron malabsorption.

Iron homeostasis requires carefully coordinated regulation of intestinal iron absorption, cellular iron import and export, and iron storage besides from enterocyte sloughing, humans have no physiologic iron excretion mechanism; therefore, the control of iron balance must occur at the level of intestinal absorption.

Hepcidin, a small peptide hormone synthesized in the liver, plays a central role in iron homeostasis, specifically in intestinal iron absorption and macrophage iron release. It negatively regulates ferroportin, causing its internalization and degradation, thus limiting iron transfer into the plasma. Hepcidin synthesis is decreased in iron-deficient states, allowing for increased ferroportin-mediated cellular iron export and increased iron absorption and plasma iron levels, and facilitating increased erythrocyte production.

Iron deficiency anemia is the end stage of a relatively long-drawn process of deterioration in the iron status of an individual. It is only the tip of the iceberg of the iron deficiency state, which may be divided into three functionally distinct stages of severity.

1. *First stage of storage iron depletion:* Iron reserve is smaller or absent. It is characterized by reduced serum ferritin or reduced iron concentration in marrow and liver tissue. Hemoglobin, serum iron transferrin concentration, and saturation are within normal limits.
2. *The second stage of iron, limited erythropoiesis:* It is transient and consists of deserved iron transportation. Hemoglobin may still be normal or may be in a lower range, but serum iron is low and TIBC is increased with normal transferrin saturation (TS) and low serum ferritin.
3. *Third stage of IDA:* The flow of iron to erythroid marrow is impaired to cause a reduction in hemoglobin concentration. This leads to progressive microcytic hypochromic anemia and low MCV. Reduced serum iron, TS, and serum ferritin levels.

Iron stores in the body such as hemosiderin in the liver and bone marrow are diminished. Thereafter the iron ferritin level falls to <10 μg/mL followed by a decrease in TIBC.

Free erythrocyte porphyrin (FEP) level increases. Microcytic hypochromic anemia occurs. The activity of iron-containing enzymes diminishes.

Intestinal iron absorption appears to be mediated by at least five physiologic regulators that primarily affect hepcidin gene transcription (dietary iron load, total body iron stores, erythropoietic demand, hypoxia, and inflammation), as well as a more recently described erythroid regulator, erythroferrone (ERFE).

■ CLINICAL FEATURES (FIG. 1)

Onset may be very insidious, and the progression of the symptoms and signs may be so gradual that they may not be noticed till hemoglobin drops as low as 3 and 4 g%. However, improved work tolerance and feeling of well-being may be noticed following treatment before hemoglobin starts rising. It occurs most frequently between the ages of 6 and 24 months and between 11 and 17 years. The peak incidence is at a younger age in preterm than in those born at term.

Symptomatology depends on the rate of fall in hemoglobin and the hemostatic adjustment of various systems in the body.

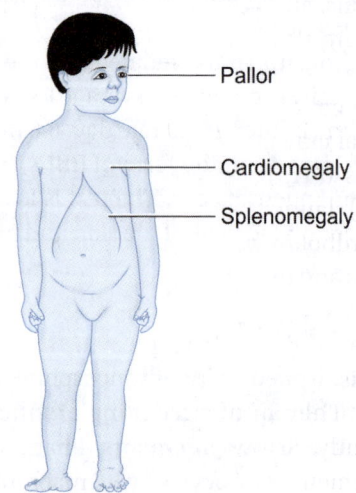

Fig. 1: Clinical features.

In severe IDA, fatigue, shortness of breath, decreased exercise tolerance, irritability, anorexia, and pallor may be noted.

Most children with iron deficiency are asymptomatic and are identified by recommended laboratory screening at 12 months of age, or sooner if at high risk. Pallor is the most important clinical sign of iron deficiency but is not usually visible until the hemoglobin falls to 7–8 g/dL. It is most readily noted as pallor of the palms, palmar creases, nail beds, or conjunctivae.

In mild to moderate iron deficiency (i.e., hemoglobin levels of 6–10 g/dL), compensatory mechanisms, including increased levels of 2,3-diphosphoglycerate and a shift of the oxygen dissociation curve, may be so effective that few symptoms of anemia aside from mild irritability are noted.

When the hemoglobin level falls to <5 g/dL, irritability, anorexia, and lethargy develop, and systolic flow murmurs are often heard. As the hemoglobin continues to fall, tachycardia and high-output cardiac failure can occur.

Gradual onset of pallor may escape notice even when hemoglobin falls to 4 and 5 g%. Blowing apical systolic murmur, recurrent infections, and occasionally slightly enlarged spleen are also well known to occur.

Pica is an unexplained but well-documented feature in children with anemia. Habitual cravings to eat unusual substances such as dirt, clay (geophagia), ice (pagophagia), laundry starch (amylophagia), salt, and cardboard are seen in almost 70–80% of patients and usually are cured by prompt iron therapy.

The onset of anemia is insidious. Pallor is a major sign. The children fail to thrive. They suffer from infection more frequently. Severe anemia leads to cardiac enlargement. Splenomegaly is present. There will be systolic and as well as diastolic flow murmur. There will be atrophy of the tongue papillae. Nails become thin, brittle, and flat. Longitudinal ridges appear on the nail. Nails become spoon-shaped and appear concave—koilonychia. There will be growth retardation. School performance and mental performance will be affected.

Iron deficiency has nonhematologic systemic effects. Both iron deficiency and iron-deficiency anemia are associated with impaired neurocognitive function in infancy. There is also an association of iron-deficiency anemia and later, possibly irreversible, cognitive defects. Given the frequency of iron deficiency and iron-deficiency anemia and the potential for adverse neurodevelopmental outcomes, minimizing the incidence of iron deficiency is an important goal.

Growth retardation—children with IDA have lower than normal weight at the time of diagnosis, attributable to anorexia, reduced synthesis of nucleic acids, and altered intestinal functions. Rapid weight gain usually follows iron therapy.

Epithelial changes koilonychia, platynychia, atrophic glossitis, angular stomatitis, cheilosis, and esophageal web (Plummer-Vinson or Paterson-Kelly syndrome), etc., are rare in children and are more common in adults. Koilonychia is the pathognomonic of IDA.

Iron deficiency has nonhematologic systemic effects. Both iron deficiency and iron-deficiency anemia are associated with impaired neurocognitive function in infancy. Iron-deficiency anemia is also associated with later, possibly irreversible, cognitive defects.

Other nonhematologic consequences of iron deficiency include *pica*, the desire to ingest nonnutritive substances, and *pagophagia*, the desire to ingest ice. The pica can result in the ingestion of lead-containing substances and result in concomitant *plumbism*.

> **ESSENTIAL DIAGNOSTIC POINTS**
> - Pallor and fatigue
> - Poor dietary intake of iron
> - Chronic blood loss
> - Microcytic hypochromic anemia
> - Responds to iron therapy

■ DIAGNOSIS

First tissue iron stores are depleted. This depletion is reflected by reduced serum ferritin, an iron-storage protein, which provides an estimate of body iron stores in the absence of inflammatory disease. Next, serum iron levels decrease, the iron-binding capacity of the serum (serum transferrin) increases, and the TS falls below normal. As iron stores decrease, iron becomes unavailable to complexes with protoporphyrin to form a home. Free erythrocyte protoporphyrins accumulate, and hemoglobin synthesis is impaired. At this point, iron deficiency progresses to iron-deficiency anemia. With less available hemoglobin in each cell, the red cells become smaller and varied in size. The variation in red cell size is measured by an increasing red cell-distribution width (RDW).

This is followed by a decrease in MCV and MCH. Developmental changes in MCV require the use of age-related standards for recognizing microcytosis. The RBC count also decreases. The reticulocyte percentage may be normal or moderately elevated, but absolute reticulocyte counts indicate an insufficient response to the degree of anemia. The blood smear reveals hypochromic, microcytic red cells with substantial variation in cell size. Elliptocytic or cigar-shaped red cells are often seen. Detection of increased soluble transferrin receptor and decreased reticulocyte hemoglobin concentration provide very useful and early indicators of iron deficiency, but their availability is more limited.

White blood cell count is normal, and thrombocytosis is often present. Thrombocytopenia is occasionally seen with iron deficiency, potentially confusing the diagnosis with bone marrow failure disorders. The stool for occult blood should be checked to exclude blood loss as the cause of iron deficiency.

A presumptive diagnosis of iron-deficiency anemia is most often made by a CBC demonstrating microcytic anemia with a high RDW, reduced RBC count, normal WBC count, and normal or elevated platelet count. Other laboratory studies, such as reduced serum ferritin, reduced serum iron, and increased TIBC, are not usually necessary unless severe anemia requires a more rapid diagnosis, other complicating clinical factors are present, or the anemia does not respond to iron therapy. An increase in hemoglobin >1 g/dL after a month of iron therapy is usually the most practical means to establish the diagnosis.

Diagnosis of severe and moderate IDA is relatively straightforward. Low levels of hemoglobin, MCV <75 m^3, MCH <28 pg, low serum iron, and TS, and high levels of TIBC and FEP will help diagnose IDA. RDW, a parameter available by particle cell counters will be high in IDA.

However, mild cases of IDA, especially those with hemoglobin concentration within 1 g% below the reference range may be difficult to diagnose. Such children show an increase in hemoglobin and a feeling of well-being when treated with iron.

> **LABORATORY SALIENT FINDINGS**
> - Decreased serum ferritin
> - Decreased transferrin saturation
> - Decreased free erythrocyte protoporphyrin
> - Decreased hemoglobin
> - Decreased MCV

Laboratory tests can be divided into tests for the plasma compartment, tests for storage iron, and tests for the RBC compartment.

The plasma compartment is tested by doing serum iron, TIBC, and TS tests. Storage iron is tested by doing serum ferritin and bone marrow iron staining. RBC compartment is tested by doing blood indices (preferably on particle cell counter) including RDW, thorough peripheral smear examination, and FEP.

Screening Tests

The best screening test for the diagnosis of anemia includes the measurement of hemoglobin concentration and hematocrit [packed cell volume (PCV)] in circulating blood. Practically speaking, one can diagnose mild anemia when hemoglobin concentration is below 10 g/dL moderate anemia between 7 and 10 g, and severe anemia below 7 g%.

Red Cell Indices

With the availability of electronic particle counters estimation of PCV, MCV, MCH, and RBC count has become accurate and reproducible. Manual determination of these red cell indices is time-consuming, variable, and poorly reproducible. A low MCV and MCH favor the diagnosis of IDA.

Reticulocyte is the most recently produced RBC in circulation. The earliest sign of IDA may be a fall in the concentration of hemoglobin in the reticulocyte. The studies have indicated that a concentration >30 pg per cell has no chance of IDA.

Red Cell Size Distribution Width

Most of the recent particle cell counters give the graph of red cell size distribution and the calculated value of the red cell distribution width. The variability in the size of RBC will lead to a broad base of the graph and increased values of RDW. It reflects the amount of anisocytosis as seen on the peripheral smear. In IDA, RBCs have greater anisocytosis and hence, increased value of RDW.

FREE ERYTHROCYTE PROTOPORPHYRIN

Protoporphyrin accumulates in the RBCs when it does not have sufficient iron to combine with, to form hemoglobin. The free erythrocyte protoporphyrin can be measured rapidly by a simple fluorescence assay performed directly on the thin film of blood on the hemoflurocytometer. FEP value in a normal person is 15.5q 8.3 µg/dL of RBC. About >80 µg/dL of RBC below the age of 4 years and >70 mg/dL of RBC above that age are significant values to detect IDA. The FEP/Hb ratio is a useful index of iron deficiency. The FEP/Hb ratio increases when iron reserve is exhausted even before anemia becomes apparent.

Confirmatory Test for Iron Deficiency Anemia

The most commonly used tests for confirming the diagnosis of IDA are serum iron, serum ferritin, and TS.

- *Serum iron* Levels of serum iron reflect the balance between the iron absorbed, iron utilized for hemoglobin synthesis, and iron released by red cell destruction and the size of the storage dept. Thus, it represents the equilibrium between iron entering and leaving the circulation. Serum iron is influenced by many physiological as well as pathological states.
- *Total iron-binding capacity* and transferrin circulating in the blood. Normally there is enough transferrin present in 100 cc of serum to bind about 250–450 µg of iron. TIBC is increased in patients with

IDA whereas it is lower in patients with anemia of chronic inflammation as the cause of anemia.

- *Serum ferritin* Iron is stored in the body in the form of ferritin and hemosiderin. A small amount of ferritin is found in blood reflecting the body's stores of iron. It is a sensitive measure of total iron stores in the body and can be determined by radioimmunoassay or by enzyme-linked immunosorbent assay (ELISA). ELISA is a simpler and less expensive method and can be performed on a microquantity of blood. Serum ferritin level <10–12 ng/mL indicates depletion of iron stores.
- *Bone marrow examination:* Bone marrow aspiration is not indicated in the diagnosis of IDA. The degree of cellularity and the proportion of myeloid erythroid normobiastic hyperplasia.
- *Bone marrow iron staining* is the most accurate method of diagnosing iron-deficiency anemia but is invasive, expensive, and usually unnecessary.

A diagnosis of iron deficiency in the absence of anemia is more challenging. Serum ferritin is a useful measure whose value is increased by also measuring C-reactive protein to help identify false-negative results because of concomitant inflammation. Tests to detect increased soluble transferrin receptors and decreased reticulocyte hemoglobin concentration may find increasing use if they become more available.

Confirmatory test for IDA.

Age (years)	Serum ferritin (ng/mL)	Transferrin saturation (%)	RBC FEP (µg/dL)
0.5–4	10	12	80
5–10	10	14	70
11–14	10	16	70
15	12	16	70

> **GENERAL FEATURES**
> - Pagophagia—desire to ingest unusual substance
> - Irritability
> - Anorexia
> - Underweight

■ DIFFERENTIAL DIAGNOSIS

Differential diagnosis of microcytic hypochromic anemia is IDA, anemia of chronic infection, thalassemia, sideroblastic anemia, and lead poisoning.

These include thalassemia, lead poisoning (plumbism), chronic infections, copper deficiency, and sideroblastic anemia.

■ TREATMENT

The regular response of iron-deficiency anemia to adequate amounts of iron is a critical diagnostic and therapeutic feature. Oral administration of simple ferrous salts (most often ferrous sulfate) provides inexpensive and effective therapy.

The therapeutic dose should be calculated in terms of elemental iron. A daily total dose of 3–6 mg/kg of elemental iron in three divided doses is adequate, with the higher dose used in more severe cases. The maximum dose would be 150–200 mg of elemental iron daily. Ferrous sulfate is 20% elemental iron by weight and is ideally given between meals with juice, although this timing is usually not critical with a therapeutic dose.

Parenteral iron preparations are only used when malabsorption is present or when compliance is poor because oral therapy is otherwise as fast, as effective, much less expensive, and less toxic. When necessary, parenteral iron sucrose, ferric carboxymaltose, and ferric gluconate complex have a lower risk of serious reactions than iron dextran, although only the latter is The United States Food and Drug Administration (US FDA)-approved for use in children.

In addition to iron therapy, dietary counseling is usually necessary. Excessive intake of milk, particularly cow's milk, should be limited. Iron deficiency in adolescent girls secondary to menorrhagia is treated with iron and menstrual control with hormone therapy.

If the anemia is mild, the only additional study is to repeat the blood count approximately 4 weeks after initiating therapy. At this point, the hemoglobin has usually risen by at least 1–2 g/dL and has often normalized. If the anemia is more severe, earlier confirmation of the diagnosis can be made by the appearance of reticulocytosis usually within 18–96 hours of instituting treatment. The hemoglobin will then begin to increase 0.1–0.4 g/dL/day depending on the severity of the anemia. Iron medication should be continued for 2–3 months after blood values formalize to reestablish iron stores. Good follow-up is essential to ensure a response to therapy.

Because a rapid hematologic response can be confidently predicted in typical iron deficiency, blood transfusion is rarely necessary. It should only be used when heart failure is imminent or if the anemia is severe with evidence of substantial ongoing blood loss. Unless there is active bleeding, transfusions must be given slowly to avoid precipitating or exacerbating congestive heart failure.

Treatment of Cause

It is important to find out the etiological factor of iron deficiency to prevent failure of therapy and recurrence of deficiency after treatment is stopped. Promotion of exclusive breastfeeding for the first 4–6 months, continuing breastfeeds for as long as possible thereafter with the introduction of proper and age-appropriate food items and prophylactic iron supplementation will prevent iron deficiency during infancy and early childhood. In older children, diet modification to improve total calories intake and iron-containing food will prevent iron deficiency. Treatment of worms, giardiasis, bleeding from any sites, and recurrent infections is a must to treat the patient adequately.

Iron supplementation: Iron can be given orally or parenterally.

Oral Iron Therapy

Oral iron therapy is cost-effective, safe, convenient, well tolerated, preferred, and advocated route of therapy.

Dose

It is given in the dose of 4–6 mg, of elemental iron/kg/day. It is ideally given as a single dose in older children or in two divided doses in younger children. It is preferably given in between meals to facilitate better absorption. Compliance in the first month of therapy is important as the majority of iron absorption occurs during this period. It is continued for at least 2–3 months after hemoglobin becomes normal to replenish stores.

The therapeutic dose should be calculated in terms of elemental iron. *A daily total dose of 3–6 mg/kg of elemental iron in one or two doses is adequate*, with the higher dose used in more severe cases. The maximum dose is 150–200 mg of elemental iron daily.

Various iron salts available include Ferrous fumarate, ferrous gluconate, ferrous sulfate-hydrous or anhydrous forms, ferric salts, ferrous glycine sulfate, and iron polymaltose complexes. Of these ferrous salts are preferred as they are better absorbed than ferric forms. Ferrous sulfate is the best as it is also cost-effective.

Nausea, vomiting, abdominal cramps, diarrhea, constipation, straining of tongue and teeth, blackish discoloration of stools, etc., are common side effects.

Parenteral Iron Therapy

Indications:
- Intolerance of oral iron
- Malabsorptive states
- Ongoing blood loss

This includes both intramuscular and IV iron therapy. The preparation available is iron dextran which is a complex of ferric hydroxide with high molecular weight dextrans in a colloidal solution containing 50 mg of elemental iron/mL.

Dose

Total dose of elemental iron (mg) = Weight (kg) × Desired increment of Hb (g/dL) × 3

Or

Iron required (mg) = Weight (kg) × 2.3 × (15–patients Hb in/dL) + (500–1,000) is given in divided doses intramuscularly or as full-dose IV therapy.

- *Intramuscular route (IM):* This is very painful and may lead to serious allergic reactions and is hence not used in children. IM injections are best given into the upper outer quadrant of a gluteal region using the Z track technique. A dose of 0.1 mL should be given as a test dose intramuscularly, and if there are no reactions within 1 hour, a full dose (to a maximum of 0.5 cc) can be given every day.
- *IV route:* There are two methods: (1) Infusion of total dose diluted in a ration of 5 mL of iron dextran complex in 100 mL of normal saline. Initially, the flow rate should be kept at 20 drops/min for 5–10 minutes and if there are no reactions, then the rate can be increased to 40–60 drops/min.
- *Bolus injection of iron dextran:* Bolus of iron dextran diluted in 20 mL of saline is given over 10–20 minutes.

Both these routes are however used after a prior sensitivity testing where 1 mL of iron dextran solution is diluted in 20 cc of normal saline and injected slowly over 10–15 minutes following which one should observe for reactions for half an hour to 1 hour.

Time after iron administration	Response
12–24 hours	Replacement of intracellular iron enzymes subjective improvement; decreased irritability; increased appetite
36–48 hours	Initial bone marrow response; erythroid hyperplasia
48–72 hours	Reticulocytosis; peaking at 5–7 days
4–30 days	Increase in hemoglobin level
1–3 months	Repletion of stores

Side-effects

Reactions can occur with both IM and IV therapy and can be either immediate or delayed.

- *Immediate reactions:* These include pain at the injection site, flushing, and metabolic taste. Such reactions are brief in duration and often are relieved by slowing the rate of injection. Severe reactions such as anaphylaxis, hypotension, cardiac arrest, headache, malaise, vomiting, and nausea should be contraindication to further doses.
- *Delayed reactions:* These include tender regional lymphadenitis, myalgia, arthralgia, fever, etc.

Though most of the reactions are mild and transient, anaphylactic reactions may be life-threatening, and hence one should always keep an injection of adrenaline, injection.

Hydrocortisone and resuscitative measures are handy before injecting, Parenteral therapy should be only given in a hospital setup.

Chronic Iron-deficiency Anemia

Chronic iron-deficiency anemia from occult bleeding may be caused by a lesion of the GIT, such as peptic ulcer, Meckel diverticulum, polyp, hemangioma, or inflammatory bowel disease. Infants can have chronic intestinal blood loss induced by exposure to whole cow's milk protein. Involved infants characteristically develop anemia that is more severe and occurs earlier than would be expected simply from an inadequate intake of iron. The ongoing loss of blood in the stools can be prevented either by breastfeeding or by delaying the introduction of whole cow's milk in the first year of life and then limiting the quantity to <24 oz/24 h. Unrecognized blood loss also can be associated with chronic diarrhea and rarely, with pulmonary hemosiderosis.

■ PREVENTION

Iron deficiency is best prevented to avoid both its systemic manifestations and anemia. Breastfeeding should be encouraged, with the addition of supplemental iron at 4 months of age. Infants who are not breastfed should only receive iron-fortified formula (12 mg of iron/L) for the first year, and thereafter cow's milk should be limited to >20–24 oz daily. This approach encourages the ingestion of foods richer in iron and prevents blood loss as a result of cow's milk—induced enteropathy.

When these preventive measures fail, routine screening helps prevent the development of severe anemia. Routine screening using hemoglobin or hematocrit is done at 12 months of age, or earlier if at 4 months of age the child is assessed to be at high risk for iron deficiency. Thereafter, screening should continue if risk factors are identified.

■ BIBLIOGRAPHY

1. Camaschella C. Iron-deficiency anemia. N Engl J Med. 2015;372(19)1832-43.
2. Eden AN, Sandoval C. Iron deficiency in infants and toddlers in the United States. Pediatr Hemtol Oncol. 2012;29(8):704-9.
3. Lozoff B, Jimenez E, Hagen J, Mollen E, Wolf AW. Poorer behavioral and developmental outcome more than 10 years after treatment for iron deficiency in infancy. Pediatrics. 2000;105(4):E51.
4. Mantadakis E. Advances in pediatric intravenous iron therapy. Pediatr Blood Cancer. 2016;63(1):11-16.
5. Powers JM, Buchanan GR. Diagnosis and management of iron deficiency anemia Hematol Oncol Clin North Am. 2014;28(4)729-45,vi-vii.
6. Shelley E, Crary Katherine Hall, Bachanan GR. Intravenous iron sucrose for children with iron deficiency failing to respond to oral iron therapy. Pediatr Blood Cancer. 2011; 56(4):615-9.
7. World Health Organization. (2001). Iron deficiency anemia: assessment, prevention, and control. [online] Available from https://www.who.int/publications/m/item/iron-children-6to23--archived-iron-deficiency-anaemia-assessment-prevention-and-control [Last accessed June, 2024].

CASE 41

Polycythemia

■ PRESENTING COMPLAINTS

A 5-day-old girl was brought with the complaint of:
- Breathlessness since 1 day
- Irritability since 6 hours
- Excessive crying since 2 hours

History of Presenting Complaints

A 5-day-old girl baby was brought to the hospital with a history of irritability, excessive crying, and breathlessness. The mother also said that her daughter was not taking feeds regularly. There was also a history of subcostal indrawing. But there was no history of cough and cold, suggestive of respiratory tract infection. There was no history of vomiting and loose motion. The child used to become silent on taken into the mother's lap.

Past History of the Patient

She was the first sibling of a nonconsanguineous marriage. The mother was hypertensive antenatally. However, the blood pressure was under control with antihypertensive medicine. She was delivered at term by normal vaginal delivery. She cried immediately after the delivery. The cry of the baby was normal. Features of intrauterine growth retardation (IUGR) were present. Her birth weight was 3 kg. There was no significant postnatal event. The baby was taking breast milk and was discharged on the third day.

CASE AT A GLANCE

Basic Findings

Length	:	45 cm (<3rd centile)
Weight	:	2.75 kg (>10th centile)
Temperature	:	37°C
Pulse rate	:	128 beats/min
Respiratory rate	:	48 breaths/min
Blood pressure	:	50/40 mm Hg

Positive Findings

History:
- Irritability
- Respiratory distress
- Hypertension in mother

Examination:
- Intrauterine growth retardation
- Plethoric child
- Tachypnea
- Tachycardia
- Tender hepatomegaly

Investigation:
- *Hemoglobin:* Increased
- *Packed cell volume (PCV):* Increased

■ EXAMINATION

On examination the child was irritable. Features of IUGR were present. The child used to be more comfortable on the mother's lap. Anterior fontanelle was normal. The ear was normal. Anthropometric measurements included the length was 45 cm (<3rd centile), the weight was 2.75 kg (>10th centile) and the head circumference was 34 cm.

The child was afebrile, the heart rate was 128 beats/min, and the respiratory rate was

48 breaths/min. The blood pressure recorded was 50/40 mm Hg. Subcostal indrawing was present.

The child looked more plethoric than normal. Icterus was present. There was no clubbing and lymphadenopathy. The cardiovascular examination revealed tachycardia and no murmur. Per abdomen examination revealed presence of hepatomegaly with about 4 cm below the costal margin. It was tender and soft in consistency. Bowel sounds were regular.

■ INVESTIGATION

- *Hemoglobin:* 22 g/dL
- *Total leukocyte count (TLC):* 7,600 cells/mm^3
- *Platelet count:* 250,000 cells/mm^3
- *Red cell count:* 8.0 × 10^6 cells/mm^3
- *PCV:* 60%
- *Serum bilirubin:* 3 mg/dL
- *Coombs test:* Negative
- *Blood group:* O-positive
- *Peripheral blood smear:* Normal
- *Cerebrospinal fluid (CSF) examination:* Normal
- *X-ray chest:* Normal

■ DISCUSSION

Polycythemia vera is also called polycythemia rubra vera, erythema, or vague Osler disease.

Polycythemia exists when the RBC count, hemoglobin level, and total RBC volume all exceed the upper limits of normal. In postpubertal individuals, an RBC mass >25% above the mean normal value (based on body surface area) or a hemoglobin level >18.5 g/dL in males) or >16.5 g/dL (in females) indicates absolute erythrocytosis.

Polycythemia is defined by venous hematocrit of >65% found in normal newborns. This is more by two standard deviations. As the central venous hematocrit rises above 65%, there are dramatic increases in viscosity. Because direct measurement of blood viscosity is not available, high hematocrit level is the best indirect indicator of hyperviscosity.

The fundamental abnormality is hyperplasia of a precursor of red cells, granulocytes, and platelets in the bone marrow. This results in excess of these cells in peripheral blood.

Monozygotic twins with placental vascular anastomoses may have unequal distribution. Hence one twin is born pale and with hypovolemia, while the other is plethoric. Neonatal polycythemia is more common with Down syndrome, Beckwith's syndrome, IUGR, and small-for-dates (SFD) babies.

Polycythemia exists when the RBC count, hemoglobin level, and total RBC volume all exceed the upper limits of normal. In postpubertal individuals, an RBC mass >25% above the mean normal value (based on body surface area) or a hemoglobin >18.5 g/dL (in males) or >16.5 g/dL (in females) indicate absolute erythrocytosis.

A decrease in plasma volume, such as occurs in acute dehydration and burns, may result in a high hemoglobin value. These situations are more accurately designated as hemoconcentration or relative polycythemia because the RBC mass is not increased, and normalization of the plasma volume restores hemoglobin to normal levels. Once the diagnosis of true polycythemia is made, sequential studies should be done to determine the underlying etiology.

Polycythemia vera is an acquired clonal myeloproliferative disorder. Although primarily manifesting as erythrocytosis, thrombocytosis, and leukocytosis can also be seen. When isolated severe thrombocytosis exists in the absence of erythrocytosis, the myeloproliferative disorder is called essential thrombocythemia. The erythropoietin receptor is normal, and serum erythropoietin levels are normal or low. In vitro cultures do not require added erythropoietin to stimulate the growth of erythroid precursors. Risk factors for the development of polycythemia vera include a family history of polycythemia vera and the presence of an autoimmune disorder, such as Crohn's disease.

Secondary polycythemia results either because of hypoxia or without hypoxia. Hypoxia may be due to an underlying disease. The most common diseases are pulmonary and cardiac disease. The infants are associated with cyanosis and clubbing with engorged retinal vessels. Secondary polycythemia without hypoxia is associated with renal disorders and tumors. This is due to increased erythropoietin production.

■ NONCLONAL POLYCYTHEMIA

Pathogenesis

Nonclonal polycythemia is diagnosed when polycythemia is caused by a physiologic process that is not derived from a single cell. Nonclonal polycythemia can be congenital or acquired (secondary).

■ CONGENITAL POLYCYTHEMIA

Lifelong or familial polycythemia should trigger a search for a congenital problem. These inherited conditions may be transmitted as dominant or recessive disorders. Autosomal dominant causes include sickle hemoglobin (HbS) that have increased oxygen affinity {P50 [partial pressure of oxygen (pO_2) in the blood at which the hemoglobin is 50% saturated] <20 mm Hg}, erythropoietin receptor mutations resulting in an enhanced effect of erythropoietin or mutations in the von Hippel–Lindau gene that result in altered intracellular oxygen sensing.

Subtle decreases in oxygen delivery to tissues may cause polycythemia. Congenital methemoglobinemia resulting from an autosomal recessive deficiency of cytochrome b5 reductase may cause cyanosis and polycythemia. Most affected individuals are asymptomatic. Neurologic abnormalities may be present in patients whose enzyme deficits are not limited to hematopoietic cells. Hemoglobin M disease (autosomal dominant) causes methemoglobinemia and can lead to polycythemia. Cyanosis may occur in the presence of as little as 1.5 g/dL of methemoglobin but is uncommon in other hemoglobin variants unless hyperviscosity results in localized hypoxemia.

■ ACQUIRED POLYCYTHEMIA

Polycythemia may be present in clinical situations associated with chronic arterial oxygen desaturation. Cardiovascular defects involving right-to-left shunts and pulmonary diseases interfering with proper oxygenation are the most common causes of hypoxic polycythemia. Clinical findings usually include cyanosis, hyperemia of the sclerae and mucous membranes, and clubbing of the fingers. As the hematocrit rises to >65%, clinical manifestations of hyperviscosity, such as headache and hypertension, may require phlebotomy. Living at high altitudes also causes hypoxic polycythemia; the hemoglobin level increases approximately 4% for each rise of 1,000 m (3,300 ft) in altitude. Partial obstruction of a renal artery rarely results in polycythemia. Polycythemia has also been associated with benign and malignant tumors that secrete erythropoietin.

Exogenous or endogenous excess of anabolic steroids also may cause polycythemia. A common spurious cause is a decrease in plasma volume, as occurs in moderate to severe dehydration.

■ CLINICAL FEATURES (FIG. 1)

The clinical picture is influenced by increased blood volume, and also by thrombotic and

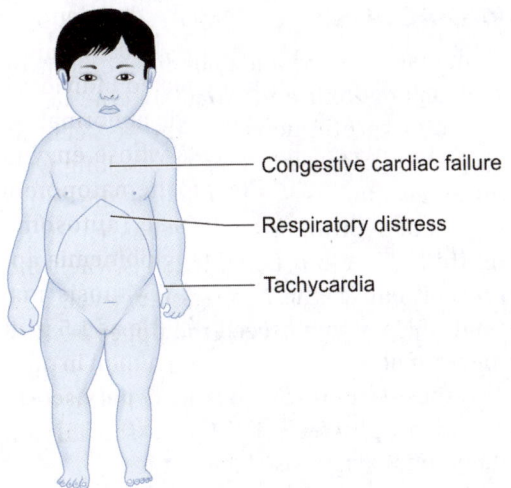

Fig. 1: Clinical features.

hemorrhagic complications. Increased blood volume produces engorgement and slowing of the circulation in many organs, and symptoms may be referred to a number of systems.

Patients with polycythemia vera usually have hepatosplenomegaly. Erythrocytosis may cause hypertension, headache, shortness of breath, and neurologic symptoms, and increase the risk of thrombosis. Granulocytosis may cause diarrhea or pruritus from histamine release. Thrombocytosis (with or without platelet dysfunction) may cause thrombosis or hemorrhage.

The infant may present with convulsion, respiratory distress, tachycardia, congestive cardiac failure (CCF), and hyperbilirubinemia. These may be associated with hypoglycemia and hypocalcemia.

Cardiovascular defects involving right to left shunts and pulmonary disease interfering with the proper oxygenation. These are the most common causes of hypoxic polycythemia. Clinical findings usually include cyanosis, hyperemia of the sclera and mucus membrane, and clubbing of the fingers. As the hematocrit rises above 65%, clinical manifestations of hyperviscosity, such as headache and hypertension occur.

■ CONGENITAL POLYCYTHEMIA

Lifelong or familial polycythemia should trigger a search for a congenital problem. These inherited conditions may be transmitted as dominant or recessive disorders. Autosomal dominant causes include HbS that have increased oxygen affinity [P50 (pO$_2$ in the blond at which the hemoglobin is 50% saturated) <20 mm Hg], erythropoietin receptor mutations resulting in an enhanced effect of erythropoietin or mutations in the von Hippel–Lindau gene that result in altered intracellular oxygen sensing. Another rare cause is an autosomal recessive 2,3-diphosphoglyceric acid deficiency, which leads to a left shift of the oxygen dissociation curve, increased oxygen affinity, and consequent polycythemia.

Subtle decreases in oxygen delivery to tissues may cause polycythemia. Congenital methemoglobinemia resulting from an autosomal recessive deficiency of cytochrome b5 reductase may cause cyanosis and polycythemia. Most affected individuals are asymptomatic. Neurologic abnormalities may be present in patients whose enzyme deficits are not limited to hematopoietic cells. Hemoglobin M disease (autosomal dominant) causes methemoglobinemia and can lead to polycythemia. Cyanosis may occur in the presence of as little as 1.5 g/dL of methemoglobin but is uncommon in other hemoglobin variants unless hyperviscosity results in localized hypoxemia.

■ ACQUIRED POLYCYTHEMIA

Polycythemia may be present in clinical situations associated with chronic arterial oxygen desaturation. Cardiovascular defects involving right-to-left shunts and pulmonary diseases interfering with proper oxygenation are the most common causes of hypoxic polycythemia. Clinical findings usually include cyanosis, hyperemia of the sclerae and mucous membranes, and clubbing of the fingers. As the hematocrit rises to >65%, clinical manifestations of hyperviscosity, such as headache and hypertension, may require phlebotomy. Living at high altitudes also causes hypoxic polycythemia; the hemoglobin level increases by approximately 4% for each rise of 1,000 m in altitude. Partial obstruction of a renal artery rarely results in polycythemia. Polycythemia has also been associated with benign and malignant tumors that secrete erythropoietin. Exogenous or endogenous excess of anabolic steroids also may cause polycythemia. A common spurious cause is a decrease in plasma volume such as in moderate to severe dehydration.

WORLD HEALTH ORGANIZATION DIAGNOSTIC CRITERIA FOR POLYCYTHEMIA VERA

Major Criteria

- Hb >18.5 g/dL (men) or Hb >16.5 g/dL (women)
  Or,
  Hb or hematocrit (Hct) >99th percentile of reference range for age, sex, or altitude of residence
  Or,
  Hb >17 g/dL (men) or Hb >15 g/dL (women) is associated with a sustained increase of 2g/dL from baseline that cannot be attributed to correction of iron deficiency.
  Or,
  Elevated red cell mass >25% above the mean normal predicted value
- Presence of *Janus kinase 2 (JAK2)* or similar mutation.

Minor Criteria

- Bone marrow trilineage myeloproliferation
- Subnormal serum erythropoietin level
- Endogenous erythroid colony growth

DIAGNOSIS

Both major criteria and one minor criteria or first major criteria and two minor criteria.

The overproduction of the red cells is responsible for symptoms. This along with an excess number of platelets is the cause of vascular thrombosis. This causes much morbidity and mortality. It exists when the red cell count, the hemoglobin level, and total RBC volume exceed the upper limit of the normal.

Measurement of total RBC volume by radioisotopic technique is essential for differential diagnosis of polycythemia.

True polycythemia is characterized by an increase of both RBC and total blood volume. Supportive laboratory abnormalities are thrombocytosis (>400.00/μc) leukocytosis, i.e., 1200/μL), increased leukocyte phosphatase level >100 μL, and increased vitamin B_{12} (>900 pg/mL).

High levels of hemoglobin and hematocrit are usual in the newborn. The normal hemoglobin at birth is 14–21 g/dL and hematocrit is 45–65%. The blood volume of the normal term infant is 70–100 mL/kg and red cell volume is 40–60 mL/kg. In polycythemia, the red cell count is increased, and hematocrit is increased to >60%. The hemoglobin level and ESR are also increased. White cell count may be normal or raised. It will be raised in polycythemia rubra.

ESSENTIAL DIAGNOSTIC POINTS
• *CNS:* Lethargy, hypotonia, irritability, and seizures
• *GIT:* Vomiting, distension, and NEC
• *Renal:* Renal vein thrombosis and acute renal failure
• *Cardiopulmonary system:* Respiratory distress, congestive cardiac failure
• Hypoglycemia
• Increase in both RBCs and total blood volume
• Hyperplasia of precursor of red cells, granulocytes, and platelets in bone marrow
• Phlebotomy, partial exchange transfusion
(CNS: central nervous system; GIT: gastrointestinal tract; NEC: necrotizing enterocolitis; RBCs: red blood cells)

LABORATORY SALIENT FINDINGS

- Increased hemoglobin
- Increased hematocrit
- Increased red cell count
- Increased ESR

Complications include bleeding, thrombosis, myelofibrosis, and acute leukemia.

GENERAL FEATURES

- Convulsions
- Hyperbilirubinemia
- Hypoglycemia
- Hypocalcemia

■ TREATMENT

Partial exchange transfusion can be performed through the umbilical venous catheter, an umbilical artery catheter, or a peripheral venous catheter. Aliquots of 5% of estimated blood volume are withdrawn and replaced either with fresh frozen plasma or normal saline. The amount of the blood volume to be replaced is calculated as follows:

$$\text{Blood volume to be exchanged} = \frac{\text{Observed hematocrit} - \text{dissolved hematocrit}}{\text{Observed hematocrit}} \times \text{blood volume} \times \text{weight(kg)}$$

For mild disease, observation is sufficient. When the hematocrit is >65–70% (hemoglobin >23 g/dL), blood viscosity markedly increases. Periodic phlebotomy may prevent or decrease symptoms, such as headache, dizziness, and exertional dyspnea. Apheresed blood should be replaced with plasma or saline to prevent hypovolemia in patients accustomed to a chronically elevated total blood volume. Increased demand for RBC production may cause iron deficiency. Iron-deficient microcytic red cells are more rigid, further increasing the risk of intracranial and other thromboses in patients with polycythemia. Periodic assessment of iron status, with treatment of iron deficiency, should be performed.

In symptomatic children, phlebotomy is aliquots of 10–15 mL/kg replaced with an equal volume of plasma or normal saline may be indicated to reduce the red cell mass and hyperviscosity. If required antiproliferative chemotherapy is considered.

Phlebotomy is the initial treatment of choice to alleviate symptoms of hyperviscosity and decrease the risk of thrombosis. Iron supplementation should be given to prevent viscosity problems from iron-deficient microcytosis or thrombocytosis. In patients with marked thrombocytosis, antiplatelet agents (e.g., aspirin) may reduce the risks of thrombosis and bleeding. If these treatments are unsuccessful or the patient has progressive hepatosplenomegaly, antiproliferative treatments (hydroxyurea, anagrelide, interferon-a) may be helpful. The use of JAK2 inhibitors is an active area of investigation. Transformation of the disease into myelofibrosis or acute leukemia is rare in children. Prolonged survival is not unusual.

■ BIBLIOGRAPHY

1. Manco-Johnson MJ. Hemostasis in neonate. NeoReviews. 2008;9(3):e119-23.
2. Remon JI, Raghavan A, Maheshwari A. Polycythemia in newborn. NeoReviews. 2011;12(1):e20-8.

CASE 42

Sickle Cell Anemia

■ PRESENTING COMPLAINTS

A 4-year-old boy was brought with the complaint of:
- Severe backache since 1 day
- Vomiting since 1 day

History of Presenting Complaints

A 4-year-old boy was brought to the pediatric casualty with a history of severe backache and vomiting since the previous night. Backache was present in his lower back. It was very severe, and that boy was finding it very difficult to get up from the sitting posture. Along with that, the child vomited. Vomiting was projectile in nature. The child had vomited all the food he had taken at night. Vomiting remained uncontrolled. The child was not tolerating any food and not even water.

The mother gave a history of a similar type of attack of back pain that occurred during the preceding months. He was admitted to the hospital for this purpose. IV fluids, analgesics, and antibiotics were given.

Past History of the Patient

He was the first sibling of a nonconsanguineous marriage. He was born at full term and delivered vaginally. He cried immediately after birth. There was no significant postnatal event. The child was exclusively breastfed for 3–4 months. Weaning started with cereals and fruits. His developmental milestones were normal. He had been completely immunized. His backache and vomiting were the main concern of the parents.

■ EXAMINATION

The boy was moderately built and nourished. He appeared pale and apprehensive. Anthropometric measurements included height

---

CASE AT A GLANCE

Basic Findings
Height	:	100 cm (50th centile)
Weight	:	15 kg (50th centile)
Temperature	:	38°C
Pulse rate	:	100 beats/min
Respiratory rate	:	20 breaths/min
Blood pressure	:	100/70 mm Hg

Positive Findings

History:
- Backache
- Vomiting
- Repeated episodes

Examination:
- Pallor
- Splenomegaly

Investigation:
- **Hemoglobin (Hb):** Decreased
- **Peripheral blood smear:** Target cells, sickled cells, nucleated red blood cells, and hypochromic microcytic anemia
- **X-ray skull:** Hair on end appearance of frontal bone

was 100 cm (50th centile), weight was 15 kg (50th centile).

The boy was febrile. The pulse rate was 100 beats/min and the respiratory rate was 20 breaths/min. The blood pressure recorded was 100/70 mm Hg. There was pallor, icterus was present, no lymphadenopathy, and no cyanosis.

Per abdomen examination revealed the enlarged spleen about 3 cm below the costal margin. It was nontender and firm in consistency. Other systemic examinations were normal.

INVESTIGATION

- *Hemoglobin:* 7 g/dL
- *TLC:* 11,200 cells/mm^3
- *ESR:* 29 mm in the first hour
- *Peripheral blood smear:* Shows hypochromic microcytic anemia, elongated crescent-shaped RBCs and target cells
- *AEC:* 400 cells/cumm
- *Serum bilirubin:* 2 mg/dL
- *X-ray skull:* Showed hair on end appearance of the frontal bone
- *X-ray chest:* Normal

DISCUSSION

An anemic child presented with a history of backache and vomiting. There were repeated attacks of backache in the last few months. On examination, the child had mild splenomegaly. A radiograph of the skull showed hair on end appearance. All these go in favor of the sickle cell crisis which is a part of sickle cell anemia (HbSS).

It is an inherited disorder. In a heterozygous state of the sickle cell trait, only one mutant chain is inherited. An amino acid sequence in the beta-peptide chain is abnormal. On the beta chain, valine is substituted for glutamic acid at position 6. The alpha chain is normal. This results in HbS.

Sickle cell disease (SCD) is the name for a group of related disorders caused by HbS. HbS is qualitatively abnormal hemoglobin caused by a point mutation of the beta-globin gene. The sixth codon of the normal *f*-globin gene, *GAG*, codes for glutamic acid. In HbS, the adenine nucleotide is replaced by thymidine, producing GTG, which is a codon for valine.

PATHOPHYSIOLOGY

Sickle hemoglobin is the result of a single base-pair change, thymine for adenine, at the sixth codon of the beta-globin gene. This change encodes valine instead of glutamine in the 6th position in the beta-globin molecule, HbSS, homozygous HbSS, occurs when both beta-globin alleles have the sickle cell mutation (beta's). The glutamine-to-valine substitution replaces hydrophilic glutamic acid with a hydrophobic valine, permitting abnormal hydrophobic interactions between adjacent deoxyhemoglobin molecules, which decreases the solubility or HbS in the deoxygenated state. Thus, as sickled RBCs traverse the circulation, cycling through oxygenated and deoxygenated states, HbS repeatedly forms rigid polymers that damage the RBC membrane, causing hemolytic anemia and, ultimately, the systemic manifestations of SCD.

Sickle cell disease refers to not only patients with HbSS, but also to compound heterozygotes where one beta-globin allele includes the sickle cell mutation and the second beta-globin allele includes a gene mutation other than the sickle cell mutation, such as hemoglobin C (HbC), beta-thalassemia, hemoglobin D (HbD), and hemoglobin O (HbO). In HbSS, HbS is commonly as high as 90% of the total hemoglobin; whereas as in SCD, HbS is >50% of all hemoglobin.

As they traverse the circulation, RBCs that contain mostly HbS go through cycles of sickling (polymerization of HbS) and unsickling (depolymerization of HbS) due to deoxygenation of HbS in the tissues and reoxygenation in the lungs. The tendency of individual RBCs to sickle is influenced by several factors including the relative concentration of HbS in the cell, the abundance of other hemoglobins that inhibit the polymerization of deoxy-HbS [notably (fetal hemoglobin (HbF)], and the degree to which the HbS is deoxygenated. When a solution of HbS is deoxygenated, there is a characteristic time delay during which no polymerization occurs, followed by a phase of rapid polymerization. In vivo, this delay allows most HbS-containing RBCs to traverse the capillary beds before polymerization and sickling occur. A small number of RBCS remain permanently sickled due to membrane damage, even when fully oxygenated. These are called irreversibly sickled cells. Hemoglobins such as F and A within the RBC inhibit or delay the polymerization of HbS.

In RBCs, the hemoglobin molecule has a highly specified conformation allowing for the transport of oxygen in the body. In the absence of globin-chain mutations, hemoglobin molecules do not interact with one another. However, the presence of HbS results in a conformational change in the hemoglobin tetramer, and, in the deoxygenated state, HbS molecules can now interact with each other forming rigid polymers that give the RBC its characteristic "sickled" shape. The lung is the only organ capable of reversing the polymers, and any disease of the lung can be expected to compromise the degree of reversibility.

Intravascular sickling primarily occurs in the postcapillary venules and is a function of both mechanical obstructions by sickled RBCs and increased adhesion between RBCs, leukocytes, and the vascular endothelium. SCD is also an inflammatory disease based on nonspecific markers of inflammation.

Hemoglobin is normally present in soluble form in the red blood corpuscle. The tendency of deoxyhemoglobin "S" to undergo polymerization is responsible for innumerable expressions of sickling syndromes. The "sol" form of hemoglobin changes to the "gel" form when "HbS" is deoxygenated. In gel form, the hemoglobin changes to small, rigid, boat-shaped objects known as "tactoids." These tactoids polymerize and form a helical structure with 14–16 tetramers in each layer. The points of contact between tactoids are along the longitudinal axis and laterally between the chains.

Sickle erythrocytes become dehydrated over time through loss of potassium and water, and this enhances the polymerization of HbS. The renal medulla is especially susceptible to damage from stickling because its hypertonicity further promotes the polymerization of HbS. The spleen and bone marrow are similarly prone to damage because their sluggish blood flows allow more time for deoxygenation and polymerization of HbS to occur in capillaries and sinusoids.

The two main pathophysiologic consequences of the polymerization of S, or sickling, are hemolysis and vaso-occlusion. Hemolysis or destruction of RBCs, in SCD occurs predominantly in the extravascular compartment. Cycles of sickling damage the RBC, especially its membrane. These damaged RBCs are recognized as abnormal and removed from circulation by the RE system.

Some intravascular hemolysis occurs as well, by microvascular trapping and destruction of adhesive and rigid sickle RBCs. The mean RBC lifespan in HbSS is dramatically shortened to 10–20 days from the normal RBC lifespan of 120 days. The rate of hemolysis in SCD usually exceeds the rate at which new RBCs can be produced by the bone marrow. Therefore, SCD is characterized by a partially compensated hemolytic anemia with significant reticulocytosis.

The two major pathophysiological mechanisms include:
1. *Hemolysis:* Sickled RBCs undergo both intravascular and extravascular hemolysis. This leads to anemia, reticulocytosis, jaundice, gallstones, and occasional aplastic crises.
2. *Vaso-occlusive:* Intermittent and chronic vaso-occlusion results in both acute exacerbation (e.g., painful crisis and stroke) and chronic disease manifestation (e.g., retinopathy and renal disease). The adhesion of sickled erythrocytes to inflamed vascular endothelium is the principal pathological component.

Normally during oxygenation in the lungs, the pO_2 is 95 torr. When oxygenated RBCs enter arterioles and capillaries in the tissues, the O_2 is released into the tissues. In venous blood, pO_2 drops to 40 torr. The equilibrium of HbS between sol and gel form is affected by O_2 tension, concentration of deoxyhemoglobin in RBC, p2-3 DPG, temperature, and presence of other hemoglobin.

Ionic changes in HbS polymerization are associated with a decrease in potassium, an increase in sodium, increase in the calcium content of the red cell. Loss of potassium and gain of sodium is due to partial failure of the adenosine triphosphatase (ATPase) pump, which regulates Na and K transport.

In addition to their shortened lifespan, sickle erythrocytes are also abnormally adhesive and have decreased flexibility. Consequently, they can adhere to and damage the endothelium of blood vessels and block the flow of blood. This microvascular obstruction, called vaso-occlusion, leads to ischemia and the interaction of different tissues. Vaso-occlusion is believed to be the main cause of acute episodes of pain that are characteristic of SCD.

Finally, SCD is also characterized by an as-yet incompletely understood vasculopathy caused by endothelial activation, abnormal interactions between the endothelium and blood cells, and reduced nitric oxide (NO) signaling. Vascular intimal proliferation results in progressive narrowing of the vessel lumen, constraining perfusion of downstream issues. This progressive stenosis, in conjunction with chronic anemia and episodic vaso-occlusion, is responsible for the chronic organ damage seen in people with SCD.

Change in Red Blood Cell Membrane

The membrane damage is pronounced with repeated cycles of sickling and unsickling, resulting in fixation of the membrane in sickled configuration leading to irreversible sickle cell formation.

Heinz bodies are aggregates of a small amount of HbS form micro-Heinz bodies. This gets attached to the cytoplasmic part of the band 3 protein of the red cell membrane. This binding results in changes on the outer side of the membrane forming antiband 3 protein antibodies contributing to a shortened lifespan of "SS" red cells.

Increased adherence to endothelium in SCD red cells has a tendency of binding endothelium. This is probably due to surface molecule receptors vascular cell adhesion molecules and fibronectin. The red cells adhere to endothelium, assume sickle shape after deoxygenation, and damage the endothelial cells leading to subendothelial infiltration and narrowing of the vessels.

Platelets aggregate over the adherent red cells and damage endothelium, causing blockage of microvasculature and ischemia of the tissue.

The homozygous state causes the SCD. It is characterized by episodes of pain, sickled RBCs, and crisis. The types of crises include vaso-occlusive crisis, anoxic crisis, and hemolytic crisis.

Under the conditions of anoxia and acidosis, the erythrocytes are deformed into sickle-shaped cells. These distorted cells block the capillaries and cause local anoxia. Anoxia leads to further sickling. This produces the blockage of the capillaries. It causes infarction in various tissues and organs. Hyperhemolytic crisis occurs in homozygous SCD which coincidentally has G6PD deficiency, which ingests the oxidant drug.

Other states such as vomiting, diarrhea, and fever produce hemoconcentration and precipitate into sludging. The sickle cells sequestered in the capillaries of the RE system are hemolyzed. The resulting anemia is associated with reticulocytes. Biliary pigment stones and gallstones are formed in long-standing cases. Hypoxia produces clubbing. Anemia leads to hyperactivity of bone marrow resulting in radiological change in bone.

Microinfarcts in the liver cause hepatomegaly and jaundice. Infarct in the spleen manifests as abdominal pain with eventual fibrosis and reduction in the spleen size.

Central nervous system infarct occurs proceeding strokes. Renal function is progressively impaired by diffuse glomerular and tubular fibrosis. Renal papillary necrosis and nephrotic syndrome occur.

Functional asplenia may begin as early as 5–6 months of age. It may precede the presence of Howell–Jolly bodies in the peripheral smear. Most children with HbSS who are >5 years old have functional asplenia with a small atrophied spleen. Splenic dysfunction causes increased susceptibility to meningitis and sepsis.

Sickle Cell Trait

The predominance of HbA within HbS trait RBCs prevents sickling under normal oxygen tensions. The hypertonicity and relative acidosis in the renal medulla can induce sickling in the kidney. Therefore, hyposthenuria and renal papillary necrosis with gross hematuria are known potential medical complications of HbS trait. Under conditions of extreme physical exertion, low oxygen tension, or both, other complications have been described in people with the HbS trait.

It is important for individuals to know that they have HbS traits because of the risk to their offspring. HbSS is an autosomal recessive disease, so if both parents have HbS traits, each of their offspring will have a 25% chance of having HbSS. Even if only one parent has the HbS trait, offspring are still at risk of having SCD if the parent without the HbS trait happens to have the HbC trait or β-thalassemia trait.

CLINICAL FEATURES (FIG. 1) AND RESPECTIVE MANAGEMENT

There are considerable variations in the manifestations of SCD. Some patients remain asymptomatic and are detected only during screening, whereas others constantly experience painful episodes. Most of the patients fall in these two extreme categories and experience intermittent clinical crises.

CLINICAL COURSE

A patient with SCD has at baseline chronic hemolytic anemia to which he or she

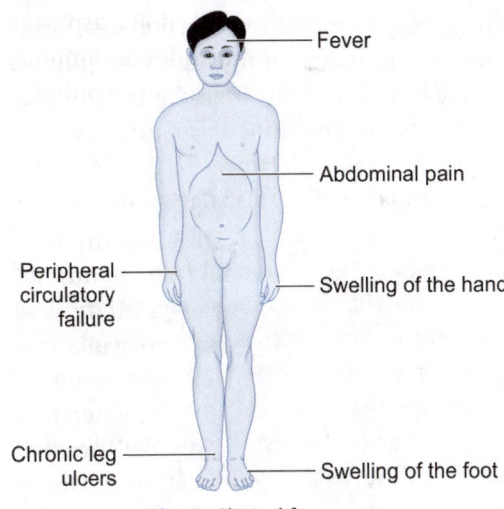

Fig. 1: Clinical features.

becomes physiologically adapted. This baseline anemic, but relatively healthy, state is called the steady state. This steady state is punctuated by intermittent, acute episodes of illness, called vaso-occlusive episodes, events, or crises, through the term crisis. Recurrent vaso-occlusion and chronic anemia also produce chronic organ damage.

At birth, newborns with HbSS disease have normal birth weight and are not anemic. Anemia and reticulocytosis usually appear between 2 and 6 months of age. Scleral icterus and a cardiac flow murmur are expected findings as a result of the anemia. Prophylactic penicillin to prevent pneumococcal sepsis should be initiated prior to the onset of splenic infarction and hyposplenism, which may begin to occur as early as 3 months of age. Before splenic infarction is complete, the spleen may be palpably enlarged.

Acute vaso-occlusive events are unusual before 6 months of age.

The first painful event is often dactylitis, which is a swelling of the hands and feet caused by vaso-occlusion in the marrow found in the bones of the digits. Dactylitis is rare beyond 3 years of age once this marrow is resorbed. Although birth weight is normal, growth retardation is commonly observed during childhood. On average, individuals with HbSS tend to be thinner and shorter than their peers, but a normal adult height can often be attained. The onset of puberty and development of secondary sex characteristics are usually delayed by 2–3 years.

Usually, children with SCD are asymptomatic up to 6 months of age. This is due to the large amount of hemoglobin "F" at birth, which has a positive correlation with a milder presentation. Mild hemolytic anemia is apparent by 3 months of age. Splenomegaly is usually detected by 6 months of age.

Children with palpable spleen within 6 months of age are at risk of developing subsequent pneumococcal septicemia. The majority of patients experience the first episode of vaso-occlusive crisis between 6 months and 6 years.

Fever and Bacteremia

By 5 years of age, most children with HbSS have complete functional asplenia. Regardless of age, all patients with HbSS are at increased risk of infection and death from bacterial infection, particularly encapsulated organisms such as *Streptococcus pneumoniae*, *Haemophilus influenzae* type b, and *Neisseria meningitidis*.

Outpatient management of fever without a source should be considered in children with the lowest risk of bacteremia and after appropriate cultures are obtained and IV ceftriaxone or another cephalosporin is given. Observation after antibiotic administration is important because children who have HbSS treated with ceftriaxone can develop severe, rapid, and life-threatening immune hemolysis.

Fever in a child with HbSS is a medical emergency, requiring prompt medical evaluation and delivery of antibiotics because of the increased risk of bacterial infection and subsequent high mortality rate. Infants with HbSS, as early as 6 months of age, develop abnormal immune function due to splenic infarction. By 5 years of age, most children with HbSS have complete functional asplenia. Regardless of age, all patients with HbSS are at increased risk of infection and death from bacterial infection, particularly encapsulated organisms, such as *S. pneumoniae*, *H. influenzae* type b, and *N. meningitidis*.

The rate of bacteremia in children with SCD, presenting with fever in busy pediatric emergency departments is <1%. Several clinical strategies have been developed to manage children with HbSS who present with fever. These vary from hospital admission for IV antimicrobial therapy to administering a third-generation cephalosporin in an emergency department or outpatient setting to patients without established risk factors for occult bacteremia.

Infections

Fatal *S. pneumoniae* sepsis occurred in 15% to 20% of children in the first 5 years of life. These infections were typically fulminant, with death occurring within 24 hours of the onset of fever. Children with SCD have an unusual vulnerability to severe pneumococcal sepsis due to their early loss of splenic RE function (functional hyposplenism) and their lack of circulating antibodies against polysaccharide-encapsulated bacteria.

In early life, the spleen, although often palpably enlarged, loses RE function because of continuous vaso-occlusive infarction. The enlarged spleen gradually becomes small and fibrotic, and it is rarely palpable after 6 years of age. The combination of hyposplenism and lack of antibodies against polysaccharide antigens accounts for the high susceptibility and the historically high frequency and mortality of pneumococcal infections in young children with HbSS.

Patients with SCD also have a predilection for osteomyelitis, perhaps because certain pathogens can survive and escape immunologic clearance in the ischemic or infarcted bone and bone marrow. *Salmonella* species cause about half the cases of osteomyelitis in SCD, and staphylococci cause most of the rest. It can be difficult to differentiate osteomyelitis from an acute painful episode that results in infarction of cortical bone. Both can cause bony tenderness, effusions, and lucencies on X-ray imaging. Even bone scans and magnetic resonance imaging (MRI) fail to distinguish between the two. Clinical features are more helpful than imaging studies in this situation. The occurrence of fever, a single locus of pain, and a positive blood culture are more consistent with a diagnosis of osteomyelitis than an acute painful episode.

Outpatient management of fever without a source should be considered in children with the lowest risk of bacteremia and after IV ceftriaxone or other cephalosporin is given. In the event that *Salmonella* spp. or *Staphylococcus aureus* bacteremia occurs, strong consideration should be given to an evaluation for osteomyelitis with a bone scan given the increased risk of osteomyelitis in children with HbSS when compared to the general population.

Sickle Cell Pain

Dactylitis, referred to as hand-foot syndrome, is often the first manifestation of pain in infants and young children with HbSS, occurring in 50% of children by their second year of life. Dactylitis often manifests with symmetric or

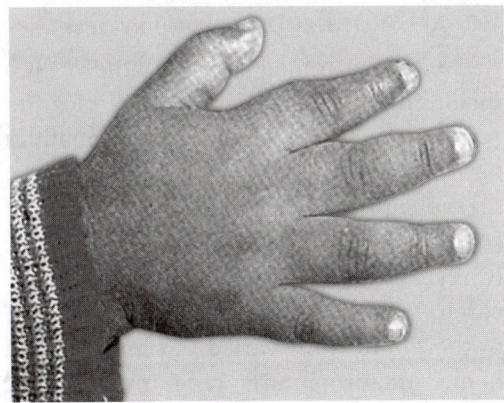

Fig. 2: Dactylitis.

unilateral swelling of the hands and/or feet (Fig. 2). Unilateral dactylitis can be confused with osteomyelitis, and careful evaluation to distinguish between the two is important because treatment differs significantly. Dactylitis requires palliation with pain medications, such as hydrocortisone, whereas osteomyelitis requires at least 4–6 weeks of IV antibiotics. Given the recent association between genotype and metabolism of codeine, a subgroup of children may not get pain relief from codeine.

Skeletal pain (bone or bone marrow infarction) with or without fever must be differentiated from osteomyelitis. Both *Salmonella* spp. and *S. aureus* cause osteomyelitis in children with HbSS, which is often in the diaphysis of long bones (in contrast to children without HbSS where osteomyelitis is in the metaphyseal region of the bone). Differentiating osteonecrosis from a vaso-occlusive crisis and osteomyelitis is often difficult; patients with osteomyelitis often have a longer duration of fever and pain, swelling of the affected area, fewer or only one location of pain and tenderness, higher WBC counts, and elevated C-reactive protein. Blood cultures, when positive, are helpful.

Magnetic resonance imaging findings suggestive of osteomyelitis include localized medullary fluid, sequestrum, and cortical defects. Ultimately, aspiration with or without biopsy and culture will be needed to differentiate the two processes.

Painful Episodes

The acute painful episode is the hallmark of SCD. It is the most common reason for medical consultation and hospitalization in this population. The pain seems to be caused by acute vaso-occlusion, primarily in bones and bone marrow, with consequent ischemia and inflammation.

Pain can occur anywhere in the body, but it is most commonly osteoarticular and juxta-vertebral. The earliest physical manifestation of HbSS is often a characteristic painful episode of dactylitis, an often symmetric swelling of the hands and feet that occurs in about 30% of children in the first 3 years of life. As the child ages, painful episodes instead involve the long bones, vertebrae, sternum, ribs, lower back, and abdomen.

The treatment of the painful episode is symptomatic and focuses on controlling the severity of the pain. Analgesia must be tailored to the degree of pain and to the patient. Moderate pain without fever or other signs of concomitant illness can usually be managed at home with hydration, analgesics, and rest. However, some pain is so severe that hospitalization for IV hydration and parenteral opioids is necessary, Overhydration is not helpful and may actually precipitate acute chest syndrome (ACS). A combination of NSAIDs and opioid analgesics, titrated to effect will usually achieve adequate pain relief.

A useful strategy in patients admitted for inpatient pain management is to initiate patient-controlled analgesia (PCA), consisting of IV opioid medication administered at a continuous (basal) rate with available on-demand (bolus) dosing under the patient's control. Frequent assessments of the number of on-demand doses requested, along with the patient's self-report of the adequacy of pain control and clinical monitoring for adverse effects of opioid therapy, can permit rapid titration to adequate analgesia, at which point the transition to oral long- and short-acting opioids can be initiated.

Patients with SCD-related pain, even severe, typically have no accompanying physical signs, such as edema and erythema, so it is important to trust the patient's report of pain and its intensity and to use this self-report to titrate analgesia. Transfusion does not relieve acute sickle cell pain, and there is currently no therapy to shorten the duration of the painful episode. The pain must be treated until the episode resolves spontaneously, which may take as long as a week. Once the pain begins to resolve, opioid therapy can be weaned relatively quickly.

Neurologic Complications

Neurologic complications associated with HbSS range from acute ischemic stroke with focal neurologic deficit to clinically silent abnormalities found on radiologic imaging. A functional definition of overt stroke is the presence of a focal neurologic deficit lasting for >24 hours and/or abnormal neuroimaging of the brain indicating a cerebral infarct on T2-weighted MRI corresponding to the focal neurologic deficit. The complications include headaches that may or may not correlate to a degree of anemia, seizures, cerebral venous thrombosis, and reversible posterior leukoencephalopathy syndrome, also referred to as posterior reversible encephalopathy syndrome (PRES).

Renal Complications

Renal disease among patients with SCD is a major comorbid condition that can lead to premature death. Seven SCD nephropathies have been identified, i.e., (1) Gross hematuria; (2) Papillary necrosis; (3) Nephritic syndrome; (4) Renal infarction; (5) Hyposthenuria; (6) Pyelonephritis; and (7) Renal medullary carcinoma. As expected, the presentation of these entities is varied but may include hematuria, proteinuria, renal insufficiency, concentrating defects, or hypertension.

Vaso-occlusive Crisis

The cardinal clinical feature of HbSS is acute vaso-occlusive pain. No written definition can describe the visual picture of a child with HbSS experiencing pain. Acute sickle cell pain is characterized as unremitting discomfort that can occur in any part of the body but most often occurs in the chest, abdomen, or extremities.

The extract etiology of pain is unknown, but the pathogenesis is initiated when blood flow is disrupted in the microvasculature by sickled cells, resulting in tissue ischemia. A vaso-occlusive crisis occurs because of blockage of microvascular circulation leading to ischemic tissue injury. There are episodes of painful crisis, which vary in intensity and duration lasting from a few days to a few weeks.

The precipitating factors include hypoxia, infection, fever, acidosis, dehydration, sleep apnea, and exposure to cold. Emotional or physical stress can be a precipitating cause. Sometimes the etiology is idiopathic. Successful treatment of painful episodes requires education of both the caregivers and patients regarding the recognition of symptoms and the optimal management strategy.

Hand–Foot Syndrome

The age of occurrence could be as early as 4 months. The prevalence is highest at 2 years of age and is rare after 5 years. Ischemic necrosis and death of active bone marrow initiate an inflammatory response, increasing intermedullary pressure.

Clinically, there is swelling over the affected small bones of the four extremities, with severe pain and tenderness. Fever is a common accompanying feature. WBC count is increased up to $15,000/mm^3$.

Radiological changes are limited to soft-tissue swelling. Cortical thinning and destruction of metatarsals, metacarpals, and phalanges follow. Usually, complete clinical and radiological recovery occurs within 2–3 weeks. Sometimes damaged epiphysis may cause premature fusion and permanent shortening of small bones. Management consists of hydration and analgesia. Blood transfusion is usually not required.

Avascular Necrosis of Femoral Head

Avascular necrosis (AVN) occurs at a higher rate among children with HbSS than in the general population and is a source of both acute and chronic pain. Most commonly, the femoral head is affected. In AVN, hip and shoulder joints can be affected, but weight-bearing makes femoral head necrosis more likely to cause severe disability. It can occur at any age after infancy; however, the incidence is high in the second or third decade. Other sites affected include the humeral head and mandible. Risk factors for AVN include HbSS disease with alpha-thalassemia trait, frequent vaso-occlusive episodes, and elevated hematocrit (for patients with HbSS).

Total collapse and destruction of the femoral head can occur after the closure of the epiphysis. The patient presents with pain in the groin and buttocks with restriction of movements of the hip joint. Radiological changes appear after a long time; MRI or radionuclide imaging can detect the earliest changes associated with pain.

Initial management may include referral to a physical therapist to address strategies to increase strength and decrease weight-bearing daily activities that may exacerbate the pain associated with AVN. Opioids are often used but usually can be tiered after the acute pain has subsided with AVN. Considerable healing and recovery can occur if AVN occurs before the closure of the epiphysis of the femoral head.

Initial treatment in children and teenagers consists of avoidance of weight bearing and judicious use of analgesics in the first 6 months. Osteotomy with rotation of the femoral head to change the weight-bearing area has also been used. In older patients with severe pain but no radiological evidence of collapse, decompression of the femoral head results in immediate pain relief. Replacement of the hip joint may be done in patients with incapacitating pain interfering with daily activities.

Abdominal Crisis

It occurs predominantly in childhood due to small infarcts of the mesentery and abdominal viscera. There is severe abdominal pain and signs of peritoneal irritation. The persistence of bowel sound differentiates it from acute abdomen requiring surgical exploration. It usually resolves in a period of 4–5 days. The management consists of bowel rest and maintenance of hydration by IV fluids.

Acute Chest Syndrome: Pulmonary Complication

It is one of the common causes of hospital admissions in patients with SCD. It is characterized by acute chest pain, dyspnea, hypoxia, fever, and prostration. Radiologically it is characterized by the appearance of new pulmonary infiltrates. X-ray changes may take several days to appear. Hematologically it is characterized by a sudden drop in hemoglobin concentration and an increase in leukocyte count and platelet count. The term "acute chest syndrome" is used because a more precise etiology is rarely documented.

Lung disease in children with HbSS is the second most common reason for hospital admission and is associated with significant mortality refers to a life-threatening pulmonary complication of SCD defined as a new radiodensity on chest radiography plus any two of the following: (1) Fever; (2) Respiratory distress; (3) Hypoxia; (4) Cough; or (5) Chest pain.

Infection is the most well-known etiology, yet only 30% of ACS episodes will have positive sputum or bronchoalveolar culture, and the most common pathogens are *S. pneumoniae*, *Mycoplasma pneumoniae*, and *Chlamydia* spp. The most frequent event preceding ACS is a painful episode requiring systemic opioid treatment. Fat emboli have been implicated as a cause of ACS, arising from infarcted bone marrow, and can be life-threatening if large amounts are released into the lungs.

Pulmonary hypertension has been identified as a major risk factor for death in adults with HbSS. The natural history of pulmonary hypertension in children with HbSS is unknown.

The causative factors are thought to be: (1) Infection, (2) in situ vaso-occlusion in lungs due to erythrocyte stasis, (3) pulmonary infarction due to immobilization from deep vein thrombus or of fat from infracted marrow, and (4) analgesic narcotic induced hypoventilation hereby enhancing sickling. In children, infectious etiology is common, whereas in adults in situ vaso-occlusion is more common.

Oxygen should be administered to patients who demonstrate hypoxia. Blood transfusion therapy using either simple or exchange (manual or automated) transfusion is the only method to abort a rapidly progressing episode of ACS.

Commonly blood transfusions are given when at least one of the following clinical features are present: Decreasing oxygen saturation, increasing work of breathing, rapid change in a respiratory effort either with or without a worsening chest radiograph, a drop in hemoglobin of 2 g/dL below their baseline, or previous history of severe ACS requiring admission to the intensive care unit.

Treatment usually consists of broad-spectrum antibiotics even in the absence of infection for prevention of secondary infection. Severe episodes should be monitored by pulse oximetry and blood gas analysis. Deterioration of pulmonary functions should be treated as an emergency and can be dramatically reversed by exchange transfusion. Oxygenation and ventilator support should be provided whenever required.

Management includes maintenance of hydration without overhydration, adequate but not excessive analgesia, good airway clearance with incentive spirometry or other measures, bronchodilators if there is any component of reactive airway disease and antibacterials. Infectious etiology is often not apparent; however, the use of empiric antibiotics active against *Pneumococcus*, *Mycoplasma*, and *Chlamydia* (typically a macrolide and a third-generation cephalosporin) is prudent. It is also important to initiate anti-influenza therapy if there is any clinical suspicion of influenza.

Corticosteroids such as dexamethasone may also be beneficial, but their role has not been demonstrated in controlled clinical trials. Supplemental oxygen can be provided as needed but should be closely monitored, as an increasing oxygen requirement is a sign of worsening disease.

Simple RBC transfusions can be helpful in interrupting disease progression, especially if anemia has worsened from the patient's baseline. Exchange transfusions may be needed for severe cases of ACS requiring significant oxygen supplementation or ventilatory support. Patients with evidence of right heart strain or respiratory distress out of proportion to findings on lung imaging should also undergo evaluation for pulmonary embolism. It is important to perform a thorough assessment of pulmonary function in patients who have experienced severe or recurrent episodes of ACS, both to assess for chronic lung damage and to identify potentially reversible airway or lung disease.

Stroke

There are five main clinical presentations of overt cerebrovascular disease in HbSS: Cerebral infarction, cerebral hemorrhage, and transient ischemic attacks (TIAs). Infarction and hemorrhage cause weakness, paralysis, aphasia, and sometimes seizures and headaches. TIAs are episodes of weakness, paralysis, or aphasia that lasts <24 hours. TIAs are likely to be overlooked in young children, but they are harbingers of overt stroke. All 3 presentations can occur at any age, but hemorrhagic stroke is more common in patients older than 20 years.

A stroke is usually preceded by a very severe headache. Rapid progressive generalized deterioration may progress to a coma. The patient may exhibit decorticate or decerebrate posturing. Associated signs of acute tissue injury due to vaso-occlusive crisis involving lungs, kidneys, and liver.

Other risk factors include anemia, painful episodes, and high white cell count. Hemorrhagic stroke presents with generalized phenomena, such as coma, headache, and convulsions.

Magnetic resonance imaging and magnetic resonance angiography (MRA) are needed to visualize cerebral infarction and stenosis of intracranial arteries. CT can be obtained more quickly than MRI, and it may be helpful when cerebral hemorrhage is strongly suspected. MRI and MRA are more sensitive for detecting ICH and infarctions in the early period.

Acute management includes exchange transfusion, careful hydration, and control of any seizures. An additional 20–30% of patients experience covert or silent cerebral infarctions (SCIs) that are not accompanied by motor signs. Both overt and covert strokes can cause neurocognitive impairment.

These patients need admission to the intensive care unit. Ventilator support with facilities for positive end-expiratory pressure (PEEP) or oscillating ventilator devices are necessary. Seizures should be controlled with anticonvulsant drugs. Exchange transfusion to reduce the HbS level to <30% should be done. A regular transfusion program designed to keep HbS <30%, lowers the recurrence rate to 10%. This should be continued for 2–5 years.

Priapism

Priapism is defined as an unwanted persistent painful erection of the penis and most commonly affects males with HbSS. The mean age of the first episode is 15 years, although priapism has been reported in children as young as 3 years. Priapism occurs in two patterns: (1) Prolonged, lasting >4 hours, or (2) stuttering, with brief episodes that resolve spontaneously but may occur in clusters and herald a prolonged event.

Both types occur from early childhood to adulthood. Most episodes occur between 3 and 9 AM. Priapism in SCD represents a low flow state caused by venous stasis from sickling of RBCs in the corpora cavernosa. Recurrent prolonged episodes of priapism are associated with impotence.

1. Recurrent acute priapism manifests with episodic short attacks, which subside spontaneously. Impotency may be sequelae.
2. Acute prolonged priapism is characterized by a very painful penile erection that does not subside for several hours. Radionuclear scan shows very low blood flow.
3. Chronic priapism may follow an acute episode or may arise de novo. The penis is semierected there is no pain. The scan shows good blood flow.

The optimal treatment for acute priapism is unknown. Acutely, supportive therapy and urology consultations are required to initiate this procedure, with appropriate input from a hematologist.

Treatment includes supportive measures such as a hot shower, short aerobic exercise, and pain medication, which are commonly used by patients at home. A prolonged episode lasting >4 hours should be treated by aspiration of blood from the corpora cavernosa followed by irrigation with dilute epinephrine to produce immediate and sustained detumescence maintenance of hydration and analgesia. Transfusion therapy is indicated if engorgement persists for 24–48 hours. In severe cases, an exchange transfusion should be done.

Surgery involving the creation of a temporary fistula between the glans and corpora cavernosa is the treatment of choice if there is no improvement 48 hours after exchange transfusion.

Sequestration Crisis

Acute splenic sequestration is a life-threatening complication occurring primarily in infants and young children with HbSS. Sequestration can occur as early as 5 weeks of age, but most often occurs in children between the ages of 6 months and 2 years. The event is characterized by the sudden trapping of blood in the spleen or less commonly in the liver. These patients bleed into their spleen. They present with sudden weakness, significant pallor with profound anemia tachycardia, tachypnea, and enormously enlarged spleen filling the abdomen.

Splenic sequestration is associated with rapid spleen enlargement causing left-sided abdominal pain and a decline in hemoglobin of at least 2 g/dL from the patient's baseline. Sequestration may lead to signs of hypovolemia as a result of the trapping of blood in the spleen; profound anemia, with total hemoglobin falling below 3 g/dL, has been reported. Reticulocyte count is markedly elevated, and thrombocytopenia is noticed. A decrease in WBC and platelet count may also be present. Sequestration may be triggered by fever, bacteremia, or viral infections. The condition must be promptly treated, as, within hours of the first sign of this disturbance hypovolemic shock and death can occur. Subacute episodes are characterized by moderate splenomegaly reduction of hemoglobin level by 2–3 g, and increased reticulocyte count.

Treatment includes early intervention and maintenance of hemodynamic stability using isotonic fluid or blood transfusions. Careful blood transfusions with RBCs are recommended to treat both the sequestration and the resultant anemia. Blood transfusion aborts the RBC sickling in the spleen and allows the release of the patient's blood cells that have become sequestered, often raising the hemoglobin above baseline values. 5 mL/kg of RBCs is recommended because the goal is to prevent hypovolemia. Blood transfusion that results in hemoglobin levels above 10 g/dL may put the patient at risk for hyperviscosity syndrome because of the risk that that patient may release the blood within the spleen.

If a child gets two or more episodes splenectomy is advised, and parents should be educated about regular palpation of the spleen enabling them to seek medical treatment in time.

Aplastic Crisis

Human parvovirus Bl9 infection poses a unique threat to patients with SCD because this infection results in temporary red cell aplasia, limiting the production of reticulocytes and causing profound anemia. Testing for the presence of human parvovirus B19 with polymerase chain reaction (PCR) testing is superior to using immunoglobulin M (IgM) and immunoglobulin G (IgG) titers. The acute exacerbation of anemia is treated conservatively using red cell transfusion when the patient becomes hemodynamically symptomatic or has a concurrent illness, such as ACS and acute splenic sequestration.

Red blood cells lifespan is greatly shortened from the normal of 120 days to 10–20 days in HbSS. Consequently, patients must chronically maintain a marked increase in RBC production by the bone marrow producing chronic reticulocytosis, to maintain a stable hemoglobin concentration compatible with life. If RBC production is impaired for even a short time, the hemoglobin concentration will fall rapidly during many viral infections and inflammatory states, erythropoiesis may be modestly reduced, resulting in relative reticulocytopenia and transiently more severe anemia. Human parvovirus BI9, the agent causing fifth disease, has especially profound effects on patients with chronic hemolytic anemia.

Parvovirus destroys early RBC precursors in the bone marrow and causes RBC aplasia for about a week The consequent erythroblastopenia and reticulocytopenia cause a dramatic and potentially life-threatening anemia, with the hemoglobin concentration falling as low as 1–2 g/dL without measurable reticulocytes. This episode of severe anemia is called an aplastic crisis. There may be variable degrees of leukopenia or thrombocytopenia due to the effects of parvovirus. Bilirubin concentration and jaundice are also acutely decreased because there are fewer sickle erythrocytes undergoing hemolysis

It is characterized by acute anemia, which may lead to readily preventable mortality in young children. The causative organism is parvovirus B19. The parvovirus has direct toxicity to erythroid precursors, colony forming unit.

The clinical features are often interrupted by sickle cell crisis due to suddenly enhanced intravascular sickling. The patient gets pain and aches in the body. Jaundice becomes pronounced. Anemia worsens and the spleen enlarges rapidly. The child would be easily fatigued. The patients present with increased fatigue, dyspnea, anemia, and few or no reticulocytes. The condition is always self-limiting with a duration of 7–10 days.

Physical growth is retarded. The onset of puberty is delayed. Clubbing of the fingers is present due to chronic anoxia. The heart size is enlarged. Hemic murmur, i.e., ejection systolic murmur is found on auscultation of the heart. Liver size is enlarged due to sinusoidal dilatation. The spleen becomes palpable at the age of 9 months and may reach up to the umbilicus. Then it shrinks due to infarction by the end of the first decade. This is functionally hyposplenic. Flow murmur and venous hum are auscultated. Dehydration may occur as their inability to concentrate urine is present. These patients are vulnerable to pneumococcal meningitis and septicemia.

The hemoglobin may drop to 2 g%. Urgent transfusion is required. Daily monitoring of reticulocyte count should be done. The parvovirus offers lifelong immunity.

The acute RBC aplasia is transient and self-limited. Spontaneous recovery begins about 1 week after the onset of reticulocytopenia due to antibody-mediated clearance of the virus. Recovery is heralded by the appearance of nucleated RBCs in the circulation, followed shortly by brisk reticulocytosis.

Transfusion of blood is the most important intervention for symptomatic or severe anemia. In contrast to acute splenic sequestration, blood must be transfused relatively slowly in patients with aplastic crisis because their blood volume is typically normal or increased as a physiologic adaption to a more slowly progressive anemia. Lifelong immunity against parvovirus prevents recurrent episodes.

GENERAL FEATURES
• Acute sickle cell dactylitis
• Hand-foot syndrome
• Priapism
• Cardiomyopathy
• Gallstone formation
• Underweight

DIAGNOSIS

The most commonly used procedures for newborn diagnosis include thin layer/isoelectric focusing (IEF) and high-performance liquid chromatography (HPLC). Some laboratories perform genetic testing on specimens demonstrating abnormal HbS. A confirmatory step is recommended, with all patients who have initial abnormal screens being retested during the first clinical visit. In addition, a CBC and Hb phenotype determination is recommended for both parents to confirm the diagnosis and to provide an opportunity for genetic counseling. Infants who may have HbS-hereditary persistence fetal hemoglobin (HbS-HPFH) but do not have full parental studies should have molecular testing for globin genotype before 12 months of age.

Beyond the immediate newborn period, the laboratory evaluation of suspected SCD should include a CBC, reticulocyte count, and examination of the peripheral blood smear. To confirm a diagnosis of SCD, however, some analysis of hemoglobin types must be performed. Abnormal HbS must be identified using at least two methods because they can be difficult to differentiate.

Because patients with SCD have chronic hemolytic anemia, they also have unconjugated hyperbilirubinemia and variable elevations of lactate dehydrogenase (LDH) and aspartate transaminase (AST). Bilirubin is a product of heme degradation, and LDH and AST are released from RBCs that undergo hemolysis. After the first year of life, the peripheral blood smear shows variable numbers of pathognomonic irreversibly sickled cells, as well as polychromatophilic cells, Howell–Jolly bodies, poikilocytes, and target cells. Howell–Jolly bodies are nuclear remnants, and their presence on the blood smear outside the immediate neonatal period is indicative of hyposplenism.

- *Peripheral smear*—contains variations of the sickbed form of RBIs **(Fig. 3)**. Target cells are in abundance. Features suggestive of accelerated erythropoiesis,

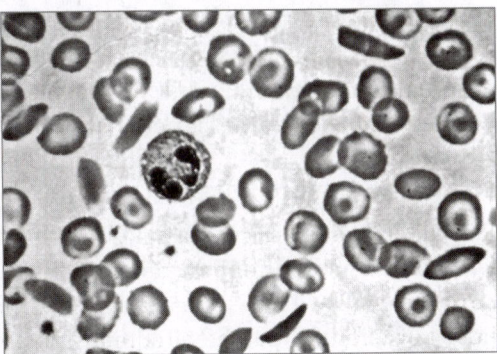

Fig. 3: Sickle cells. *(For color version, see Plate 2)*

such as polychromatophils, basophilic stippling, and normoblasts are prominent. Reticulocyte count ranges from 5 to 30%. Heinz bodies, Howell–Jolly bodies are present. WBC count ranges from 8,000 to 20,000/mm^3.

- *Coagulation profile*—platelet count is increased—factor 8, factor 13, fibrinogen, fibrinolytic activity, beta-thromboglobulin are increased factor 12, prekalikrein are decreased. Alterations in the coagulation system are thought to be responsible for occlusive complications of the SCD either directly or in the formation of fibrin strands and platelet aggregation. They may modulate the cell-vessel interaction.
- *Sickling test*—the principle is, that maneuvers used to extract oxygen, cause red cells with HbS to assume a sickle shape. Whereas cells lacking HbS maintain normal configuration. This can be achieved by sealing a blood drop under a cover slip to exclude oxygen, or, by adding an agent, such as 2% Na$^-$ metabisulfite.
- *Solubility test*—blood containing HbS is added to a buffered solution of a reducing agent, such as sodium dithionite. Deoxy HbS is precipitated and solution becomes turbid. However other hemoglobin such as HbC-Georgetown, HbI, Hb Barts, and unstable HbS are also precipitate by this test.

Both the above tests are screening tests. Diagnosis of a neonatal screening of high-risk population should be cloned for SCD. Antenatal diagnosis can be done at 8–10 weeks of gestation, with chorionic vials biopsy, or amniocentesis.

> **LABORATORY SALIENT FINDINGS**
> - Anemia
> - Reticulocytosis
> - *Peripheral blood smear:* Sickle cells, Heinz bodies, and Howell–Jolly bodies
> - Sickling test, solubility tests

Definite diagnosis is done by: Electrophoresis of blood lysate on cellulose acetate at alkaline pH 8.6. Certain hemoglobin variants have the same electrophoretic mobility as that of HbS on cellulose acetate electrophoresis. For their differentiation:

- Citrate agar electrophoresis at an acidic pH
- IEF
- Globin chain electrophoresis should be done

■ DIFFERENTIAL DIAGNOSIS

Differential diagnoses include rheumatic fever, rheumatoid arthritis, osteomyelitis, and leukemia.

> **ESSENTIAL DIAGNOSTIC POINTS**
> - Genetic mutation leads to abnormal beta-globin chain
> - Anemia, elevated reticulocyte count, and jaundice
> - Recurrent musculoskeletal or abdominal pain
> - Splenomegaly in early childhood
> - High risk of bacterial sepsis
> - Hemoglobin electrophoresis = HbS > HbA
> - Dactilitis (painful hand or foot swelling)
>
> (HbA: hemoglobin A; HbS: sickle hemoglobin)

TREATMENT

General Management

Treatment is aimed at preventing serious complications. Administration of a polyvalent pneumococcal vaccine may be beneficial. Prophylactic penicillin is highly effective in preventing serious pneumococcal infections. Oral penicillin can be given starting from 4 months of age. By 5 years of age, this can be discontinued.

Prompt parenteral antibiotics are given for infants and young children with acute onset of high fever.

Preventive care and family education about the potential complications of SCD are important components of SCD management. To this end, the primary care clinician or the hematologist should stress the importance of adherence to penicillin prophylaxis and the standard childhood immunization schedule to prevent early infection. The clinician should also provide anticipatory guidance about surveillance for fever, respiratory distress, pallor, jaundice, splenic enlargement, and neurologic abnormalities, all of which could represent the onset of significant complications of SCD. Early intervention and prompt medical care may be critical in averting life-threatening or severely debilitation morbidities if such symptoms emerge.

There are three main disease-modifying treatments that can reduce the overall severity of SCD or cure it, including: (1) hydroxyurea, (2) chronic transfusions, and (3) hematopoietic stem-cell transplantation (HSCT).

Hydration

High incidence of hyposthenuria, reduced fluid intake, and increased insensible water loss make them prone to dehydration. Loss of electrolytes may lead to red cell dehydration precipitating the sickling process. The fluid requirement is usually increased by 50% of the usual maintenance fluid requirement. Monitoring of electrolytes is necessary.

Drugs for Severe Pain

Painful episodes or acute crisis is managed with oral acetaminophen alone or with codeine. Severe episodes may require hospitalization and parenteral administration of narcotics. Anti-inflammatory agents, especially ketorolac are very useful. Dehydration or acidosis should be rapidly corrected by IV fluids. Transfusion of RBCs can provide relief to disabling chronic pain. For children with stroke, cardiomyopathy, and other complications, long-term transfusion regimens are a mainstay. PRBCs are used for spleen sequestration. Splenectomy is indicated if there are repeated episodes of pain.

Bone marrow transplantation from a normal donor is helpful. Chemotherapy is helpful to stimulate HbF synthesis. The damage includes hydroxyurea and butyrate.

- Injection morphine 0.1–0.15 mg/kg/3 hourly; oral morphine 0.3–0.6 mg/kg/3 hourly
- Injection meperidine 0.75–1.5 mg/kg/dose/3 hourly; oral meperidine 1.5 mg/kg/dose/3 hourly

Drugs for Mild Pain

- *Codeine:* 0.5–1 mg/kg/dose/4 hourly/orally
- *Aspirin:* 10 mg/kg/dose/orally enhances analgesia if given with narcotic
- *Ibuprofen:* 5–10 mg/kg/dose 8 hourly/orally
- *Acetaminophen*: 10 mg/kg/day/orally/4 hourly enhances analgesia with narcotic
- *Naproxen*: 10 mg/kg/day orally
- *Indomethacin*: 1–3 mg/day/6 hourly/orally

Hydroxyurea

Hydroxyurea, a myelosuppressive agent, is the only drug proven effective in reducing the frequency of painful episodes. In a large clinical trial of adults with HbSS, hydroxyurea was found to decrease the rate of hospitalization for painful episodes by 50% and the rate of ACS and blood transfusion by almost 50%. Follow-up of the original trial found that adults taking hydroxyurea had shorter hospital stays and required less pain medication during hospitalization. In children with HbSS, a safety feasibility trial of hydroxyurea demonstrated that hydroxyurea was safe and well tolerated in children >5 years of age. Infants treated with hydroxyurea also experienced fewer episodes of pain, dactylitis, and ACS, and were less often hospitalized or received a blood transfusion. Despite being a myelosuppressive agent, the infants treated with hydroxyurea did not experience increased rates of bacteremia or serious infection.

The typical starting dose of hydroxyurea is 15–20 mg/kg given once daily, with an incremental dosage increase every 8 weeks of 5 mg/kg, and if no toxicities occur, up to a maximum of 35 mg/kg/dose. The infant hydroxyurea study found young children could safely be started at 20 mg/kg/day without increased toxicity. Achievement of the therapeutic effect of hydroxyurea can require several months, and for this reason, inpatient initiating of hydroxyurea is not optimal.

Role of Blood Transfusion

Red blood cell transfusions are frequently used in the management of children with HbSS, both in the treatment of acute complications such as ACS, aplastic crisis, splenic sequestration, and acute stroke and to prevent surgery-related ACS and first stroke in patients.

Patients with SCD are at increased risk of developing alloantibodies to less common red cell surface antigens after receiving even a single transfusion. Its addition to standard cross-matching for major blood group antigens (A, B, O, and RhD), more extended matching should be performed to identify donor units that are C-, E-, and Kell-antigen negative. Some centers have begun to perform full RBC phenotyping for patients receiving chronic blood transfusions.

Three methods of blood transfusion therapy are used in the management of acute and chronic complications associated with HbSS: Automated erythrocytapheresis, manual exchange transfusion (phlebotomy of a set amount of patient's blood followed by rapid administration of donated PRBCs), and simple transfusion.

Automated erythrocytapheresis is the preferred method for patients requiring chronic blood transfusion therapy because there is a minimum net iron balance after the procedure, followed by manual exchange transfusion. Simple transfusion therapy is the least preferable method for regular blood transfusion therapy because this strategy results in the highest net-positive iron balance after the procedure. Despite being the preferred method, erythrocytapheresis is less frequently performed because of the requirement of technical expertise, large venous access, multiple units of matched RBCs, and an available cytapheresis machine.

Blood transfusion in SCD should be used as sparingly as possible, and only for specific indications, which are as follows:
- Severely anemic patients
- Sudden fall of hemoglobin as seen in sequestration crisis.

- Acute of suspected cerebrovascular accidents
- Multiorgan failure syndrome
- ACS or other acute lung disease where actual oxygenation cannot be maintained near normal even after oxygen therapy and the process is progressive despite of antibiotics given.
- Children who have had a cerebrovascular accident, to prevent further similar attacks.
- Chronic CCF in conjunction with other treatments.

Chronic Transfusion

Chronic transfusion programs entail regular, usually monthly, transfusions of PRBCs aimed to maintain the percentage of HbS in the blood at <30%. Transfusion may consist of simple top-off transfusions, phlebotomy transfusions in which a volume of blood is removed before transfusion of nonsickle erythrocytes, or automated exchange transfusion (erythrocytapheresis) in which the patient's erythrocyte mass is continuously removed and replaced with nonsickle erythrocytes. Chronic transfusions are effective at preventing most complications of SCD, but the most common indications are primary and secondary stroke prophylaxis.

Complications of transfusions include iron overload and the need for chelation therapy, alloimmunization, and transfusion-transmitted infections. Iron chelation to prevent toxicity from transfusional iron overload is described below in the section on therapy for thalassemia.

Preparation for surgery for children with SCD requires a coordinated effort between the hematologist, surgeon, and primary care provider. ACS and pain are the two most common postoperative complications, with ACS being a significant risk factor for postoperative death. Blood transfusion prior to surgery for children with HbSS is recommended to raise the hemoglobin level preoperatively to no >10 g/dL, although benefit also may be seen at lower hemoglobin values.

Hematopoietic Stem-Cell Transplantation

Hematopoietic stem-cell (or bone marrow) transplantation is the only cure for SCD. Widespread use of transplantation is limited by the lack of donor availability and toxicities of the procedure. Transplantation is safest when hematopoietic stem cells are obtained from a human leukocyte antigen (HLA)-matched sibling without SCD, but only 10% of patients actually have a potential donor. The use of alternative donors is an area of ongoing study.

The only cure for HbSS is transplantation with HLA-matched hematopoietic stem cells from a sibling or unrelated donor. The most common indications for transplant are recurrent ACS and stroke. Sibling-matched stem cell transplantation has a lower risk for graft-versus-host disease than unrelated donors.

Excessive Iron Stores

The primary toxic effect of blood transfusion therapy relates to excessive iron stores, which can result in organ damage and premature death. Excessive iron stores develop after 100 mL/kg of red cell transfusion or about 10 transfusions.

The primary treatment of excessive iron stores resulting from RBC transfusion requires iron dictation using medical therapy. The three chelating agents are commercially available and approved for use in transfusional iron overload. Deferoxamine is administered subcutaneously five of seven nights/week for 10 hours a night. Deferasirox is an effervescent tablet that is dissolved in liquid and taken by mouth daily, and deferiprone is available in tablets taken orally a day. The US-FDA approved deferasirox, the newest orally administered, chelator, for use in patients aged >2 years.

Drugs Augmenting Hemoglobin F Synthesis

Fetal hemoglobin does not copolymerize with HbS, and interferes with bonding of the tactoids. Agents augmenting HbF synthesis thus offer a protective effect against gelation (5-azacytidine, hydroxyurea, and butyric acid analogs).

Antisickling Agents

These can be covalent and noncovalent. Covalent agents act at various sites of the globulin chain to decrease deoxy HbS gelation or to increase oxygen affinity of hemoglobin or by both mechanisms. They bind to hemoglobin irreversibly. Examples are cyanales.

Noncovalent agents bind reversibly with hemoglobin. They reduce the gelation of HbS by interference with hydrophobic bonds between hemoglobin tetramers. An example is urea.

LONG-TERM MORBIDITIES
- Chronic lung disease
- Renal failure
- Congestive cardiac failure
- Retinal damage
- Chronic leg ulcer
- Aseptic necrosis of hip and shoulder
- Poor growth

■ BIBLIOGRAPHY

1. Chou ST, Fasano RM. Management of patients with sickle cell disease using transfusion therapy: guidelines and complications. Hematol Onco Clin North Am. 2016;30(3):591-608.
2. Meier ER, Rampersad A. Pediatric sickle cell disease: past successes and future challenges. Pediatr Res. 2017;81(1):249-58.
3. National Heart Lung and Blood Institute. (2014). Evidence-based management of sickle cell disease: Expert panel report, 2014. [online] Available from https://www.nhlbi.nih.gov/health-topics/evidence-based-management-sickle-cell-disease [Last accessed June, 2024].
4. Steinberg MH. Management of sickle cell disease. N Engl J Med. 1999;340(13):1021-30.
5. Yawn BP, Buchanan GR, Afenyi-Annan AN, Ballas SK, Hassell KL, James AH, et al Management of sickle cell disease: summary of the 2014 evidence-based report by expert panel members. JAMA. 2014;312(10):1033-48.

CASE 43

Thalassemia

■ PRESENTING COMPLAINTS

An 8-month-old girl was brought with the complaint of:
- Not taking feeds since 2 months
- Not gaining weight since 2 months
- Distension of abdomen since 1 month
- Sweating at the time of feeding since 15 days

History of Presenting Complaints

An 8-month-old child was brought to the pediatric outpatient department with a history of not gaining weight and distension of the abdomen since the last 2 months. The mother said that there was no significant weight gain in the last 2 months. The mother also revealed the history that her daughter was not taking feed properly. There was a history of sweating at the time of feeding. She also noted that there was distension in the abdomen. The child was shown to the family doctor, and she was diagnosed as anemic, and iron preparation was given. But the mother concluded all these treatments were in vain.

Past History of the Patient

She was the second sibling of a non-consanguineous marriage. She was born at term with normal delivery. She cried immediately after the delivery. The birth weight of the baby was 2.9 kg. The child started taking breast milk. The child was breastfed exclusively for 3 months. Later weaning started with cereals as per the guidance of the family doctor.

The developmental milestones were normal. The child developed neck control by 3 months. She was sitting with support for

CASE AT A GLANCE

Basic Findings
Height	:	72 cm (50th centile)
Weight	:	7 kg (10th centile)
Temperature	:	37°C
Pulse rate	:	110 beats/min
Respiratory rate	:	20 breaths/min
Blood pressure	:	70/50 mm Hg

Positive Findings

History:
- Failure to thrive
- Abdominal distension
- Sweating

Examination:
- Depressed nasal bridge
- Prominent frontal bone
- Pallor
- Hepatosplenomegaly

Investigation:
- *Hemoglobin:* Decreased
- *Red blood cells:* Decreased
- *Reticulocytes:* Increased
- *Peripheral blood smear:* Microcytic hypochromic anemia and basophil stippling
- *X-ray skull:* Widening of the diploic space

6 months. Now she was sitting independently. She had developed a social smile by 2 months.

EXAMINATION

On examination, the child was active, alert, and was moderately built and nourished. She was playing with the toys on the examination table. There was a depressed nasal bridge. A prominent frontal lobe was present. The anterior fontanelle was normal. Anthropometric measurements included a length was 72 cm (50th centile) and a weight was 7 kg (10th centile). The head circumference was 39 cm.

The child was afebrile, the pulse rate was 110 beats/min, and the respiratory rate was 20 breaths/min. The blood pressure recorded was 70/50 mm Hg. There was pallor, no icterus, no lymphadenopathy, no edema, and no cyanosis.

Per abdomen examination revealed the presence of mild distension, liver was palpable about 3 cm below the costal margin. It was nontender and soft in consistency. The spleen was palpable about 2 cm. It was nontender, and firm in consistency. The cardiovascular system and respiratory systems were normal.

INVESTIGATION

- *Hemoglobin:* 5 g/dL
- *RBC count:* $5.5 \times 10^6/mm^3$
- *PCV:* 47%
- *Reticulocyte count:* 1.5%
- *MCV:* 78 μm^3
- *MCH:* 30 pg
- *MCHC:* 34%
- *Serum iron:* 200 μg/dL (normal range: 22–184 μg/dL)
- *Serum bilirubin:* 3 mg/dL
- *Peripheral blood smear:* Showed microcytic hypochromic anemia. Basophil stippling was present
- *X-ray of the skull:* Showed widening of the diploic space, absence of the outer table, and generalized radial striations

DISCUSSION

It is a heterogeneous disorder recessively inherited resulting from various mutations of the genes that code for globin chains of hemoglobin, leading to reduced or absent synthesis of globin chains, and when beta-chain synthesis is affected, it is called beta-thalassemia.

The thalassemia syndrome is a heterogeneous group of hereditary disorders of reduced hemoglobin synthesis. There is diminished or absent normal globin chain production. Normally, four alpha-globin genes are expressed to make the tetrameric globin protein, which then combines with hem moiety to make the predominant hemoglobin that is found in red cells.

The thalassemias are quantitative disorders of hemoglobin. Thalassemia occurs when there is decreased synthesis of generally structurally normal globin proteins. Like qualitative disorders of hemoglobin, quantitative disorders of hemoglobin can also be subdivided by the particular globin that is affected, e.g., there can be alpha-thalassemias and beta-thalassemias.

In α-thalassemia, there is an absence or reduction in α-globin action usually due to deletions of α-globin genes. Normal individuals have four α-globin genes; the more genes affected, the more severe the disease. α-thalassemia indicates no α-chains produced from that chromosome (-alpha-/). α-thalassemia produces a decreased amount of the α-globin chain from that chromosome (-alpha/). Primary pathology in thalassemia syndromes stem from the quantity of β-globin produced, whereas the primary pathology in sickle cell disease is related to the quality of b-globin produced.

Two related features contribute to the sequelae of β-thalassemia syndromes: inadequate β-globin gene production leading to decreased levels of normal HbA and unbalanced α- and β-globin chain production leading to ineffective erythropoiesis. In β-thalassemia -globin chains are in excess to non-α-globin chains, and α-globin tetramers (α) are formed and appear as RBC inclusions. The free-globin chains and inclusions are very unstable, precipitate in RBC precursors, damage the RBC membrane, and shorten RBC survival, leading to anemia and increased erythroid production. This results in a marked increase in erythropoiesis, with early erythroid precursor death in the bone marrow.

Clinically, this is characterized by a lack of maturation of erythrocytes and an inappropriately low reticulocyte count. This ineffective erythropoiesis and the compensatory massive marrow expansion with erythroid hyperactivity characterize β-thalassemia. Due to the low or absent production of β-globin, the α-chains combine with γ-chains, resulting in HbF ($\alpha_2\gamma_2$) being the dominant hemoglobin. In addition to the natural survival effect, the γ-globin chains may be produced in increased amounts, regulated by genetic polymorphisms. The δ-chain synthesis is not usually affected in β-thalassemia or β-thalassemia trait, and therefore patients have a relative or absolute increase in hemoglobin A2 (HbA2) production ($\alpha_2\delta_2$).

GENETICS AND PATHOPHYSIOLOGY

Mutations that decrease the synthesis of alpha-globins cause beta-thalassemia; mutations that decrease the synthesis of beta-globins cause beta-thalassemia. In general, alpha-thalassemias are caused by deletions of deoxyribonucleic acid (DNA) affecting the alpha-globin alleles; whereas, beta-thalassemias are caused by point mutations affecting the beta-globin alleles. There are also distinct embryonic, fetal, and minor adult analogs of the alpha-globins and beta-globins, all of which are encoded by separate genes.

Depending on the number of genes that are deleted, the production of polypeptide chains is diminished. The result is ineffective erythropoiesis, precipitation of unstable hemoglobin, and hemolysis as a result of intramedullary RBC destruction. If the synthesis of X-chain is suppressed, all three normal hemoglobin are reduced. If the beta chains are suppressed, then the production of adult hemoglobins is affected. This is the most common form of thalassemia.

Thalassemia refers to a group of genetic disorders of globin chain reduction in which there is an imbalance between the alpha-globin and beta-globin chain production. Beta-thalassemia syndromes result from a decrease in beta-globin chains, which results in a relative excess of alpha-globin chains. Beta-thalassemia refers to the absence of production of the beta-globin.

Beta-thalassemia major refers to the severe beta-thalassemia patient who requires early transfusion therapy and often is homozygous for the beta mutation. Beta-thalassemia intermedia is a clinical diagnosis of a patient with a less severe clinical phenotype that usually does not require transfusion therapy in childhood.

Carriers with a single beta-globin mutation are generally asymptomatic, except for microcytosis and mild anemia. In alpha-thalassemia, there is an absence or reduction in alpha-globin production.

Normal individuals have four alpha-globin genes. The primary pathology in thalassemia syndromes stem from the quantity of globin produced. In contrast, the primary pathology in SCD is related to the quality of beta-globin produced.

■ PATHOPHYSIOLOGY

Two related features contribute to the sequelae of beta-thalassemia major: Inadequate beta-globin gene production leading to decreased levels of normal HbA and unbalanced alpha and beta-globin chain production. In beta-thalassemia major, alpha-globin chains are in excess to nonalpha-globin chains, and alpha-globin tetramers (alpha$_4$) are formed and appear as red cell inclusions. The free alpha-globin chains and inclusions are very unstable, precipitate in red cell precursors, damage the red cell membrane, and shorten red cell survival leading to anemia and increased erythroid production.

In the alpha-thalassemia syndromes, two genes with two maternal and two paternal alleles control alpha-globin production, which varies from complete absence (hydrops fetalis) to only slightly reduced (alpha-thalassemia silent carrier). In the alpha-thalassemia syndromes, an excess of beta and gamma-globin chains are produced. These excess chains form Bart hemoglobin (Gamma$_4$) in fetal life and HbH (beta$_4$) after birth. These abnormal tetramers are nonfunctional HbS with very high oxygen affinity. They do not transport oxygen and result in extravascular hemolysis. A fetus with the most severe form of alpha-thalassemia (hydrops fetalis) develops in utero anemia and fetal loss because HbF production requires sufficient amounts of alpha-globin. In contrast, infants with beta-thalassemia major become symptomatic only after birth when HbA predominates and insufficient beta-globin production manifests in clinical symptoms.

In homozygous thalassemia major, severe thalassemia genes are inherited from both parents, and the production of β-chains is markedly reduced. In heterozygous individuals, a normal β chain is inherited along with the thalassemia β-gene or mild β-thalassemia gene.

Production of beta peptide chains is suppressed. Gamma and delta chains may be enhanced. A part of the latter combines with normally produced chains and forms an excess of HbF. Most of the alpha chains are destroyed in the bone marrow. Hence, there is ineffective erythropoiesis. Increased erythropoiesis results in expansion of the medullary cavity of various bones.

It is characterized by an imbalance in the production of α and β-globin polypeptide chains of hemoglobin.

- In alpha-thalassemia, alpha-chain synthesis is decreased. In beta-thalassemia, beta-chain synthesis is decreased.
- Excessive alpha-chains precipitate in the red cell membrane and damage it. This leads to premature red cell destruction both in the bone marrow and peripheral circulation, particularly in the RE system of the spleen (ineffective erythropoiesis and hemolysis).
- Synthesis of gamma chain persists after fetal life.
- Increased HbF with its high affinity for oxygen leads to tissue hypoxia, which in turn stimulates erythropoietin secretion leading to both medullary and extramedullary erythropoiesis— expansion of bone marrow space causing a characteristic hemolytic facies with frontoparietal and occipital bossing, malar prominence and malocclusions of teeth, and complications that include distortion

of ribs and vertebrae and pathological fracture of the long bones, splenomegaly and its complication hypersplenism, hepatomegaly, gallstones, and chronic leg ulcers.

Hypertrophy of the erythropoietic tissue occurs in medullary and extramedullary locations. The bones become thin and pathological fracture may occur. Massive expansion of the marrow of the skull and face produces characteristic facies.

Extramedullary hematopoiesis produces enlargement of the liver and spleen. The breakdown of endogenous or transfused red cells produces the release of iron. This iron is deposited in various organs producing hemosiderosis.

CLINICAL FEATURES (FIG. 1)

Clinical heterogeneity results from variability in the number of gene deletions particularly in alpha thalassemia. As a rule, the greater the number of deletions, the more the symptoms.

The infants are born normally. The child becomes paler after 4–6 months. Mostly it may be mistaken for IDA. But this will not respond to iron therapy. There will be hepatosplenomegaly. The abdomen will be protuberant. After 1 year mongoloid facies will develop. There will be frontal bossing of the skull. Prominent frontal and parietal eminences, straight forehead, hypertrophy of maxilla, prominent malar eminence, depressed nasal bridge, and puffy eyelids. Teeth will be malformed.

If not treated, children with homozygous beta-thalassemia usually become symptomatic from progressive hemolytic anemia, with profound weakness and cardiac decompensation during the second 6 months of life. Depending on the mutation and degree of HbF production, transfusions in β-thalassemia major are necessary beginning in the second months to the second year of life, but rarely later.

The developing signs of ineffective erythropoiesis such as growth failure, bone deformities secondary to marrow expansion, and hepatosplenomegaly are important variables in determining transfusion initiation.

The classic presentation of children with severe disease includes thalassemic facies (maxilla hyperplasia, flat nasal bridge, and frontal bossing), pathologic bone fractures, marked hepatosplenomegaly, and cachexia and is now primarily seen in countries without access to chronic transfusion therapy.

In nontransfused patients with severe ineffective erythropoiesis, marked splenomegaly can develop with hypersplenism and abdominal symptoms. The features of ineffective erythropoiesis include expanded medullary spaces (with massive expansion of the marrow of the face and skull producing the characteristic thalassemic fades), extramedullary hematopoiesis, and higher metabolic needs.

Chronic transfusion therapy dramatically improves the quality of life and reduces the complications of severe thalassemia.

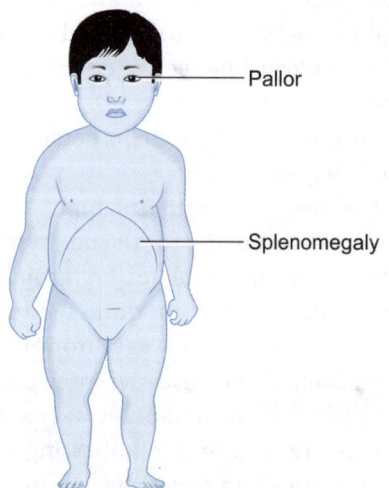

Fig. 1: Clinical features.

Transfusion-induced hemosiderosis becomes the major clinical complication of transfusion-dependent thalassemia. Each mL of packed red cells contains 1 mg of iron.

Liver hemosiderosis develops after 1 year of chronic transfusion therapy and is followed by iron deposition in the endocrine system. This leads to a high rate of hypothyroidism, hypogonadotropic gonadism, growth hormone deficiency, hypoparathyroidism, and diabetes mellitus.

Physical growth is markedly retarded. These develop intermittently due to infection. The course of illness depends upon the severity of the disease. Deaths may occur in a few years of life due to severe anemia, cardiac, and liver failure. However, with current management, they can lead near normal life.

Pallor, hemosiderosis, and jaundice combine to produce a characteristic greenish-brown complexion. The liver and spleen is enlarged. Growth is impaired in older children. Puberty is delayed, because of secondary endocrine abnormalities. Diabetes mellitus results from pancreatic siderosis and intractable arrhythmias, chronic CCF are caused by myocardial siderosis.

Infants with serious beta-thalassemia disorders have progressive anemia after the newborn period. Microcytosis, hypochromia, and targeting characterize the RBCs. Nucleated RBCs, marked anisopoikilocytosis, and relative reticulocytopenia are typically seen. The hemoglobin level falls progressively often to <6 g/dL unless transfusions are given. The reticulocyte count is commonly <8% and is inappropriately low compared to the degree of anemia caused by ineffective erythropoiesis. The unconjugated serum bilirubin level is usually elevated, but other chemistries may be initially normal. Even if the child does not receive transfusions, iron eventually accumulates with elevated serum ferritin and TS. Evidence of bone marrow hyperplasia can be seen on radiographs.

GENERAL FEATURES
• Severe progressive anemia
• Hemosiderosis
• Jaundice
• Arrhythmias
• Impaired growth
• Diabetes mellitus

The thalassemias can be described simply by two independent nomenclatures: genetic and clinical. Genetic nomenclature refers to the causative mutation, such as α-thalassemia and β-thalassemia, indicating mutations of the α- and β-globin genes, respectively. The clinical nomenclature divides the thalassemias into, the asymptomatic, carrier or trait state (thalassemia minor), severe transfusion-dependent anemia (thalassemia major), and everything in between (thalassemia intermedia)

The clinical feathers of beta thalassemia include:

- *Thalassemia minor:* Minimal or no anemia; microcytosis, elevated RBC count.
- *Thalassemia intermedia:* Microcytic, anemia, growth, failure, hepatosplenomegaly, hyperbilirubinemia, and thalassemic facies (frontal bossing, mandibular malocclusion, and prominent malar eminences), develop between the age of 2 and 5 years.
- *Thalassemia major (Cooley's anemia):* Severe anemia, hepatosplenomegaly, and growth failure.

DIAGNOSIS

The level of the hemoglobin is reduced. The hemoglobin level falls progressively to <6 g/dL unless transfusions are given. The reticulocyte count is commonly <8% and is inappropriately low when compared to the degree of anemia as a result of ineffective erythropoiesis. HbF level has increased. Total erythrocyte count is low. Reticulocyte count is raised. Hematocrit is reduced, and microcytosis (MCV), hypochromia (MCH), and targeting characterize the red cells.

The peripheral blood smear shows microcytic hypochromic anemia. Anisocytosis and poikilocytosis are present. Fragmented red cells and early intermediate and late erythroblasts are seen. Nucleated red cells marked anisopoikilocytosis, and relative reticulocytopenia are typically seen. Marked basophil stippling is seen. Reticulocyte count ranges from 2 to 4%.

The bone marrow is hypercellular with erythroid hyperplasia, with an increased number of stippled erythroblasts and sideroblasts. Myeloid ratio is reversed. Hemosiderin deposits in the marrow are increased.

The unconjugated serum bilirubin level is usually elevated. Bone marrow hyperplasia can be seen on radiographs. Hemoglobin electrophoresis is diagnostic. HbF is increased in the patient and HbA2 is over 3.4% in both parents.

The fragility of the cells on exposure to hypotonic saline is decreased. Serum bilirubin level is moderately elevated. It depends upon the rate of hemolytic activity. Serum iron levels are high. Serum ferritin levels are markedly raised.

LABORATORY SALIENT FINDINGS
• Reduced hemoglobin • Increased fetal hemoglobin • Reduced hematocrit • MCV, MCH, or MCHC are low • Hypercellular bone marrow, erythroid hyperplasia • Microcytic hypochromic anemia
(MCH: mean corpuscular hemoglobin; MCHC: mean corpuscular hemoglobin concentration; MCV: mean corpuscular volume)

Earliest bone changes occur in small bones of the hand. A medullary portion is widened and the bony cortex is thinned out. There will be a coarse trabecular pattern in the medulla.

Diploic spaces in the skull are widened. Interrupted porosity gives hair an end appearance on the radiography of the skull. The frontal bones appear thickened.

Radiological findings include the widening of the medulla due to bone marrow hyperplasia, thinning of the cortex, and trabeculation in the long bones and metacarpals and metatarsals. Skull X-ray shows a "hairs-on-end" appearance.

Periodic tests for organ dysfunction are necessary which include serum glutamic oxaloacetic transaminase (SGOT), serum glutamate pyruvate transaminase (SGPT), serum bilirubin, serum calcium, endocrinal studies, etc.

■ DIFFERENTIAL DIAGNOSIS

- Iron deficiency anemia (IDA
- Sickle cell anemia
- Hookworm infestation
- Methemoglobinemia

ESSENTIAL DIAGNOSTIC POINTS
• Quantitative reduction in globin synthesis • Expansion of fascial bones-extramedullary hematopoiesis • Microcytic hypochromic anemia • No response to iron therapy • Marked hepatosplenomegaly

■ TREATMENT

The thalassemia trait (thalassemia minor) requires no treatment. The lifelong hypochromic, microcytic anemia neither requires nor responds to iron supplementation. Establishing a diagnosis of thalassemia trait will prevent repeated unnecessary diagnostic tests and inappropriate treatment with iron. It is important, however, to counsel individuals with either alpha- or betathalassemia traits regarding the risk of having offspring with a significant hemoglobinopathy. The risk of clinically significant alpha-thalassemia disease is dependent on both the exact genotype of the individual and that of the partner. Individuals with the β-thalassemia trait can also be affected by spring with significant variability in disease severity depending on the severity of each parent β-thalassemia mutation. Additionally, individuals with the β-thalassemia trait can have offspring with other hemoglobinopathies, such as sickle β-thalassemia and hemoglobin E (HbE)-β-thalassemia, depending on the partner's carrier status.

Patients with thalassemia intermedia, by definition, do not require regular or chronic transfusions of RBCs. However, intermittent simple transfusions may be needed in the event of illness or complications. For example, infection with parvovirus (the cause of erythema infectiosum or fifth disease) causes an aplastic crisis that may require transfusion. Other causes of worsening anemia include infection and drug-mediated hemolysis, splenectomy may benefit patients who develop significant hypersplenism with severe anemia. Cholecystectomy may be necessary for symptomatic cholelithiasis caused by pigmented gallstones or cholecystitis. Sometimes chelation therapy for iron overload is needed for older individuals, especially if they have received multiple transfusions.

By definition, patients with thalassemia major are transfusion dependent. Historically, transfusions were given sparingly and did not effectively prevent many of the consequences of severe anemia and marrow expansion. More vigorous transfusion programs designed to maintain a minimum hemoglobin concentration of 10 g/dL or higher (hypertransfusion) were instituted.

Generally, modern chronic transfusion regimens are given to alleviate severe anemia and to suppress and greatly diminish ineffective erythropoiesis. When started early in life and continued thereafter, chronic transfusions can prevent bony and dental abnormalities, decrease extramedullary hematopoiesis, normalize growth and development, and prolong and improve quality of life.

Transfusions are usually given monthly and sometimes more frequently to maintain a nadir hemoglobin concentration in the 9.5–10 g/dL range. The risks of blood transfusions include alloimmunization, hemolytic and nonhemolytic transfusion reactions, transfusion-transmitted infections, and iron overload.

Transfusion Therapy

Before initiating chronic transfusions, the diagnosis of transfusion-dependent β-thalassemia should be confirmed by both clinical and laboratory parameters. β-thalassemia major is a clinical diagnosis that requires the integration of laboratory findings and the clinical course.

The long-term observation of the clinical characteristics, such as growth, bony changes, and hemoglobin, are necessary to determine chronic transfusion therapy.

Transfusion therapy in thalassemia has two goals:
1. To prevent anemia.
2. To suppress endogenous erythropoiesis to avoid ineffective erythropoiesis.

Blood transfusion is mandatory for all children with thalassemia major and for those children with thalassemia intermedia who cannot maintain hemoglobin above 7 g% or those who show evidence of growth retardation, severe bony changes. Regular blood transfusions are presently the mainstay of treatment of thalassemia major.

Cross-matched triple saline-washed packed cells are transfused to avoid transfusion reactions as saline washing minimizes reactions due to the depletion of leukocytes and plasma proteins. If a cold centrifuge that is required is not available, then simple packed cells may be given. Other means of decreasing sensitization include the use of leukocyte filters and frozen cells.

Transfusion regimen may be (1) a low transfusion regimen when hemoglobin is maintained around 7-10 g% and (2) hypertransfusion: Hemoglobin. Level 10-12 g% and supertransfusion, when hemoglobin maintained, is above 12-14 g%.

The popular transfusion regimen of today is a hypertransfusion regime which aims at maintaining mean hemoglobin levels at 12.5 g/dL and pretransfusion levels not <10 g%. Such a regimen permits normal growth and physical activities, suppresses erythropoiesis, thus preventing skeletal changes and GI iron absorption, and also inhibits extramedullary hemopoiesis, thereby preventing splenomegaly and hypersplenism. With this regime, the requirement of blood is high only at the start of therapy and does not produce an iron overload more than the low transfusion regime.

Guidelines for Transfusion Therapy

Patients at risk for transfusion therapy should have an extended red cell phenotype and/or genotype. Patients should receive red cells depleted from leukocytes and matched for, at least, D, C, c, E, e, and Kell antigens.

Transfusions should generally be given at intervals of 3-4 weeks, with the goal being to maintain a pretransfusion hemoglobin level of 9.5-10.5 g/dL. Ongoing monitoring for transfusion-associated transmitted infections (hepatitis A, hepatitis B, hepatitis C, and HIV), alloimmunization, annual blood transfusion requirements, and transfusion reactions is essential.

Amount and Frequency of Transfusion

It is desirable that patients receive not >10 cc packed cells/kg/day, which raises hemoglobin level by about 3.5 g/dL. In most patients, a transfusion of about 10 cc of PRBC/kg every third week is adequate to maintain the pretransfusion baseline hemoglobin level desired 10-11 g/dL.

Rate of transfusion should be 5-7 mL/kg body weight/h to avoid a sudden increase in blood volume. In patients with cardiac insufficiency transfusions may have to be given every second week and sometimes every week and prolong the duration of transfusion by decreasing the rate to 1-3 mL/kg/h not >5 mL/kg/h.

Transfusions should preferably be given on an outpatient basis, at intervals of 2-4 weeks. Blood to be transfused should be crossmatched using Coombs sera to minimize reactions. Blood should be taken from a voluntary donor and should be screened for hepatitis B antigen, syphilis, malaria, and HIV and also for hepatitis C virus (HCV) antibodies.

The patients should be assessed annually for mean hemoglobin levels maintained, overall blood requirement, physical growth, and development, evidence of hypersplenism, antibody development, and iron overload. On average, the annual blood requirement is 180-200 mL/kg. However, if the requirement exceeds this level, hypersplenism or the development of antired cell antibodies have to be considered.

Neocyte Transfusion

This concept of transfusing thalassemic children with young red cells (neocytes). In conventionally used units of blood, red cells have a survival of 60 days. The mean age of a neocyte is 12 days, they survive in the recipient for 90 days, thus reducing the amount of blood required and prolonging the interval between two transfusions. Neocyte exchange transfusion though have been tried, are found to be impracticable.

Iron Overload Monitoring

Excessive iron stores from transfusion cause many of the complications of β-thalassemia major. Accurate assessment of excessive iron stores is essential to optimal therapy. Serial serum ferritin levels are a useful screening technique in assessing iron balance trends, but results may not accurately predict quantitative iron stores. Under treatment or over treatment of presumed excessive iron stores can occur in managing a patient based on serum ferritin alone.

Iron loading is monitored by serum tests of iron stores (ferritin) liver biopsy, and iron quantitation by. MRI can be used to estimate iron deposition in the liver, pancreas, and heart. After about 200 mL/kg of RBCs have been transfused, chelation is usually necessary.

Iron Overload and Chelation Therapy

Two factors contribute to iron overload in thalassemic children which are as follows:
1. Enhanced GI absorption of iron
2. Transfusional siderosis normal body iron content is 3–5 g; whereas, in a thalassemic child, it could be around 0.75 g/kg.

Transfusional iron overload leads to the deposition of iron in the heart leading to cardiomyopathy and irregularity of heartbeats, in the pancreas, in the islet of Langerhans leading to diabetes, in the liver and spleen leading to hepatosplenomegaly, hepatic fibrosis and cirrhosis of the liver, in the pituitary glands leading to growth retardation, delayed puberty character, in the thyroid and parathyroid gland leading to subclinical or clinical organ dysfunction, and in the skin leading to bronze or black discoloration of the skin.

Increased susceptibility to bacterial infection especially *Yersinia* with iron overload, because the relatively high serum iron levels may favor bacterial growth, or because of blockage of the mononuclear phagocyte system by the excessive red cell destruction.

Iron accumulation in the myocardium can lead to death, either by involving the conducting tissues or by causing intractable cardiac failure due to cardiomyopathy.

Iron-chelation therapy should start as soon as the patient becomes significantly iron-overloaded. In general, this occurs after 1 year of transfusion therapy and correlates with serum ferritin >1,000 ng/mL and/or a liver iron concentration of >2,500 μg/g dry weight.

There are three available iron chelators (deferoxamine, deferasirox, and deferiprone); each varies in its route of administration, pharmacokinetics, adverse events, and efficacy. Many patients require combination chelation therapy at various points in their illness. The overall goal is to prevent hemosiderosis-induced tissue injury and avoid chelation toxicity. This requires close monitoring of the patients. In general, chelation toxicity increases as iron stores decrease.

Deferoxamine is the most studied iron chelator; it has an excellent safety and efficacy profile. Desferrioxamine (DFO) is a hydroxylamine compound produced by *Streptomyces pilosus*. A single gram of DFO is able to bind 85 mg of iron. DFO should be started before the age of 3-5 years.

It requires subcutaneous, or IV, administration because of a half-life of <30 minutes, necessitating administration of at least 8 hours daily, 5-7 days/week. Deferoxamine is initially started at 20 mg/kg and can be increased to 60 mg/kg, in heavily iron-overloaded patients. Given on a daily basis for a minimum of five to six times per week, it is given subcutaneously over 6-8 hours using an infusion pump. The daily dose of Desferal is about 30-70 mg/kg and should be tailored according to the needs of the patient. In general, the goal is to keep the serum ferritin level below 1,000 ng/mL.

The major problem with deferoxamine is noncompliance because of the route of administration. Adverse side effects include ototoxicity, retinal changes, and bone dysplasia with truncal shortening.

The oral iron chelator deferasirox is commercially available in patients on Desferal, 70% have switched to deferasirox because it is orally available. Deferasirox has a half-life of >16 hours and requires once-a-day administration of a dispersal tablet in water. The initial dose is 20 mg/kg with gradual escalation to 30 mg/kg. The most common side effects are GI symptoms.

Deferiprone (Ferriprox), an oral iron chelator has a half-life of approximately 3 hours and requires 25 mg/kg three times a day. Deferiprone, a small molecule, effectively enters cardiac tissue and may be more effective than other chelators in reducing cardiac hemosiderosis. The most serious side effect of deferiprone is transient agranulocytosis, which occurs in 1% of patients. The use of deferiprone requires weekly WBC counts.

It mobilizes iron from transferring, ferritin, and hemosiderin. *Dose:* 50-100 mg/kg/body weight. Physical examination particularly of the joints and CBC including platelet count must be done regularly when a child is on deferiprone (L1) therapy.

With recent advances in chelation therapy especially with the availability of oral chelating drugs like deferiprone (L1) compliance has remarkably improved. The cost of therapy has reduced considerably and hence even in developing countries, many children are able to use the drug.

Deferoxamine, in combination with deferiprone, is routinely used in patients with increased cardiac iron. Combination therapy of deferoxamine and deferasirox may also be efficacious in similar patients.

Role of Vitamin C

Ascorbic acid deficiency increases insoluble iron hemosiderin. Vitamin C helps in the conversion of hemosiderin into ferritin from which iron can be chelated.

- High doses of vitamin C can lead to increased free radical reaction and lipid peroxidation resulting in tissue damage, rapid cardiac decompensation, and even death.
- The addition of vitamin C 100 mg daily prior to DF therapy increases iron excretion.
- 60% of DFO chelated iron is excreted in urine, and 40% in stool.

Hydroxyurea

Hydroxyurea, a DNA antimetabolite, increases stress erythropoiesis, which results in increased HbF production. It has been most successfully used in SCD and in some patients with β-thalassemia intermedia.

Hydroxyurea therapy in thalassemia intermedia may have other benefits including decreasing the vascular disease associated with thalassemia intermedia. The initial starting dose for thalassemia intermedia is 10 mg/kg and because these patients are more sensitive to toxicity than SCD, higher doses are used with great caution.

Hydroxyurea, a DNA antimetabolite, increases HbF production. It has been most successfully used in SCD and in some patients with β-thalassemia intermedia. Studies in β-thalassemia major are limited. In many parts of the world, hydroxyurea therapy is used in β-thalassemia intermedia patients. Even though increases in HbF levels are observed, they do not predictively correlate with an increase in total hemoglobin in these patients. In general, there appears to be a mean increase in hemoglobin of 1 g/dL (range: 0.1–2.5 g/dL). Hydroxyurea therapy in thalassemia intermedia is associated with a reduced risk of leg ulcers, pulmonary hypertension, and extramedullary hematopoiesis. The initial starting dose for thalassemia intermedia is 10 mg/kg and may be escalated to 20 mg/kg/day. Patients with β-thalassemia are at increased risk of developing cytopenias with hydroxyurea use, which may prevent dose escalation. Close monitoring of the CBC with differential is required.

Hematopoietic Stem-cell Transplantation

Stem cell (or bone marrow) transplantation is the only cure for thalassemia. About >1,000 transplants have been done worldwide. Transplantation is safest when hematopoietic stem cells are obtained from an HLA-identical sibling (without thalassemia), but only 25% of siblings will be HLA identical. The use of alternative donors is an area of ongoing study.

For well-chelated children without liver disease, event-free survival at 5 years after transplantation is 85–95%, depending on the report. Results are considerably worse in adults and in patients who are poorly compliant with chelation and have hepatic disease. The relatively high immediate mortality associated with transplantation stands in contrast to the many years of reasonably normal life that can be obtained with appropriate transfusion and chelation therapies, which makes the decision to accept transplantation difficult for many families.

Most success has been in children younger than 15 years of age without excessive stores and hepatomegaly who undergo sibling HLA-matched allogeneic transplantation. All children who have an HLA-matched sibling should be offered the option of bone marrow transplantation. Alternative transplantation regimens for patients without donors are experimental and have variable success.

Splenectomy

With the advent of hyper and supertransfusion therapy, splenomegaly and hypersplenism have become a rarity and hence splenectomy is usually not needed in these patients.

Splenectomy may be required in thalassemia patients who develop hypersplenism. These patients have a falling steady state hemoglobin and/or a rising transfusion requirement. Overall, splenectomy is less frequently used as a therapeutic option.

If the child has already developed splenomegaly and signs of hypersplenism and is above 5 years of age, splenectomy is indicated. The indication for splenectomy is an increase in the yearly requirement of packed cells more than double the basal requirement, i.e., packed cells 200 cc/kg/year or more. A decrease in WBC and platelet count is a late manifestation of hypersplenism.

There is an increased recognition of serious adverse effects of splenectomy beyond infection risk. In thalassemia intermedia, splenectomized patients have a marked increased risk of venous thrombosis, pulmonary hypertension, leg ulcers, and SCIs compared to nonsplenectomized patients.

There is an increased risk of bacterial sepsis following splenectomy, especially in young children. Hence antibacterial prophylaxis with pneumococcal vaccination is necessary. There is also evidence that splenectomy increases the risk of thrombosis and, perhaps, pulmonary hypertension.

All children needing splenectomy should receive pneumococcal vaccine, *H. influenzae* vaccine, and meningococcal vaccine 4–6 weeks prior to surgery or earlier. In endemic areas, prophylactic antimalarial treatment may be given to prevent malaria.

Prophylactic penicillin therapy must be continued lifelong after splenectomy. Episodes of infection should be treated promptly, and newer broad-spectrum antibiotics may be empirically started to prevent septicemia and other complications. If necessary, these children should be hospitalized. Blood culture and antibiotic sensitivity must be performed to guide treatment.

Bone Marrow Transplantation

A ray of hope for a permanent cure and a better future for children with genetic disorders has brightened with the rapid advancement in the techniques and the success of bone marrow transplantation.

The principles of bone marrow transplantation in thalassemia are: (1) To destroy and prevent regeneration of defective stem cells, (2) sufficient immune suppression for good engraftment of normal marrow, (3) to infuse stem cells with a normal gene for β-chain globin, and (4) to prevent graft versus host disease (GVHD) with high dose therapy of busulfan, cyclophosphamide, total body irradiation, and other modalities.

The three most important adverse prognostic factors for survival and event-free survival are as follows:
1. Presence of hepatomegaly (liver >2 cm below costal margin)
2. Portal fibrosis
3. Iron overload

Bone marrow transplantation is most successful in patients who are young, properly transfused, well-chelated, and in good clinical shape without hepatomegaly.

Gene Manipulations

It has been tried to increase the production of HbF and to prevent the precipitation of unpaired hemoglobin chains. Augmenting the production of γ-chain reduces the imbalance of the globin chain and increases the synthesis of HbF, and thus lessening the severity of the disease. Those drugs being tried are 5-azacytidine, hydroxyurea, butyrate derivatives, ICL670, HBED, dimethyl HBED, and pyridoxal isonicotinoyl hydrazone (PIH).

Hydroxyurea has been found to increase HbF levels. It is not found to be useful in thalassemia major. However, it has been found to help in the prolongation of intervals in blood transfusion and in alleviating symptoms of children with HbSS and thalassemia intermedia.

Butyrates

Butyrates are found naturally increased in diabetic mothers. Their babies at birth have

100% HbF. This drug is given IV infusion slowly over 6–8 hours in doses of 200–400 mg/kg/day and has been shown to increase in HbF by 8–12% and rise in hemoglobin by 2–3 g%. The problem with this drug is the tedious IV route. Oral analog Na Butyrate is useful in some patients to sustain the response after IV therapy. The side effects are few and include nausea, vomiting, electrolyte disturbances, and occasional seizures.

ICL-670

During the last couple of years, the new synthetic oral chelator ICL-670A has given a ray of hope. It belongs to the tridentate triazole group and is undergoing a phase III trial.

Iron is chelated both from RE cells as well as parenchymal organs. It also has the ability to prevent myocardial cell iron uptake and remove iron directly from myocardial cells. Iron excretion is predominantly fecal. It excretes iron from both RE cells and parenchymal cells of various organs and chelated iron excreted by the liver through the bile. The only side effects reported include mild abdominal pain, GI discomfort, constipation, and skin rash. No changes in auditory, visual (ocular), or cardiac functions were observed. It also has the ability to prevent myocardial cell iron uptake, remove the iron directly from myocardial cells, and exchange the iron with DFO. Coadministration of ICL 670 with injection DFO has a synergic effect and helps in reducing the dose of both the drugs thus improving the compliance and cost of the treatment as is done with oral chelation therapy with deferiprone.

■ BIBLIOGRAPHY

1. Nadkarni A, Gorakshakar AC, Krishnamoorthy R, Ghosh K, Colah R, Mohanty D. Molecular pathogenesis and clinical variability of beta-thalassemia syndromes among Indians. Am J Hemotol. 2001;68(2): 75-80.
2. Northern California Thalassemia Centre. Standard Guidelines for Management of Thalassemia 2012. [online] Available from httthalassemia.com/SOC/index,aspx. [Last accessed June, 2024].
3. Piel FB, Weatherall DJ. The α-thalassemias. NEngl J Med. 2014;371(20):1908-16.
4. Steinberg MH, Forget BG, Higgs DR. Disorders of hemoglobin: Genetics, Pathophysiology, and clinical management, 2nd edition. Cambridge, United Kingdom: Cambridge University Press; 2009.

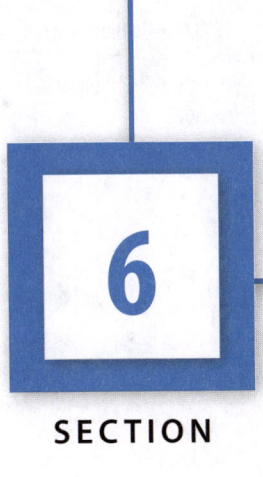

SECTION 6

Renal System

- Case 44 **Acute Poststreptococcal Glomerulonephritis**
- Case 45 **Hemolytic Uremic Syndrome**
- Case 46 **Nephrotic Syndrome**
- Case 47 **Urinary Tract Infection**

CASE 44

Acute Poststreptococcal Glomerulonephritis

■ PRESENTING COMPLAINTS

A 6-year-old boy was brought with the complaint of:
- Skin lesions since 2 weeks
- Puffiness of face since 1 week
- Passing high-colored urine since 2 days

History of Presenting Complaints

A 6-year-old boy was brought to pediatric outpatient department with history of puffiness of face around the eyes since 1 week. His mother noticed swelling around his eyes. This used to be more in morning. The swelling used to reduce as the day passes on. There was no history of swelling of lower limbs of the body.

This was associated with history of passing high-colored urine. There was no history of burning sensation while passing the urine. There was no history of increased frequency of micturition.

Past History of the Patient

He was the elder sibling of nonconsanguineous marriage. He was born at full term by normal delivery. He cried immediately after delivery. His birth weight was 3 kg. He was exclusively on breast milk for 3 months. Later weaning was started and he was on family food by 15 months. His developmental milestones were normal. He was immunized completely. His performance at school was good.

> **CASE AT A GLANCE**
>
> **Basic Findings**
> Height : 124 cm (95th centile)
> Weight : 20 kg (70th centile)
> Temperature : 37°C
> Pulse rate : 86 beats/min minute
> Respiratory rate : 20 breaths/min
> Blood pressure : 100/80 mm Hg
>
> **Positive Findings**
> *History:*
> - Puffiness of face
> - High-colored urine
> - 2-week old skin lesions
>
> *Examination:*
> - Periorbital edema
> - Healed skin lesions
> - Raised blood pressure
>
> *Investigation:*
> - *ESR:* Raised
> - *BUN:* Raised
> - *Creatinine:* Raised
> - *ASLO:* Significant
> - *Urine:* Albumin, RBCs, granular casts, 10–12 pus cells observed
> - *X-ray chest:* Showed pulmonary venous congestion and cardiomegaly.
>
> (ASLO: antistreptolysin O; BUN: blood urea nitrogen; ESR: erythrocyte sedimentation rate; RBCs: red blood cells)

There was development of oozing skin lesions treated with the course of antibiotics and local antiseptic ointment. There was no history of fever, convulsions, suggestive of oliguria, sore throat, and breathlessness.

EXAMINATION

On examination, the body was moderately built and moderately nourished. He was alert. There were healed pyogenic skin lesions. Anthropometric measurements included, the height was 124 cm (95th centile), and the weight was 20 kg (70th centile).

Child was afebrile and the pulse rate was 86 beats/min and regular. Respiratory rate was 20 breaths/min. Blood pressure recorded was 100/80 mm Hg in right upper limb. Pallor was present. Periorbital edema was present. There was no clubbing and no lymphadenopathy. All the systemic examinations were normal.

INVESTIGATION

- *Hemoglobin:* 8 g/dL
- *Total leukocyte count (TLC):* 8,700 cells/cumm
- *Platelet count:* 2,00,000 cells/cumm
- *Erythrocyte sedimentation rate (ESR):* 32 mm in first hour
- *Blood urea nitrogen (BUN):* 40 mg/dL
- *Serum creatinine:* 4 mg/dL
- *Hepatitis B surface antigen (HbSAg):* Negative
- *Antistreptolysin O (ASLO):* 200 Todd units
- *Complement level:* C_3 decreased
- *Serum potassium:* 4 mEq/L
- *Serum sodium:* 130 mEq/L
- *Peripheral blood smear:* Normocytic hypochromic anemia
- *Serum bilirubin:* 1.3 mg/dL
- *Pus for culture and sensitivity:* No growth
- *Urine examination:* Albumin present granular casts, plenty of red blood cells (RBCs) and 10–12 pus cells were present
- *X-ray chest:* Pulmonary venous congestion and cardiomegaly

DISCUSSION

A school going child developed sudden onset of puffiness of the face. This was more around the face. This was also associated with history of high-colored urine probably hematuria. There was significant history of treatment for pyodermic lesions about 2 weeks back.

On examination, there was periorbital edema and moderately raised blood pressure. All these findings make a diagnosis of acute poststreptococcal glomerulonephritis (APSGN). This is supported by raised blood urea level and serum creatinine level.

Group A β-hemolytic streptococcal infections are common in school-age children and is more common in boys and can lead to the postinfectious complication of acute glomerulonephritis (AGN). Acute poststreptococcal glomerulonephritis (APSGN) is a classic example of the acute nephritic syndrome characterized the sudden onset of gross hematuria, edema, hypertension, and insufficiency.

Acute glomerulonephritis is characterized by a relatively abrupt onset of variable degrees of hematuria, edema, hypertension, oliguria along with diminished glomerular filtration rate (GFR), salt, and fluid retention and circulatory congestion.

ETIOLOGY

Acute glomerulonephritis may follow infection with a variety of microorganisms, when it is called "postinfectious". AGN occurring after β-hemolytic streptococcal infection is the most common type in children, accounting for approximately 80% cases. However, many other bacterial, viral, and parasitic pathogens may also induce acute postinfectious glomerulonephritis (PIGN). Identifying a specific causative pathogen often is difficult, because the infection usually precedes the nephritis by a few weeks. Other agents responsible for nephritis are influenza A, coxsackie, echovirus, Epstein–Barr virus, *Staphylococcus* and pneumococcus. AGN may occur as part of a systemic disease, and acute nephritic features may be observed in acute interstitial nephritis.

Poststreptococcal GN commonly follows streptococcal pharyngitis during cold-weather months and streptococcal skin infections or pyoderma during warm-weather months. APSGN has been shown to be nephritogenic following pharyngitis (strain 3, 4, 12, 18, 25, and 49) or impetigo (strains 2, 49, 55, 57, and 60). It is extremely rare for APSGN and acute rheumatic fever (associated with M strains 1, 3, and 12) to occur simultaneously in the same patient. Although epidemics of nephritis have been described in association with throat (serotypes M1, M4, M25, and some strains of M12) and (serotype M49) infections, this disease is most commonly sporadic.

■ PATHOLOGY

Glomeruli appear enlarged and relatively bloodless and show diffuse mesangial cell proliferation, with an increase in mesangial matrix. Neutrophil infiltration is striking in early stages. The capillary basement membrane and the arterioles do not show significant abnormality. Epithelial cell proliferation and crescents are uncommon. In a very small proportion of cases, however, extensive crescentic changes are present, which is associated with a rapidly progressive course and a poor prognosis.

Polymorphonuclear leukocyte infiltration is common in glomeruli in the early stage of the disease. Crescents and interstitial inflammation may be seen in severe cases, but these changes are not specific for poststreptococcal GN. The glomerular abnormalities are very characteristic. Proliferative and exudative changes are uniformly distributed. Glomeruli are enlarged and the lobular pattern is accentuated. There is proliferation of both endothelial and mesangial cells with obliteration of capillary lumen giving the glomeruli a "bloodless" appearance.

Immunofluorescence examination shows granular deposits of immune complexes immunoglobulin G (IgG) and C3 along the capillary walls and in the mesangium. C1q and C4 deposits may also be seen. Electron microscopy shows electron-dense subepithelial deposits or "humps". These are more striking, early, and tend to disappear after 6 weeks. IgG has been demonstrated in these deposits. Immunofluorescence microscopy reveals a pattern of "lumpy-bumpy" deposits of immunoglobulin and complement on the glomerular basement membrane and in the mesangium. On electron microscopy, electron-dense deposits, or humps are observed on the epithelial side of the glomerular basement membrane.

The histological abnormalities resolve rapidly, and within 6-8 weeks there is considerable decrease in exudative changes. Mild mesangial hypercellularity may persist for 1-2 years but eventually disappears. Capillary loops are narrowed. Glomeruli appear enlarged and ischemic changes are seen. There will be proliferation of mesangial cells and infiltration of neutrophils in glomeruli.

■ PATHOGENESIS

The precise nature of the antigen–antibody complex that causes nephritis remains unclear. The latency period between the acute infection and the onset of nephritis represents the time required to generate sufficient IgG antistreptococcal antibodies to trigger immune complex formation.

Morphologic studies and a depression in the serum complement (C3) level provide strong evidence that ASPGN is mediated by immune complexes. Circulating immune complex formation with streptococcal antigens and subsequent glomerular deposition is thought to be less likely a pathogenic mechanism. Group A streptococci possess M proteins, and nephritogenic strains related to the M protein serotype.

Although epidemics of nephritis have been described in association with throat (serotypes M1, M4, M25, and some strains of M12) and skin (serotype M49) infections, this disease is most commonly sporadic.

Although several streptococcal antigens have been identified in the glomerular immune deposits, two proteins are of particular interest, based on currently available evidence. First is the cationic cysteine proteinase exotoxin B that colocalizes with complement and IgG within glomerular subepithelial immune deposits. The presence of circulating anti-streptococcal B antibodies is a strong evidence of a recent nephritogenic streptococcal infection. Second is the nephritis-associated plasmin receptor, a protein that does not colocalize with glomerular immune deposits but is associated with increased intraglomerular plasmin activity and is thought to facilitate immune complex formation and inflammation.

Additional antigens are of interest and suggest that a group of streptococcal proteins may be involved in the initiation and progression of glomerular injury. It is currently thought that the target streptococcal antigen is initially trapped within glomeruli, with subsequent immune complex formation occurring in situ in the kidney. Once glomerular immune deposits are formed, the alternative and lectin complement pathways are activated, followed by neutrophil infiltration and glomerular damage. APSGN is an "exudative" GN characterized by the presence of many intraglomerular neutrophils. Pyuria and even white cell casts may be observed in the urinary sediment.

Postinfectious:
- Streptococci, staphylococci, *Treponema pallidum, Salmonella* typhi, leptospirosis.
- *Plasmodium malaria, Toxoplasma,* filarial
- Hepatitis B and C, cytomegalovirus, parvovirus, Ebstein–Barr virus
- Associated with severe infections; infection of shunts, prostheses, bacterial endocarditis

Systemic vasculitis:
- Henoch–Schonlein purpura, systemic lupus erythematosus
- Microscopic polyarteritis, Wegener's granulomatosis

Others:
- Membranoproliferative glomerulonephritis
- Immunoglobulin A (IgA) nephropathy
- Hereditary nephropathy
- Acute interstitial nephritis

GLOMERULONEPHRITIS WITH HYPOCOMPLEMENTEMIA

- Poststreptococcal
- Subacute bacterial endocarditis
- Shunt nephritis
- Systemic lupus erythematosus
- Membranoproliferative
- Other postinfectious causes

■ CLINICAL FEATURES (FIG. 1)

Onset of the disease is sudden. It usually affects children between the ages of 5 and 12 years and is rare below the age of 3 years. A male preponderance is reported. Patients usually are afebrile with a latency period of 1–2 weeks after having pharyngitis and 3–6 weeks after having a skin infection.

There will be puffiness of face with periorbital swelling. Edema is usually the result of salt and water retentions. Some degree of oliguria is usually associated, but anuria is infrequent and if persistent suggests rapidly progressive glomerulonephritis (GN). If the fluid intake has been unrestricted, the edema may increase to involve the hands and legs.

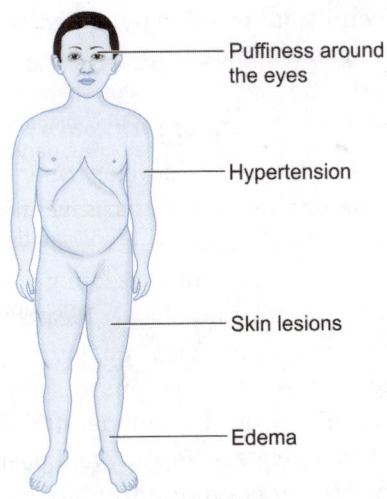

Fig. 1: Clinical features.

- Puffiness around the eyes
- Hypertension
- Skin lesions
- Edema

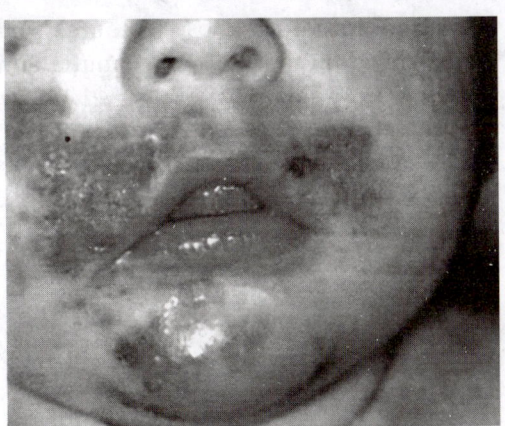

Fig. 2: Impetigo. *(For color version, see Plate 2)*

Gross hematuria (30–50%) will be associated. Urine is typically reddish-brown or smoky or cola-colored. Hematuria is defined as the presence of more than five RBCs per high-power field (HPF) on at least two performed urine analysis. GN is the most important cause of asymptomatic hematuria. Almost all the patients have microscopic hematuria.

In some cases pharyngitis may be mild and have gone unnoticed. Active or healed lesions of impetigo **(Fig. 2)** may be present when AGN develops. During an epidemic of streptococcal throat infection, many subclinical cases occur who have only microscopic hematuria.

The severity of kidney involvement varies from asymptomatic-microscopic hematuria with normal renal function to gross hematuria with acute renal failure (ARF). Depending on the severity of renal involvement, patients can develop various degrees of edema, hypertension, and oliguria. Patients are at risk for developing encephalopathy and/or heart failure secondary to hypertension or hypervolemia. Hypertensive encephalopathy must be considered in patients with blurred vision, severe headaches, altered mental status, or new seizures. Respiratory distress, orthopnea, and cough may be symptoms of pulmonary edema and heart failure. Peripheral edema typically results from salt and water retention and is common; nephrotic syndrome (NS) develops in a minority (<5%) of childhood cases. Nonspecific symptoms such as malaise, lethargy, abdominal pain, or flank pain are common.

The acute phase generally resolves within 6–8 weeks. Although urinary protein excretion and hypertension usually normalize by 4–6 weeks after onset, persistent microscopic hematuria can persist for 1–2 years after the initial presentation.

Mild hypertension is usually present. The nonspecific symptoms such as malaise, lethargy, abdominal pain, and fever are common. The severity of the renal involvement varies from asymptomatic microscopic hematuria with normal renal function to ARF.

In most cases, there is a history of sore throat or pyoderma. The latent period is 7–14 days in the former and 2–4 weeks in the latter.

The severity of poststreptococcal glomerulonephritis (PSGN) is variable and mild cases may just have microscopic hematuria with slight proteinuria. Those at the other end of the spectrum may have oligoanuria and severe hypertension.

> **ESSENTIAL DIAGNOSTIC POINTS**
> - Edema
> - Proteinuria—1+
> - Transient hypertension
> - Oliguria
> - *Urinalysis:* Dysmorphic red blood cells (RBCs), red cell casts

The urine often has a unique color or tea color. Rapidly progressive GN can occur, but only rarely. Although many patients have significant proteinuria and a slightly depressed serum albumin level (at least in part due to intravascular volume expansion), fewer than 5% of symptomatic patients develop frank NS. Severe complications, including pulmonary hemorrhage and cerebrovascular accidents, have been reported and can require kidney biopsy to distinguish APSGN from systemic vasculitis or Goodpasture syndrome.

■ ATYPICAL PRESENTATIONS

The child may present with one or more of the complications of AGN. A history of sore throat and gross hematuria may be absent and the edema mild. Occasionally, urinalysis may not show significant abnormality. A correct diagnosis and prompt management are crucial.

Acute Pulmonary Edema

Expansion of extracellular volume may lead to congestive heart failure and pulmonary edema. There is dyspnea and restlessness. The blood pressure is high, but in later stages when heart failure and shock supervene, there may be hypotension. A chest X-ray film typically shows mild cardiomegaly and features of pulmonary edema. Often the condition is wrongly diagnosed as bronchopneumonia or myocarditis.

Hypertensive Encephalopathy

Children with AGN may develop hypertensive encephalopathy at comparatively lower levels of blood pressure. Drowsiness and convulsions may be the presenting features, and may resemble encephalitis. Measurement of blood pressure and urinalysis is diagnostic.

Hypertension is common (60-80%) but usually is mild to moderate; rarely, hypertensive encephalopathy and posterior reversible encephalopathy syndrome (PRES) can develop, even without a significant elevation in the serum creatinine concentration. Echocardiographic evidence of left ventricular dysfunction is a common finding in children hospitalized with APSGN.

Acute Renal Failure

In occasional cases, oligoanuria and azotemia are the chief features, and gross hematuria and edema may be absent.

Nephrotic Syndrome

A mixed picture of AGN and nephritic syndrome may be present. The child has gross hematuria, hypertension, generalized edema, and heavy proteinuria. In such cases, the glomerular lesions are invariably severe and extensive crescent formation may be present.

■ COMPLICATIONS

Complications include those occurring as a consequence of hypertension such as hypertensive encephalopathy and congestive cardiac failure. Other complications include hyperkalemia, hyperphosphatemia, hypocalcemia, acidosis, seizures, and uremia.

Features of delayed resolution:
- Oliguria, hypertension and/or azotemia persisting for past 2 weeks
- Gross hematuria persisting for 3-4 weeks
- Low C3 levels beyond 6-8 weeks
- Persistent hematuria or proteinuria beyond 6-12 months

GENERAL FEATURES
• Rapid onset
• Hematuria
• Convulsions
• Sore throat

■ DIAGNOSIS

The serum C3 level usually is below 50% of normal levels in patients with APSGN. 10% of APSGN patients have normal C3 level at the time of assessment. In patients with other forms of acute PIGN, this percentage is even higher. The serum C3 level typically returns to normal within 8-12 weeks after APSGN. Urinalysis generally shows hematuria, proteinuria, and cellular casts (both red and white cells); rarely, patients may have a normal urinalysis.

Urinalysis demonstrates RBCs, often in association with RBC casts, proteinuria, and polymorphonuclear leukocytes. A mild normochromic anemia may be present from hemodilution and low-grade hemolysis.

Confirmation of the diagnosis requires clear evidence of a prior streptococcal infection. A positive throat culture report might support the diagnosis or might represent the carrier state. A rising antibody titer to streptococcal antigen(s) confirms a recent streptococcal infection.

A fresh, uncentrifuged urine specimen should be examined for casts as these disintegrate on standing and centrifugation. Hyaline and granular casts also may be seen.

The ASLO titer is commonly elevated after a pharyngeal infection but rarely increases after streptococcal skin infections. Evidence of preceding streptococcal infection is indicated by a rise in ASLO titer, which is elevated in 60-80% cases. Early antibiotic treatment may attenuate this response. The rise in ASLO titer begins 1-3 weeks after the streptococcal infection, reaches a peak in 3-5 weeks and then falls to insignificant levels in 6 months.

The best single antibody titer to document cutaneous streptococcal infection is the anti-dexyribonuclease B (anti-DNase B) level. Serologic evidence for streptococcal infections is more sensitive than the history of recent infections and far more sensitive than positive bacterial cultures obtained at the time of onset of acute nephritis.

Gross hematuria is present in a majority of moderate-to-severe cases. Proteinuria is usually mild; occasionally it may be in the nephrotic range. Microscopic examination shows dysmorphic red cells, red cell casts, and neutrophils. In initial stages, urine may contain a large number of neutrophils, which is often mistakenly regarded to indicate urinary tract infection (UTI).

The levels of blood area and creatinine are elevated. In patients with ARF, there may be hyponatremia, hyperkalemia, and acidosis.

Chest X-ray is indicated in those with signs of heart failure or respiratory distress, or physical examination findings of a heart gallop, decreased breath sounds, rales, or hypoxemia. A chest X-ray film may show cardiomegaly and pulmonary congestion. Anemia and hypolbuminemia are secondary to renal sodium and water retention with consequent hemodilution.

Renal function studies show a decrease in GFR and renal blood flow, increased distal tubular readsorption of sodium and water leading to hypervolemia, and expansion of extracellular volume. The levels of plasma renin and aldosterone are decreased. These abnormalities are exactly opposite to those observed in minimal-change nephrotic syndrome (MCNS) with edema.

> **LABORATORY SALIENT FINDINGS**
>
> - *Urinalysis:* Dimorphic RBCs, red cell casts
> - BUN, creatinine: Raised
> - *Serum C3 and C4:* Decreased
> - *Streptococcal serology:* ASLO-raised
> - *Serum albumin:* Decreased
> - Throat culture, skin culture if lesions present
> - ANA, anti-DNA antibodies
>
> (ANA: antineutrophil antibody; ASLO: antistreptolysin O; BUN: blood urea nitrogen; RBCs: red blood cells)

Magnetic resonance imaging of the brain is indicated in patients with severe neurologic symptoms and can demonstrate PRES in the parieto-occipital areas on T2-weighted image.

The serum C3 level is significantly reduced in >90% of patients in the acute phase, and returns to normal 8–12 weeks after onset. Serum C5 levels are mildly reduced but those of C4 are normal. Persistent hypocomplementemia is rare in PSGN and suggests an alternative condition such as membranoproliferative GN (MPGN), lupus nephritis, or GN related to endocarditis or occult abscesses. The degree of C3 depression is not related to the severity of the disease.

Renal biopsy should be considered only in the presence of ARF, NS, absence of evidence of streptococcal infection, or normal complement levels. In addition, renal biopsy is considered when hematuria and proteinuria, diminished renal function, and/or a low C3 level persist >2 months after onset.

Renal biopsy is not required in typical cases of PSGN, except when the serum complement remains depressed or if renal function is severely impaired making the diagnosis questionable. The following **Box 1** summarizes the situations where a biopsy is indicated. The biopsy is done to assess prognosis or detect the presence of other underlying glomerular diseases such as systemic vasculitis, lupus erythematosus, or MPGN.

> **BOX 1:** Indications for renal biopsy in acute glomerulonephritis (AGN).
>
> - *Systemic features:* Fever, rash, joint pain, heart disease
> - Absence of serologic evidence of streptococcal infection; normal level of C3
> - Mixed picture of AGN and nephritic syndrome
> - Severe anemia, very high levels of blood urea or anuria requiring dialysis
> - *Delayed resolution:*
>   – Oliguria, hypertension and/or azotemia persisting past 2 weeks
>   – Gross hematuria persisting past 3–4 weeks
>   – Low C3 levels beyond 6–8 weeks
>   – Persistent hematuria or proteinuria beyond 6–12 months

Immunofluorescence microscopy reveals lumpy-bumpy deposits of immunoglobulin and complement in the glomerular basement membrane and mesangium. Peripheral blood smear shows normocytic hypochromic type of anemia. This is because of hemodilution.

■ DIFFERENTIAL DIAGNOSIS

- Nephrotic syndrome
- Hemolytic uremic syndrome (HUS)
- UTI
- Anaphylactoid purpura
- Angioneurotic edema
- Insect bite

■ TREATMENT

Treatment of AGN includes strict bed rest, management of hypertension and congestive cardiac failure. During the acute phase, patients may need to be hospitalized for observation and treatment of hypertension, edema, oliguria, elevated serum creatinine, or electrolyte abnormalities. Intake of sodium, potassium, and protein should be restricted. Urine output should be correctly measured. Fluid intake should be restricted to an amount equal to insensible losses and 24-hour urine output.

Acute poststreptococcal glomerulonephritis is an acute disease that resolves without specific medical therapy. Close monitoring and supportive care are essential to manage the acute nephritis syndrome until the glomerular injury spontaneously resolves. If not previously administered, antibiotics should be given to prevent the spread of the nephritogenic strain of streptococcus to other individuals. Penicillin may be administered for 7 days if active pyoderma or residual pharyngitis is present. Antibiotic therapy has no influence on the course of the disease but may prevent spread of streptococcal infection from patients with positive cultures.

Hypertension usually is not severe and can be managed with short-acting calcium channel blockers. Moderate-to-severe hypertension with or without encephalopathy usually responds to treatment with nifedipine and frusemide. Beta (β)-adrenergic blockers such as atenolol and angiotensin-converting enzyme (ACE) inhibitors such as enalapril are also useful in lowering blood pressure.

Circulatory congestion and edema can be treated with restriction of salt and water and judicious use of diuretics. In patients having acute pulmonary edema and shock, appropriate supportive measures should be promptly instituted. Dopamine or dobutamine should be infused and ventilatory support may be needed. Frusemide should be given intravenously in a dose of 4–6 mg/kg.

If oliguria is present and the level of blood urea is elevated, dietary protein should be appropriately restricted.

In patients with more severe acute kidney injury (AKI), hyperkalemia, hyperphosphatemia, and acidosis are likely to occur and will require medical management. Corticosteroids and cytotoxic agents have no substantiated therapeutic role, although there is limited anecdotal evidence of benefit for patients with rapidly progressive GN associated with crescents on biopsy. This is such a rare presentation that performing prospective clinical trials to evaluate the benefit of such therapies is impossible.

■ COURSE AND PROGNOSIS

Spontaneous improvement should begin within 1 week, with the gross hematuria, oliguria, azotemia, and hypertension generally resolving within 4 weeks; low C3 within 2 months; proteinuria by 6 months; and gross hematuria rapidly clears but microscopic hematuria may be detected for 6–12 months or longer. APSGN in children has been considered a completely reversible disease, which is still generally true. In the exceptional patient with crescentic disease, prolonged oliguria, and massive proteinuria, recovery may not be complete. Proteinuria subsides earlier, but orthostatic or intermittent proteinuria may be observed. Such urinary abnormalities are of no significance. Occasionally mild-to-moderate hypertension may persist for a few weeks.

The long-term prognosis of PSGN in children is excellent. Even patients with severe disease completely recover; the only exception is the presence of extensive glomerular crescentic lesions. Since immunity to streptococcal M-protein is type-specific and long-lasting and nephritogenic serotypes are limited in number, and recurrent episodes of PSGN are rare. Penicillin prophylaxis is not recommended.

Children with AGN without evidence of a preceding streptococcal infection should be closely followed for several years with periodic urine examinations and measurements of blood pressure. Renal biopsy may be considered if mild-to-moderate proteinuria persists or if there is a decline in renal function.

■ BIBLIOGRAPHY

1. Eison TM, Ault BH, Jones DP, Chesney RW, Wyatt RJ. Post streptococcal acute glomerulonephritis in children: clinical features and pathogenesis. Pediatr Nephrol. 2011;26(2)165-80.
2. González E, Gutiérrez E, Galeano C, Chevia C, de Sequera P, Bernis C, et al.; Grupo Madrileño De Nefritis Intersticiales. Early steroid treatment improves the recovery of renal function in patients with drug-induced acute interstitial nephritis. Kidney Int. 2008; 73:940-6.
3. Master Sankar Raj V, Gordillo R, Chand DH. Overview of C3 glomerulopathy. Front Pediatr. 2016;4:45.

CASE 45

Hemolytic Uremic Syndrome

■ PRESENTING COMPLAINTS

A 5-year-old girl was brought with the complaint of:
- Cough and cold since 3 days
- Loose motions since 3 days
- Abdominal pain since 1 day
- Headache since 1 day
- Nausea since 1 day
- Abnormal movement of limb since 1 hour

History of Presenting Complaints

A 5-year-old girl was brought to the casualty with history of sudden onset of nausea, abdominal pain, and headache. Abdominal pain was present in upper abdomen. The pain was not related to food intake. There was no radiation of pain. The child was complaining of headache. Headache was nonspecific. She had been treated for cough and cold a week back. The medicine used was paracetamol. The girl had loose motion about 3 days back. She was passing loose motion about 6–7 times a day. Loose motion was foul-smelling and was associated with blood stain. The condition of the child was worsening despite of parenteral ampicillin. She developed convulsions involving both the upper and lower limbs. The convulsions were of generalized type.

Past History of the Patient

She was the second sibling of nonconsanguineous marriage. She was born at term by normal delivery. She cried immediately after the delivery. There was no significant postnatal event. She was completely immunized. There was no delay in developmental milestones. Her performance at school was good. There was past history of similar attack.

CASE AT A GLANCE

Basic Findings
Height	:	108 (50th centile)
Weight	:	17 kg (60th centile)
Temperature	:	37°C
Pulse rate	:	120 beats/min
Respiratory rate	:	30 breaths/min
Blood pressure	:	70/50 mm Hg

Positive Findings
History:
- Cough and cold
- Abdominal pain
- Headache
- Loose motions
- Convulsions

Examination:
- Pale toxic look
- Mild distended abdomen
- Abdominal tenderness
- Hepatomegaly

Investigation:
- Hemoglobin (Hb): 5.4 g/dL
- Bilirubin: Increased
- Hyperkalemia
- Blood urea: Increased

EXAMINATION

The girl was moderately built and moderately nourished. There were signs of moderate dehydration. She was in distress and looking sick. Anthropometric measurements included her height 108 cm (50th centile) and her weight 17 kg (60th centile).

She was febrile, the pulse rate was 120 beats/min, and the respiratory rate was 30 breaths/min. The blood pressure recorded was 70/50 mm Hg. Pallor was present. There was no lymphadenopathy, no icterus, and no cyanosis.

Per abdomen examination revealed presence of mild distension. Tenderness was present all over the abdomen. Hepatomegaly was present about 3 cm below the costal margin in the midclavicular region. It is firm in consistency and nontender. Bowel sounds were sluggish. Respiratory system revealed presence of crepitations at the base of right lung.

INVESTIGATION

- *Hemoglobin:* 5.4 g/dL
- *Total leukocyte count (TLC):* 12,300 cells/cumm
- *Packed cell volume (PCV):* 30%
- *Platelet count:* 2,00,000 cells/cumm
- *Blood urea:* 42 mg/dL
- *Serum creatinine:* 1 mg/dL
- *K:* 6.2 mEq/L
- *Na:* 100 mEq/L
- *Peripheral blood smear:* Showed burr cells
- *X-ray chest:* Moderate cardiomegaly, bilateral increased hilar and pulmonary shadow
- *Ultrasound abdomen:* Mild hepatomegaly

DISCUSSION

Hemolytic uremic syndrome (HUS) is the most common cause of ARF in young children. It has common features to systemic disease as well as thrombotic thrombocytopenic purpura (TTP) and cutaneous signs.

It is characterized by the triad of microangiopathic hemolytic anemia, thrombocytopenia, and acute renal insufficiency. The possibility of a genetic form of the disease should be considered in any child with an atypical presentation.

The most common form of HUS is caused by Shiga toxin-producing *Escherichia coli* (STEC), which causes prodromal acute enteritis and is commonly termed STEC-HUS or diarrhea-associated HUS. In the subcontinent of Asia and in southern Africa, the toxin of *Shigella dysenteriae* type 1 is causative, whereas in Western countries, verotoxin producing *E. coli* or STEC is the usual cause. STEC-HUS accounts for about 90% of all HUS cases in childhood.

Shiga toxin-producing *E. coli* has been spread by person-to-person contact within families or childcare centers. A rare but distinct entity of infection-triggered HUS is related to neuraminidase-producing *Streptococcus pneumoniae*. HUS, typically severe, develops during acute infection with this organism, typically manifesting as pneumonia with empyema. A thrombotic microangiopathy (TMA), similar to HUS or TTP, also can occur in patients with untreated human immunodeficiency virus (HIV) infection and influenza infection.

Genetic forms of HUS (atypical, non-diarrheal) compose the second major category of the disease. Inherited deficiencies of either von Willebrand factor-cleaving protease (ADAMTS13) or complement factor H, I, or B can cause HUS. A specific genetic defect has not been identified in approximately 50% of familial cases transmitted in classic Mendelian autosomal dominant or recessive patterns. Some of these may be due to cobalamin C mutations. A major feature characteristic of genetic forms of HUS is the absence of a preceding diarrheal prodrome. Genetic forms of HUS can be indolent and unremitting once they become manifest, or they can have a relapsing pattern precipitated by an infectious illness. The latter feature likely explains the association of many infectious agents with HUS, particularly in reports published before the recognition of the unique pathophysiology of STEC and neuraminidase-producing pneumococci in causing HUS.

Two broad subgroups of HUS are recognized. The first is most commonly seen in infants and young children. It is associated with diarrheal prodrome. It has also been called as typical HUS. HUS is the most common glomerular disease to cause severe AKI in a previously healthy young child. Most children with HUS (90%) have an antecedent diarrheal illness caused by a strain of *E. coli* that produces a Shiga-like toxin. This group of patients had been formerly classified as having diarrhea-associated HUS (D+HUS), and this disorder is now known as Shiga toxin-producing *E. coli*-associated (STEC+) HUS.

It more frequently follows an episode of gastroenteritis caused by enterohemorrhagic strain of *E. coli*. It has also been associated with other bacteria such as *Shigella, Salmonella, Campylobacter, S. pneumoniae*. The viruses responsible for this are coxsackie, influenza, and Epstein–Barr viruses.

Several serotypes of *E. coli* can produce the toxin. Disease commonly is transmitted by undercooked meat or unpasteurized (raw) milk. HUS develops during acute infection with this organism, typically manifesting as pneumonia with empyema. A TMA, similar to HUS or TTP, also can occur in patients with untreated HIV infection. Second form is not associated with antecedent HUS. It usually follows a bacterial or viral infection. It may result from hypertensive encephalopathy and convulsions. Fluid retention occurs secondary to fluid overload because of oliguria and anuria leading to cardiac failure.

It has been associated with systemic lupus erythematosus (SLE), malignant hypertension, and preeclampsia. The picture of HUS may be mimicked by sepsis, when complicated by consumption coagulopathy, especially in young infants. Such cases should be distinguished from HUS. HUS may resemble ITP. Whereas TMA and the resulting hemolytic anemia and thrombocytopenia are common to both of these disorders; their typical profiles are very different.

The features of HUS occasionally may be seen in association with a wide variety of conditions such as bacterial and viral infections, malignancies, collagen diseases, renal transplantation, and malignant hypertension, but these are uncommon in children.

Hemolytic uremic syndrome is occasionally seen following invasive *S. pneumoniae* infection, in which there is damage to endothelium from streptococcal neuraminidase. That leads to exposure of crypted Thomsen–Friedenreich antigen and absorption of natural circulating antibodies.

■ PATHOLOGY

The basic lesion of HUS is termed (TMA). Glomerular TMA is very characteristic of HUS, and similar lesions are only seen in allograft glomerulopathy and in some forms of chronic rejection. Early lesions are best demonstrated on electron microscopy. The endothelial cells are swollen with increase in intracytoplasmic organelles.

There is peripheral extension of mesangial cell cytoplasm and matrix into capillary wall with narrowing of lumen. Mesangial cells are hypertrophied with increase in rough endoplasmic reticulum and lipid droplets. Finely granular fibrillar material similar to that seen in subendothelial space is present in the mesangium.

Intralobular and arcuate arteries show a mixture of fibrous endarteritis and fibrinoid necrosis. Interlobar arteries are not involved. The glomeruli are superficial, cortex looks ischemic with splitting of capillary wall, widening of subendothelial space and wrinkling of glomerular basement membrane.

Early glomerular changes include thickening of the capillary walls caused by swelling of endothelial cells and accumulation of fibrillar material between endothelial cells and the underlying basement membrane, causing narrowing of the capillary lumens. Platelet–fibrin thrombi are often seen in glomerular capillaries.

PATHOGENESIS OF HEMOLYTIC UREMIC SYNDROME

The familial recessive and dominant forms of HUS, including the inherited deficiencies of ADAMTS13 and regulators of the complement cascade, probably predispose patients to developing HUS but do not cause the disease per se, because these patients might not develop HUS until later childhood or even adulthood. In such cases, HUS is often triggered by an inciting event such as an infectious disease. The absence of ADAMTS13 impairs cleavage of von Willebrand factor multimers, which enhances platelet aggregation. Factor H plays a central role in complement regulation, primarily arresting the amplification and propagation of complement activation. It is possible that mild endothelial injury that would normally resolve instead evolves to an aggressive microangiopathy because of the inherited deficiencies of these factors.

Microvascular injury with endothelial cell damage is characteristic of all forms of HUS. Normally the vascular endothelial lining presents a nonreactive surface to circulating blood cells. Thus, intravascular activation of platelets is prevented. This property is related to the negative charge on the endothelial cell surface, which repels negatively charged platelets and red cells, and also to their synthesis of platelet and coagulation-inhibiting factors (such as prostacyclin, plasminogen activator, and heparin sulfate).

In the diarrhea-associated form of HUS, enteropathic organisms produce either Shiga toxin or the highly homologous Shiga-like verotoxin, both of which directly cause endothelial cell damage. Shiga toxin can directly activate platelets to promote their aggregation. In pneumococcal-associated HUS, neuraminidase cleaves sialic acid on membranes of endothelial cells, red cells, and platelets to reveal the underlying cryptic Thomsen–Friedenreich (T) antigen Endogenous immunoglobulin M (IgM) recognizes the T antigen and triggers the microvascular angiopathy.

Following severe dysentery Shiga toxin enters the circulation and leads to endothelial injury in the microvasculature. Neutrophils may have a role in endothelial injury and oxidant damage may be important. There is localized coagulation and deposition of platelet thrombi and fibrin in glomeruli. Involvement of other organs, e.g., pancreas and brain may occur.

The initial changes of glomeruli include thickening of the capillary walls and narrowing of capillary lumina and widening of mesangium. There will be subendothelial and mesangial deposition of granular and amorphous material. Fibrin thrombi can be found in glomerular capillaries and arterioles and may lead to cortical necrosis. There will be partial and total sclerosis of the glomeruli. Ischemia will result as a result of vascular involvement. Concentric intimal proliferation of the arteries and arterioles lead to vascular occlusion.

In each form of HUS, capillary and arteriolar endothelial injury in the kidney leads to localized thrombosis, particularly in glomeruli causing a direct decrease in glomerular filtration. Progressive platelet aggregation in the areas of microvascular injury results in consumptive thrombocytopenia. Microangiopathic hemolytic anemia results from mechanical damage to RBCs as they pass through the damaged and thrombotic microvasculature.

A perturbation in the coagulant–anticoagulant status, following cytotoxin-mediated endothelial cell injury, may lead to coagulation in capillaries and other inflammatory events. Platelets are highly reactive cells, which can be activated by a variety of stimuli such as contact with damaged endothelium, immune complexes, endotoxin, fibrin, platelet-activating factor and other vasoactive agents.

Release of von Willebrand factor antigen from the endothelial cells by a cytopathic effect might explain the abnormalities of this factor in the plasma of HUS patients and may be related to platelet agglutination and thrombocytopenia.

Abnormalities of coagulation and increased blood levels of fibrin degradation products (FDP), suggesting disseminated intravascular coagulation (DIC) may be present in dysentery-associated HUS. Localized coagulation evidenced by the presence of fibrin thrombi and platelets in glomerular capillaries is a constant feature.

■ CLINICAL FEATURES (FIG. 1)

The syndrome is most common in children under the age of 4 years. The onset is preceded by gastroenteritis and less commonly by upper respiratory tract infection. This is followed in about 5–10 days by sudden onset of pallor, irritability, weakness, lethargy, and oliguria. This is seen commonly in summer months and may occur in small epidemics. Encephalopathy and more serious extrarenal manifestation can occur. It is uncommon. But hemorrhagic colitis is common.

Hypertension is usually present. Uncommon features include gross hematuria, petechiae and purpura, jaundice, and convulsions. Renal involvement is usually severe. With prolonged oliguria and anuria, complication of ARF may present HUS with no diarrhea mostly seen in older children. Many have heavy proteinuria and gross hematuria. Severe hypertension is usually present.

Hemolytic uremic syndrome can occur in adolescents and adults. In HUS caused

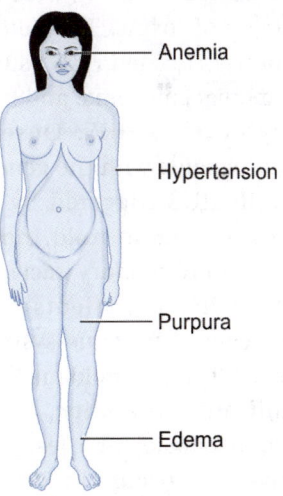

Fig. 1: Clinical features.

by toxigenic *E. coli* onset occurs a few days after onset of gastroenteritis with fever vomiting, abdominal pain, and diarrhea. The prodromal intestinal symptoms may be severe and require hospitalization, but they can also be relatively mild and considered trivial. The diarrhea is often bloody but not necessarily so. Following the prodromal illness, the sudden onset of pallor, irritability, weakness, and lethargy heralds the onset of HUS.

In patients with HUS following shigellosis, dysentery is usually severe and persistent and may continue well beyond the development of HUS. In those not related to shigellosis, there is a prodrome of diarrhea, which is mild or severe and often bloody, and may subside by the time HUS develops. Patients presenting late may show more severe neurological involvement with convulsions and occasionally focal abnormalities. In those with prolonged oliguria or anuria (which correlate with the severity of renal injury) complications of ARF may be present.

Oliguria can be present in early stages but may be masked by ongoing diarrhea, because the prodromal enteritis often overlaps the onset of HUS, particularly with ingestion of large doses of toxins. The patients with pneumococci-associated HUS usually are ill with pneumonia, empyema, and bacteremia when they develop HUS. Onset can be insidious in patients with the genetic forms of HUS, with HUS triggered by a variety of illnesses, including mild, nonspecific gastroenteritis or respiratory tract infections.

The majority of patients with HUS have some central nervous system (CNS) involvement. Most have mild manifestations, with significant irritability; lethargy, or nonspecific encephalopathic features. Severe CNS involvement occurs in 20% of cases. Seizures and significant encephalopathy are the most common manifestations in those with severe CNS involvement, resulting from focal ischemia secondary to microvascular CNS thrombosis. Small infarctions in the basal ganglion and cerebral cortex have also been reported, but large strokes and intracranial hemorrhage are rare. Hypertension may produce an encephalopathy and seizures.

Intestinal complications can be protean and include severe inflammatory colitis, ischemic enteritis, bowel perforation, intussusception, and pancreatitis. Patients can develop but petechiae and significant or severe bleeding is rare despite very low platelet counts. Besides intestinal complications (pseudomembranous colitis, perforation, and intussusception) that are more common in post-dysenteric HUS, involvement of the liver, heart, endocrine and exocrine pancreas, and muscles has also rarely been observed. However, most patients who recover do not appear to have residual functional impairment of organs other than the kidney.

> **ESSENTIAL DIAGNOSTIC POINTS**
> - Microangiopathic microcytic anemia
> - Thrombocytopenia
> - Renal insufficiency
> - Purpuric rashes
> - Diarrhea
> - Disseminated intravascular coagulation (DIC)
> - Oliguria

■ DIAGNOSIS

The diagnosis is made by the combination of microangiopathic hemolytic anemia with schistocytes, thrombocytopenia, and some degree of kidney involvement. The anemia can be mild at presentation, but rapidly progresses. Thrombocytopenia is an invariable finding in the acute phase, with platelet counts usually 20,000–100,000/mm^3.

Partial thromboplastin and prothrombin times are usually normal.

The diagnosis of the syndrome is supported by findings of microangiopathic hemolytic anemia, thrombocytopenia, and ARF. The peripheral blood smear shows helmet cells, burr cells, and fragmented RBCs. Plasma hemoglobin levels are elevated and plasma haptoglobin levels are diminished. The reticulocytes are moderately elevated. White cell count may be elevated, and thrombocytopenia is seen.

The Coombs test is negative, with the exception of pneumococci-induced HUS, where the Coombs test is usually positive. Leukocytosis is often present and significant. Urinalysis typically shows microscopic hematuria and low-grade proteinuria. The renal insufficiency can vary from mild elevations in serum BUN and creatinine to acute, anuric kidney failure.

Hemolytic anemia: Peripheral blood smear characteristically shows broken and deformed RBC. Fragmentation of red cells results from mechanical damage as these cells traverse the abnormal microvasculature through a meshwork of fibrin stands. Increased oxidant damage to RBC membrane may also play a role. Bacterial neuraminidase and phospholipase C can injure endothelial cells, RBC, and platelets.

Thrombocytopenia: Platelet counts are almost invariably decreased and return to normal in 2–3 weeks. There is enhances platelet consumption; their destruction is chiefly related to contact with damaged vascular endothelium the products of platelet injury cause chemotaxis of neutrophils. Serum levels of serotonin and platelet factor IV are increased.

Leukocytosis: Neutrophilic leukocytosis is a very common finding in HUS, especially in the post-dysenteric form. Activated neutrophils release lysosomal enzymes and reactive oxygen radicals that can cause or aggravate endothelial cell damage.

Coagulation: Normal levels of fibrinogen and normal fibrinogen turnover in HUS suggest absence of DIC. Raised levels of FDP indicate activation of the fibrinolytic system. Endothelial injury leads to release of large von Willebrand factor polymers that cause platelet aggregation and increased formation of platelet thrombi. Normal levels of fibrinogen rules out DIC. Raised level of FDP indicates activation of fibrinolytic system. Serum concentration of potassium may be low. Urinalysis shows red cells and occasional casts.

Biochemistry: Biochemical changes indicative of renal dysfunction are present. Serum concentration of potassium may be low initially in some cases, possible as a result of gastrointestinal losses during the diarrheal prodrome. Urinalysis shows red cells and occasional casts.

Renal biopsy: This shows endothelial cells are swollen and separated from the basement membrane with accumulation of foamy material in the subendothelial space. The capillary lumen is narrowed by swollen endothelial cells, blood cells, and fibrin thrombi. Arterioles may show similar changes. Patchy or extensive renal cortical necrosis may be present.

In patients with STEC-HUS, establishing etiology requires either stool culture or polymerase chain reaction (PCR) for STEC or ELISA for Shiga toxin. Serum complement C3 levels are low in some patients with atypical HUS and abnormalities of the complement system. Detailed analysis of components of the alternative complement pathway and its regulators is recommended in all patients with atypical HUS.

LABORATORY SALIENT FINDINGS
- Hemolytic anemia
- Thrombocytopenia
- Leukocytosis
- Negative Coombs test
- Abnormal renal biochemical parameters

GENERAL FEATURES
- Hematuria
- Altered sensorium
- Oliguria

DIFFERENTIAL DIAGNOSIS

- Disseminated intravascular coagulation
- AGN
- Trauma
- Anaphylactoid purpura

COMPLICATIONS

Complications include anemia, acidosis, hyperkalemia, fluid overload, congestive cardiac failure, hypertension, and uremia. CNS manifestation includes irritability seizures and coma. Colitis and diabetes mellitus are common.

TREATMENT

The primary approach that has substantially improved acute outcome in HUS is early recognition of the disease, monitoring for potential complications, and meticulous supportive care. Supportive care includes careful management of fluid and electrolytes, including prompt correction of volume deficit, control of hypertension, and early institution of dialysis if the patient becomes significantly oliguric or anuric, particularly with hyperkalemia.

Early intravenous (IV) volume expansion before the onset of oligoanuria may be nephroprotective in diarrhea-associated HUS; red cell transfusions are usually required as hemolysis can be brisk and recurrent until the active phase of the disease has resolved. Packed RBCs must be infused slowly or during dialysis, with careful monitoring of the patient's blood pressure. Platelet transfusions should be avoided unless the patients are actively bleeding or the transfusions are needed in preparation for an invasive procedure.

In pneumococci-associated HUS, it is critical that any administered red cells be washed before transfusion to remove residual plasma, because endogenous IgM directed against the revealed T antigen can play a role in accelerating the pathogenesis of the disease.

There is no evidence that any therapy directed at arresting the disease process of the most common, diarrhea-associated form of HUS provides benefit. However, attempts have been made using anticoagulants, antiplatelet agents, fibrinolytic therapy, plasma therapy, immune globulin, and antibiotics. Prompt treatment of causative pneumococcal infection is important. In adults who were treated with azithromycin demonstrated more rapid elimination of the organism.

Plasma infusion or plasmapheresis has been proposed for patients suffering with severe manifestations of HUS with serious CNS involvement. It is specifically contraindicated in those with pneumococcal-associated HUS as it could exacerbate the disease. Treatment in this epidemic included plasma exchange in most of the adult patients, as well as the use of eculizumab.

Plasma therapy can be of substantial benefit to patients with identified deficits of ADAMTS13 or factor H. It may also be considered in patients with other genetic forms of HUS, such as the undefined familial (recessive or dominant) form or sporadic but recurrent HUS. In contrast to its use in STEC-HUS, eculizumab shows great promise in the treatment of atypical HUS, including HUS occurring following renal transplantation. Whether it should be combined with plasma therapy or used as a primary treatment of atypical HUS, is still undetermined.

Most patients with diarrhea-associated HUS recover completely with little risk of long-term sequelae. Patients with hypertension, any level of renal insufficiency, or residual urinary abnormalities persisting a year after an episode of diarrhea-positive HUS (particularly significant proteinuria) require careful follow-up. Patients who have recovered completely with no residual urinary abnormalities after 1 year, are unlikely to have long-term sequelae. Because of some report of late sequelae in such patients, annual examinations with a primary physician are still warranted.

More than 90% of the patients will survive with aggressive management of ARF in acute phase. These recover back to normal renal functions. Treatment involves anticoagulants and primarily heparin. Fibrinolytic therapy will help to dissolve intrarenal thrombi. Plasmapheresis and/or administration of fresh frozen plasma has been recommended.

Eculizumab is an anti-C5 antibody that inhibits complement activation, a pathway that contributes to active disease in some forms of atypical familial HUS; this pathway may contribute to the process in STEC-HUS. Eculizumab is approved by the Food and Drug Administration (FDA) for the treatment of atypical HUS.

While initial reports suggested that eculizumab provided benefit in patients with diarrhea-associated HUS, subsequent systematic analysis showed no benefit from either plasma exchange or eculizumab.

In enteritis-related (D+) cases, no specific therapy has been beneficial. Anticoagulation, antiplatelet, and fibrinolytic agents, infusion of fresh frozen plasma and plasma exchange, administration of vitamin E (for its antioxidant action) and infusion of immune globulin are not effective. Adequate supportive care including early and repeated dialysis to prevent and treat complications of renal failure, correction of anemia, control of hypertension, prevention and treatment of infections, and nutritional support are the mainstay of management.

Neurological dysfunction and hypertension may result from increased intracranial pressure or cerebral microangiopathy with normal intracranial pressure. A careful evaluation is necessary with computed tomography (CT) scanning. In post-dysenteric cases, prolonged dysentery and, occasionally, its surgical complications interfere with oral feeding and lead to severe malnutrition. Parenteral nutrition, modified to the requirements of ARF, may be instituted.

Peritoneal dialysis not only controls the manifestation of uremic state but also promotes the recovery by removing an inhibitor, i.e., plasminogen activates inhibitor of fibrinolysis from the circulation, thus allowing endogenous fibrinolytic mechanisms to dissolve vascular thrombi. Recurrence of the disease is rare.

■ PROGNOSIS

With optimal management most patients with D+HUS recover. The death rate in the acute stage is about 5–10%, from infections and serious complications especially of the CNS. Significant return of renal function seldom occurs in those with TMA of majority of the glomeruli or extensive renal cortical necrosis. Almost 30–40% patients who recover from the acute illness are left with impaired renal function or persistent urinary abnormalities.

BIBLIOGRAPHY

1. Davin JC, Coppo R. Henoch-Schönlein purpura nephritis in children. Nat Rev Nephrol. 2014;10(10):563-73.
2. Nayer A, Asif A. Atypical hemolytic-uremic syndrome: A clinical review. Am J Ther. 2016;23(1)151-8.
3. Trachtman H. HUS and TTP in Children. Pediatr Clin North Am. 2013;60(6):1513-26.

CASE 46

Nephrotic Syndrome

■ PRESENTING COMPLAINTS

A 3-year-old boy was brought with the complaint of:
- Irritability since 3 weeks
- Not taking feeds since 3 weeks
- Swelling of the face and limb since 10 days
- Decrease urine output since 10 days

History of Presenting Complaints

A 3-year-old boy was brought to the hospital with history of swelling in face and limbs. Mother also complained that the child was passing decreased amount of urine. Mother had noticed that her son was not well since almost 3 weeks. In the beginning, she had noticed that the boy used to be more irritable and was not taking food at all. After 1 week she noticed swelling of face, especially around the eye. The swelling used to be more in morning and used to disappear as day passes on. Later, she noticed that swelling started to appear all over the body. The child was not passing sufficient amount of urine as he was passing previously. There was no history of increased frequency of micturition. There was no history of burning sensations of micturition. There was no history of allergy or insect bite.

Past History of the Patient

The child was the second sibling of nonconsanguineous marriage. He was born at full term by normal delivery. He cried immediately after delivery. There was no significant postnatal event. He was on breast milk immediately after delivery. His developmental milestones were normal. He had been completely immunized. His performance at school was good.

■ EXAMINATION

The boy was moderately built and moderately nourished. Anthropometric measurements

CASE AT A GLANCE	
Basic Findings	
Height	: 106 cm (80th centile)
Weight	: 16 kg (95th centile)
Temperature	: 38°C
Pulse rate	: 110 beats/min
Respiratory rate	: 22 breaths/min
Blood pressure	: 70/50 mm Hg
Positive Findings	
History:	
• Generalized swelling	
• Decreased amount of urine	
• Tiredness	
Examination:	
• Anasarca	
• Increased weight	
• Absence of breath sounds	
Investigation:	
• *Cholesterol:* Increased	
• *Triglycerides:* Decreased	
• *Serum albumin:* Decreased	
• *Serum complement:* Decreased	
• *Urine albumin:* +++	

included the height 106 cm (80th centile) and the weight 16 kg (95th centile). He was afebrile, pulse rate was 110 beats/min, and the respiratory rate was 22 breaths/min. Blood pressure recorded was 70/50 mm Hg. There was no pallor, but there was generalized edema, which was pitting in nature.

Per abdomen examination revealed presence of abdominal wall edema. There was no free fluid and no organomegaly. Respiratory system revealed absence of breath sounds on right lower lobe. It was stony dull to percuss. Cardiovascular system was normal.

■ INVESTIGATION

- *Hemoglobin:* 12.2 g/dL
- *TLC:* 7,600 cells/cumm
- *ESR:* 36 mm in the first hour
- *AEC:* 540 cells/cumm
- *Serum cholesterol:* 300 mg/dL
- *Triglycerides:* 50 mg/dL
- *Serum albumin:* 3 g/dL
- *Urine:* Albumin +++
- *Sugar:* Nil
- *Microscopy:* Normal

■ DISCUSSION

Here the boy has presented with the history of generalized edema, oliguria, and presence of protein in urine, which suggests nephrotic syndrome (NS). The diagnosis is supported by increased level of cholesterol and decreased level of triglycerides. Serum protein levels are decreased.

Nephrotic syndrome is a common renal disease. It is characterized by massive proteinuria, hypoalbuminemia, and edema. Hyperlipidemia is usually associated with hematuria, hypertension, and renal functional impairment. Heavy proteinuria is the basic abnormality leading to hypoproteinemia.

The resultant fall in plasma oncotic pressure is responsible for hypovolemia. This stimulates aldosterone functions which in turn enhances sodium retention.

Nephrotic syndrome is the clinical manifestation of glomerular diseases associated with heavy (nephrotic range) proteinuria. Nephrotic-range proteinuria is defined as proteinuria >3.5 g/24 h or a urine protein: creatinine ratio >2. The triad of clinical findings associated with NS arising from the large urinary losses of protein are hypoalbuminemia (<2.5 g/dL), edema, and hyperlipidemia (cholesterol >200 mg/dL).

Nephrotic syndrome is not a disease but a constellation of clinical findings common to several glomerular disorders. By definition, it comprises proteinuria >50 mg/kg per 24 hours, hypoalbuminemia (serum albumin <3.0 g/dL), and hyperlipidemia (elevated very-low-density lipoprotein, intermediate-density lipoprotein, low-density lipoprotein, and triglycerides).

■ ETIOLOGY

Most children with NS have a form of primary or idiopathic NS. Glomerular lesions associated with idiopathic NS include minimal-change disease (the most common), focal segmental glomerulosclerosis (FSGS), membranoproliferative GN (MPGN), C3 glomerulopathy, and membranous nephropathy (MN). These etiologies have different age distributions. Nephritic syndrome may also be secondary to systemic diseases such as SLE, Henoch–Schönlein purpura, malignancy (lymphoma and leukemia), and infections (hepatitis, HIV, and malaria). Rarely the disorder may be congenital as in syphilis and other intrauterine infections, and Finnish type of NS. A number of hereditary proteinuria syndromes are caused by mutations in genes that encode critical protein components of the glomerular filtration apparatus.

The clinical and biochemical features of nephritic syndrome result from heavy proteinuria (>40 mg/m^2/h to 1 g/m^2/24 h). Hypoalbuminemia, lowered plasma oncotic pressure, and edema follow sustained loss of large amounts of protein in urine. Hyperlipidemia and other abnormalities such as raised plasma aldosterone and antidiuretic hormone levels are prominent in patients having massive proteinuria and anasarca.

■ PATHOLOGY

In minimal-change nephrotic syndrome (approximately 85% of total cases of NS in children) **(Fig. 1)**, the glomeruli appear normal or show a minimal increase in mesangial cells and matrix. Findings on immunofluorescence microscopy are typically negative, and electron microscopy simply reveals effacement of the epithelial cell foot processes. More than 95% of children with minimal-change disease respond to corticosteroid therapy.

Mesangial proliferation is characterized by a diffuse increase in mesangial cells and matrix on light microscopy. Immunofluorescence microscopy might reveal trace to 1+ mesangial IgM and/or immunoglobulin A (IgA) staining. Electron microscopy reveals increased numbers of mesangial cells and matrix as well as effacement of the epithelial cell foot processes. Approximately 50% of patients with this histologic lesion respond to corticosteroid therapy.

In FSGS, glomeruli show lesions that are both focal (present only in a proportion of glomeruli) and segmental (localized to >1 intraglomerular tufts). The lesions consist of mesangial cell proliferation and segmental scarring on light microscope.

Idiopathic NS can be clearly separated into minimal-change steroid-responsive type. Others with significant glomerular histological lesions are mostly nonresponsive to prednisolone.

Heavy proteinuria is almost due to "glomerular" cause, following alterations of the selective properties of the glomerular capillary wall. As a result proteins that are not normally filtered, or filtered in very small amounts such as albumin pass readily into the urinary space and are excreted in the urine.

■ PATHOGENESIS

Role of the Podocyte

The underlying abnormality in NS is an increased permeability of the glomerular capillary wall, which leads to massive proteinuria and hypoalbuminemia. The podocyte plays a crucial role in the development of proteinuria and progression of glomerulosclerosis. It is a highly differentiated epithelial cell located on the outside of the glomerular capillary loop. Foot processes are extensions of the podocyte that terminate on the glomerular basement membrane. The foot processes of a podocyte interdigitate with those from adjacent podocytes and are connected by a slit called

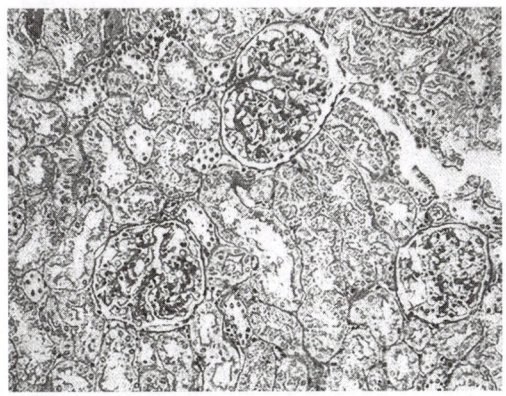

Fig. 1: Minimal change nephrotic syndrome. *(For color version, see Plate 2)*

the slit diaphragm. The podocyte functions as structural support of the capillary loop, is a major component of the glomerular filtration barrier to proteins, and is involved in synthesis and repair of the glomerular basement membrane. The slit diaphragm is one of the major impediments to protein permeability across the glomerular capillary wall. Slit diaphragms are not simple passive filters; they consist of numerous proteins that contribute to complex signaling pathways and play an important role in podocyte function. Important component proteins of the slit diaphragm include nephrin, podocin, CD2AP, and alpha-actinin 4. Podocyte injury or genetic mutations of genes producing podocyte proteins may cause nephrotic-range proteinuria.

In idiopathic, hereditary, and secondary forms of NS, there are immune and non-immune insults to the podocyte that lead to foot process effacement of the podocyte, a decrease in number of functional podocytes, and altered slit diaphragm integrity. The end result is increased protein "leakiness" across the glomerular capillary wall into the urinary space.

Role of the Immune System

Minimal-change nephrotic syndrome (MCSN) may occur after viral infections and allergen challenges. It has also been found to occur in children with Hodgkin lymphoma and T-cell lymphoma. That immunosuppression occurs with drugs such as corticosteroids and cyclosporine provides indirect additional evidence that the immune system contributes to the overall pathogenesis of the NS.

In MCNS light microscopy does not disclose significant abnormalities and glomerular deposits of immune reactants are not seen on immunofluorescence examination. Serum levels of complement (C3) are normal and circulating immune complexes are absent. There is indirect evidence that immunologic mechanisms may be involved in the pathogenesis of MCNS.

The remissions that occasionally follow measles, presence of allergy in some cases, and response to immunoactive agents (corticosteroids, immunosuppressive, and immunomodulatory drugs) suggest an underlying immune dysfunction.

In MCNS urinary protein mainly consists of albumin, whereas with significant glomerular lesions larger protein molecules (IgG, other globulins) are also detected. The amount of urinary protein excretion in MCNS is also related to the level of serum albumin. With prolonged heavy loss of protein, the serum levels fall to very low levels and thus the total amount of urine protein loss declines. While hypoalbuminemia essentially results from heavy urinary losses, increased gastrointestinal losses and perturbed protein metabolism may also contribute.

Hyperlipidemia is due to increased hepatic synthesis of beta lipoprotein and decreased lipoprotein lipase activity. Multiple factors are responsible for hypercoagulable state. Blood viscosity secondary to hyperlipidemia, platelet adhesiveness, altered coagulation factors and clotting inhibitors, increased fibrinogen, and decreased antithrombin levels are responsible for hypercoagulable state.

■ CLINICAL CONSEQUENCE

Edema

Edema is the most common presenting symptom of children with NS. Despite its almost universal presence, there is uncertainty as to the exact mechanism of edema formation. There are two opposing theories: The underfill hypothesis and the overfill hypothesis that have been proposed as mechanisms causing nephrotic edema.

The underfill hypothesis is based on the fact that nephrotic-range proteinuria leads to a fall in the plasma protein level with a corresponding decrease in intravascular oncotic pressure. This leads to leakage of plasma water into the interstitium, generating edema. As a result of reduced intravascular volume, there is increased secretion of vasopressin and atrial natriuretic factor, which, along with aldosterone, result in increased sodium and water retention by the tubules. Sodium and water retention therefore occur as a consequence of intravascular volume depletion.

This hypothesis does not fit the clinical picture of some patients with edema caused by NS who have clinical signs of intravascular volume overload, not volume depletion. Treating these patients with albumin alone may not be sufficient to induce a diuresis without the concomitant use of diuretics. Also, reducing the renin–aldosterone axis with mineralocorticoid receptor antagonists does not result in a marked increase in sodium excretion. With the onset of remission of MCNS, many children will have increased urine output before their urinary protein excretion is measurably reduced.

The overfill hypothesis postulates that NS is associated with primary sodium retention, with subsequent volume expansion and leakage of excess fluid into the interstitium. There is accumulating evidence that the epithelial sodium channel in the distal tubule may play a key role in sodium reabsorption in NS. The clinical weaknesses of this hypothesis are evidenced by the numerous nephrotic patients who present with an obvious clinical picture of intravascular volume depletion: Low blood pressure, tachycardia, and elevated hemoconcentration. Furthermore, amiloride, an epithelial sodium channel blocker, used alone is not sufficient to induce adequate diuresis.

The goal of therapy should be a gradual reduction of edema with judicious use of diuretics, sodium restriction, and cautious use of IV albumin infusions, if indicated.

Hyperlipidemia

There are several alterations in the lipid profile in children with NS, including an increase in cholesterol, triglycerides, low-density lipoprotein, and very-low-density lipoproteins. The high-density lipoprotein level remains unchanged or is low. Hyperlipidemia is thought to be result of increased synthesis as well as decreased catabolism of lipids.

Increased Susceptibility to Infections

Children with NS are especially susceptible to infections such as cellulitis, spontaneous bacterial peritonitis, and bacteremia. This occurs as a result of many factors, particularly hypoglobulinemia as a result of the urinary losses of IgG. In addition, defects in the complement cascade from urinary loss of complement factors (predominantly C3 and C5), as well as alternative pathway factors B and D, lead to impaired opsonization of microorganisms.

Children with NS are at significant increased risk for infection with encapsulated bacteria and in particular, pneumococcal disease. Spontaneous bacterial peritonitis presents with fever, abdominal pain, and peritoneal signs. Although pneumococcus is the most frequent cause of peritonitis, gram-negative bacteria also are associated with a significant number of cases. Children with NS and fever or other signs of infection must be evaluated aggressively, with appropriate cultures drawn and should be treated promptly and empirically with antibiotics. Peritoneal leukocyte counts >250 are highly suggestive of spontaneous had peritonitis.

Hypercoagulability

Nephrotic syndrome is a hypercoagulable state resulting from multiple factors: Vascular stasis from hemoconcentration and intravascular volume depletion, increased platelet number and aggregability, and changes in coagulation factor levels. There is an increase in hepatic production of fibrinogen along with urinary losses of antithrombotic factors such as antithrombin III and protein S. Deep venous thrombosis may occur in any venous bed, including the cerebral venous sinus, renal vein, and pulmonary veins. The clinical risk is low in children (2–5%) compared to adults, but has the potential for serious consequences.

■ CLINICAL FEATURES (FIG. 2)

The NS of childhood has been divided into three broad groups: Congenital/infantile, primary (inherited or idiopathic), and secondary. Only 10–15% of children have an identifiable secondary cause for their NS.

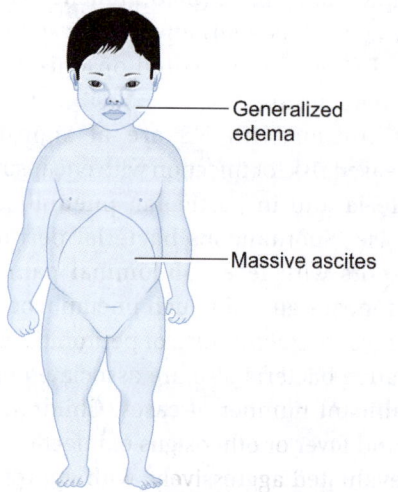

Fig. 2: Clinical features.

Congenital NS is defined as heavy proteinuria, hypoproteinemia, and edema starting within 3 months after birth. It is rare. Cases are caused either by genetic defects, especially nephrin and podocin or by a perinatal infection. The Finnish type of congenital NS is caused by a nephrin gene mutation and is not accompanied by extrarenal malformations. Most of these children are born prematurely, with a birth weight ranging between 1.5 and 3.5 kg. The placental weight is >25% of the newborn weight in practically all cases.

In congenital NS, renal histology shows cystic tubular dilatation as the prominent feature. With increasing edema urine output may fall. The blood pressure is usually normal. Infection may be present. Hydrothorax and hydrocele may be present.

Proteinuria begins in utero and is detectable in the first urine sample after birth. Microscopic hematuria and normal creatinine values during the first months are typical. Heavy protein loss (up to 100 g/L) results in oliguria and severe edema it not treated. Hyperlipidemia, hypothyroidism, and hypogammaglobulinemia are present, due to urinary losses of lipoproteins, thyroid-binding globulins, and immunoglobulin.

By ultrasound, the kidneys are large: With increased cortical echogenicity and indistinct corticomedullary borders. The glomerular histopathology can vary and include minimal change, mesangial expansion, FSGS, or diffuse mesangial sclerosis, and the findings overlap in different entities. If congenital infections are ruled out, genetic analysis is the preferred method för establishing a definitive diagnosis.

For congenital NS, immunosuppression is not recommended. Conservative management of edema with sodium and fluid restriction and intermittent IV albumin and loop diuretics can usually keep these patients out of the hospital. The management of these patients also includes a hypercaloric diet, thyroid hormone replacement, monitoring tor thrombotic episodes, and prompt management of infectious complications.

The outcome of these patients without major extrarenal manifestations is comparable with those of other patient groups after kidney transplantation. Judicious use of ACE is and indomethacin to limit glomerular filtration and subsequent protein losses can allow for adequate growth until the children are large enough to get a kidney transplant. However, other patients require unilateral or bilateral nephrectomy and chronic dialysis as a bridge to kidney transplant.

Primary NS is the occurrence of the constellation of clinical findings that define NS in the absence of an identifiable causative agent or disease. Primary NS is classified into four categories based on biopsy findings: MCNS, MCNS with proliferative changes, FSGS, and MN. Although it is still debated, one theory is that MCNS and FSGS represent different ends in the spectrum of the same disease rather than distinct disorders. From a prognostic perspective, the histologic pattern is less important than is the responsiveness to corticosteroids. Most children with steroid-sensitive-disease have MCNS, so patients with new-onset NS do not undergo routine kidney biopsy at the time of diagnosis.

The idiopathic NS is more common in boys than in girls (2:1) and most commonly appears between the ages of 2 and 6 years. However, it has been reported as early as 6 months of age and throughout adulthood. MCNS is present in 85–90% of patients <6 years of age.

The initial episode of idiopathic NS, as well as subsequent relapses, usually follows minor infections and, uncommonly, reactions to insect bites and bee stings.

Most patients (95%) initially present with dependent edema that is most obvious in the eyelids, scrotum, and labia. Early morning swelling of the eyelids (periorbital edema) is a common occurrence. The onset is insidious with swelling around the eyes and facial puffiness. In some cases an upper respiratory tract infection may be associated. The swelling gradually increases to involve the extremities and abdomen and if untreated may become massive. Mild diarrhea is common, probably due to intestinal edema **(Figs. 3A and B)**.

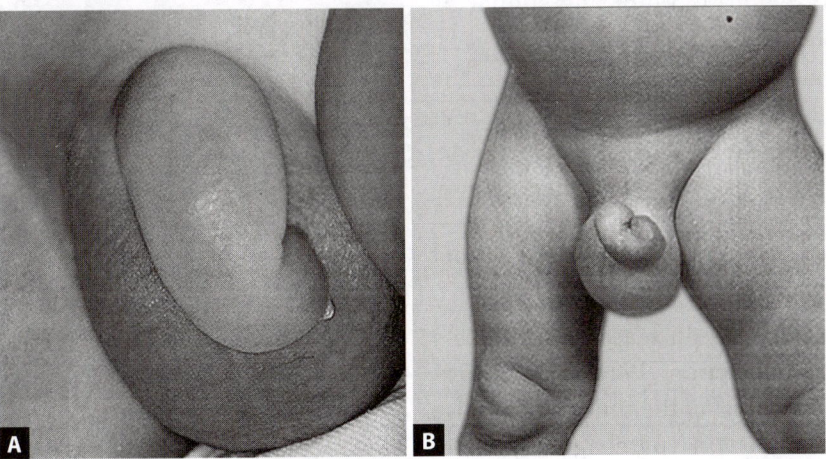

Figs. 3A and B: Edema.

Occasionally, generalized swelling over the body may develop acutely and be associated with gross hematuria and oliguria. Such cases present a mixed picture of nephritic syndrome and acute nephritis. They would require urgent detailed investigations including a renal biopsy.

Nephrotic syndrome can initially be misdiagnosed as an allergic disorder because of the periorbital swelling that decreases throughout the day. With time, the edema becomes generalized, with the development of ascites, pleural effusions, and genital edema. Anorexia, irritability, abdominal pain, and diarrhea are common. Important features of minimal-change idiopathic NS are the absence of hypertension and hematuria (the so-called nephritic features).

Blood pressure should be repeatedly recorded with appropriate cuff with massive edema. It may be elevated. Hypovolemia stimulates several vasoconstricting mechanisms that lead to hypertension. The blood pressure level returns to normal with remission. Features of systemic disorder, i.e., fever, joint pain, hepatosplenomegaly causing secondary nephritic syndrome should be looked for.

Several factors may contribute to the increased risk of having cardiovascular disease and stroke; they include hypertension, the use of steroids, systemic inflammation, and the atherogenic plasma lipid profile. In particular, plasma cholesterol and lipoprotein levels are high.

The patients have increased susceptibility to bacterial infection. Peritonitis is frequently seen. Most of the time it is because of pneumococcus. Hypercoagulable state produces renal vein thrombosis.

ESSENTIAL DIAGNOSTIC POINTS
• Protienuria
• Hypoalbuminemia
• Edema
• Hyperlipedemia
• Hematuria

DIAGNOSIS

The child should be examined to detect any associated infection. Blood pressure should be repeatedly measured with appropriate sized cuff. In MCNS the blood pressure is normal but occasionally in patients with massive edema it may be elevated.

Confirming the Diagnosis of Nephrotic Syndrome

The diagnosis of NS is confirmed by urinalysis with the first morning urine protein:creatinine ratio and serum electrolytes, blood urea nitrogen (BUN), creatinine, albumin, and cholesterol levels; an evaluation to rule out secondary forms of NS (children >10 years) by the complement C3 level, antinuclear antibody, double-stranded DNA; hepatitis B and C and HIV in high-risk populations; and kidney biopsy (for children >12 years, who are less likely to have MCNS).

It is likely that hypovolemia in such cases stimulates several vasoconstricting mechanisms that lead to hypertension. The blood pressure levels return to normal with remission. Features of a systemic disorder (fever, rash, joint pains, hepatosplenomegaly, lymphadenopathy), causing secondary nephritic syndrome, should be looked for.

Urinalysis

The diagnosis of NS is confirmed by urinalysis with first morning urine protein:creatinine ratio and serum electrolytes, BUN, creatinine, albumin, and cholesterol levels.

The urinalysis reveals 3+ or 4+ proteinuria, and microscopic hematuria present in 20% of children. Measurement of 24-hour urinary protein is not essential. Protein excretion of >4 $mg/m^2/h$ on a timed urine collection is considered abnormal. In children with nephrosis, it exceeds >40 $mg/m^2/h$. A urine protein/urine creatinine ratio of >0.5 in children below 2 years old and of >0.2 in older children is considered significant. A spot urine protein creatinine ratio should be > 2.0.

Careful and repeated microscopic examination of persistent microscopic hematuria suggests the likelihood of significant renal histologic lesion. Urine should be cultured to exclude UTI. Hyalin and granular casts may be present.

Blood Examination

Blood is examined for the levels or urea, creatinine, electrolytes, proteins and cholesterol. In MCNS, blood urea levels are within normal range (unless the edema is massive with associated oliguria); elevated levels suggest the presence of significant renal histologic lesions. The level of serum albumin is decreased below 2.5 g/dL and that of cholesterol increased above 250 mg/dL. The severity of these abnormalities is related to the duration of heavy proteinuria. Severe anasarca and massive edema are often associated with serum albumin level of below 1.5 g/dL and cholesterol >500 mg/dL.

Serum sodium levels are occasionally decreased, suggesting pseudohyponatremia related to profound hyperlipidemia. Low serum sodium levels in these situations do not require correction; serum IgG levels are usually low and those of IgM are raised. Serum C3 levels are decreased in a significant proportion of patients with MPGN.

An X-ray film of chest and a Mantoux test should be done. An ultrasound evaluation of kidney and urinary tract should also be performed.

Indications for renal biopsy:
- Persistent hematuria, high blood urea or creatinine
- Patients who fail to get remission with 2-4 weeks of daily treatment with prednisolone
- FSGS
- Mesangial proliferative GN
- MPGN

GENERAL FEATURES
- Insidious onset
- Oliguria
- Albuminemia

■ DIFFERENTIAL DIAGNOSIS
- Congestive cardiac failure
- Angioneurotic edema
- Kwashiorkor
- Malabsorption syndrome
- Filariasis
- GN
- UTI

LABORATORY SALIENT FINDINGS
- Hypoalbuminemia
- Hyperlipidemia
- Proteinuria
- Hemuturia

■ TREATMENT

The treatment includes management of initial episode, management of relapse, and management of complications.

Management of Initial Episode

Clinical and laboratory evaluation identifies children likely to have MCNS. In such cases, a standard course of prednisolone is instituted. The onset of nephritic syndrome beyond the age of 8-10 years, presence of gross or persistent microscopic hematuria, hypertension, and raised serum creatinine levels indicate the presence of a significant glomerular lesion. Renal biopsy should be carried out in these patients.

Children with presumed MCNS, prednisone, or prednisolone should be administered as a single daily dose of 60 mg/m^2/day or 2 mg/kg/day to a maximum of 60 mg daily for 4-6 week followed by alternate-day prednisone (starting at 40 mg/m^2 qid or 1.5 mg/kg qid) for a period ranging from 8 weeks to 5 months, with tapering of the dose. When planning the duration of steroid therapy, the side effects of prolonged corticosteroid administration must be kept in mind. Treatment with corticosteroids results in abolition of proteinuria (remission) usually by 10-14 days, diuresis, and loss of edema.

The parents should be given an explanation of the condition and the importance of compliance with the treatment. The side effects of prednisolone and the need for prolonged initial therapy should be made clear.

Infusion of 25% albumin solution in dose of 0.5-1 g/kg of albumin over 1-2 hours and followed by a potent diuretic such as furosemide (1-4 mg/kg/day in two divided doses) alone or with an aldosterone antagonist/spironolactone (2-3 mg/kg/day in two divided doses) can be used to induce diuresis in a child not responding to furosemide alone.

Children with their first episode of NS and mild-to-moderate edema may be managed as outpatients. Children with onset of uncomplicated NS between 1 and 8 years of age are likely to have steroid-responsive MCNS, and steroid therapy may be initiated without a diagnostic renal biopsy. Children with features that make MCNS less likely (gross hematuria, hypertension, renal insufficiency, hypocomplementemia, or age <1 year or >12 years) should be considered for renal biopsy before treatment.

Approximately 80-90% of children respond to steroid therapy. Response is defined as the attainment of remission within the initial 4 weeks of corticosteroid therapy. Remission consists of a urine protein:creatinine ratio of <0.2 or <1+ protein on urine dipstick for 3 consecutive days. The vast majority of children who respond to prednisone therapy do so within the first 5 weeks of treatment.

Most patients respond to prednisolone with complete disappearance of proteinuria by the end of the second week of therapy and only a minority will respond after 4 weeks of treatment. Persisting proteinuria after 4-6 weeks of therapy defines initial steroid resistance.

Children in their first episode should be treated for at least 3 months, with an increase in benefit being demonstrated for up to 6-7 months is likely to result in a longer remission and fewer relapses without an increase in serious adverse events. Based on these observations, a regimen of a prolonged duration of alternate-day therapy with tapering doses of prednisolone will be adopted.

In a very small proportion of cases, there may be no relapse or a single relapse. In most cases, however, relapses and remissions over a varying period of time are the rule. Relapses are more frequent in younger children. Various terms used to describe the patterns of response of NS to a standard regimen of corticosteroids are listed in **Table 1**.

Of patients who respond to prednisolone, 25-40% have infrequent relapses (an occasional patient may get one or two

TABLE 1: Pattern of response to corticosteroid therapy.

Remission	Protein-free urine (urine protein negative or trace or <4 mg/m²/h) for 3 consecutive days
Relapse	Proteinuria (urine protein 3+ or more) for 3 consecutive days
Infrequent relapse	A responder who relapses but has 3 or less relapses within 1 year
Frequent relapse	A relapser who has two relapses or more within 6 months of the initial episode or more than three relapses within any 12-month period
Steroid-dependent	Occurrence of two consecutive relapses during alternate-day prednisolone therapy or within 2 weeks of its discontinuation
Initial resistance	Absence of remission despite 6 weeks of initial steroid treatment
Late responder	Patient with initial resistance, who responds at some time after initial treatment
Late resistance	Initial responder, who subsequently fails to respond to steroid therapy

relapses followed by permanent cure), 40% have frequent relapses, and the remainder show steroid dependence.

> **INDICATIONS FOR SECONDARY THERAPY**
> - Not responding initial dose of prednisolone
> - Frequent relapsers
> - Affected by side effects steroids
> - Nonresponders to prednisolone during relapses

The current definition of steroid-responsiveness is response within 8 weeks. Once the urine becomes negative for protein, the prednisone is switched to alternate days and tapered over the course of 6 weeks or longer. The total duration of daily and alternate-day steroid therapy used to treat the initial episode influences the subsequent relapse rate. However, three recent, well-designed clinical trials showed no significant reduction in the risk of having a relapse when extending the therapy past 3 months. Alternate-day dosing of prednisone during the taper has been shown in pediatrics to cause less growth suppression.

Almost 50% of children with steroid-sensitive nephrotic syndrome (SSNS) experience several relapses. There is no agreement on a standard protocol for treating relapses. A commonly used protocol is prednisone 60 mg/kg/day until the urine is free of protein for 5–7 days; this is followed by alternate-day therapy that is tapered over several weeks.

Prednisolone Dependence

About 20% patients respond to prednisolone but require its continued daily administration for maintenance of remission. They promptly relapse when either the dosage of prednisolone is reduced or the medication stopped. Some of these patients may be managed with relatively higher doses of prednisolone given on alternate days.

When a child with NS develops two consecutive relapses during steroid therapy or when the ability to achieve and/or remain in remission from NS requires administration of corticosteroids (relapse within 14 days of its cessation), then the child is considered to be steroid-dependent. Patients with steroid-dependent nephrotic syndrome (SDNS) may also fit the definition for having frequently relapsing nephrotic syndrome (FRNS), and similarly to FRNS, the potential adverse effects of the cumulative steroid doses required to maintain remission exceed presumed benefits of achieving remission of NS. MCNS is the most common cause of SDNS. Before initiating steroid-sparing therapies, a biopsy may be performed.

Steroid Resistance

Steroid resistance is defined as the failure to achieve remission after 8 weeks of corticosteroid therapy.

Steroid-resistant nephrotic syndrome (SRNS) is defined as a failure to achieve remission after 6–8 weeks of full-dose daily prednisone. Approximately 15–20% of children with idiopathic NS will develop disease that is resistant to steroids. In addition, a small subset of patients who initially are responsive to steroids do evolve into having SRNS.

Because MCNS is less common and FSGS is more common in this population, a biopsy is recommended for steroid-resistant patients prior to initiating alternative therapies. Genetic testing also is performed by many nephrologists for patients with SRNS, especially those who present at younger than 2 years of age or when there is a positive family history of NS.

Children with steroid-resistant NS require further evaluation, including a diagnostic kidney biopsy, evaluation of kidney function, and quantitation of urine protein excretion (in addition to urine dipstick testing). Steroid-resistant NS is usually caused by FSGS (80%), MCNS, or MPGN.

Steroid-resistant NS, and specifically FSGS, is associated with a 50% risk for end-stage kidney disease within 5 years of diagnosis if patients do not achieve a partial or complete remission. Children reaching end-stage kidney disease have a greatly reduced life expectancy compared to their peers.

A renal biopsy is carried out in all steroid resistant patients to determine the pattern of the underlying glomerular lesion. Minimal change, mesangial proliferative GN, FSGS, MPGN and MN account for most of these cases.

A small proportion of patients with MCNS have initial steroid resistance. Of these almost 40% respond to treatment with a 12-week course of cyclophosphamide (2–2.5 mg/kg/day). Those who subsequently relapse may respond to corticosteroids.

RELAPSE OF NEPHROTIC SYNDROME

Relapse of NS is defined as a urine protein:creatinine ratio of >2 or protein on urine dipstick testing for 3 consecutive days. Relapses are common, especially in younger children, and are often triggered by upper respiratory or gastrointestinal in feet ions. Relapses are usually treated in a manner similar to the initial episode, except that daily prednisone courses are shortened.

Frequent Relapsers (Frequently Relapsing Nephrotic Syndrome)

If a child with NS experiences frequent relapses (two or more relapses within 6 months of initial response or four or more relapses within any 12-month period), then the potential adverse effects of cumulative steroid doses required to achieve remission begin to exceed the presumed benefits of maintaining remission of the NS.

Treatment of Relapse

An upper respiratory infection, or occasionally some other infection, often precipitates a relapse. Sometimes mild-to-moderate proteinuria occurs with such infections. Urine protein does not usually exceed 2+ (although occasionally even 3+/4+ may be observed or 3 or 4 days) and lasts for a week or so. Such brief episodes of spontaneously resolving mild proteinuria may not be regarded as relapses.

The relapse is treated with prednisolone 2 mg/kg daily in two divided doses (single-daily dose is equally effective) until the urine is protein free for 3 consecutive days, which usually takes 10–14 days. Thereafter prednisolone is given at a dose of 1.5 mg/kg on alternate days for 4 weeks and then stopped.

Long-term Alternate-day Prednisolone

Prednisolone given as a single early morning dose on every alternate day for several months is often effective in maintaining a remission or reducing the number of relapses. Thus, a dose of 0.5–0.25 mg/kg on alternate days for 9–12 months or longer should be the initial regimen for children with frequent relapses. It has few side effects and does not seem to interfere with growth. Breakthrough relapses are treated with the standard therapy of relapse.

Long-term, Low Dose, Daily Prednisolone

A few studies suggest that daily administration of a small dose of prednisolone (0.25 mg/kg/day) or hydrocortisone for 1 year or more may maintain a patient in remission. However, because of concern with physical growth, this regimen has not been widely used.

Patients with frequent relapses (FRNS) who show persistence or development of steroid toxicity need treatment with alternative drugs.

The possibility of medication non-compliance, including use of lower than recommended prednisone doses, and the presence of occult infections (dental infections or sinusitis) should always be considered in patients with frequent relapses. Although some nephrologists perform kidney biopsy on children after diagnosis of frequently relapsing NS (FRNS), nearly all have proven to be minimal-change disease.

In cases of FRNS, the alternate-day dose can be tapered to a "threshold dose" (a dose below which relapses occur) to reduce the number of relapses and the total cumulative dose of steroid therapy. This dose is often in the range of 15–20 mg/kg and is continued for 12–18 months.

Steroid-sparing strategies have also been developed to treat FRNS. One strategy involves alkylating agents such as oral cyclophosphamide for 8–12 weeks, which is generally well tolerated with minimal risk of gonadal toxicity (total cumulative dose <200 mg/kg). Chlorambucil also is effective but is used less widely because of the risk of seizures. The alkylating agent is ideally started after induction of remission (to minimize the risks of developing infections and hemorrhagic cystitis) and is used in combination with low-dose prednisone. Other steroid-sparing strategies used for treatment include a 6-month course of oral MME, B-cell depletion with rituximab, and calcineurin inhibitors.

Patients having frequent relapses and requiring repeated courses of prednisolone often develop serious steroid toxicity. Important side effects include severe cushingoid features (obesity, hirsutism, striae), hypertension, impaired glucose tolerance, posterior subcapsular lenticular opacities, emotional problems, and growth retardation. Institution of an alternative regimen is required in patients with frequent relapses. Serious complications of corticosteroid therapy should not be allowed to develop.

As in FRNS, the alternate-day oral corticosteroid can be tapered to the threshold dose. Other steroid-sparing strategies used for treatment include a 6-month course of B-cell depletion with rituximab, calcineurin inhibitors, and vincristine. Children with SDNS do not respond as well to alkylating agents as does the FRNS subgroup. Patients with SDNS tend to also be medication-dependent to maintain a sustained remission.

A helpful assessment is the steroid threshold, i.e., the minimum corticosteroid dosage at which relapses have occurred. This should not be confused with the dosage used to treat the relapse. The maintenance dose should be continued for a period of 9–12 months or longer, provided there are no major side effects.

Levamisole

Levamisole, an immunomodulatory agent without anti-inflammatory effect, has been successfully employed in patients with frequent relapses and steroid dependence. A dose of 2–2.5 mg/kg administered on alternate days for 1–2 years or longer has been found to be effective in about 50–60% cases, with a marked reduction in the relapse rate. Initially, prednisolone 0.75–1 mg/kg is given along with levamisole, and after a few weeks its dose is gradually decreased. In 20–30% cases prednisolone can be stopped and levamisole alone is sufficient. There is a strong tendency for relapses to recur when levamisole is discontinued.

Neutropenia may occur in 2% of cases, monitoring of blood leukocyte counts is advised every 2–4 months.

Alkylating Agents: Cyclophosphamide

The role of alkylating agents in treating SRNS is unclear, but a subset of patients will respond, especially those who had at least a partial response to prednisone therapy. Combined treatment with high-dose corticosteroids (oral prednisone with or without IV pulse steroids) and alkylating agents have induced a partial or complete remission in 30–60% of patients in some case series, but these protocols are associated with significant morbidity and should be limited to patients with well-preserved kidney function. Even a partial response is associated with a better outcome.

Alkylating agents, chiefly cyclophosphamide and chlorambucil, may induce long-lasting or rarely permanent remission in children with FRNS. Either of these drugs is administered after inducing a remission with the standard prednisolone treatment.

A 12-week course of cyclophosphamide at a dosage of 2–2.5 mg/kg/day along with alternate-day prednisolone (1–1.2 mg/kg) results in prolonged remission in a majority of patients. The results are better in older children. The use of chlorambucil has been more limited than that of cyclophosphamide. The dose of chlorambucil is 0.2–0.3 mg/kg/day along with alternate-day prednisolone (1 mg/kg) for 12 weeks. Both of these agents cause leukopenia, nausea, and vomiting. Blood examination is done every 2 weeks and if the total white cell count falls below 4,000/mm^3 the drug is withheld till the counts reach normal levels.

Cyclosporine

Cyclosporine A (CsA) causes specific and reversible inhibition of T-helper lymphocytes. It also inhibits production and release of lymphokines including interleukin-2. CsA is mainly employed in organ transplantation, but it has been found to be effective in a variety of immunologically mediated disorders and in nephritic syndrome.

Cyclosporine A (CsA) is effective in inducing and sustaining remission in 75–80%

of patients with SRNS and has had a major impact in a small group of patients debilitated by the disease and steroid toxicity and in some patients who have had a poor response to cyclophosphamide.

The dose of CsA is 3–5 mg/kg/day (100–150 mg/m^2/day), which may achieve whole blood trough levels of 150–250 ng/mL. CsA is preferably combined initially with alternate-day prednisolone (for 12–20 weeks) and is given for 1 year or longer.

Cyclosporine A levels must be carefully monitored, and some recommend repeat kidney biopsy to evaluate the degree of interstitial fibrosis if therapy is continued for longer than 18 months. Unfortunately, relapses commonly occur once CsA is discontinued. Mild side effects frequently occur and include hypertension, gingival hypertrophy, and hirsutism.

Mycophenolate Mofetil

Mycophenolate mofetil (MMF) is a potent, reversible inhibitor of inosine monophosphate dehydrogenase, an enzyme required for de novo purine synthesis. Long-term treatment with this medication appears to be promising in patients with difficult nephritic syndrome, with no risks of nephrotoxicity, hepatotoxicity of neurotoxicity, or cosmetic side effects. The dose of MMF is 20–25 mg/kg per day in two divided doses.

Other Therapies

Cyclosporine in combination with alternate-day prednisolone may induce remission in 60–70% patients of steroid resistant MCNS and 30–40% of those with FSGS. Most patients who respond do so within 3 months of therapy. The treatment is carried out for 1–2 years. Other drugs that may have some benefit include nitrogen mustard and tacrolimus (FK 506).

Tacrolimus appears to be equally effective, avoids the development of the hirsutism and gingival hypertrophy associated with CsA treatment, and is now more commonly used in many programs. Starting doses of 0.05–0.1 mg/kg/dose twice daily are usually adjusted to achieve goal predose blood levels of 4–10 mg/mL. Steroid- and calcineurin-inhibitor-resistant patients rarely respond to the other known immunosuppressant medications, including cytotoxic agents, rituximab, and MMF.

GENERAL SUPPORTIVE MANAGEMENT

Besides specific therapy, control of edema, prevention and treatment of infections, and the general care of the child and management of psychological problems are crucial.

Dietary Management

Patients with NS often present with anasarca, either initially or during relapses. They may show evidence of prolonged, severe protein deficiency such as a greatly reduced muscle mass and infections. In such cases, a high-protein diet should be encouraged along with supplements of vitamins and micronutrients.

There is little doubt that the high-protein diet and rise in serum albumin will increase proteinuria, but no evidence to indicate that all ingested protein is lost. Conversely, severe reduction of dietary protein (often advised by indigenous practitioners) decreases proteinuria, at the expense of extreme reduction of serum albumin and muscle mass. In MCNS proteinuria is resolved within 10–14 days with corticosteroid therapy and a high-protein diet is continued to replete body protein.

During daily administration of prednisolone dietary salt should be restricted, to decrease the tendency to hypertension. The 12-week prednisolone regimen may lead to excessive weight gain, and in this period fat intake should be curtailed.

Calcium and vitamin D supplements are required in patients with persistent heavy proteinuria due to SRNS. Diuretic-induced losses of potassium may be replaced by potassium supplements.

Edema

Children with severe symptomatic edema, including large pleural effusions, ascites, or severe genital edema, should be hospitalized. In addition to sodium restriction (<1,500 mg daily), water/fluid restriction may be necessary if the child is hyponatremic. A swollen scrotum may be elevated with pillows to enhance fluid removal by gravity. Diuresis may be augmented by the administration of loop diuretics (furosemide), orally or intravenously, although extreme caution should be exercised. Aggressive diuresis can lead to intravascular volume depletion and an increased risk for ARF and intravascular thrombosis.

When a patient has severe generalized edema with evidence of intravascular volume depletion (e.g., hemoconcentration, hypotension, tachycardia), IV administration of 25% albumin (0.5–1.0 g albumin/kg) as a slow infusion followed by furosemide (1–2 mg/kg/ dose IV) is sometimes necessary.

In MCNS, edema occurs due to massive proteinuria, hypoalbuminemia, reduction in plasma oncotic pressure, and leakage of fluid into the interstitial space. Hypovolemia and decreased effective arterial volume lead to activation of compensatory mechanisms (e.g., secondary hyperaldosteronism) that result in salt and water retention. Other mechanisms may be responsible in patients with nonminimal lesions and reduced renal function.

Early treatment of relapse and judicious use of diuretics will ensure that the child does not develop more than a slight edema.

Diuretics

Frusemide and Bumetanide

Frusemide and bumetanide (called loop diuretics) are very potent diuretics with their principal site of action on the thick ascending limb (TAL) of the loop of Henle, where 25–30% of the filtered sodium and chloride is normally reabsorbed.

On oral administration of frusemide, the onset of action is within 1 hour with a peak action between 1 and 2 hours and duration of action of 6–8 hours. With IV injection, the action starts within 5 minutes, the peak is within 30 minutes, and the duration is of 2 hours.

Thiazides

Thiazides are organic anions that are also secreted into the proximal nephron. They inhibit sodium reabsorption in the distal convoluted tubule chiefly by inhibiting the Na-Cl transporter. They have no action on the ascending limb of loop of Henle. Onset of action is within 2 hours with a peak at 4 hours and the effect persists for 6–12 hours. Side effects include hypokalemia, hyponatremia, hypokalemic alkalosis, and hypomagnesemia.

Metolazone

Metolazone belongs to the thiazide class of diuretics. It blocks sodium chloride reabsorption in proximal and early distal nephron sites by unknown mechanisms. Since the major tubular site for phosphate reabsorption is the proximal tubule, the phosphaturia associated with metolazone administration exceeds that with thiazides.

Spironolactone

Spironolactone, a specific pharmacological antagonist of aldosterone, acts through competitive binding to receptors of aldosterone dependent Na-K exchange sites in the principal cells of cortical collecting ducts. Spironolactone is rapidly absorbed.

Triamterene and Amiloride

These potassium-sparing agents block the sodium channel in the principal cell of cortical collecting duct, inhibiting sodium reabsorption.

Dyslipidemia

Dyslipidemia should be managed with a low-fat diet. Dietary fat intake should be limited to <30% of calories with saturated fat intake <10% calories. Dietary cholesterol intake should be <300 mg/day.

Infections

If there is suspicion of infection, a blood culture should be drawn prior to starting empiric antibiotic therapy. In the case of spontaneous bacterial peritonitis, peritoneal fluid should be collected if there is sufficient fluid to perform a paracentesis and sent for cell count, Grain stain, and culture. The antibiotic provided must be of broad enough coverage to include pneumococcus and gram-negative bacteria. A third-generation cephalosporin is a common choice of IV antibiotic.

Thromboembolism

Studies to delineate a specific underlying hypercoagulable state are recommended. Anticoagulation therapy in children with thrombotic events appears to be effective—heparin, low-molecular-weight heparin, and warfarin are therapeutic options.

Obesity and Growth

Glucocorticoids may increase the body mass index in children who are overweight when steroid therapy is initiated, and these children are more likely to remain overweight. Anticipatory dietary counseling is recommended. Growth may be affected in children who require long-term corticosteroid therapy. Steroid-sparing strategies may improve linear growth in children who require prolonged courses of steroids.

■ COMPLICATIONS

- Massive anasarca with ascites and serious effusions
- Serious infections such as peritonitis and extensive cellulites
- Flare up of tuberculosis
- Severe hypovolemia that may lead to ARF especially when complicated by gastroenteritis and other infections
- Thrombosis (both arterial and venous) of major vessels, including cerebral venous sinuses.

Management of Complications

- *Edema:* It is controlled with salt reduction and oral dose of hydrochlorothiazide (1–2 mg/kg day) or frusemide. Sometimes furosemide along with spironolactone is used.
- *Infection:* Nephrotic state and corticosteroid therapy makes susceptible to infections. This can be with S. pneumoniae, gram-negative organism and varicella, peritonitis, pneumonia, and meningitis.
- *Thrombotic complications:* These include renal, pulmonary, and cerebral vein thrombosis.
- *ARF:* Appropriate preventive measures and judicious fluid replacement is required.

IMMUNIZATIONS IN CHILDREN WITH NEPHROTIC SYNDROME

To reduce the risk of serious infections in children with NS, give full pneumococcal vaccination (with 13-valent conjugant vaccine and 23-valent polysaccharide vaccine—influenza vaccination) annually to the child and their household tacts; defer vaccination with live vaccines until the prednisone is below either 1 mg/kg daily or 2 mg/kg on alternate days.

BIBLIOGRAPHY

1. Ellis D. Pathophysiology, evaluation, and management of edema in childhood nephrotic syndrome. Front Pediatr. 2016; 3:111.
2. Gulati A, Bagga A, Gulati S, Mehta KP, Vijayakumar S. Guidelines for the management of steroid resistant nephrotic syndrome. Indian Pediatr. 2009;46:35-47.
3. Lombel RM, Hodson EM, Gipson DS: Kidney Disease: Improving Global Outcomes. Treatment of steroid-resistant nephrotic syndrome in children: new guidelines from KDIGO. Pediatr Nephrol. 2013;28(3): 409-14.
4. Lombel RM, Gipson DS, Hodson EM: Kidney Disease: Improving Global Outcomes. Treatment of steroid resistant nephrotic syndrome in children: new guidelines. Pediatr Nephrol. 2013;28(3):415-26.
5. Sinha A, Menon S, Bagga A. Nephrotic syndrome: State of the Art. Curr Pediatr Rep. 2015;3:43-61.

CASE 47

Urinary Tract Infection

■ PRESENTING COMPLAINTS

A 4-year-old girl was brought with the complaint of:
- Fever since 2 days
- Abdominal pain since 2 days
- Increased frequency of urine since 1 day

History of the Presenting Complaints

A 4-year-old girl was brought to the pediatric outpatient department by her mother with the history of fever, abdominal pain, and increased frequency of the micturition. Her mother had noticed the fever since 2 days of moderate-to-high degree, with no associated chills and rigors. The child used to be relieved temporarily by paracetamol. Her mother also revealed that her daughter is complaining of the pain in the abdomen. It was diffuse more so in the lower abdomen. She also told her daughter is passing the urine very frequently. The amount of the urine used to be small. She was crying while passing the urine. Her mother had also noticed that her daughter had nausea.

Past History of the Patient

The child was the only sibling of the non-consanguineous marriage. She was born at term with the normal vaginal delivery. The birth weight was 3 kg. She started taking the breast milk immediately.

CASE AT A GLANCE

Basic Findings
Height : 100 cm (75th centile)
Weight : 15 kg (50th centile)
Temperature : 39°C
Pulse rate : 126 beats/min
Respiratory rate : 22 breaths/min
Blood pressure : 70/50 mm Hg

Positive Findings
History:
- Fever
- Abdominal pain
- Increased frequency of urine
- Nausea

Examination:
- Febrile
- Sign of mild dehydration
- Abdominal tenderness

Investigation:
- Total leukocyte count (TLC) increased
- *Urine:* Albumin ++
  - *Pus cells:* 18–20 cells/HPF (high-power field)
  - *Red blood cells (RBCs):* 2–4 cells/HPF
- *Urine culture and sensitivity:* Yields *Escherichia coli*

There was no significant postnatal event. She was discharged on the third day. Child was exclusively on breast milk for the first 3 months. Later weaning was started with cereals and vegetables. The child was on family food by 18 months. Her development milestones were normal. She had been immunized completely.

EXAMINATION

The child was moderately built and nourished. She was looking sick. Signs of moderate dehydration were present. Anthropometric measurements included the height 100 cm (75th centile) and weight 15 kg (50th centile).

The child was febrile 39°C, and pulse rate was beats/min. The respiratory rate was 22 breaths/min. Blood pressure recorded was 70/50 mm Hg. There was no pallor, no edema, no clubbing, and no lymphadenopathy.

Per abdomen examination revealed diffuse tenderness at the lower abdomen. There was no organomegaly. Bowel sounds were regular. Cardiovascular and respiratory system were normal.

INVESTIGATION

- *Hemoglobin:* 11 g/dL
- *TLC:* 18,000 cells/cumm
- *Differential leukocyte count (DLC):* $P_{80} L_{18} M_2$
- *ESR:* 20 mm in the first hour
- *Urine routine:* Albumin ++
- *Sugar:* Nil
- *Pus cells:* 18–20 cell/HPF
- *RBC:* 2–4 cells/HPF
- *Urine culture and sensitivity:* Yields *E. coli*
- *Ultrasound abdomen:* No abnormality detected (NAD)

DISCUSSION

Urinary tract infections imply invasion of urinary tract by pathogens, which may involve the upper or lower tract depending on the infection in the kidney, or bladder and urethra.

Urinary tract infections constitute a common cause of morbidity in association with abnormalities of the urinary tract and contribute to long-term complications, including hypertension and chronic renal failure. Prompt detection and treatment of UTI and complicating factors are of utmost importance.

The incidence of UTI in the term neonate is approximately 1% and in the preterm 3%, both with male preponderance (male-to-female ratio of 5:1) during infancy.

Obstructive lesions may be found in 10% of boys investigated for UTI and 30–40% patients show vesicoureteral reflux (VUR). The occurrence of UTI below 2 years of age, delay in starting treatment, and presence of VUR or obstruction are the chief risk factors associated with renal scarring.

PATHOGENESIS AND PATHOLOGY

The pathogenesis of UTI depends on a complex interaction between bacterial and host factors. The urinary tract is normally a sterile environment with nearby bacterial reservoirs in the distal urethra, periurethral region, perianal region, perineum, and vagina. With normal hydration and spontaneous voiding, the urinary flow through the distal urethra helps to prevent bacterial ascension into the bladder. Maintenance of normal flora prevents more virulent strains from colonizing the gut and the periurethral area; an individual's microbiome may be influenced by age, hormones, recent antibiotic use, hygiene, or spermicides.

E. coli is the most common uropathogen and causes about 80% of all UTIs; other common Gram-negative uropathogens include *Klebsiella, Proteus, Enterobacter,* and *Citrobacter*. Common Gram-positive uropathogens include *Staphylococcus saprophyticus, Enterococcus,* and rarely, *Staphylococcus aureus*.

Urinary tract infections are caused primarily by colonic bacteria. In girls, 75–90% of all infections are caused by *E. coli*, followed by *Klebsiella* spp. and *Proteus* spp. Although *E. coli* is also the most common organism in males, some series report that in boys older than 1 year of age, *Proteus* is as common a cause as *E. coli*, others report a preponderance of Gram-positive organisms in boys *S. saprophyticus* and *Enterococcus* are pathogens in both sexes. Adenovirus and other viral infections also can occur, especially as a cause of cystitis with gross hematuria.

Proteus and *Pseudomonas* are associated with recurrent UTI, instrumentation, and nosocomial infections. Pathogens of low virulence and fungi may be causative in patients who are immunocompromised. *Candida albicans* infections are particularly seen in preterm infants.

In the neonatal period, renal parenchymal infection is due to hematogenous spread. Acute bacterial pyelonephritis may cause or follow septicemia. At all other ages, bacteria reach the urethra and bladder through the ascending route and ureters and kidney through VUR. Bacteria infecting the urinary tract generally arise from the bowel.

Nearly all UTIs are ascending infections. The bacteria arise from the fecal flora, colonize the perineum, and enter the bladder via the urethra. In uncircumcised boys, the bacterial pathogens arise from the flora beneath the prepuce. In some cases, the bacteria causing cystitis ascend to the kidney to cause pyelonephritis.

The majority of UTIs are initiated by bacteria that ascend the urethra and adhere to the mucosal lining of the bladder; a hematogenous source that seeds the urinary tract is much less common but is also possible. The pathogenesis of UTI is based in part on the presence of bacterial pili or fimbriae on the bacterial surface. There are two types of fimbriae, type I and type II. Type I fimbriae are found on most strains of *E. coli*. Because attachment to target cells can be blocked by D-mannose, these fimbriae are referred to as mannose-sensitive. They have no role in pyelonephritis. The attachment of type II fimbriae is not inhibited by mannose, and these are known as mannose-resistant. These fimbriae expressed by only certain strains of *E. coli*. The receptor for type II fimbriae is a glycosphingolipid that is present on both the uroepithelial cell membrane and RBCs. Because these fimbriae can be agglutinated by erythrocytes, they are known as *P fimbriae*. Bacteria *P fimbriae* are more likely to cause pyelonephritis.

Following adhesion, the bacteria may invade across the mucosal barrier and trigger an inflammatory host reaction. White blood cells (WBCs) are then recruited to respond to the bacterial invasion, resulting in leukocytes appearing in the urine (pyuria). The inflammatory response results in the typical symptoms of cystitis including dysuria, urinary frequency, and urgency. Between 76% and 94% of pyelonephritogenic strains of *E. coli* have *P fimbriae*, compared with 19–23% of cystitis strains.

Bacteria that reach the urinary bladder are expelled with micturition. However, because of very rapid bacterial multiplication normal voiding cannot eliminate all bacteria. A small number may remain in a moist film lining the bladder mucosa and are destroyed by the intrinsic defense of the bladder epithelial cells. Other defense mechanisms include secretory IgA in urine and blood group antigens in secretions that impede bacterial adhesion.

Infected urine then stimulates an immunologic and inflammatory response. The result can cause renal injury and scarring. Children of any age with a febrile UTI can have acute pyelonephritis and subsequent renal scarring, but the risk is highest in those younger than 2 years of age.

Symptomatic UTI occurs when local bladder defense mechanisms are overcome by virulence of invading bacteria. Whenever bladder emptying is not complete and there is residual urine, the likelihood of UTI is increased. Primary disturbances of bladder function with incomplete evacuation are often present in children with recurrent UTI in whom no anatomical abnormalities of the urinary tract or VUR can be demonstrated.

There can be mechanical, anatomic, or structural risk factors that promote UTI. Indwelling catheters breach the separation between urinary tract and colonized body surface. Congenital genitourinary anomalies indicated by dilation anywhere along the urinary tract often present with UTI, because there has been obstruction to normal antegrade urine flow. On the other hand, if during gestational development there was abnormal migration of the Wolffian ducts resulting in VUR. VUR increases the risk of pyelonephritis by promoting bacterial ascension to the kidneys.

Throughout childhood, adolescence, and adulthood, females are at higher risk for UTI than males. In contrast, during the early part of the first year of life, boys have a higher incidence of UTI than girls. After the first year of life, the incidence of UTI in males drops and rises in females. Uncircumcised boys have up to 12 times the risk of UTI than circumcised boys. Factors such as dysfunctional voiding, constipation, sexual activity, and bladder catheterization increase the risk of UTI.

■ PREDISPOSING FACTORS

A variety of conditions lead to an increased predisposition to UTI. These include obstructive uropathy, stones in urinary tract, incomplete emptying of bladder with residual urine, constipation, and threadworm infestation. UTI are 10 times more common in noncircumcised infants.

> **RISK FACTORS FOR URINARY TRACT INFECTION (UTI)**
> - Premature infants
> - Immunodeficiency disease
> - Systemic disease
> - Urinary tract abnormalities
> - Renal calculi
> - Neurogenic bladder
> - Voiding dysfunction
> - Chronic severe constipation
> - Family history of UTI
> - Girl <5 years with history of (H/o) UTI

The greatly increased incidence of UTI in girls after infancy may be related to the short female urethra, which permits easy entry of bacteria into the bladder. However, uncircumcised boys also have a high incidence of UTI despite their long urethra. Bacterial colonization may be an important factor. Babies born of mothers with bacteriuria during pregnancy develop rapid colonization by uropathogens and have a higher incidence of UTI.

Broad-spectrum antibiotic therapy for minor infections, such as, upper respiratory tract infections, may abolish the normal bacterial flora of perineum and allow colonization by more virulent organisms, thus predisposing to UTI.

Breastfeeding has been found to protect infants against UTI during the first 6 months of life. Human milk provides anti-adhesive factors in the urine and stabilizes intestinal flora with less pathogenic enteropathogens. Bacterial properties play a major role in UTI. Adhesion of bacteria to the epithelial cells is a prerequisite for their further multiplication and induction of inflammation.

■ CLINICAL FEATURES (FIG. 1)

The manifestations of UTI are related to the age and the severity of the infection. Features of the physical examination that should be emphasized include: (1) An accurate measurement of blood pressure (hypertension may be present in patients who have chronic renal disease); (2) general growth and development (failure to thrive may be a sign or chronic or recurrent UTI); and (3) a careful abdominal examination which might reveal tenderness or a mass caused by either an enlarged bladder or an obstructed urinary tract). An effort should be made to elicit the finding of costovertebral angle tenderness in children of all ages. The perineum should be inspected carefully to search for signs of irritation, scars, signs of trauma, labial adhesions, or evidence of vulvovaginitis. A rectal examination should be considered to detect masses or poor sphincter tone, which might be associated with a neurogenic bladder. The lower back should be observed for any lipoma, sinus, pigmentation, or tuft of hair that may be evidence of an occult myelodysplasia.

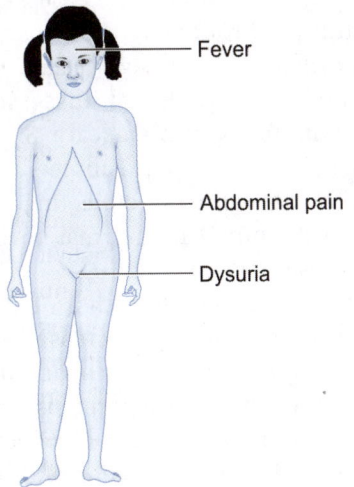

Fig. 1: Clinical features.

Neonates and Infants

In neonates, acute pyelonephritis presents with features of sepsis such as lethargy, seizures, shock, unstable temperature and persistence of physiological jaundice. Nonspecific symptoms including failure to thrive, vomiting, and diarrhea may be caused by UTI.

Urine may be foul-smelling. In infants, unexplained fever may be the only symptom of acute pyelonephritis. UTI in infants below 1 year of age is indicative of acute pyelonephritis.

The presence of UTI should be strongly considered in infants and young children, below 2 years of age having unexplained fever. Approximately 3–5% of such children, girls more than boys, with fever and no obvious source of infection on physical examination have UTI. Infants and young children are at higher risk for acute renal injury from UTI. Further the risk of renal damage increases exponentially with the number of such episodes.

GENERAL FEATURES
• Lethargy
• Seizures
• Shock
• Unstable temperature
• Jaundice
• Burning micturation
• Prolonged voiding
• Hypogastric pain
• Rigors and chills

Older Children

Dribbling, prolonged voiding, straining, crying during micturition and poor urinary stream indicate an abnormality of the distal urinary tract. Diurnal incontinence, urgency, frequency, and squatting suggest voiding dysfunction. Dysuria, frequent voiding, and hypogastric pain suggest cystitis.

Fever, chills and rigors, and flank pain indicate renal parenchymal involvement. Gross hematuria occasionally may be present. The presence of fever is regarded as indicative of pyelonephritis. Because of therapeutic implications, it is useful to clinically differentiate between UTI involving renal parenchyma (pyelonephritis) from that confined to the bladder and urethra.

Patients with urinary stasis (mechanical or neurogenic) having UTI from urea-splitting organisms, usually *Proteus* but also *Klebsiella*, are at risk of developing hyperammonemia and encephalopathy.

Recurrent Urinary Tract Infection

Some children usually girls in the school age-group, with an anatomically and functionally normal urinary tract may develop recurrent lower tract, afebrile UTI. The risk of renal scarring in these patients is low. Some of these children may have symptoms of bladder instability, such as urge incontinence or squatting.

Complicated Urinary Tract Infection

It implies the presence of either anatomical abnormalities (e.g., obstruction, VUR) or functional abnormalities (e.g., neurogenic bladder, voiding dysfunction). These have symptoms that are consistent with pyelonephritis and have infections with more virulent organisms such as *Proteus, Pseudomonas* species.

The two basic forms of UTIs (defined as symptoms and a positive culture) are *pyelonephritis* and *cystitis*.

Pyelonephritis

Pyelonephritis is characterized by any or all of the following: Abdominal, back, or flank pain; fever; malaise; nausea; vomiting; and, occasionally, diarrhea. Fever may be the only manifestation; particular consideration should occur for a temperature >39°C without another source lasting >24 hours for males and >48 hours for females. Newborns can show nonspecific symptoms, such as poor feeding, irritability, jaundice, and weight loss.

Pyelonephritis is the most common serious bacterial infection in infants younger than 24 months of age, who have fever without an obvious focus. Involvement of a renal parenchyma is termed acute pyelonephritis, whereas if there is no parenchymal involvement, the condition may be termed pyelitis. Acute pyelonephritis can result in renal injury, termed pyelonephritic scarring.

Renal abscess typically occurs following hematogenous spread with *S. aureus* or can occur following a pyelonephritic infection caused by the usual uropathogens. Most abscesses are unilateral and right-sided and can affect children of all ages. Both acute lobar nephronia and renal abscess are associated with an increased risk of renal scarring.

Perinephric abscess can occur secondary to contiguous infection in the perirenal area (e.g., vertebral osteomyelitis, psoas abscess) or pyelonephritis that dissects to the renal capsule. It differs from renal abscess in that it is diffuse throughout the capsule and is not walled off, although it can develop septations. As with renal abscesses, the most common organisms are *S. aureus* and *E. coli*. A perinephric abscess may not communicate with the collecting system, and, thus, abnormal findings may not be seen on urinalysis or culture.

Other findings vary, such as irritability, poor feeding, vomiting, decreased urinary output, and clinical evidence of dehydration. Infants with acute pyelonephritis usually have high fever without other localizing features; since their clinical presentation of UTI tends to be nonspecific.

Cystitis

Cystitis is the most common clinical manifestation of infection of the urinary tract. Classic symptoms include urgency, frequency, or dysuria. Children may also have a history of difficulty in initiating the urinary stream. Occasionally, children may complain of abdominal or suprapubic pain. If fever is present, it is usually low grade. The urine may be foul-smelling and cloudy.

Cystitis indicates that there is bladder involvement; symptoms include dysuria, urgency, frequency, suprapubic pain, incontinence, and malodorous urine. Cystitis does not cause fever and does not result in renal injury. Malodorous urine is not specific for a UTI.

Acute hemorrhagic cystitis often is caused by *E. coli*; it also has been attributed to adenovirus types 11 and 21. Adenovirus cystitis is more common in boys; it is self-limiting, with hematuria lasting approximately 4 days cystitis with hematuria. On imaging, typically there are multiple solid bladder masses that consist histologically of inflammatory infiltrates with eosinophils. Ureteral dilation with hydronephrosis also is common.

Interstitial cystitis is characterized by irritative voiding symptoms such as urgency, frequency, and dysuria, and bladder and pelvic pain relieved by voiding with a negative urine culture.

If bacteria ascend from the bladder to the kidney, acute pyelonephritis can occur. Normally, the simple and compound papillae in the kidney have an antireflux mechanism that prevents urine in the renal pelvis from entering the collecting tubules. However, some compound papillae, typically in the upper and lower poles of the kidney, allow intrarenal reflux. Infected urine stimulates an immunologic and inflammatory response, causing renal injury and scarring. Children of any age with a febrile UTI can have acute pyelonephritis and subsequent renal scarring, but the risk is highest in those younger than 2 years of age.

The child is trying to retain urine to stay dry, yet the bladder may have uninhibited contractions forcing urine out. The resulting high-pressure, turbulent urine flow and incomplete bladder emptying both increase the likelihood of bacteriuria. Bowel–bladder dysfunction can arise in school-age children who refuse to use the school bathroom, creating a state of urinary retention. Obstructive uropathy resulting in hydronephrosis increases the risk of UTI because of urinary stasis. Specifically, patients who require clean intermittent catheterization due to neurogenic bladder dysfunction are at high risk for UTI, often from organisms with more antibiotic resistance. Constipation with fecal impaction can increase the risk of UTI, because it can cause bladder dysfunction.

Asymptomatic Bacteriuria

Asymptomatic bacteriuria refers to a condition in which there is a positive urine culture without any manifestations of infection. It is most common in girls.

ESSENTIAL DIAGNOSTIC POINTS
• Fever with rigors and chills
• Pain abdomen
• Vomiting
• Hematuria
• Pyuria
• Dehydration

■ DIAGNOSIS (FLOWCHART 1)

Urine Examination

The specimen should be transported to laboratory as early as possible. The urine

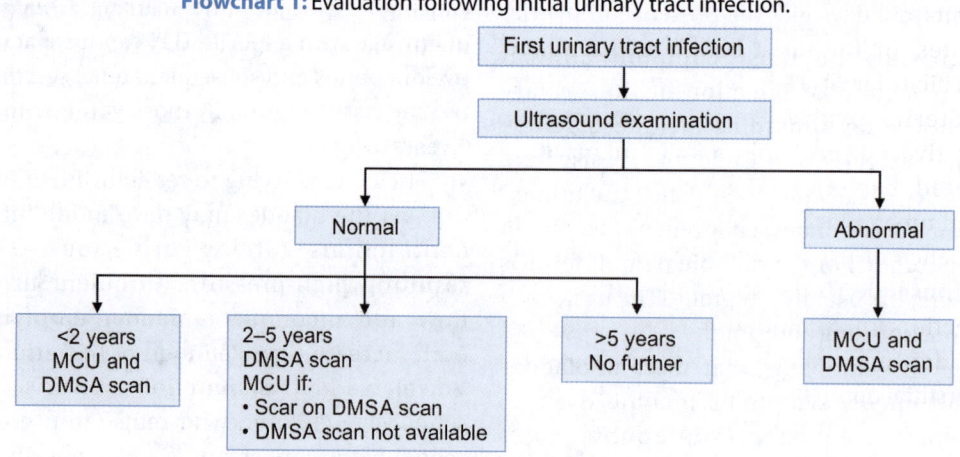

Flowchart 1: Evaluation following initial urinary tract infection.

(DMSA: dimercaptosuccinic acid; MCU: micturating cystourethrogram)

is tested for protein and sugar, examined microscopically and cultured. There may be mild proteinuria in UTI.

Urine Microscopy

An uncentrifuged specimen is examined in a counting chamber. More than 10 WBC/mm^3 are abnormal. The urine specimen may be centrifuged in standard manner (10 mL spun at the rate of 5,000 rpm for 5 minutes, supernatant decanted off, and sediment resuspended in the remaining 0.5 mL). Febrile UTI is usually associated with pyuria (>5 white cells/HPF in a centrifuged urine sample or more than 10 white cells/mm^3 in uncentrifuged urine).

Microscopic hematuria is common in acute cystitis, but microhematuria alone does not suggest UTI. WBC casts in the urinary sediment suggest renal involvement, but in practice these are rarely seen. If the child is asymptomatic and the urinalysis result is normal, it is unlikely that there is a UTI. However, if the child is symptomatic, a UTI is possible, even if the urinalysis result is negative, and the urine culture should be monitored.

Detection of leukocytes (>5 WBC/HPF in centrifuged urine) and bacteria on microscopic examination of a carefully collected fresh sample of urine suggests UTI. Enhanced urinalysis using uncentrifuged urine sample for leukocyturia (>10 WBC/mm^3) in Neubauer counting chamber along with Gram staining of sediment for bacteria is useful.

Pyuria (leukocytes on urine microscopy) suggests infection, but infection can occur in the absence of pyuria; this finding is more confirmatory than diagnostic. A WBC count on urinalysis above 3–6 WBCs/HPF is indicative of infection with a likelihood ratio of 10 in a symptomatic child. Conversely, pyuria can be present without UTI. Asymptomatic bacteriuria can also have pyuria.

Nitrites and leukocyte esterase (LE) are often positive in infected urine. Bacteria generally require 4 hours for metabolism of nitrates to nitrites. Nitrites may not be detected in cases of UTI, if the organism does not convert nitrates to nitrites (most notably enterococcus) or if the child has urinary frequency, where there may not be enough time for the conversion to nitrites. In febrile infants <60 days old, the presence of pyuria, nitrites, or LE has a high sensitivity and specificity for a UTI.

Sterile pyuria (positive leukocytes, negative culture) may occur in partially treated bacterial UTIs, viral infections, renal tuberculosis, renal abscess, UTI in the presence of urinary obstruction, urethritis as consequence of a sexually transmitted infection inflammation near the ureter or bladder (appendicitis, Crohn's disease), or interstitial nephritis (eosinophils).

Urine Culture

The criteria for the diagnosis of UTI depend on the method of collection of urine. On culture of urine collected by a standard midstream clean catch specimen, a colony count of $>10^5$ CFU/mL should be documented. A colony count below 10^4 is usually due to urinary contamination unless the child has polyuria or has received antimicrobial therapy. If urine sample is obtained by suprapubic aspiration (e.g., infants), any number of pathogens indicate UTI. On samples collected by urethral catheterization, a colony count of $>5 \times 10$ CFU/mL indicates UTI.

If the culture shows >50,000 colonies of a single pathogen (suprapubic or catheter sample), or if there are 10,000 colonies and the child is symptomatic, the child is considered to have a UTI. In a bag sample, if the urinalysis result is positive, the patient is symptomatic, and there is a single organism cultured with a colony count >100,000, there is a presumed UTI. If any of these criteria are not met, confirmation of infection with a catheterized sample is recommended.

Definitions of positive or negative cultures are dependent on the method of urine collection and the patient's clinical status. On culture, a colony count of $>10^5$/mL organisms of a single species is considered confirmatory of UTI. Counts between 10^4 and 10^5/mL may require reevaluation. Bacterial counts $<10^5$/mL are significant if symptoms of UTI are present. The colony counts may be low if the urine is very dilute or antibiotic therapy has been started. Infants have a smaller bladder capacity and void frequently and therefore may have low colony counts.

The presence of even a few bacteria on a suprapubic specimen is abnormal **(Table 1)**.

Dipstick Tests

Urinary bacteria convert nitrate to nitrite, which can be detected as a color change on chemically coated paper strips. The intensity of color change is proportional to the number of bacteria in the urine. Similarly production of esterase by neutrophils in the urine can be detected by chemical methods.

TABLE 1: Diagnosis of urinary tract infection.

Method of collection	Colony count (per mL)	Probability of infection
Suprapubic aspiration	Any number	99%
Urethral catheterization	$>10^5$	95%
	10^4–10^5	Very likely
	10^3–10^4	Suspicious; repeat
	$<10^3$	Unlikely
Midstream void	$>10^4$	Very likely
	$>10^5$	90–95%
	10^4–10^5	Suspicious; repeat
	$<10^4$	Unlikely

Dipstick tests based on nitrite reduction and detection of LE correlate well with urine culture.

In a febrile infant or a child with symptoms suggestive of UTI, a urinalysis suspicious for UTI may include the presence of bacteria or WBCs on microscopy or the presence of LE or nitrites on dipstick. Nitrites result from the conversion of dietary nitrates to nitrites by Gram-negative enteric bacteria such as *E. coli* and require about 4 hours in the bladder. A false-negative nitrite on a dipstick may be due to insufficient bladder time in young children who frequently empty their bladders in <4 hours or due to infection with bacteria that do not convert dietary nitrates to nitrites (e.g., *Enterococcus, Pseudomonas, Acinetobacter*, and *S. saprophyticus*). LE is an enzyme found in WBCs and is a surrogate marker for WBCs in the urine. LE has a specificity of about 78%; accordingly, false-positive results may be observed. The presence of bacteria on a Gram stain of a sample of fresh, uncentrifuged urine correlates with 10 CFUs/mL but requires more equipment and expertise than dipsticks.

Blood Tests

With acute renal infection, leukocytosis, neutrophilia, and elevated serum ESR, procalcitonin, and C-reactive protein are common. However, these are all nonspecific markers of inflammation, and their elevation does not prove that the child has acute pyelonephritis. With a renal abscess, the WBC count is markedly elevated to >20,000–25,000/mm³. An elevated serum procalcitonin level is associated with pyelonephritis and a high risk of renal scarring. Because sepsis is common in pyelonephritis, particularly in infants and in any child with obstructive uropathy, blood cultures should he drawn before starting antibiotics if possible.

> **LABORATORY SALIENT FINDINGS**
> - Pyuria
> - Albuminuria
> - Hematuria
> - Leukocytosis
> - *Urine:* Culture and sensitivity
> - *Ultrasonography (USG)* Abdomen
> - Radionuclide imaging

■ IMAGING STUDIES

In view of the high incidence of abnormalities of the kidney and urinary tract that are associated with UTI, it is essential that imaging studies be done. Earliest detection of VUR is particularly important since in the presence of severe VUR, UTI may lead to renal parenchymal scarring. Posterior urethral valves are commonly detected in male infants with UTI.

Structural abnormalities of the kidney and bladder dilatation can be detected on ultrasonographic evaluation, but a micturating cystourethrogram (MCU) needs to be done to look for VUR and examine the distal urinary tract.

Ultrasonography

It is an excellent, but observer-dependent method. The anatomy of the kidney and urinary tract can be satisfactorily examined. The interpretation of findings requires more expertise in neonates and infants.

Intravenous Pyelography (Excretory Urogram)

This study provides sharper details and is a good indicator of kidney function. However, because of the hazards of radiocontrast agent and the high dose of radiation, the intravenous pyelography (IVP) is not performed provided a good ultrasonographic examination can be done.

Micturating Cystourethrogram

A micturating cystourethrogram (MCU) is necessary to detect VUR and evaluate the distal urinary tract, especially for posterior urethral valve. It also gives useful information on bladder dynamics as assessed by the filling and emptying of bladder and the amount of residual urine. MCU is done by introducing the radiocontrast medium into the bladder through a thin catheter, or directly through suprapubic puncture. The child's cooperation is necessary; an infant may be scared and unable to empty the bladder fully.

Micturating cystourethrogram is generally performed, with strict aseptic precautions, after the urine has been sterile for 3–4 weeks. Concern that obtaining a MCU too soon after a UTI may result in a false-positive study for VUR is ill founded. Firstly, children who have VUR only when they have cystitis do have a significant problem, since reflux causes scarring by allowing bacteria to ascend. Secondly, it is rare for VUR to be detected during UTI and then to disappear following treatment.

Catheterization of the urinary tract, during MCU, carries the risk of introducing bacteria into the urinary tract. Antibiotic prophylaxis (oral cotrimoxazole in full dosage, first dose 12 hours before the procedure and three doses thereafter, or parenteral gentamicin 30 minutes before the procedure) reduces the risk of iatrogenic infections.

Radionuclide Imaging

Dimercaptosuccinic acid (DMSA) scan: It is superior to ultrasonography and IVP in detecting renal parenchymal scarring. It can also detect acute pyelonephritis, when decreased areas of tracer uptake are seen without distortion or normal renal outline.

INDICATIONS FOR IMAGING STUDIES
- Episode of acute pyelonephritis
- Boys with their first urinary tract infection (UTI)
- Girls <3 years old with their first UTI
- Girls >3 years old with second UTI
- Family history of (H/o) UTI-related features

Direct radionuclide cystourethrogram (DRCG): Instead of the radiocontrast agent, a radionuclide is introduced into the bladder. This procedure is more sensitive in detecting VUR, but the grading of VUR cannot be done. As it exposes the child to less radiation, it can be employed for follow-up studies.

■ TREATMENT

For febrile UTI, the length of treatment should be 7–14 days. In an otherwise healthy child with suspected afebrile acute cystitis and without a history of recurrent UTI, a shorter course may be sufficient.

Oral and parenteral antibiotics are equally efficacious treatment for a UTI: The latter is indicated if the patient is either toxic or vomiting or if there are no oral options available **(Tables 2 and 3)**.

Infection with *Enterococcus* is more common during early infancy; accordingly, antibiotic coverage for neonates should

TABLE 2: Empiric parenteral antibiotics.

Agent	Dosage
Ceftriaxone	75 mg/kg/day
Cefotaxime	150 mg/kg/day, divided every 6–8 hours
Ceftazidime	100–150 mg/day, divided every 8 hours
Gentamicin	7.5 mg/kg/day, divided every 8 hours
Tobramycin	5 mg/kg/day, divided every 8 hours
Piperacillin	300 mg/kg/day, divided every 6–8 hours

TABLE 3: Empiric oral antibiotics.

Agent	Dosage
Amoxicillin–clavulanate	20–40 mg/kg/day, divide in three doses
Trimethoprim–sulfamethoxazole	6–12 mg/kg trimethoprim and 30–60 mg/kg sulfamethoxazole/day divided in two doses
Sulfisoxazole	120–150 mg/kg/day, divided in one dose
Cefixime (third generation)	8 mg/kg/day
Cetpodoxime (third generation)	10 mg/kg/day, divided in two doses
Cefprozil (second generation)	30 mg/kg/day, divided in two doses
Cefuroxime (second generation)	20–30 mg/kg/day, divided in two doses
Cephalexin (first generation)	50–100 mg/kg/day, divided in four doses
Nitrofurantoin	5–7 mg/kg/day, divided in four doses

include IV ampicillin. Broader coverage should also be considered for patients with recent antibiotic exposure, recent hospitalization, or history of genitourinary anomaly, because they are at risk for infection with drug-resistant bacterial species. Increased coverage includes antipseudomonal penicillins, beta-lactam/beta-lactamase inhibitor combinations, fluoroquinolones, second- or third- or fourth-generation cephalosporins, and carbapenems. Fluoroquinolones are not a first-line consideration but are an effective choice when *Pseudomonas aeruginosa* is suspected or proven to be the cause of infection.

Infants below 3 months of age and children with complicated UTI should initially receive parenteral antibiotics. The risk of recurrent UTI is highest 3–6 months after the index infection. Parents should be educated regarding this possibility and encouraged to seek prompt treatment if a fever or symptomatic UTI develops again. Besides a recent UTI, risk factors for recurrent UTI include bladder and bowel dysfunction (voiding dysfunction and constipation) and congenital anomalies.

The urgency of treatment is particularly important in neonates and infants who should preferably be hospitalized to ensure supportive measures, such as fluid therapy and control of pyrexia. Neonates and infants should receive parenteral antibiotics such as a combination of ampicillin and gentamicin, or cefotaxime or ceftriaxone.

Parenteral antibiotic therapy is also required, initially, in older children who have complicated UTI for the first 48–72 hours. Once the clinical condition improves and the oral intake is satisfactory, antibiotics may be given orally. Careful monitoring and repeated clinical examinations are required.

Children over 1 year, who are accepting feeds by mouth and are not toxic, may be treated with oral medications such as amoxicillin, cefaclor, cephalexin, or cotrimoxazole have rendered them less effective than others. Cephalexin has no activity against *Proteus vulgaris* and *Pseudomonas*. Norfloxacin and ciprofloxacin are broad-spectrum quinolones, which are active against *E. coli, Klebsiella pneumoniae, Proteus mirabilis* and *P. aeruginosa*. They should not be used as first-line agents and reserved for serious infections.

If treatment is initiated before the results of a culture and sensitivities are available, a 3- to 5-day course of therapy with trimethoprim–sulfamethoxazole (TMP-SMX) or trimethoprim is effective against many strains of *E. coli*. Nitrofurantoin (5–7 mg/kg/24 h in 3–4 divided doses) also is effective and has the advantage of being active against *Klebsiella* and *Enterobacter* organisms. Amoxicillin (50 mg/kg/24 h) also is effective as initial treatment but has a high rate of bacterial resistance.

Acute cystitis should be treated promptly to prevent possible progression to pyelonephritis. If the symptoms are severe, presumptive treatment is started pending results of the culture. If the symptoms are mild or the diagnosis is doubtful, treatment can be delayed until the results of culture are known, and the culture can be repeated if the results are uncertain.

If treatment is initiated before the results of a culture and sensitivities are available, a 3- to 5-day course of therapy with TMP-SMX (6-12 mg TMP/kg/day in two divided doses) or trimethoprim is effective against many strains of *E. coli*. Nitrofurantoin (5-7 mg/kg/24 h in three to four divided doses) also is effective and has the advantage of being active against *Klebsiella* and *Enterobacter* organisms. Amoxicillin (50 mg/kg/24 h in two divided doses) also may be effective as initial treatment but has a high rate of bacterial resistance. A course of antibiotics for 7-14 days that is capable of reaching significant tissue levels is preferable for pyelonephritis; oral and parental routes are equally efficacious. For hospitalized children, parenteral treatment with ceftriaxone (50 mg/kg/24 h, not to exceed 2 g) or cefepime (100 mg/kg/24 h q 12 hours) or cefotaxime (100-150 mg/kg/24 h in three to four divided doses) is recommended.

In acute febrile infections suggesting clinical pyelonephritis 7-14 days course of broad-spectrum antibiotics capable of reaching significant tissue levels is preferable. Children who are dehydrated, are vomiting, are unable to drink fluids, are 1 month of age or younger, have complicated infection, or in whom urosepsis is a possibility should be admitted to the hospital for IV rehydration and IV antibiotic therapy.

Initial oral antibiotic options include cephalosporins, amoxicillin-clavulanate, or TMP-SMX. Sulfonamides should be avoided in premature infants or newborns younger than 4 weeks given the risk of hyperbilirubinemia, jaundice, and kernicterus. Nitrofurantoin does not reach adequate concentrations in tissue, so it is not a good option if pyelonephritis is suspected. Nitrofurantoin should also be avoided in neonates and those with renal insufficiency, liver dysfunction, and glucose-6-phosphate dehydrogenase deficiency.

Parenteral treatment with ceftriaxone (50-75 mg/kg/24 h, not to exceed 2 g) or cefotaxime (100 mg/kg/24 h), or ampicillin (100 mg/kg/24 h) with an aminoglycoside such as gentamicin (3-5 mg/kg/24 h in 1-3 divided doses) is preferable. The potential ototoxicity and nephrotoxicity of aminoglycosides should he considered; serum creatinine should be obtained before initiating treatment, and daily through gentamicin levels should be obtained during therapy. Treatment with aminoglycosides is particularly effective against *Pseudomonas* spp., and alkalinization of urine with sodium bicarbonate increases its effectiveness in the urinary tract.

Oral third-generation cephalosporins such as cefixime are as effective as parenteral ceftriaxone against a variety of Gram-negative organisms other than *Pseudomonas*, and these medications are considered by some authorities to be the treatment of choice for oral outpatient therapy.

The oral fluoroquinolone ciprofloxacin is an alternative agent for resistant microorganisms, particularly *Pseudomonas*, in patients older than age 17 years. It also has been used on occasion for short-course therapy in younger children with *Pseudomonas* UTI.

Levofloxacin is an alternative quinolone with a good safety profile in children. However, the clinical use of fluoroquinolones in children should be used with caution because of potential cartilage damage.

In some children with a febrile UTI, intramuscular injection of a loading dose of ceftriaxone followed by oral therapy with a third-generation cephalosporin is effective. A urine culture 1 week after the termination of treatment of a UTI ensures that the urine is sterile but is not routinely needed. A urine culture during treatment almost invariably is negative.

In a child with recurrent UTIs, identification of predisposing factors is beneficial. Antimicrobial prophylaxis using trimethoprim or nitrofurantoin once a day is another approach to this problem. It is unnecessary in most children with recurrent UTIs in the absence of severe reflux. Prophylaxis with TMP-SMX, amoxycillin, or cephalexin can also be effective, but the risk of breakthrough UTI may be higher because bacterial resistance may be induced.

RESPONSE TO TREATMENT

With appropriate treatment the urine becomes sterile after 24 hours and microscopic examination of urine does not show bacteriuria, although neutrophils may persist for a few days. Within 2–3 days the symptoms disappear. Failure to respond to therapy suggests: (1) nonsensitivity of the pathogens; (2) presence of complicating factors; or (3) noncompliance. If the expected clinical response does not occur with 2 days of antimicrobial therapy, another urine specimen should be cultured and an ultrasonography performed to exclude complicating factors.

PREVENTING RECURRENT URINARY TRACT INFECTION (TABLE 4)

Prophylactic antibiotics are administered to young infants. The medication is given as single bedtime dose. Long-term antibiotic prophylaxis is recommended in patients with VUR and in those with frequent febrile UTI (three or more episodes in a year), even if the urinary tract is normal. Circumcision reduces the risk of recurrent UTI in infant boys and might have benefits inpatients with high-grade VUR.

GENERAL MEASURES AND SURVEILLANCE

INDICATIONS FOR PROPHYLACTIC ANTIBIOTICS
- Infants or children on treatment and waiting for laboratory reports
- Children with known urological abnormalities
- Adolescent with recurrent urinary tract infection (UTI)

TABLE 4: Antibiotics for prophylaxis.

Drug	Dosage (mg/kg/day)	Remarks
Cotrimaxazole	1–2 of trimethoprim	Maintain adequate fluid intake; avoid in infants <6 weeks age and G6-PD (glucose-6-phosphate dehydrogenase) deficiency
Nitrofurantoin (NFT)	1–2	Considerable GI upset; contraindicated in G6-PD deficiency, infants <3 months and renal insufficiency; efficacy reduced with decreasing renal function; does not interfere with intestinal flora; bacterial resistance is rare
Cephalexin	10–12	Use in young infants where use of NFT and cotrimaxazole is restricted

ANTIBIOTICS FOR PROPHYLAXIS
- Trimethoprim/sulfamethoxazole
- Nitrofurantion
- Sulfisoxazole
- Nalidixic acid
- Methenamine mandelate

RISK FACTORS FOR PERMANENT RENAL DAMAGE
- Younger age
- Obstruction
- Vesicoureteral reflux (VUR)
- Recurrent infections
- Pyelonephritis
- Nephrolithiosis
- Delay in diagnosis and initiation of therapy

BIBLIOGRAPHY

1. Awais M, Rehman A, Baloch NU, Khan F, Khan N. Evaluation and management of recurrent urinary tract infections: state of art. Expert Rev Anti Infect Ther. 2015;13(2):209-31.
2. Garcia-Roig ML, Kirsch AJ. Urinary tract infection in the setting of vesicourethral reflux. F1000Res. 2016;5:F1000 Faculty Rev-1552.
3. Indian Society of Pediatric Nephrology; Vijayakumar M, Kanitkar M, Nammalwar BR, Bagga A. Revised statement on management of urinary tract infections. Indian Pediatr. 2011;48:709-17.
4. Subcommittee on Urinary Tract Infection; Steering Committee on Quality Improvement and Management; Roberts KB. Urinary tract infection: clinical practice guideline for the diagnosis and management of the initial UTI in febrile infants and children 2 to 24 months. Pediatrics. 2011;128(3):595-610.
5. Traisman ES. Clinical management of urinary tract infections. Pediatr Ann. 2016;45(4):e108-11.

SECTION 7

Central Nervous System

- Case 48 Acute Hemiplegia of Childhood
- Case 49 Cerebral Palsy
- Case 50 Duchenne Muscular Dystrophy
- Case 51 Epilepsy
- Case 52 Febrile Convulsions
- Case 53 Guillain–Barré Syndrome
- Case 54 Hydrocephalus
- Case 55 Meningitis
- Case 56 Meningomyelocele

CASE 48

Acute Hemiplegia of Childhood

■ PRESENTING COMPLAINTS

A 4-year-old girl was brought with the complaints of:
- Fever since 3 days
- Vomiting since 2 days
- Abnormal movements of left upper limb and lower limb since 1 day
- Not able to move on left side of the body since morning

History of Presenting Complaints

A 4-year-old girl was brought by mother with a history of not being able to move the left upper and lower limb since she got up in the morning. Mother has noticed the complete weakness on the left side. Mother gave the history of tonic–clonic convulsions on the left side in the previous evening. For the same, she showed the daughter to her family doctor. There were about 2–3 such attacks each lasting 5–8 minutes in the night. As mother noticed that her daughter was not able to move the left side of the limbs, she rushed to the hospital.

Mother also gave the history of fever since 3 days. Fever was of moderate-to-high degree and intermittent which used to be relieved by paracetamol. These was a history of vomiting since the previous day. The child had projectile type of vomiting. Child had vomited about 3–4 times.

CASE AT A GLANCE

Basic Findings
Height	: 97 cm (75th centile)
Weight	: 14 kg (50th centile)
Temperature	: 39°C
Pulse rate	: 126 beats/min
Respiratory rate	: 26 breaths/min
Blood pressure	: 50/70 mm Hg

Positive Findings

History:
- Convulsion
- Fever
- Vomiting
- Weakness in left limbs

Examination:
- Moderate dehydration
- Altered sensorium
- Left upper and lower limb hypotonia
- Deep tendon reflexes (DTR) absent
- Signs of meningitis

Investigation:
- *Total leukocyte count (TLC):* Raised
- *Cerebrospinal fluid (CSF):* Turbid and polymorphs cell present

Past History of the Patient

The child was the only sibling of the non-consanguineous marriage. She was born at full term by vaginal delivery. Her birth weight was 3 kg. She started taking breast milk immediately after the birth. There was no significant postnatal event. Weaning was started at 4th month and completed by

1 year. She was immunized completely. All the developmental milestones were normal.

■ EXAMINATION

The girl was moderately built and nourished. There were finding of moderate dehydration. The anthropometric measurements included that the height was 97 cm (75th centile) and weight was 14 kg (50th centile).

The child was febrile (39°C). The pulse rate was 126 beats per minute and respiratory rate was 26 breaths per minute. The blood pressure recorded was 70/50 mm Hg. There was neither pallor, nor lymphadenopathy, cyanosis, and clubbing.

There was altered sensorium but was responding to the oral command sluggishly. She was responding to painful stimulus by resisting the stimulus. There was complete flabbiness on the left upper and lower limbs. She was not at all moving to the painful stimulus. Deep tendon reflexes (DTR) were absent. Neck rigidity and Kernig's sign were present. There were signs of meningitis. Other systemic examinations were normal.

■ INVESTIGATION

- *Hemoglobin:* 12 g/dL
- *Total leukocyte count (TLC):* 14,600 cells/mm^3
- *Differential leukocyte count (DLC):* P_{68} L_{28} E_2 M_2
- *Erythrocyte sedimentation rate (ESR):* 36 mm in the 1st hour
- *Platelet count:* 1.6 lakh/mm^3
- *X-ray chest:* Normal
- *Mantoux test:* Negative
- *Cerebrospinal fluid (CSF) examination:* Turbid, elevated cell count mainly consists of polymorphs; Sugar was 20 mg/dL; Gram stain negative
- *Computed tomography (CT) scan:* Inflammatory changes present
- *Electroencephalogram (EEG):* Normal
- *Magnetic resonance angiogram (MRA):* Normal

■ DISCUSSION

These signs and symptoms are often due to the cerebrovascular disorders. There will be often history of ear, throat, and mastoid infection. This is associated with cardiac disease or hematological disorders. This will help to determine the cause of the acute hemiplegia.

Ischemic and hemorrhagic strokes result in the loss of neurologic function of the corresponding injured regions of the brain. It is a common cause of neonatal seizures and cerebral palsy, and stroke often leads to permanent cognitive and motor deficits. Stroke is often under recognized in children, particularly during the acute period. Prompt recognition and treatment may potentially reduce morbidity and mortality rates.

The incidence of stroke in childhood ranges from 2–13 per 100,000 children per year. For unclear reasons, childhood arterial ischemic stroke is more common in boys than girls. In neonates, the occurrence of stroke is greater than that of childhood stroke and occurs in approximately 1 in 4,000 births. Neonatal nontraumatic hemorrhagic stroke has an estimated incidence of 1.1 per 1,000 live births.

Stroke is classified broadly into two types: Ischemic and hemorrhagic stroke. Ischemic stroke occurs when a thrombotic or embolic occlusion creates loss of perfusion to an area of the central nervous system (CNS). Bleeding occurring into brain parenchyma is classified as hemorrhagic stroke. Ischemic stroke occurs more commonly than the hemorrhagic stroke.

In pediatric patients, strokes are additionally classified based on age. Perinatal strokes, sometimes referred to as neonatal strokes, occur in infants up to 28 days of age. In older infants and children up to age 18 years, this disease is referred to as childhood stroke. This distinction is important because risk factors, treatments, and outcomes are different in these two groups of pediatric patients.

■ CAUSES

The causes of acute hemiplegia of childhood are as follows:
- Cerebrovascular occlusive disease
  - Venous thrombosis of sinus
  - Arterial thrombosis
  - Cerebral embolism
- Intracranial hemorrhage
  - Arteriovenous (AV) malformation
  - Hypertension
  - Sturge–Weber syndrome
  - Trauma
- Inflammatory granuloma
- Cerebral abscess
- Meningitis
- Intracranial space occupying lesion.

■ RISK FACTORS

Many risk factors are associated with childhood stroke. The most common risk factors for arterial ischemic stroke in childhood are cardiac disease (congenital or acquired), hemoglobinopathies such as sickle cell disease, and arterial dissection. Other risk factors include prothrombotic states, infection, autoimmune diseases, drug use, trauma, and radiation exposure. A risk factor for stroke is identifiable in the majority of children with stroke.

Heart disease, both congenital and acquired, is the most common risk factor identified in patients with childhood strokes. The highest risk time for stroke seems to be during periprocedural or perioperative time frames. The role in childhood stroke of common cardiac abnormalities such as patent foramen ovale and mitral valve prolapse is unknown, but complex cardiac conditions that greatly alter hemodynamics carry an increased risk of thrombus formation.

Infectious diseases that have been associated with ischemic and hemorrhagic stroke include meningitis, tonsillitis, otitis media, and viral infections such as varicella infection, which may cause areas of focal vascular narrowing or may cause an inflammatory vasculitis leading to stroke. The incidence of stroke related to infection has decreased dramatically with improvements in vaccination strategies and antimicrobial therapy.

Numerous types of vasculopathies are associated with childhood stroke and include dissection, moyamoya vasculopathy, postviral arteriopathy, radiation-induced arteriopathy, vasculitis, and fibromuscular dysplasia. There are genetic risk factors for some vasculopathies.

Hypercoagulable states, many of which are inherited thrombophilias, are often seen associated with stroke in the young patients. They include antithrombin deficiency, protein C deficiency, protein S deficiency, prothrombin gene mutations, anticardiolipin antibodies, and lupus anticoagulant.

Sickle cell diseases, specifically hemoglobin SS disease (sickle cell anemia) and sickle cell β thalassemia, are one of the most common causes of stroke in the pediatric population. The highest risk population has the genotype hemoglobin SS. Sickle cell disease is considered a hypercoagulable state. The risk of hemorrhagic stroke in this population increases with age, with more frequent presentation in late adolescence and early adulthood. Children with sickle cell disease have an increased risk of aneurysm development, and often aneurysms are multiple when they develop. Consultation with a hematologist is essential in this situation, as these children may be started on chronic transfusion therapy for primary stroke prevention.

■ CLINICAL FEATURES (FIG. 1)

Childhood stroke is defined as stroke occurring after 28 days of age until the age of 18 years. Approximately 55% are reported to be ischemic, and the remaining 45% are hemorrhagic strokes.

The mode of onset varies with the cause. Children with stroke present similarly to adults. Focal motor symptoms such as monoparesis, hemiparesis, or rarely, quadriparesis may result. Focal sensory loss can occur. Vision loss affecting or both eyes may occur and may manifest as visual field defects. Slurred speech, or dysarthria, is a common symptom reflecting motor impairment of speech production. Aphasia, which is loss of expressive or receptive language fluency, is seen typically in infarcts of the dominant hemisphere or rarely, in regions of the thalamus.

Maximum neurological signs with the sudden onset will be associated with emboli. Seizures are frequently associated. Head and neck rigidity will be associated with intracranial hemorrhage and infection. The relatively late onset is seen with cerebrovascular thrombosis.

There is circumduction of the walking. The movements of the upper extremities are asymmetric. There will be lateral propping reaction. This is the protective reaction by the child from falling, i.e., extension of the arm. This happens when the child is pushed from sitting position.

This reaction is asymmetric in spastic hemiplegia. Absence of the propping reaction in infants after the age of 8–9 months is

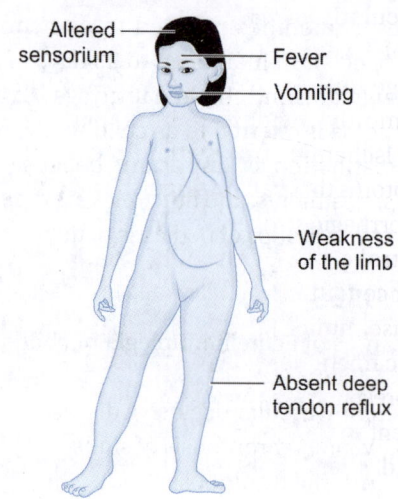

Fig. 1: Clinical features.

always abnormal. Multifocal seizures, raised intracranial pressure (ICP), and vomiting are common features of superior sagittal sinus thrombosis.

Arterial occlusions are associated with hemiparesis and seizures. These generally occur within 2 years. These seizures are very difficult to control with medication. Hemiparesis, cerebral hemihypertrophy, and cerebral porencephaly may result.

Specific pattern of motor deficit is seen with cortical lesions. This depends upon the vascular distribution of the artery. Seizures and cortical necrosis are usual. Aphasia is common or dominant in left-sided lesion. Lack of attention for objects is seen with parietal lesions.

Other symptoms include motor incoordination, gait ataxia, diplopia, vertigo, and, rarely, altered levels of consciousness. Although these symptoms can occur in isolation, they more typically occur in combination. Some patients may experience weakness of the palatal musculature and develop dysphagia, or poor ability to swallow. Seizures occur more commonly with stroke in childhood than with stroke in adulthood, particularly in children younger than the age of 1 year. Although symptoms such as change in levels of consciousness are more commonly seen in hemorrhagic rather than ischemic stroke, there are no specific symptoms that can distinguish ischemic from hemorrhagic strokes.

Stroke-like symptoms can be seen in other conditions such as acute demyelinating disease, tumor, Todd's paralysis, and hemiplegic migraine. However, a study evaluating the presence of stroke mimics when children present to the hospital with stroke symptoms found that stroke mimics were present only 20% of the time. Numerous studies have shown a delay in diagnosing stroke in childhood. Prompt recognition of this disease is necessary because of the emergent need to potentially stabilize the patient.

GENERAL FEATURES
- Altered sensorium
- Nausea and vomiting
- Headache
- Signs of meningitis
- Spasticity
- Seizures
- Aphasia

ESSENTIAL DIAGNOSTIC POINTS
- Sudden in onset
- Seizures
- Raised intracranial pressure (ICP)
- Gait disturbances: Circumduction
- Aphasia
- Cerebral hemihypertrophy
- Cerebral porencephaly

Cortical lesions are characterized by the specific pattern of motor deficit, depending on the vascular distribution of the artery involved. Seizures and cortical sensory loss are usual.

In the left-sided lesion, aphasia is a dominant clinical feature. The child finds difficulty in reading, writing, and comprehension. Organization of space and body image are affected. In right parietal lessons, the child exhibits lack of attention for objects on his/her left side. He/she may ignore the left side of a picture placed before him/her or may not even recognize his/her left hand. He/she has difficulty in copying simple figures (indicating constructional apraxia). He/she gets lost easily and confuses directions given to him/her because of spatial disorganization.

Corona radiata lesions produce the hemiplegia, which is generally complete and seizures are absent. With internal capsule affection, hemiplegia is complete, often with sensory loss.

Midbrain involvement includes hemiplegia that affects the contralateral side and paralysis of 3rd and 4th cranial nerves of the same side (Weber syndrome).

Hemiplegia affects the opposite side and involves paralysis of 6th and 7th cranial nerves on the same side (Millard–Gubler syndrome) with the affection of the pons.

Contralateral hemiplegia with ipsilateral involvement of lower cranial nerves is noted in the involvement of Medulla oblongata.

■ DIAGNOSIS

The evaluation requires accurate history, thorough clinical examination, investigations, and neuroimaging. A patient presenting with stroke should be investigated in a systematic fashion. All patients coming with acute onset neurological deficit should first undergo neuroimaging. Magnetic resonance imaging (MRI) is the investigation of choice since a CT scan cannot pick up an infarct in early stage. In case MRI cannot be done, a plain CT scan is mandatory. This will help to differentiate between infarction and hemorrhage and rule out other diagnosis.

Magnetic resonance imaging is a valuable tool for evaluation of stroke and should be used as a first-line investigation, but it is expensive, less readily available, and more time consuming. Diffusion-weighted MRI is even more sensitive than conventional MRI. The other advantage of MRI is that MRA and MR venography (MRV) can be done at the same time if necessary. This helps to elucidate, noninvasively, the vascular anatomy of cerebral vessels and demonstrates stenosis or occlusion in ischemia and vascular malformation in cases with hemorrhage. Hence, it helps to obviate the need for invasive cerebral angiography in majority of patients. Imaging of the cervical and proximal intracranial arterial vasculature should be performed in all children with arterial ischemic stroke.

The diagnostic evaluation in a patient with stroke is aimed at confirming the diagnosis of cerebrovascular disease, defining the extent, identifying the type of stroke (ischemic or hemorrhagic), and determining the vascular territory (large vessel vs. small vessel) and, if possible, identifying the underlying etiology of stroke.

The stroke-like picture can be seen in variety of conditions and the diagnosis of cerebrovascular disease has to be confirmed by neuroimaging. The causes of stroke in children are varied and it is important to identify the underlying cause as it has implications on the management, future recurrences, prognosis, and even genetic counseling of the family.

After confirming the existence of infarct or hemorrhage, one should investigate further to determine the etiology of stroke. All patients should have a thorough cardiac examination, chest X-ray, electrocardiogram, and echocardiogram as underlying heart disease is a very common cause of stroke in the pediatric population. If transthoracic echocardiography is noncontributory and the suspicion of cardiac source of embolism is high, then the patient should be subjected to transesophageal echocardiography.

Cerebrospinal fluid analysis is mandatory in a stroke patient with unexplained fever or signs of central nervous infections.

> **LABORATORY SALIENT FINDINGS**
> - Evaluation of predisposing illness
> - MCV, MCH, serum iron
> - CSF lactate and pyruvate
> - Chest X-ray and ECG
> - Neurological workup
> - CT scan, EEG, and MR angiography.
> - Lumbar puncture
>
> (CSF: cerebrospinal fluid; CT: computed tomography; ECG: electrocardiogram; EEG: electroencephalography; MR: magnetic resonance; MCH: mean corpuscular hemoglobin; MCV: mean corpuscular volume)

■ TREATMENT

Any patient, regardless of age, presenting with symptoms of stroke requires emergent medical evaluation. Initial management, as with any patient with a medical emergency, includes assessment and stabilization of airway, breathing, and circulation. Continuous cardiac and pulse oximetry monitoring should be instituted, and oxygen should be administered when necessary.

A detailed neurologic examination should be performed. Laboratory studies ordered during the assessment of a child with stroke may include complete blood count, prothrombin time, partial thromboplastin time, fibrinogen, blood glucose, electrolyte panels, type and screen, hemoglobin profile, and markers for thrombophilia.

Neuroimaging is essential to distinguish between hemorrhagic and ischemic stroke and to differentiate between stroke and stroke mimics. CT of the brain is performed in the emergency setting to evaluate for signs of hemorrhage. Ischemic stroke may not always be apparent on CT of the brain, particularly if the CT is obtained early in the clinical course. MRI of the brain is used to differentiate between stroke and other causes of focal neurologic deficits.

Magnetic resonance angiography of the head and neck is often used as a noninvasive method to evaluate arterial abnormalities. MRV of the head is used with ischemic or hemorrhagic infarcts that are not localized to typical arterial distributions. CT angiography and venography are alternative imaging modalities that may be used for children who are unable to undergo MRI.

Ischemic or hemorrhagic stroke causing hydrocephalus or severe mass effect may require neurosurgical intervention for decompression. Hemicraniectomy and other decompressive surgical techniques are used frequently in the acute and subacute ischemic stroke period in adults presenting with signs and symptoms of severe mass effect due to their ischemic stroke, typically because of large territory infarctions of the middle cerebral artery or cerebellar infarctions. Early neurosurgical consultation for hemorrhagic infarctions and for ischemic lesions associated with significant mass effect is recommended.

Treatment of Hemorrhagic Stroke

Because of the risk of rapid deterioration in patients with hemorrhagic stroke, rapid diagnosis and stabilization are crucial. Focal or generalized seizures have been reported and these children may benefit from prophylactic antiepileptic medications. Investigations for the etiology of hemorrhage, such as arterial venous malformations (AVMs), intracranial aneurysms, or hemophilia, are warranted. AVMs and intracranial aneurysms may require conventional angiography to diagnose and may necessitate neurosurgical treatments or treatments by interventional radiology. Factor replacement therapy for hemophilia is useful to prevent future hemorrhage in this population, and long-term management with a hematologist is necessary.

Treatment and Prevention of Ischemic Stroke

Treatment of ischemic stroke is classified as either primary or secondary stroke prevention. The goal of primary stroke prevention is to prevent a first stroke occurrence. Secondary stroke prevention is targeted at preventing stroke recurrence.

For the primary stroke prevention, children with sickle cell disease should be screened from approximately age of 2 years with transcranial Doppler ultrasound looking for evidence of intracranial stenosis. Elevated doppler velocities of ≥ 200 cm/s indicate an increased risk of having a stroke. Studies in this population have shown that they may benefit from chronic transfusion therapy. Growing evidence indicates the use of hydroxyurea as a potential agent for primary stroke prevention in children with elevated Doppler velocities.

For the secondary stroke prevention, few data in pediatrics are available. The choice of antithrombotic therapy used for prevention depends on the etiology of infarction. Aspirin therapy is used frequently to prevent recurrent stroke, unless there are complicated cardiac or prothrombotic disorders associated with ischemic stroke. In the setting of complex cardiac or prothrombotic risk factors that carry a high risk of stroke recurrence, anticoagulation with warfarin or low molecular-weight heparin is often recommended. Collaboration with hematology experts is often used in this setting.

In the management of acute ischemic stroke in adults, intravenous tissue plasminogen antigen and intra-arterial therapies with thrombolytic medications and mechanical clot-retrievers are used emergently within the first few hours of the onset of stroke symptoms to recanalize the thrombosed artery, restore perfusion, and prevent or limit permanent ischemic damage. In adult ischemic stroke, these therapies have been shown to reduce morbidity and mortality rates; they do, however, carry a risk of intracerebral hemorrhage.

■ PROGNOSIS

It is worse for patients below 3 years of age, especially with respect to seizures and mental retardation. There will be atrophy of hemiplegic side and post hemiplegic athetosis may be seen.

Cerebral hemiatrophy with the flattening of the skull and porencephaly secondary to parenchymal damage may occur.

Complex cardiac disease, vasculopathy, and specific prothrombotic risk factors such as elevated lipoprotein and protein deficiencies have been associated with risk of recurrence. Patients with hemorrhagic stroke have a higher risk of mortality compared with patients with ischemic stroke. Permanent neurologic deficits are common, most commonly hemiparesis and neuropsychological deficits, and are reported in between 40% and 80% of childhood stroke survivors.

■ CONCLUSION

Perinatal and childhood strokes, although rare diseases, are life-threatening and disabling conditions, leading to a potentially long lifetime of disability in the survivors. Much of what is known in stroke in the pediatric population is gathered from small cohorts of patients. At this time, because of the paucity of data, the guidelines for treatment are often based on research findings in adult stroke. It is essential to identify stroke promptly in this population to reduce morbidity and mortality rate. Further research in the management of stroke in infants and children is vital.

■ BIBLIOGRAPHY

1. Carpenter J, Tsuchida T. Cerebral sinovenous thrombosis in children. Curr Neurol and Neurosci Rep. 2007;7:139-46.
2. Goldenberg NA, Bernard TJ. Pediatric arterial ischemic stroke. Pediat Clin N. 2008; 55(2):320-3.
3. Nelson KB, Lynch JK. Stroke in newborn infants. Lancet Neurol. 2004;3(3):150-8.

CASE 49

Cerebral Palsy

■ PRESENTING COMPLAINTS

An 18-month-boy was brought with the complaints of:
- Abnormal walking since 15 days
- Not swinging the hands during walking since 15 days
- Delayed developmental milestone since birth

History of Presenting Complaints

An 18-month-old boy was brought to hospital with history of abnormal gait. Mother had noticed this as her child had started walking about 15 days back. Mother had also told that all other motor developmental milestones were delayed. She had also noticed the difference of the stance of the left upper limb. The left arm was abducted at the shoulder and flexed at the elbow. The left hand was not swinging during walking.

Past History of the Patient

The boy was the first sibling of consanguineous marriage. The boy was born at full term. Fetal condition was normal in the latent and early phase of the labor. Fetal distress was noted in later part of delivery. Hence, the baby was extracted by emergency lower segment caesarean section (LSCS). Apgar score at 1 minute was 6/10. Child had to be intubated and needed resuscitation to establish spontaneous respiration. This took around 10 minutes. Apart from this, child became normal and recovered with no other postnatal events. The birth weight was 2.6 kg. The child was discharged after 10 days. He was taking breastfeeds at the time of discharge. He was breastfed exclusively till the age of 4 months and gradually brought to the family food at the age of 15 months. During this time, he never had any major health problem. All the developmental milestones were delayed. He started walking without support at the age of 17 months. Then his mother noticed the abnormal gait and brought him to the

CASE AT A GLANCE

Basic Findings
Height	: 82 cm (90th centile)
Weight	: 11 kg (80th centile)
Temperature	: 37°C
Pulse rate	: 110 beats/min
Respiratory rate	: 18 breaths/min
Blood pressure	: 60/40 mm Hg

Positive Findings

History:
- Abnormal gait
- Fetal distress
- Asphyxia
- Delayed motor milestones

Examination:
- Spasticity
- Abnormal gait
- Delayed milestones

Investigation:
- No abnormality detected (NAD)

hospital. The child had been immunized completely.

EXAMINATION

The boy was moderately built and nourished. He was alert and playing with toys on the examination table. He was not moving his left hand properly while playing. His anthropometric measurements included his height of 82 cm (90th centile), his weight of 11 kg (80th centile), and the head circumference of 47 cm. Anterior fontanelle (AF) was open and tense. He was afebrile, the pulse rate was 110 beats per minute, the respiratory rate was 18 breaths per minute. Blood pressure recorded was 60/40 mm Hg. There was no pallor, no icterus, no lymphadenopathy, and no edema.

Left arm was abducted at the shoulder and flexed at the elbow. It was swinging during walking and movement on left side was less. These were suggestive of spastic hemiplegic gait. Vision and hearing were normal. There was no cranial nerve involvement and no sensory deficits. All other systemic examinations were normal.

INVESTIGATION

- *Hemoglobin:* 10 g/dL
- *TLC:* 8,900 cells/mm^3
- *Platelet count:* 3,00,000 cells/mm^3
- *X-ray chest:* Normal
- *X-ray skull:* Normal
- *ECG:* Normal
- *EEG:* No significant finding
- *CT scan brain:* Normal

DISCUSSION

Cerebral palsy (CP) is a persistent disorder of movement and posture, as a result of nonprogressive disorder of immature brain. CP is unique as it involves static lesion upon which maturation and development are superimposed. Its manifestations depend on the stage of development, and thus may appear to change over time. It is frequently accompanied by epilepsy, sensory impairment, and mental retardation.

Infants with very low birth weight have a significant increase in the risk of CP compared to normal birth weight children. Very premature infants (<28 weeks) are also much more likely to have CP than term infants, which is thought to be related to the immature germinal matrix leading to increased risk of ischemic or hemorrhagic injury.

The motor disorders are often accompanied by disturbances of sensation, perception, cognition, communication, and behavior as well as by epilepsy and secondary musculoskeletal problems. CP is caused by a broad group of developmental, genetic, metabolic, ischemic, infectious, and other acquired etiologies that produce a common group of neurologic phenotypes. CP has historically been considered as static encephalopathy, but some of the neurologic features of CP, such as movement disorders and orthopedic complications, including scoliosis and hip dislocation can change or progress over time. Many children and adults with CP function at a high educational and vocational level, without any sign of cognitive dysfunction.

RISK FACTORS

Prematurity

Risk factors for cerebral palsy in preterm infants include premature rupture of membranes, chorioamnionitis, monochorionic twin placentation and respiratory distress syndrome, bronchopulmonary dysplasia, and abnormal findings on cranial ultrasound—periventricular leukomalacia (PVL) and ventriculomegaly (**Box 1**).

> **BOX 1:** Risk factors for cerebral palsy (CP).
>
> - Prenatal:
>   - Infections—TORCH
>   - Fetal anoxia
>   - Maternal diabetes
>   - Hypertension
>   - Maldevelopment of brain
> - Perinatal:
>   - Asphyxia
>   - Prematurity
>   - APH
>   - Drugs
>   - Birth Trauma
> - Postnatal:
>   - CNS infections
>   - Trauma
>   - Toxins, for example, lead
>   - Anoxia due to cardiac arrest, drowning
>   - Intracranial bleed
>
> [APH: Antepartum hemorrhage; CNS: central nervous system; TORCH: Toxoplasmosis, others (syphilis, varicella zoster, and parvovirus B19), rubella, cytomegalovirus, and herpes]

Asphyxia

In preterm infants, a strong relationship between spastic diplegia and hypoxic–ischemic encephalopathy (HIE) induced PVL has been demonstrated. The association of hypoxia and CP in term infants is much harder to substantiate.

Infections

Intrauterine viral infections such as rubella herpes simplex and cytomegalovirus cause central nervous system (CNS) injury. It will manifest as CP with spastic quadriplegia as the most common type. Approximately 10% of infants infected with cytomegalovirus will manifest with CP.

Prenatal Abnormalities

Maternal disorders which can interfere with normal fetal nutrition and oxygenation such as placental infarction, intrauterine infections, and congenital malformations of the brain including neuronal migration defects and cerebral dysgenesis can manifest as CP. Facial dysmorphism and presence of minor malformations point to prenatal origin of CP.

Biochemical Abnormalities

Kernicterus is a classic example of biochemical abnormality causing CP. Besides Rh incompatibility, bilirubin encephalopathy can occur in low-birth-weight children with additional risk factors, for example, sepsis. CP following kernicterus has distinct clinical features such as choreoathetosis, sensorineural hearing loss, enamel dysplasia, and upward gaze palsy.

Postnatal Causes

Viral and bacterial infections of CNS are major risk factors. Gastroenteritis with hypernatremic dehydration and accidental injuries are other common causes of CP.

Perinatal problems such as prolonged difficult delivery and antepartum hemorrhage are observed in a significant proportion of children with tetraplegia. Intrauterine infections and congenital malformations of brain are also associated with this type of CP.

Classification of Cerebral Palsy

> **ESSENTIAL DIAGNOSTIC POINTS**
>
> - Chronic static impairment of muscle tone
> - Nonprogressive neuromuscular disorder
>   - Hyperreflexia
>   - Microcephaly
>   - Ataxia
>   - Involuntary movements

■ CLASSIFICATION

The classification of CP is given in **Box 2**.

> **BOX 2:** Classification of cerebral palsy (CP).
>
> - Tone and topography:
>   - *Spasticity:* Quadriplegia, diplegia, and hemiplegia
>   - *Dyskinetic:* Choreoathetosis and dystonic
>   - Ataxic
>   - Mixed
>   - Hypotonic
> - Severity:
>   - *Mild:* Physical findings but no limitation in ordinary activities
>   - *Moderate:* Definite difficulty in daily activity and need for assistive devices
>   - *Severe:* Moderate-to-great limitation in everyday activity

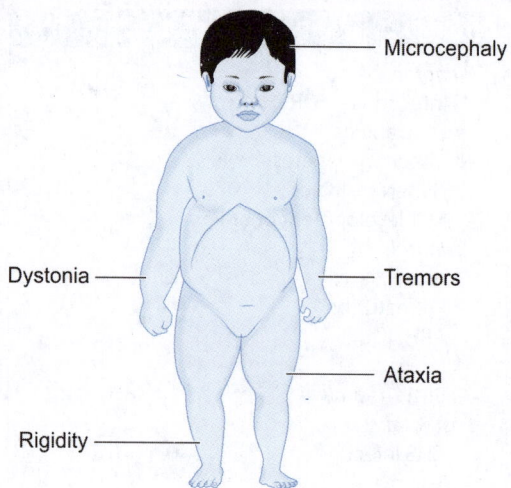

Fig. 1: Clinical features.

PATHOLOGY

Pathological changes include cerebral atrophy, porencephaly, and degeneration of basal ganglia. Gliosis or contralateral hemiparesis results from vascular occlusion.

CLINICAL FEATURES (FIG. 1)

Clinical Types and Manifestations

Cerebral palsy is difficult to diagnose during the 1st year of life because:
- Hypotonia is more common than hypertonia and spasticity.
- Early abundance of primitive reflexes may confuse clinical picture.
- Limited variety of volitional movements is available for evaluation.

Clinical features of CP are given in **Figure 1**. POSTER criteria of CP are given in **Box 3**.

Spastic Cerebral Palsy

The most common form is spastic CP. This comprises about 65% of the CP patients. This is due to the involvement of motor cortex and pyramidal system. They may have spastic quadriparesis, diplegia, and hemiparesis. Early features include abnormal persistence of neonatal reflexes.

They are often hyperexcitable and have a firm grasp reflex. Spasm of adductor muscles manifests as scissoring of the lower limbs. The stretch reflexes are brisk. They may suffer from pseudobulbar palsy, and some may be ataxic.

In neonatal period, hypotonia, lethargy, and feeding difficulties are the cause of concern. Therefore, baby looks almost normal for 2–3 months although there is delay in motor milestones. Gradually, hypotonia disappears and child shows generalized increase in tone. The evaluation varies but reaches the spastic stage by the age of 2–3 years. Upper limbs are less affected as compared to lower limbs. Hence, locomotion is more impaired compared to manipulation **(Figs. 2 to 4)**.

Spasticity is characterized by increased muscle tone, stereotyped and limited patterns of movements, decreased active and passive range of movements, the tendency to develop contractures and deformities, the persistence of primitive and tonic reflexes, and poor development of postural reflex mechanism.

Spasticity refers to the quality of increased muscle tone, which increases with the speed

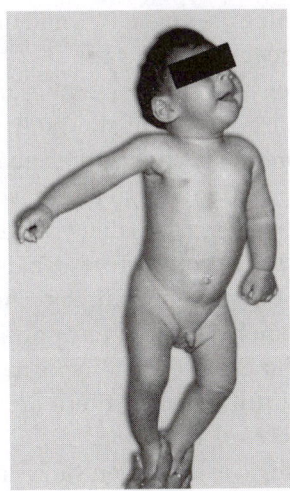

Fig. 2: Cerebral palsy with microcephaly.

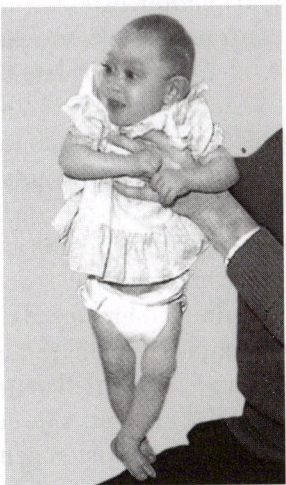

Fig. 3: Cerebral palsy.

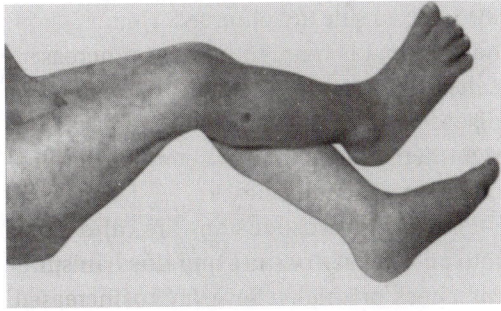

Fig. 4: Scissoring of lower limb.

of passive muscle stretching and is greatest in antigravity muscles. It is apparent in the affected extremities, particularly at the ankle, causing an equinovarus deformity of the foot. An affected child often walks on tiptoe because of the increased tone in the antigravity gastrocnemius muscles, and the affected upper extremity assumes a flexed posture when the child runs. Ankle clonus and a Babinski sign may be present, the DTR are increased, and weakness in the hand and foot dorsiflexors is evident.

Infants with spastic hemiplegia have decreased spontaneous movements on the affected side and show hand preference at a very early age. The arm is often more involved than the leg and difficulty in hand manipulation is obvious by 1 year of age. Walking is usually delayed until 18–24 months of age, and a circumductive gait is apparent. Examination of the extremities may show growth arrest, particularly in the hand and thumbnail, especially if the contralateral parietal lobe is abnormal, because extremity growth is influenced by this area of the brain.

Spastic Diplegia

Spastic diplegia is common in premature infants, and patients with diplegic CP usually will have low tone for the first few months, followed by increased muscle tone that is more apparent in their legs than their arms. These patients, if ambulatory, will often toe walk. Contractures commonly develop in the hips and hamstrings.

Spastic diplegia is bilateral spasticity of the legs that is greater than in the arms. Spastic diplegia is strongly associated with damage to the immature white matter during the vulnerable period of immature oligodendroglia between 20–34 weeks of gestation.

The first clinical indication of spastic diplegia is often noted when an affected infant begins to crawl. The child uses the arms in a normal reciprocal fashion but tends to drag the legs behind more as a rudder (commando crawl) rather than using the normal four-limbed crawling movement. If there is paraspinal muscle involvement, the child may be unable to sit.

Examination of the child reveals spasticity in the legs with brisk reflexes, ankle clonus, and a bilateral Babinski sign. When the child is suspended by the axillae, a scissoring posture of the lower extremities is maintained. Walking is significantly delayed, the feet are held in a position of equinovarus, and the child walks on tiptoe.

Severe spastic diplegia is characterized by disuse atrophy, impaired growth of the lower extremities, and disproportionate growth with normal development of the upper torso. The prognosis for normal intellectual development for these patients is good, and the likelihood of seizures is minimal. Such children often have learning disabilities and deficits in other abilities, such as vision, because of disruption of multiple white matter pathways that carry sensory as well as motor information.

The most common neuropathologic finding in children with spastic diplegia is PVL, which is visualized on MRI in more than 70% of cases. MRI typically shows scarring and shrinkage in the periventricular white matter with compensatory enlargement of the cerebral ventricles.

Spastic Quadriplegia

Spastic quadriplegia is the most severe form of CP because of marked motor impairment of all extremities and the high association with intellectual disability and seizures. Swallowing difficulties are common as a result of supranuclear bulbar palsies, often leading to aspiration pneumonia. The most common lesions seen on pathologic examination or on MRI scanning are severe PVL and multicystic cortical encephalomalacia.

Diffuse spasticity (sometimes more prominent on one side of the body than the other) is present in patients with quadriplegic CP. These patients typically have truncal dystonia, intellectual disability, hyperreflexia, and progressive contractures leading to loss of range of motion in all limbs. This type of CP is commonly seen in term or near-term infants who experience a hypoxic ischemic injury at birth or when there are bilateral large-vessel strokes.

Neurologic examination shows increased tone and spasticity in all extremities, decreased spontaneous movements, brisk reflexes, and plantar extensor responses. Flexion contractures of the knees and elbows are often present by late childhood. Associated developmental disabilities, including speech and visual abnormalities, are particularly prevalent in this group of children. Children with spastic quadriparesis often have evidence of athetosis and may be classified as having mixed CP.

The associated sensory deficit may be as detrimental to ultimate function as is spasticity and motor deficit. The child often ignores the affected side. Perpetual and learning problems, astereognosis, and seizures are common associated problems.

Sensory deficits of cortical type such as two-point discrimination and astereognosis on the affected side are observed. Homonymous hemianopia is frequently present but rarely cause a disability. Speech and language disorders are seen with both left as well as right hemiplegia. Mental retardation is less common in hemiplegic CP.

On ventral suspension, the infant goes into an extensor posture and does not reflex his knees or thighs. Severely handicapped children may be in a position of opisthotonus.

They may have variable degree of mental and visual handicaps and behavioral problems. Seizures are common in all infants and require treatment.

> **BOX 3:** POSTER criteria of cerebral palsy (CP).
>
> - *Posturing:* Abnormal movements
> - Oropharyngeal problems
> - Strabismus
> - *Tone:* Hyper/hypo
> - *Evolutional maldevelopment:* Persistence of primitive reflexes
> - *Reflexes:* Increased deep tendon reflexes/persistent Babinski reflex
>
> Any of the these criteria suggest cerebral palsy (CP)

Dyskinetic Cerebral Palsy

When injury is predominantly to the deep gray matter, such as in kernicterus, the patient's predominant symptoms will be abnormal movements. They can include dystonia, chorea, athetosis, and myoclonus.

This pattern of CP is often noticed around the first birthday as the movements are typically exacerbated by voluntary motor activities (reaching, crawling, and walking). Patients with dyskinetic syndromes will also often have speech abnormalities. Symptoms tend to be exacerbated by stress, fatigue, anxiety, or intercurrent illness.

Athetoid CP, also called choreoathetoid, extrapyramidal, or dyskinetic CP, is less common than spastic CP and makes up approximately 15–20% of patients with CP. Affected infants are characteristically hypotonic with poor head control, marked head lag, and develop variably increased tone with rigidity and dystonia over several years.

The term dystonia refers to the abnormality of tone in which muscles are rigid throughout their range of motion and involuntary contractions can occur in both flexors and extensors leading to limb positioning in fixed postures. Unlike spastic diplegia, the upper extremities are generally more affected than the lower extremities in extrapyramidal CP.

Feeding may be difficult, and tongue thrust, and drooling may be prominent. Speech is typically affected because the oropharyngeal muscles are involved. Speech may be absent or sentences are slurred, and voice modulation is impaired. Generally, upper motor neuron signs are not present, seizures are uncommon, and intellect is preserved in many patients.

The choreoathetoid CP is associated with neonatal hyperbilirubinemia and the pathologic correlate is selective involvement of central grey nuclei. The dystonic type is associated with hypoxia and neuropathologic correlate is status marmoratus—marbled appearance of basal ganglia, which results from diffuse gliosis.

Associated problems include severely impaired speech and oral–motor problems. High-frequency hearing loss is common in patients with dyskinetic CP related to erythroblastosis fetalis. Intelligence is normal in most of the patients and epilepsy is less common in this type. Speech is usually impaired due to the involvement of buccopharyngeal muscles and drooling may be a major problem.

Ataxic Cerebral Palsy

Ataxic CP motor disorder is cerebellar ataxia due to nonprogressive lesion of brain. The etiology of pure ataxic CP is different from other types in which genetic factors are important. Developmental anomalies of cerebellum are often seen on neuroimaging.

There is initial stage of hypotonia and delayed motor milestones. This is followed by the appearance of truncal ataxia and intention tremor or the ataxic stage. It is characterized by low postural tone and disturbed equilibrium. Wide-based gait imbalances on standing are noted.

Typical nystagmus is not common but strabismus and poor eye tracking may be seen in some cases. Ataxia is often accompanied with spastic diplegia. Associated problems include delay and articulation defects in speech, intellectual impairment, and epilepsy.

Mixed-type Cerebral Palsy

Mixed-type CP is a term used to indicate any child who shows features of more than one type of CP. The most common combination is that of spastic diplegia with dyskinesia. Children with ataxic form often have diplegia—ataxic diplegia. Hypotonic CP is a transient stage in infancy in the evolution of spasticity or dyskinetic variety of CP.

Hypotonic Syndrome

Initially after a hypoxic injury, neonates will typically exhibit low muscle tone, which often progresses over time to spasticity. It may be difficult initially to detect reflexes in hypotonic infants. Prematurity can also cause delayed milestones, so using corrected gestational age and performing serial assessments is important. If hypotonia persists, patients will continue to have diminished or absent reflexes, marked weakness of the legs, and arms with low muscle tone more pronounced than weakness. This is the rarest type of CP. It is important in these patients to exclude similar diagnoses including lower motor neuron diseases, metabolic disorders, neurodegenerative diseases, or genetic conditions that predispose to low tone such as Down syndrome, Prader–Willi syndrome, and Angelman syndrome.

BOX 4: Associated problems in children with cerebral palsy.
- *Neurological:*
  - Mental retardation
  - Cortical sensory deficits
  - Visual and hearing problems
  - Epilepsy
  - Communication disorders
- *Gastrointestinal:*
  - Oropharyngeal dysphagia
  - Gastroesophageal reflux
  - Constipation
  - Malnutrition
  - Drooling of saliva
- *Orthopedic:*
  - Equinus
  - Hip subluxation/dislocation
  - Scoliosis
  - Hamstring contracture
- *Miscellaneous:*
  - Sleep problems
  - Lower urinary tract dysfunction
  - Emotional and behavioral problems

Associated problems in children with CP are given in **Box 4**.

GROSS MOTOR DELAYS ASSOCIATED WITH CEREBRAL PALSY
- Unable to bring both the hands together by the age of 4 months
- Head lag persisting beyond 6 months
- No volitional rolling by 6 months
- Unable to sit without support by 8 months
- No hands to knee crawling by 12 months

GENERAL FEATURES
- Presence of primitive reflexes
- Quadriplegia
- Diplegia
- Pseudobulbar palsy

DIAGNOSIS

A thorough history and physical examination should preclude a progressive disorder of the CNS, including degenerative diseases, metabolic disorders, spinal cord tumor, or muscular dystrophy. The possibility of anomalies at the base of the skull or other disorders affecting the cervical spinal cord needs to be considered in patients with little involvement of the arms or cranial nerves.

The diagnosis is suspected when early growth and development is delayed. Evaluation includes perinatal history, detailed neurological and developmental examination, electroencephalogram (EEG), psychomotor, and sensory evaluation. Precise etiological diagnosis should be sought for the progressive lesion.

An MRI scan of the brain is indicated to determine the location and extent of structural lesions or associated congenital malformations. MRI scan of the spinal cord is indicated if there is any question about spinal cord pathology. If the MRI is abnormal, the location and degree of abnormalities are considered as to whether they are consistent with the clinical presentation. If migrational abnormalities are present, consideration should be made for a genetic cause. When the distribution of damage is concerning for a, vascular lesion, coagulopathy workup should be performed, and the patient should be referred for hematology. In the case of normal imaging, further evaluation should be pursued in order to ensure that a mimic of CP, for example a genetic or metabolic disorder or neuromuscular disease, is not present. There are rare cases of "MRI-negative" CP, but it should be a diagnosis of exclusion. Additional studies may include tests of hearing and visual function.

In spastic hemiplegia, the MRI is far more sensitive than cranial CT scan for most lesions seen with CP, although a CT scan may be useful for detecting calcifications associated with congenital infections.

The most common neuropathologic finding in children with spastic diplegia is PVL, which is visualized on MRI in more than 70% of cases. MRI typically shows scarring and shrinkage in the periventricular white matter with compensatory enlargement of the cerebral ventricles.

In spastic quadriplegia, the most common lesions seen on pathologic examination or on MRI scanning are severe PVL and multicystic cortical encephalomalacia. Neurologic examination shows increased tone and spasticity in all extremities, decreased spontaneous movements, brisk reflexes, and plantar extensor responses.

In athetoid CP, also called *choreoathetoid, extrapyramidal CP,* the MRI scan shows lesions in the globus pallidus bilaterally. Extrapyramidal CP can also be associated with lesions in the basal ganglia and thalamus caused by metabolic genetic disorders such as mitochondrial disorders and glutaric aciduria. MRI scanning and possibly metabolic testing are important in the evaluation of children with extrapyramidal CP to make a correct etiologic diagnosis. In patients with dystonia who have a normal MRI, it is important to have a high level of suspicion for dihydroxyphenylalanine (DOPA)-responsive dystonia (Segawa disease), which causes prominent dystonia that can resemble CP.

Genetic evaluation should be considered in patients with congenital malformations (chromosomes) or evidence of metabolic disorders (e.g., amino acids, organic acids, MR spectroscopy). In addition to the genetic disorders mentioned earlier that can present as CP, the urea cycle disorder arginase deficiency is a rare cause of spastic diplegia, and a deficiency of sulfite oxidase or molybdenum cofactor can present as CP caused by perinatal asphyxia. Tests to detect inherited thrombophilic disorders may be indicated in patients in whom an in utero or neonatal stroke is suspected as the cause of CP.

Inborn errors of metabolism such as aminoaciduria should be excluded by chromatography of the plasma and urine. The diagnosis of the CP should be suspected if child with low birth weight, perinatal insult has increased tone and feeding difficulties.

Electroencephalogram

Infants with CP are at higher risk than the general population to have seizures, and up to 50% of patients, depending on the location of their lesion and type of CP, will have at least one seizure in their lifetime: Evaluation for seizure predisposition with EEG is not routinely indicated in patients with CP; thus, consideration of EEG should be on a case-by-case basis.

Genetic Testing

Genetic testing is not indicated routinely in patients with CP. However, in individuals in whom the neonatal course or imaging is not consistent with symptomatology, in patients with regression, or in families with a strong history of children with a diagnosis of CP, referral to genetics should be placed. Typical testing will include chromosome microarray, often followed by whole-exome sequencing, although more targeted testing may be performed based on the patient's phenotype.

LABORATORY SALIENT FINDINGS

- Magnetic resonance imaging (MRI)
- *Computed tomography (CT) scan:* Periventricular calcification
- Immunoglobulin G (IgG), IgM, and antibody levels
- *Blood:* Amino acids, lactate, pyruvate, and ammonia concentrate
- *Urine:* Amino acids and organic acids

■ DIFFERENTIAL DIAGNOSIS

Differential diagnosis involves the following:
- Hydrocephalus with subdural effusion
- Intracranial space occupying lesion (ICSOL)
- Muscular dystrophy
- Ataxia telangiectasia
- Leukodystrophies
- Spinal cord lesions

■ TREATMENT

Progress has been made in both prevention of CP before it occurs and treatment of children with the disorder. Preliminary results from controlled trials of magnesium sulfate given intravenously to mothers in premature labor with birth imminent before 32-week gestation showed significant reduction in the risk of CP at 2 years of age.

To treat a child with CP, one must evaluate the different possible malfunctions of the system. Ability to relate sensory input to motor input forms the basis of posture control development. Coupling visual and nonvisual information is crucial to developing and maintaining movements. The therapy aims at:
- Reduction of spasticity
- Prevention of abnormal posture
- Prevention of contractures and deformities
- Inhibition of primitive reflexes and facilitation of normal patterns of movement
- Stimulation of sensory, cognitive, and perceptual functions

While neurodevelopmental therapy has the widest appeal all over, many therapists use an eclectic approach to treatment. They first evaluate the patient's deficits and needs and then choose a variety of modalities from the established modalities, tailoring it to the needs of the child.

Children with spastic diplegia are treated initially with the assistance of adaptive equipment, such as walkers, poles, and standing frames. If a patient has marked spasticity of the lower extremities or evidence of hip dislocation, consideration should be given to performing surgical soft-tissue procedures that reduce muscle spasm around the hip girdle, including an adductor tenotomy or psoas transfer and release.

A rhizotomy procedure in which the roots of the spinal nerves are divided produces considerable improvement in selected patients with severe spastic diplegia. A tight heel cord in a child with spastic hemiplegia may be treated surgically by tenotomy of the Achilles tendon.

Quadriplegia is managed with motorized wheelchairs, special feeding devices, modified typewriters, and customized seating arrangements. The function of the affected extremities in children with hemiplegic CP can often be improved by therapy in which movement of the good side is constrained with casts while the impaired extremities perform exercises, which induce improved hand and arm functioning. This constraint-induced movement therapy is effective in patients of all ages.

■ MEDICAL MANAGEMENT

Respiratory

Individuals with CP are at a high risk for aspiration, and lung disease often is a cause of significant morbidity and mortality. Factors that increase the risk of choking include poor swallowing, increased secretions, scoliosis, and airway obstruction. It is important to obtain proper studies such as swallow studies to evaluate for aspiration, sleep studies to evaluate for central or obstructive sleep apnea, and routine films for scoliosis monitoring to ensure that appropriate interventions are being performed. Patients may benefit from chest physiotherapy and bronchodilators to help with clearance of secretions, noninvasive respiratory support such as continuous positive airway pressure (CPAP) or bilevel positive airway pressure (BIPAP) to help with sleep-disordered breathing, and scoliosis surgery to help with restrictive lung disease. Medications for secretions and reflux can also help to prevent aspirations.

Circulatory

Patients can have issues with their peripheral circulation as a result of poor mobility and will often have cold or discolored extremities. Congenital heart disease can lead to neonatal stroke, which can predispose to CP. Patients with neonatal stroke also may have a coagulopathy leading to their symptoms and should undergo hematologic evaluation.

Gastrointestinal

Swallowing difficulty is a common problem in patients with CP for several reasons. During the infancy period, patients may have issues in coordinating a strong suck and swallow. As patients get older, swallowing issues may lead to a pooling of secretions and profuse drooling. It is important to perform swallow studies and modify diet as needed to help prevent aspiration. Medications such as glycopyrrolate or scopolamine can also be helpful to treat drooling; and in some individuals with refractory secretions, botulinum toxin injections or ablation of the salivary glands is indicated.

Constipation is another frequent issue, often due to immobility and dehydration. Patients may also have constipation as a side effect of medications used to help decrease secretions. Use of conservative measures such as prune juice, medications such as laxatives or stool softeners, or in some cases suppositories or enemas is helpful in maintaining a normal bowel regimen.

Nutrition

Failure to thrive is another common issue due to increased metabolic demand in the spastic patient, swallowing issues as noted earlier, and decreased gastric motility leading to prolonged feeding times. Growth parameters need to be monitored closely, and evaluation by a nutritionist is often indicated. Some patients require a gastrostomy tube either due to lengthy time required for meals, aspiration with oral intake, or difficulty in maintaining a healthy weight. Avoidance of malnutrition is important as this increases risk for development of illness, fractures, and skin breakdown, and can lead to a decrease in life expectancy.

Neurologic

The neurologic status of patients with CP varies widely, from individuals with normal intelligence and no seizures to patients who are profoundly intellectually disabled and have medically refractory epilepsy. The location and extent of the anatomic lesion in the brain may be helpful in some cases to predict the degree of neurologic involvement, although it is important to prognosticate on a case-by-case basis.

Almost half of patients with CP will have epilepsy, most commonly patients with hemiplegic or quadriplegic syndromes. EEGs must be obtained to evaluate patients with suspected seizures, and appropriate anti-epileptic medications should be prescribed. Some medications such as the benzodiazepines can be used for the dual purpose of managing muscular tone and preventing seizures. Side effects of medications should be monitored closely as many seizure medications can cause cognitive slowing drowsiness, or anorexia, which often exacerbates pre-existing problems in patients with CP.

Abnormal movements, including myoclonic jerks, startle myoclonus, opisthotonic posturing, chorea, and athetosis, are seen frequently in patients with CP. Some of the movements may mimic seizures, and therefore differentiating between a movement disorder and seizure disorder often requires prolonged EEG monitoring. Treatment for movement disorders can include oral medications or, in some refractory cases, deep brain stimulation.

Intellectual disability can occur in as many as half of patients with CP. It is important to discern whether a true intellectual disability is present or whether a communication difficulty is preventing the patient from performing at his or her full ability. Dysarthria, present in many patients, can make it very difficult for patients to express themselves, and these patients benefit greatly from augmentative communication devices. Assessment by developmental pediatricians is helpful to establish developmental quotient and appropriate school modifications. Patients may also have associated hearing and vision deficits, and screening should be performed so that interventions can be performed at an early age. Evaluation for attention deficit disorders, autistic spectrum disorders, and mood disorders may also be indicated.

Genitourinary

Issues with urination, including incontinence and retention, can be the result of intellectual disability, poor voluntary muscle control, mobility issues, or inability to process sensory feedback. If urinary continence is achieved, it may be delayed. Some patients will require intermittent catheterization to prevent sequelae of urinary retention, which can include increased risk for urinary tract infections, overflow incontinence, and kidney damage from vesicoureteral reflux.

Medications used to treat other symptoms can cause urologic symptoms (e.g., urinary retention with anticholinergic medications for treatment of drooling or dystonia and renal stones with certain antiepileptic medications).

Musculoskeletal

Patients with CP, especially those who are unable to ambulate, are at risk for developing contractures, bony deformities, and joint pain. Exercise, if possible, is helpful to prevent these changes. Treatment for increased muscle tone with stretching, medications, injections, and braces is also helpful to preserve range of motion. It is important to perform surveillance imaging of the spine and hips to evaluate for scoliosis and hip dislocation, which can be a source of discomfort. Osteopenia and fractures are another risk, and patients are often treated with vitamin D and calcium to help improve bone density. Bisphosphonates are another option but are not widely used due to side-effect concerns.

Orthopedic

The judgement of when to operate and the type of procedure to be used is the key to orthopedic care. For hip subluxation, abduction splinting or surgery may be required. This consists of adductor tenotomies/myotomies.

Osteotomies may be necessary in advanced cases. Achilles tendon contracture is treated by bracing, casting, or surgical procedure. Treatment of scoliosis can be nonoperative such as bracing or by surgical stabilization, depending on the severity.

Neurosurgery

The disability in children with CP is often attributed to concomitant spasticity. Partial division of posterior lumbar roots or selective dorsal rhizotomy (SDR) has become a common surgical treatment to reduce spasticity. The technique involves bilateral isolation of the posterior roots from L2 to S1 and stimulation of each root with electromyography (EMG) and direct observation of sustained muscle contraction in order to decide which rootlets to divide.

Rehabilitation

For a child with CP, infancy is the time during which process of rehabilitation is set on a firm footing since it is during this crucial period that the parents are likely to raise concern regarding the child's development. The medical professionals play an important role in communicating the diagnosis and counseling parents regarding treatment. The goal of rehabilitation is to achieve promotion of motor and functional development and independence as far as possible in activities of daily living and to prepare the child for schooling depending upon his mental status.

Physiotherapy

The physiotherapists help in improving the motor and functional skills and locomotion as well as prevention of contractures and deformities. Physiotherapy aims at reducing abnormal patterns of movements and posture and to promote the normal ones so as to enable the child to gain maximal functional independence. The rationale for early physiotherapy in CP is based on plasticity of brain.

The role of physiotherapy and occupational therapy is closely linked, and both must work for the same goal. The occupational therapist advises the parents on activities of daily living such as bathing, feeding, and dressing.

Speech Therapy

The speech therapist also helps in developing an effective feeding program along with occupational therapist. Appropriate positioning of head and jaw is basic to both feeding and speech. The inhibition of abnormal oral reflexes is necessary for feeding. Speech therapists employ auditory stimulation and work for improvement in muscle control required for feeding and articulation.

MEDICATIONS

Antiepileptic Drugs

A very high incidence of West syndrome has been observed in patients with spastic quadriplegia. The guidelines of stopping the therapy are similar to the general population but only 1/5th of the patients may achieve remission and withdrawal of medication. Tigabine—a newer antiepileptic drug (AED) has been shown to bring about seizure control as well as reduction in spasticity with improvement in function.

Antispasticity Drugs

Several drugs have been used to treat spasticity, including the benzodiazepines and baclofen. These medications have beneficial effects in some patients but can also cause side effects such as sedation for benzodiazepines and lowered seizure threshold for baclofen. Several drugs can be used to treat spasticity, including oral diazepam (0.01–0.3 mg/kg/day, divided bid or qid), baclofen (0.2–2 mg/kg/day, divided bid or tid) or dantrolene (0.5–10 mg/kg/day, bid). Small doses of levodopa (0.5–2 mg/kg/day) can be used to treat dystonia or DOPA-responsive dystonia. Artane (trihexyphenidyl, 0.25 mg/day, divided bid or tid and titrated upward) is sometimes useful for treating dystonia and can cause increase in use of the upper extremities and vocalizations. Reserpine (0.01–0.02 mg/kg/day, divided bid to a maximum of 0.25 mg daily) or tetrabenazine (12.5–25.0 mg, divided bid or tid) can be useful for hyperkinetic movement disorders including athetosis or chorea.

- *Baclofen:* 10–15 mg in 3 divided doses, maximum 40–60 mg
- *Tizanidine:* 2–4 mg/day in 3–4 divided doses, maximum of 35 mg/day
- *Diazepam:* 0.2–0.8 mg/kg/day in 3–4 divided doses

Antispasticity drugs like baclofen, dantrolene, and diazepam bring limited benefit because although these reduce spasticity, there is no improvement in coordination. Baclofen works primarily at spinal cord level through a presynaptic gamma-aminobutyric acid (GABA) receptor-GABA subtype.

Intrathecal Baclofen

For severely affected children who have significant side effects with antispasticity drugs or who have persistent and severe spasticity despite maximal doses, intrathecal baclofen may be an option and is an effective intervention.

Side effects include lethargy, confusion, hypotonia, and catheter-related complications.

It is started at the dose of 2.5 mg twice daily and increased every 3–5 days up to 2 mg/kg (maximum 70 mg) divided in 3– 4 doses. It is important to strike a balance between relaxation and spasticity so that child does not lose his functional capacity secondary to excessive relaxation.

Botulinum Toxin

Botulinum toxin is used in patients who have increased muscle tone that interferes with function or is likely to lead to joint contracture with growth. For patients with diffuse hypertonia, botulinum toxin can be injected into multiple muscles to treat the main foci of the generalized spasticity. Ideally, only two or three muscles will require treatment at one time. The patient should be reevaluated 6–8 weeks after treatment.

The effect typically lasts 3–8 months, after which treatment can be repeated.

Medication for Excessive Salivation

Oral physiotherapy and use of ice cubes are most effective. In case of nonresponse, glycopyrrolate (0.5–1 mg/day), transdermal scopolamine, and botulinum toxin can be used. Benztropine may be used in patients with excessive drooling.

Medications for Dystonia

Levodopa may be tried in cases with severe athetosis. Athetosis in dyskinetic CP may respond to treatment with benzodiazepines also. Trihexyphenidyl and carbamazepine may be useful in patients with severe dystonia. Since all these drugs are accompanied with side effects, these medications should be used only in patients in whom involuntary movements are persistent and disabling.

- *Trihexyphenidyl* (0.2–1 mg/kg/day) given in 3–4 divided doses is useful in dystonia. Other drugs that can be useful include gabapentin, baclofen, and diazepam. In refractory cases, deep brain stimulation (DBS) and pallidotomy may be useful in selected cases.
- *Tetrabenazine* (12.5–50 mg/day) may be used for choreoathetoid movements.

■ PROGNOSIS

Parents of the affected child generally want to know whether and when the child will be able to walk and what the future holds for him/her. The type and severity of CP are useful guides in predicting ambulation.

Most children with spastic hemiplegia have walked by 2 years and all walked by 3 years. Similarly, all children with ataxic CP will walk much later than those with spastic hemiplegia. Of children with spastic diplegia, 65% will walk unassisted and 20% with the help of assistive devices.

Children with quadriparesis have a poorer prognosis. The presence of primitive reflexes at 2 years was highly associated with nonambulatory skills at 8 years. All children who can sit by 2 years will eventually walk.

■ BIBLIOGRAPHY

1. Aneja S. Evaluation of a child with cerebral palsy. Indian J Pediatr. 2004;71(7):627-34.
2. Blair E. Epidemiology of cerebral palsies. Orthop Clin North Am. 2010;41(4):441-55.
3. Gulati S, Sondhi V. Cerebral palsy: An Overview. Indian J Pediatr. 2018;85(11):1006-16.
4. Novak I, Hines M, Goldsmith S, Barclay R. Clinical prognostic messages from a systematic review on cerebral palsy. Pediatrics. 2012;130(5):e1285-312.
5. Quality Standards Subcommittee of the American Academy of Neurology and the Practice Committee of the Child Neurology Society; Delgado MR, Hirtz D, Aisen M, Ashwal S, Fehlings DL, McLaughlin J, et al. Practice parameter: pharmacologic treatment of spasticity in children and adolescents with cerebral palsy (an evidence-based review): report of the Quality Standards Subcommittee of the American Academy of Neurology and the Practice Committee of the Child Neurology Society. Neurology. 2010;74(4):336-43.
6. Rethlefsen SA, Ryan DD, Kay RM. Classification systems in cerebral palsy. Orthop Clin North Am. 2010;41(4):457-67.

CASE 50

Duchenne Muscular Dystrophy

■ PRESENTING COMPLAINTS

A 6-year-old boy was brought with the complaints of:
- Abnormal walking posture since 2 years
- Difficulty in getting up since 2 months

History of Presenting Complaints

A 6-year-old boy was brought to the hospital with history of abnormal gait. Parents noticed that their son's gait was not normal. Gait was becoming more abnormal as the days passed. Mother informed that her son found very difficult to get up from the sitting-up posture. He was taking the help of the objects to get up. He was not able to play or run as other kids were doing. Parents also told that they noticed this abnormal gait when he was 2 years old.

Past History of the Patient

He was the elder sibling of nonconsanguineous marriage. He was born at term by normal delivery. He cried immediately after the delivery. He had transient tachypnea which settled by itself within 24 hours. The birth weight of the child was 3 kg. The child was on breast milk immediately after the delivery. He was on breast milk exclusively for 3 months. Weaning was started at the age of 4 months. He was on family food by the age of 10 months. Mother had noticed that he had difficulty in climbing the stairs. He was not able to run or hop. He used to frequently fall.

CASE AT A GLANCE

Basic Findings
Height	: 114 cm (50th centile)
Weight	: 18 kg (60th centile)
Temperature	: 37°C
Pulse rate	: 110 beats/min
Respiratory rate	: 20 breaths/min
Blood pressure	: 70/50 mm Hg

Positive Findings

History:
- Abnormal gait

Examination:
- Hypertrophy of calf muscles
- Proximal muscle weakness

Investigation:
- Creatine phosphokinase (CPK): 1,000 U/L
- Lactate dehydrogenase (LDH): 800 U/L
- Muscle biopsy: Suggestive of primary muscle disorders

■ EXAMINATION

On examination the child was moderately built and nourished. He was sitting on the table with his hands supporting on the thighs. Anthropometric measurements included that the height was 114 cm (50th centile), the weight was 18 kg (60th centile). He was afebrile. The pulse rate was 110 beats per minute. The respiratory rate was 20 breaths per minute. The blood pressure recorded was 70/50 mm Hg. There was no pallor, no lymphadenopathy, and no edema.

His posture showed marked lumbar lordosis. There were hypertrophied calf muscles. The child had difficulty in getting up from the sitting posture. He had flat foot. He was making use of his own thigh and furniture to get up from the sitting posture. There was symmetrical proximal muscle weakness. All the systemic examinations were normal.

■ INVESTIGATION

- *Hemoglobin:* 12 g/dL
- *TLC:* 6,000 cells/mm^3
- *ESR:* 26 mm in the first hour
- *CPK:* 1,000 U/L
- *LDH:* 800 U/L
- *Muscle biopsy:* Suggestive of primary muscular disease

■ DISCUSSION

The boy presented with history of abnormal gait with delayed motor milestones, and symmetrical proximal muscle weakness gives the suspicion of Duchenne muscular dystrophy (DMD). The diagnosis is again supported by presence of hypertrophied calf muscle and lordosis. Laboratory investigations such as CPK and LDH levels are grossly elevated. Muscle biopsy suggests primary muscular disease.

Duchenne muscular dystrophy is the most common hereditary neuromuscular disease affecting all races and ethnic groups. Its characteristic clinical features are progressive weakness, intellectual impairment, hypertrophy of the calves, and proliferation of connective tissue in muscle. The incidence is 1 in 3,600 liveborn infant boys. This disease is inherited as an X-linked recessive trait. The abnormal gene is at the Xp21.1–p21.2 locus and is one of the largest genes. Becker muscular dystrophy (BMD) is a disease that is fundamentally similar to DMD, with a genetic defect at the same locus, but clinically it follows a milder and more protracted course, the associated pathological changes in the muscles are due to deficiency of protein dysmorphia.

Despite the X-linked recessive inheritance in DMD, approximately 30% of cases are new or de novo mutations, and the mother is not a carrier. The female carrier state usually shows no muscle weakness but due to skewed X-inactivation, about 8% of carrier females are manifesting carriers with some weakness, although typically milder than is seen in affected males. These symptomatic females are explained by the Lyon hypothesis, in which the normal X chromosome becomes inactivated and the one with the gene deletion is active. The full clinical picture of DMD has occurred in several females with Turner syndrome in whom the single X chromosome must have had the *Xp21* gene deletion.

The molecular defects in the dystrophinopathies vary and include intragenic deletions, duplications, or point mutations of nucleotides.

Phenotypic or clinical variations are explained by the alteration of the translational reading frame of messenger RNA (mRNA), which results in unstable, truncated dystrophin molecules and severe, classic DMD; on the other hand, mutations that preserve the reading frame still permit translation of coding sequences further downstream on the gene and produce a semifunctional dystrophin, expressed clinically as DMD.

■ CLINICAL FEATURES (FIG. 1)

Duchenne muscular dystrophy is the most common hereditary neuromuscular disease. It is inherited as X-linked recessive trait.

Infant boys are rarely symptomatic at birth or in early infancy, although some are

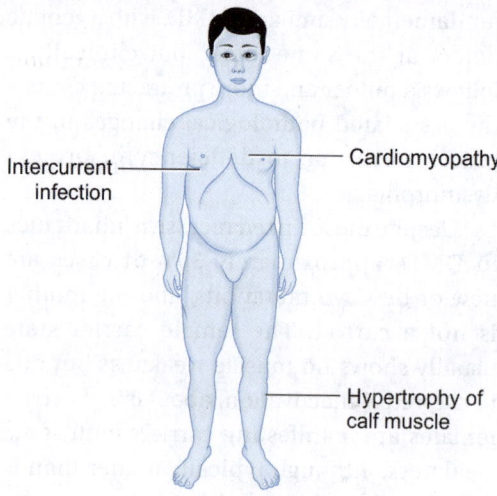

Fig. 1: Clinical features.

mildly hypotonic. Early gross motor skills, such as rolling over, sitting, and standing, are usually achieved at the appropriate ages or may be mildly delayed.

Early development of the child is normal or slightly delayed. Poor head control in the infancy may be the first sign of weakness. Hip girdle weakness may be seen in subtle forms at the age of 2 years. By the age of 2 years, child may appear clumsy while walking. Hypertrophy of the calf muscle may be observed at the age of 4–5 years. The older children may assume lordotic postures. When standing to compensate gluteal muscle weakness, waddling gait, difficulty in climbing the stair, and hypertrophy of calf muscles are the common presentation. Enlargement of the calves (pseudohypertrophy) and wasting of thigh muscles are classic features. The enlargement is caused by hypertrophy of some muscle fibers, infiltration of muscle by fat, and proliferation of collagen. After the calves, the next most common site of muscular hypertrophy is the tongue, followed by muscles of the forearm. Other muscles which get hypertrophied are deltoid and brachioradialis.

Early in the disease, the hypertrophied muscles are often strong, but later the muscles become weak. The hypertrophied calf muscles are stronger than the anterior leg muscles. Hence, toe walking will be there. This leads to the contraction of heel cord.

Weakness of pelvic muscles produces waddling lordotic gait and difficulty in rising from the floor. When gets up from the floor, the patient first rolls to prone position, kneels and then arises himself to stand by pushing his hands against shin, knee, and thighs. He stands up, he climbs upon his own body by supporting it with his hands—Gowers's sign **(Fig. 2)**. It indicates weakness in pelvic girdle muscle.

Gower's sign is often evident by the age of 3 years and is fully expressed by the age of 5–6 years. A Trendelenburg gait, or hip waddle, appears at this time. Common presentations in toddlers include delayed walking, falling, toe walking, trouble running or walking upstairs, developmental delay and, less often, malignant hyperthermia after anesthesia.

> **ESSENTIAL DIAGNOSTIC POINTS**
> - Delayed motor milestones
> - Symmetrical proximal muscle weakness
> - Lordosis
> - Gowers's sign
> - Increased CPK and LDH levels
> - Cardiomyopathy
> - No mental debility
>
> (CPK: creatine phosphokinase; LDH: lactate dehydrogenase)

Forced vital capacity is reduced in these patients due to scoliosis. These children are more prone to develop aspiration pneumonitis due to esophageal reflux because of distortion of diaphragm.

In the late teens or early 20s respiratory failure may occur as a result of increasing nocturnal hypoventilation and hypoxia.

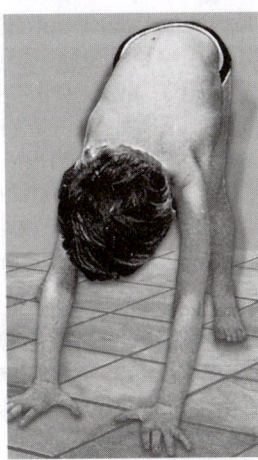

Fig. 2: Gowers's sign.

Higher incidences of emotional disturbances are seen. It is accompanied by cerebral atrophy as demonstrated by CT scan.

Cardiomegaly, persistent tachycardia and cardiomyopathy are constant features. ECG changes are often present. Severe peripheral circulatory failure may follow aspiration. Facial features include wide arch of mandible with wide separation of teeth which may be due to macroglossia.

Cardiomyopathy, including persistent tachycardia and myocardial failure, are seen in 50–80% of patients with this disease. The severity, if cardiac involvement, does not necessarily correlate with the degree of skeletal muscle weakness. Some patients die early of severe cardiomyopathy while still in ambulatory stage, and others in terminal stages of the disease. However, in patients with DMD, patients may develop worsening of cardiomyopathy and even develop severe heart failure despite still being ambulant. Smooth muscle dysfunction, particularly of the gastrointestinal tract, is a minor, but often overlooked, feature.

Contractures most often involve the ankles, knees, hips, and elbows. As upper extremity weakness progresses, contractures are also seen in neck lateral rotation, shoulders, and fingers. Scoliosis is common in patients with DMD. Scoliosis usually progresses more rapidly after the child becomes nonambulatory and may be uncomfortable or painful. After the calves, the next most common site of muscular hypertrophy is the tongue, followed by muscles of the forearm. Abnormalities of the muscle are demonstrated using muscle MR techniques to assess signal, water content, fat fractions, and even MR spectroscopy profiles. Fasciculations of the tongue do not occur. The voluntary sphincter muscles rarely become involved.

Ambulation is important not only for postponing psychological depression but also to prevent scoliosis. Scoliosis often becomes rapidly progressive after confinement to wheelchair. There is a tendency to walk on toes and calf muscles are prominent, and hence indicating pseudohypertrophy.

Ankle jerks are brisk and knee jerks are sluggish. They resemble clinically chronic spinal atrophy, dermatomyositis, limb girdle, and muscular dystrophy.

The relentless progression of weakness continues into the second decade. The function of distal muscles is usually relatively well enough preserved, allowing the child to continue using eating utensils, a pencil, and a computer keyboard. Respiratory muscle involvement is expressed as a weak and ineffective cough, frequent pulmonary infections, and decreasing respiratory reserve. Pharyngeal weakness can lead to episodes of aspiration, nasal regurgitation of liquids, and nasal voice quality. The function of the extraocular muscles remains well preserved. Incontinence due to anal and urethral sphincter weakness is an uncommon and very late event.

Death in boys with DMD occurs in the late teens to 20s. The causes of death are respiratory failure during sleep, intractable heart failure, pneumonia, or, occasionally, aspiration and airway obstruction.

> **GENERAL FEATURES**
> - Appears clumsy while walking
> - Falls easily
> - Difficulty in climbing up the stairs
> - Gowers's sign
> - Weakness of pelvic girdle muscle

■ DIAGNOSIS

Polymerase chain reaction (PCR) for the dystrophin gene mutation is the primary test, if the clinical features and serum CPK are consistent with the diagnosis. If the blood PCR is diagnostic, muscle biopsy may be deferred. If it is normal and clinical suspicion is high, the more specific dystrophin immunocytochemistry is performed on muscle biopsy sections. This detects the 30% of cases that do not show PCR abnormalities.

The muscle biopsy is diagnostic and shows characteristic changes. Myopathic changes include endomysial connective tissue proliferation, scattered degenerating and regenerating myofibers, foci of mononuclear inflammatory cell infiltrates as a reaction to muscle fiber necrosis, mild architectural changes in still, functional muscle fibers, and many dense fibers. These hypercontracted fibers probably result from segmental necrosis at another level allowing calcium to enter the site of breakdown of the sarcolemmal membrane and trigger a contraction of the whole length of the muscle fiber. Calcifications within myofibers are correlated with secondary β-dystroglycan deficiency.

The serum CPK level is consistently greatly elevated in DMD, even in presymptomatic stages, including at birth. The usual serum concentration is 15,000–35,000 IU/L (normal <160 IU/L). A normal serum CK level is incompatible with the diagnosis of DMD, although in terminal stages of the disease, the serum CPK value may be considerably lower than it was a few years earlier because there is less muscle to degenerate. Other lysosomal enzymes present in muscle, such as aldolase and aspartate aminotransferase, are also increased but are less specific.

Cardiac assessment is done by echocardiography, ECG and chest radiography. ECG shows minor abnormalities in 70% of cases.

Electromyogram (EMG) shows characteristic myopathic features and a normal interference pattern. There is no spontaneous activity at rest and low amplitude, short duration polyphasic motor units on stimulation.

Muscle biopsy shows a wider-than-normal variation in fiber diameter, internal nuclei opaque fibers, and increased fat and connective tissues.

The same methods of deoxyribonucleic acid (DNA) analysis from blood samples may be applied for carrier detection in female relatives at risk, such as sisters and cousins, and to determine whether the mother is a carrier or whether a new mutation occurred in the embryo. Prenatal diagnosis is possible as early as the 12th week of gestation by sampling chorionic villi for DNA analysis by southern blot or PCR. In cases of aborted fetuses with DMD, muscle demonstrates abnormal dystrophin staining by immunohistochemistry.

> **LABORATORY SALIENT FINDINGS**
> - Elevated CPK
> - Elevated LDH
> - ECG and Echocardiography
> - Chest X-ray
> - Electromyogram
> - Muscle biopsy
>
> (CPK: creatine phosphokinase; ECG: electrocardiography; LDH: Lactate dehydrogenase)

Carrier detection: 10% of carriers at least manifest a few clinical signs with varying degree of muscle weakness due to ionization, 45X chromosomal status, or autosomal translocation. Muscle biopsy may reveal myopathic changes in one third of carriers.

Chorionic villus sample taken around 10 weeks of gestation is subjected for rapid fetal sexing as well as DNA studies.

DIFFERENTIAL DIAGNOSIS

- Polyneuritis
- Chronic spinal muscular atrophy
- Dermatomyositis
- Myelopathies

TREATMENT

There is no medical cure for this disease. Much can be done to treat complications and to improve the quality of life of affected children. Cardiac decompensation often responds initially well to digoxin. Pulmonary infections should be promptly treated. Patients should avoid contact with children who have obvious respiratory or other contagious illnesses. Immunizations for influenza virus and other routine vaccinations are indicated.

Preservation of a good nutritional state is important. DMD is not a vitamin-deficiency disease, and therefore excessive doses of vitamins should be avoided. Adequate calcium intake is important to minimize osteoporosis in boys confined to a wheelchair, and fluoride supplements may also be given, particularly if the local drinking water is not fluoridated.

Physiotherapy delays but does not always prevent contractures. At times, contractures are actually useful in functional rehabilitation. If contractures prevent extension of the elbow beyond 90° and the muscles of the upper limb no longer are strong enough to overcome gravity, the elbow contractures are functionally beneficial in fixing an otherwise flail arm and in allowing the patient to eat and write. Surgical correction of the elbow contracture may be technically feasible, but the result may be deleterious. Physiotherapy contributes little to muscle strengthening because patients usually are already using their entire reserve for daily function, and exercise cannot further strengthen involved muscles. Excessive exercise can actually accelerate the process of muscle fiber degeneration.

EXONDYS 51 (eteplirsen) is an exon 51 skipping antisense oligonucleotide approach that binds RNA and skips over the defective exon, restoring the reading frame, thereby producing a shorter but potentially functional dystrophin protein. This only applies to patients with mutations amenable to this repair (~13% of patients). It is given as a weekly IV infusion.

Another recommended treatment of patients with DMD involves the use of prednisone, prednisolone, deflazacort, or other steroids. Glucocorticoids decrease the rate of apoptosis or programmed cell death of myotubes during ontogenesis and can decelerate the myofiber necrosis in muscular dystrophy. Strength usually improves initially, but the long-term complications of chronic steroid therapy, including considerable weight gain and osteoporosis, can offset this advantage or even result in greater weakness than might have occurred in the natural course of the disease.

Nevertheless, some patients with DMD treated early with steroids appear to have an improved long-term prognosis in muscle and myocardial outcome, as well as short-term improvement in muscle strength, and steroids can help keep patients ambulatory for more years than expected without treatment.

Initiation of steroids is indicated when a child shows a plateau in development and/or a regression in motor development as compared with peers. One protocol gives prednisolone (0.75 mg/kg/day) for the first 10 days of each month to avoid chronic complications. Deflazacort, administered as 0.9 mg/kg/day, may be more effective than prednisolone. Fluorinated steroids, such as dexamethasone or triamcinolone, should be avoided because they induce myopathy by altering the myotube abundance of ceramide.

Alternative protocols for steroid administration include weekend-only dosing, alternate-day regimens, or 10-day-on/10-day-off regimens; the daily regimen has been the preferred regimen based upon comparative studies.

Newer therapies include exon skipping using antisense oligonucleotides. Phase 3 trails have shown significant clinical benefits. Eteplirsen has Food and Drug Administration (FDA) approval.

■ BIBLIOGRAPHY

1. Birnkrunt DJ, Bushby K, Bann CM, Apkon SD, Blackwell A, Brumbaugh D, et al.; DMD Care Considerations Working Group. Diagnosis and management of Duchenne muscular dystrophy, part 1: Diagnosis, and neuromuscular, rehabilitation, endocrine, and gastrointestinal and nutritional management. Lancet Neurol. 2018;17(3): 251-67.
2. Bushby K, Finkel R, Birnkrant DJ, Case LE, Clemens PR, Cripe L, et al; DMD Care Considerations Working Group. Diagnosis and management of Duchenne muscular dystrophy, part 1: diagnosis, and pharmacological and psychosocial management. Lancet Neurol. 2010;9(1): 77-93.
3. Darras BT, Urion DK, Ghosh PS. Dystrophinopathies. In: Adam MP, Feldman J, Mirzaa GM (Eds). Seattle (WA): University of Washington, Seattle; 1993-2024. [online] Available from: https://www.ncbi.nlm.nih.gov/books/NBK1119/ [Last accessed June, 2024].
4. Thornton CA. Myotonic dystrophy. Neurol Clin. 2014;32(3);7705-19.

CASE 51

Epilepsy

■ PRESENTING COMPLAINTS

An 8-year-old boy was brought with the complaints of:
- Cough and cold since 1 week
- Fever since 1 week
- Headache since 1 week
- Abnormal movements of limbs since 2 hours

History of Presenting Complaints

An 8-year-old boy was brought to pediatric casualty department with a history of abnormal movements involving both upper limb and lower limb. There was also uprolling of eyeballs. According to the mother, her son became unconscious simultaneously with abnormal movements. That was associated with froth in the mouth. According to the mother, her son has been treated for cough, cold, and fever about 10 days back. She also recollected that her son got repeated attacks of headache recently. There was no history of similar attacks before.

Past History of the Patient

The patient was the second child of a consanguineous marriage. He was delivered at full term by normal vaginal delivery. Delivery was uneventful. He was on breastfeed exclusively for 6 months. Later, weaning was started, and he was on family food by 10 months. He had been completely immunized. His developmental milestones were normal. His scholastic performance was good. His sister was 11-year-old and maintained good health.

■ EXAMINATION

On examination, the boy was moderately built and nourished. He had tonic and clonic movements of the upper limb and lower limb

---

CASE AT A GLANCE

Basic Findings
Height	: 126 cm (70th centile)
Weight	: 22 kg (50th centile)
Temperature	: 37°C
Pulse rate	: 110 beats per minute
Respiratory rate	: 24 breaths per minute
Blood pressure	: 90/70 mm Hg

Positive Findings

History:
- Abnormal movements
- Uprolling of eyeballs
- Unconscious

Examination:
- Convulsions
- Tongue bite
- Crepitation in chest
- Abdominal distension
- Normal nervous system

Investigation:
- *Chest X-ray:* Shows patchy pneumonitis
- *EEG:* Shows random spikes

with uprolling of eyeball and froth in mouth at the time of admission. His convulsions were brought under control by the casualty medical officer.

He was drowsy after the attack of convulsion was brought under control. He was responding to painful stimulus by resisting it.

Anthropometric measurements included the height of 126 cm (70th centile) and weight of 22 kg (50th centile). He was afebrile. His pulse was 110 beats per minute and respiratory rate was 24 breaths per minute. The blood pressure recorded was 90/70 mm Hg.

There was no pallor, no edema, and no lymphadenopathy. There was tongue bite. Respiratory system revealed presence of crepitations at basal region. Abdominal examination revealed presence of mild distension. There was no hepatosplenomegaly.

The CNS examination revealed a normal mental function. No cranial nerve was involved. No motor or sensory involvement was found. There were no meningeal signs.

■ INVESTIGATION

- *Hemoglobin:* 12 g/dL
- *TLC:* 6,700 cells/mm^3
- *DLC:* P_{80} L_{18} E_2
- *ESR:* 22 mm in 1st hour
- *Blood sugar:* 98 g/dL
- *Serum calcium:* 8 mg/dL
- *Chest X-ray:* Patchy pneumonitis
- *EEG:* Shows random spikes followed by slow waves.
- *CT scan:* Normal

■ DISCUSSION

An 8-year-old boy presented with tonic-clonic type of seizures without having any history suggestive of any infection associated with abnormal EEG findings will help come to the diagnosis of generalized tonic–clonic type of convulsion, i.e., epilepsy.

Seizures are common neurological disorder in pediatric age group. It occurs in 3–5% of children. A seizure or convulsion is defined as paroxysmal involuntary disturbance of brain function that may be manifested as an impairment or loss of consciousness, abnormal motor activity, behavioral abnormalities, sensory disturbances, or autoimmune dysfunction. Some seizures are characterized by abnormal movements without loss of impairment of consciousness.

Epilepsy is defined as recurrent seizures unrelated to fever or to an acute cerebral insult. The highest incidence of epilepsy is in the 1st year of life. It decreases after that age. The second peak is seen in second decade of life, explaining the higher prevalence of epilepsy reported in adolescence. Generalized epilepsy accounts for most of the newly diagnosed cases in the first 5 years of life. After that, partial epilepsy accounts for 50% or more of the newly identified epilepsies.

■ CLASSIFICATION

Etiologically, seizure disorders can be classified into two broad groups: Provoked seizures and unprovoked seizures. Provoked seizures occur in response to an insult to the CNS (e.g., infection and head injury) or in association with severe systemic insult (uremia and hypoglycemia).

Seizures can be further divided into the following types:
- Partial seizures
  - Simple partial (consciousness retained)
    - Motor
    - Sensory
    - Autonomic
  - Complex partial (consciousness impaired)
  - Simple partial, followed by impaired consciousness

- Consciousness impaired at onset
- Partial seizures with secondary generalization
■ Generalized seizures
  - Absence
    ♦ Typical
    ♦ Atypical
  - Generalized tonic–clonic
    ♦ Tonic
    ♦ Clonic
    ♦ Myoclonic
    ♦ Atonic
    ♦ Infantile spasm

■ CLINICAL FEATURES (FIG. 1)

Idiopathic Generalized Epilepsies (IGEs)

In 1989, International League Against Epilepsy (ILAE) defined the criteria of idiopathic generalized epilepsies (IGEs) as follows: IGEs are forms of generalized epilepsies in which all seizures are initially generalized (absences, myoclonic jerks, and generalized tonic-clonic seizures), with an EEG impression that is a generalized, bilateral, synchronous symmetrical discharge.

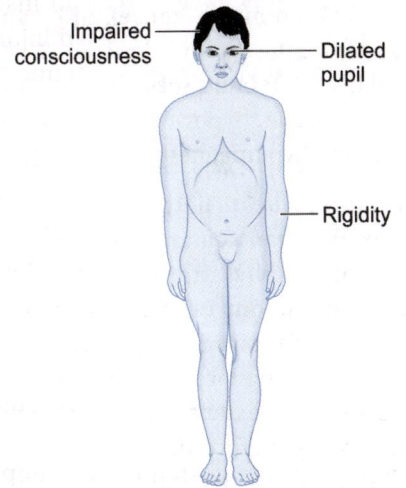

Fig. 1: Clinical features.

The patient has a normal interictal state, without neurological or neuroradiological signs. In general, interictal EEGs show normal background activity and generalized discharges, such as spikes and polyspike waves (>3 Hz). The discharges are increased by slow sleep. The various syndromes of IGEs differ mainly in age of onset.

GENERAL FEATURES
• Abnormal motor activity
• Behavioral abnormality
• Sensory abnormality
• Autoimmune dysfunction

Benign neonatal familial convulsions, benign neonatal convulsions, and benign myoclonic epilepsy in infancy are the IGEs. The onset is either during the first few days of life or during 1st or 2nd year of life as the name indicates.

Partial Seizures

Partial seizures predominantly involve a focal area of brain and the presence of a focal epileptic abnormality in the interictal EEG is a strong evidence of a partial seizure disorder. These can be nonlesional or lesional epilepsies depending on whether an underlying anatomic abnormality related to the seizure activity is found on imaging procedure, preferably a MRI. The nonlesional group includes benign childhood partial epilepsies while the lesional group includes various etiologies.

Simple partial seizures (SPS): The movements are characterized by asynchronous clonic or tonic movements. They tend to involve face, neck, and extremities. Automatisms do not occur. But some patients complain of aura in the form of chest discomfort and headache. This may be the only manifestation of seizure. The distinguishing characteristics of SPS is that patients remain conscious and may talk during the seizure. No postictal phenomenon follows the event. EEG may show spikes or sharp waves unilaterally or bilaterally or a multifacial spike pattern.

Complex partial seizures (CPS): These may begin with a SPS with or without an aura followed by impaired consciousness. Onset may coincide with altered consciousness. The aura may comprise vague, unpleasant feelings and epigastric discomfort. The presence of aura always indicates a focal onset of seizure. There may be brief blink stare or a sudden cessation or a pause in activity that is frequently overlooked by parents. The period of altered consciousness may be brief and infrequent. Only an experienced observer or an EEG may be able to identify the event.

Automatisms are a common feature of CPS. It occurs in approximately 50–75% cases. The frequency of automatism is more in older children. Automatisms develop after the loss of consciousness and may persist into postictal state. But these are not recalled by child. The automatic behavior observed in infant is characterized by lip smacking, chewing, swallowing, and excessive salivation.

Radiographic studies including CT scans and especially MRIs are most likely to identify an abnormality in temporal lobe of the child with CPS.

Generalized Seizures

Absence seizures: Simple typical absence petit mal are characterized by a sudden cessation of motor activity or speech with blank facial expression and flickering of eyelids. These are uncommon before age of 5 years. It is more prevalent in girls. These are not associated with aura. They rarely persist longer than 30 seconds. They are not associated with postictal state. These features differentiate from CPS. EEG shows a typical 3 per second spike and generalized wave discharge.

Generalized tonic–clonic seizures (GTCS): These are extremely common. It may follow partial seizure with the focal onset. They may be associated with aura. Patients suddenly lose consciousness, shrill piercing cry, and rolling back eyeballs can occur. Entire body musculature undergoes tonic contractions. They rapidly became cyanotic and associated with apnea. The clonic phase of the seizure is heralded by rhythmic clonic contractions alternating with relaxation of all muscle groups. The clonic phase occurs toward the end of the seizure unusually lasts for few minutes. During the seizure child may bite their tongue. Loss of sphincter control particularly the bladder is common during GTCS.

Neonatal Seizures

Poor myelination and incomplete dendrite arborization result in clinical seizures. Neonatal seizures may be subtle, multifocal clonic, focal clonic, generalized tonic, and myoclonic events.

Subtle seizures may manifest as eye blinking, fluttering, and buccolingual movements. The common causes are hypoxic ischemic encephalopathy, sepsis, and bacterial meningitis. Metabolic seizures may be due to hypoglycemia, hypocalcemia, dyselectrolytemia, and hypomagnesemia.

Myoclonic seizures: These are characterized by three important features: Spasms, mental retardation, and hysarrhythmia. Spasms are abrupt contractions of less than 2 seconds in duration followed by sustained tonic contraction lasting for 2–10 seconds. Spasms can be flexor or extensor or both, typically occurring just before or on awakening or just before sleep. Hypsarrhythmia is the EEG feature in which all normal activity is replaced by asynchronous large amplitude slow waves mixed with multifocal spikes and sharp waves.

An underlying etiology is found in 85% patients (symptomatic group), which results from prenatal, perinatal, or postnatal insults. In 10–15%, the cause is not known (cryptogenic group) and this group carries a better prognosis. Areas of focal hypometabolism on positron emission tomography (PET) were reported with normal MRI.

Juvenile myoclonic epilepsy: It is a genetically inherited disorder with onset around the puberty. Bilateral symmetrical jerks of short duration involving mainly arms and shoulder are seen. Consciousness is not lost and most attacks occur on awakening. Generalized tonic–clonic or absence seizures may be associated. Sleep deprivation precipitates attacks. EEG shows bilateral multispikes and wave pattern.

Lennox–Gastaut Syndrome (LGS): It is characterized by three main characteristics:
1. *A triad of seizure types:* Axial tonic spasms, atonic seizures, and atypical absences
2. EEG abnormalities consisting of diffuse slow (2–2.5 Hz) and spike-wave discharges when awake, bursts of 10 Hz rhythms in sleep, and generalized 3 Hz spike-wave discharges (petit mal variant) on awakening
3. Slowing and plateauing of cognitive development

Lennox–Gastaut syndrome accounts for 3% of childhood epilepsy. Usually, they are idiopathic or cryptogenic. Symptomatic cases (with definable etiology) are rare. LGS manifests in children aged 1–8 years. Onset can be with any one of the seizure types described but other seizure types such as myoclonic. GTCS or partial seizures are frequently associated with this syndrome. Seizure frequency is high and status epilepticus is frequent, and it is seen in over two-thirds of cases. Carbamazepine (CBZ) is most effective for tonic seizures and sodium valproate (VPA) for atypical absences. The effect of lamotrigine and ethosuximide is long-lasting. In occasional cases vigabatrin and gabapentin are effective.

> **ESSENTIAL DIAGNOSTIC POINTS**
> - Recurrent nonfebrile seizures
> - Often, interictal electroencephalographic (EEG) changes
> - Classified as focal partial onset and generalized

■ INVESTIGATION

Estimation of glucose and calcium and screening tests for neurometabolic causes usually suffice.

The interictal EEG is not always abnormal for inpatients with epilepsy. The yield from routine EEG can be increased by repeating waking recording, recording during sleep, and by using activating techniques: Hyperventilation, photic stimulation, and specific trigger in reflex epilepsies.

When the nature of attack is uncertain to determine the seizure type, videotelemetry EEG is used. EEG shows slow random spikes followed by slow waves in tonic, clonic type. In absence seizures a 3 per second spike and slow wave or multiple spike discharges are seen. Myoclonic seizure is characterized by grossly chaotic record with very tall waves often exceeding 200 millivolts with the frequency of 1–2 per second. Absence of electrical activity suggests subdural hematoma.

Special electrodes: Nasopharyngeal, anterior temporal, and sphenoidal electrodes can be used when routine EEG has not shown epileptiform discharges. Use of intracranial electrodes is indicated in patients with medically intractable epilepsy undergoing presurgical evaluation.

Imaging in Epilepsy

Magnetic resonance imaging, CT scan, and functional imaging with single-photon emission computed tomography (SPECT) or PET are used to evaluate an epileptic child. These are indicated in partial seizures, seizures with focal neurological deficits, dysmorphic features, and focal EEG abnormalities. Findings may include atrophies, inflammatory, malformations, neoplasia, and vascular malformation.

Neuroimaging, either CT or MRI, is necessary in all cases of partial epilepsy, neonatal onset seizures, seizure onset after 20 years of age, generalized seizures not responsive to therapy, and in the presence of focal neurological signs.

Magnetic resonance imaging is useful in defining etiology like small focal pathologies, migration disorders, and malformation. MRI is preferred imaging modality for the investigation of epilepsy. It can detect hippocampal sclerosis and neuronal migration disorders. MRI is essential in intractable CPS with CT negative or unclear, seizures with focal neurological signs and CT negative or unclear, and during presurgical evaluation.

Single-photon emission computed tomography: The epileptic focus is imaged interictally in the region of reduced cerebral blood flow. A significant asymmetry of cerebral blood flow has been noted in about 50% of cases in temporal lobe epilepsy. Due to poor sensitivity and specificity interictal SPECT studies have little role in routine investigation in pediatric procedure.

Positron emission tomography: It has a superior spatial resolution. Interictally, the epileptic focus is an area of reduced glucose metabolism. Partial seizures are associated with increase in both regional cerebral blood glucose metabolism and blood flow. The current role of SPECT and PET is useful when high-quality MRI has not shown a relevant structural abnormality in patients who are the candidates for surgical treatment.

> **LABORATORY SALIENT FINDINGS**
> - *Lumbar puncture:* CSF analysis
> - PCR for herpes
> - CT scan
> - MRI
> - SPECT or PET scan
> - Serum Calcium, PO_4, glucose, BUN, amino acid screen
>
> (BUN: blood urea nitrogen; CSF: cerebrospinal fluid; CT: computed tomography; PCR: polymerase chain reaction; PET: positron emission tomography; PO_4: phosphate ion; SPRECT: single-photon emission computed tomography)

■ TREATMENT

The decision to treat a child with an AED depends on the frequency of seizures, epilepsy syndrome, and neurological findings. The decision to treat a single unprovoked seizure should be individualized. Numerous attempts have been made to predict accurately the risk of epilepsy developing after the first unprovoked seizure.

Treatment may not be recommended after a single brief GTCS but necessary after a cluster of seizures or an episode of status epilepticus. A child with severe physical and learning difficulties who develops infrequent myoclonic or atypical absence (CPS) seizures may not require AED, but a child with normal intelligence, frequent absences, and GTCS on wakefulness may require treatment. Once an AED is started, the objective is to achieve complete seizure control without side effects and to use the most appropriate formulation for the child (**Table 1**).

The choice of AED and prognosis of epilepsy depend on the identification of

TABLE 1: Pediatric dosages of anticonvulsant drugs.

Drugs	Usual total daily dosage (mg/kg/day)	Doses per day
Acetazolamide	10–20	2
Carbamazepine	10–25	2/3
Clobazam	0.5–1.5	2
Clonazepam	0.1–0.3	2/3
Ethosuximide	15–35	2(3)
Gabapentin	15–30	3
Lamotrigine	0.5–3.0	2
Nitrazepam	0.5–1	2/3
Phenobarbitone	4–10	2
Phenytoin	4–15	2(1)
Sodium valproate	15–60	2
Vigabatrin	20–100	2

the epileptic syndrome or seizure type (Table 2). Once the most appropriate AED has been selected, it should be used alone (monotherapy) and in the lowest dose that control the seizures without producing unacceptable side effects.

Neonates, infants, and children under the age of 2 years frequently require higher doses than older children, because of a higher rate of drug metabolism. If initial seizure control is suboptimal, the AED dosage should be increased gradually until either seizure control is achieved or unacceptable side effects develop. If side effects occur before seizure control, the child will require substitution with a different drug or an additional AED (polytherapy).

If initial seizure control occurs with first AED and next most appropriate AED and once

TABLE 2: Drugs of first, second, and third choices in the treatment of various seizure types/epilepsies.

	First	Second	Third
Primary generalized			
Tonic–clonic	Sodium valproate	Lamotrigine	• Carbamazepine • Phenytoin
Myoclonic	Sodium valproate	Lamotrigine	• Clonazepam • Ethosuxximide • Phenobarbiton
Tonic	Sodium valproate	Lamotrigine	• Phenytoin • Clobazam • Phenobarbitone
Absence	Sodium valproate	• Lamotrigine • Ethosuximide	• Clobazam
Partial (simple/complex)	Carbamazepine	• Sodium valproate • Vigabatrin	• Lamotrigine • Gabapentin • Phenytoin • Clobazam • Acetazolamide
Infantile spasms	Vigabatrin	• Sodium valproate • Nitrazepam (ACTH)	• Lamotrigine • Prednisone

(ACTH: adrenocorticotropic hormone)

complete seizure control is achieved, the first drug can be withdrawn after a seizure-free period of 2–3 months.

If the initial AED is wholly ineffective, the first drug should be replaced with second one simultaneously, maintaining monotherapy. Polytherapy with two AEDs may result in additional (even complete) seizure control in another 5–10% of children. But the problems of polytherapy are pharmacokinetic interactions—potentially reducing the effectiveness of each drug, difficulty in interpreting the effect of each drug, cumulative toxicity, and increased risk of idiosyncratic toxic interactions.

The currently recommended first-line drugs in treating majority of childhood epilepsies are VPA and CBZ. Most pediatric epilepsy syndromes are associated with generalized seizures, and hence VPA is the drug of choice. Syndromes associated with partial seizures are less common and CBZ is the preferred AED. Though adrenocorticotropic hormone (ACTH) has been used for the treatment of infantile spasms of West syndrome, vigabatrin or VPA should be the drugs of first choice.

Phenytoin and phenobarbitone are useful only when the other drugs have failed and where seizure control is the major priority. The use of benzodiazepines is restricted because of acute toxicity, development of tolerance, or tachyphylaxis, hence rarely, if ever, is used as the initial AED.

Stopping Antiepileptic Drug Treatment

As many as 70–80% of the patients on AED treatment will eventually become seizure free. Drug withdrawal can be considered after a patient has been seizure free for 3 or more years. The risk of relapse remission is about 20% overall. Since the safety of drug withdrawal cannot be guaranteed in any one case, the relative risks of continued drug intake against the risk of further seizures inherent in drug withdrawal should be discussed. If a decision to withdraw medication is made, discontinuation of the treatment should be undertaken slowly, over a period of months, to minimize the risks of relapse.

New Antiepileptic Drugs

Newer antiepileptic drugs are given in **Table 3**.

Felbamate, which blocks N-methyl-D-asparate (NMDA) receptor, is indicated for adjunctive treatment of partial seizures, generalized seizures, infantile spasms, and LGS. The initial recommended dose of felbamate as adjunctive therapy in children was 15–45 mg/kg/day.

Gabapentin, a GABA analog, is indicated for adjunctive treatment of partial and secondarily generalized seizures.

The optimal therapeutic dose of gabapentin in pediatric patients ranges from 30 to 90 mg/kg/day with higher doses being necessary for refractory partial epilepsy. A reduction rate of more than 50% in partial or generalized seizures was seen in 34.4% patients with 6.25% becoming seizure free in an open-label, add-on study of gabapentin.

Lamotrigine blocks voltage-dependent sodium channels (**Table 4**). Used as adjunctive therapy of partial seizures, it has a specific role in the treatment of LGS. Effective maintenance doses in children are 1–15 mg/kg/day. Dosing is markedly influenced by concomitant therapy. Even monotherapy with lamotrigine is found to be effective. It has been shown to be effective to treat juvenile myoclonic epilepsy and infantile spasms.

Tiagabine selectively inhibits the reuptake of GABA into neurons and glia. It is indicated for adjunctive therapy of partial seizures or as monotherapy. Dosing in children should

TABLE 3: Seizure/epilepsy type and effective antiepileptic drugs (AEDs) used.

Antiepileptic drug	Partial	Primary generalized	Infantile spasm	Lennox–Gastaut syndrome	Myoclonic	Absence
Felbamate	+	+	+	+	+	+
Gabapentin	+	+/–	–	–	–	–
Lamotrigine	+	+	?	+	+	+
Oxcarbazepine	+	+/–	–	–	–	–
Vigabatrin	+	+/–	+	+/–	–	+/–

Note: + Efficacious; – No efficacy proven; +/– Mixed results among population; ? Needs further evaluation

TABLE 4: Lamotrigine dose recommendations (mg/day) for children.

Concurrent AED	Weeks 1 and 2	Weeks 3 and 4	Usual maintenance dose
EIAED	2.0 mg/kg/day	5.0 mg/kg/day	5–15 mg/kg/day
Monotherapy	0.5 mg/kg/day	1.0 mg/kg/day	2–8 mg/kg/day
Valproic acid	0.2 mg/kg/day	0.5 mg/kg/day	1–5 mg/kg/day

(EIAED: enzyme-inducing antiepileptic drug; AED: antiepileptic drug)

begin with 0.1 mg/kg/day for first 2 weeks and increased by 0.1 mg/kg/day every 2 weeks until an optimal effect is reached. The most common adverse events are somnolence, dizziness, and headache.

Topiramate is useful both as monotherapy and adjunctive drug in the treatment of LGS, infantile spasms, and refractory partial seizures. It acts by three mechanisms, i.e., blocking the voltage-dependent sodium channels, potentiation of GABA-mediated effects, and antagonism of excitatory glutamate receptors. The initial dose is 1 mg/kg/day with target maintenance doses of 3–6 mg/kg/day and can even be increased up to 10 mg/kg/day according to the need. The side effects include somnolence, fatigue, abnormal thinking, headache, diplopia, ataxia, psychomotor slowing, speech difficulty, paresthesia, impaired concentration, and confusion. Weight loss and nephrolithiasis are the other side effects.

Vigabatrin is a specific, reversible GABA aminotransaminase inhibitor. In children, it has been proved to be safe and efficacious in the treatment of partial seizures, generalized seizures, and in some patients with LGS. It is particularly useful in the treatment of infantile spasms. Vigabatrin is the drug of choice especially in symptomatic cases with tuberous sclerosis. 50% respond in a few days. Steroids (ACTH or prednisolone) are tried for nonresponders or relapsing cases. VPA and benzodiazepines also control infantile spasms in 50–60% of cases.

Epilepsy Surgery

Epilepsy surgery is becoming an increasingly used therapy for young children and infants with severe, medically intractable seizures. The most commonly performed surgery in older children is temporal lobe resection while nontemporal lobe resections, corpus callosotomies, and hemispherectomies are more commonly performed in younger children. Surgery should be considered early in the course of the catastrophic seizure disorders of childhood—infantile spasms such as Sturge-Weber syndrome and Rasmussen's encephalitis.

■ PROGNOSIS

The idiopathic epilepsies with partial seizures (Rolandic epilepsy, partial childhood epilepsy with occipital paroxysms) have a good prognosis for spontaneous remission and for control with medication. The prognosis for remission for childhood absence epilepsies is about 80% with appropriate therapy while control is poor with juvenile absence epilepsies. The remission rate for juvenile myoclonic epilepsy is 70-80% with continued therapy. However, after discontinuation of the medication, seizures recur in about 70% of the patients.

The incidence of intractable seizures is high with symptomatic epilepsies with static or progressive disorders. Symptomatic West syndrome has a bad prognosis while cryptogenic form has a favorable prognosis. Similarly, the prognosis of LGS varies according to whether it has a cryptogenic or symptomatic background. In Landau-Kleffner syndrome, though the prognosis for disappearance of seizures is favorable, the prognosis for aphasia is poor. The prognosis for reflex epilepsies is good both with appropriate AED therapy and avoidance of the specific precipitating stimuli. Febrile seizures are age limited and improvement occurs with time.

■ STATUS EPILEPTICUS

Status epilepticus is defined as two or more seizures without regaining consciousness in between or a continuous seizure lasting for more than 5 minutes. Physiologically, status epilepticus is defined as recurrent seizures without complete normalization of neurochemical and physical homeostasis in the brain between seizures. Children with prior neurological abnormalities are more susceptible.

The etiology of status epilepticus varies. Status epilepticus can occur in the setting of an acute illness, in patients with established epilepsy, or for the first time as unprovoked seizures.

Remote symptomatic, acute symptomatic, and febrile seizures are the major causes of status epilepticus in most children while the cause for status epilepticus is unknown in 24-39% of the children. Progressive encephalopathy is the cause in 2-6% of the cases. Overall mortality varies from 3-10% with almost all fatalities associated with acute CNS insults or progressive neurologic disorders.

Neurologic sequelae in children with idiopathic or febrile status is rare. Neurologically normal children with status epilepticus as their first unprovoked seizure have the same risk of experiencing subsequent seizures of any type as children who present with a brief first seizure.

The risk of recurrent episodes of convulsive status is 50% in neurologically abnormal children but very low in normal children. The favorable outcome of status epilepticus in children may be related to the therapy and the resistance of the immature brain to damage from seizures.

Management of Status Epilepticus

The goals in the management of status epilepticus include stopping seizure activity as quickly as possible to protect the neurons from seizure-induced damage and allowing full recovery from the episode of status epilepticus.

The general measures include stabilization of airway, with adequate respiratory support, and maintenance of blood pressure.

Then the blood sample should be collected for evaluation of hematological and serum chemistry parameters and determination of AED levels.

Plasma glucose should be determined and glucose should be given only in the presence of documented hypoglycemia. Hyperpyrexia should be corrected. Status-induced transient acidosis should not be corrected as the pH rapidly normalizes once status epilepticus is controlled. Supplement oxygen may be helpful.

Emergency Drug Treatment

Premonitory Stage

Diazepam 0.25–0.5 mg/kg IV or 0.5 to 0.75 mg/kg/rectally, repeated once 15 minutes later if status continues to threaten or lorazepam 0.1 mg/kg IV bolus if seizures continue or status develops.

Stage of Early Status

Lorazepam 0.1 mg/kg IV bolus (if not given earlier) is given if status continues after 30 minutes.

Stage of Established Status

Phenobarbital IV infusion of 15–20 mg/kg at a rate of <100 mg/min or phenytoin IV infusion of 20 mg/kg at a rate of <25 mg/min if status continues after 30–60 minutes.

Stage of Refractory Status

General anesthesia with either propranolol 2 mg/kg IV bolus, repeated if necessary, and then followed by a continuous infusion of 5–10 mg/kg/hour, initially to 1–3 mg/kg/hour when seizures have been controlled for 12 hours, the drug dosages should be slowly tapered over 12 hours or thiopental 100–250 mg IV bolus given over 20 seconds, with further 50 mg boluses every 2–3 minutes until seizures are controlled, followed by a continuous IV infusion to maintain a burst suppression pattern on the EEG (usually 3–5 mg/kg/hour). Thiopental should be slowly withdrawn 12 hours after the last seizure.

> **CAUSES OF REFRACTORY EPILEPSY**
> - Inadequate serum level of drug
> - *Drug toxicity:* Phenytoin
> - *Metabolic:* Inborn errors
> - Incorrect identification
> - Paradoxical reaction of medications

BIBLIOGRAPHY

1. Abend NS, Loddenkemper T. Management of pediatric status epilepticus. Curr Treat Options Neurol. 2014;16(7):301.
2. Chu-Shore CJ, Thiele EA. New drugs for pediatric epilepsy. Semin Pediatr Neurol. 2010;17(4):214-23.
3. Fenichel GM. Paroxysmal disorders. Clinical Peditric Neurology: A Signs and Symptoms Approach, 7th edition. Amsterdam, Netherlands: Elsevier Saunders; 2013.
4. Frank LM, Shinnar S, Hesdorffer DC, Shinnar RC, Pellock JM, Gallentine W, et al. Cerebrospinal fluid findings in children with fever-associated status epilepticus: Results of the consequences of prolonged febrile seizures (FEBSTAT) study. J Pediatr. 2012; 161(6):1169-71.
5. Ostrowsky K, Arzimanoglou A. Outcome and prognosis of status epilepticus in children. Semin Pediatr Neurol. 2010;17(3):195-200.

CASE 52

Febrile Convulsions

■ PRESENTING COMPLAINTS

A 10-month-old girl was brought with the complaint of:
- Cough and cold since 3 days
- Fever since 2 days
- Irritable since 1 day
- Abnormal movements and uprolling of the eyeball since 20 minutes

History of Presenting Complaints

A 10-month-old girl was brought to the casualty with a history of convulsions. Convulsion was generalized. It involved both upper and lower limbs. It was tonic and clonic type with uprolling of eyeballs. According to the mother, the convulsions lasted for 5 minutes. By the time child came to hospital, there were no convulsions. But the child was irritable. Mother also told that her daughter had been getting treatment for cough, cold, and fever since two days by the family doctor.

Past History of the Patient

The patient was the first sibling of a non-consanguineous marriage. She was born at full term by normal delivery. Her birth weight was 3 kg. There was no significant postnatal event. The child started to take the breastfeeds immediately. She was on breast milk exclusively for 3 months. Weaning was started as per the advice of the family doctor from 4th month onward. Developmental milestones were normal. There was no family history of convulsions. There was no history of similar illness.

■ EXAMINATION

On examination, the child was moderately built and moderately nourished. She was alert, irritable, and crying. Anthropometric

---

CASE AT A GLANCE

Basic Findings
- Length : 72 cm (75th centile)
- Weight : 8.5 kg (75th centile)
- Temperature : 39°C
- Pulse rate : 130 beats/min
- Respiratory rate : 32 breaths/min
- Blood pressure : 60/40 mm Hg

Positive Findings

History:
- Convulsions
- Fever
- Cough and cold

Examination:
- Irritable child
- Febrile
- Convulsions

Investigation:
- Anemia
- TLC: 16,000 cells/cumm
- CSF: Normal
- CT scan: Normal

measurements included that the length of the child was 72 cm (75th centile) and the weight was 8.5 kg (75th centile). The head circumference was 42 cm.

The child was febrile—39°C. The pulse rate was 130 beats per minute, the respiratory rate was 32 breaths per minute. The blood pressure recorded was 60/40 mm Hg. There was pallor, no lymphadenopathy, no edema, and no cyanosis.

There were signs of rhinitis. Throat examination was normal. Respiratory system revealed the presence of crepitations at base of the lung. All other systemic examinations were normal. Pupils were round, reactive, and dilated. There was no involvement of motor and sensory systems. There was no cranial nerve involvement.

■ INVESTIGATION

- *Hemoglobin:* 9 g/dL
- *TLC:* 16,000 cells/mm^3
- *DLC:* P_{80} L_{18} M_2
- *ESR:* 18 mm at the 1st hour
- *CSF:* Normal
- *CT scan:* Normal

■ DISCUSSION

The child had convulsions lasting for 5 minutes. The convulsions are of generalized and clonic–tonic type. At the time of convulsion, the child had fever as a result of the upper respiratory tract infection. There was no loss of consciousness and postictal drowsiness. As the CNS examination and CT scan were normal, the diagnosis of febrile convulsion was made.

Febrile seizures (FSs) are seizures that occur between the ages of 6 months and 6 years with a temperature of 38°C (100.4°F) or higher, that are not the result of CNS infection or any metabolic imbalance, and that occur in the absence of a history of prior afebrile seizures.

A simple FS is a primarily generalized, usually tonic–clonic, attack associated with fever lasting for a maximum of 15 minutes and not recurrent within a 24-hour period. A complex FS is more prolonged (>15 minutes), focal, and/or reoccurs within 24 hours. Febrile status epilepticus is a FS lasting longer than 30 minutes. Some use the term simple "febrile seizure plus" for those with recurrent FSs within 24 hours. Most patients with simple FSs have a very short postictal state and usually return to their baseline normal behavior and consciousness within minutes of the seizure. But it is frequent if the temperature rises abruptly. There are two types of febrile convulsions: One is simple typical febrile convulsions, and the second is atypical febrile convulsions.

■ PATHOPHYSIOLOGY OF FEBRILE SEIZURES

Several hypotheses have been proposed to explain the causation of FSs. It is believed that in genetically predisposed children, an increase in brain temperature leads to perturbation of temperature-sensitive ion channels that in turn cause increased neuronal firing. Moreover, interleukin-1β acts as both a pyrogen and seizure provocator, acting at the glutamate pathway. Interleukin-1β is also an NMDA agonist. Last, but not the least, hyperthermia-induced brain alkalosis is also believed to result in neuronal excitability.

■ CLINICAL FEATURES (FIG. 1)

By definition, FSs occur between the ages of 6 months and 6 years. Although there are exceptions, children of ages that fall outside this range are less likely to have FSs.

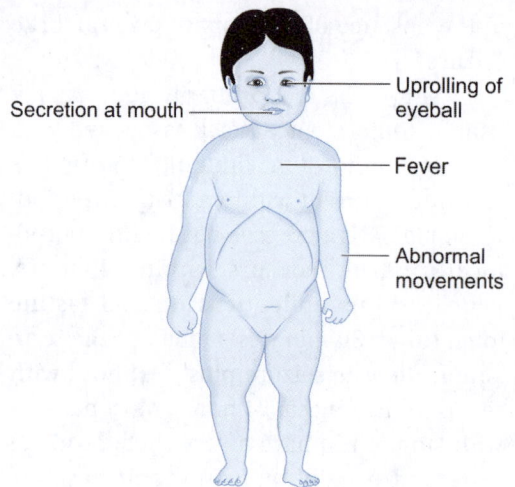

Fig. 1: Clinical features.

A high incidence of epilepsy has been reported in children over 6 years of age with FSs and these seizures have been called epileptic seizures precipitated by fever. These children have other risk factors for the development of epilepsy.

The most commonly associated illnesses are upper respiratory infections, gastrointestinal infections, otitis media, and roseola. A viral infection is implicated in more than 80% of cases. The primary human herpes virus types 6 and 7 have recently been implicated as possible specific causal agents. A bacterial pathogen was suspected in children with FSs. Shigellosis is a bacterial gastrointestinal infection associated with FSs.

Simple versus Complex Febrile Seizures

The idea of separating FSs into simple and complex subgroups originated from the description of clinical risk factors that predicted a much higher probability of chronic epilepsy according to seizure subtype. The risk factors include:
- Seizure for >15 minutes
- Focal seizure manifestation
- More than 1 seizure in 24 hours
- Abnormal neurologic status
- Afebrile seizure in a parent or sibling.

Simple FSs occur within 24 hours of the onset of the temperature. These seizures usually last for about <10 minutes. The convulsions are generalized type. But more than one episode may occur. There are no postictal neurological deficits. There may be a family history of febrile convulsions. EEG will be normal. There may be no further seizures. 3–10% of the children may develop recurrent seizures. These are commonly seen between the ages of 6 months and 6 years.

Atleast 80% of FSs are generalized and simple. However, a FS can be of partial or different generalized type. In addition, tonic, clonic, and even atonic episodes may characterize FSs. Some children have multiple seizures within a 24-hours period. Prolonged seizures have been reported in children. One-half of these seizures lasted >30 minutes. Febrile status epilepticus occurs more commonly in girls with focal seizures.

Convulsions due to organic neurological damage are precipitated with fever as the cerebral threshold for the seizure is reduced with the elevation of the temperature. Infections of the CNS are important causes of convulsion associated with fever. Atypical febrile convulsions include unilateral seizure, multiple convulsions in the same febrile illness, Todd's paralysis, and status epilepticus.

When complex FSs occur, the risk of epilepsy increases to 50%, when all risk factors are present. The exact mode of inheritance of FSs is uncertain. A positive family history can be elicited in 25–40% of children. Some studies show a high concordance rate in monozygotic versus dizygotic twins. In a large family with multiple affected individuals, linkage has been made to a locus on chromosome 8q13-21.

One-third of children with FSs experience a second episode. The most important identified risk factor is the age of onset. Studies have confirmed that 50% of children younger than 1 year of age experienced a recurrence. Additional risk factors include a history of FSs in a first degree consanguineous, seizures induced by low-grade fever, and a brief duration between the onset of fever and the convulsion.

The greatest concern for the family following their child's FS is the risk of developing epilepsy, which is defined as two unprovoked seizures. The presence of a family history of epilepsy, neurodevelopmental retardation, and atypical episode of attacks increases the recurrent risk of febrile episodes and subsequent epilepsy. Three risk factors for unprovoked seizures were identified in these study are:

- Abnormal neurologic examination prior to the first FS
- A history of afebrile seizure in a parent or sibling
- A complex first FS

The risk of developing into epilepsy in febrile convulsions is more if the attack has lasted for more than 30 minutes, the convulsion is focal, or there are abnormal EEG findings.

ESSENTIAL DIAGNOSTIC POINTS

- Fever
- Abnormal movements of limbs and body
- Child is unconscious
- No postictal residuals
- More common between 6 months and 6 years

GENERAL FEATURES

- Fever
- Generalized convulsion
- Common between 6 months and 6 years

DIAGNOSIS

Electroencephalogram

In many cases, if an electroencephalogram (EEG) is indicated, it is delayed until or repeated after more than 2 weeks have passed. An EEG should, therefore, generally be restricted to special cases in which epilepsy is highly suspected, and generally, it should be used to delineate the type of epilepsy rather than to predict its occurrence. If an EEG is done, it should be performed for atleast 20 minutes in wakefulness and in sleep according to international guidelines to avoid misinterpretation and drawing of erroneous conclusions.

At times, if the patient does not recover immediately from a seizure, then an EEG can help distinguish between ongoing seizure activity and prolonged postictal period, sometimes termed a nonepileptic twilight state. EEG can also be helpful in patients who present with febrile status epilepticus because the presence of focal slowing pattern present on the EEG obtained within 72 hours of the status has been shown to be highly associated with MRI evidence of acute hippocampal injury.

Blood Studies

Blood studies (serum electrolytes, calcium, phosphorus, magnesium, and complete blood count) are not routinely recommended in the workup of a child with a first simple FS. Blood glucose should be determined in children with prolonged postictal obtundation or with poor oral intake (prolonged fasting).

Serum electrolyte values may be abnormal in children after a FS, but this should be suggested by precipitating or predisposing conditions elicited in the history and reflected in abnormalities of the physical examination. If clinically indicated (e.g., in a history or physical examination suggestive of dehydration), these tests should be performed. A low sodium level is associated with a higher risk of recurrence of the FS within the following 24 hours.

Lumbar puncture (LP) should be done for CSF analysis. This may help to diagnose intracranial infection. LP should be performed in children under the age of 18 months with the first attack of febrile convulsions.

The most important aspect of diagnosis is to rule out an underlying infection of the CNS. Seizures associated with meningitis are usually brief generalized, tonic–clonic seizures similar to simple FSs.

> **LABORATORY SALIENT FINDINGS**
> - Evaluation of underlying cause of fever
> - Electroencephalogram (EEG)
> - Computed tomography (CT) scan
> - Magnetic resonance imaging (MRI)
> - *Lumbar puncture:* Cerebrospinal fluid (CSF) analysis

■ TREATMENT

Temperature Control

Because the majority of FSs are simple, the physician will assess the child in the postictal state to determine the etiology of the fever. The initial step should be to measure the temperature and if the child is still febrile, attempts should be made to lower it to avoid recurrences. The acetaminophen (15 mg/kg/dose) should be given every 4–6 hours when the rectal temperature exceeds 37.9°C; if the child is vomiting, acetaminophen may be given rectally. Anti-inflammatory drugs can also be used.

In a prospective study, which compared the efficacy of acetaminophen syrup (10 mg/kg/dose) with that of ibuprofen syrup (5 mg/kg/dose), children treated with ibuprofen had a significantly greater seizure reduction.

Treatment of Acute Attack

The drug of choice is diazepam, which can be given parenterally at doses of 0.5–1 mg/kg. Its short half-life is preferable as compared to the prolonged effects of parenteral phenobarbital. In cases where FSs recur frequently, it is appropriate to provide the rectal diazepam to shorten the duration of seizures.

This condition should be managed by prompt reduction of temperature. The intravenous line should be started to maintain hydration and to give anticonvulsant medications. Injection of diazepam (0.2–0.3 mg/kg dose), slow intravenous, with the maximum dose of 5 mg/dose is given to control convulsions. Phenobarbitone can be given in the dose of 20 mg/kg. When given intravenously, action starts in 5–10 minutes, but the peak concentration in brain is reached in 30–60 minutes. Paraldehyde can be tried per rectally. It is diluted with olive oil when given per rectally.

If the seizure lasts for longer than 5 minutes, acute treatment with diazepam, lorazepam, or midazolam is needed. Rectal diazepam is often prescribed to be given at the time of recurrence of FSs lasting longer than 5 minutes.

Alternatively, buccal or intranasal midazolam may be used and is often preferred by parents. Intravenous benzodiazepines, phenobarbital, phenytoin, or valproate may be needed in the case of febrile status epilepticus. If the parents are very anxious concerning their child's seizures, intermittent oral diazepam (0.3 mg/kg every 8 hour during fever) or intermittent rectal diazepam (0.5 mg/kg, administered as a rectal suppository every 8 hour), can be given during febrile illnesses. Intermittent oral nitrazepam, clobazam, and clonazepam (0.1 mg/kg/day) have also been used. Such therapies help to reduce, but do not eliminate, the risks of recurrence of FSs.

Other therapies have included continuous phenobarbital (4-5 mg/kg/day in 1 or 2 divided doses) and continuous valproate (20-30 mg/kg/day in 2 or 3 divided doses). In the vast majority of cases, it is not justified to use continuous therapy owing to the risk of side effects and lack of demonstrated long-term benefits, even if the recurrence rate of FSs is expected to be decreased by these drugs.

Antipyretics can decrease the discomfort of the child but do not reduce the risk of having a recurrent FS, probably because the seizure often occurs as the temperature is rising or falling. Chronic antiepileptic therapy may be considered for children with a high risk for later epilepsy. Currently, available data indicate that the possibility of future epilepsy does not change with or without antiepileptic therapy. Iron deficiency is associated with an increased risk of FSs, and thus screening for that problem and treating it appears appropriate.

Prophylaxis

Recurrence risk is 12% if there are no risk factors. It is 75-100% if there are risk factors. The risk factors include disadvantages of social environment, seizure disorder of any type in first-degree relative, onset before the age of 15 months, complex FSs, and suboptimal neurodevelopment. Prophylaxis is indicated in children with one or more risk factors. Three groups of anticonvulsants may be effective in preventing FSs: Barbiturates, benzodiazepines, and valproic acid.

Phenobarbital

Until recently, phenobarbital was considered the drug of choice for the prophylaxis of FSs. When therapeutic levels of the drugs were maintained, it led to a significant reduction in the risk of recurrence. However, phenobarbital is poorly tolerated and compliance is problematic. Daily administration of phenobarbital results in hyperkinesis, moodiness, irritability, sleep disturbances, and decreased intelligence.

Benzodiazepines

As a result of their pharmacokinetic properties, benzodiazepines can be effective when used to prevent FSs intermittently. They are rapidly absorbed and have a short, effective half-life. Both oral diazepam and nitrazepam have been effective in preventing FS recurrences compared to placebo, even in children at high risk for FSs. However, side effects, such as ataxia, somnolence, agitation, irritability, and lethargy, should be expected.

Valproic Acid

Valproic acid has been reported to be effective against FSs. Because of the risk of serious side effects such as liver failure in young children, valproic acid is not recommended as preventive therapy for FSs. However, in children with mixed febrile and afebrile seizures and children with a clear underlying epileptic syndrome, valproic acid is the drug of choice.

Continuous prophylaxis is advised in children with CNS disease, recurrent atypical seizures, and family history of epilepsy. The drugs used are sodium valproate (10-20 mg/kg/day) or phenobarbitone (3-5 mg/kg/day). The duration of therapy is 1-2 years or 6 years of age whichever comes earlier. Carbamazepine and phenytoin are ineffective.

■ FUTURE RISK OF EPILEPSY

Children with simple FSs have 1% risk of developing epilepsy by the age of 7 years (same as the general population) and 2.4% by 25 years of age

Children who have had multiple simple FSs are younger than 12 months at the time of their first FS and have a family history of epilepsy are at higher risk.

Risk of epilepsy after complex FSs depends on the number of complex features:
- With 1 complex feature: 6–8%
- With 2 complex features: 17–22%
- With 3 and more features: 49%

Risk factors for developing subsequent epilepsy include family history of epilepsy, any neurodevelopmental problem, prolonged or focal FSs, and febrile status epilepticus.

PARENT EDUCATION

Control of fever with antipyretic treatment may limit recurrences, and although initial temperature rise can be missed, the same applies for intermittent benzodiazepine treatment. The bottom line is that parents must feel comfortable with the final decision and treatment should not be imposed. There is no evidence that preventing new FSs is associated with a more favorable prognosis than shortening the duration of seizures.

CONCLUSION

Febrile seizures are a frequent and benign disorder. In more than 80% of children, they represent the expression of a genetically inherited response to fever. For these children, no treatment is required, and parents should be reassured. Rarely, FSs represent early evidence for later epilepsy.

The majority of children with risk factors for later epilepsy do not develop recurrent unprovoked seizures. EEG is not predictive of later epilepsy in children with FSs. Benzodiazepines can be used to shorten the duration of FSs, particularly if families live in remote areas and do not have access to immediate care. Only very rarely should daily prophylactic anticonvulsant therapy be considered for use in children with FSs.

BIBLIOGRAPHY

1. Frank LM, Shinnar S, Hesdorffer DC, Shinnar RC, Pellock JM, Gallentine W, et al. Cerebrospinal fluid findings in children with fever associated status epilepticus: results of the consequences of prolonged febrile seizures (FEBSTAT) study. J Pediatr. 2012;161(6):1169-71.
2. Shinnar S, Hesdorffer DC, Nordli DR Jr, Pellock JM, O'Dell C, Lewis DV, et al. Phenomenology of prolonged febrile seizures: results of the FEBSTAT study. Neurology. 2008;71(3):170-6.
3. Subcommittee on Febrile Seizures; American Academy of Pediatrics. Neurodiagnostic evaluation of the child with simple febrile seizure. Pediatrics. 2011;127(2):389-94.

CASE 53

Guillain–Barré Syndrome

PRESENTING COMPLAINTS

A 12-year-old boy was brought with the complaints of:
- Headache since 1 week
- Vomiting since 2 days
- Unable to walk and move the lower limbs since 1 day

History of Presenting Complaints

A 12-year-old boy was brought to the hospital with a history of headaches and vomiting. Headache was diffuse and stabbing in nature. Headache never used to be relieved by analgesics. It was associated with vomiting. Vomiting was insidious in nature. There was also a history of pain in lower back and in the arms. His mother had noticed that her son was having difficulty in walking. The boy was finding it very difficult to move his lower limbs. Boy complained that he was feeling pins and needles in the legs. 2 weeks back, the child had cough, cold, and fever. This was treated by his family doctor.

Past History of the Patient

He was the eldest sibling of a consanguineous marriage. The boy was born at full term by normal delivery. His birth weight was 3 kg. He was on breastfeeds immediately after the delivery. There were no significant postnatal events. His developmental milestones were normal. His performance at school was good.

CASE AT A GLANCE

Basic Findings
- Height : 138 cm (40th centile)
- Weight : 36 kg (50th centile)
- Temperature : 38°C
- Pulse rate : 96 beats/min
- Respiratory rate : 20 breaths/min
- Blood pressure : 90/70 mm Hg

Positive Findings

History:
- Headache
- Vomiting
- Difficulty in walking
- Pain in the back

Examination:
- Hypotonia
- Gross motor weakness in legs
- Gradual deterioration

Investigation:
- *Cerebrospinal fluid examination:* Moderate increase in protein and pleocytosis

EXAMINATION

On examination, the boy was moderately built and moderately nourished. Anthropometric measurements included that his height was 138 cm (40th centile) and his weight was 36 kg (50th centile).

He was febrile. The pulse rate was 96 beats per minute, the respiratory rate was 20 breaths per minute. The blood pressure recorded was 90/70 mm Hg. There was no pallor, no lymphadenopathy, no cyanosis, and no clubbing.

There was considerable weakness in the lower limbs. There was gross motor weakness in the legs. But there was no wasting. Generalized hypotonia was present. No tendon reflexes could be elicited. The left arm was also involved and he was unable to lift a spoon. His condition involved the trunk muscles and arms leading to complete paraplegia. Bilateral facial weakness was present. The boy even developed difficulty in swallowing. Hence, the nasogastric tube was given. Later, he required mechanical ventilation.

INVESTIGATION

- *Hemoglobin:* 12 g/dL
- *TLC:* 9,600 cells/mm
- *DLC:* P_{70} L_{25} M_0 E_4 B_1
- *ESR:* 30 mm in the 1st hour
- *Mantoux test:* Negative
- *Cerebrospinal fluid examination:* Moderate increase in protein (60 mg/dL); Pleocytosis (50–100 cells/mm^3)
- *CT scan:* Normal

DISCUSSION

The boy developed paresthesia in both lower limbs and in the left arm after a viral infection. Gradually, it made him unable to walk around as a result of muscle weakness and hypotonia. Later, it involved all the limbs producing quadriplegia. There is also involvement of the trunk muscles producing respiratory distress.

The Guillain–Barré syndrome (GBS) is an acute, monophasic, demyelinating neuropathy in which abnormal immune responses are directed against peripheral nerves. There will be an antecedent viral infection 2 weeks before the onset of weakness. It usually follows a viral infection such as infectious mononucleosis, mumps, measles, coxsackie, and influenza. Respiratory tract infections are most common and the remainder are mainly gastrointestinal infections. Enteritis caused by specific strains of *Campylobacter jejuni* is the inciting disease.

The basic myelin protein is altered and rendered immunogenic by the infection. This immune mechanism may cause demyelination. *Campylobacter* infection has been strongly associated with severe forms and acute motor axonal neuropathy (AMAN) syndrome. Other subtypes include acute inflammatory demyelinating polyneuropathy (AIDP), acute motor and sensory axonal neuropathy (AMSN), and Miller Fisher syndrome (MFS).

The paralysis usually follows a nonspecific gastrointestinal or respiratory infection by approximately 10 days. The original infection might have caused only gastrointestinal (especially *Campylobacter jejuni* but also *Helicobacter pylori*) or respiratory tract (especially *Mycoplasma pneumoniae*) or systemic (Zika virus) symptoms. Consumption of undercooked poultry, unpasteurized milk, and contaminated water are the main sources of gastrointestinal infections. GBS is reported following the administration of vaccines against rabies, influenza, and poliomyelitis (oral) and following the administration of conjugated meningococcal vaccine, particularly serogroup C. Additional infectious precursors of GBS include mononucleosis, Lyme disease, cytomegalovirus, and *H. influenzae* [for the (MFS)].

ESSENTIAL DIAGNOSTIC POINTS
- Delayed hypersensitivity and T-cell mediated antiganglioside antibodies
- Nonspecific respiratory and gastrointestinal symptoms
- Symmetric weakness of lower limbs, trunk, and face
- *Ataxia, ophthalmoplegia and cranial nerves:* IX, XI, III, VI

PATHOLOGY

The pathologic findings are characterized by a marked segmental demyelination. In some cases, there is an early antibody attack on myelin, whereas in others the process is mainly inflammatory. Both processes lead to a macrophage response that causes myelin destruction.

It is characterized by symmetric weakness of the muscles, diminished reflexes, and sensory involvement, i.e., usually paresthesia. Neurological manifestations usually begin after the viral illness that has already subsided. It is probably due to the fact that peripheral lymphocytes are sensitized to a protein component of the myelin. These migrate into the peripheral nerve and cause myelin breakdown.

CLINICAL FEATURES (FIG. 1)

Guillain-Barré syndrome is an autoimmune disorder often considered a postinfectious polyneuropathy involving mainly motor but also sensory and sometimes autonomic nerves.

The onset is gradual and progresses over days or weeks, the process plateaus in 1-28 days. Particularly in cases with an abrupt onset, tenderness on palpation and pain in muscles are common in the initial stages. Affected children are irritable. Weakness can progress to inability or refusal to walk and later to flaccid tetraplegia. The maximal severity of weakness is usually reached by 4 weeks after onset.

Initial symptoms include numbness and paresthesia, followed by weakness. There may be associated neck, back, buttock, and leg pain. Weakness usually begins in the lower extremities and progressively involves the trunk, the upper limbs, and, finally, the bulbar muscles—a pattern known as Landry ascending paralysis. Proximal and distal muscles are involved relatively symmetrically, but asymmetry is found 9% of patients.

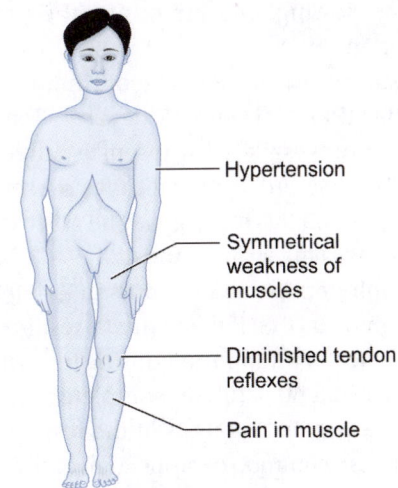

Fig. 1: Clinical features.

Characteristically, it is symmetric, although minor differences between the sides are not rare. In about 50% of patients, the weakness is mostly distal, whereas in about 15% the proximal muscles are more extensively involved.

Paresthesias occur in some cases. Cranial nerve palsies can appear at any time during the illness. The facial nerve is involved most commonly. Oculomotor and other cranial nerve involvement is also seen occasionally.

Weakness progresses over days or weeks, the clinical nadir occurring in less than 4 weeks. Approximately 60% of children lose the ability to walk at some point in their illness; a small proportion progress to flaccid tetraplegia.

Bulbar involvement occurs in about 50% of cases and can result in respiratory insufficiency. Dysphagia and facial weakness can be the signs of impending respiratory failure, interfering with saliva control and swallowing, and increasing the risk of aspiration.

Urinary retention or incontinence is a complication in about 20% of cases. Tendon reflexes are diminished or absent usually early in the course but are sometimes preserved until later, and this finding may be misleading in arriving at an early diagnosis.

Respiratory paralysis occurs in 20–30% of children with GBS. If the patients' respiratory function can be supported during the critical time of profound paralysis, complete recovery can be expected. Paralysis of the respiratory muscles is a common complication in severely involved patients, but even in the absence of respiratory symptoms vital capacity can be impaired.

The autonomic nervous system may also be involved in some cases. Profuse sweating hypertension, postural hypotension, cardiac arrhythmias, and gastrointestinal dysfunctions are manifestations of autonomic dysfunction.

There is associated facial weakness and sometimes bulbar palsy may occur. It may occur at any age after 6 months. But it is commonly seen between the age group of 5 and 9 years.

Distal sensory loss may be detectable and sensory ataxia can occasionally dominate the picture. Tendon reflexes are absent. Occasionally, extensor plantar responses are found. Headache, neck pain, back pain, and limb pain are common in acute phase.

Subtypes of GBS include AIDP and AMAN; these are distinguished by findings on nerve conduction studies and an associated pattern of antiganglioside antibodies. Localized forms of GBS also occur and include a pattern of facial diplegia with paresthesias and a pattern of pharyngeal-cervical-brachial weakness. MFS is an uncommon GBS variant associated with acute external (and occasionally internal) ophthalmoplegia, ataxia, and areflexia. The 6th cranial nerve is most often involved in MFS. Although areflexia is seen in MFS, patients have no or only very mild lower extremity weakness, compared with GBS.

Chronic inflammatory demyelinating polyradiculoneuropathy (CIDP), sometimes called chronic inflammatory relapsing polyneuritis, is a more chronic, slowly progressive, acquired inflammatory neuropathy with some clinical overlap with GBS.

Symptoms such as weakness and paresthesia develop over more than 4–6 weeks, recur intermittently (relapsing), or progress slowly over periods of months to years. Weakness is generally both proximal and distal, and variably severe. Hyporeflexia or areflexia is almost universal.

This variant of GBS is characterized by external ophthalmoplegia, ataxia, and areflexia. Bilateral facial paresis and internal ophthalmoplegia are other manifestations. Symptoms remain severe for 1–2 weeks before recovery starts. Recovery is generally complete. At present, it is a matter of dispute whether it should be distinguished from brain stem encephalitis.

The clinical course is usually benign and spontaneous recovery begins within 2-week. Most patients regain full muscular strength, although some are left with residual weakness. The tendon reflexes are usually the last function to recover. The improvement usually follows a gradient inverse to the direction of involvement, with the recovery of bulbar function first and lower extremities weakness resolving last.

Congenital GBS is very rare, manifesting as generalized hypotonia, weakness, and areflexia in an affected neonate, fulfilling all electrophysiologic and cerebrospinal fluid (CSF) criteria and in the absence of maternal neuromuscular disease. Treatment is not always required.

■ DIAGNOSIS

A CSF study is essential for diagnosis. An elevation in the CSF protein content is characteristic. This exceeds 45 mg/dL in 88% of affected children and rises to its maximum by 4–5 weeks, thereafter gradually returning to normal. The CSF cell count is usually normal. Fewer than 10 leucocytes/mm^3 may be found. Significant pleocytosis (100+ cells/mm^3) occurs in about 5% of patients. They disappear rapidly for CSF; CSF glucose is normal. The results of bacterial culture are negative and viral culture rarely isolates specific viruses.

Nerve conduction studies and electromyography are sensitive to early signs of peripheral nerve inflammation in GBS. Motor and sensory nerve conduction velocities are reduced to a variable extent, reflecting the patchy nature of nerve involvement in this disorder, which is also reflected in the presence of focal conduction block and dispersed responses.

Motor nerve conduction velocities are greatly reduced, and sensory nerve conduction time is often slow. Electromyography shows evidence of acute denervation of muscle. Serum creatine kinase level may be mildly elevated or normal. Antiganglioside antibodies, mainly against GM$_1$ and GD$_I$, are sometimes elevated in the serum in GBS, particularly in cases with primarily axonal rather than demyelinating neuropathy and suggest that they might play a role in disease propagation and/or recovery in some cases. Muscle biopsy is not usually required for diagnosis; specimens appear normal in early stages and show evidence of denervation atrophy in chronic stages. Sural nerve biopsy tissue shows segmental demyelination, focal inflammation, and Wallerian degeneration, but also is usually not required for diagnosis.

Serologic testing for *Campylobacter* and *Helicobacter* infection helps establish the cause if the results are positive but does not alter the course of treatment. Stool cultures are rarely positive because the infection is self-limited and only occurs for about 3 days, and the neuropathy follows the acute gastroenteritis.

Spiral MRI scanning is indicated if the clinical picture suggests the possibility of spinal cause for acute flaccid weakness, for example, spinal angioma, hydromyelia, spinal trauma, epidural abscess, or spinal tumor.

GENERAL FEATURES

- Diminished reflexes
- Paresthesia
- Facial cranial nerve involvement
- Involvement of autonomous nervous system
- Postural hypotension

LABORATORY SALIENT FINDINGS

- *Cerebrospinal fluid (CSF) analysis:* Cytoalbuminologic dissociation, high protein, normal glucose, immunoglobulin G (IgG) may be raised
- Nerve conduction velocities markedly decreased
- *Search for the cause:* Infection intoxication and autoimmune disease
- Electromyogram
- Spiral nerve biopsy

■ DIFFERENTIAL DIAGNOSIS

Differential diagnosis includes poliomyelitis, polymyositis, transverse myelitis, and cerebellar ataxia. Acute dermatitis causes diagnostic confusion, but the doubt is clarified by CPK enzymes. The toxicology screening should be done for lead, arsenic, thallium, and mercury.

■ TREATMENT

Treatment of GBS is mainly symptomatic. The potential paralysis of the respiratory muscles should be considered in each patient, and therefore the facilities for tracheostomy and mechanical respiration should be readily available.

Chronic and intermittent forms of polyneuritis appear to show a clear-cut response to steroids. High-dose pulsed methylprednisolone given intravenously is successful in some cases.

The natural course of the disease is self-limited. There will be a gradual recovery in the majority of the patients. In some patients, there will be severe paralysis at onset. It may be associated with respiratory muscles involvement. These patients definitely require treatment. Supportive therapy includes assisted ventilation. Tracheostomy should be done if necessary.

Patients in the early stages of this acute disease should be admitted to the hospital for observation because the ascending paralysis can rapidly involve respiratory muscles during the next 24 hours. Respiratory efforts (negative inspiratory force and spirometry) must be monitored to prevent respiratory failure and respiratory arrest. Patients with a slow progression might simply be observed for stabilization and spontaneous emission without treatment.

Rapidly progressive ascending paralysis is treated with intravenous immunoglobulin (IVIG), administered for 2, 3, or 5 days. A commonly recommended protocol for IVIG is 0.4 g/kg/day for 5 consecutive days, but some studies suggest that larger doses are more effective (1 g/kg/day for 2 consecutive days) and related to improved outcomes. A good response is seen with IVIG administered at the doses of 200–300 mg/kg/day for 5–10 days. Response is good if the treatment is given within 3–4 days. Recovery is complete but takes about 6 months to 2 years for restoration of full function.

Plasmapheresis has also been recommended. Controlled studies have confirmed that plasmapheresis shortens the interval to independent ambulation and the duration of mechanical ventilation, and thus plasmapheresis was recommended. Plasmapheresis and/or immunosuppressive drugs are alternatives if IVIG is ineffective. Steroids are effective. Supportive care, such as respiratory support, prevention of decubitus ulcers in children with flaccid tetraplegia, nutritional support, management, prevention of deep vein thrombosis, and treatment of secondary bacterial infections, is important.

Neuropathic pain in GBS should be treated aggressively with narcotic analgesics, where necessary, and with medications such as gabapentin. CIDP can be treated with either oral or pulsed steroids or IVIG, with refractory cases often requiring the use of other immunosuppressive medications.

An important part of the general support of the child with GBS is physiotherapy. This should be started during convalescence, and both active and passive exercises should be graduated as recovery progress.

■ PROGNOSIS

The clinical course is usually benign and spontaneous recovery begins within 2–3 weeks. Most patients regain full muscular strength, although some are left with residual weakness. The tendon reflexes are usually the last function to recover. Improvement usually follows a gradient opposite direction of involvement—bulbar function recovering first, and lower extremity weakness resolving last. Bulbar and respiratory muscle involvement can lead to death if the syndrome is not recognized and treated. Although the prognosis is generally good and the majority of children recover completely, three clinical features are predictive of poor outcome with sequelae: Cranial nerve involvement, intubation, and maximum disability at the time of presentation. The electrophysiologic features of conduction block are predictive of good outcomes.

Long-term follow-up studies of patients who recover from an attack of GBS reveal that many do have some permanent axonal loss, with or without residual clinical signs of chronic neuropathy. Easy fatigue is one of the most common chronic symptoms, but it is not the rapid fatigability of muscles seen in myasthenia gravis. Most patients with the axonal form of GBS had a slow recovery over the first 6 months and could eventually walk, although some required years to recover. Electromyography and nerve conduction velocity electrophysiologic studies do not necessarily predict the long-term outcome.

■ BIBLIOGRAPHY

1. Dumitru D, Amato A, Zwarts M. Acquired neuropathies. Electrodiagnostic Medicine, 2nd edition. Philadelphia: Hanley and Belfus; 2002.
2. Hughes RAC. Give or take? Intravenous immunoglobulin or plasma exchange for Guillain-Barré syndrome. Crit Care. 2011; 15(4):174.
3. Ryan MM. Pediatric Guillain-Barré syndrome. Curr Opin Pediatr. 2013;25(6):689-93.
4. Yuki N, Hartung HP. Guillain-Barré syndrome. N Eng J Med. 2012;366(24);2294-304.

54 CASE

Hydrocephalus

■ PRESENTING COMPLAINTS

An 8-month-old boy was brought with the complaints of:
- Big head since 2 months
- Vomiting since 1 week

History of Presenting Complaints

An 8-month-old boy was brought to the pediatric casualty with a history of bouts of vomiting. It has started 6–8 hours back. It was projectile in nature. Vomitus contained ingested food material, sometimes yellowish in color. The mother revealed a similar attack of vomiting about 3 days back. For that child had taken treatment from a general practitioner. But there was no loose motion. According to mother, her child was irritable. She had noticed that the head of the child was bigger than the other children of the same age group. There was no history of altered sensorium and convulsions.

Past History of the Patient

He was the first sibling of consanguineous marriage. He was born at term. He had been delivered by lower segment cesarean section (LSCS) for cephalopelvic disproportion. He cried immediately after the delivery. The birth weight was 2.5 kg. The head circumference was 36 cm. The length was 50 cm. He started taking breast milk. There was no significant postnatal event. He was exclusively breastfed for 3–4 months. Weaning started later with cereals and fruits gradually. His developmental milestones are a bit delayed. He had been completely immunized.

■ EXAMINATION

The child was moderately built and moderately nourished. These were signs of moderate dehydration. The head appeared larger with a prominent forehead. White part of the sclera was visible above the pupil, i.e.,

CASE AT A GLANCE

Basic Findings

Length	: 70 cm (85th centile)
Weight	: 8 kg (50th centile)
Head circumference	: 50 cm
Temperature	: 37°C
Pulse rate	: 116 beats per minute
Respiratory rate	: 20 breaths per minute
Blood pressure	: 70/50 mm Hg

Positive Findings

History:
- Vomiting
- Lower segment cesarean section delivery
- Delayed milestones

Examination:
- Large head
- Sunset sign
- Anterior fontanelle was large
- Prominent scalp veins

Investigation:
- *CT scan:* Uniform dilatation of the ventricle
- *Hemoglobin:* Decreased

sunset sign. The atrial fibrillation (AF) was large. There was splaying of sagittal suture. Transillumination test was positive.

The anthropometric measurements included the length of 70 cm (85th centile), the weight of 8 kg (50th centile). The head circumference was 50 cm.

The child was afebrile, pulse rate was 116 beats per minute, and respiratory rate 20 breaths per minute. Blood pressure was recorded 70/50 mm Hg. There was no pallor, no lymphadenopathy, and no clubbing.

■ INVESTIGATION

- *Hemoglobin:* 9 g/dL
- *TLC:* 9,600 cells/mm^3
- *ESR:* 26 mm in the 1st hour
- *Cerebrospinal fluid examination:* Normal
- *Plain X-ray skull:* Normal
- *CT scan:* Uniform dilatation of the ventricle

■ DISCUSSION

The child was brought to the hospital with a history of projectile vomiting and not taking feeds usually suggests some intracranial infection. This is again supported by the large AF and sunset sign. Other findings such as a large head, splaying of the sagittal suture, positive transillumination, and cracked pot or Macewen's sign (hearing of cracked pot on percussion of the head) helped in the diagnosis of hydrocephalus.

Hydrocephalus is an excessive accumulation of cerebrospinal fluid (CSF) in the head. The hydrocephalus is usually caused by a disturbance of the CSF flow or its absorption.

Physiology of Cerebrospinal Fluid Circulation

Hydrocephalus represents a diverse group of conditions that result from impaired circulation and/or absorption of CSF or, in rare circumstances, from increased production of CSF by a choroid plexus papilloma.

The CSF is formed primarily in the ventricular system by the choroid plexus, which is situated in the lateral, third, and fourth ventricles. Although most CSF is produced in the lateral ventricles, approximately 25% originates from extrachoroidal sources, including the capillary endothelium within the brain parenchyma. There is active neurogenic control of CSF formation because adrenergic and cholinergic nerves innervate the choroid plexus. Stimulation of the adrenergic system diminishes CSF production, whereas excitation of the cholinergic nerves may double the normal CSF production rate. In a normal child, approximately 20 mL/h of CSF is produced. The total volume of CSF approximates 50 mL in an infant and 150 mL in an adult. Most of the CSF is extraventricular. The choroid plexus forms CSF in several stages through a series of intricate steps; a plasma ultrafiltrate is ultimately processed into a secretion called the CSF.

Cerebrospinal fluid flow results from the pressure gradient that exists between the ventricular system and venous channels. Intraventricular pressure may be as high as 180 mmH$_2$O in the normal state, whereas the pressure in the superior sagittal sinus is in the range of 90 mmH$_2$O. Normally, CSF flows from the lateral ventricles through the foramina of Monro into the 3rd ventricle. It then traverses the narrow aqueduct of Sylvius which is approximately 3 mm long and 2 mm in diameter in a child to enter the fourth ventricle. The CSF exits the fourth ventricle through the paired lateral foramina of Luschka and the midline foramen of Magendie into the cisterns at the base of the brain.

Hydrocephalus resulting from the obstruction within the ventricular system is called obstructive or noncommunicating hydrocephalus. The CSF then circulates from the basal cisterns posteriorly through the cistern system and over the convexities of the cerebral hemispheres. CSF is absorbed primarily by the arachnoid villi through tight junctions of their endothelium by the pressure forces that were noted earlier. CSF is absorbed to a much lesser extent by the lymphatic channels directed to the paranasal sinuses, along nerve root sleeves, and by the choroid plexus itself. Hydrocephalus resulting from obliteration of the subarachnoid cisterns or malfunction of the arachnoid villi is called nonobstructive or communicating hydrocephalus.

The primary function of CSF is to provide buoyancy and allow the brain to float, protecting it from repetitive trauma whenever the head moves. Movement of CSF through the foramen magnum compensates for the changes that occur in cerebral blood volume with each heartbeat. Slow circulation of CSF from the ventricular system of the brain into the subarachnoid space is achieved by arterial pulsation in brain and choroid plexus and by changes in venous pressure responding to respiration, change in posture, exercise, and coughing.

Cerebrospinal fluid absorption access to the arachnoid granulations is passive and depends upon the pressure gradient between CSF and the superior sagittal sinus and the outflow resistance.

Cerebrospinal fluid is produced by active transport of Na+ ions and passive transfer of water with Na+ across the choroid plexus from the vascular compartment to the cerebral ventricle. From the lateral ventricle, it moves via the foramen of Monro, third ventricle, aqueduct of sylvius, fourth ventricle, and foramen of Luschka and Magendie into the subarachnoid cistern. It is reabsorbed into the circulation through arachnoidal granulations (arachnoid villi) in the subarachnoid space.

The conventional model holds that CSF flows through the aqueduct, fourth ventricle and foramina of Luschka and Magendie to the cisterna magna. From there the CSF flows over the surface of the cerebral hemispheres to be reabsorbed into the blood stream via the arachnoid granulations which contain the arachnoid villi.

Pathophysiology of Hydrocephalus

The major physiological abnormality in hydrocephalus is an imbalance of normal CSF formation and impaired absorption due to obstruction in flow of CSF. If CSF is retained within the cranial cavity, the intracranial pressure (ICP) must increase unless compensatory mechanisms are available; with increased ICP, any additional fluid is forced into alternate pathways for absorption.

Obstruction to CSF flow leads to the reversal of the transependymal movement of ventricular fluid into the periventricular white matter and is associated with a reduction in the local cerebral blood flow resulting in demyelination and progressive gliosis, if left untreated.

With acute hydrocephalus, the initial ventricular dilatation is accompanied by high ICP. Later, ICP subsides to remain modestly raised (10–15 mm Hg) but ventriculomegaly progresses.

Choroid plexus papilloma is the only condition in which excess production has been adequately documented to produce hydrocephalus otherwise any lesion that isolates the CSF-producing structures from major sites of absorption will result in excessive accumulation of CSF within that part of the ventricular system. During the 1st year of life, the most common causes are developmental abnormalities of brain.

Obstructive, also known as noncommunicating, hydrocephalus occurs when the CSF flow is blocked along the ventricles or along a passage connecting the ventricles, causing ventricular dilation proximal to the point of blockage. Obstruction may be congenital or acquired. Congenital hydrocephalus is estimated to occur at a rate of 1–2 per every 1,000 live births. Aqueductal stenosis, due to stenosis of the Sylvian aqueduct connecting the third and fourth ventricles, is the most frequent cause of congenital hydrocephalus. Aqueductal stenosis results from an abnormally narrow aqueduct of Sylvius that is often associated with branching or forking. In a small percentage of cases, aqueductal stenosis is inherited as a sex-linked recessive trait. These patients occasionally have minor neural tube closure defects, including spina bifida occulta. Other etiologies include complications of myelomeningoceles and Chiari malformations that obstruct CSF outflow from the fourth ventricle. Acquired causes of obstructive hydrocephalus frequently are posterior fossa tumors, including medulloblastomas, astrocytomas, or ependymomas.

Intrauterine viral infection can also produce aqueductal stenosis followed by hydrocephalus and mumps meningoencephalitis has been reported as a cause in a child. A vein of Galen malformation can expand to become large and because of its midline position, obstruct the flow of CSF. Lesions or malformations of the posterior fossa are prominent causes of hydrocephalus, including posterior fossa brain tumors, Chiari malformation, and the Dandy-Walker syndrome.

Nonobstructive, or communicating, hydrocephalus may be the result of excess CSF production or decreased absorption, which causes the dilation of the entire ventricular system. Increased production of CSF may occur in the case of a choroid plexus papilloma. Decreased absorption may result from central nervous system (CNS) hemorrhage infection, inflammation, or increased venous pressure.

Nonobstructive or communicating hydrocephalus most commonly follows a subarachnoid hemorrhage, which is usually a result of intraventricular hemorrhage in a premature infant. Blood in the subarachnoid spaces can cause obliteration of the cisterns or arachnoid villi and obstruction of CSF flow. Pneumococcal and tuberculous meningitis have a propensity to produce a thick, tenacious exudate that obstructs the basal cisterns, and intrauterine infections can also destroy the CSF pathways. Leukemic infiltrates can seed the subarachnoid space and produce communicating hydrocephalus.

In preterm infants, intraventricular hemorrhages (IVHs) commonly lead to hydrocephalus. Preterm infants have IVH as a complication. Other sources of hemorrhage, including ruptured arteriovenous malformations, ruptured aneurysms, trauma, or bleeding disorders, may cause hydrocephalus by decreasing reabsorption at the arachnoid villi.

Congenital infections, such as TORCH [Toxoplasmosis, others (syphilis, varicella zoster, and parvovirus B19), rubella, cytomegalovirus, and herpes] infections, as well as acquired bacterial or viral meningitis, may lead to decreased absorption of CSF and hydrocephalus. Increased venous pressure, as seen in the vein of Galen malformations, may lead to decreased resorption of CSF and hydrocephalus. Arnold-Chiari malformation is an important cause of communicating hydrocephalus which occurs in association with spina bifida, meningocele, and meningomyelocele.

ESSENTIAL DIAGNOSTIC POINTS

- Increased volume of cerebrospinal fluid (CSF) with progressive ventricular dilatation
- Hemorrhage, infection, tumors, and congenital malformation
- Macrocephaly and increased rate head growth
- Impaired extra ocular movements
- Hypertonia of lower limbs and generalized hyperreflexia
- Papilledema and optic atrophy in infants

■ CLINICAL FEATURES (FIG. 1)

Clinical presentation of hydrocephalus is variable and depends on many factors including the age at onset, the nature of the lesion causing obstruction, and the duration and rate of increase of the ICP.

Neonate/Infant

In an infant, an accelerated rate of enlargement of the head is the most prominent sign **(Fig. 2A)**. In addition, the AF is wide open and bulging, and the scalp veins are dilated. The forehead is broad, and the eyes might deviate downward because of impingement of the dilated suprapineal recess on the brainstem tectum, producing the setting sun eye sign. Long-tract signs, including brisk tendon reflexes, spasticity, clonus (particularly in the lower extremities), and Babinski sign, are common owing to stretching and disruption of the corticospinal fibers originating from the leg region of the motor cortex.

Head circumference at birth is about 34 cm for term infant. The head circumference normally grows by 2 cm/month for the first 3 months of the life and 1 cm/month for 4–6 months and 0.5 cm/month up to 1 year of life.

Accurate serial recording of the head circumference is essential for early diagnosis of hydrocephalus and should be supported by serial ultrasonography (USG). An increase in the head circumference in the first 3 months of life >1 cm every fortnight should arouse suspicion of hydrocephalus. Brain grows very rapidly in the first few weeks of life and therefore sagittal and coronal sutures may be separated up to 0.5 cm. This physiological separation disappears after the first fortnight of life. Persistent widening of squamoparietal sutures is not physiological and should arouse suspicion of hydrocephalus. Accurate serial recording of head circumference is required for early diagnosis of neonatal hydrocephalus. Widening of squamoparietal suture is not physiological and should be considered as a suspicion of hydrocephalus.

In neonates, rapid head enlargement may be asymptomatic until irritability, poor appetite, vomiting, and poor head control develop. Regular and accurate head circumference measurements are important in infants to detect hydrocephalus before clinical symptoms appear.

In hydrocephalus, the open fontanelle feels tense and fusion of the sutures is delayed, resulting in an enlarged head. The scalp veins become dilated because of raised ICP.

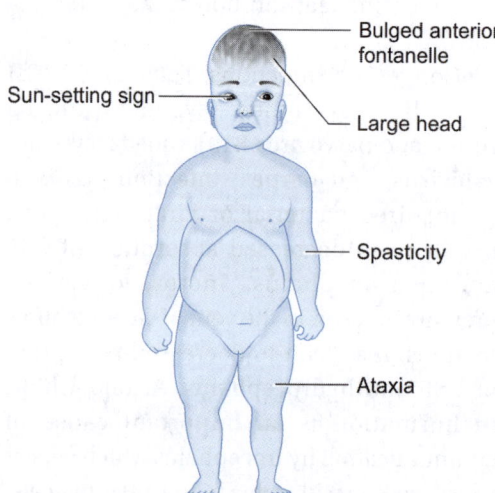

Fig. 1: Clinical features.

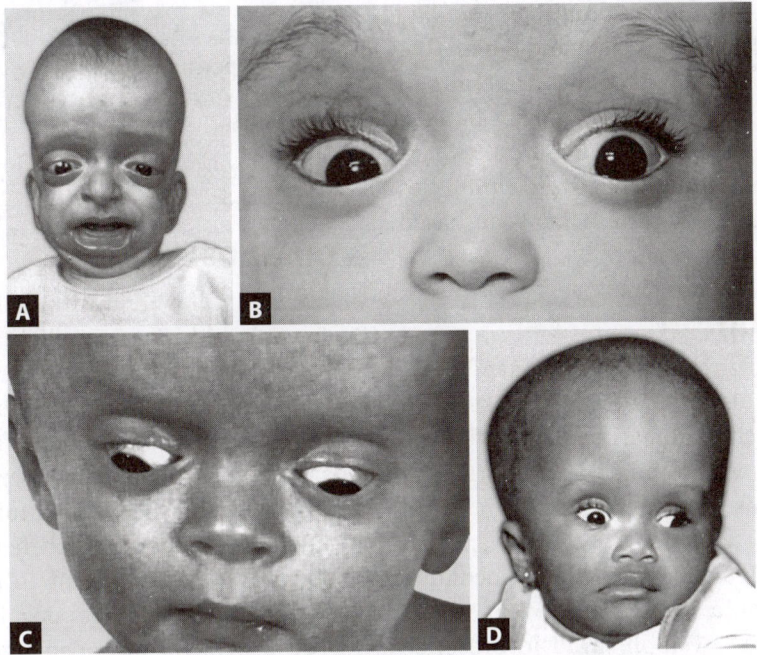

Figs. 2A to D: Hydrocephalus. (A) Enlarged head; (B to D) Setting sun sign.

Late signs include the following:
- The tympanitic sound obtained on percussing the vault of the thinned hydrocephalic skull—Macewen's sign, i.e., resonant note on percussions of the skull is noted
- The scalp vein becomes dilated because of raised ICP.
- Brilliant transillumination
- The "setting sun" sign (paralysis of upward gaze and prominence of the upper part of the sclera resulting from pressure of the dilated third ventricle on the tectum of mid-brain) **(Figs. 2B to D)**.
- Papilledema is unusual in infants.

Older Children

In an older child, the cranial sutures are less accommodating, so the signs of hydrocephalus may be subtler. Irritability, lethargy, poor appetite, and vomiting are common to both age groups, and headache is a prominent symptom in older patients. A gradual change in personality and deterioration in academic productivity suggest a slowly progressive form of hydrocephalus. With regard to other clinical signs, serial measurements of the head circumference often indicate an increased velocity of growth. Percussion of the skull might produce a cracked pot sound or Macewen's sign, indicating separation of the sutures. A foreshortened occiput suggests Chiari malformation, and a prominent occiput suggests the Dandy–Walker malformation. Papilledema, abducens nerve palsies, and pyramidal tract signs, which are most evident in the lower extremities, are apparent in many cases.

In older children, once the sutures begin to fuse, patients may present with raised ICP. Headache often is worse early in the morning. Other symptoms include nausea, vomiting, blurred vision, and later drowsiness leading to depressed conscious state and death. Gait abnormalities are due to the stretching of paracentral corticospinal fibers of the parietal cortex by expanding lateral ventricle. More nerve fibers that serve the lower extremities are compressed early producing wide-based waddling gait.

■ EXAMINATION

Examination includes careful inspection, palpation, and auscultation of the skull and spine. The occipitofrontal head circumference is recorded and compared with previous measurements. The size and configuration of the AF are noted, and the back is inspected for abnormal midline skin lesions, including tufts of lipoma, or angioma that might suggest spinal dysraphism. The presence of a prominent forehead or abnormalities in the shape of the occiput can suggest the pathogenesis of the hydrocephalus. A cranial bruit is audible in association with many cases of vein of Galen arteriovenous malformation. Transillumination of the skull is positive with massive dilation of the ventricular system or in the Dandy-Walker syndrome. Inspection of the eyegrounds is mandatory because the finding of chorioretinitis suggests an intrauterine infection, such as toxoplasmosis, as a cause of the hydrocephalus. Papilledema is observed in older children but is rarely present in infants because the cranial sutures separate as a result of the increased pressure.

Child appears spastic or ataxic with gradual deterioration of the mental activity. Associated symptoms include headache, nausea and vomiting, irritability, apathy, and drowsiness. Limbs become spastic because of stretching of cortical fibers. Distortion of the brainstem may lead to bradycardia, systemic hypertension, and altered respiration.

GENERAL FEATURES
• Resonant percussion of skull
• Dilated scalp veins
• Papilledema
• Spastic
• Ataxia

■ DIAGNOSIS

Investigation of a child with hydrocephalus begins with the history. Familial cases suggest X-linked or autosomal hydrocephalus secondary to aqueductal stenosis. A past history of prematurity with intracranial hemorrhage, meningitis, or mumps encephalitis is important to ascertain. Multiple café-au-lait spots and other clinical features of neurofibromatosis point to aqueductal stenosis as the cause of hydrocephalus.

The head might appear enlarged (and can be confused with hydrocephalus) secondary to a thickened cranium resulting from chronic anemia, rickets, osteogenesis imperfecta, and epiphyseal dysplasia. Chronic subdural collections can produce bilateral parietal bone prominence. MRI has revealed the common occurrence of benign external hydrocephalus, a growth-limited condition where intervention is rarely required.

Various metabolic and degenerative disorders of the CNS produce megalencephaly as a result of abnormal storage of substances within the brain parenchyma. These disorders include lysosomal diseases (Tay-Sachs disease, gangliosidosis, and the mucopolysaccharidoses), the aminoaciduria (maple syrup urine disease), and the leukodystrophies (metachromatic leukodystrophy, Alexander disease, and Canavan disease).

In addition, cerebral gigantism (Sotos syndrome), other overgrowth syndromes, and neurofibromatosis arc characterized by increased brain mass. Familial megalencephaly is inherited as an autosomal dominant trait and is characterized by delayed motor milestones and hypotonia but normal or near-normal intelligence Measurement of parents' head circumferences is necessary to establish the diagnosis.

Cerebrospinal Fluid

Analysis of CSF, both biochemistry and cellular components, can provide additional information related to the cause of hydrocephalus and may aid in directing therapy. In neonates and premature infants, elevation of red cell counts and xanthochromia, usually in association with low CSF glucose and elevated protein, suggest the diagnosis of intraventricular hemorrhage.

Radiography

Plain X-rays in infants with hydrocephalus will reveal frontal bossing as well as macrocephaly. Separation of sutures is easily seen in older children but can be difficult in neonates. Enlargement of posterior fossa suggests possibility of Dandy–Walker's syndrome. In older children, a silver beaten appearance is early seen which is attributed to cortical impression against the inner table of the skull.

Ultrasonography

Transfontanelle USG is useful in neonates because it is noninvasive and repeatable. Lateral ventricular size and morphology are easily ascertained. Third ventricular size and shape is typically demonstrated, although delineation of the anatomy of the recess is variable. Ultrasound studies are less reliable for surface lesions, e.g., hydranencephaly, subdural or epidural collections, and for subarachnoid hemorrhage. The visualization of fourth ventricle is usually difficult.

Computed Tomography

Visualization of entire ventricular system by CT provides valuable information about pathogenesis or cause. Moderate degrees of ventricular asymmetry are common in both normal and hydrocephalic brain. Dilatation of occipital and temporal horns tends to occur prior to marked enlargement of the frontal horns. Space occupying lesions of brain are easily seen after contrast administration.

If no areas of abnormal enhancement are visualized, the location of the ventricular obstruction will be indicated by the status of the fourth ventricle. If the fourth ventricle is normal or small, the obstruction is presumed to be proximal to this site, suggesting a diagnosis of aqueductal stenosis. Dilatation of the fourth ventricle suggests distal obstruction either at the outflow foramina of the fourth ventricle or within the subarachnoid pathways. Inoculation of contrast agent directly into the CSF by either lumbar puncture (LP) or by direct ventricular tap provides additional detail and may be of value in situations where exact location of obstruction is needed.

Magnetic Resonance Imaging

The MRI studies provide more finer details if ventricular system is not available by CT scans. Small obstructing lesions about the foramen of Monro or aqueduct of Sylvius and cyst of cysticercus larvae in fourth ventricle, often isodense on CT, are seen by MRI. MRI is helpful in complex cases to define multiple congenital lesions and anatomy at the foramen magnum. Dynamic MRI can image the pattern of pulsatile CSF flow.

Electroencephalography

The electroencephalography (EEG) is rarely of diagnostic value unless the hydrocephalus is accompanied by seizures. EEG is important in differentiating the absence of cerebral cortex (severe hydrocephalus). Significant therapeutic and prognostic differences exist between these two entities.

Intracranial Pressure Monitoring

A saline-filled catheter or catheter-tipped transducer inserted into the lateral ventricle, brain, or subdural space records a pulsatile pressure of 0–10 mm Hg relative to the foramen of Monro when patient is lying flat. As a mass or the ventricles enlarge within the skull, the mean ICP rises, and spontaneous periodic waves become more pronounced particularly during rapid-eye-movement sleep.

LABORATORY SALIENT FINDINGS
• X-ray of skull • CT scan • Ultrasonography • Magnetic resonance imaging (MRI) • Electroencephalography • *Lumbar puncture:* Cerebrospinal fluid (CSF) analysis

■ DIFFERENTIAL DIAGNOSIS

Megalencephaly refers to the increase in volume of brain parenchyma. There are no signs of increased ICP. The ventricles are neither large, nor under increased pressure. Causes include Hurler syndrome, metachromatic leukodystrophy and Tay-Sachs disease.

Chronic subdural hematoma causes large head, mostly located in the parietal region without prominent scalp veins or sun setting sign. Large head size is also observed in hydranencephaly, rickets, achondroplasia, hemolytic anemia, and familial macrocephaly.

The differential diagnoses of hydrocephalus include megalencephaly, chronic subdural hematoma, cerebral atrophy, and brain tumor.

■ TREATMENT

Therapy for hydrocephalus depends on the cause. Medical management, including the use of acetazolamide and furosemide, can provide temporary relief by reducing the rate of CSF production, but long-term results have been disappointing. Most cases of hydrocephalus require extracranial shunts, particularly a ventriculoperitoneal shunt.

The cause of hydrocephalus should be treated, and the obstruction of CSF outflow should be relieved as early as possible.

Carbonic anhydrase inhibitors (e.g., acetazolamide) decrease CSF production and in conjunction with corticosteroids or diuretics help to control hydrocephalus in premature infants until they are well enough to undergo surgery. In patients where hydrocephalus may be transient (e.g., after subarachnoid hemorrhage), temporary CSF diversion may be carried out using a ventricular or lumbar catheter with careful control of the drainage pressure to avoid rerupture of any aneurysm.

In patients with noncommunicating hydrocephalus and where it is assumed that the subarachnoid space remains patent, a transventricular, endoscopic third ventriculostomy may be performed, with puncture of the floor of the third ventricle and drainage of the CSF into the basal cisterns.

Endoscopic third ventriculostomy has evolved as a viable approach and criteria have been developed for its use, but the procedure might need to be repeated to be effective. Ventricular shunting may be avoided with this approach.

The major complications of shunting are occlusion (characterized by headache, papilledema, emesis, and mental status changes) and bacterial infection (fever, headache, and meningismus), usually caused by *Staphylococcus*. With meticulous preparation, the shunt infection rate can be reduced to <5%. The results of intrauterine surgical management of fetal hydrocephalus have been poor (possibly because of the high rate of associated cerebral malformations in addition to the hydrocephalus) except for some promise in cases of hydrocephalus associated with fetal meningomyelocele.

Cerebrospinal fluid is usually drained form the ventricular cistern via a ventricular catheter (a valve with reservoir mechanism and a distal catheter) into the peritoneal cavity (historically almost every cavity and hollow organ in the body has been used).

Lumboperitoneal shunts are used to drain fluid from the lumbar subarachnoid space to the peritoneal cavity in some patients with communicating hydrocephalus and in those with benign intracranial hypertension. These shunts usually work well a few months only, and where they are successful, may be associated with symptomatic secondary herniation of the cerebellar tonsils. It is helpful to insert a separate ventricular access device at the time of shunt procedure because it facilitates investigation if complications ensue.

Surgical intervention may not be required if hydrocephalus gets arrested spontaneously. Medical management include acetazolamide given in dose of 50 mg/kg/day. It diminishes CSF production in mild-to-moderate degree of hydrocephalus. Oral glycerol and isosorbide have also been used.

Surgical intervention is needed if size of the head enlarges rapidly or associated with progressive symptoms such as impairment of visions or if life is affected before irreparable damage occurs.

In congenital obstructive hydrocephalus, a ventriculoarterial or ventriculoperitoneal shunt should be done. This will help to drain the CSF directly into circulation or into peritoneal cavity. As child grows in size, it may be necessary to revise the shunt, using a longer tube.

Acute hydrocephalus may be managed by repeated LP.

■ COMPLICATIONS

The decision to insert a shunt is clear where there is active, progressive hydrocephalus, supported by radiological evidence of ventriculomegaly. However, the presence of ventriculomegaly in the absence of any supporting features does not mean that there is active hydrocephalus, and a shunt may be dangerous. Under these circumstances, more detailed investigations, often repeated over months or years, are necessary. The incidence of epilepsy attributable to shunt insertion is small. Trauma to the brain during shunt insertion is uncommon provided appropriate techniques are used.

Underdrainage (malfunction): The highest risk of underdrainage is in the 1st year (30%). It is usually caused by a gradual occlusion of the ventricular catheters by choroids plexus.

Plain radiographs can demonstrate disconnection. A CT brain scan is the best investigation for suspected underdrainage, especially if the scan can be compared with one infection. Contamination most often occurs at the time of insertion; 70% of infections appear within 1 month of insertion.

Many organisms may be responsible but the most common is *Staphylococcus epidermidis*. Aspiration of CSF from the shunt reservoir, under neurosurgical guidance, gives the best yield for the assessment of contamination, but its absence does not exclude shunt infection.

Overdrainage: The gravity effect caused by the hydrostatic column of CSF between the inlet and outlet of a shunt may cause some shunts to overdrain, particularly in tall patients. The siphon effect may produce slit-ventricle syndrome, subdural hematomas, enysted fourth ventricle, or postshunt craniosynostosis. Antisiphon devices and flow-regulating valves have been developed to reduce the incidence of these complications.

Slit-ventricle syndrome: In children with functioning CSF shunt, symptoms of raised ICP may develop, which is characterized by small ventricles as determined by CT scan. It is believed that the ability of the ventricles to expand is impaired. The reduction in brain compliance has been attributed to subependymal gliosis.

Several causes have been suggested for slit-ventricle syndrome such as intermittent ventricular catheter, obstruction between the collapsed walls of the lateral ventricles, overdrainage of CSF, and intracranial hypertension with normal functioning shunt. Evaluation of the shunt is required before appropriate treatment is given.

■ FOLLOW-UP

In a well child or adult, routine outpatient follow-up may be a waste of time because complications most commonly occur between visits. Careful instructions must be given to the family about the symptoms and signs that may suggest malfunction.

■ PROGNOSIS

Prognosis depends on the underlying condition and type of hydrocephalus. In a group of newly diagnosed babies with treated nontumoral hydrocephalus, 70% would be expected to attend a normal school and have a normal IQ.

Prognosis depends on the cause of the dilated ventricles and not on the size of the cortical mantle at the time of operative intervention, except in cases in which the cortical mantle has been severely compressed and stretched. Hydrocephalic children are at increased risk for various developmental disabilities. The mean intelligence quotient is reduced compared with the general population, particularly for performance tasks as compared with verbal abilities. Many children have abnormalities in memory function. Vision problems are common, including strabismus, visuospatial abnormalities, visual field defects, and optic atrophy with decreased acuity secondary to increased ICP.

■ BIBLIOGRAPHY

1. Fisayo A, Bruce BB. Overdiagnosis of idiopathic intracranial hypertension. Neurology. 2016; 86(4):341-50.
2. Haridas A, Tomita. Hydrocephalus in children: Clinical features and diagnosis. UpToDate. 2018;3:1-27.
3. Kumar R, Bansal A. Approach and management of children with raised intracranial pressure. J Pediatr Crit Care. 2015;2(3):13-24.
4. Mazzola CA, Choudhri AF, Auguste KI, Limbrick DD Jr, Rogido M, Mitchell L, et al. Pediatric hydrocephalus systemic literature review and evidence-based guidelines. Part 2: Management of posthemorrhagic hydrocephalus in premature infants. J Neurosurg Pediatr. 2014;14:8-23.

CASE 55

Meningitis

PRESENTING COMPLAINTS

A 3-year-old girl was brought with the complaint of:
- Fever since 4 days
- Not taking feeds since 2 days
- Vomiting since 1 day
- Abnormal movements since 5 minutes

History of Presenting Complaints

A 3-year-old girl was brought by the mother with the history of convulsions since morning.

CASE AT A GLANCE	
Basic Findings	
Height	: 95 cm (75th centile)
Weight	: 13 kg (50th centile)
Temperature	: 39°C
Pulse rate	: 124 beats/min
Respiratory rate	: 22 breaths/min
Blood pressure	: 70/50 mm Hg
Positive Findings	
History:	
• Convulsions	
• Fever	
• Altered sensorium	
Examination:	
• Altered sensorium	
• Meningeal signs	
• DTR exaggerated	
Investigation:	
• *ESR:* Raised	
• *CSF:* Turbid, polymorph cells present	

(CSF: cerebrospinal fluid; DTR: deep tendon reflexes; ESR: erythrocyte sedimentation rate)

Her mother gave the history that her daughter developed tonic–clonic convulsions about 30 minutes back. It involved both the upper and lower limbs. The convulsions were continuous for 5 minutes. Later she was taken to nearby clinic. Convulsions were brought under control by intravenous administration of diazepam. After that the doctor referred the child to the hospital for further management.

Her mother also gave history of fever since 4 days. Fever was moderate-to-high degree and intermittent, which used to be relieved by antipyretics. She had also noticed that the child was inactive and was not taking feeds properly since 3 days. There was history of vomiting since previous day. Child had vomited about two to three times. The vomiting was projectile in nature.

Past History of the Patient

The child was the only sibling of nonconsanguineous marriage. She was born at full term by normal delivery. Her birth weight was 3 kg. She started taking breast milk immediately after delivery. There was no significant postnatal event. Weaning was started in the fourth month and completed by 1 year. She was immunized completely and all the developmental milestones were normal.

EXAMINATION

The girl was moderately built and nourished. She was in altered sensorium. She was not responding to oral commands. She was responding to the painful stimulus by resisting it. Anthropometric measurements included the height 95 cm (75th centile) and the weight 13 kg (50th centile). There were signs of moderate dehydration.

The child was febrile 39°C. The pulse rate was 124 beats/min. The respiratory rate was 22 breaths/min regular. Blood pressure recorded was 70/50 mm Hg. There was no pallor, no lymphadenopathy, no cyanosis, and no clubbing.

Higher mental functions could not be elicited as child was in altered sensorium status. She was not responding to oral commands. She was responding to the painful stimulus by resisting the stimulus. There was no motor and sensory involvement. No cranial nerve was involved. Hypertonia was present. DTR were exaggerated. Neck rigidity was present and Kernig's sign was present. Other systemic examinations were normal.

■ INVESTIGATION

- *Hemoglobin:* 11.5 g/dL
- *TLC:* 12,000 cells/cumm
- *DLC:* $P_{68} L_{28} E_2 M_2$
- *ESR:* 30 mm in the first hour
- *X-ray chest:* Normal
- *Mantoux test:* Negative
- *CSF examination:* Turbid elevated cell count mainly polymorphs; blood sugar was 20 mg/dL
- *Gram stain:* NAD

■ DISCUSSION

Child came to the hospital with history of convulsions, fever, and altered sensorium. The meningeal signs were present. As the history of the illness is of short duration, the diagnosis goes in favor of pyogenic bacterial meningitis.

Bacterial meningitis is one of the most potentially serious infections occurring in infants and older children. This infection is associated with a high rate of acute complications and risk of long-term morbidity. The incidence of bacterial meningitis is sufficiently high in febrile infants that it should be included in the differential diagnosis of those with altered mental status and other evidence of neurologic dysfunction.

■ ETIOLOGY

The most common causes of bacterial meningitis in children older than 1 month of age are *Streptococcus pneumoniae* and *Neisseria meningitidis*. Bacterial meningitis caused by *S. pneumoniae* and *Haemophilus influenzae* type b has become much less common in developed countries since the introduction of universal immunization against these pathogens begins at 2 months of age. Infection caused by *S. pneumoniae* or *H. influenzae* type b must be considered in incompletely vaccinated individuals or those in developing countries. Those with certain underlying immunologic [human immunodeficiency virus (HIV) infection, immunoglobulin G (IgG) subclass deficiency] or anatomic (splenic dysfunction, cochlear defects or implants) disorders also may be at increased risk of infection caused by these bacteria.

Bacterial meningitis remains a common disease. The important factors include age, status of host immune system, and colonization of the nasopharynx with potential pathogens.

During the neonatal period, Gram-negative bacilli (principally *Escherichia coli*), other Enterobacteriaceae, Group B streptococci, *Pseudomonas* sp., *Listeria monocytogenes* are the major causative agents.

From 1–3 months of age, the common causes are group B streptococci, the Gram-negative organisms become less common while *H. influenzae*, *N. meningitidis* begins to appear.

From 3 months to 3 years of age, *H. influenzae* is the most common cause of meningitis followed by *S. pneumoniae*.

The risk for the development of neonatal meningitis includes prematurity, septicemia, and prolonged rupture of the membrane (PROM).

Alterations of host defense resulting from anatomic defects or immune deficits also increase the risk of meningitis from less common pathogens such as *Pseudomonas aeruginosa*, *Staphylococcus aureus*, coagulase-negative staphylococci, *Salmonella* species, anaerobes, and *L. monocytogenes*. Patients with diminished host resistance are responsible for development of meningitis.

Bacteria enters the cerebrospinal fluid (CSF) by hematogenous route, direct extension, or by direct implantation of bacteria. The pathological steps include nasopharyngeal colonization, cell invasion, blood stream invasion crossing the blood–brain barrier and entry in CSF, and survival and replication of subarachnoid space.

ACUTE BACTERIAL MENINGITIS BEYOND THE NEONATAL PERIOD

The risk of pneumococcal meningitis is increased in children with congenital or acquired CSF leak across a mucocutaneous barrier, such as a lumbar dural sinus, cranial or midline facial defects (cribriform plate), fistulas of the middle ear (stapedial foot plate) or inner ear (oval window, internal auditory canal, cochlear aqueduct), or CSF leakage as a result of basilar or other skull fracture.

PATHOGENESIS AND PATHOPHYSIOLOGY

The organisms causing neonatal meningitis are usually acquired during passage down the birth canal, from the mother or the nursery environment. Colonization of the nasopharynx, umbilicus, and gastrointestinal tract precedes invasion of the bloodstream and meninges.

For the most common cause of meningitis, the bacteria must first attach to the epithelial cells in the nasopharynx. *H. influenzae* and *N. meningitidis* have pili, which attach to the specific receptors on host cells, the bacteria must evade the local secretary mucosal IgA antibody. All the major bacterial pathogens causing meningitis have IgA proteases that disarm IgA, thereby clearing the way to attachment.

The bacteria must pass through these cells and access the bloodstream. Once in the blood stream, the bacteria must survive the immune mechanism and arrive at CNS capillaries. The most common organism causing bacterial meningitis are able to avoid these host defenses in the bloodstream by virtue of their antiphagocytic and anticomplement nature of their polysaccharide capsule.

Most cases of bacterial meningitis are hematogenous in origin, thus bacterial agents reach, invade, and replicate in the CSF. These pathological steps include:
- Nasopharyngeal colonization
- Nasopharyngeal epithelial cell invasion
- Bloodstream invasion
- Bacteremia with intravascular survival
- Crossing of the blood brain barrier and entry into the CSF
- Survival and replication in the subarachnoid space

Bacteria enters the CSF by any one of the, namely several, possible routes:
- *Hematogenous:* Most common route through which bacteria enters the CSF; there occurs seeding of the subarachnoid space from a distant focus of infection or spontaneous bacteremia from nasopharyngeal colonization with the pathogen.
- Direct extension of the invading bacteria into the subarachnoid space
- Direct implantation of the bacteria into the subarachnoid space either due to trauma or surgical event.

From the CNS capillaries, the bacteria must penetrate the blood–brain barrier and cross into the subarachnoid space. The bacteria enter the CSF via capillaries in the choroid plexus of the lateral ventricles. Once in the CSF, it can multiply freely, because the CSF is virtually devoid of complement, antibody, and phagocytic cells. Even with the emergence of inflammation and the ingress of cells, complement, and antibody into the CSF, the infection generally continues to progress.

Interstitial brain edema is the main pathological change. Brain edema is further induced by presence of arachidonic acid and its metabolites. These are released from the damaged cells of CNS and by the fatty acids released from polymorphonuclear leukocytes. The specific adhesion molecule causes adhesion to those epithelial cells and further provokes disruption of blood–brain barrier. All these factors lead to the increase in brain edema and decrease in the perfusion of the brain due to increased ICP and endothelial cell vasculitis and thrombosis. The final outcome of these processes is ischemic damage to the CNS.

The leptomeninges are infiltrated with inflammatory cells. The cortex of the brain shows edema, exudate, and proliferation of microglia. Ependymal cells are destroyed purulent exudate, which collect at the base of the brain. Exudate may block foramina of Luschka and Magendie and produces hydrocephalus. Permanent neurological sequela results from infarction, necrosis, and hydrocephalus. Deaths may occur as result of endotoxic shock.

A meningeal purulent exudate of varying thickness may be distributed around the cerebral veins, venous sinuses, convexity of the brain, and cerebellum, and in the sulci, sylvian fissures, basal cisterns, and spinal cord. Ventriculitis with bacteria and inflammatory cells in ventricular fluid may be present (more often in neonates), as subdural effusions and, rarely, empyema. Perivascular inflammatory infiltrates may also be present, and the ependymal membrane may be disrupted.

Vascular and parenchymal cerebral changes characterized by polymorphonuclear infiltrates extending to the subintimal region of the small arteries and veins, vasculitis, thrombosis of small cortical veins, occlusion of major venous sinuses, and necrotizing arteritis producing subarachnoid hemorrhage. Cerebral infarction, resulting from vascular occlusion because of inflammation, vasospasm, and thrombosis, is a frequent sequelae.

Inflammation of spinal nerves and roots produces meningeal signs, and inflammation of the cranial nerves produces cranial neuropathies of optic, oculomotor, facial, and auditory nerves. Increased ICP also produces oculomotor nerve palsy because of the presence of temporal lobe compression of the nerve during tentorial herniation. Abducens nerve palsy may be a nonlocalizing sign of elevated ICP.

Increased ICP is a result of cell death (cytotoxic cerebral edema), cytokine-induced increased capillary vascular permeability (vasogenic cerebral edema), and, possibly, increased hydrostatic pressure (interstitial cerebral edema) after obstructed reabsorption of CSF in the arachnoid villus or obstruction of the flow of fluid from the ventricles. ICP may exceed 300 mm H_2O; cerebral perfusion may be further compromised if the cerebral perfusion pressure (mean arterial pressure – ICP) is <50 cm H_2O as a result of systemic hypotension with reduced cerebral blood flow. The syndrome of inappropriate antidiuretic hormone secretion (SIADH) may produce excessive water retention and potentially increase the risk of elevated ICP.

Hydrocephalus can occur as an acute complication of bacterial meningitis. It most often takes the form of a communicating hydrocephalus caused by adhesive thickening of the arachnoid villi around the cisterns at the base of the brain. Thus, there is interference with the normal resorption of CSF. Less often, obstructive hydrocephalus develops after fibrosis and gliosis of the aqueduct of Sylvius or the foramina of Magendie and Luschka.

Raised CSF protein levels are partly a result of increased vascular permeability of the blood–brain barrier and the loss of albumin-rich fluid from the capillaries and veins traversing the subdural space. Continued transudation may result in subdural effusion, usually found in the later phase of acute bacterial meningitis.

Recurrent meningitis may be associated with pilonidal sinus, CSF rhinorrhea, traumatic lesion of cribriform plate, and ethmoidal sinus or congenital fistula.

Damage to the cerebral cortex may be a result of the focal or diffuse effects of vascular occlusion (infarction, necrosis, lactic acidosis), hypoxia, bacterial invasion (cerebritis), toxic encephalopathy (bacterial toxins), elevated ICP, ventriculitis, and transudation (subdural effusions). These pathologic factors result in the clinical manifestations of impaired consciousness, seizures, cranial nerve deficits, motor and sensory deficits, and later psychomotor retardation.

Rarely, meningitis may follow bacterial invasion from a contiguous focus of infection such as paranasal sinusitis, otitis media, mastoiditis, orbital cellulitis, or cranial or vertebral osteomyelitis or may occur after introduction of bacteria via penetrating cranial trauma, dermal sinus tracts, or meningomyelocele.

■ CLINICAL FEATURES (FIG. 1)

The clinical signs and symptoms of meningitis vary greatly depending on the age of the child and duration of the illness. The disease may have acute or insidious presentation.

Acute presentation is with headache, fever, and altered mental status. While insidious in presentation, the illness develops over several days to a week and then to pneumonia. Sinusitis and otitis media are present more commonly.

The onset of acute meningitis has two predominant patterns. The more dramatic and, fortunately, less common presentation is sudden onset with rapidly progressive

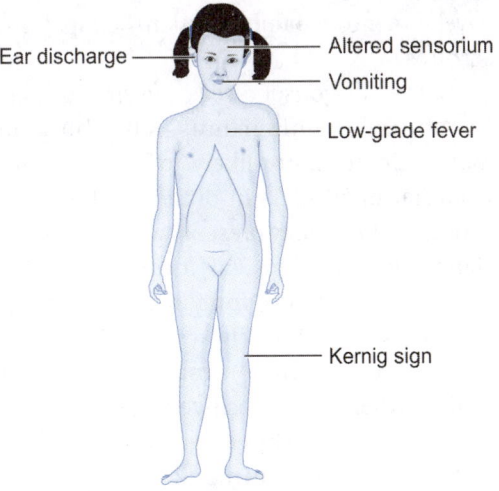

Fig. 1: Clinical features.

manifestations of shock, purpura, disseminated intravascular coagulation, and reduced levels of consciousness often resulting in progression to coma or death within 24 hours. More often, meningitis is preceded by several days of fever accompanied by upper respiratory tract or gastrointestinal symptoms, followed by nonspecific signs of CNS infection, such as increasing lethargy and irritability.

Alterations of mental status are common among patients with meningitis and may be the consequence of increased ICP, cerebritis hypotension; manifestations include irritability, lethargy, stupor obtundation, and coma. Comatose patients have a poor prognosis.

The common and classic triad of fever, headache, and stiff neck is quite variable depending upon the age-group and virulence of the organisms. The factors other than age that determine the clinical manifestations include the degree of meningeal infection and inflammation, the presence of increased ICP (headache, vomiting, bulging fontanelle, papilledema): The occurrence of vasculitis or venous thrombosis (hemiparesis, other focal neurological deficits, seizures), and the development of subdural effusion (hemiparesis, seizures).

In the later-onset disease, fever, seizures, irritability, meningismus, and bulging fontanelle are more likely to be observed. Bacterial meningitis in older children and young adults usually presents with the classic signs and symptoms of fever, headache, photophobia, nausea, vomiting, and meningismus. Fever is almost always present.

Meningeal irritation may be suggested by the presence of a positive Brudzinski sign and Kernig sign. These signs of meningeal irritation are seen in up to 50% of older children and 90% of adults. Lethargy and confusion are more common in bacterial than with viral meningitis and the altered mental status is a consistent finding in older children. Headache is usually intense and severe. With pneumococcal meningitis, and associated pulmonary, ear or sinus infection is often found.

Focal neurological deficit (cranial neuropathies, seizures, hemiparesis) may relate to cerebritis or CNS infarction secondary to large-vessel vasculitis or dural sinus thrombosis. Focal deficit should prompt investigation for brain abscess, subdural effusion, or empyema.

Convulsions occur in 20–30% of children with meningitis. The seizures are usually generalized and do not necessarily indicate a poor prognosis. Focal seizure and focal neurological signs indicate the possible presence of cortical venous or arterial thrombosis with cortical infarct and suggest a less favorable prognosis. Seizures that occur on presentation or within the first 4 days of onset are usually of no prognostic significance. Seizures that persist after the fourth day of illness and those that are difficult to treat may be associated with a poor prognosis.

Febrile seizures are common with streptococcal meningitis and *H. influenzae* meningitis. Convulsions occurring during an upper respiratory tract infection are common and must be distinguished from convulsions occurring with meningitis.

In older children LP is unnecessary after a febrile convulsion, if meningitis is not suspected clinically. However, in children under 18 months of age in whom the signs of meningitis are subtle, CSF examination may be necessary to exclude meningitis. Ataxia may be the presenting feature with *H. influenzae* meningitis.

Cutaneous manifestations are an important early clue to some form of meningitis **(Fig. 2)**.

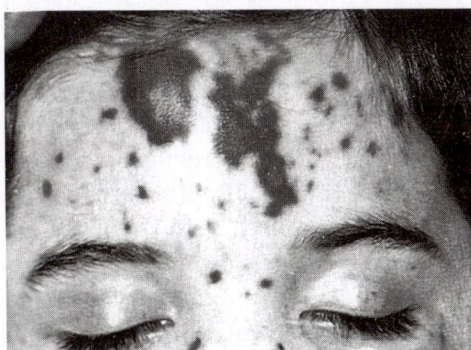

Fig. 2: Purpuric rash of meningococcus.
(For color version, see Plate 2)

A rapidly spreading purpuric rash is characteristic of meningococcal septicemia, but is also occasionally seen with pneumococcal or *H. influenzae* sepsis.

Papilledema due to raised ICP is an uncommon finding in acute bacterial meningitis but if present, it indicates subdural effusion, empyema, or brain abscess. Cranial nerves VI, VII, IV, and VIII are most commonly affected during acute bacterial meningitis.

Symptoms and signs found in newborn are vacant stare, irritability and drowsiness, persistent vomiting with fever, poor tone, poor cry, shock and circulatory collapse, refusal to feed, fever or hypothermia, convulsions, and tremors. Petechial hemorrhages on the skin and mucous membrane are seen in meningococcal meningitis.

The diagnosis is more difficult in the neonatal period and in young infants when the signs are subtle and nonspecific. Fever is present in only half of neonates with meningitis. Lethargy, disinterest in feeding, vomiting or diarrhea, jaundice, and respiratory distress are common presenting features. Irritability and abnormal muscle tone are present in one-third of neonates with meningitis. Convulsions and a bulging fontanelle are late manifestations. As no sign is specific for meningitis, a high index of suspicion is necessary in assessing any ill neonate or infant.

Sepsis hypotension, hypoxemia, and increased ICP all contribute to the reduction of the perfusion of CNS. Fluid restriction has been recommended as a management of SIADH. A reasonable approach is to give two-thirds of daily fluid maintenance volume.

ESSENTIAL DIAGNOSTIC POINTS
• Fever • Headache with projectile vomiting • Altered sensorium, irritability • Convulsions • Meningeal irritation signs • CSF findings • CT scan • MRI • Focus of infection
(MRI: magnetic resonance imaging; CSF: cerebrospinal fluid; CT: computed tomography)

GENERAL FEATURES
• Loss of appetite • Papilledema • Motor deficits

DIAGNOSIS

As early diagnosis of meningitis is extremely important it should be suspected in any child with lethargy, unconsciousness, inability to feed, stiff neck and seizures. It is important to note that the absence of fever or meningeal signs does not exclude the diagnosis of bacterial meningitis.

Blood cultures should be performed in all patients with suspected meningitis. Blood culture reveals the responsible bacteria in up to 80–90% of cases of meningitis. Elevations of the C-reactive protein, ESR, and procalcitonin have been used to differentiate bacterial causes (usually elevated) from viral causes of meningitis.

Cerebrospinal Fluid Examination

The diagnosis of acute pyogenic meningitis is confirmed by analysis of the CSF, which typically reveals microorganisms on Gram stain and culture, a neutrophilic pleocytosis, elevated protein, and reduced glucose concentrations. LP should be performed when bacterial meningitis is suspected.

Acute bacterial meningitis should be suspected in children presenting with a brief history of fever, irritability, photophobia, headache, vomiting, convulsions, and altered sensorium. Diagnosis should be substantiated by examination of the CSF.

Contraindications for an immediate LP include (1) evidence of increased ICP (other than a bulging fontanel), such as third or sixth cranial nerve palsy with a depressed level of consciousness, or hypertension and bradycardia with a respiratory abnormalities; (2) severe cardiopulmonary compromise requiring prompt resuscitative measures for shock or in patients in whom positioning for the LP would further compromise cardiopulmonary function; and (3) infection of the skin overlying the site of the LP.

Gram stain and culture of the CSF will result in identification of the bacteria in most cases of bacterial meningitis. CSF and blood culture should be taken before initiating antibiotics. **Table 1** shows the typical CSF finding in bacterial meningitis. The CSF is usually cloudy and contains several hundreds to thousands of WBC, predominantly polymorphonuclear leukocytes. CSF leukocytosis of greater than 10,000 cells/cumm should suggest the presence of brain abscess or parameningeal abscess with rupture into subarachnoid space.

Cerebrospinal fluid glucose concentration is usually low in bacterial meningitis (i.e., <50% of simultaneous serum concentration) with levels ranging from <10 mg/dL to 50 mg/dL. The ratio of CSF/serum glucose in bacterial meningitis should be <0.3 but no higher than 0.5. CSF protein concentrations are elevated (usually greater than 100 mg/dL). If there is marked protein concentration, a subarachnoid block of CSF flow should be suspected.

Rapid Diagnostic Tests

The development of rapid tests of CSF for the detection of specific bacterial antigens or the presence of endotoxin from Gram-negative bacteria has helped in establishing the diagnosis of bacterial meningitis.

Rapid diagnostic tests may be used to distinguish between viral, bacterial, and tuberculous meningitis based on antigen or antibody demonstration, e.g., countercurrent immunoelectrophoresis, latex particle agglutination, coagglutination, enzyme-linked immunosorbent assay (ELISA), and other techniques. Besides being rapid, they are unaltered by previous antibiotic usage. Latex agglutination and ELISA have sensitivity and specificity of almost 80%. PCR is used for diagnosis of infection with herpes simplex, enteroviruses, meningococci, and tuberculosis.

TABLE 1: Cerebrospinal fluid (CSF) characteristics in acute bacterial meningitis.

Characteristics	Bacterial meningitis
CSF cells counts (cells/cumm)	Polymorphonuclear >5–10,000
CSF glucose	<10–50 mg/dL
CSF/serum glucose ratio	0.3–0.5
CSF protein	100–500 mg/dL
CSF Gram stain/culture	90% positive

The available diagnostic tests include latex particle agglutination (LPA) kits that contain antisera directed against the specific capsular antigens of *H. influenzae, S. pneumoniae, N. meningitidis*, coagulation tests (COA), and counter immunoelectrophoresis (CIE) tests are also of use. These tests have sensitivity and specificity between 50% and 90%.

INDICATIONS FOR COMPUTED TOMOGRAPHY (CT) SCAN
• Prolonged irritability • Prolonged obtundation • *Seizures:* Third day of therapy • Focal seizures • Focal neurologic deficits • Increasing head circumference • Recurrence of disease

Computed tomography scanning/MRI is useful in patients with raised ICP or with focal neurological signs and in these may reveal the presence of brain abscess, subdural effusion, hydrocephalus, infarction secondary to vasculitis or dural sinus thrombosis. Inflammation of the meninges can be demonstrated with contrast CT scan or MRI. The role of CT or MRI in meningitis is to exclude other CNS lesions or sequelae of bacterial meningitis.

LABORATORY SALIENT FINDINGS
• *Lumbar puncture:* CSF analysis • Serological, immunological nucleic detection (PCR) test • CT scan • MRI • Brain biopsy
(CSF: cerebrospinal fluid; CT: computed tomography; MRI: magnetic resonance imaging; PCR: polymerase chain reaction)

■ ORGANISM IDENTIFICATION

CSF Grain stain: It is quick, reliable, and inexpensive; positivity depends on the number of organisms in the CSF—at least 10^5 colony forming units/mL of CSF is required. The yield is markedly increased by examining fresh centrifuged sediment of the CSF.

Acridine orange: It stains the nucleic acid of some bacteria so that they appear bright red orange under a fluorescent microscope. It stains the intracellular bacteria better than the Gram stain and may be positive even when the Gram stain is negative.

Cerebrospinal fluid culture: A positive CSF culture is the gold standard for organism identification, High positivity (75%) reported from developed countries is not seen in developing countries because of prehospital antibiotic therapy, delayed plating, and inadequate storage and transport of CSF.

Samples from other site of infection: Samples from other sites of infection such as pleural fluid, cellulitis, aspiration of petechiae in suspected meningococcemia, and urine in young infants should also be collected for organism identification.

■ DIFFERENTIAL DIAGNOSIS

Meningism: This may occur in inflammatory cervical lesions, apical pneumonia, and in toxemia due to typhoid and influenza. There are no neurological signs and the CSF is normal.

Partially treated bacterial meningitis: If the child has received prior antibiotics, the CSF becomes sterile. Biochemistry may be altered and pleocytosis persists, though type of cellular response changes. It poses a difficult problem in the differential diagnosis from tuberculous meningitis and aseptic meningitis. The onset, clinical course, rapid diagnostic tests, and other ancillary investigations may be useful.

Aseptic meningitis: The clinical and laboratory profile is similar to pyogenic meningitis.

The CSF pressure is elevated and shows mild pleocytosis and moderate increase in protein with near normal sugar. The CSF lactic acid is not elevated. No organisms are cultured.

Tuberculous meningitis: The onset is insidious with lethargy, low-grade fever, irritability, vomiting and weight loss. Features of meningeal irritation are less prominent and course of the illness is prolonged. Neurological features include seizures, gradually progressive unconsciousness, cranial nerve deficits, motor deficits and visual involvement. Features of hydrocephalus and decerebration are relatively common. Evidence of systemic tuberculosis and family contact should be looked for. Mantoux test may be positive and there may be evidence of tuberculosis elsewhere. CSF shows 100–500 cells, with majority of lymphocytes: Sugar is less reduced than in pyogenic meningitis and protein is elevated.

Cryptococcal meningitis: It usually occurs in an immunocompromised host. There is low-grade fever, mild cough, and pulmonary infiltration. Meningeal involvement has a gradual onset with a protracted course. The clinical features are not specific. The CSF shows the fungus as thick-walled budding yeast cells, surrounded by a large gelatinous capsule in India ink preparation. The organism grows well in Sabouraud medium.

Viral encephalitis: It has acute onset with early disturbances of sensorium, raised ICP, and variable neurological deficit. The CSF is clear and may show mild pleocytosis; there is mild elevation of protein and normal sugar. PCR for viral antigens and rising CSF antibody titers are useful diagnostic clues,

Subarachnoid hemorrhage: Sudden headache and sensorial alteration occur without preceding fever. The course of illness is rapid and signs of meningeal irritation are marked. CT scan is diagnostic. CSF reveals crenated RBCs.

Lyme disease: It is an infection of CNS with *Borrelia burgdorferi*, a tick-borne spirochete. Patients develop encephalopathy, polyneuropathy, leukoencephalitis, and hearing loss.

■ COMPLICATIONS

Complication of acute bacterial meningitis can develop early in the course of disease or it may be a long-term late sequelae. Apart from early and late meningeal complications, systemic complications can develop during the illnesses and are associated with high mortality and require specific therapeutic intervention.

Main neurological complications developing during the course of illness are ventriculitis, subdural effusion, neurological deficits, such as, hemiparesis, quadriparesis, cranial nerve palsy, hydrocephalus, hearing loss, arachnoiditis, and mental retardation.

Late complications and sequelae are mental retardation, seizures, sensory neural hearing loss, visual impairment, behavioral problems, motor deficit, ataxia, and hydrocephalus.

■ TREATMENT

Treatment of acute pyogenic meningitis falls into two categories. Antibacterial chemotherapy and specific measures designed to reverse systemic and neurological complications. The ideal antibiotic for a bacterial pathogen causing meningitis is the one that:
- Penetrates the blood–brain carrier and achieve CSF concentration at least 10 times greater than the minimal bactericidal concentration for the organisms
- Is nontoxic to the patient

- Is bactericidal and not bacteriolytic
- Does not promote emergence of resistance and sterilizes the CSF quickly.

Initial Antibiotic Therapy

The initial (empirical) choice of therapy for meningitis in immunocompetent infants and children is primarily influenced by the antibiotic susceptibilities of *S. pneumoniae*. In contrast, most strains of *N. meningitidis* are sensitive to penicillin and cephalosporins, although rare resistant isolates have been reported. Approximately 30–40% of isolates of *H. influenzae* type b produce beta-lactamases and, therefore, are resistant to ampicillin. These beta-lactamase-producing strains are sensitive to the extended-spectrum cephalosporins.

Based on the substantial rate of resistance of *S. pneumoniae* to beta-lactam drugs, vancomycin (60 mg/kg/24 h, given every 6 hours) is recommended as part of initial empirical therapy. Because of the efficacy of third-generation cephalosporins in the therapy of meningitis caused by sensitive *S. pneumoniae*, *N. meningitidis*, and *H. influenzae* type b, cefotaxime (300 mg/kg/24 h, given every 6 hours) or ceftriaxone (100 mg/kg/24 h administered once per day or 50 mg/kg/dose, given every 12 hours) should also be used in initial empirical therapy. Patients allergic to beta-lactam antibiotics and >1 month of age can be treated with chloramphenicol, 100 mg/kg/24 h, given every 6 hours.

If *L. monocytogenes* infection is suspected, as in young infants or those with a T-lymphocyte deficiency, ampicillin (200 mg/kg/24 h, given every 6 hours) also should also be given because cephalosporins are inactive against *L. monocytogenes*. Intravenous trimethoprim–sulfamethoxazole is an alternative treatment for *L. monocytogenes*.

If a patient is immunocompromised and Gram-negative bacterial meningitis is suspected, initial therapy might include ceftazidime and an aminoglycoside or meropenem **(Table 2)**.

TABLE 2: Recommended antibiotics for initial treatment of meningitis in different age-groups.

Age-group	Drug	Dose (mg/kg/day)	
		0–7 days	7–28 days
Neonates	Ampicillin	100–150	150–200
	And		
	Gentamicin	5	7.5
	Or		
	Ampicillin	100–150	150–200
	And		
	Cefotaxime	100	150–200
	Or		
	Ceftazidime	60	90
Infants and children	Ampicillin	200–300	
	And		
	Chloramphenicol	75–100	
	Or		
	Third-generation cephalosporin		
	Cefotaxime	200	
	Ceftriaxone	100	
	Ceftazidime	150	

In neonatal bacterial meningitis, the list of likely pathogens is covered by regimen of ampicillin and gentamycin. The use of third-generation cephalosporins alone (cefotaxime, ceftriaxone, ceftazidime) dose not adequately treat the *Enterococcus* or *Listeria*. Therefore, the combination of ampicillin and gentamycin is appropriate until the infecting pathogen has been defined by culture. Since the blood–brain barrier has not fully formed at this age, aminoglycosides enter the CSF in adequate concentration via the intravenous route.

Intraventricular administration of gentamycin is indicated if the meningitis process is unresponsive and that too when the gram-negative bacteria are unresponsive to newer cephalosporins. The routine and direct instillation of aminoglycosides intraventrically should be avoided in neonatal meningitis because of the worse morbidity and mortality associated with this route of administration.

Seizures are common during the course of bacterial meningitis. Immediate therapy for seizures includes intravenous diazepam (0.1–0.2 mg/kg/dose) or lorazepam (0.05–0.10 mg/kg/dose), and careful attention is paid to the risk of respiratory suppression. Serum glucose, calcium, and sodium levels should be monitored. After immediate management of seizures, patients should receive phenytoin (15–20 mg/kg loading dose, 5 mg/kg/24 h maintenance) to reduce the likelihood of recurrence. Phenytoin is preferred to phenobarbital, because it produces less CNS depression and permits assessment of a patient's level of consciousness. Serum phenytoin levels should be monitored to maintain them in the therapeutic range (10–20 µg/mL). The subsequent oral dose of 5 mg/kg/day for 3–4 weeks is advised. If the child is unconscious feeding is done through nasogastric tube.

In older children and adults, use of the newer third-generation cephalosporins is recommended in the initial empiric regimen and when the pathogen has been defined and its antibiotic sensitivity known, therapy may be simplified. Penicillin G is the drug of choice for the pneumococcus and meningococcus. *H. influenzae, S. pneumoniae*, and *N. meningitidis* are sensitive to cephalosporins.

In the patients with severely immunocompromised host, the additional pathogen to cover is *Listeria*. For *Listeria*, trimethoprim/sulfamethoxazole may be the antibiotic of choice.

The duration of antibiotic treatment for neonatal meningitis has been 2–3 weeks. If intraventricular antibiotics are used, a daily dose of 3–5 days is usually sufficient to sterilize the CSF compartment. The duration of antimicrobial therapy given via the intravenous route for the treatment of most cases of bacterial meningitis is 7–10 days. Longer duration of therapy (2–3 weeks) is recommended for staphylococcal and Gram-negative bacillary meningitis.

Therapy for uncomplicated penicillin-sensitive *S. pneumoniae* meningitis should be for 10–14 days with a third-generation cephalosporin or intravenous penicillin (400,000 U/kg/24 h, given every 4–6 hours). If the isolate is resistant to penicillin and the third-generation cephalosporin, therapy should be completed with vancomycin. Intravenous penicillin (300,000 U/kg/24 h) for 5–7 days is the treatment of choice for uncomplicated *N. meningitidis* meningitis.

Uncomplicated *H. influenzae* type b meningitis should be treated for 7–10 days. Patients who receive intravenous or oral antibiotics before LP and who do not have an identifiable pathogen, but do have evidence of an acute bacterial infection on the basis of their CSF profile should continue to receive therapy with ceftriaxone or cefotaxime for 7–10 days. If focal signs are present or the child does not respond to treatment, a parameningeal focus may be present and a CT or MRI scan should be performed.

Meningitis caused by *Escherichia coli* or *P. aeruginosa* requires therapy with a third-generation cephalosporin active against the isolate in vitro. Most isolates of *E. coli* are sensitive to cefotaxime or ceftriaxone and most isolates of *P. aeruginosa* are sensitive to ceftazidime. Gram-negative bacillary meningitis should be treated for 3 weeks or for at least 2 weeks after CSF sterilization, which may occur after 2–10 days of treatment.

> **MINIMUM DURATION OF THERAPY**
> - *Meningococcal meningitis:* 5 days
> - *Haemophilus influenzae meningitis:* 7–10 days
> - *Pneumococcal meningitis:* 10 days
> - *Group B streptococcal meningitis:* 14–21 days
> - *Listeria monocytogenes meningitis:* 14–21 days
> - *Gram-negative bacilli meningitis:* 21 days

Supportive Therapy

Sepsis, hypotension, hypoxemia, and increased ICP all contribute to a reduction in perfusion of the CNS.

Supportive measures to maintain an adequate circulation to the CNS should include reversal of hypoxemia and hypercarbia; intubation and ventilatory support may be necessary for this purpose. Increased partial pressure of arterial carbon dioxide ($PaCO_2$) causes cerebral vasodilatation and thereby worsens ICP. Hyperventilation may be beneficial by causing vasoconstriction and thus reducing cerebral blood volume and decreasing ICP.

Fluid restriction during the first several days in bacterial meningitis has been recommended as a management of the SIADH. A reasonable approach is to give approximately two-thirds of the daily fluid maintenance volume.

Mannitol (0.5 g/kg given intravenously over 20 minutes) can be used to decrease cerebral edema by osmotic movement of fluid from edematous brain tissue to the intravascular compartment. Mannitol can be given repeatedly over a 24 hours period to a total maximum dose of 2 g/kg. Dexamethasone may reduce vasogenic brain edema by a direct effect on vascular endothelial cells.

Subdural effusion develops in 15–30% of patients with bacterial meningitis who are <2 years old. The effusions are usually benign and need not be surgically drained unless they are causing a clinically significant increase in ICP. Subdural empyema is treated by drainage of the subdural space. Hydrocephalus is treated by shunt.

Corticosteroids

Rapid killing of bacteria in the CSF effectively sterilizes the meningeal infection but releases toxic cell products after cell lysis (cell wall endoxin) that precipitate the cytokine-mediated inflammatory cascade. The resultant edema formation and neutrophilic infiltration may produce additional neurologic injury with worsening of CNS signs and symptoms. Therefore, agents that limit production of inflammatory mediators may be of benefit to patients with bacterial meningitis.

Corticosteroids appear to have maximum benefit if given 1–2 hours before antibiotics are initiated. They also may be effective if given concurrently with or soon after the first dose of antibiotics. Complications of corticosteroids include gastrointestinal bleeding, hypertension, hyperglycemia, leukocytosis, and rebound fever after the last dose.

Glucocorticoids have been shown to decrease the inflammatory response in the subarachnoid space and has marked influence on cytokine generation. Data support the use of intravenous dexamethasone, 0.15 mg/kg/dose given every 6 hourly for 5 days, in the treatment of children older than 6 weeks with acute bacterial meningitis caused by *H. influenzae* type b. It is useful in preventing hearing loss and short-term neurological sequel. Among children with meningitis caused by *H. influenzae* type b, corticosteroid recipients have a shorter duration of fever, lower CSF protein and lactate levels, and a reduction in sensorineural hearing loss. Adjunctive dexamethasone therapy is potentially beneficial in children particular those with *H. influenzae* disease. The mechanism of the beneficial effect of steroid is not completely clear.

Specific Antibiotic Therapy

- *Meningococci:* Penicillin 4–5 lakh units/kg/day 4 hourly; cefotaxime 200 mg/kg/day 8 hourly; ceftriaxone 150 mg/kg/day 12 hourly
- *H. influenzae:* Ceftriaxone, cefotaxime, ampicillin 300 mg/kg/day intravenously 6 hourly
- *Pneumococcus:* Cefotaxime or ceftriaxone
- *Staphylococci:* Vancomycin is used

PROGNOSIS

The morbidity and mortality is associated with bacterial meningitis are clearly related to host (age, immune status), the organism (virulence factors), and the adequacy of therapy. Untreated bacterial meningitis is usually fatal.

Mortality rates in neonates with Gram-negative bacillary meningitis is 50%. Mortality rates for *H. influenzae* is 3–5% and *N. meningitidis*, *S. pneumoniae*. The mortality with group B streptococci meningitis is related with the age of onset. Pneumococcal meningitis carries the greatest risk of hearing impairment and highest mortality than with any other organism.

BIBLIOGRAPHY

1. Brouwer MC, McIntyre P, Prasad K, van de Beek D. Corticosteroids for acute bacterial meningitis. Cochrane Database Syst Rev. 2015;2015(9):CD004405.
2. Kim KS. Acute bacterial meningitis in infants and children. Lancet Infect Dis. 2010; 10:32-42.
3. Lehman RK, Schor NF. Neurologic evaluation. In: Kliegman RM, Stanton BF, St. Geme III JW, Schor NF, Behrman RE (Eds). Nelson Textbook of Pediatrics, 19th edition. United Kingdom: Elsevier Health Sciences; 2011. p. 1998.
4. Wootton SH, Aguilera E, Salazar L, Hemmert AC, Hasbun R. Pathogen identification in patients with meningitis. Ann Clin Microbiol Antimicrob. 2016;15:26.

CASE 56

Meningomyelocele

■ PRESENTING COMPLAINTS

New born male baby was brought with the complaint of:
- Swelling in the lower back since birth

History of Presenting Complaints

A 1-day-old male baby was brought to neurosurgery department with history of swelling at the lower back. The resident doctor who attended the delivery noticed the small swelling in the midline at the lower back. He thought it as the defect in the vertebral arch or the neural tube and hence referred to neurosurgical department. The child passed urine and meconium. The movements in all the limbs were normal.

Past History of the Patient

He was the first child of nonconsanguineous marriage. He was born at full term and delivered by cesarean section. The indication for the section was breech presentation. The child cried immediately after the delivery. Small swelling was noticed at the back. The child had all the neonatal reflexes satisfactory. He started taking breast milk. He had transient tachypnea, which settled by itself within 24 hours.

■ EXAMINATION

The boy was moderately built and nourished. He was active and sleeping. All the neonatal reflexes were satisfactory. He had good swallowing, sucking, and rooting reflexes. He had passed urine without dribbling. He had passed meconium.

Anthropometric measurements included the length 49 cm (25th centile), the weight 3 kg (25th centile), and the head circumference 36 cm. There was neither pallor nor edema. He was afebrile. The heart rate was 136 beats/min, the respiratory rate was 28 breaths/min, blood pressure recorded was 50/30 mm Hg.

There was a midline defect in skin of the back. The defect was covered by transparent membrane. It appeared as a small swelling.

CASE AT A GLANCE

Basic Findings
- Length : 49 cm (25th centile)
- Weight : 3 kg (25th centile)
- Temperature : 37°C
- Pulse rate : 136 beats/min
- Respiratory rate : 28 breaths/min
- Blood pressure : 50/30 mm Hg

Positive Findings

History:
- Small swelling at lower back
- Transient tachypnea
- Breech presentation

Examination:
- Small midline defect

Investigation:
- No abnormality detected (NAD)

Under the transparent membrane neural tissue was attached to inner surface. Other systemic examination was normal.

■ INVESTIGATION

- *Hemoglobin:* 14 g/dL
- *TLC:* 9,800 cells/cumm
- *CT scan of head:* Normal
- *MRI of the spine:* Normal

■ DISCUSSION

Meningomyelocele is the midline defect **(Figs. 1 and 2)** of the skin, vertebral arch, and neural tube. It is usually in the lumbosacral region. It is evident at birth as a skin defect over the back bordered laterally by bony prominences of unfused neural arches of the vertebrae.

Folate is intricately involved in the prevention and etiology of neural tube defects (NTDs). Folate functions in single-carbon transfer reactions and exists in many chemical forms. Folic acid (pteroylmonoglutamic acid, which is the most oxidized and stable form of folate, occurs rarely in food but is the form used in vitamin supplements and in fortified food products, particularly flour.

Most naturally occurring folates (food folate) are pteroylpolyglutamates, which contain 1–6 additional glutamate molecules joined in a peptide linkage to the y-carboxyl of glutamate. Folate coenzymes are involved in DNA synthesis, purine synthesis, generation of formate into the formate pool, and amino acid interconversion; the conversion of homocysteine to methionine provides methionine for the synthesis of S-adenosylmethionine (SAMe, an agent important for in vivo methylation). To be effective, folic acid supplementation should be initiated before conception and continued until at least the 12th week of gestation, when neurulation is complete.

Disorders of neural tube formation can involve defects in primary neurulation, closure of the anterior or posterior neuropore, or failure in the development of the lower spinal cord, which may be present before 28 days of gestation. This leads to defects in the spinal cord, dura, meninges, cranium, and vertebrae as well as the dermal coverings. Open neural tube defects, the most common being the myelomeningocele, are characterized by failure of the surface ectoderm to close over the neural elements leaving meninges and spinal cord exposed.

However, disorders in neural tube formation include a wide array of disorders including cranioschisis (total failure

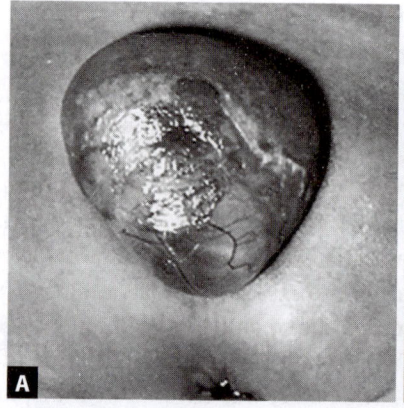 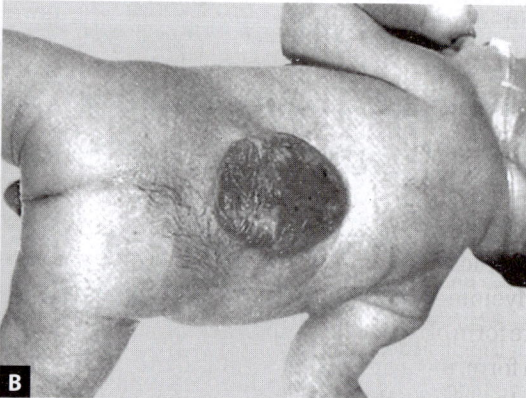

Figs. 1A and B: (A) Meningomyelocele; (B) Myelomeningocele. *(For color version, see Plate 3)*

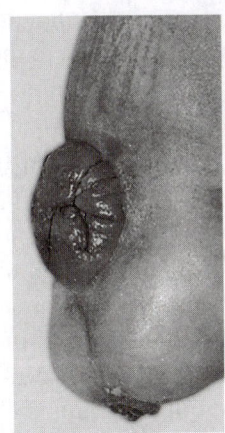

Fig. 2: Meningomyelocele.
(For color version, see Plate 3)

of neurulation), anencephaly (defects in cranial neural tissue development), and encephalocele (herniation of brain or meninges through a cranial defect), as well as occult spinal dysraphisms (skin-covered defects of vertebrae and dermal structures with subtle or absent neural abnormalities).

The defect is usually covered by transparent membrane. This may have neural tissue attached to the inner surface. CSF leaks from this membrane initially. But soon after the birth, drying of the membrane prevents it. As the CSF accumulates membrane bulges. This eventually forms large sac.

Neural tube defects result from a combination of environmental risk factors in addition to genetic causes. 70–80% of all cases are the result of environmental/gene interactions, with the rest being related to aneuploidies, duplications, or deletions. The most common risk factors include folic acid deficiency, fetal exposure to drugs such as valproic acid, and gestational diabetes.

Myelomeningocele represents the most severe form of dysraphism, i.e., called aperta or open form, involving the vertebral column and spinal cord, which occurs with an incidence of approximately 1 in 4,000 live births.

Mutations in the genes encoding the enzymes involved in homocysteine metabolism may play a role in the pathogenesis of meningomyelocele. These enzymes include 5,10-methylenetetrahydrofolate reductase, cystathionine beta-synthase, and methionine synthase.

Children will have a complex, multifaceted congenital disorder of structure that represents dysraphic state (a defective closure of the embryonic neural groove). It is characterized anatomically as follows:
- Presence of unfused or excessively separated vertebral arches of the bony spine
- Cystic dilation of the meninges that surround the spinal cord
- Cystic dilation of spinal cord itself
- Hydrocephalus and the spectrum of congenital cerebral abnormalities

■ CLINICAL FEATURES (FIG. 3)

Myelomeningocele produces dysfunction of many organs and structures, including the skeleton, skin, and gastrointestinal and genitourinary tracts, in addition to the peripheral nervous system and the CNS. A myelomeningocele may be located anywhere along the neuraxis, but the lumbosacral region accounts for at least 75% of the cases. The extent and degree of the neurologic deficit depend on the location of the myelomeningocele and the associated lesions. A lesion in the low sacral region causes bowel and bladder incontinence associated with anesthesia in the perineal area but with no impairment of motor function. Newborns with a defect in the midlumbar or high lumbothoracic region typically have either a saclike cystic structure covered by a thin layer of partially epithelialized tissue or an exposed flat neural placode without overlying tissues. When a cyst or membrane is present,

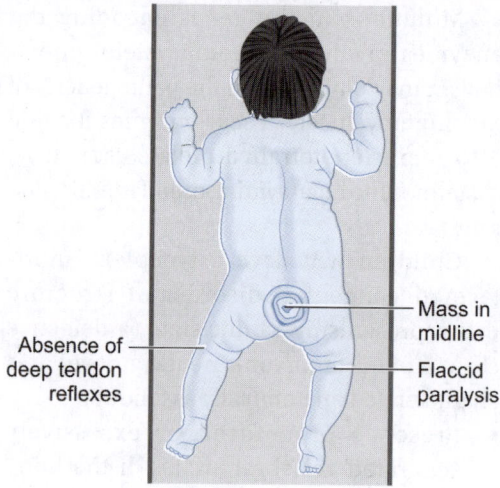

Fig. 3: Clinical features.

remnants of neural tissue are visible beneath the membrane, which occasionally ruptures and leaks CSF.

Infants with myelomeningocele typically have increased neurologic deficit as the myelomeningocele extends higher into the thoracic region. These infants sometimes have an associated kyphotic gibbus that requires neonatal orthopedic correction. Patients with a myelomeningocele in the upper thoracic or cervical region usually have a very minimal neurologic deficit and, in most cases, do not have hydrocephalus. They can have neurogenic bladder and bowel.

In most (80%) of the cases, meningomyelocele is associated with a type II Arnold–Chiari malformation. There will be maldevelopment and downward displacement of the cerebellum, 4th ventricle, and medulla oblongata. Hydrocephalus occurs as a result of aqueductal stenosis. The associated deformities of the meningomyelocele include dislocated hips, talipes equinovarus, and atrophy of the tongue.

Examination of the infant shows a flaccid paralysis of the lower extremities, an absence of DTR, a lack of response to touch and pain, and a high incidence of lower-extremity deformities (clubfeet, ankle and/or knee contractures, and subluxation of the hips). Some children have constant urinary dribbling and a relaxed anal sphincter. Other children do not leak urine and in fact have a high-pressure bladder and sphincter dyssynergy, thus, myelomeningocele above the midlumbar region tends to produce lower motor neuron signs because of abnormalities and disruption of the conus medullaris and above spinal cord structures.

Neurological assessment should be done. This is to determine the severity of the functional defect. Pin prick over the legs and trunk will help to know the upper level of the spinal cord dysfunction. Defective innervation of the bladder is indicated by urinary dribbling. Patulous anal sphincter and lack of anal reflex indicate defective perianal region. The denervated limbs are patulous.

Diagnosis of open neural tube defects is suspected early in the second trimester of pregnancy if elevated serum levels of alpha fetoprotein are detected. Open neural tube defects are also diagnosed prenatally through the routine use of fetal USG. Changes in the head shape (lemon sign) and cerebellum (banana sign) are often the presenting findings on fetal ultrasound. Early prenatal diagnosis is crucial in order to allow, families the opportunity to plan the pregnancy, including considering the option of fetal surgery, which can be performed between 19 and 26 weeks of gestation. Prenatal diagnosis is also beneficial in order to plan for delivery at an institution.

GENERAL FEATURES

- Bladder incontinence
- Congenital midline defect
- Lack of response to touch and pain.

DIFFERENTIAL DIAGNOSIS
- Spina bifida occulta
- Meningocele
- Encephalocele

TREATMENT

Management and supervision of a child and family with a myelomeningocele require a multidisciplinary team approach, including surgeons, other physicians, and therapists, with one individual (often a pediatrician) acting as the advocate and coordinator of the treatment program.

Careful evaluation and reassessment of the genitourinary system is an important component of management. Latex-free catheters and gloves must be used to prevent development of latex allergy. Periodic urine cultures and assessment of renal function, including serum electrolytes and creatinine as well as renal scans, vesiculourethrograms, renal ultrasonograms, and cystometrograms, are obtained according to the risk status and progress of the patient and the results of the physical examination.

Although incontinence of fecal matter is common and is socially unacceptable during the school years, it does not pose the same organ.

In utero surgical closure of a spinal lesion has been successful. There is a lower incidence of hindbrain abnormalities and hydrocephalus (fewer shunts) as well as improved motor outcomes.

Postnatal treatment remains the safest treatment option for both mother and child with open neural tube defects. Infants are usually delivered at term by cesarean section to prevent potential injury to the exposed neural elements during a vaginal birth. Broad-spectrum antibiotics are started after delivery, a moist sterile dressing is applied to the back, and baseline neurologic assessment and head ultrasound are performed.

Surgery is often done within a day or so of birth but can be delayed for several days (except when there is a CSF leak) to allow the parents time to begin to adjust to the shock and to prepare for the multiple procedures and inevitable problems that lie ahead. Evaluation of other congenital anomalies and renal function can also be initiated before surgery. Most pediatric centers aggressively treat the majority of infants with myelomeningocele. After repair of myelomeningocele, most infants require a shunting procedure for hydrocephalus. If symptoms or signs of hindbrain dysfunction appear, early surgical decompression of the posterior fossa is indicated. Clubfeet can require taping or casting, and dislocated hips may require operative procedures.

Hydrocephalus

Aqueductal gliosis can also give rise to hydrocephalus. As a result of neonatal meningitis or a subarachnoid hemorrhage in a premature infant, the ependymal lining of the aqueduct is interrupted and a brisk glial response results in complete obstruction. Intrauterine viral infections can also produce aqueductal stenosis followed by hydrocephalus, and mumps meningoencephalitis has been reported as a cause in a child. A vein of Galen malformation can expand to become large and, because of its midline position, obstruct the flow of CSF. Lesions or malformations of the posterior fossa are prominent causes of hydrocephalus, including posterior fossa brain tumors, Chiari malformation, and the Dandy–Walker syndrome.

Nonobstructive or communicating hydrocephalus most commonly follows a subarachnoid hemorrhage, which is usually a result of IVH in a premature infant. Blood in the subarachnoid spaces can cause obliteration of the cisterns or arachnoid villi and obstruction of CSF flow.

Therapy for hydrocephalus depends on the cause. Medical management, including the use of acetazolamide and furosemide, can provide temporary relief by reducing the rate of CSF production, but long-term results have been disappointing. Most cases of hydrocephalus require extracranial shunts, particularly a ventriculoperitoneal shunt.

Endoscopic third ventriculostomy has evolved as a viable approach and criteria have been developed for its use, but the procedure might need to be repeated to be effective. Ventricular shunting may be avoided with this approach. The major complications of shunting are occlusion (characterized by headache, papilledema, emesis, mental status changes) and bacterial infection (fever, headache, meningismus), usually caused by *Staphylococcus epidermidis*. With meticulous preparation, the shunt infection rate can be reduced to <59%. The results of intrauterine surgical management of fetal hydrocephalus have been poor (possibly because of the high rate of associated cerebral malformations in addition to the hydrocephalus) except for some promise in cases of hydrocephalus associated with fetal meningomyelocele.

Open neural tube defects are one of the most common causes of pediatric hydrocephalus in the world. Prior to the introduction of fetal surgery, approximately 80% of patients with a myelomeningocele required treatment for hydrocephalus, and the most common treatment is the implantation of a CSF ventriculoperitoneal shunt. Shunts are an effective treatment; however, they have a very high failure rate, especially in infants, in whom the failure rate is 30% in the first year. Endoscopic third ventriculostomy with choroid plexus coagulation is a reemerging alternative treatment for hydrocephalus that does not rely on an implant and has a moderate success rate in the myelomeningocele population.

Chiari II Malformations

Open neural tube defects almost always result in Chiari II malformations. It is defined by the caudal herniation of the cerebellar vermis, brain stem, and fourth ventricle into the spinal canal, and it is associated with a variety of other changes in the brain and skull due to the persistent leak of CSF through the open neural tube defect. Most Chiari II malformations are asymptomatic or mildly symptomatic and respond to treatment with a CSF shunt. This is the leading cause of death in patients following treatment for a myelodysplastic syndrome. Treatment for this condition includes tracheostomy, gastric tube, and cervical decompressive laminectomies for palliation.

Cognitive Development

The brain development of children with myelomeningocele is affected by the presence of the Chiari II malformation. Cognition can be further affected by complications of hydrocephalus and by shunt infections, especially those that occur during infancy. Most individuals with myelomeningoceles have cognition in the normal range but with averages of first standard deviation below the general population. Early intervention is crucial in the first years of life. Therapeutic goals are best integrated into the family routine.

Lower Extremity Paraparesis

Lower extremity weakness occurs in varying degrees with neural tube defects, and is much more common with open defects. Infants with the ability to flex their hips and extend their knees have the best prognosis for ambulation with or without orthotics. Early evaluation and intervention by a physical medicine and rehabilitation specialist maximizes the potential for ambulation.

Neurogenic Bowel and Bladder

Neurogenic bowel and bladder leads to incontinence in nearly all individuals with open neural tube defects. Bowel and bladder dysfunction is related to the lack of communication of the lower sacral nerves with the CNS. Bladder pressures are often high secondary to bladder sphincter dysfunction, and poor drainage leads to stasis and risk of infection. Lack of proper bladder care can lead to the deterioration of the upper urinary tract and the development of renal disease.

Careful evaluation and reassessment of the genitourinary system are some of the most important components of the management. Periodic urine cultures and assessment of renal function including serum electrolytes and creatinine as well as renal vesiculourethrograms, renal USG, and cystometrograms are obtained according to the risk status and progress of the patient and the results of the physical examinations.

Although incontinence of fecal matter is common and is socially, unacceptable during the school years, it does not pose the same organ damaging risks as urinary dysfunction.

Management of the neurogenic bladder involves routine clean intermittent catheterization to drain the bladder and the use of anticholinergic drugs to decrease bladder irritability and pressures. Antibiotic prophylaxis is also helpful for those with vesicoureteral reflux. These treatment modalities also help with the achievement of continence.

The neurogenic bowel presents with poor motility and sphincter control, leading to incontinence. Constipation and fecal impaction are common. Fecal impaction can lead to encopresis, with the passage of liquid stools, which is often misinterpreted by patients and their families as diarrhea. Management of the bowel involves the use of laxatives and a high-fiber diet to prevent constipation. Continence is best achieved through the use of suppositories or enemas daily.

Orthopedic Issues

Joint and spine complications are common such as scoliosis, talipes equinovarus, hip dislocation, and contractures. Paralysis with resulting unbalanced muscle strength around joints leads to various deformities. Management involves maximizing the potential for ambulation and independence. Scoliosis is common in higher level lesions, but rapidly progressing curves warrant an evaluation for a tethered cord. Surgical intervention is also directed at maintenance of proper positioning in braces and wheelchairs to prevent skin breakdown and pressure ulcer development.

■ PROGNOSIS

For the child born with defect treated aggressively, mortality rate is approximately 10–15% and death occurs before the age of 1–4 years. 70% of survivors have normal intelligence.

Because myelomeningocele is a chronic disabling condition, periodic and consistent multidisciplinary follow-up is required for life. Renal dysfunction is one of the most important determinants of mortality.

Prognosis depends upon the extent of motor deficits and status of bladder innervation, and also associated cerebral anomalies. Most infants die during early childhood from complications of therapy such as hydrocephalus and chronic renal failure. Without surgery 90% of the affected infants die in their first year.

PREVENTION

Although there have been many advancements in the care for patients with spina bifida over the years, none are as effective as prevention. Neural tube defects are not completely preventable; however, the addition of folic acid to the food supply has lowered the incidence of spina bifida significantly. Women of childbearing age should take folic acid supplementation to prevent open neural tube defects; mothers of children with spina bifida should take high doses of folic acid if they plan on becoming pregnant again. Current recommendations are 400 ug of folic acid daily for all women of childbearing ages and 4 mg daily for women who have had a previously affected pregnancy.

BIBLIOGRAPHY

1. Adzick NS, Thom EA, Spong CY, Brock JW 3rd, Burrows PK, Johnson MP, et al.; MOMS Investigators. A randomized trial of prenatal versus postnatal repair of myelomeningocele. N Engl J Med. 2011;364(11);993-1004.
2. Menkes JH, Moser FG. Neurological examination of child and infant. In: Menkes JH, Sarnat HB, Maria BL (Eds). Child Neurology, 7th edition. United Kingdom: Lippincott Williams & Wilkins; 2006. pp. 1-29.
3. Phadke SR, Puri RD, Ranganath P. Prenatal screening of genetic disorders. Indian J Med Res. 2017;146(6):686-99.
4. SOGC Genetics Committee; Wilson RD, Audibert F, Brock JA, Campagnolo C, Carroll J, Cartier L, et al.; Society of Obstetricians and Gynaecologists of Canada. Prenatal screening, diagnosis, and pregnancy management of fetal neural tube defects. J Obstet Gynaecol Can. 2014;36(10):927-42.

SECTION 8

Endocrine System

- Case 57 **Ambiguous Genitalia**
- Case 58 **Congenital Adrenal Hyperplasia**
- Case 59 **Cushing's Syndrome**
- Case 60 **Diabetes Insipidus**
- Case 61 **Diabetes Mellitus**
- Case 62 **Hypothyroidism**
- Case 63 **Precocious Puberty**
- Case 64 **Undescended Testes**

CASE 57

Ambiguous Genitalia

■ PRESENTING COMPLAINTS

A newborn baby was brought with the complaint of:
- Abnormality in external genitalia since birth

History of Presenting Complaints

A baby was noticed at birth to be having ambiguous genitalia. The baby was the first child of a nonconsanguineous marriage. The age of the mother was 24 years, and the age of the father was 27 years. The child was born at full term by normal delivery. The mother did not have any antenatal check-ups. She was not on any medication throughout the pregnancy. She went into labor spontaneously. She delivered about 12 hours of labor. The child cried immediately after the delivery. The child did not require any resuscitation. There was no family history of ambiguous genitalia.

■ EXAMINATION

On examination, the child was active, alert, and normally built. There were no dysmorphic facial features. The color of the baby was pink. Anthropometric measurements included, the length of the child was 50 cm (50th centile), the weight of the child was 3 kg (50th centile), and the head circumference was 3 cm.

CASE AT A GLANCE

Basic Findings
Length	: 50 cm (50th centile)
Weight	: 3 kg (50th centile)
Temperature	: 37°C
Pulse rate	: 120 beats/min
Respiratory rate	: 30 breaths/min
Blood pressure	: 60/40 mm Hg

Positive Findings

History:
- Ambiguous genitalia

Examination:
- Hepatomegaly
- Small phallus
- Perineal hypospadias
- Labia fused
- Palpable symmetric gonads

Investigation:
- *Hemoglobin:* Decreased
- *Serum cortisol:* Increased
- *17-hydroxyprogesterone:* Raised
- *Urinary 17-ketosteroids:* Raised
- *Karyotype:* 46 XY

The child was afebrile. The pulse rate was 120 beats/min. The respiratory rate was 30 breaths/min. The blood pressure recorded was 60/40 mm Hg.

There was pallor, no cyanosis, and no lymphadenopathy. There was no edema and no icterus. Per abdomen examination revealed a soft abdomen, liver was palpable about 2 cm below the costal margin. The baby had a small phallus, perineal hypospadias, and labia were fused. Two symmetrical gonads about 1 cm were palpable in the labioscrotal folds.

■ INVESTIGATION

- *Hemoglobin:* 9 mg/dL
- *Total leukocyte count (TLC):* 9,000 cells/mm^3
- *Serum electrolytes:*
  - *Na:* 140 mEq/L
  - *K:* 5 mEq/L
  - *Cl:* 100 mEq/L
- *Serum glucose:* 80 mg/dL
- *Serum cortisol:*
  - 30 µg/dL: 8 AM
  - 20 µg/dL: 6 PM
- *17-hydroxy progesterone:* 5 nmol/L
- *Karyotype:* 46 XY
- *Urinary 17-ketosteroids:* 40 mg/24 h

■ DISCUSSION

Ambiguous genitalia is defined as a discrepancy between external genitalia and internal gonads.

The definition of atypical or ambiguous genitalia, in a broad sense, is in any case in which the external genitalia do not appear completely male or completely female. Although there are standards for genital size dimensions, variations in the size of these structures do not always constitute ambiguity.

An understanding of the embryology of sexual differentiation is essential for the investigation of sexual ambiguity. The sex-determining region of the human Y chromosome during the critical phase determines the differentiation of the germinal ridge between 7 and 8 weeks of gestation. The resultant testicular tissue contains seminiferous and Sertoli cells. This produces the Müllerian inhibiting factor. Functional ovaries are not required for female internal genital organs.

Because there is no Müllerian inhibitory substance (MIS) the gonads are ovaries and not testes, the uterus, tubes, and ovaries develop. It results from the exposure of the female fetus to excessive exogenous and endogenous androgens during intrauterine life. The changes consist principally of virilization of the external genitals, i.e., clitoral hypertrophy and labioscrotal fusion. The causes are congenital adrenal hyperplasia (CAH), aromatase deficiency virilizing maternal tumors, and administration of androgenic drugs to women during pregnancy.

Anti-Müllerian hormone (AMH) causes the Müllerian ducts to regress; in its absence, they persist in the uterus, fallopian tubes, cervix, and upper vagina. AMH activation in the testes may require the steroidogenic factor-1 (*SF-1*) gene by about 8 weeks of gestation the Leydig cells of the testis begin to produce testosterone. During this critical period of male differentiation, testosterone secretion is stimulated by placental human chorionic gonadotropin (hCG) which peaks at 8–12 weeks. In the latter half of pregnancy, lower levels of testosterone are maintained by luteinizing hormone (LH) secreted by the fetal pituitary. Testosterone produced locally initiates the development of the ipsilateral Wolffian duct into the epididymis, vas deferens, and seminal vesicle.

Development of the external genitalia also requires dihydrotestosterone (DHT), the more active metabolite of testosterone. DHT is produced largely from circulating testosterone and is necessary to fuse the genital folds to form the penis and scrotum. DHT is also produced via an alternative biosynthetic pathway from androstanediol, and this pathway must be intact for normal and complete prenatal virilization to occur.

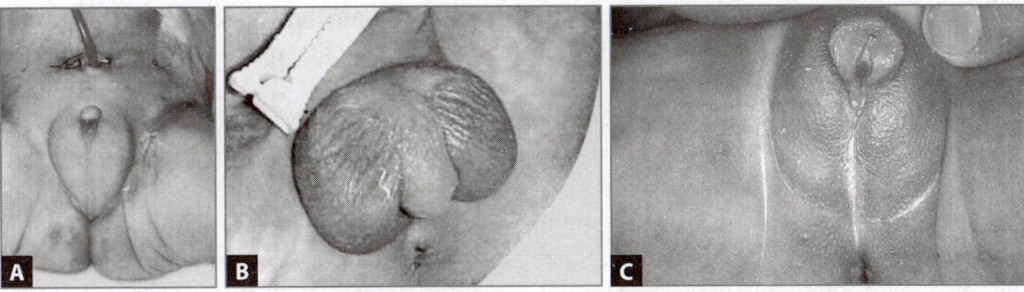

Figs. 1A to C: (A and B) Ambiguous genitalia and (C) Abnormal genitalia—CAH.

A functional androgen receptor, produced by an X-linked gene, is required for testosterone and DHT to induce these androgen effects.

In the XX fetus with normal long and short arms of the X chromosome, the bipotential gonad develops into an ovary by about the 10–11th week. This occurs only in the absence of sex-determining region on the Y chromosome (SRY), testosterone, and AMH and requires a normal gene in the dosage sensitive.

A female external phenotype **(Figs. 1A to C)** develops in the absence of fetal gonads. However, the male phenotype development requires androgen production and action. Estrogen is unnecessary for normal prenatal sexual differentiation, as demonstrated by 46,XX patients with aromatase deficiency and by mice without estradiol receptors.

Development of the male phenotype is potentially more complex. It requires a Y chromosome and, specifically, an intact *SRY* gene, which, in association with genes such as *SOX9*, *SF-1*, Wilms' tumor 1 (WT1), and others, directs the undifferentiated gonad to become a testis. Aberrant recombinations may result in X chromosomes carrying SRY, resulting in XX males, or Y chromosomes that have lost SRY, resulting in XY females.

A variety of abnormalities in chromosomal distribution, gonadal differentiation, gonadal function, testosterone synthesis, and action, or adrenal function can lead to aberrant development of internal and external genital structures. These abnormalities can be divided into four categories.

Abnormalities in Normal Gonadal Differentiation

These abnormalities usually result from an abnormality in the number of sex chromosomes. Klinefelter syndrome with a 47,XXY karyotype, is associated with a male phenotype but with poorly functioning testes. Turner syndrome with a 45,XO karyotype is associated with a female phenotype but with streak ovaries (gonadal dysgenesis).

Mosaic forms of gonadal dysgenesis that contain a Y-bearing cell line have variable ambiguous internal and external phenotypes.

Idiopathic testicular failure prior to the completion of sexual differentiation results in ambiguous genitalia (incomplete virilization).

True hermaphroditism with the presence of both testicular and ovarian tissue, is rare and associated with external genitalia that range from fully masculine to almost completely feminine.

Abnormalities in Testosterone Synthesis or Action

These disorders are generally present as micropenis, genital ambiguity, or complete absence of male external genitalia in an XY individual. Testicular tissue is present and therefore, internal structures are Wolffian.

Disorders in this category include enzymatic defects in testosterone synthesis (such as 12-ketoreductase deficiency) or defects in the conversion of testosterone to DHT (5-alpha reductase deficiency). Since the gonads and adrenal glands share common enzymes of steroid hormone production, some of the enzymatic defects associated with male genital ambiguity may also affect the production of cortisol and aldosterone, leading to symptoms of CAH or salt wasting.

Defects in testosterone action result from absent or defective androgen receptors (androgen insensitivity) and depending on the resultant degree of defect in androgen binding, the genital phenotype can range from relatively mild male ambiguity to complete female external development.

Disorders of Adrenal Androgen Production

These disorders can cause genital ambiguity in both XY and XX individuals. Excessive adrenal androgen production secondary to an enzyme defect in cortisol synthesis (i.e., CAH) is the cause of 95% inappropriate virilization in 46,XX newborns. It is a rare cause of genital ambiguity in XY individuals.

Miscellaneous

Various syndromes such as VATER (vertebrae, anus, heart, trachea, esophagus, renal, and limbs), Denys–Drash, and Smith–Lemli–Opitz, have a wide variety of congenital anomalies including genital ambiguity. Maternal exposure to androgens or androgen antagonists is a rare cause of genital ambiguity in newborns.

Differentiation of the urogenital sinus and external genitalia in males is dependent on testosterone and specifically DHT in the first 14 weeks. The practical implications are as follows:

- *Genetic:* Usually signified by karyotype.
- *Gonadal:* Testes, ovaries, or incompletely differentiated gonads.
- *Phenotypic:* Complete male differentiation being dependent on intact testosterone and migration inhibitory factor (MIF) pathways.

Female Pseudohermaphroditism

The genotype is XX and gonads are ovaries. The external genitalia are virilization. This occurs if there is exposure of the female fetus to androgens during sexual differentiation. This can be because of maternal medication, maternal virilization tumor—arrhenoblastoma, or adrenal androgen production.

Male Pseudohermaphroditism

The genotype XY, but external genitalia are incompletely virilized, ambiguous, or completely female.

True

Both the ovaries and testicular tissues are present. The clinical picture resembles male or female pseudohermaphroditism. The majority of them have 46,XX karyotypes.

Partial Androgen Insensitivity

This diagnosis depends upon the confirmation that tests are morphologically normal. They are capable of testosterone synthesis and the 5α-reductase step is intact. HCG stimulation with the androgen analysis in plasma and urine samples are used to assess the Leydig cell reserves and integrity of the testosterone and DHT pathways.

If no gonads had been palpable, as occurs in most cases of ambiguous genitalia, the most likely diagnosis would have been CAH.

When the gonads can be found, they are invariably testes, their development may range from rudimentary to normal. Because the process of normal virilization in the fetus is complex, there are many varieties of male hermaphroditism.

The presence of two equal gonads means the patient is likely to be a boy with karyotype 46,XY. These will be insensitive to testosterone or impaired biosynthesis to testosterone. When the defect is complete the patient is phenotypically female, but the partial defect produces ambiguous genitalia with palpable two gonads. This is the most common cause of male pseudohermaphroditism.

If the testosterone synthesis is impaired by an enzyme defect male informal genitalia do not develop because of lack of DHT. The gonadal biopsy is indicated to distinguish these conditions.

■ CLINICAL FEATURES (FIG. 2)

There is a spectrum of characters ranging from almost complete feminization of the external genitalia to an apparently normal male with oligospermia. In more severe form, the key discussion is whether the phallus has sufficient erectile tissue to allow for growth and a satisfactory male role.

A palpable gonad in the scrotum **(Fig. 3)** is nearly always testes. If no gonad is palpable and external genitalia appear ambiguous, such a newborn is likely to be female with virilization due to the production of excess nongonadal androgen.

External genitalia in male children may be incompletely developed. The testes may be undescended. The genital swelling that forms the scrotal fold may not fuse in the middle and superficially looks like labia major. The size of the penis may be small. This has to be differentiated from the enlarged clitoris.

If the perineal urethra does not fuse, the perineal hypospadias results in female infants with ambiguous genitalia. There may be a single external opening both for the urethra and vagina. The presence or absence of urethra can be determined by rectal examination. Genetic abnormalities may be associated with other anomalies, such as renal agenesis, anal anomalies, Wilms' tumor, and aniridia.

The phallus must meet two major criteria to classify as micropenis:
1. The phallus must be normally formed, with the urethral meatus located on the head of the penis and the penis positioned in an appropriate relationship

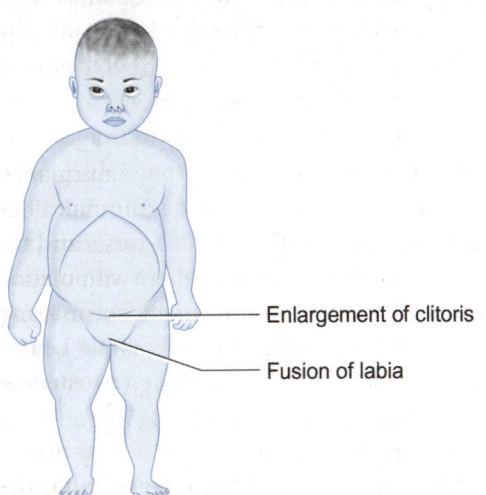

Fig. 2: Clinical features.

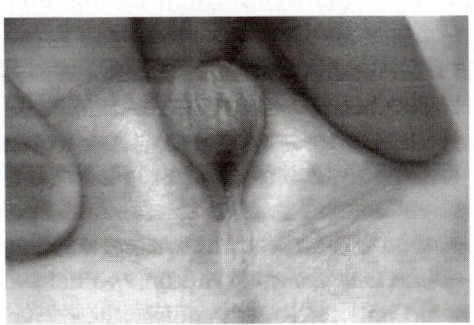

Fig. 3: Palpable gonad in the scrotum.

to the scrotum and other pelvic structures. If these features are not present, then the term *micropenis* should be avoided.
2. The phallus must be >2.5 standard deviations below the appropriate mean of age. For a term newborn, this means that a penis <2 cm in a stretch length is classified as a micropenis.

It is essential that the phallus be measured appropriately. This entails the use of a rigid ruler pressed firmly against the public symphysis, depressing the suprapubic fat pad as much as possible. The phallus is grasped gently by its lateral margins and stretched. The measurement is taken along the dorsum of the penis. Note should be made of the breadth of the phallic shaft. Micropenis must be recognized early in life so that appropriate diagnostic tests can be done.

Causes of Micropenis

Regression of the Müllerian system, a fusion of the labioscrotal folds, and migration of the urethral meatus occur during the first trimester of gestation, further growth of the phallus during the second and third trimester is dependent on the production of testosterone in response to fetal LH. Growth hormone (GH) also enhances penile length in utero. Thus, the following disorders can result in micropenis:
- *Hypothalamic/pituitary dysfunction:* Isolated Kallmann syndrome, Prader–Willi syndrome, septooptic dysplasia, and testicular dysfunction or failure.
- *Testicular dysfunction or failure:* Intra-uterine testicular torsion and testicular dysplasia.
- *Complex (testicular and/or pituitary) or idiopathic:* Robinow syndrome, Klinefelter syndrome, and other X polysomies.
- Partial androgen resistance

> **GENERAL FEATURES**
> - Incompletely developed genitalia
> - Penis may be small
> - Single external opening both for urethra and vagina

■ DIAGNOSIS

The appearance of the external genitalia is rarely diagnostic of a particular disorder and thus does not often allow distinction among the various forms of disorders of sex development. The most common forms of 46,XX disorders of sex development are virilizing forms of CAH. It is important to note that in 46,XY disorders of sex development, the specific diagnosis is not found in up to 50% of cases; partial androgen insensitivity syndrome and pure gonadal dysgenesis are common identifiable etiologies in XY disorders of sex development.

The six most common diagnoses accounted for 50% of the cases. These included virilizing CAH, androgen insensitivity syndrome, mixed gonadal dysgenesis, clitoral/labial anomalies, hypogonadotropic hypogonadism, and 46,XY small-for-gestational-age males with hypospadias.

The relative lack of established diagnoses in 46,XY disorders of sex development disorders of sex development and the resulting lack of specific management emphasizes the need for thorough diagnostic evaluations. These include biochemical characterization of possible steroidogenic enzymatic defects in each patient with genital ambiguity. The parents need counseling about the potentially complex nature of the baby's condition, and guidance as to how to deal with their well-meaning but curious friends and family members.

The evaluation and management should be carried out by a multidisciplinary team of experts that includes pediatric endocrinology, pediatric surgery/urology, pediatric radiology, newborn medicine, genetics, and psychology. Once the sex of rearing has been agreed on by the family and team, treatment can be organized. Genetic counseling should be offered when the specific diagnosis is established.

After a complete history and physical exam, the common diagnostic approach includes multiple steps, described in the following outline. These steps are usually performed simultaneously rather than waiting for the results of one test prior to performing another, because of the sensitive and sometimes urgent nature of the condition. Careful attention to the presence of physical features other than the genitalia is crucial, to determine if a diagnosis of a particular multisystem syndrome is possible.

Diagnostic tests include the following:
- *Karyotype*, with a rapid determination of sex chromosomes (in many centers this is available within 24–48 hours)
- *Other blood tests:*
  - Screen for CAH: Cortisol biosynthetic precursors and adrenal androgens (particularly 17-hydroxyprogesterone (17-OHP) and androstenedione for 21-hydroxylase deficiency (21-OHD), the most common form).
  - Screen for androgens and their biosynthetic precursors.
  - Screen for gonadal response to gonadotropin in patients suspected of having testicular gonads: Stimulation with injections of hCG; measure testosterone and DHT before and after hCG.
  - Molecular genetic analyses for SRY and other Y-specific loci
  - Gonadotropin levels

Both testosterone and estrogen estimation are useful in the diagnosis of intersex states.

HCG stimulation tests by intramuscular injection for 3–5 days help to determine the enzymatic deficiency. Basal gonadotropin levels are elevated in primary testicular disease and androgen resistance syndrome, Turner syndrome, and gonadotropin receptor defect. The level is low in hypothalamic and pituitary defects.

Plasma testosterone/DHT ratio is elevated in 5-α-reductase deficiency. A gonadal biopsy is indicated if the karyotyping is 46,XX.

A rectal examination is done for the evaluation of the presence of the vaginal pouch, uterus, and prostate.

Bone age is advanced in CAH and delayed in gonadal dysgenesis and hypopituitarism.

A retrograde genitourethrogram is done to identify urogenital sinus. Pelvic ultrasonography, computed tomography (CT), or magnetic resonance imaging (MRI) is helpful to evaluate internal genitalia, undescended gonads, and adrenal anomalies.

- *The internal anatomy of patients with ambiguous genitalia* can be defined with one or more of the following studies:
  - Voiding cystourethrogram
  - Endoscopic examination of the genitourinary tract
  - Pelvic ultrasound; renal and adrenal ultrasound
  - Pelvic CT or MRI
  - Exploratory laparoscopy

LABORATORY SALIENT FINDINGS
• Bone age
• Retrograde genitourethrogram
• Pelvic ultrasonography
• CT scan
• MRI
• *Genetic studies:* Chromosomal analysis
• Measurement of adrenal steroids
• Measurement of testosterone and dihydrotestosterone
(CT: computed tomography; MRI; magnetic resonance imaging)

> **ESSENTIAL DIAGNOSTIC POINTS**
> - Presence of gonadal structure in labioscrotal fold
> - Gonads found in the inguinal canal
> - Phallic size and location urethral meatus
> - Presence of midline abnormalities

■ DIFFERENTIAL DIAGNOSIS

- CAH
- Precocious puberty
- Reifenstein syndrome
- Leydig cell agenesis
- Tumor of adrenal

■ TREATMENT

In male pseudohermaphroditism, a trial of exogenous testosterone depo injection (25 mg) monthly for 3 months can be used to judge whether there is an adequate increase in stretched penile length.

If the female role is agreed upon, management includes genitoplasty with reconstruction of the vagina (uterus and fallopian tube are absent). Removal of testes is advised to avoid masculinization in puberty. Estrogen replacement is introduced from the age of 12 years.

Surgical Management of Ambiguous Genitals

Significantly virilized females usually undergo surgery between 2 and 6 months of age. If there is severe clitoromegaly, the clitoris is reduced in size, with partial excision of the corporal bodies and preservation of the neurovascular bundle; however, moderate clitoromegaly may become much less noticeable even without surgery as the patient grows. Vaginoplasty and correction of the urogenital sinus usually are performed at the time of clitoral surgery; revision in adolescence is often necessary.

■ BIBLIOGRAPHY

1. Ahmed SE, Rodie M. Investigation and initial management of ambiguous genitalia. Best Pract Res Clin Endocrinol Metab. 2010; 24(2):197-218.
2. MacLaughlin DT, Donahoe PK. Sex determination and differentiation. N Engl J Med. 2004;350(4):367-78.

Congenital Adrenal Hyperplasia

CASE 58

■ PRESENTING COMPLAINTS

A 3-week-old boy was brought with the complaint of:
- Vomiting since 2 weeks
- Not taking proper feeds since 1 week

History of Presenting Complaints

A 3-week-old boy was brought to the hospital early in the morning with the history that the child was not taking feeds. The mother complained that her son was not taking feeds properly and not sucking satisfactorily. His mother also told him that he was vomiting. The child had several bouts of vomiting. Vomitus used to contain the milk in curdled form. He was exclusively on breast milk.

Past History of the Patient

He was the second sibling of a nonconsanguineous marriage. He was born at full term by normal delivery. He cried immediately after the delivery. The birth weight was 3.25 kg. The head circumference was 35 cm. There was no significant postnatal event. He started taking breast milk regularly. The child was discharged on the fifth day. He had transient physiological jaundice.

■ EXAMINATION

On examination, the child was moderately built and nourished. There were signs of moderate dehydration. The anterior fontanelle was sunken. He was lying flaccid on the examination table. Anthropometric measurements included, length was 54 cm (75th centile), weight was 3 kg (10th centile), and head circumference was 35 cm.

The child was afebrile. The pulse rate was 116 beats/min and the respiratory rate was 30 breaths/min. The blood pressure recorded was 60/50 mm Hg. Pallor was present. No edema, no icterus, and no lymphadenopathy. Per abdomen revealed the presence of mild distension. There was no organomegaly, and other systemic examinations were normal.

CASE AT A GLANCE

Basic Findings
- Length : 54 cm (75th centile)
- Weight : 3 kg (10th centile)
- Temperature : 37°C
- Pulse rate : 116 beats/min
- Respiratory rate : 30 breaths/min
- Blood pressure : 60/50 mm Hg

Positive Findings

History:
- Feeding problems
- Vomiting

Examination:
- Dehydration

Investigation:
- Hyponatremia
- Hyperkalemia
- *Hydrocortisone challenge test:* Increased 17-hydroxyprogesterone levels

INVESTIGATION

- *Hemoglobin:* 10 g/dL
- *TLC:* 7,000 cells/mm^3
- *Erythrocyte sedimentation rate (ESR):* 22 mm in the first hour
- *Blood urea:* 16 mg/dL
- *Plasma testosterone:* 15 nmol (normal range: 9.5–30 nmol/L)
- *Plasma cortisol:*
  - 6 μg/dL at 8 AM
  - 2 μg/dL at 6 PM
- *Serum aldosterone:* 5 ng/dL
- *Serum electrolyte:*
  - Na: 118 mEq/L
  - K: 4 mEq/L
  - HCO_3: 12 mEq/L
- *Plasma 17-OHP:* 650 nmol/L
- *Urine routine:* Normal
- *Hydrocortisone challenge test for urinary 17-hydroxy-progesterone:* 488 nmol (normal range <15 nmol)
- *Ultrasound abdomen:* To rule out hydronephrosis and bladder obstruction.

DISCUSSION

A 3-week-old boy presented with a history of feeding problems and persistent vomiting with severe dehydration. This is also associated with hyponatremia and hyperkalemia with raised 17-OHP levels. These findings suggest CAH.

It is inherited as an autosomal recessive trait. It is a group of defects in steroid synthesis, is characterized by a deficiency of adrenocortical hormones on one hand and an excess of steroid precursors on the other hand. As most steroidogenic enzymes are expressed in the adrenal, their disorders tend to be lumped under the term CAH.

Most disorders of adrenal steroidogenesis are not characterized by adrenal hyperplasia. One form of CAH, 21-OHD, accounts for >90% of cases and is found in all ethnic groups. The other disorders are rare and tend to be found in isolated genetic clusters. Because each steroidogenic enzyme has multiple activities and many extra-adrenal tissues contain enzymes that have similar activities, the complete elimination of a specific adrenal enzyme may not result in the complete elimination of its steroidal products from circulation.

Aldosterone and Cortisol Deficiency

Because both cortisol and aldosterone require 21-hydroxylation for their synthesis, both hormones are deficient in the most severe, salt-wasting form of the disease. This form constitutes approximately 70% of cases of classic 21-OHD. The signs and symptoms of cortisol and aldosterone deficiency.

Congenital adrenal hyperplasia differs from other causes of primary adrenal insufficiency in that precursor steroids accumulate proximal to the blocked enzymatic conversion. Because cortisol is not synthesized efficiently, adrenocorticotropic hormone (ACTH) levels are high, leading to hyperplasia of the adrenal cortex and levels of precursor steroids that may be hundreds of times normal. In the case of 21-OHD, these precursors include 17-OHP and progesterone.

Prenatal Androgen Excess

The most important problem caused by the accumulation of steroid precursors is that 17-OHP is shunted into the pathway for androgen biosynthesis, leading to high levels of androstenedione that are converted outside the adrenal gland to testosterone. This problem begins in affected fetuses by 8–10 weeks of gestation and leads to abnormal genital development in females.

This is manifested by enlargement of the clitoris and by partial or complete labial fusion. The vagina usually has a common opening with the urethra (urogenital sinus). The clitoris may be so enlarged that it resembles a penis; because the urethra opens below this organ, some affected females may be mistakenly presumed to be males with hypospadias and cryptorchidism.

Postnatal Androgen Excess

Signs of androgen excess include rapid somatic growth and accelerated skeletal maturation. Thus, affected patients are tall in childhood, but premature closure of the epiphyses causes growth to stop relatively early, and adult stature is stunted. Muscular development may be excessive. Pubic and axillary hair may appear, and acne and a deep voice may develop. The penis, scrotum, and prostate may become enlarged in affected males; however, the testes are usually prepubertal in size so that they appear small relative to the enlarged penis. Occasionally, ectopic adrenocortical cells in the testes of patients become hyperplastic similar to the adrenal glands, producing testicular adrenal rest tumors (TARTs). The clitoris may become further enlarged in affected females. Although the internal genital structures are female, breast development and menstruation may not occur unless the excessive production of androgens is suppressed by adequate treatment.

Genotyping is clinically available and may help to confirm the diagnosis, but it is expensive and may take weeks. Because the gene conversions that generate most mutant alleles may transfer more than one mutation, at least one parent should also be genotyped to determine which mutations lie on each allele.

Five distinct varieties have been identified. They are:
1. 21-OHD
2. 11-hydroxylase deficiency
3. 3 beta-hydroxysteroid dehydrogenase deficiency
4. 20,22 desmolase deficiency
5. 17-hydroxylase deficiency

Congenital adrenal hyperplasia is due to defects in enzymatic sequence and converts cholesterol to cortisol, aldosterone, and sex steroids. These defects may manifest as:
- Masculinization of female
- Under masculinization of male
- Acute crisis in salt-losing type
- Failure to thrive
- Hypertension
- Postnatal virilization with growth acceleration.

Autosomal recessive enzyme defects involved in adrenal steroidogenesis are common. Defects in cortisol biosynthesis with resultant increased ACTH secretion occur during fetal life. ACTH excess subsequently results in adrenal hyperplasia with increased production of various adrenal hormone precursors, including androgens, and increased urinary excretion of their metabolites. Increased pigmentation, especially of the scrotum, labia majora, and nipples frequently results from excessive ACTH secretion.

Often there is a family history of unexplained death in infancy. Female newborn infants show virilization of external genitalia resulting from 11 or 21-OHD. In its severe form, excess adrenal androgen production beginning in the first trimester of fetal development results in virilization of the female infant and life-threatening hypovolemic, hyponatremic shock (adrenal crisis) in the newborn.

Patients with 21-OHD indicate that the clinical type (salt-wasting versus nonsalt wasting) is usually consistent within a family and that a close genetic linkage exists between the *21-hydroxylase* gene and the human leukocyte antigen (HLA) complex on chromosome 6.

The diagnosis of 21-OHD is suggested by genital ambiguity in females, a salt-losing episode in either sex or rapid growth, and virilization in males or females. Plasma 17-OHP is markedly elevated (>2,000 ng/dL after 24 hours of age in an otherwise healthy full-term infant) and hyperresponsive to stimulation with ACTH. Additional measurement of 11-deoxycortisol, 17-OHP, dehydroepiandrosterone (DHEA), and androstenedione distinguishes among the forms of CAH and testicular tumors that also produce 17-OHP. Similarly, ACTH will induce a substantial rise in serum 21-deoxycortisol in all forms of 21-OHP, but not in normal, providing a useful adjunctive test when this steroid can be measured.

Female pseudohermaphroditism can be caused by factors other than enzyme deficiencies. These factors include virilizing maternal conditions or related hormones taken by the mother during the first trimester of pregnancy. In such cases, the condition does not progress after birth, and cortisol deficiency with abnormal steroidogenesis is not present.

Male pseudohermaphroditism may occur in children with 17,20-desmolase deficiency because that enzyme is necessary for normal androgen biosynthesis. Male pseudohermaphroditism can also be a consequence of androgen receptor abnormalities.

Virilization of the female or male fetus may result from tumors of the adrenal gland, ovary, or testes or from nonclassic CAH later in life. Symptoms begin after birth and progress until treated.

Congenital adrenal hyperplasia is usually classified as part of a spectrum of three typical presentations that result from varying degrees of enzyme activity.

Salt-wasting Congenital Adrenal Hyperplasia

About >90% of CAH cases are caused by 21-OHD. This P450 enzyme (CYP21, P450c21) hydroxylates progesterone and 17-OHP to yield 11-deoxycorticosterone (11-DOC) and 11-deoxycortisol, respectively. These conversions are required for the synthesis of aldosterone and cortisol, respectively. Both hormones are deficient in the most severe "salt-wasting" form of the disease.

Patients with the most severe form (salt-wasting CAH) have aldosterone deficiency due to an inability to convert progesterone to DOC. This results in severe hyponatremia (Na often <110 mEq/L), hyperkalemia (K often >10 mEq/L), and acidosis (pH often <7.1) with concomitant hypotension, shock, cardiovascular collapse, and death in an untreated newborn infant; this usually develops during the second week of life.

Cortisol deficiency results from the inability to convert 17-OHP to 11-deoxycortisol. This impairs postnatal carbohydrate metabolism and worsens cardiovascular collapse because a permissive action of cortisol is required for full pressor action of catecholamines. Low fetal cortisol stimulates corticotropin (ACTH) secretion, which stimulates adrenal growth and stimulates the steroidogenic steps upstream, leading to the accumulation of 17-OHP and other steroids that can be converted to testosterone.

Affected females are often diagnosed at birth because of genital virilization. Males are undiagnosed at birth and either come to medical attention due to screening or during a salt-losing crisis, typically in the second week of life. Following initial fluid and electrolyte resuscitation, the mineralocorticoids and glucocorticoids can be replaced orally and the genital virilization can be corrected surgically.

Drug doses require frequent adjustment in the growing child, and there is also considerable individual variability in what constitutes physiologic replacement.

Simple Virilizing Congenital Adrenal Hyperplasia

Slightly less severely affected patients are able to synthesize adequate amounts of aldosterone but have elevated levels of androgens of adrenal origin; this is termed "simple virilizing disease."

Virilized females with elevated 17-OHP concentrations who do not suffer a salt-losing crisis have the "simple virilizing" form of CAH. Males with this disorder often escape diagnosis until ages 3–7 years, when they come to medical attention because of early development of pubic, axillary, and facial hair, and phallic growth. In contrast to boys with true central precocious puberty, when sexual precocity is caused by CAH, the testes remain of prepubertal size because they have not been stimulated by gonadotropins. These children grow rapidly and are tall for age when diagnosed, but their bone ages are advanced, so that their ultimate adult height is invariably compromised.

When treatment is begun at several years of age, suppression of adrenal testosterone secretion may remove tonic inhibition of the hypothalamus, occasionally resulting in true central precocious puberty, requiring treatment with a gonadotropin-releasing hormone (GnRH) agonist. High concentrations of ACTH in some poorly treated boys may stimulate the enlargement of adrenal rests in the testes. These enlarged testes are usually nodular, unlike the homogeneously enlarged testes in central precocious puberty. Because the adrenal normally produces 100–1,000 times as much cortisol as aldosterone, mild defects in P450c21 are less likely to affect mineralocorticoid secretion than cortisol secretion. Thus, patients with simple virilizing CAH simply have a less severe disorder of P450c21. This is reflected physiologically by the increased plasma renin activity seen in these patients after moderate salt restriction.

Nonclassic Congenital Adrenal Hyperplasia

Patients with the nonclassic disease have relatively mildly elevated levels of androgens and may be asymptomatic or have signs of androgen excess at any time after birth. Very mild forms of CAH are common, evidenced by hirsutism, virilism, menstrual irregularities, and decreased fertility in adult women (so-called late-onset CAH). However, sometimes there may be no phenotypic manifestations other than an increased response of plasma 17-OHP to an intravenous ACTH test.

■ CLINICAL FEATURES (FIG. 1)

- *In females:* In the female with potentially normal ovaries and uterus, virilization occurs and sexual development is therefore along heterosexual lines. The abnormality of the external genitalia may vary from mild enlargement of the clitoris to complete fusion of the labioscrotal folds, forming a scrotum, a penile urethra, a penile shaft, and enlargement of the clitoris to form a normal-sized glans **(Fig. 2)**.

  It is associated with some degree of masculinization at birth. It is expressed as an enlarged clitoris and varying degrees of labial fusion. The vagina has a common opening with the urethra. The internal genital organs are those of a normal female. The severity of virilization is greater in salt-losing CAH.

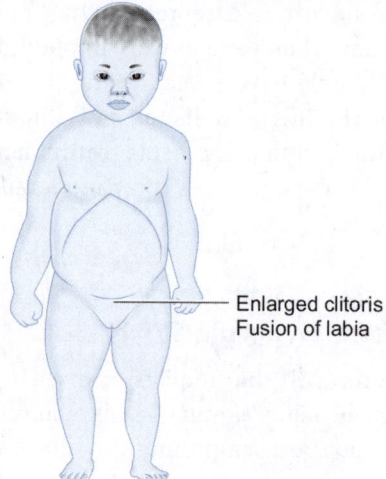

Fig. 1: Clinical features.
— Enlarged clitoris
Fusion of labia

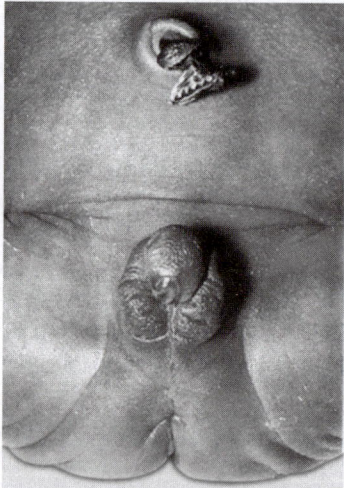

Fig. 2: Congenital adrenal hyperplasia.
(For color version, see Plate 3)

Signs of adrenal insufficiency (salt loss) may be present during the first days of life (typically in the first or second week). In rare cases, adrenal insufficiency does not occur for months or years. When the enzyme defect is milder, salt loss may not occur and evidence of virilization predominates (simple virilizing form).

In untreated, non-salt losing 21-OHD or 11-hydroxylase deficiency, growth rate, and skeletal maturation are accelerated and patients may become muscular. Pubic hair appears early (often before the second year); acne may be excessive; and the voice may deepen. Excessive pigmentation may develop.

- *In males:* In males, sexual development proceeds normally. The male infant usually appears normal at birth but may present with a salt-losing crisis in the first 2–4 weeks of life. In milder forms, a salt-losing crisis may not occur. In this circumstance, enlargement of the penis and increased pigmentation may be noted during the first few months.

In males, there is premature isosexual development. Somatic precocity may appear within the first 6 months of life and develop more gradually becoming evident at the age of 4–5 years. Enlargement of penis and scrotum, acne, and deep voice are noted. Muscles are well developed, and bone age is advanced. Muscles are well developed. Bone age is advanced for chronological age. Although affected patients are tall in early childhood, premature closure of epiphyses causes the growth to stop relatively early. Adult stature is shunted. The testes are normal in size and appear relatively smaller in proportionate to the size of the penis.

Urinary excretion of 17-ketosteroids and pregnanetriol is increased. In 21-OHD, plasma 17-OHP levels are increased. In 11-hydroxylase deficiency, serum levels of the compounds and DOC (deoxycortisol) are elevated **(Table 1)**.

Other symptoms and signs are similar to those seen in females. The testes are soft and not enlarged except in the rare male in whom aberrant adrenal cells (adrenal rests) are present in the testes and produce unilateral or bilateral enlargement, often asymmetric.

TABLE 1: Clinical and laboratory findings in adrenal enzyme defects resulting in CAH.

Enzyme deficiency	Urinary 17-ketosteroids	Elevated plasma metabolite	Plasma androgens	Aldosterone	Hypertension/ salt loss	External genitalia
20,22-desmolase	↓↓↓	–	↓↓↓	↓↓↓	–/+	Males: Ambiguous Females: Normal
3β-ol-dehydrogenase	↑↑ DHEA	17-OH-Pregnenolone (DHEA)	↑ DHEA	↓↓↓	–/+	Males: Ambiguous Females: Possible virilized
17-hydroxylase	↓↓↓	Progesterone	↓↓	Normal to ↑	+/–	Males: Ambiguous Females: Normal
21-hydroxylase	↑↑↑	17-OHP	↑↑	↓↓	–/+	Males: Normal Females: Virilized
11-hydroxylase	↑↑	11-deoxycortisol	↑↑	↓↓ Deoxycorticosterone	+/–	Males: Normal Females: Virilized
17,20-desmolase	↓↓↓	17-hydroxy-steroids	↓↓	Normal	–/–	Males: Ambiguous Females: Normal

(DHEA: dehydroepiandrosterone; 17-OHP: 17-hydroxyprogesterone)

In the male fetus with 21-OHD, the additional testosterone produced in the adrenals has no phenotypic effect. In a female fetus, the testosterone inappropriately produced by the adrenals of the affected female fetus causes varying degrees of virilization of the external genitalia [disordered sexual development (DSD)]. This can range from mild clitoromegaly with or without posterior fusion of the labioscrotal folds to complete labioscrotal fusion that includes a urethra traversing the enlarged clitoris. These infants have normal ovaries, fallopian tubes, and a uterus, but their external genitalia may be sufficiently virilized so that they appear to be male, resulting in errors of sex assignment at birth.

In the rare, isolated defect of 17,20-desmolase activity, ambiguous genitalia may be present because of the compromise in androgen production.

ESSENTIAL DIAGNOSTIC POINTS

- Pseudohermaphroditism in females, with urogenital sinus, enlargement of clitoris, or other evidence of virilization
- Salt losing crisis in infant males or increased precocity in older males with infantile testes
- Increased linear growth in young children, advancement of skeletal maturation
- *Urinary and plasma androgen elevation:* Plasma 17-hydroxyprogesterone and urinary pregnanetriol concentration increased

DIAGNOSIS

17-OHP is normally high in cord blood but falls to normal newborn levels after 12–24 hours, thus, assessment of 17-OHP levels should not be made in the first 24 hours of life. In general, when testing is done on full-term infants >24 hours after birth, the screening is reliable. Pediatricians should become familiar with local assays and the values found in premature infants, which may be read as false positives for

21-OHD. Premature infants and term infants under severe stress (e.g., with cardiac or pulmonary disease) typically have persistently elevated 17-OHP concentrations with normal 21-hydroxylase.

Diagnosis of salt wasting form is established by demonstration of extreme elevation of 17-OHP levels (10,000–20,000 ng/dL, normal <90 ng/dL) in the presence of clinical and laboratory features of adrenal insufficiency. 17-OHP levels are elevated to a lesser extent in those with simple virilizing and nonclassic forms.

Diagnosis of 21-OHD is most reliably established by measuring 17-OHP before and 30 or 60 minutes after an intravenous bolus of 0.125–0.25 mg or 0.25 mg intramuscular injection of synacthen ACTH. On short synacthen (also ACTH) stimulation test, serum 17-OHP and DHEA rise more than two- to threefolds but there is no significant elevation of serum cortisol. Basal levels are usually >2,000 ng/dL and there will be an increase to >5,000–10,000 ng/dL after ACTH in CAH. Patients with nonclassical CAH typically have normal to mildly elevated basal levels, but supranormal responses to ACTH stimulation. The cortisol response to ACTH is subnormal in patients with classical CAH and is normal in patients with nonclassical CAH.

Patients with salt-losing disease have typical laboratory findings associated with cortisol and aldosterone deficiency, including hyponatremia, hyperkalemia, metabolic acidosis, and often hypoglycemia, but these abnormalities can take 10–14 days or longer to develop after birth. Blood levels of 17-OHP are markedly elevated. However, levels of this hormone are high during the first 2–3 days of life even in unaffected infants and especially if they are sick or premature. Blood levels of cortisol are usually low in patients with the salt-losing type of disease. They are often normal in patients with simple virilizing disease but inappropriately low in relation to the ACTH and 17-OHP levels.

In addition to 17-OHP, levels of androstenedione and testosterone are elevated in affected females; testosterone is not elevated in affected males, because normal infant males have high testosterone levels compared with those seen later in childhood. Levels of urinary 17-ketosteroids and pregnanetriol are elevated but are now rarely used clinically because blood samples are easier to obtain than 24-hour urine collections. ACTH levels are elevated but have no diagnostic utility over 17-OHP levels. Plasma levels of renin are elevated, and serum aldosterone is inappropriately low for the rennin level. However, renin levels are high in normal infants in the first few weeks of life.

- *Blood and urine:* Hormonal studies are essential for accurate diagnosis. With adrenal tumors, secretion of DHEA is greatly elevated, and determining plasma concentrations of DHEA sulfate may be useful in the differential diagnosis.
- *Genetic studies:* When available, rapid chromosomal diagnosis should be obtained in any newborn with ambiguous genitalia. A buccal smear and karyotype are done to determine the gender of infants.
- *Radiograph:* Adrenal ultrasonography, CT scanning, and MRI may be useful in defining pelvic anatomy or enlarged adrenals or in localizing an adrenal tumor. Vaginograms using contrast material and pelvic ultrasonography may be helpful in delineating the internal anatomy of a newborn with ambiguous genitalia.

Prenatal diagnosis can be done by estimation of 17-ketosteroids, pregnanetriol, and 17-OHP in amniotic fluid or by genotyping HLA typing of amniotic cells obtained by chorion villus sampling. Neonatal screening can be performed by heel prick blood 17-OHP estimation.

Newborn Screening

Because 21-OHD is often undiagnosed in affected males until they have severe adrenal insufficiency, many countries have instituted newborn screening programs. These programs analyze 17-OHP levels in dried blood obtained by heelstick and absorbed on filter paper cards; the same cards are screened in parallel for other congenital conditions, such as hypothyroidism and phenylketonuria. Potentially affected infants are typically quickly recalled for additional testing electrolytes and repeat 17-OHP determination) at approximately 2 weeks of age. Infants with salt-wasting disease often have abnormal electrolytes by this age but are usually not severely ill. Thus, screening programs are effective in preventing many cases of adrenal crisis in affected males. The nonclassic form of the disease is not reliably detected by newborn screening, but this is of little clinical significance because adrenal insufficiency does not occur in this type of 21-OHD.

GENERAL FEATURES
- Virilization at birth
- Children grow tall
- Failure to thrive
- Advanced bone age

LABORATORY SALIENT FINDINGS
- Hormonal studies
- Secretion of DHEA increased
- *Genetic studies:* Chromosomal analysis
- Adrenal ultrasonography
- CT scan
- MRI
- Pelvic ultrasonography

(CT; computed tomography; DHEA: dehydroepiandrosterone; MRI: magnetic resonance imaging)

DIFFERENTIAL DIAGNOSIS
- Precocious puberty
- Pyloric stenosis
- Intestinal obstruction
- Hypothyroidism
- Virilizing tumor

TREATMENT

Medical Treatment

Treatment in CAH consists of normalizing growth velocity and skeletal maturation using the smallest dose of glucocorticoids that will suppress adrenal function.

Glucocorticoids

Cortisol deficiency is treated with glucocorticoids. Treatment also suppresses the excessive production of androgens by the adrenal cortex and thus minimizes problems, such as excessive growth and skeletal maturation, and virilization. This often requires larger glucocorticoid doses than are needed in other forms of adrenal insufficiency, typically 15–20 mg/m^2/24 h of hydrocortisone daily administered orally in three divided doses. Affected infants usually require dosing at the high end of this range. Double or triple doses are indicated during periods of stress, such as infection or surgery. Between 50% and 60% of the daily dose should be given in the late evening to suppress the early morning ACTH rise. Dosage is adjusted to maintain a normal growth rate and a normal rate of skeletal maturation.

Glucocorticoid treatment must be continued indefinitely in all patients with classic 21-OHD but may not be necessary for patients with nonclassic disease unless signs of androgen excess are present. Therapy must be individualized. It is desirable to maintain linear growth along percentile lines; crossing to higher height percentiles may suggest undertreatment; whereas, loss of height percentiles often indicates overtreatment with glucocorticoids. Overtreatment is also suggested by excessive weight gain. Pubertal development should be monitored by periodic examination and skeletal maturation is evaluated by serial radiographs of the hand and wrist for bone age.

Hormone levels, particularly 17-OHP, and androstenedione, should be measured early in the morning, before taking the morning medications, or at a consistent time in relation to medication dosing. In general, desirable 17-OHP levels are in the high-normal range or several times normal; low-normal levels can usually be achieved only with excessive glucocorticoid doses.

Menarche occurs at the appropriate age in most girls in whom good control has been achieved; it may be delayed in girls with suboptimal control.

Children with a simple virilizing disease, particularly males, are frequently not diagnosed until 3–7 years of age, at which time skeletal maturation maybe 5 years or more in advance of chronological age. In some children, especially if the bone age is 12 years or more, spontaneous central (i.e., gonadotropin-dependent) puberty may occur when treatment is instituted because therapy with hydrocortisone suppresses the production of adrenal androgens and thus stimulates the release of pituitary gonadotropins if the appropriate level of hypothalamic maturation is present. This form of superimposed true precocious puberty may be treated with a gonadotropin hormone-releasing hormone analog, such as leuprolide.

Males with 21-OHD who have had inadequate corticosteroid therapy may develop TARTs, which usually regress with increased steroid dosage. Testicular MRI, ultrasonography, and color flow Doppler examination help define the character and extent of the disease. Testis-sparing surgery for steroid-unresponsive tumors has been reported.

A variety of serum and urine androgens have been used to monitor the adequacy of therapy, including 17-OHP, androstenedione, and urinary pregnanetriol. In adolescent females, normal menses are a sensitive index of the adequacy of therapy.

Mineralocorticoids

Fludrocortisone in a dose of 0.05–0.15 mg is given orally once a day or in two divided doses. Periodic monitoring of blood pressure is recommended to avoid overdosing.

Patients with salt-wasting disease (i.e., aldosterone deficiency) require mineralocorticoid replacement with fludrocortisone. Infants may have very high mineralocorticoid requirements in the first few months of, life, usually 0.1–0.3 mg daily in two divided doses but occasionally up to 0.4 mg daily, and often require sodium supplementation (sodium chloride, 8 mmol/kg) in addition to the mineralocorticoid.

Older patients and children are usually maintained with 0.05–0.1 mg daily of fludrocortisone. In some patients, simple virilizing disease may be easier to control with a low dose of fludrocortisone in addition to hydrocortisone even when these patients have normal aldosterone levels in the absence of mineralocorticoid replacement.

Therapy is evaluated by monitoring vital signs; tachycardia and hypertension are signs of overtreatment with mineralocorticoids. Serum electrolytes should be measured frequently in early infancy as therapy is adjusted. Plasma renin activity is a useful way to determine the adequacy of therapy;

it should be maintained in or near the normal range but not suppressed.

Children with salt wasting and those with elevated plasma renin activity, require increased salt intake and mineralocorticoid. In the first 24 hours of dehydration, 4–8 g of sodium chloride is needed for the replacement. In infants, 9-alpha-fluorocortisone acetate is given in the dose of 0.05–0.1 mg/day in addition.

Surgical Treatment

Consultation with a urologist experienced with female genital reconstruction is indicated in affected females as soon as possible during infancy.

Feminizing genitoplasty is undertaken in a staged manner. The enlarged clitoris is resected within the first year. Vaginoplasty is undertaken after some time.

COURSE AND PROGNOSIS

When therapy is initiated in early infancy, abnormal metabolic effects and progression of masculinization can be avoided. Treatment with glucocorticoids permits normal growth, development, and sexual maturation.

However, if not adequately controlled, CAH results in sexual precocity and masculinization throughout childhood. Affected individuals will be tall as children but short as adults because the rate of skeletal maturation is excessive and leads to premature closure of epiphyses.

If treatment is delayed or inadequate until somatic development is over 12–14 years as determined by skeletal maturation (bone age), true central sexual precocity may occur in males and females.

Patient education stressing lifelong therapy is important to ensure compliance in adolescence and later life.

■ BIBLIOGRAPHY

1. Auchus RJ. Steroid 17-hydroxylase and 17,20-lyase deficiencies, genetic and pharmacologic. J Steroid Biochem Mol Biol. 2017; 165(Pt A):71-8.
2. Bose HS, Sugawara T, Strauss JF 3rd, Miller WL; International Congenital Lipoid Adrenal Hyperplasia Consortium. The pathophysiology and genetics of congenital lipoid adrenal hyperplasia. N Engl J Med. 1996; 335(25):1870-8.
3. Miller WL. Disorders in the initial steps of steroid hormone synthesis. J Steroid Biochem Mol Biol. 2017;165(Pt A):18-37.
4. Speiser PW, White PC. Congenital adrenal hyperplasia. N Engl J Med. 2003;349(8): 776-88.

CASE 59

Cushing's Syndrome

■ PRESENTING COMPLAINTS

A 10-year-old was presented with complaint of:
- Fever since 3 days
- Abdominal pain since 2 days

History of Presenting Complaints

A 10-year-old girl presented with a history of abdominal pain. Abdominal pain was present on the right side of the loin. According to the girl, the abdominal pain was radiating from the loin to the inner part of the thigh. The pain was of severe type. It was associated with a moderate degree of fever. Fever was of intermittent type associated with chills and rigor. There was no history of suggestive urinary and bladder disturbances.

Past History of the Patient

She was the eldest sibling of a nonconsanguineous marriage. She was delivered at full term by normal delivery. Her birth weight was 3.25 kg. She was on breastfeeds immediately after the delivery. She was exclusively on breastfeeds for the first 3 months. Later weaning was started with cereals and fruits. She was on family food for 18 months. Her developmental milestones were normal. She was completely immunized. She was overweight despite of strict diet control. Her weight increased markedly in the last 6 months. The younger sibling was a 6-year-old healthy boy.

■ EXAMINATION

The girl was very obese. She was looking unhappy. Her anthropometric measurements included, her height was 133 cm (50th centile), and her weight was 38 kg (90th centile). She was febrile, 38°C. Her pulse

---

CASE AT A GLANCE

Basic Findings
Height	:	133 cm (50th centile)
Weight	:	38 kg (50th centile)
Temperature	:	38°C
Pulse rate	:	110 beats/min
Respiratory rate	:	22 breaths/min
Blood pressure	:	140/96 mm Hg

Positive Findings

History:
- Abdominal pain
- Fever
- Obese

Examination:
- Obese
- Prominent cheeks
- Hypertension
- Buffalo hump

Investigation:
- *Urine:* Suggestive of urinary tract infection (UTI)
- *Plasma cortisol:* Increased
- *Serum androgen:* Increased
- *Urinary 17-hydroxycorticosteroids:* Increased
- *Urinary 17-ketosteroids:* Increased

rate was 110 beats/min, and her respiratory rate was 22 breaths/min. The blood pressure recorded was 140/96 mm Hg.

There was no pallor, no lymphadenopathy, and no edema. The face was round with prominent cheeks. Hypertrichosis on the face was present. Acnes were present. Other systemic examinations were normal.

■ INVESTIGATION

- *Hemoglobin:* 13 g/dL
- *TLC:* 16,000 cells/cumm
- *Absolute eosinophil count (AEC):* 750 cells/mm^3
- *Blood urea:* 40 mg/dL
- *Serum electrolytes:*
  - *Na:* 150 mEq/dL
  - *K:* 2.5 mEq/dL
- *Plasma cortisol:*
  - 30 µg/dL at 8 AM
  - 20 µg/dL at 6 PM
- *Serum androgen:* 3 nmol/L (Normal: 1.08–2.26 nmol/l)
- *Urine routine:*
  - 10–20 white blood cells (WBCs)/high power field (HPF)
  - Protein++
  - Red cells+++
  - Albumin++
- *Urinary 17-hydroxycorticosteroids:* 20 mg/dL/24 h (Normal range: 2–8 mg/dL/24 h)
- *Urinary 17-ketosteroids:* 26 mg/dL/24 h (Normal range: 4–13 mg/dL/24 h)

■ DISCUSSION

The girl presented with urinary tract infection, obesity, the presence of acne, and systemic hypertension. These clinical features make the diagnosis of Cushing syndrome.

Cushing syndrome is the result of abnormally high blood levels of cortisol or other glucocorticoids. Iatrogenic Cushing syndrome results from the administration of supraphysiologic quantities of glucocorticoids. Early signs of glucocorticoid excess include increased appetite, weight gain, and growth arrest without delayed bone age.

The genes causing nodular adrenocortical hyperplasia that have been identified thus far all produce overactivity of the ACTH signaling pathway either by constitutively activating G, a (McCune–Albright syndrome), by reducing the breakdown of cyclic adenosine monophosphate (cAMP) and thus increasing its intracellular levels [mutations of phosphodiesterase 8B (PDE8B) or PDE11A], or by disrupting the regulation of the cyclic adenosine monophosphate-dependent enzyme, protein kinase A (PRKAR1A mutations).

Chronic glucocorticoid excess in children results in typical Cushingoid facies, but the centripetal fat distribution characteristic of the adult Cushing disease is seen only in long-standing disease. Mineralocorticoid excess is characterized by hypertension, but patients receiving low-sodium diets (e.g., newborns) are not hypertensive, as mineralocorticoids increase blood pressure by retaining sodium and increasing intravascular volume.

Moderate hypersecretion of adrenal androgens is characterized by mild signs of virilization; substantial hypersecretion of adrenal androgens is characterized by accelerated growth, increased bone age, increased muscle mass, acne, hirsutism, and deepening of the voice. Cushing disease designates hypercortisolism from the pituitary and over-production of corticotropin (ACTH). Other causes include adrenal adenoma, adrenal carcinoma, multinodular adrenal hyperplasia, and ectopic ACTH syndrome.

■ ETIOLOGY

Cushing syndrome is nonspecific. It may result from excessive secretion of adrenal steroids autonomously (adenoma or carcinoma), from excessive ACTH secretion from the pituitary (Cushing disease) or from ectopic sources, or from chronic exposure to pharmacologic doses of glucocorticoids. ACTH-independent Cushing syndrome with nodular hyperplasia and adenoma formation occurs in cases of McCune–Albright syndrome. The symptoms begin in infancy and childhood.

In children under age 12 years, Cushing syndrome is usually iatrogenic (secondary to pharmacologic doses of ACTH or one of the glucocorticoids). It may rarely be due to an adrenal tumor, adrenal hyperplasia, an adenoma of the pituitary gland, or even more rarely, an extrapituitary (ectopic) ACTH-producing tumor from the bronchus, thymus, and pancreas.

The most common cause of Cushing syndrome is prolonged exogenous administration of glucocorticoid hormones, especially at the high doses used to treat lymphoproliferative disorders. This rarely represents a diagnostic challenge, but the management of hyperglycemia, hypertension, weight gain, linear growth retardation, and osteoporosis often complicates therapy with corticosteroids.

The most common etiology of endogenous Cushing syndrome in children older than 7 years of age is Cushing disease, in which excessive ACTH secreted by a pituitary adenoma causes bilateral adrenal hyperplasia. Patients with these tumors often exhibit signs of hypercortisolism along with signs of hypersecretion of other steroids, such as androgens, estrogens, and aldosterone. Such adenomas are often too small to detect by imaging techniques and are termed microadenomas. They consist principally of chromophobe cells and frequently show positive immunostaining for ACTH and its precursor, proopiomelanocortin.

Adrenocorticotropic hormone-dependent Cushing syndrome may also result from ectopic production of ACTH, although this is uncommon in children. Ectopic ACTH secretion in children is associated with islet cell carcinoma of the pancreas, neuroblastoma or ganglioneuroblastoma, hemangiopericytoma, Wilms' tumor, and thymic carcinoid. Hypertension is more common in the ectopic ACTH syndrome than in other forms of Cushing syndrome, because of very high cortisol levels.

Adrenocorticotropic hormone-independent Cushing syndrome with nodular hyperplasia and adenoma formation occurs rarely in cases of McCune–Albright syndrome, with symptoms beginning in infancy or childhood.

Several syndromes are associated with the development of multiple autonomously hyperfunctioning nodules of adrenocortical tissue, rather than single adenomas or carcinomas. In many cases, they are caused by mutations in genes in the cAMP-mediated signaling pathway by which ACTH normally regulates cortisol secretion. Primary pigmented nodular adrenocortical disease (PPNAD) is a distinctive form of ACTH-independent Cushing syndrome. It may occur as an isolated event or, more commonly, as a familial disorder with other manifestations. The adrenal glands are small and have characteristic multiple, small (<4 mm in diameter), pigmented (black) nodules containing large cells with cytoplasm and lipofuscin; there is cortical atrophy between the nodules. This adrenal disorder occurs as a component of Carney complex, an autosomal dominant disorder also consisting of centrofacial lentigines and blue nevi; cardiac and cutaneous myxomas; pituitary, thyroid, and testicular tumors; and pigmented melanotic schwannomas.

CLINICAL FEATURES (FIG. 1)

Cushing syndrome is characterized by obesity with associated hypertension. It occurs as a result of the maintenance of abnormally high blood levels of cortisol by hyperfunction of the adrenal cortex. In infants, it is most commonly caused by a functioning adrenocortical tumor. PPNAD is also the cause among infants and children. In children above 7 years, bilateral adrenal hyperplasia is the cause. It may be because of the ectopic production of ACTH.

Signs of Cushing syndrome have been recognized in infants younger than 1 year of age. The disorder appears to be more severe, and the clinical findings are more flagrant in infants than in older children. The face is rounded, with prominent cheeks and a flushed appearance (moon facies). Generalized obesity is common in younger children. In children with adrenal tumors, signs of abnormal masculinization occur frequently; accordingly, there may be hirsutism on the face and trunk to pubic hair, acne, deepening of the voice, and enlargement of the clitoris in girls. Growth is impaired, with length falling below the third percentile, except when significant virilization produces normal or even accelerated growth. Hypertension is common and may occasionally lead to heart failure. An increased susceptibility to infection may also lead to sepsis.

> **ESSENTIAL DIAGNOSTIC POINTS**
> - Truncal adiposity with thin extremities
> - Moon facies, muscle wasting, weakness, plethora
> - Easy bruising, purplish striae, decreased growth rate, delayed skeletal maturation
> - Hypertension, osteoporosis, glycosuria
> - Elevated serum and urine adrenocorticosteroids; low serum potassium levels; eosinopenia, lymphopenia

Prolonged exogenous administration of corticotropin or hydrocortisone or its analog results in clinical pattern. Clinical manifestations are due to gluconeogenesis, which leads to protein catabolism and accumulation of fat. These children have rounded faces with prominent flushed cheeks and double chins, i.e., moon facies. Growth is retarded and blood pressure is elevated. Hypertension may lead to heart failure. Increased susceptibility to infection may produce septicemia. These children are easily fatigued with weakness and personality changes.

In older children, gradual onset of obesity, short stature, deceleration, or cessation of growth may be the only early manifestation of purplish striae on hips, abdomen, and thigh are common. Older children most often have more severe obesity of the face and trunk. Buffalo hump and generalized obesity, signs of abnormal masculinization are seen. There may be hypertrichosis trunk compared with the extremities. Deepening of the voice, acne, and enlargement of the clitoris are seen in girls. Pubertal development may be delayed. Amenorrhea may occur in girls. Weakness, headache, and emotional lability may be

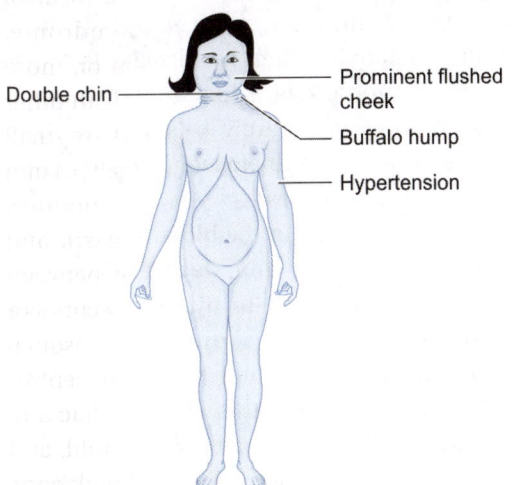

Fig. 1: Clinical features.

prominent. Hypertension and hyperglycemia usually occur; hyperglycemia may progress to frank diabetes. Osteoporosis is common and may cause pathologic fractures.

The earliest, most reliable indicators of hypercortisolism in children are weight gain and growth arrest. The obesity of pediatric Cushing disease is initially generalized rather than centripetal. Psychological disturbances, including compulsive overachieving behavior and emotional lability, are distinct from depression typically seen in adults. There can be a substantial degree of bone loss and undermineralization. Cushing syndrome caused by adrenal carcinoma or ectopic ACTH syndrome can follow a rapid fulminant course.

GENERAL FEATURES
• Rounded face
• Growth is retarded
• Fatigue

■ DIAGNOSIS

Blood

- *Plasma cortisol concentrations*: These are elevated, with a loss of the normal diurnal variation in cortisol secretion. Determination of cortisol levels between midnight and 2 AM may be a sensitive indicator of loss of variation.
- *Serum chloride and potassium concentrations:* These values may be lowered. Serum sodium and bicarbonate concentrations may be elevated (metabolic alkalosis).
- *Serum ACTH concentrations:* ACTH concentrations are slightly elevated with adrenal hyperplasia (Cushing disease), decreased in cases of adrenal tumor, and greatly increased with ACTH-producing pituitary or extrapituitary tumors.
- *The leukocyte count:* This measurement shows polymorphonuclear leukocytosis with lymphopenia and eosinophil count is low. The erythrocyte count may be elevated.

Urine

- *Urinary-free cortisol excretion:* This value is elevated. This is currently considered the most useful initial diagnostic test.
- *Urinary 17-hydroxycorticosteroid excretion (excretion products of the glucocorticoids):* This value is elevated.
- *Urinary 17-ketosteroid excretion:* This is usually elevated in association with adrenal tumors.
- *Glycosuria:* This finding may be present.

Response to Dexamethasone Suppression Testing

There is diminished suppression of adrenal function after a small dose (0.5 mg) of dexamethasone. In *low dose dexamethasone test* 0.5 mg of dexamethasone is given every 6 hours for 2 days. The levels of urinary 17-OHS will fall below 1.5 mg/m^2/24 h. Serum ACTH levels may be increased. The larger doses of dexamethasone cause suppression of adrenal activity when the disease is due to adrenal hyperplasia. Adenomas and adrenal carcinomas may rarely be suppressed by large doses of dexamethasone (4–16 mg/day in four divided doses).

Cortisol levels in the blood are normally highest at 8 AM and decrease to <50% by midnight except in infants and young children in whom a diurnal rhythm is not always established. In patients with Cushing syndrome, this circadian rhythm is lost; midnight cortisol levels > 4.4 µg/dL strongly suggest the diagnosis. It is difficult to obtain diurnal blood samples as part of an outpatient evaluation, but cortisol can be measured in saliva samples, which can be obtained at home at the appropriate times of day. Elevated nighttime salivary cortisol levels raise suspicion for Cushing syndrome.

A glucose tolerance test is often abnormal but is of no diagnostic utility. Levels of serum electrolytes are usually normal, but potassium may be decreased, especially in patients with tumors that secrete ACTH ectopically.

The next step is to decide whether Cushing's syndrome is ACTH-dependent or independent by the estimation of plasma ACTH.

If circulating ACTH is suppressed to <10 pg/mL, it suggests ACTH-independent Cushing's syndrome, most likely a clue to adrenal cause.

Radiograph

It is to determine the anatomical site of a lesion by radiological investigations.

Once ACTH-independent Cushing's syndrome is confirmed, adrenal CT or MRI should be performed to detect the type of adrenal lesion—unilateral or bilateral, or benign adenoma or carcinoma.

Pituitary imaging may demonstrate pituitary adenoma. This can be used in conjunction with pituitary venous sampling for localization of ACTH-secreting adenomas. Adrenal imaging (e.g., CT scan) may demonstrate adenoma or bilateral hyperplasia.

Radionuclide studies of the adrenals may be useful in complex cases. Sellar tomography is indicated though the pituitary cell is usually normal. The thymic shadow is absent because excessive cortisol produces the involution.

Osteoporosis (evident first in the spine and pelvis) with compression fractures may occur in advanced cases, and skeletal maturation is usually delayed. Osseous maturation is usually moderately retarded but may be normal. Osteoporosis is common. Pathological fractures are noted.

Computed tomography detects virtually all adrenal tumors larger than 1.5 cm in diameter. MRI may detect ACTH-secreting pituitary adenomas, but many are too small to be seen; the addition of gadolinium contrast increases the sensitivity of detection. Bilateral inferior petrosal blood sampling to measure concentrations of ACTH before and after corticotropin-releasing hormone administration may be required to localize the tumor when a pituitary adenoma is not visualized; this is not routinely available in many centers, and moreover may be of decreased specifically in children.

■ DIFFERENTIAL DIAGNOSIS

Differential diagnosis includes obesity, precocious puberty, and Frohlich's syndrome.

■ TREATMENT

In all cases of primary adrenal hyperfunction due to a tumor, surgical removal is indicated. ACTH should be given preoperatively and postoperatively to stimulate the nontumorous contralateral adrenal cortex, which is generally atrophied.

Glucocorticoids should be administered parenterally in pharmacologic doses during and after surgery until the patient is stable. Supplemental oral glucocorticoids, potassium, salt, and mineralocorticoids may be necessary until the suppressed contralateral adrenal gland has recovered, sometimes over a period of several months.

If a pituitary adenoma does not respond to treatment or if ACTH is secreted by an ectopic metastatic tumor, the adrenal glands may need to be removed. This can often be accomplished laparoscopically.

Adrenalectomy may lead to increased ACTH secretion by an unresected pituitary adenoma, evidenced mainly by marked hyperpigmentation; this condition is termed Nelson syndrome.

If the lesion is a benign cortical adenoma unilateral adrenalectomy is indicated. If the adenoma is bilateral, then the treatment of choice is subtotal adrenalectomy. Transsphenoidal pituitary microsurgery is the treatment of choice in Cushing's disease.

Management of patients undergoing adrenalectomy requires adequate preoperative and postoperative replacement therapy with a corticosteroid. Tumors that produce corticosteroids usually lead to atrophy of the normal adrenal tissue, and replacement with cortisol (10 mg/m^2/24 h in three divided doses after the immediate postoperative period) is required until there is the recovery of the hypothalamic-pituitary-adrenal axis. Postoperative complications may include sepsis, pancreatitis, thrombosis, poor wound healing, and sudden collapse, particularly in infants with Cushing syndrome. Substantial catch-up growth, pubertal progress, and increased bone density occur, but bone density remains abnormal and adult height is often compromised.

Transsphenoidal pituitary microsurgery is the treatment of choice for pituitary Cushing disease in children. The overall success rate with follow-up of <10 years is 60–80%. Low postoperative serum or urinary cortisol concentrations predict long-term remission in the majority of cases. Relapses are treated with reoperation or pituitary irradiation.

Cyproheptadine, a centrally acting serotonin antagonist that blocks ACTH release, has been used to treat Cushing disease in adults; remissions are usually not sustained after discontinuation of therapy.

Pasireotide, a somatostatin analog, can inhibit ACTH secretion and is approved for use in adults with persistent disease after surgery or in whom surgery is contraindicated.

Irradiation of the pituitary gland may be considered. Cyproheptadine blocks the ACTH release and can be tried with Cushing's disease. Patients with metastasis are treated with mitotane (o,p'-DDD) or cisplatin.

If a pituitary adenoma does not respond to treatment or if ACTH is secreted by an ectopic metastatic tumor, the adrenal glands may need to be removed. This can often be accomplished laparoscopically Adrenalectomy may lead to increased ACTH secretion by an unresected pituitary adenoma, evidenced mainly by marked hyperpigmentation; this condition is termed *Nelson syndrome*.

BIBLIOGRAPHY

1. Joshi SM, Hewitt RJ, Storr HL, Rezajooi K, Ellamushi H, Grossman AB, et al. Cushing's disease in children and adolescents: 20 years of experience in a single neurosurgical center. Neurosurgery. 2005;57(2):281-5.
2. Keil MF, Zametkin A, Ryder CB, Lodish M, Stratakis CA. Cases of psychiatric morbidity in pediatric patients after remission of Cushing syndrome. Pediatrics. 2016;137(4): e20152234.
3. Lodish M, Stratakis CA. A genetic and molecular update on adrenocortical causes of Cushing syndrome. Nature Rev Endocrinal. 2016;12(5):255-62.
4. Storr HL, Savage MO. Management of endocrine disease: Paediatric Cushing's disease. Euro J Endocrinol. 2015;173(1):R35-45.

CASE 60

Diabetes Insipidus

■ PRESENTING COMPLAINTS

A 3-year-old girl was brought with the complaint of:
- Frequency of micturition since 6 months
- Passing large amounts of urine since 6 months
- Bed wetting since 6 months

History of Presenting Complaints

A 3-year-old girl was brought by the mother with a history of passing large quantities of urine since 6 months. The mother said that her daughter will pass urine more frequently and she passes large quantities of urine every time. There was no history of a burning sensation while passing the urine. The mother also revealed that her daughter drinks lots of water and she even passes urine in the nighttime.

Past History of the Patient

She was the only sibling of the nonconsanguineous marriage. She was born at full term by normal delivery. Her birth weight was 3 kg. She started taking breast milk immediately after the delivery. There was no significant postnatal event. Weaning was started in the fourth month and completed by 1 year. She was immunized completely and all the developmental milestones were normal.

CASE AT A GLANCE	
Basic Findings	
Height	: 90 cm (50th centile)
Weight	: 12 kg (50th centile)
Temperature	: 37°C
Pulse rate	: 120 beats/min
Respiratory rate	: 20 breaths/min
Blood pressure	: 70/50 mm Hg
Positive Findings	
History:	
• Passing large amounts of urine	
• Drinks lots of water	
• Nocturia	
Examination:	
• No abnormality detected (NAD)	
Investigation:	
• *Urine specific gravity:* 1001	
• *Urine osmolality:* 100 mOsm/kg water	
• *Urine routine:* NAD	

■ EXAMINATION

The girl was moderately built and nourished. She was sitting comfortably and was very cooperative. Anthropometric measurements included a height of 90 cm (50th centile), and a weight was 12 kg (50th centile). There were signs of mild dehydration.

The child was afebrile. The pulse rate was 120 beats/min. The respiratory rate was 20 breaths/min. The blood pressure recorded was 70/50 mm Hg. There was no pallor, no lymphadenopathy, no cyanosis, and no clubbing.

All the system examinations were normal.

INVESTIGATION

- *Hemoglobin:* 11 g/dL
- *TLC:* 9,000 cells/mm^3
- *Differential leukocyte count (DLC):* $P_{68}L_{28}E_2M_2$
- *ESR:* 20 mm in the first hour
- *Urine-specific gravity:* 1.001
- *Osmolality:* 100 mOsm/kg water
- *Urine routine:*
  - Albumin—nil
  - Sugar—nil
  - Microscopy—normal
- *Skull X-ray:* No abnormality detected (NAD)
- *Chest X-ray:* NAD

DISCUSSION

Diabetes insipidus (DI) results from a lack of antidiuretic hormone (ADH) or arginine vasopressin (AVP), from neurohypophysis. The deficiency may be partial, complete, or transient.

Diabetes insipidus manifests clinically with polyuria and polydipsia and can result from either vasopressin deficiency [central diabetes insipidus (CDI)] or vasopressin insensitivity at the level of the kidney [nephrogenic diabetes insipidus (NDI)]. Both CDI and NDI can arise from inherited defects of congenital or neonatal onset or can be secondary to a variety of causes.

Vasopressin, secreted from the posterior pituitary, is the principal regulator of tonicity, its release is largely stimulated by increased plasma tonicity. Vasopressin exerts its principal effect on the kidney via vasopressin 2 (V2) receptors located primarily in the collecting tubule, the thick ascending limb of the loop of Henle, and the periglomerular tubules.

Activation of the V2 receptor results in an increase in intracellular cAMP, which leads to the insertion of the aquaporin-2 water channel into the apical (luminal) membrane. This allows water movement along its osmotic gradient into the hypertonic inner medullary interstitium from the tubule lumen and excretion of concentrated urine.

The human V2 receptor gene is located on the long arm of the X chromosome (Xq28) at the locus associated with *congenital, X-linked, vasopressin-resistant DI*. In contrast to aquaporin-2, aquaporin-3, and aquaporin-4 are expressed on the basolateral membrane of the collecting duct cells and aquaporin-1 is expressed in the proximal tubule. These channels may also contribute to urinary concentrating ability.

CENTRAL DIABETES INSIPIDUS

Causes of Central Diabetes Insipidus

Congenital
- Optic nerve hypoplasia (septooptic dysplasia)
- Ectopic or absent pituitary
- Other midline craniofacial defects

Familial
- Autosomal dominant
- Autosomal recessive
- Wolfram syndrome (DIDMOAD)-autosomal recessive

Acquired
Postoperative (with triple-phase response).

Neoplasms
- Craniopharyngioma
- Germinoma
- Pinealoma
- Optic glioma

Metastatic Tumors
- Leukemias
- Infiltrative/autoimmune
- Sarcoidosis

Trauma
Transection of the stalk

Drugs
- Ethanol
- Phenytoin
- Opiate antagonists

Septic Shock (Infarction)
- Sheenan syndrome (postpartum hemorrhage)
- Hypoxic brain injury

Infections
- Basal meningitis
- Encephalitis
- Aneurysm and cysts

Central diabetes insipidus, a result of vasopressin deficiency, is caused by defects in hypothalamic vasopressin synthesis, packaging, or transport along the neurohypophyseal tract to the posterior pituitary gland.

Genetic causes of vasopressin deficiency are rare and include inherited mutations in the vasopressin structural gene, defects in the neurophysin protein, and the MOAD [diabetes insipidus, diabetes mellitus (DM), optic atrophy, and deafness] syndrome.

Central diabetes insipidus can result from multiple etiologies, including genetic mutations in the vasopressin gene; trauma (accidental or surgical) to vasopressin neurons; congenital malformations of the hypothalamus or pituitary neoplasms; infiltrative, autoimmune, and infectious diseases affecting vasopressin neurons or fiber tracts; and increased metabolism of vasopressin.

Autosomal dominant CDI usually occurs within the first 5 years of life and results from mutations in the vasopressin gene. CDI can result from multiple etiologies, including genetic mutations in the vasopressin gene; trauma (accidental or surgical) to vasopressin neurons; congenital malformations of the hypothalamus or pituitary; neoplasms; infiltrative, autoimmune, and infectious diseases affecting vasopressin neurons or fiber tracts; and increased metabolism of the vasopressin. In approximately 10% of children with CDI, the etiology is idiopathic.

Midline brain abnormalities such as septooptic dysplasia and holoprosencephaly may also be associated with CDI. Accidental or surgical trauma to the axons of the vasopressin-containing neurons can lead to transient or permanent DI. The triphasic response following surgery refers to an initial phase of transient DI, lasting for 12–48 hours, followed by a second phase of syndrome of inappropriate ADH secretion, lasting up to 10 days, which may be followed by permanent DI. The initial phase may be the result of local edema interfering with normal vasopressin secretion; the second phase results from unregulated vasopressin release from dying neurons, whereas in the third phase, permanent DI results if >90% of the neurons have been destroyed.

Hypothalamic tumors and infiltrative diseases occur in s significant number of children who present with DI. In patients with craniopharyngiomas, DI usually develops only after surgical intervention. This is in contrast to germinomas in which DI is often the presenting symptom.

Trauma to the base of the brain and neurosurgical intervention in the region of the hypothalamus or pituitary are common causes of CDI. The triphasic response following surgery refers to an initial phase of transient DI, lasting 12–48 hours, followed by a second phase of syndrome of inappropriate antidiuretic hormone secretion (SIADH), lasting up to 10 days, which may be followed by permanent DI. The initial phase may be the result of local edema interfering with normal vasopressin secretion; the second phase results from unregulated vasopressin release from dying neurons, whereas in the third phase, permanent DI results if > 90% of the neurons have been destroyed.

Germinomas and pinealomas typically arise in this region and are among the most common primary brain tumors associated with DI. Hematologic malignancies, such as acute myelocytic leukemia, can cause DI via infiltration of the pituitary stalk and sella.

Germinomas may be undetectable by MRI for several years; consequently, children with unexplained DI should have regularly repeated MRI scans. Infiltrative diseases such as histiocytosis and lymphocytic hypophysitis are other causes of DI in children. In these conditions, as well as germinomas, MRI scans characteristically show a thickening or a mass within the infundibular stalk.

Langerhans cell histiocytosis and lymphocytic *hypophysitis* are common types of infiltrative disorders causing CDI, with hypophysitis as the cause in 50% of cases of idiopathic CDI.

Drugs associated with the inhibition of vasopressin release include ethanol, phenytoin, opiate antagonists, halothane, and a-adrenergic agents.

Wolfram syndrome, which includes DI, DM, optic atrophy, and deafness, also results in vasopressin deficiency. Mutations in two genes, which give rise to endoplasmic reticulum proteins, are associated with this condition. Congenital brain abnormalities such as optic nerve hypoplasia syndrome with agenesis of the corpus callosum, the Niikawa–Kuroki syndrome, holoprosencephaly, and familial pituitary hypoplasia with absent stalk may be associated with CDI and defects in thirst perception (adipsia). Empty sella syndrome, possibly resulting from unrecognized pituitary infarction, can be associated with DI in children.

NEPHROGENIC DIABETES INSIPIDUS

Nephrogenic diabetes insipidus is a disorder in which the collecting tubule is unresponsive to vasopressin.

Urine osmolality ranges from 50 to 1,200 mOsm/kg in adults and from 50 to 500 mOsm/kg in neonates. The urine osmolality is dependent on the formation of a hypertonic medullary interstitium and the secretion of vasopressin. Vasopressin binds to the V2 receptor and acts on the collecting tubule to increase passive water transport through the insertion of water channels (designated aquaporin-2) by exocytotic insertion into the luminal membrane, which increases collecting tubule water permeability. The hypertonic medullary interstitium is formed by the countercurrent system.

Causes of Nephrogenic Diabetes Insipidus

Congenital

- *X-linked NDI* results from inactivating mutations of the vasopressin V2 receptor, arginine vasopressin receptor 2 (AVPR2).

    Congenital autosomal recessive NDI results from defects in the aquaporin-2 gene, *AQP2*. An autosomal *dominant form of NDI* is associated with processing mutations of the *AQP2* gene.

- Acquired NDI can result from hypercalcemia or hypokalemia and is associated with lithium, demeclocycline, foscarnet, clozapine, amphotericin, methicillin, and rifampin.

Congenital
- X-linked V2 receptor defect
- Autosomal dominant aquaporin-2 defect
- Autosomal recessive aquaporin-2 defect

Acquired
- Metabolic
- Hypercalcemia
- Hypercalciuria
- Hypokalemia

Renal Diseases
- Polycystic kidney disease
- Medullary cystic kidney
- Sickle cell nephropathy (disease/trait)
- Chronic pyelonephritis
- Acute tubular necrosis
- Obstructive uropathy

Drugs
- Lithium
- Demeclocycline
- Amphotericin B
- Foscarnet
- Rifampin

Nephrogenic diabetes insipidus is attributed to the inability of the kidney to respond to ADH. A psychogenic form of polydipsia with associated polyuria is attributed to compulsive water drinking. DI with DM, optic atrophy, and deafness is known as Wolfram syndrome or MOAD syndrome.

Nephrogenic (vasopressin-insensitive) DI can result from genetic or acquired causes. Genetic causes are less common but more severe than acquired forms of NDI. The polyuria and polydipsia associated with genetic NDI usually occur within the first several weeks of life but may only become apparent after weaning or with longer periods of nighttime sleep. Many infants initially present with fever, vomiting, and dehydration. Failure to thrive may be secondary to the ingestion of large amounts of water, resulting in caloric malnutrition. Longstanding ingestion and excretion of large volumes of water can lead to nonobstructive hydronephrosis, hydroureter, and megabladder.

Congenital X-linked NDI results from inactivating mutations of the vasopressin V2 receptor. Congenital autosomal recessive NDI results from a defect in the *AQP2* gene. An autosomal dominant form of NDI is associated with processing mutations of the *AQP2* gene.

Acquired NDI can result from hyperkalemia or hypokalemia. Impaired renal concentrating ability can also be seen with ureteral obstruction, chronic renal failure, polycystic kidney disease, medullary cystic disease, Sjogren syndrome, and sickle cell disease.

CLINICAL FEATURES (FIG. 1)

The onset of DI is often abrupt with polyuria and intense thirst. The affected child typically has nocturia or enuresis and cannot go through the night without drinking water. Cold water is typically the preferred fluid. Dehydration may occur if fluid intake is not sufficient to keep up with urine losses or if there is concomitant damage to the normal thirst mechanism.

In infants, symptoms may also include failure to thrive, vomiting, constipation, and unexplained fevers. It is especially difficult to recognize polyuria and polydipsia in a young

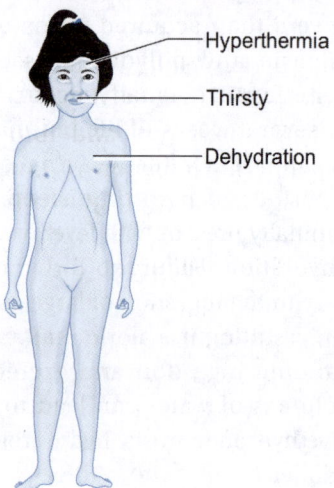

Fig. 1: Clinical features.

GENERAL FEATURES
- Growth retardation
- Passing large quantities of water
- Nocturnal enuresis
- Poor appetite

ESSENTIAL DIAGNOSTIC POINTS
- Polydipsia and polyuria
- Urine specific gravity <1.010
- Inability to concentrate urine after fluid restriction
- Hyperosmolality of plasma
- Subnormal plasma arginine vasopressin (AVP) concentration
- Responsiveness to AVP administration

infant on an ordinary feeding regimen and the infant may present with severe dehydration, circulatory collapse, and convulsions. Familial DI may have a more insidious onset and a slowly progressive course.

Nephrogenic diabetes insipidus can present in the first week of life with irritability, vomiting, and unexplained fever. The infant will have repeated episodes of hypernatremic dehydration, which may be accompanied by seizures, until the diagnosis is made, and therapy is initiated. Many infants with NDI initially present with fever, vomiting, and dehydration, often leading to an evaluation for infection. They may also have growth failure and mental retardation. Intracerebral calcification of the frontal lobes and basal ganglia is common in children with X-linked NDI.

Repeated episodes of hypernatremia can result in intellectual impairment. Patients often fail to thrive due to their need to ingest water at the expense of food. The enormous urine volumes can result in urinary tract dilatation.

■ DIAGNOSIS

Initial investigations should include testing for urine sugar and early morning specific gravity or osmolality. Blood gas, urea, electrolytes, calcium, and creatinine should be estimated. High plasma osmolality (>300 mOsm/kg or serum sodium >146 mmol/L) and low urine osmolality (<300 mOsm/kg and urine specific gravity <1.005) suggest the diagnosis of DI, which needs further classification on the basis of response to AVP. Patients with normal plasma osmolality and low urine osmolality (<800 mOsm/kg) should undergo a water deprivation test. Urinary osmolality >800 mOsm/kg (specific gravity >1.010) excludes DI.

Often the distinction between CDI and NDI titers is a water deprivation test or desmopressin (DDAVP) test. During the water deprivation test foot minimum (3–6 hours, children with CDI and NDI fail to concentrate urine and plasma >300 mOsm/kg; whereas, there is urinary concentration in children with compulsory water drinking. If there is a concentration of urine following DDAVP (5 µg intranasal), the cause is primary AVP deficiency. Failure to concentrate urine and absence of response to DDAVP indicates NDI.

Water Deprivation Test

The test is indicated in children with polyuria, low urinary osmolality, and normal plasma osmolality. The aim is to increase plasma osmolality above 300 mOsm/kg to allow an opportunity for maximal renal concentration. Renal failure and renal tubular acidosis (RTA) should be excluded before the test. A water deprivation test is not required in the presence of hypernatremia. The test should be done on an inpatient basis due to the risk of dehydration. Water deprivation starts early in the morning. The child should be weighed, and target weight loss calculated (5% of total body weight). Body weight, urine output, and urine and blood osmolality should be monitored hourly. The test should be stopped when urine osmolality increases above 800 mOsm/kg or the specific gravity is >1.010.

Since this excludes DI, plasma osmolality increases above 300 mOsm/kg or serum sodium is above 146 mEq/L (target achieved) or weight loss is >5% (risk of dehydration). Urine osmolality below 300 mOsm/kg in the presence of plasma osmolality above 300 mOsm/kg confirms DI. These patients should be evaluated further with response to vasopressin. Children with urine osmolality between 300 and 800 mOsm/kg with plasma osmolality above 300 mOsm/kg may have partial CDI or NDI.

The child should be observed carefully during the water deprivation test to ensure compliance and to prevent severe dehydration. Administration of DDAVP, DDAVP (10 µg intranasal) raises the urine osmolality. Failure to concentrate urine and absence of response to DDAVP indicate NDI. Definitive tests of renal function are indicated in them.

Vasopressin Response Test

This test is performed for the differentiation of complete CDI from NDI. Urine osmolality is measured one and four hours after vasopressin injection (0.1 unit/kg). An increase in urine osmolality by >50% of baseline levels is diagnostic of CDI while a smaller increase suggests NDI.

Once the diagnosis of CDI has been established as explained earlier MRI should be obtained. MRI is not very helpful in distinguishing CDI from NDI but will help establish the underlying cause of CDI. The posterior pituitary "bright spot" is diminished or absent in both forms of DI, normal in primary polydipsia, and decreased in SIADH. In patients with CDI who have normal brain MRI on diagnosis, serial imaging over time should be obtained as the cause may be evident years later. Quantitative measurement of the beta subunit of hCG, often secreted by germinomas and pinealomas, should be performed in children with idiopathic or unexplained CDI.

For the postsurgical patient, it is important to differentiate the normal increased diuresis from CDI. Serum osmolality will be high in acute postsurgical CDI, whereas it will be low or normal in cases of polyuria due to the normal diuresis of intraoperative fluids. The intraoperative fluid record should also help distinguish between these two possibilities. In patients with coexisting vasopressin and cortisol deficits, symptoms of DI may be masked because cortisol deficiency impairs renal free water clearance. In such cases, glucocorticoid therapy may precipitate polyuria, leading to the diagnosis of DI.

Radiologic Studies

Magnetic resonance imaging may reveal evidence for intracranial tumors such as calcification, enlargement of sella, erosion of clinoid process, and increased width of suture lines, or evidence of reticuloendotheliosis, such as rarefaction. MRI also can demonstrate the absence of a bright hyperintense spot in hypothalamic-pituitary lesions.

X-ray of the skull may reveal evidence for intracranial tumors such as calcification, enlargement of sella, erosion of clinoid process, and increased width of suture lines, and evidence of reticuloendotheliosis, such as rarefaction. CT or MRI scans are indicated for evaluation of the posterior pituitary.

> **LABORATORY SALIENT FINDINGS**
> - Hypotonic urine and hypertonic serum
> - *Urine specific gravity:* <1.010; osmolality <300 mOsm/kg
> - Serum AVP concentration
> - MRI scan to evaluate for tumors or infiltrative process
> - CT scan
> - X-ray of the skull
>
> (AVP: arginine vasopressin CT: computed tomography; MRI: magnetic resonance imaging)

TREATMENT OF CENTRAL DIABETES INSIPIDUS

Fluid Therapy

With an intact thirst mechanism and free access to oral fluids, a person with complete DI can maintain plasma osmolality and sodium in the high normal range, although at great inconvenience.

Neonates and young infants are often best treated solely with fluid therapy, given their requirement for large volumes (3 L/m^2/24 h) of nutritive fluid. The use of vasopressin analogs in patients with obligate high fluid intake is difficult given the risk of life-threatening hyponatremia. The use of diluted parenteral and lyophilized long-acting vasopressin analog DDAVP has been successfully administered to infants with CDI both subcutaneously and orally without causing severe hyponatremia.

Vasopressin Analogs

Treatment of CDI in older children is best accomplished with the use of DDAVP. DDAVP is available (onset 15–30 minutes). The intranasal preparation of DDAVP (2.5–10 µg/0.1 mL every 12 hourly) can be administered by rhinal tube (allowing dose titration) or by nasal spray. Use of DDAVP oral tablets requires at least a 10-fold increase in the dosage compared with the intranasal preparation. Oral dosages of 25–300 µg every 8–12 hours are safe and effective in children. The appropriate dosage and route of administration are determined empirically based on the desired length of antidiuresis and patient preference.

Aqueous Vasopressin

Central diabetes insipidus of acute onset the following neurosurgery is best managed with continuous administration of synthetic aqueous vasopressin. Under most circumstances, total fluid intake must be limited to 1 L/m^2/24 h during antidiuresis. A typical dosage for intravenous vasopressin therapy is 1.5 mL/kg/h, which results in a blood vasopressin concentration of approximately 10 µg/mL. Vasopressin concentrations >1,000 µg/mL should be avoided because they can cause cutaneous necrosis, rhabdomyolysis, cardiac rhythm disturbances, and hypertension: Postneurosurgical patients treated with vasopressin infusion should be switched from intravenous to oral fluids as soon as possible to allow thirst sensation, if intact, to help regulate osmolality.

Neurogenic diabetes insipidus is treated by administration of DDAVP, an analog of ADH given as a nasal spray. The usual dose is 5–10 µg daily either as a single dose or divided into two doses. Children under 2 years require lesser doses (0.15–0.50 µg/kg). An oral preparation of DDAVP (0.2 mg) is also available now.

Oral administration of chlorpropamide 20 mg/kg/24 hours in two divided doses may reduce polyuria and polydipsia in partial deficiency. Hypoglycemia is a major side effect. Chlorpropamide potentiates the residual secretion of ADH and also has an effect on the thirst center.

TREATMENT OF NEPHROGENIC INSIPIDUS

The treatment of acquired NDI focuses on eliminating, if possible, the underlying disorder, such as offending drugs, hypercalcemia, hypokalemia, and ureteral obstruction. Congenital NDI is often difficult to treat. The main goals are to ensure the intake of adequate calories for growth and to avoid severe dehydration. Even with the early institution of therapy, however, growth failure, and developmental disabilities are common.

Nephrogenic Diabetes Insipidus

The solute load should be decreased, and sufficient water should be given to prevent dehydration. Hydrochlorothiazide 0.5–1.5 mg/kg/day reduces urinary volume as a paradoxical effect. Addition of indomethacin 1–2 mg/kg/24 hours is beneficial in some. Chloropropamide is not useful in NDI.

Pharmacologic approaches to the treatment of NDI include the use of thiazide diuretics which are intended to decrease the overall urine output. Thiazides appear to induce a state of mild volume depletion by enhancing sodium excretion at the expense of water and by causing a decrease in the glomerular filtration rate, which results in proximal tubular sodium and water reabsorption. Indomethacin and amiloride may be used in combination with thiazides to further reduce polyuria, high dose DDAVP therapy, in combination with indomethacin, has been used in some subjects with NDI. This treatment could prove useful in patients with genetic defects in the V2 receptor associated with a reduced binding affinity for vasopressin.

BIBLIOGRAPHY

1. Bockenhauer D, Bichet DG. Pathophysiology, diagnosis and management of nephrogenic diabetes insipidus. Nat Rev Nephrol. 2015; 11(10)576-88.
2. Di Lorgi N, Allegri AE, Napoli F, Calcagno A, Calandra E, Fratangeli N, et al. Central diabetes insipidus in children and young adults: Etiological diagnosis and long-term outcome of idiopathic cases. J Clin Endocrinol Metab. 2014;99(4):1264-72.
3. Fenske W, Allolio B. Clinical review: current state and future perspectives in the diagnosis of diabetes insipidus: a clinical review. J Clin Endocrinol Metab. 2012;97(10):3426-37.
4. Vyas A, Menon RK. Growth Hormone deficiency and resistance. PG Textbook of Pediatrics, 2nd edition. New Delhi: Jaypee Brothers Medical Publishers (P) Ltd; 2017. pp. 2676-80.

CASE 61

Diabetes Mellitus

■ PRESENTING COMPLAINTS

A 6-year-old boy was brought with the complaints of:
- Loss of weight since 6 months
- Tiredness since 6 months
- Increased frequency of urine since 6 months

History of Presenting Complaints

A 6-year-old boy was brought to the pediatric outpatient department with the history of drastic loss of weight since last 6 months. His mother was very much worried about the loss of weight. Mother gave the history that his son was weighing about 22 kg 6 months back, now he has reduced to 18 kg. She revealed that she had noticed that her son was more frequently passing the urine. There was no burning sensation. She also told that her son gets up in the night to pass urine. Mother informed that her son's eating habits were normal. Of late, she noticed tiredness in her son for which she showed him to the family doctor who advised some B-complex syrup. She also pointed out the school absenteeism from the last 3 months.

Past History of the Patient

The boy was the elder sibling of nonconsanguineous marriage. He was born at full term by normal delivery. He cried immediately after the delivery. His birth weight was 3 kg. He was exclusively on breast milk for the first 3 months. Later, weaning was started and he was on family food by 15 months. His developmental milestones were normal. He was immunized completely. School absenteeism was present since last 3 months.

■ EXAMINATION

The boy was moderately built and poorly nourished. He was conscious and looking tired.

CASE AT A GLANCE

Basic Findings
Height	: 124 cm (95th centile)
Weight	: 15 kg (50th centile)
Temperature	: 37°C
Pulse rate	: 86 beats/min
Respiratory rate	: 20 breaths/min
Blood pressure	: 90/70 mm Hg

Positive Findings

History:
- Loss of weight
- Polyuria
- School absenteeism

Examination:
- Poorly nourished
- Evidence of recent loss of weight
- Pallor

Investigation:
- *Hemoglobin:* 9 g/dL
- *RBS:* 300 mg/dL
- *FBS:* 130 mg/dL
- *Urine:* Sugar++
  Ketone bodies+++

Anthropometric measurements included the height of 124 cm (95th centile), the weight was 15 kg (50th centile).

Child was afebrile. The pulse rate was 86 beats per minute. Respiratory rate was 20 breaths per minute. Blood pressure recorded was 90/70 mm Hg. There was pallor. Presence of folded skin indicating recent weight loss were present. All the systemic examination were normal.

■ INVESTIGATION

- *Hemoglobin:* 9 g/dL
- *TLC:* 8,700 cells/mm^3
- *DLC:* $P_{72}L_{18}E_6M_2B_2$
- *ESR:* 26 mm in the 1st hour
- *Random blood sugar (RBS):* 300 mg/dL
- *Fasting blood sugar (FBS):* 130 mg/dL
- *Urine:*
  - Albumin++
  - Sugar+++
  - Ketone bodies+
  - 1–2 red blood cells (RBCs)/HPF
  - 6–7 pus cells/HPF

■ DISCUSSION

History of weight loss since last 6 months along with normal food intake. There was history of nocturia. This along with the laboratory findings of presence of sugar and ketone bodies and raised blood glucose level clinches the diagnosis of diabetes mellitus (DM).

Diabetes mellitus is a chronic disease caused by deficiency of insulin, which is secreted by the beta cells of pancreas. The illness is characterized by hyperglycemia and glucosuria. Diabetes may also result from defects of insulin action. The disease causes long-term damage, dysfunction, or failure of various organs including the eyes, kidneys, nerves, heart, and blood vessels.

■ CLASSIFICATION

Diabetes is usually classified as type I and type 2. Type I diabetes is usually a disease of young people, and thus much more frequent in children. Children with type I diabetes have to rely on lifelong insulin therapy. Thus, this type was also known as insulin-dependent DM (IDDM). Type 2 was previously known as non-insulin-dependent DM (NIDDM). Other distinguishing features of types 1 and 2 diabetes are given in the **Table 1**.

Type 1A diabetes occurs from immunologic damage to the insulin-producing β-cells of the pancreatic islets. The damage occurs gradually over months or years in most people and symptoms do not appear until about 90% of the pancreatic islets have been destroyed. The immunologic damages have a genetic predisposition and are probably affected by environmental factors.

There is an association with human leukocyte antigen-DR3 (HLA-DR3) and HLA-DR4, and about 95% of white diabetic children have at least one of these HLA types. The presence of aspartic acid on position 57 of the DQ β chain of the HLA complex is associated with protection from type 1 diabetes.

Islet cell antibodies (ICA), insulin, "64 K" or glutamic acid decarboxylase (GAD), ICA512 (IA-2), and other antibodies are present in the serum of over 90% of patients who will develop type 1A diabetes for months to years prior to diagnosis. These antibodies are probably the effect and not the cause of islet β-cell destruction.

The etiology of type 2 diabetes has been related to a number of genetic alterations. All have the common denominator of a reduced sensitivity to insulin.

■ PATHOGENESIS

Pathogenesis is multifactorial. Genetic alterations located on chromosome 6 may

TABLE 1: Distinguishing features of type 1 and 2 diabetes.

Features	Type 1	Type 2
Onset	Rapid and obvious	Slow and insidious
Age of onset	Before 30 years	After 30 years
Obesity	No role	Predisposing
Association with HLA DR3 and 4	2.5 times	Equal to normal
Family history	10%	Strong
Concordance in identical twins	25–50%	Nearly 100%
Anti-islet cell antibody	>80%	<5%
Ketoacidosis	Frequent	Absent
Microvascular complications	Rare at onset	May be present
Need for insulin	Universal	Uncommon

(HLA: human leukocyte antigen)

initiate β-cell damage. Autoimmune destruction of β-cells has been demonstrated in children with type 1 DM.

Environmental factors trigger the onset of autoimmunity in genetically susceptible individuals. Infections (mumps, coxsackie virus B3 and B4, and cytomegalovirus), toxins (rodenticides and nitrosamines), and early introduction of cow's milk protein may be important factors in the subsequent development of diabetes in genetically susceptible individuals.

■ CLINICAL FEATURES (FIG. 1)

Clinical features manifest only when more than 90% of the pancreatic β-cell synthesis and release capacity has been destroyed or effectively inactivated.

GENERAL FEATURES
• Fatigue
• Loss of weight
• Failure to thrive

Initial symptoms include polyuria, polydipsia, polyphagia, and fatigue. Diabetic ketoacidosis (DKA) supervenes in more than half of the children.

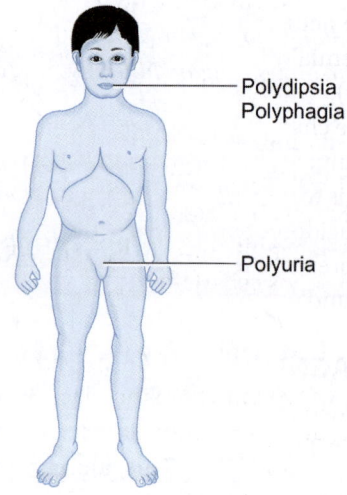

Fig. 1: Clinical features.

The final stage is total diabetes, which refers to complete β-cell destruction with no capacity of endogenous insulin synthesis or release. This is irreversible.

Total diabetes is considered to have reached when the insulin requirement of a preadolescent has plateaued at approximately 0.8 units/kg/day and in an adolescent at about 1.0 units/kg/day.

Suspect DM in a child with the classical triad of polyuria, polydipsia, and polyphagia.

Random plasma glucose concentration >200 mg/dL on 2 separate occasions with symptoms of diabetes suggests the diagnosis. Fasting plasma glucose levels >126 mg/dL on 2 occasions are also suggestive of the diagnosis of diabetes.

In a patient who presents with the classical symptoms of polyuria, thirst, and weight loss, the diagnosis of diabetes is straightforward, and requires only the demonstration of hyperglycemia. In a child with an accidental finding of glycosuria, one must differentiate DM from renal glycosuria or Fanconi syndrome. Ketonuria can occur in starvation, and in adolescents, after an alcohol binge on an empty stomach. Both these conditions will not be accompanied by hyperglycemia and ketonemia will be mild (not positive in dilute serum).

The child presenting with acidosis must be differentiated from other causes of metabolic acidosis with increased anion gap, like uremia, lactic acidosis, and salicylate poisoning. Every child presenting in a coma must have a blood sugar and urine ketone to detect DKA.

DIAGNOSIS

Diagnostic criteria for diabetes mellitus are given in **Table 2**.

TABLE 2: Diagnostic criteria for diabetes mellitus: Any one to be fulfilled.

	Prediabetes	Diabetes
Fasting plasma glucose	100–125 mg/dL	≥126 mg/dL
2 hours PG during OGTT	140–199 mg/dL	≥200 mg/dL
Hemoglobin A1C (HbA1C)	5.7–6.4%	≥6.5%
Random plasma glucose		≥200 mg/dL

(OGTT: oral glucose tolerance test; PG: postload glucose)

DIFFERENTIAL DIAGNOSIS OF POLYURIA

Differential diagnosis of polyuria are as follows:
- *Diabetes mellitus:* It presents with polydipsia, polyphagia, recurrent infections, and weight loss in addition to polyuria.
- *Renal disorders:* Polyuria is common in obstructive uropathy and is often the presenting feature of tubular disorders like RTA, Bartter syndrome, and Gitelman syndrome. These conditions are associated with severe failure to thrive and rickets.
- *Inefficient aldosterone action:* These include adrenal insufficiency, isolated aldosterone deficiency, or aldosterone resistance. They present with hyponatremia, hyperkalemia, and dehydration. The condition may be lethal. Failure to thrive is common. Pigmentation is characteristic of adrenal insufficiency. Polyuria and salt wasting in the neonatal period should prompt evaluation for CAH. Genital ambiguity in girls may be the only clue to this diagnosis.
- *Excessive water drinking (psychogenic polydipsia):* The condition is extremely rare and is a diagnosis of exclusion.

ESSENTIAL DIAGNOSTIC POINTS
• Polyuria, polydipsia, and weight loss
• Hyperglycemia and glucosuria with without ketonuria

COMPLICATIONS

Complications can be classified as acute, intermediate, and chronic.

The acute complications include ketoacidosis and hypoglycemia. These are usually reversible.

Intermediate complications include lipoatrophy, growth failure, impaired intellectual development, and hypoglycemia unawareness. These are potentially reversible.

Chronic complications are irreversible and are due to micro and macrovascular pathology. These include retinopathy, neuropathy, and nephropathy. The following section will discuss two most common acute complications, i.e., hypoglycemia and DKA.

Hypoglycemia

Hypoglycemia is defined as blood glucose levels <60 mg/dL. It is characterized by adrenergic symptoms such as sweating, pallor, trembling, and tachycardia. Untreated, this may progress to drowsiness, confusion, coma, and seizures. The diagnosis should be confirmed by a quick blood test. Simple carbohydrates like sugar, glucose, honey, fruit juice, or carbonated drinks may be offered immediately. An unconscious child should be given intravenous 25% dextrose (2–4 mL/kg) or glucagon (0.5 mg in children and 1.0 mg in adolescents) intramuscularly.

LABORATORY SALIENT FINDINGS
• Random blood glucose level >300 mg/dL. • Fasting blood glucose level >200 mg/dL • Ketonuria

Diabetic Ketoacidosis

Diabetic ketoacidosis is the most common and severe manifestation of diabetes. It occurs as a result of insulin deficiency with concomitant increased production of the stress hormones, glucagon, cortisol, and GH. The prime responses include increased gluconeogenesis, glycogenolysis, and ketone body production as well as decreased glycogen synthesis.

Clinical Features

Precipitating factors for DKA include intercurrent illness, trauma, and obscure infection. Manifestations include symptoms of hyperglycemia and ketoacidosis such as polyuria, nocturia, polydipsia, polyphagia, weight loss, lethargy, weakness, nausea, vomiting, change in level of consciousness, increased respiratory rate with Kussmaul breathing, and abdominal pain. The child is acidotic and has deep rapid breathing with severe dehydration. Blood pressure, pulse rate, skin turgor, and body weight should be taken to evaluate dehydration.

Diagnosis

Criteria for confirmation of diagnosis of DKA include ketonuria, ketonemia, blood glucose >250 mg/dL, blood pH <7.3 and serum bicarbonate <20 mEq/L. Serum potassium levels may be high. Urinalysis may reveal the presence of glucose and acetoacetate/acetone.

ESSENTIAL DIAGNOSTIC POINTS OF DIABETIC KETOACIDOSIS
• Triad of metabolic derangement include hyperglycemia, ketonuria, and acidosis • Abdominal pain may mimic appendicitis • Hyperventilation can mimic pneumonia • Administer insulin promptly to prevent ketone and acid production • Total body potassium is usually significantly diminished • Cerebral edema is the most common cause of death • Avoid excess fluid therapy because of the risk of cerebral edema

Managing Ketoacidosis

The aim of management should be to restore normal hemodynamic status, normal acid-base balance, and slowly correct blood glucose to a range that is not acutely dangerous.

The main strategies of therapy include: (i) Replacement of water and electrolytes and (ii) starting insulin. Replacement of fluid is essential for maintaining hemodynamic stability and to prevent lactic acidosis and poor perfusion.

Fluid Therapy

- Immediately secure a venous access and obtain blood samples for counts, sugar, urea, sodium, potassium, etc. An arterial sample should be taken for blood gas and pH estimation.
- Start IV fluids. The initial fluid should be normal saline (0.9%) IV given in a dose of 20 mL/kg within the 1st hour of diagnosis.
- After 1 hour, continue with normal (0.45%) saline till signs of severe dehydration disappear. Infusion of maintenance fluids and deficit should be given over 24–36 hours.
- Monitor blood glucose levels hourly. Obtain simultaneous urine samples for documentation of glucosuria and ketonuria. When blood sugar falls to 300 mg/dL or less, 5% dextrose should be added to the infusate.
- Once the child has passed urine, add potassium (40 mEq/L of IV fluids). Potassium replacement is important because potassium shifts from extracellular to intracellular compartment during treatment.
- *Correction of acidosis:* Bicarbonate therapy is usually not necessary. Insulin therapy inhibits ketogenesis and stimulates the metabolism of ketone bodies. Bicarbonate is necessary if there is impending ventilatory and circulatory compromise.

Insulin

- *Start insulin:* Give an initial bolus dose of 0.1 unit/kg IV followed by a continuous IV infusion at a rate of 0.1 unit/kg/h. In infants, the dose may be reduced to 0.05 unit/kg/h. The aim is to decrease blood glucose by 50 to 100 mg/dL every hour.
- If there is no significant reduction in blood sugar, the dose can be increased to 0.2 units/kg/h.
- The usual practice is to add 1 unit/kg of insulin in 100 mL of 0.9% saline and administer at a rate of 10 mL/h (1 unit/kg/h).
- The IV tubing should be flushed with insulin prior to starting the infusion to avoid binding of insulin to plastic surfaces and reduced delivery of insulin.
- Reduce the dose rate to 0.5 unit/kg/h when acidosis clears (pH >7.3) and blood glucose reaches 200 mg/dL. Urine ketones are not a good guide for monitoring insulin dose.
- The insulin infusion can be discontinued when the blood glucose levels fall into a normal range. However, it should be continued till 30 minutes after the administration of subcutaneous insulin.

Monitoring

- Meticulously monitor the vital signs, state of consciousness, blood glucose, and urine ketones till IV infusion is terminated.
- Monitor electrolyte and pH every 2–4 hours.
- Urine output should be checked every 4 hours.
- Watch for cerebral edema. This may occur due to rapid correction of hyperglycemia and hyperosmolality, excessive use of alkali, high doses of insulin, and overhydration.

Chronic Complications

In the past, about 30–40% of persons with type 1 diabetes eventually developed renal failure or loss of vision. Factors that greatly reduce this likelihood are longitudinal Hemoglobin A levels in a good range, maintenance of blood pressure below the 90th percentile for age.

Annual retinal examinations and urine microalbumin measurements are important for children aged 10 years or older who have diabetes for 3 years or longer. Data now show that the use of angiotensin-converting enzyme inhibitors may reverse or delay kidney damage when it is detected in the microalbuminuria stage (20–300 μg/min). Similarly, laser treatment to coagulate proliferating capillaries prevents bleeding and leakage of blood into the vitreous fluid or behind the retina. This treatment helps to prevent retinal detachment and to preserve useful vision for many people with proliferative diabetic retinopathy.

The aim of immediate therapy is to restore fluid volume and return acid-base status to normal, and not to achieve stable euglycemia. When the patient is ready to take orally, with a blood pH of <7.3 and glucose <300 mg/dL, switch from IV to subcutaneous insulin. Start regular insulin (0.5 units/kg/day) in newly diagnosed children <5 years and 1.0 unit/kg/day in older children. Subsequently, the child can be started on a split-mix regime.

BIBLIOGRAPHY

1. Dabelea D, Mayer-Davis EJ, Saydah S, Imperatore G, Linder B, Divers J, et al. Prevalence of type 1 and type 2 diabetes in children and adolescents from 2001 to 2009. JAMA. 2014;311(17):1778-86.
2. Diabetes Control and Complications Trial Research Group; Nathan DM, Genuth S, Lachin J, Cleary P, Crofford O, Davis M, et al. The effect of intensive treatment of diabetes on the development and progression of long-term complications on insulin-dependent diabetes mellitus. N Engl J Med. 1993;329(14):977-86.
3. Meléndez-Ramirez LY, Richards RJ, Cefalu WT. Complications of type 1 diabetes. North Am Clin. 2010;39:625-40.
4. Pickup JC. Insulin-pump therapy for type 1 mellitus. N Engl J Med. 2012;366(17):1616-24.
5. Redondo MJ, Eisenbarth GS. Genetic control of autoimmunity in type 1 diabetes and associated disorders. Diabetologia. 2002;45(5):605-22.
6. Wolfdorf JI, Craig ME, Daneman D, Dunger D, Edge J, Lee W, et al. Diabetic ketoacidosis in children and adolescents with diabetes. Pediatr Diabetes. 2009;10 Suppl 12:118-33.

CASE 62

Hypothyroidism

■ PRESENTING COMPLAINTS

A 5-month-old girl was brought with the complaints of:
- Constipation since birth
- Delayed developmental milestones since 3 months

History of Presenting Complaints

A 5-month-old girl was brought to the pediatric outpatient department with history of constipation and delayed developmental milestones. Mother gave the history that her child was passing motion once in 3 or 4 days since her birth. Now, she was passing once in a week. Sometimes, child may require laxatives. The child was passing stools sometimes like pellets. Child had not developed neck control. Social smile was not present. But she was responding to local noise or commands. Mother had noticed that her developmental milestones were much delayed as compared to elder sibling.

Past History of the Patient

The girl was second sibling of a nonconsanguineous marriage. She was born at term and delivered by cesarean section. The indication of the section was nonprogression of the labor. The birth weight of the child was 3.5 kg. Child started taking breast milk immediately after birth. Child had prolonged physiological jaundice for which child had received phototherapy.

CASE AT A GLANCE

Basic Findings
Length	: 62 cm (80th centile)
Weight	: 7 kg (50th centile)
Temperature	: 36°C
Pulse rate	: 110 beats/min
Respiratory rate	: 26 breaths/min
Blood pressure	: 60/50 mm Hg

Positive Findings

History:
- Constipation
- Delayed motor development
- No social smile
- Prolonged physiological jaundice

Examination:
- Depressed nasal bridge
- Open mouth
- Protruding tongue
- Broad hand

Investigation:
- *Triiodothyronine (T3) and thyroxine (T4):* Decreased
- *Thyroid stimulating hormone (TSH):* Increased
- *X-ray delayed:* Delayed ossification of acetabular roofs

■ EXAMINATION

On examination, the child was well built and nourished. She was lying on the examination table. She was not as active as the other children of her age. She was not moving on sideways. There was depressed nasal bridge. The mouth was kept open with protruding tongue. The hands were broad and fingers were short. Anthropometric measurements included that the length was 62 cm

(80th centile), the weight was 7 kg (50th centile), and the head circumference was 40 cm.

The child was afebrile. The heart rate was 110 beats per minute, the respiratory rate was 26 breaths per minute. The blood pressure recorded was 60/50 mm Hg. There was no pallor, no edema, no icterus, and no lymphadenopathy. Other systemic examinations were normal.

■ INVESTIGATION

- *Hemoglobin:* 13 g/dL
- *TLC:* 7,600 cells/mm^3
- *DLC:* $P_{68} L_{28} M_2 B_2$
- *ESR:* 18 mm at first hour
- *Triiodothyronine (T3) level:* 60 ng/dL (62–200 ng/dL)
- *Thyroxine (T4) level:* 4 µg/dL (4.5–12.0 µg/dL)
- *Thyroid-stimulating hormone (TSH):* 0.10 IU/dL (0.30–5.5 IU/mL)
- *X-ray of the body:* Showed the delayed ossification of the acetabular roof

■ DISCUSSION

Hypothyroidism is a common endocrinal disorder of the childhood. This can appear after a period of normal thyroid function, then the disorder is named as acquired hypothyroidism. The cretinism is used to denote congenital hypothyroidism. Congenital hypothyroidism may be familial or sporadic, goitrous, and nongoitrous.

■ ETIOLOGY

Primary Hypothyroidism

- *Thyroid dysgenesis:* It is the most common cause of permanent congenital hypothyroidism, accounting for 80–85% of cases In approximately 33% of cases of dysgenesis, no thyroid tissue is present (agenesis). In the other 66% of infants, rudiments of thyroid tissue are present, either in the normal position (hypoplasia) or in an ectopic location any where along the embryologic path of descent of the thyroid.
- *Defects in thyroid hormone synthesis (dyshormonogenesis):* A variety of defects in the biosynthesis of thyroid hormone account for 15% of cases of permanent congenital hypothyroidism detected by neonatal screening programs (1 in 30,000–50,000 live births). These defects are usually transmitted in an autosomal recessive manner. Because the thyroid gland responds normally to elevated TSH stimulation, a goiter is almost always present. When the synthetic defect is incomplete, the onset of hypothyroidism may be delayed for years.
- *Defective iodide transport:* Defective iodide uptake is very rare and is caused by mutations in the sodium–iodide symporter (NIS) responsible for concentrating iodide in the thyroid gland. In this disorder, the mechanism for concentrating iodide is defective in the thyroid and salivary glands. In contrast to other defects of thyroid hormone synthesis, uptake of radioiodine and pertechnetate is low. A reduced saliva:serum ratio of $_{123}$I will support the diagnosis, which is confirmed by finding a mutation in the NIS gene. This condition responds to treatment with large doses of potassium iodide, but treatment with levothyroxine (L-T4) is preferable.
- *Pendred syndrome:* It is an autosomal recessive disorder composed of sensorineural deafness and goiter. Pendred syndrome is caused by a mutation in the chloride-iodide transport protein pendrin (SLC26A4) that is expressed

in the thyroid gland and the cochlea. Pendrin allows transport of iodide across the apical membrane of the follicular cell into the colloid where it undergoes organification and incorporation into the tyrosine residues on thyroglobulin.

- *Defects of iodine organification:* These are the most common type of thyroid hormone synthetic defects. After iodide is taken up by the thyroid, it is rapidly oxidized to reactive iodine, which is then incorporated into tyrosine residues on thyroglobulin. These reactions are catalyzed by the critical enzyme thyroperoxidase (TPO) and require locally generated H_2O_2 and hematin (a cofactor).
- *Defects of thyroglobulin synthesis:* Defects of thyroglobulin synthesis are characterized by congenital hypothyroidism with goiter and absent or low levels of circulating thyroglobulin. More than 40 different mutations in the thyroglobulin gene (TG) have been described.
- *Defects in deiodination:* Monoiodotyrosine and diiodotyrosine are normally released from thyroglobulin along with T4 and T3. The *IYD* gene (formerly *DEHAL1*) encodes the thyroidal enzyme iodotyrosine deiodinase, which deiodinates these intermediates and allows the liberated iodide to be recycled into thyroid hormone synthesis.
- *Defects in thyroid hormone transport:* Passage of thyroid hormone into the cell is facilitated by specific plasma membrane transporters.
- *Thyrotropin receptor-blocking antibodies:* Maternal TSH receptor-blocking antibodies (TRBAbs) cause about 29% of cases of congenital hypothyroidism detected by neonatal screening programs (1 in 50,000-100,000 infants). Transplacentally acquired maternal TRBAb inhibits binding of TSH to its receptor in the neonate.
- *Radioiodine administration:* Neonatal hypothyroidism can occur when radioiodine is administered as treatment for Graves' disease or thyroid cancer to a mother during (a usually unrecognized) pregnancy. The fetal thyroid is capable of trapping iodide by 70–75 days of gestation, therefore a pregnancy test must be performed in any woman of childbearing age before iodine-131 is given, regardless of menstrual history or reported history of contraception. Administration of radioactive iodine to lactating women is also contraindicated because it is excreted in breast milk.

Hypothyroidism results from deficient production of thyroid hormone, either from a defect in the gland itself (primary hypothyroidism) or a result of reduced TSH stimulation (central or hypopituitary hypothyroidism). The disorder may be manifested from birth (congenital) or acquired (juvenile hypothyroidism). When symptoms appear after a period of apparently normal thyroid function, the disorder may be truly acquired or might only appear so as a result of one of a variety of congenital defects in which the manifestation of the deficiency is delayed.

Most cases of congenital hypothyroidism are not hereditary and result from thyroid dysgenesis (**Box 1**). Some cases are familial, these are usually caused by one of the inborn errors of thyroid hormone synthesis (dyshormonogenesis) and may be associated with a goiter.

Although there are many causes of hypothyroidism in the newborn, most cases result from hypoplasia or aplasia of the thyroid gland, radioiodine therapy at the pregnancy, thyrotropin deficiency, and defective synthesis of T4. In 85% of cases, it is thyroid dysgenesis. In 10–15% cases, it is inborn errors of thyroid hormone synthesis. They are inherited as autosomal recessive traits. Most infants with congenital hypothyroidism are detected by newborn screening programs in the 1st few weeks after birth, before obvious clinical symptoms and signs develop.

Of the genetically determined enzymatic defects that cause hypothyroidism, only Pendred syndrome (a defect in iodide organification with congenital nerve deafness) has distinguishing clinical features. In children who have enzymatic defects, thyroid enlargement is usually not present in the newborn period but occurs within the first two decades of life. Although thyroid function tests (including radioactive iodide uptake studies) may be helpful in diagnosis, final clarification of the defect generally requires chromatographic fractionation of iodinated compounds in the serum, urine, and thyroid tissue.

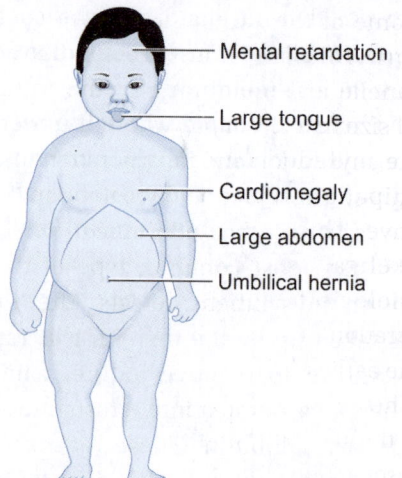

Fig. 1: Clinical features.

> **BOX 1:** Causes of congenital hypothyroidism.
> - *Primary:* Agenesis/dysgenesis, ectopic, and dyshormonogenesis
> - *Secondary:* Hypopituitarism and hypothalamic abnormality
> - *Other:* Transient and maternal factors (e.g., goitrogen ingestion and iodide deficiency)

■ CLINICAL FEATURES (FIG. 1)

Most infants with congenital hypothyroidism **(Fig. 2)** are asymptomatic at birth, even if there is complete agenesis of the thyroid gland. This situation is attributed to partial transplacental passage of maternal T4, which provides fetal levels that are approximately 33% of normal at birth. Despite this maternal contribution, hypothyroid infants still have a low serum T4 and elevated TSH level, and so will be identified by newborn screening programs.

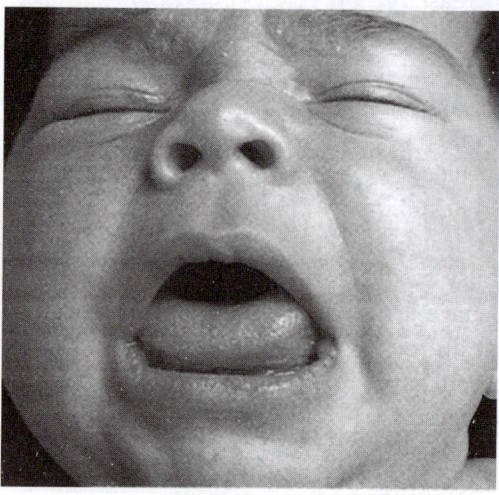

Fig. 2: Congenital hypothyroidism.

Clinical features may not be obvious for several weeks after birth. It is twice as common in girls as in boys. The infants may be significantly heavier at birth than the normal newborn infants. Most of the time, symptoms are subtle but can include lethargy, hoarse cry, feeding problems, constipation, macroglossia, umbilical hernia, large fontanels, hypotonia, dry skin, hypothermia, and prolonged jaundice. Some newborns with thyroid dyshormonogenesis can have a palpable goiter.

Some of the earlier signs of congenital hypothyroidism are patent posterior fontanelle and wide-open cranial sutures. Head size may be slightly increased because of the myxedema of brain. There may be constipation, which may not respond to laxative. This is attributed to in utero lag in skeletal maturation. Prolongation of physiologic jaundice, caused by delayed maturation of glucuronide conjugation, may be the earliest sign.

The severity of the findings in patients with thyroid deficiency depends on the age at onset and degree of deficiency. Congenital hypothyroidism is associated with an increased risk for congenital malformations when compared to the general population. The most commonly affected system is the heart, but the gastrointestinal tract, kidneys, urinary tract, and skeletal system are also affected.

Respiratory difficulties, partly caused by the large tongue, include apneic episodes, noisy respirations, and nasal obstruction. Some infants may develop respiratory distress syndrome. Affected infants cry little, sleep much, have poor appetites, and are generally sluggish. There may be constipation that does not usually respond to treatment.

Characteristic coarse facial features appear at the age of 8–10 weeks. These include puffy face, swollen eyelid, widely separated eyes, narrow palpebral fissure, broad nose with depressed bridge, and open mouth with broad thick protuberant tongue. The neck is short and thick. Supraclavicular pad of fat may be present. The voice is hoarse. The muscles are flaccid and hypotonic. They are lethargic and less active. Feeding difficulties occur due to the presence of large tongue and include apneic episodes, noisy respiration, and nasal obstruction. These infants will have constipation and hypothermia is common.

The skin may be dry, thick, scaly, and coarse with a yellowish tinge due to excessive deposition of carotene. The hair is dry, coarse and brittle (variable), and may be excessive. Lateral thinning of the eyebrows may occur. The axillary and supraclavicular fat pads may be prominent in infants.

The muscles are usually hypotonic, but in rare instances generalized muscular pseudohypertrophy occurs (Kocher-Debré-Sémélaigne syndrome). Affected older children can have an athletic appearance because of pseudohypertrophy, particularly in the calf muscles. Its pathogenesis is unknown; nonspecific histochemical and ultrastructural changes seen on muscle biopsy return to normal with treatment. Males are more prone to development of the syndrome, which has been observed in siblings born from a consanguineous mating. Affected patients have hypothyroidism of longer duration and severity.

The abdomen is large and umbilical hernia may be present. The temperature is subnormal, often less than 35°C and the skin may be cold and mottled. Edema of the genitalia and extremities may be present. The pulse is slow, heart murmur and cardiomegaly, and asymptomatic pericardial effusion are common.

Child's growth will be stunted, the extremities are short, and the head size is normal or even increased. The anterior fontanel is large, and the posterior fontanel may remain open. The eyes appear far apart, and the bridge of the broad nose is depressed. The palpebral fissures are narrow, and the eyelids are swollen. The mouth is kept open, and the thick broad tongue protrudes. The neck is short and thick, and there may be deposits of fat above the clavicles and between the neck and shoulders. The hands are broad, and the fingers are short. Retardation in physical and mental development becomes evident by 3–6 months of age. The degree of physical and mental retardation increases with age. Social smile is delayed. Dentition and skeletal maturation are significantly delayed. Refractory anemia is common.

Some infants with mild congenital hypothyroidism have normal thyroid function at birth and are not identified by newborn screening programs. In particular, some children with ectopic thyroid tissue (lingual, sublingual, and subhyoid) produce adequate amounts of thyroid hormone in a variable length of time (even years) until the abnormal thyroid tissue fails. Affected children come to clinical attention because of a growing mass at the base of the tongue or in the midline of the neck, usually at the level of the hyoid.

ESSENTIAL DIAGNOSTIC POINTS

- Growth retardation and diminished physical activities
- Impaired tissue perfusion
- Constipation
- Thick tongue and hoarseness
- Poor muscle tone
- Anemia and intellectual retardation
- Low thyroid hormone concentration
- TSH levels are elevated

CAUSES OF HYPOTHYROIDISM

The causes of hypothyroidism are as follows:
- Thyroid dysgenesis
  - Thyroid aplasia
  - Thyroid hypoplasia
  - Thyroid ectopy
- Thyroid dyshormonogenesis
- Resistance to TSH
- Defect in thyroid hormone transport
- Resistance to thyroid hormone action
- Central hypothyroidism
- Transient hypothyroidism
- T4-binding globulin deficiency

Acquired hypothyroidism is caused mainly by lymphocytic thyroiditis, autoimmune thyroiditis, irradiation, and the histiocytic infiltration of the thyroid and drugs. The drugs include iodine and amiodarone.

The clinical features include constipation, cold intolerance, increased need of sleep, and delayed closure of epiphyses. Osseous maturation is delayed. This is an indication of the duration of hypothyroidism. Younger children will have pseudoprecocious puberty and galactorrhea. Head and visual problems are also noted. They usually have hyperplastic enlargement of the pituitary gland often with suprasellar extension. Sometimes only clinical evidence may be short stature. The ratio between the upper segment and lower segment is increased.

Growth changes include short stature, infantile skeletal proportions with relatively short extremities, infantile naso-orbital configuration (bridge of nose flat, broad and underdeveloped, and eyes seem to be widely spaced), delayed epiphysial development, delayed closure of fontanelles, and retarded dental eruption. Treatment of acquired hypothyroidism may not result in the predicted final adult target height. Menometrorrhagia may occur in older girls, and galactorrhea resulting from the stimulation of prolactin secretion or elevated thyrotropin-releasing hormone (TRH) has been reported.

GENERAL FEATURES

- Large baby
- Prolonged physiological jaundice
- Constipation
- Feeding problems
- Apneic episodes
- Noisy breathing
- Delayed dentition

DIAGNOSIS

The diagnosis of primary hypothyroidism is confirmed by the presence of low serum T4 and elevated serum TSH values. Estimation of free T4 and T3 is also available. TSH is an extremely sensitive index of primary hypothyroidism. Presence of thyroglobulin in the serum is also indicative of functioning thyroid tissue.

Thyroid antibody studies—anti-thyroglobulin (ATG) and antimitochondrial (AMA) or antiperoxidase antibodies (APO) in particular—help in identifying autoimmune basis of the disease. Fine needle aspiration cytology (FNAC) is helpful.

Initial investigations in a child with high TSH levels should include evaluation of radionuclide uptake and thyroid ultrasound to confirm the presence of thyroid gland. Thyroid dysgenesis should be diagnosed if no thyroid tissue is visualized on ultrasound. Radiotracer uptake study with radioactive iodine or technetium (Tc) should be done as soon as the diagnosis of primary congenital hypothyroidism has been established. Children with absent radiotracer uptake but normal thyroid on ultrasound could be suffering from defects in iodine transport, TSH receptor defects, or transplacental passage of TSH blocking antibody. Increased radioactive tracer uptake is indicative of iodine deficiency or dyshormonogenesis. Children with low TSH levels should be worked up for other pituitary defects.

Serum cholesterol and carotene are usually elevated in childhood but may be low or normal in infants. Cessation of therapy in previously treated hypothyroidism produces a marked rise in serum cholesterol levels in 6–8 weeks. Urinary creatinine excretion is decreased, and urinary hydroxyproline is low.

Circulating autoantibodies to thyroid constituents may be present. Serum GH may be decreased, with subnormal human growth hormone (HGH) response to insulin-induced hypoglycemia and arginine stimulation in children with severe primary hypothyroidism.

Radiograph

Retardation of osseous development can be shown radiographically at birth in approximately 60% of congenitally hypothyroid infants and indicates some deprivation of thyroid hormone during intrauterine life. The distal femoral and proximal tibial epiphyses, normally present at birth, are often absent. In undetected and untreated patients, the discrepancy between chronologic age and osseous development increases. The epiphyses often have multiple foci of ossification. Deformity (beaking) of the 12th thoracic or 1st or 2nd lumbar vertebra is common. X-rays of the skull shows large fontanels and wide sutures. Intrasutural (Wormian) bones are common. The sella turcica is often enlarged and round; in rare instances, there may be erosion and thinning. Formation and eruption of teeth can be delayed. Cardiac enlargement or pericardial effusion may be present.

Skeletal maturation (bone age) is delayed. Centers of ossification, especially of the hip, may show multiple small centers or a single stippled, porous, or fragmented center (epiphysial dysgenesis). Vertebrae may show anterior beaking. Coxa vara and coxa plana may occur.

Electrocardiogram

The electrocardiogram may show low-voltage P and T waves with diminished amplitude of QRS complexes and suggest poor left ventricular function and pericardial effusion. Echocardiography can confirm a pericardial effusion. The electroencephalogram often shows low voltage. In children older than

2 years of age, the serum cholesterol is usually elevated. Cardiac enlargement may be present.

Scintigraphy with radioactive iodine may help to identify the etiology. FNAC is useful if thyroid continues to grow in spite of L-T4.

Scintigraphy can help to define the underlying cause in infants with congenital hypothyroidism, but treatment should not be delayed to obtain such imaging. I-sodium iodide is superior to Tc-sodium pertechnetate for this purpose. Scintigraphy will demonstrate an ectopic thyroid gland, but the absence of uptake in disorders of the TSH receptor (including TRBAb) or NIS may be mistaken for thyroid agenesis. On the other hand, ultrasonographic examination of the thyroid can document presence or absence of an anatomically normal gland, but it can miss some ectopic glands detectable by scintigraphy.

> **LABORATORY SALIENT FINDINGS**
> - FT3 and FT4 levels are decreased
> - Serum TSH levels are elevated
> - Serum cholesterol and carotene are raised
> - Serum GH may be reduced
> - Urinary creatinine excretion is decreased
> - Bone age is delayed
> - Cardiomegaly is common
>
> FT3: free triiodothyronine; FT4: free thyroxine; GH: growth hormone; TSH: thyroid-stimulating hormone.

Screening Programs for Neonatal Hypothyroidism

Either cord blood or postnatal sample at 48–72 hours should be collected for screening.

Strategy of second screening may be required in the following conditions:

- Preterm neonates (<37 weeks); low-birth-weight (LBW), and very-low-birth-weight (VLBW) neonates
- Ill and preterm neonates admitted to neonatal intensive care unit (NICU); specimen collection within the first ½–24 hours of life
- Multiple births, particularly in cases of same-sex twins

The repeat specimen should be collected after 2 weeks of age or 2 weeks after the first screening test was carried out.

Primary TSH screen is more sensitive and specific for the diagnosis of primary congenital hypothyroidism compared to T4 screen. Primary TSH screening may fail to detect central congenital hypothyroidism.

The TSH measured from a dried blood spot (DBS) is expressed in whole blood units while the venous TSH is expressed in serum units. (2.2 × whole blood units = serum units).

Congenital hypothyroidism should be diagnosed by neonatal screening within 10 days of birth. It may be recognized clinically during the 1st month of life or may be so mild that it remains unrecognized clinically for months. Adequate treatment started as soon as possible—but certainly before the end of the 1st month of life—gives a better prognosis with respect to intellectual performance later in life.

Blood is collected onto filter paper and sent to a centralized laboratory for testing. The initial test performed varies among states:

- Initial TSH assay
- Initial T4 assay with follow-up TSH if the T4 is <10%
- Simultaneously TSH and T4 are done which is the most optimal method.

It is advisable that each practicing general pediatrician and pediatric subspecialist should know their own state's method in order to be able take into account possible limitations. Regardless of method, the vast majority of infants with primary hypothyroidism are detected. However, each method has its disadvantages. Initial TSH assay tends to miss central hypothyroidism or infants with delayed primary hypothyroidism in whom TSH rises later. Initial TSH testing tends to detect subclinical hypothyroidism.

Evaluation and Diagnosis

Infants with abnormal newborn screening results need to be brought in to the pediatrician urgently. At this visit, besides physical examination, the infant should have the following blood work done: TSH, total T4, and free T4. The decision for treatment is based on these results. If these results confirm congenital hypothyroidism, the infant should be started on treatment and referred to a pediatric endocrinologist.

- Patients with elevated serum TSH and low and free T4 levels have primary congenital hypothyroidism, and treatment needs to be started immediately.
- Patients with elevated TSH but normal total and free T4 levels have subclinical hypothyroidism. This can be caused by an ectopic or hypoplastic thyroid gland or dyshormonogenesis. One can monitor these infants with serial blood tests tor a few weeks; however, if the TSH does not normalize after 4 weeks of life, it is appropriate to initiate treatment in order to not compromise brain development.
- Patients with a low or normal serum TSH and low total and free T4 have central hypothyroidism. These infants need to be evaluated for adrenal insufficiency (among other pituitary hormones) prior to initiating treatment with thyroid hormone. If adrenal insufficiency is present and thyroid hormone treatment is initiated, these patients may go into adrenal crisis.
- Patients with normal TSH, normal free T4, but low total T4 likely have thyroxine-binding globulin (TBG) deficiency. TBG deficiency is an X-linked recessive disorder, occurring in 1 in 4,000 newborns, predominantly males. This condition does not need treatment.

■ DIFFERENTIAL DIAGNOSIS

Differential diagnosis includes Turner syndrome, Down syndrome, gargoylism, and Pendred syndrome.

■ TREATMENT

Levothyroxine given orally is the treatment of choice. The recommended initial starting dose is 10–15 µg/kg/day (totaling 37.5–50.0 µg/day for most term infants) **(Table 1)**. The starting dose can be tailored to the severity of hypothyroidism. Rapid normalization of thyroid functions been demonstrated to be important in achieving optimal neurodevelopmental outcome. Newborns with more severe hypothyroidism as judged by a serum T4 <5 mU/L and/or imaging studies confirming aplasia, should be started at the higher end of the dosage range.

Levels of serum T4 or free T4 and TSH should be monitored at recommended intervals (every 1–2 months in the first 6 months of life, and then every 2–4 months between

TABLE 1: Initial dose of levothyroxine (L-T4).

Age	L-T4 dose (µg/kg/day)
0–3 months	10–15
4–6 months	8–10
7–12 months	6–8
1–5 years	5–6
6–12 years	4–5
12 years/puberty incomplete	2–3
12 years/puberty complete	1.7

6 months and 3 years of age). The goals of treatment are to maintain the serum free T4 or total T4 in the upper half of the reference range for serum TSH in the reference range for age, optimally 0.5–2.0 mU/L. The dose of L-T4 on a weight basis gradually decreases with age.

Levothyroxine-sodium Na-L-thyroxine is the treatment of choice for juvenile hypothyroidism. The initial dosage is based on age and is adjusted to maintain serum TSH in the normal range. In central hypothyroidism, serum TSH is not a reliable euthyroid marker, and serum T4 should be maintained in the upper half of the normal range for age.

Delay in diagnosis, failure to correct initial hypothyroxinemia rapidly, inadequate treatment, and poor compliance in the first 2–3 years of life result in variable degrees of brain damage. Without treatment, the affected infants are profoundly intellectually challenged and growth retarded. When onset of hypothyroidism occurs after 2 years of age, the outlook for normal development is much better even if diagnosis and treatment have been delayed, indicating how much more important thyroid hormone is to the rapidly growing brain of the infant.

PROGNOSIS

Prognosis without treatment leads to mentally deficit dwarfs. The treatment with thyroid hormone results in linear growth, osseous maturation, and sexual development. Infants detected and started with treatment in the 1st month of life will have normal intelligence quotient (IQ) at 6 years.

BIBLIOGRAPHY

1. Ford G, LaFranchi SH. Screening for congenital hypothyroidism. Best Pract Res Clin Endocrinol Metab. 2014;28:175-87.
2. Léger J, Olivieri A, Donaldson M, Torresani T, Krude H, van Vliet G, et al. European Society for Paediatric Endocrinology consensus guidelines on screening, diagnosing, and management of congenital hypothyroidism. J Clin Endocrinol Metab. 2014;99(2):363-84.
3. Schmaltz C. Thyroid hormones in neonate: An overview of physiology and clinical correlation. Adv Neonatal Care. 2012;12(4): 217-22.
4. Van der Sluijs Veer L, Kempers MJ, Wiedijk BM, Last BF, Grootenhuis MA, Vulsma T. Evaluation of cognitive and motor development in toddlers with congenital hypothyroidism diagnosed by neonatal screening. J Dev Behav Pediatr. 2012;33(8):633-40.

CASE 63

Precocious Puberty

■ PRESENTING COMPLAINTS

A 6-year-old boy was brought with the complaints of:
- Early development of secondary sexual characters since 6 months
- Large penis since 6 months
- Frequent erection since 6 months

History of Presenting Complaints

A 6-year-old boy was referred to the hospital because of early development of secondary sexual characters. Father had noticed that the size of penis of his son was bigger over the last 6 months. Father had also noticed that his son was having frequent erection and he had developed pubic hair.

Past History of the Patient

He was the eldest sibling of nonconsanguineous marriage. He was delivered at full term by normal delivery. His birth weight was 3 kg. There was no significant postnatal event. He was bottle-fed since birth. His developmental milestones were normal, and the child had been completely immunized.

At the time of joining the play home, i.e., at the age of 3 years, he was of the average height. Later, his parents noted that he seemed to grow excessively and always was in need of new shoes. By the age of 6 years, he was tallest in class. Neither the teacher nor the parents noted any change in behavior. His health was generally good apart from several episodes of acute otitis media in infancy. He used to complain of headache occasionally.

He had 3-year-old sister who was normal. There was no family history of sexual precocity or hyperthyroidism.

CASE AT A GLANCE

Basic Findings
Height	: 129 cm (>97th centile)
Weight	: 22 kg (75th centile)
Temperature	: 37°C
Pulse rate	: 96 beats/min
Respiratory rate	: 20 breaths/min
Blood pressure	: 100/80 mm Hg

Positive Findings

History:
- Bigger penis
- Erection
- Pubic hair
- Physical growth was faster.

Examination:
- Full muscular boy
- Acne and pubic and axillary hair
- Single café-au-lait spot

Investigation:
- *Plasma 17-hydroxyprogesterone:* Raised
- *Plasma dehydroepiandrosterone (DHEA) sulphate:* Raised
- *Plasma androsterone:* Raised

EXAMINATION

The child was a tall muscular boy. He was well nourished. Anthropometric measurements included that the height was 129 cm (>97th centile) and the weight was 22 kg (75th centile). Pubic and axillary hair were present. There was a single circular café-au-lait spot of 5 mm in diameter on his left arm. Acne were present.

He was afebrile. The pulse rate was 96 beats per minute and respiratory rate was 20 breaths per minute. Blood pressure recorded was 100/80 mm Hg. There was no pallor, no lymphadenopathy, and no cyanosis.

Secondary sexual characters were present. His penis was big. The testes were 2 mL in volume and equal in size and consistency. Other systemic examinations were normal.

INVESTIGATION

- *Hemoglobin:* 11.8 g/dL
- *TLC:* 5,800 cells/mm^3
- *ESR:* 26 mm in 1st hour
- *LH level:* 6 U/L (Normal range: 0.2–4.9 U/L)
- *Follicle-stimulating hormone (FSH) level:* 5 U/l (Normal range: 1.8–3.2 U/L)
- *Plasma 17-hydroxyprogesterone:* 2.05 nmol/L (Normal range: <0.32–1.05 nmol/L)
- *Plasma DHEA sulphate:* 4.00 nmol/L (Normal range: 1.09–2.83 nmol/L)
- *Plasma androsterone:* 5.3 nmol/L (Normal range: 1.74–3.48 nmol/L)
- *Abdominal ultrasound:* Normal

DISCUSSION

The 6-year-old boy had rapid growth and penile enlargement. Physical examination revealed acne and pubic and axillary hair. These findings are consistent with activation of the hypothalamus–pituitary–gonadal (HPG) axis—true precocious puberty. It can also be due to exogenous androgens—pseudoprecocious puberty.

Precocious puberty is defined as onset of puberty earlier than the norms for gender and race or ethnic background (2.5 standard deviation below the population mean).

Puberty is precocious if onset of breast development occurs before the age of 8 years and menarche occurs before the age of 10 years in girls, and testicular enlargement starts before the age of 9 years in boys **(Figs. 1 and 2)**. The variation in the age of the onset of puberty in normal children, particularly of different ethnicities, makes this definition somewhat arbitrary. Genetic and environmental factors affect the onset of the puberty. The course is extremely variable. The tendency for the early onset of puberty is present in case of constitutional precocity. CAH is autosomal recessive, while associated neurofibromatosis and tuberous sclerosis are inherited as autosomal dominant disorders and are the causes of precocious puberty.

Depending on the primary source of the hormonal production, precocious puberty may be classified as central (also known

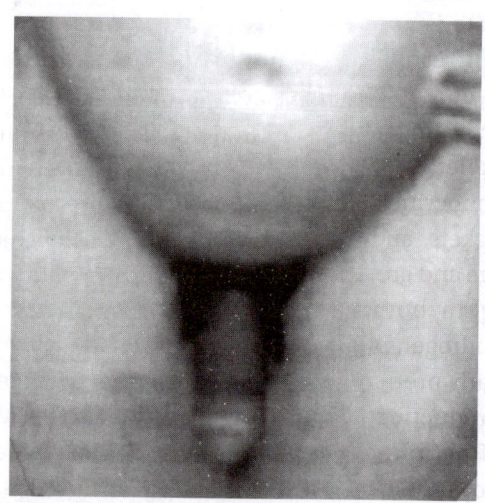

Fig. 1: True precocious puberty—male.

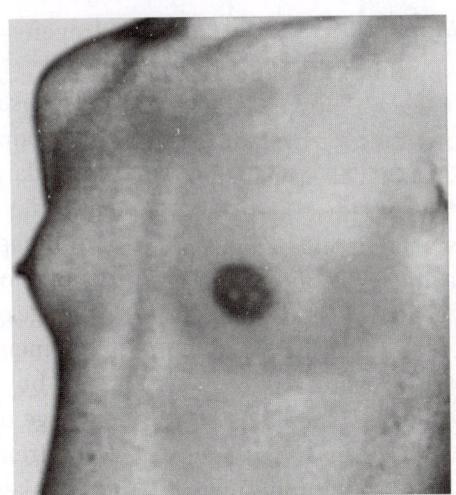

Fig. 2: Precocious puberty—female.

as gonadotropin-dependent, or true) or peripheral (also known as gonadotropin-independent or precocious pseudopuberty). The mixed type of precocious puberty occurs commonly in conditions such as CAH, McCune-Albright syndrome (MAS), and familial male-limited precocious puberty, when the bone age reaches the pubertal range (10.5–12.5 years).

In girls, fluctuating pubertal development and vaginal bleeding due to hyperestrogenic state is common. The condition is usually self-resolving and there is no treatment. Recurrent ovarian cyst, MAS, somatic activating mutation of stimulatory G protein, skeletal (multiple fibrous dysplasia) and endocrine abnormalities (hyperthyroidism, rickets, and GH excess), and delayed bone age and growth are characteristics.

In boys, this is caused by increased androgen production by testis and adrenals, with prepubertal LH levels. Adrenal overproduction due to CAH is the chief cause of peripheral precocious puberty (PPP) in boys. hCG-secreting tumors of the liver, mediastinum, or brain may present with PPP.

CLASSIFICATION OF SEXUAL PRECOCITY

Early pubertal development is classified as central or peripheral depending on the trigger for puberty.

- *Central precocious puberty (CPP) or true or gonadotropin-dependent precocious puberty:* It results from premature activation of HPG axis.
- *Peripheral precocious puberty or pseudo- or gonadotropin-independent precocious puberty with incomplete or partial pubertal development* results from the production of sex steroids and it is not influenced by HPG axis.
- *Mixed type:* CPP may be triggered in children with PPP, when the advanced state of somatic and skeletal maturation is reached due to premature release of adrenal or gonadal steroids, for example, CAH, MAS, and familial male-limited precocious puberty.
- *Incomplete form of pubertal variants:* Premature thelarche, premature menarche, premature pubarche, adolescent gynecomastia in boys, and macroorchidism.

Central Precocious Puberty (Gonadotropin-dependent)

Central precocious puberty is defined by the onset of breast development before the age of 8 years in girls and the onset of testicular development (volume >4 mL) before the age of 9 years in boys, as a result of the early activation of the HPG axis. It occurs 5–10 fold more frequently in girls than in boys and is usually sporadic.

Although the clinical course is variable, three main patterns of pubertal progression can be identified. Most females (particularly those younger than 6 years of age at the onset) and a large majority of males have rapidly progressive puberty, characterized by rapid physical and osseous maturation, leading to a loss of height potential. An increasing percentage of females (older than 6 years of age at the onset with an idiopathic form), and rarely males, have a slowly progressive variant, characterized by parallel advancement of osseous maturation and linear growth, with preserved height potential.

True CPP results from an increase in GnRH secretion at a younger age than normal. Most cases are idiopathic, but given that organic causes include brain tumors, further evaluation is typically indicated. Hypothalamic hamartoma, neuronal migration defects, craniopharyngioma, hydrocephalus, and tuberculous meningitis are important causes. These disorders are associated with increase in testicular volume and elevated basal and GnRH-stimulated LH. Precocious puberty occurs more frequently among girls than among boys, but central nervous system (CNS) tumor as a cause of precocious puberty is more common among boys than among girls.

Central precocious puberty is always isosexual and stems from HPG activation with ensuing sex hormone secretion and progressive sexual maturation. In PPP, some of the secondary sex characters appear, but there is no activation of the normal HPG interplay. In the latter group, the sex characteristics may be isosexual or heterosexual (contrasexual).

Idiopathic Central Precocious Puberty

If no CNS tumor or additional diagnosis is determined, and if no family tendency toward early puberty exists, idiopathic CPP is diagnosed. This is a diagnosis of exclusion in which patients manifest all the endocrine findings of normal puberty, but at an earlier age. Progress may be slow and continuous or waxing and waning. Girls are more frequently affected than boys.

Central Nervous System Disorders

Hamartomas of the tuber cinereum are the most common CNS lesions causing CPP. They are composed of ectopic hypothalamic tissue, which usually contains GnRH in its neurons; thus, the hamartoma functions as a supplemental hypothalamus that operates outside of the normal inhibitory effects of the CNS on GnRH secretion. They do not enlarge and are not associated with a mass effect, but they can be associated with gelastic or laughing seizures, petit mal seizures, or grand mal seizures. They have a characteristic nonenhancing appearance on MRI, so biopsy is rarely required.

Elevated intracranial pressure caused by hydrocephalus or a subarachnoid cyst can cause precocious puberty, which is reversed by release of the elevated intracranial pressure. Fetal or childhood CNS infections, such as tuberculosis and brain abscess, can cause precocious puberty, as can cerebral vascular accidents and CNS trauma (including birth trauma). Developmental delay from various causes, including static cerebral encephalopathy, can cause precocious adrenarche or complete CPP. Congenital defects of the CNS such as septo-optic dysplasia may cause CPP.

Additional Causes of Central Precocious Puberty

Exposure to high serum concentrations of sex steroids leads to early maturation of the hypothalamic-pituitary axis with CPP even after the primary cause of increased exposure is treated. This may occur after glucocorticoid treatment is initiated for long-untreated virilizing CAH. Likewise, children with androgen-secreting tumors that are removed after years of virilization can subsequently have true CPP.

Although approximately 90% of girls have an idiopathic form, a structural CNS abnormality can be demonstrated in up to 75% of boys with CPP.

- *Evidence of a CNS mass:* Examination of optic fundus for possible increased intracranial pressure; visual fields testing for evidence of optic nerve compression by a hypothalamic or pituitary mass
- *Evidence of androgenic influence:* Presence of acne and facial and axillary hair; increased muscle bulk and definition; extent of other body/pubic hair; in boys increased scrotal rugation accompanied by thinning and pigmentation of penile elongation; in girls clitoromegaly
- *Evidence of estrogenic influence:* Increase in size of breast tissue and nipple/areolar contouring; change in vaginal mucosa color (increased estrogen causes cornification of vaginal epithelium with color change form prepubertal shiny red to more opalescent pink); change in labia minor (becomes more prominent and visible between the labia majora as puberty progresses).
- *Evidence of gonadotropic stimulation:* Testicular enlargement >2.5 cm in length or >4 mL in volume (preferably measured using a Prader orchidometer of labeled volumetric beads); pubertal development without testicular enlargement usually suggests adrenal pathology.
- *Evidence of other mass:* Asymmetric testicular enlargement; hepatomegaly; abdominal mass.

Peripheral Precocious Puberty (Gonadotropin-independent)

In PPP, some of the secondary sex characteristics appear, but there is no activation of the normal HPG interplay. In this group, the sex characteristics may be isosexual or heterosexual (contrasexual). PPP can induce maturation of the HPG axis and trigger the onset of central puberty.

Unregulated sex steroid secretion is the major cause of PPP in both sexes, although boys with hCG-secreting tumors will also have PPP since the hCG stimulates the testes to produce testosterone. Laboratory analysis in PPP reveals elevation in testosterone or estrogen and low or suppressed levels of pituitary gonadotropins. However, elevation of hCG (which would cause a positive pregnancy test) occurs in the case of ectopic hCG secretion. The only tissues that can secrete sex steroids are the gonads and adrenal glands, which are the final common pathways to sex steroid secretion.

Boys

The hCG-secreting tumors can lead to sexual precocity, since high levels of hCG will stimulate the LH receptor, leading to gonadotropin-independent increases in testosterone secretion. hCG does not stimulate the seminiferous tubules, so testicular enlargement is less than that occurs with normal puberty or CPP. hCG-secreting tumors include germ cell tumors (such as seminomas, dysgerminomas, yolk sac tumors, and teratomas) and hepatoblastomas and hepatomas. Boys with 47,XXY Klinefelter syndrome have an increased incidence of hCG-secreting mediastinal germ cell neoplasms.

Virilizing CAH due to 21-hydroxylase or 11-beta-hydroxylase deficiency will result in excessive androgen secretion. In boys, untreated CAH causes virilization without testicular enlargement, due to androgen secretion solely from the adrenal glands. Because gonadotropins are suppressed, the testes can be small for age or for the degree of virilization. The classical form manifests during infancy in males with normal male genital appearance but salt loss occurring in about 50% of cases. Without salt loss, the condition can present as GnRH-independent isosexual precocity in boys later in infancy. Additionally, a TART composed of ACTH-responsive tissue located in the testes (a common ectopic location for adrenal tissue) may enlarge in individuals with CAH, usually in teenagers or adults, resulting in a testicular mass and excessive androgen secretion.

Virilizing adenomas and carcinomas of the adrenal gland secrete large amounts of DHEA and dehydroepiandrosterone sulfate (DHEAS), which is peripherally converted to more potent androgens. When the adrenal gland is the cause of the virilization, the testes remain prepubertal in size. Leydig cell tumors are rare among boys but manifest as irregular enlargement of testis or, more rarely, both testes.

Premature Leydig and germinal cell maturation (or male limited precocious puberty or testotoxicosis) is a rare and self-limited dominant condition of boys. Often, a family history of affected fathers or uncles can be determined. The condition results from an activating mutation in the 7-transmembrane domain of the LH receptor, rendering it constitutionally activated such that it constantly stimulates testosterone production even in the absence of LH. Affected boys will virilize but have only minimal enlargement of the testes because there is predominant stimulation of Leydig cells and relatively less enlargement of the seminiferous tubules.

Familial cortisol resistance syndrome leads to a compensatory increase in ACTH secretion, which increases glucocorticoid secretion; because there is resistance to glucocorticoids, there is no manifestation of excess glucocorticoid effect despite elevated circulating glucocorticoids. However, as there is an increase in ACTH, adrenal androgen secretion rises, causing premature adrenarche and virilization.

Girls

Gonadotropin-independent: Isosexual precocity among girls can be caused by ovarian cysts or neoplasms, exposure to exogenous estrogens, or abnormalities of the adrenal glands. Serum gonadotropin concentrations are suppressed, while serum estradiol levels are elevated. Prepubertal girls normally have small ovarian follicular cysts, but some cysts enlarge and secrete sufficient estrogen to cause breast development and even withdrawal bleeding. The estrogen levels are usually at pubertal values, but occasionally very high levels characteristic of tumors is encountered. Occasionally, recurrent cyst formation can occur. Surgical resection is rarely indicated.

Several neoplasms can cause gonadotropin-independent isosexual precocity among girls. Granulosa cell tumors of the ovary are rare but can be discovered by bimanual examination. Gonadoblastomas can arise in streak gonads found in gonadal dysgenesis and secrete estrogen or even testosterone. These tumors are benign but can harbor malignant ovarian tumors. Estrogen-secreting adrenal neoplasms are infrequent compared with those that secrete androgens. Tumors that secrete hCG cause no physical pubertal changes in girls due to endocrine effects alone as hCG is the biological equivalent to LH in its activity and does not stimulate estradiol secretion.

Causes of Gonadotropin-releasing Hormone-independent Sexual Precocity among Boys and Girls (Mixed)

McCune-Albright syndrome involves the triad of café-au-lait macules, polyostotic fibrous dysplasia of the skeleton, and autonomous endocrine function, caused by activating mutations of the stimulatory G-protein subunit of the adenyl cyclase system. Because these are somatic cell mutations that are not in the germline, the disease affects some organs while skipping others, leading to the variable manifestations. Patients may have autonomous hyperactivity of the somatotropes (acromegaly or gigantism), thyroid cells (thyrotoxicosis), parathyroid glands, adrenal glands (Cushing syndrome), and/or gonads. Precocious puberty is the most common endocrine finding and results from a constitutively active LH receptor.

Van Wyk–Grumbach syndrome is characterized by severe hypothyroidism, delayed bone age, and sexual precocity with reversal to a prepubertal state following thyroid hormone replacement therapy. It appears to be due to the cross-reaction of the elevated TSH on FSH receptors. Girls may have breast development and menstrual flow, and boys may have enlargement of the testes as the result of enlargement of the seminiferous tubules. Because of the severe hypothyroidism, these patients may present with precocious puberty but will paradoxically have a delayed bone age. The pituitary gland may enlarge and erode the sella turcica in a manner incorrectly suggesting a tumor because of increased TSH secretion and thyrotroph hyperplasia. Once hypothyroidism is controlled, sexual precocity reverts and the sella turcica becomes smaller.

Peutz–Jeghers syndrome is an autosomal dominant condition characterized by intestinal hamartomatous polyp formation in association with a distinctive pattern of skin and mucosal hyperpigmentation. Cancer incidence is increased, including gonadal tumors, which may result in sexual precocity in children.

The classification scheme for precocious puberty is as follows:
- *Central (or complete) isosexual precocious puberty (GnRH-dependent sexual precocity or premature activation of the hypothalamic pulse generator):*
    - Familial or constitutional CPP
    - Idiopathic true precocious puberty
    - *CNS tumors:*
        * Hamartoma of the tuber cinereum
        * Optic glioma
        * Hypothalamic astrocytoma
        * Craniopharyngioma
        * Ependymoma
    - *Other CNS disorders:*
        * Encephalitis
        * Static encephalopathy
        * Brain abscess
        * Sarcoid or tubercular granuloma
        * Head trauma
        * CNS surgery
        * Hydrocephalus
        * Arachnoid cyst
        * Myelomeningocele
        * Vascular lesion
        * Cranial irradiation
- *Peripheral (or incomplete) isosexual precocity (hypothalamic GnRH independent):*
    - *Boys:*
        * Gonadotropin-secreting tumors
        * hCG-secreting-CNS tumor
        * Increased androgen production by the adrenal gland or testes
        * CAH (CYP21 and CYP11B1 deficiency)
        * Virilizing adrenal neoplasm
        * Leydig cell adenoma
        * Premature Leydig and germ cell maturation (testotoxicosis)
        * Cortisol resistance syndrome
    - *Girls:*
        * Ovarian cyst
        * Estrogen-secreting ovarian or adrenal neoplasm

- *Both sexes:*
  - MAS
  - Peutz–Jeghers syndrome
  - Severe primary hypothyroidism
  - Exogenous exposures

■ CLINICAL FEATURES (FIG. 3)

Boys

In boys, there will be enlargement of pubis and testes, appearance of pubic hair, acne, and frequent erections occur. Voice deepens and linear growth is accelerated.

In precocious development, increase in growth rate and growth of pubic hair are the common presenting signs. Testicular size may differentiate true precocity, in which the testes enlarge, from pseudoprecocity (most commonly due to CAH), in which the testes usually remain small. There are some exceptions; for example, testicular enlargement may occur in pseudoprecocity of long-standing due to secondary activation of central precocity from prolonged elevation of androgen levels. Tumors of the testes are associated with asymmetric testicular enlargement.

A boy who exhibits symmetrically enlarging testes of homogenous consistency is likely to have CPP. Patients with gonadotropin-independent Leydig and germ cell maturation tend to have a small degree of testicular enlargement, while boys with adrenal androgen excess (as in the case of enzyme defects or tumors) or an exogenous androgen source will have nonenlarging testes. Laboratory evaluation will reveal elevated testosterone and gonadotropin levels in CPP, while gonadotropins will be low or prepubertal in PPP. If testosterone is elevated but gonadotropins are suppressed, an hCG-secreting tumor is possible and β-hCG should be measured. The modern β-hCG assay does not cross-react with LH. MRI should subsequently be invoked to determine the tumor location.

Girls

Sexual development may begin at any age and generally follows the sequence observed in normal puberty. In girls, early menstrual cycles may be more irregular than they are with normal puberty. The initial cycles are usually anovulatory, but pregnancy has been reported. In boys, testicular biopsies have shown stimulation of all elements of the testes, and spermatogenesis has been observed. In affected girls and boys, height, weight, and osseous maturation are advanced. The increased rate of bone maturation results in early closure of the epiphyses, and the ultimate stature is less than it would have been otherwise.

Spontaneously regressive or unsustained CPP is quite rare. This variability in the natural course of sexual precocity underscores the need for longitudinal observation at the onset of sexual development, before treatment is considered.

In the girls, the first sign is the development of breast. Pubic hair may appear

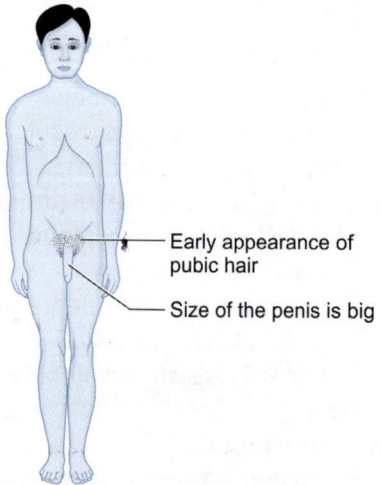

Fig. 3: Clinical features.

simultaneously and more often appears later. Other signs include development of external genitalia, appearance of axillary hair, and onset of menstruation follow. The initial cycles are anovulatory.

A girl with early breast development may have premature thelarche, CPP, or gonadotropin-independent PPP. If pubic hair development is present in appropriate amount for the degree of breast development, then CPP is likely. Laboratory evaluation begins with measurement of high-sensitivity basal or GnRH-stimulated levels of LH. If the LH is pubertal, CPP is considered, and cranial magnetic MRI is usually indicated. If LH is not pubertal, serum estradiol levels are measured. If serum estradiol is not elevated, a diagnosis of premature thelarche is made. If elevated, an ultrasound of the uterus and ovary should be performed.

In practice, most providers obtain FSH, LH, and estradiol levels simultaneously to expedite the workup and minimize number of blood draws.

A girl with early pubic hair without concurrent breast development may have benign premature adrenarche, late-onset CAH, or a virilizing tumor **(Figs. 4A and B)**. The evaluation begins with determination of DHEAS levels. If significantly elevated, virilizing adrenal tumors need to be considered.

In both girls and boys, height, weight, and bone maturity are advanced. The increased rate of ossification results in early closure of the epiphyses.

GENERAL FEATURES

• Girls
  – Breast enlargement
  – Early appearance of pubic hair
• Boys
  – Enlarged penis
  – Increased testicular size

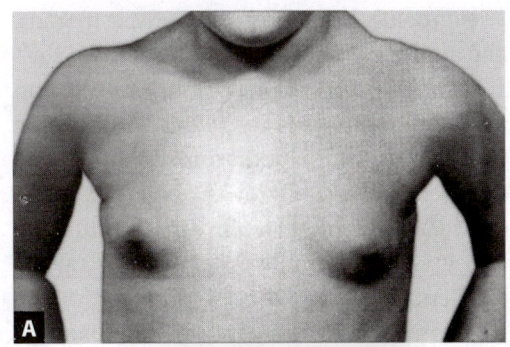
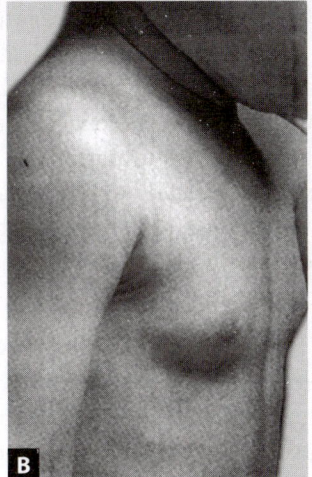

Figs. 4A and B: (A) Thelarche; (B) Premature thelarche.

■ DIAGNOSIS

A detailed history and clinical evaluation are helpful in arriving at a diagnosis and directing investigations.

Aims of evaluation include confirmation of diagnosis, identification of underlying etiology, and determination of prognosis and treatment.

Clinical: History should include the onset, progression, and extent of puberty. Idiopathic CPP usually presents between 6 and 7 years of age. The earlier the onset, the greater is the likelihood of an underlying organic cause. Hypothalamic hamartoma and familial testotoxicosis present very early in the first

3 years of life. Exposure to steroids, estrogens, and androgens should be enquired.

Family history of precocious puberty and early menarche points toward idiopathic CPP. Features of hypothyroidism should be assessed. Advanced growth is characteristic of precocious puberty; growth retardation indicates hypothyroidism or concomitant GH deficiency.

Examination of vaginal mucosa for estrogen effect provides clues regarding the pubertal status of the patient. Red, glistening mucosa suggests lack of estrogens while pink mucosa with mucus is indicative of estrogen effect. Abdominal examination for adrenal or ovarian mass should be done. Features of MAS include café-au-lait spots, polyostotic fibrous dysplasia, bony deformities, and polyendocrinopathy.

Pubertal progression: In idiopathic CPP, the rate of progression may sometimes be very slow with menarche occurring up to 5 years after breast development. Rapid progression of puberty is seen in androgen producing tumors, ovarian cysts, and some CNS masses such as hypothalamic hamartoma.

Accelerated growth is a feature of both CPP and PPP but is not seen in pubertal variants. Irregular vaginal bleeding is more common in functioning ovarian tumors and hypothalamic hamartoma. History of CNS infection suggested by headaches, visual disturbances, personality changes, developmental delay, and seizures would suggest a neurologic disorder.

Investigations: Assessment of pubertal status is based on basal or stimulated gonadotropin levels. Pooled gonadotropin levels are preferred due to their pulsatile secretion. LH is a better indicator compared to FSH as LH levels increase significantly during puberty. LH levels in the pubertal range with LH/FSH ratio more than one is suggestive of development of puberty.

It is recommended that all boys with precocious pubertal development and all girls with the following features should be evaluated for the mechanism and potential for progression of puberty:
- Precocious puberty stage 3 or higher
- Precocious puberty stage 2 with additional criteria such as increased growth velocity
- Evidence of CNS dysfunction or PPP

Hormonal evaluation:
- *Sex steroids:*
  - In girls, *serum estradiol* levels are not very helpful in determining the stage of puberty. Levels overlap between normal prepuberty, early puberty, precocious puberty, and premature thelarche. Levels >20 pg/mL suggest that puberty has started. Markedly elevated levels (>100 pg/mL) are seen in estrogen secreting ovarian tumors and sometimes in follicular cysts.
  - In boys, *serum testosterone* levels <30 ng/mL are generally prepubertal; although in some laboratories, levels of 10–30 ng/mL may indicate early puberty. Testosterone levels may be very high related to the stage of puberty in boys with primary gonadotropin excess.
- *Serum gonadotropins:* Gonadotropin levels are elevated in CPP and suppressed in PPP. Basal serum FSH and LH are of limited value in early puberty. But random LH estimated by sensitive third-generation assays is a good screening test for CPP. A level of <0.1 IU/L is prepubertal and 0.3 IU/L or more is pubertal. Random FSH levels are not helpful in discriminating between prepubertal and pubertal children.

- *GnRH-stimulation tests* are more helpful in distinguishing CPP from PPP. In CPP, an LH-predominant response is seen. An increase in FSH levels much more than LH indicates that the child is prepubertal. In PPP, gonadotropin levels do not rise in response to GnRH stimulation.
- *Serum DHEAS* levels are elevated in premature adrenarche and can be very high in virilizing adrenal problems.
- *Serum 17-hydroxyprogesterone (17-OHP)* and the response to ACTH or serum 11-deoxycortisol may be required to rule out CAH.
- *Serum hCG levels* should be measured, if an hCG-secreting tumor is suspected in boys.
- *Thyroid hormone* studies are helpful in suspected hypothyroidism.

Radiology

- *Bone age:* Skeletal maturation is advanced in all cases of precocious puberty, except if associated with hypothyroidism, but remains normal in the incomplete forms. It is also helpful in predicting adult height.
- *CT or MRI of brain:* To determine the etiology of CPP
- *Pelvic and abdominal sonography:* It is done to evaluate the size and morphology of the uterus, ovaries, and adrenals. This is essential in PPP to find the cause. In CPP, the size of the uterus is increased (>2 mL in volume or >3.4 cm in length) and an endometrial shadow is seen. The ovaries will also be enlarged bilaterally and may show multiple small follicular cysts.
- *Testicular sonography:* If a tumor is suspected.
- *Skeletal survey:* In suspected cases of MAS.
- *Advanced bone age:* >2 years ahead of chronological age suggestive of PPP, while normal bone age indicates slowly progressive puberty retarded growth and skeletal maturation are diagnostic of hypothyroidism. Pubertal LH levels are suggestive of gonadotropin-dependent precocious puberty and should be followed with an MRI of brain. Girls with prepubertal LH levels should undergo ultrasound of ovary and adrenals (for ovarian cyst and adrenal tumor) and skeletal survey (for fibrous dysplasia in MAS).

Basal serum LH and FSH concentrations are usually not in the pubertal range in boys with true sexual precocity, but the LH response to GnRH-stimulation testing is pubertal (>10 IU/L). Sexual precocity caused by CAH is usually associated with abnormal concentrations of DHEA, androstenedione, 17-OHP (in CAH due to 21-hydroxylase deficiency), 11-deoxycortisol (in CAH due to 11-hydroxylase deficiency), or a combination of these steroids.

Serum hCG concentrations can identify the presence of an hCG-producing tumors (e.g., CNS dysgerminoma and hepatoma) in boys who present with apparent true sexual precocity (i.e., accompanies by testicular enlargement) but suppressed gonadotropins following luteinizing hormone-releasing hormone (LHRH).

> **LABORATORY SALIENT FINDINGS**
> - Increased LH response to GnRH-stimulation test
> - Abnormal plasma concentration of dehydroepiandrosterone (DHEA), androstenedione, 17-hydroxyprogesterone (17-OHP)
> - Serum hCG concentration may be elevated
> - Ultrasonography is useful to detect hepatic, presacral, and testicular tumor
>
> (hCG: human chorionic gonadotropin; LH: luteinizing hormone; GnRH: gonadotropin-releasing hormone)

DIFFERENTIAL DIAGNOSIS

Differential diagnosis involves the following:
- Hypothyroidism
- MAS

- Virilizing tumor
- Granulosa cell tumor
- CAH

TREATMENT

Specific therapy should be provided whenever possible. Treatment of idiopathic true precocious puberty in boys is similar to that in girls. Treatment of MAS of familial Leydig cell hyperplasia with agents that block steroid synthesis (e.g., ketoconazole), an antiandrogen (e.g., spironolactone), or a combination of both has been successful.

If the underlying cause is amenable to neurosurgery, it should be removed. Highly potent long-acting analogue of GnRH are used. Triptorelin and leuprolide are depot preparations administered intramuscularly every month. GnRH analogue helps to increase the ultimate height.

The pseudoprecocious puberty is caused by estrogen producing granulosa cell tumor, CAH, and MAS. Underlying cause should be treated.

Medroxyprogesterone acetate is given in the dose of 100 mg/m^2 every 2–3 month by intramuscular injection. Oral dose is 10 mg twice daily is given. Cyproterone acetate given in the dose of 75–100 mg/m^2/day in 2–3 divided dose is helpful for stopping cyclical bleeding. Ketoconazole is also used to suppress peripheral gonadal hormone secretion.

Long-acting formulations of GnRH agonists, which maintain fairly constant serum concentrations of the drug for weeks or months, constitute the preparations of choice for treatment of CPP.

The available preparations include:
- Leuprolide acetate (Ld), in a dose of 0.25–0.3 mg/kg (minimum 7.5 mg) intramuscularly, once every 4 weeks.
- Longer-acting preparations of depot leuprolide, allowing for injections (11.25–30.0 mg intramuscularly), every 90 days
- Histrelin, a subcutaneous 50 mg implant with effects lasting 12 months.

Other preparations such as D-Trp-GnRH-goserelin acetate are approved for treatment of precocious puberty. Recurrent sterile fluid collections at the sites of injections are an uncommon local side effect and occur in less than 1–3% of patients treated with depot leuprolide.

Other available treatment options, usually reserved for children who cannot tolerate the products listed above, include subcutaneous injections of aqueous leuprolide, given once or twice daily (total dose 60 μg/g/24 h), or intranasal administration of the GnRH-1 agonist nafarelin, 800 μg bid. The potential for irregular compliance with daily administration, as well as the variable absorption of the intranasal route for nafarelin, may limit the long-term benefit of the latter preparations on adult height.

Congenital adrenal hyperplasia is managed with hydrocortisone and fludrocortisone. Surgery is done for adrenal and testicular tumors; radiotherapy is effective in hCG-secreting tumors. Aromatase inhibitors and antiandrogens are indicated in testotoxicosis.

Treatment results in decrease of the growth rate, generally to age-appropriate values, and an even greater decrease of the rate of osseous maturation. Some children, particularly those with greatly advanced (pubertal) bone age, may show marked deceleration of their growth rate and a complete arrest in the rate of osseous maturation.

Treatment results in enhancement of the predicted height, although the actual adult height of patients followed to epiphyseal closure is approximately 1 SD less than their mid-parental height. In girls, breast development may regress in those with Tanner stages development. Most commonly, the size of the breasts remains unchanged in girls with stages III-V development or may even increase slightly because of progressive adipose tissue deposition. The amount of glandular tissue decreases. Pubic hair usually remains stable in girls, or may progress slowly during treatment, reflecting the gradual increase in adrenal androgens. Menses, if present, cease. Isolated thelarche is usually present around the age of 12 years and show gradual regression by 5 years. Isolated adrenarche is the premature development of pubic hair and acne in absence of breast development or menarche. Most of them are normal variants and does not require any treatment. Isolated menarche, i.e., vaginal bleeding without breast development, requires evaluation of local causes (infection, foreign body, sexual abuse, or tumors).

Pelvic sonography demonstrates a decrease of the ovarian and uterine size. In boys, there is decrease of testicular size, variable regression of pubic hair, and decrease in the frequency of erections. Except for a reversible decrease in bone density (of uncertain clinical significance), no serious adverse effects of GnRH analogs have been reported in children treated for sexual precocity.

If treatment is effective, the serum sex hormone concentrations decrease to prepubertal levels (testosterone, <10–20 ng/dL in males; estradiol, <5–10 pg/mL in females). The serum LH and FSH concentrations, as measured by sensitive immunometric assays, decrease to <1 IU/L in most patients, although rarely does the LH return to truly prepubertal levels (<0.1 IU/L).

Surgical management for endocrine purposes is not usually indicated, as the lesion is responsive to GnRH agonists. Surgery for seizure management is sometimes indicated. CNS tumors can cause other symptoms, such as headache, abnormalities of vision, optic atrophy, and diabetes insipidus, and thus a thorough neurologic examination and review of systems must be a part of the evaluation of a child sexual precocity.

Radiation therapy is most commonly associated with gonadotropin deficiency but may also cause CPP even if the treated tumor does not cause precocious puberty. Higher doses of radiation may be more likely to cause GnRH deficiency, whereas lower doses may lead to CPP or hypogonadotropic hypogonadism. When radiation causes CPP, the resultant growth acceleration can mask radiation-induced GH deficiency. When both occur, treatment with combined GH and GnRH agonist may be necessary to achieve a normal range of adult height.

■ BIBLIOGRAPHY

1. Abreu AP, Dauber A, Macedo DB, Noel SD, Brito VN, Gill JC, et al. Central precocious puberty caused by mutations in the imprinted gene MKRN3. N Engl J Med. 2013;368(26):2467-75.
2. Albrecht L, Styne D. Laboratory testing of gonadal steroids in children. Pediatr Endocrinol Rev. 2007;5 Suppl 1:599-607.
3. Biro FM, Lucky AW, Huster GA, Morrison JA. Pubertal staging in boys. J Pediatr. 1995;127(1):100-2.
4. Fuqua JS. Treatment and outcome of precocious puberty: An update. J Clin Endocrinol Metab. 2013;98(6):2198-207.
5. Rogol AD. Sex steroids, growth hormone, leptin, and pubertal growth spurt. Endocr Dev. 2010;17:77-85.
6. Styne DM. Disorders of puberty. Pediatric Endocrinology: A Clinical Handbook. Switzerland: Springer International Publishing; 2016.

CASE 64

Undescended Testes

■ PRESENTING COMPLAINTS

A 2-year-old boy was brought with the complaint of:
- Absence of testes since birth

History of Presenting Symptoms

A 2-year-old boy was brought to the pediatric outpatient department with absence of testis on the left side. His mother recollects her memory that she has noticed it at the time of the birth and brought that to the attention of the pediatrician. But the pediatrician assured and asked to wait till 1 year, and to consider the evaluation if it remains like that. The testis on the right side was present and normal in size.

CASE AT A GLANCE	
Basic Findings	
Height	: 89 cm (>90th centile)
Weight	: 12 kg (above 75th centile)
Temperature	: 36°C
Pulse rate	: 98 beats/min
Respiratory rate	: 20 breaths/min
Blood pressure	: 60/46 mm Hg
Positive Findings	
History:	
• Absence of the testes	
Examination:	
• Absence of the testis in the left scrotum	
Investigation:	
• Normal	

There was no history of other congenital anomalies.

Past History of the Patient

The child was the only sibling of consanguineous marriage. He was born at full term by normal delivery. He was on breast milk as soon as possible and was on breast milk exclusively for first 4 months. Later weaning was started with advice of the family doctor. His developmental milestones were normal. He had been immunized completely.

■ EXAMINATION

On examination, the child was moderately built and nourished. He was playing with toys on the examination table. He was unaware of the reason for which he was brought to the hospital. Anthropometric measurements included the height 89 cm (>90 centile) and the weight 12 kg (above 75th centile).

He was afebrile. The heart rate was 98 beats/min and respiratory rate was 20 breaths/min. Blood pressure recorded was 60/46 mm Hg. The child was pale, there was no lymphadenopathy, no clubbing, and no edema.

Per abdomen examination revealed, soft abdomen with no organomegaly. There was absence of testis on the left side. On the right side, the testis was present and normal in size. Other systemic examinations were normal.

INVESTIGATION

- *Hemoglobin:* 9 g/dL
- *TLC:* 9,800 cells/cumm
- *ESR:* 26 mm in the first hour
- *AEC:* 440 cells/dL
- *X-ray abdomen:* Normal
- *Abdominal scan:* Revealed no significant finding

DISCUSSION

Cryptorchism (undescended testes) is a common disorder in children. It may be unilateral or bilateral and may be classified as ectopic or true cryptorchidism. Approximately 3% of term male newborns have an undescended testes at birth, with a higher proportion among premature infants, because testicular descent occurs at 7-8 months of gestation, 30% of premature male infants have an undescended testis, and the incidence is 14% at term.

Spontaneous descent occurs secondary to a temporary testosterone surge during the first 2 months, which also results in significant penile growth. In over 50% of these patients, the testes descend by the third month, and by age of 1 year 80% of all undescended testes are in the scrotum. If the testis has not descended by 4 months, it will remain undescended. Cryptorchidism is bilateral in 10% of cases.

Secondary cryptorchidism follows the repair of inguinal hernia. Further descent may occur through puberty, the later perhaps stimulated by endogenous gonadotropins.

Cryptorchidism can occur in an isolated fashion or may be associated with other findings. Abnormalities in the hypothalamic-pituitary-gonadal (HPG) axis predispose to cryptorchism. Androgen biosynthesis or receptor defects may also predispose to cryptorchidism and undervirilization.

Ectopic testes are presumed to develop normally but are diverted as they descend through the inguinal canal. They are sub-classified on the basis of their location. Surgery is indicated once the diagnosis is established.

The true undescended testis is found along normal paths of descent and processus vaginalis is usually patent. The ectopic testis has completed its course of descent through inguinal canal. But it ends up in subcutaneous location. The usual site is lateral to external inguinal ring, i.e., below the subcutaneous fascia.

Undescended testes are usually in inguinal canal. Ectopic testis is in superficial inguinal pouch or perineum. In a newborn, with bilateral nonpalpable testes, one should suspect virilized female with CAH. The diagnosis of bilateral cryptorchism in an apparently male newborn should never be made until ruling out the possibility that the child is actually a fully virilized female with potentially fatal salt-losing CAH.

PATHOGENESIS

The process of testicular descent is regulated by an interaction between hormonal and mechanical factors, including testosterone, DHT, mullerian-inhibiting factor, the gubernaculum, intra-abdominal pressure, and the genitofemoral nerve. The testis develops at 7-8 weeks of gestation. At 10-11 weeks, the Leydig cells produce testosterone, which stimulate differentiation of the Wolffian (mesonephric) duct into the epididymis, vas deferens, seminal vesicle, and ejaculatory duct. At 32-36 weeks, the testis, which is anchored at the internal inguinal ring by the gubernaculum, begins its process of descent. The gubernaculum distends the inguinal canal and guides the testis into the scrotum. Following testicular descent, the patent processus vaginalis (hernia sac) normally involute.

True cryptorchism is thought in most cases to be the result of dysgenesis.

Cryptorchid testes frequently have a short spermatic artery, poor blood supply, or both. Although early scrotal positioning of these testes will obviate further damage related to intra-abdominal location, the testes generally remain abnormal, spermatogenesis is rare, and the risk of malignant neoplasm is increased. These testes should probably be removed if spermatogenesis does not occur after a reasonable period of observation.

These are histologically normal at birth. By the end of second year, the number of germ cells in the affected testis is severely reduced. Delayed germ cell maturation and number, hyalinization of seminiferous tubules, reduced Leydig cell number are typical. These changes are progressive over time if testes remain undescended. Surgical correction at the early age results in greater possibility of fertility. The patient with cryptorchidism has 20-40% increased risk of malignant tumor in the third or fourth decade.

■ CLINICAL FEATURES (FIG. 1)

Cryptorchidism is the most common congenital abnormality of the genitourinary tract. Most cryptorchid testes are undescended, but some are absent (due to agenesis or atrophy).

True undescended testes: Testes found along normal path of descent but have not reached scrotum.

Ectopic testes: Testes are found outside normal path of descent and outside the scrotum.

Retractile testes: These are normally descended testes, found in a suprascrotal position due to an overactive cremasteric reflex.

Ascending testes or acquired undescended testes: These are usually iatrogenic.

Undescended testes are classified as abdominal (nonpalpable), peeping (abdominal but can be pushed into the upper part of the inguinal canal), inguinal, gliding (can be pushed into the scrotum but retracts immediately to the pubic tubercle), and ectopic (superficial inguinal pouch or, rarely, perineal). Most undescended testes are palpable just distal to the inguinal canal over the pubic tubercle.

A disorder of sex development should be suspected in a newborn phenotypic male with bilateral nonpalpable testes, as the child could be a virilized girl with CAH. In a boy with midpenile or proximal hypospadias and a palpable undescended testis, disorder of sexual development is present in 15% and the risk is 50% if the testis is nonpalpable.

The consequences of cryptorchidism include poor testicular growth, infertility, testicular malignancy, associated hernia, torsion of the cryptorchid testis, and the possible psychologic effects of an empty scrotum.

The undescended testis is normal at birth histologically, but pathologic changes can be demonstrated by 6-12 months. Delayed germ cell maturation, reduction in germ cell number, hyalinization of the seminiferous tubules, arid reduced Leydig cell number are typical; these changes are progressive

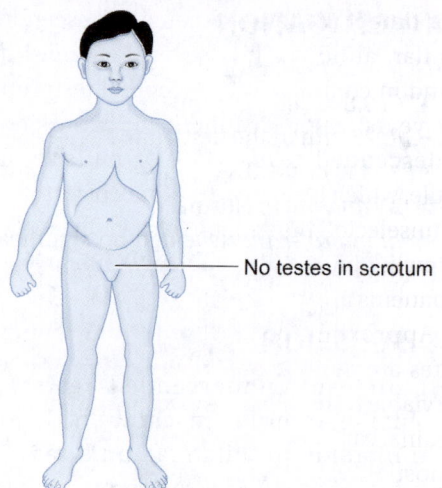

Fig. 1: Clinical features.

over time if the testis remains undescended. Similar, although less severe, changes are found in contralateral descended testis after 4-7 years. After treatment for a unilateral undescended testis, 85% of patients are fertile, which is slightly <90% rate of fertility in an unselected population of men. In contrast following bilateral orchiopexy, only 50-65% of patients are fertile.

Approximately 10% of undescended testes are nonpalpable testes. Of these, 50% are viable testes in the abdomen or high in the inguinal canal and 50% are atrophic or absent, almost always in the scrotum, secondary to spermatic cord torsion in utero (vanishing testes). If the nonpalpable testis is abdominal, it will not descend after 3 months of age. Although sonography often is performed to try to identify whether the testes is present, it rarely changes clinical management, because the abdominal testis and atrophic testis are not identified on sonography.

The risk of a germ cell malignancy developing in an undescended testis is four times higher than in the general population and is approximately 1 in 80 with a unilateral undescended testis and in 40-50 for bilateral undescended testes. Testicular tumors are less common if the orchiopexy is performed before 10 years of age, but they still occur, and adolescents should be instructed in testicular self-examination. The peak age for developing a testis tumor is 15-45 years.

An acquired or ascending undescended testis occurs when a male has a descended testis at birth but during childhood, usually between 4 and 10 years of age, the testis does not remain in the scrotum.

Retractile testes may be misdiagnosed as undescended testes. Boys older than age 1 year often have a brisk cremasteric reflex, and if the child is anxious or ticklish during scrotal examination, the testis may be difficult to manipulate into the scrotum. Boys should be examined with their legs in a relaxed frog-leg position, and if the testis can be manipulated into the scrotum comfortably, it is probably retractile. It should be monitored every 6-12 months with follow-up physical examinations, because it can become an acquired undescended testis.

Overall, as many as one-third of males with a retractile testis develop an acquired undescended testis requiring orchiopexy, and males younger than 7 years of age at diagnosis of a retractile testis are at greatest risk. Although definitive data are not available, it is generally thought that males with a retractile testis are not at increased risk for infertility or malignancy.

The most common tumor developing in an undescended testis in an adolescent or adult is a seminoma (65%); after orchiopexy, nonseminomatous tumors represent only 65% of testis tumors. Orchiopexy seems to reduce the risk of seminoma. Whether early orchiopexy reduces the risk of developing cancer of the testis is controversial, but it is uncommon for testis tumors to occur if the orchiopexy performed before the age of 2 years. The contralateral scrotal testis is not at increased risk of malignancy.

Plasma testosterone concentrations may be obtained after hCG stimulation to confirm the presence or absence of abdominal testes. The child with bilaterally undescended testes should be evaluated for sex chromosome abnormalities; evaluation should include consideration of the possibility that the child is a virilized female.

LABORATORY SALIENT FINDINGS

- Concentration of testosterone after human chorionic gonadotropin (hCG) stimulation test
- Chromosome analysis
- Ultrasonography of abdomen

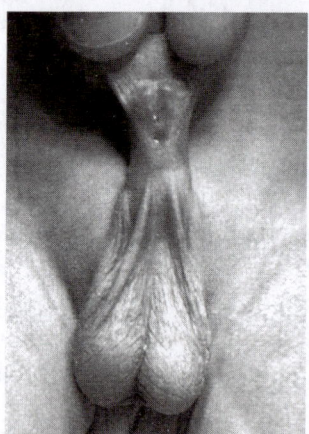

Fig. 2: Penoscrotal hypospadias and genital ambiguity.

Indirect inguinal hernia always accompanies undescended testes. It is important to differentiate true undescended testis from retractile or ectopic testis due to therapeutic and prognostic implications. Poorly developed scrotum and inability to bring down the testis to the scrotal sack suggests true descended testis. Retractile testis is an otherwise fully descended testis that has an active cremasteric reflex, which retracts it into the groin.

Penoscrotal hypospadias and genital ambiguity **(Fig. 2)** is suggestive of disorders of androgen production or action. The hCG stimulation test should be done in boys with bilateral nonpalpable testis to differentiate abdominal testis from anorchia.

GENERAL FEATURES
• Testes will be in inguinal canal
• Small scrotum
• Infertility in adult

■ DIFFERENTIAL DIAGNOSIS

In palpating for the testes, the cremasteric reflex may be elicited, with a resultant ascent of the testes into the inguinal canal or abdomen (pseudocryptorchidism). To prevent this, the fingers first should be placed across the abdominal ring and the upper portion of the inguinal canal, obstructing ascent.

Examination while the child is in the squatting position or in a warm bath is also helpful. No treatment for retractile testes is necessary and the prognosis for testicular descent and competence is excellent.

■ TREATMENT

The congenital undescended testis should be treated surgically by 9–15 months of age. With anesthesia by a pediatric anesthesiologist, surgical correction at 6 months is appropriate, because spontaneous descent of the testis will not occur after 4 months of age. Most testes can be brought down to the scrotum with an orchiopexy, which involves an inguinal incision, mobilization of the testis and spermatic cord, and correction of an indirect inguinal hernia.

Surgical Treatment

Undescended testes rarely descend after 6–10 months, hence orchidopexy should be timely performed as early as possible after *10 months* of age to prevent progressive loss of germ cells. Undescended testes can undergo torsion at any age and emergency surgery is warranted in case of acute pain with redness.

Open orchidopexy is the standard of treatment for palpable undescended testes.

Diagnostic laparoscopy is recommended for all nonpalpable undescended testes.

For nonpalpable undescended testes, sometimes the testes can become palpable under general anesthesia and surgical approach can be changed to standard inguinal orchidopexy. Diagnostic laparoscopy can reveal absent, dysplastic, or atrophic testes, which is excised and sent for biopsy. If intra-abdominal testes are identified, either a single-stage laparoscopic orchidopexy or staged Fowler–Stephen (FS) procedure is done, based on the length of the vessels. First stage of FS orchidopexy involves clipping and division of spermatic vessels. Collaterals developed from cremasteric and vassal vessels. Testes mobilized and fixed in scrotum in second stage.

Late presenters: Current recommendation is to try preserving the testes irrespective of the age of presentation. The main aim of surgery in these patients is to make it palpable for early detection of malignancy and preserve hormonal function.

The congenital undescended testis should be treated surgically by 9–15 months of age. With anesthesia by a pediatric anesthesiologist, surgical correction at 6 months is appropriate, because spontaneous descent of the testis will not occur after 4 months of age. Most testes can be brought down to the scrotum with an orchiopexy, which involves an inguinal incision, mobilization of the testis and spermatic cord, and correction of an indirect inguinal hernia. In some boys with a testis that is close to the scrotum, a prescrotal orchiopexy can be performed. In this procedure, the entire operation is performed through an incision along the edge of the scrotum. Often the associated inguinal hernia also can be corrected with this incision. Advantages of this approach over the inguinal approach include shorter operative time and less postoperative discomfort. The risk of malignancy is 4–10 times higher.

In boys with a nonpalpable testis, diagnostic laparoscopy is performed in most centers. This procedure allows safe and rapid assessment of whether the testis is intra-abdominal. In most cases, orchiopexy of the intra-abdominal testis located immediately inside the internal inguinal ring is successful, but orchiectomy should be considered in more difficult cases or when the testis appears to be atrophic. A two-stage orchiopexy sometimes is needed in boys with a high abdominal testis. Boys with abdominal testes are managed with laparoscopic techniques at many institutions.

Treatment of bilateral undescended testes is identical to the treatment of unilateral undescended testes when the testes are palpable. When testes are not palpable then the serum testosterone levels are measured before and after giving hCG. If testosterone level rises, abdominal exploration and orchidopexy should be undertaken.

Hormonal Treatment

Gonadotropin therapy (hCG) has been used in the treatment for cryptorchism but is not generally successful. Hormone treatment can be useful in the identification and descent of retractile testes or to evaluate for the presence of testicular tissue. Various treatment regimens have been used, ranging from 250 to 1,000 IU given twice weekly for 5 weeks and will generally cause descent of retractile testes.

Androgen treatment (e.g., depot testosterone) is indicated as replacement therapy in the male child, who lacks functional testes beyond the normal age of puberty.

■ BIBLIOGRAPHY

1. Eisenberg JM; Center for Clinical Decisions and Communications Science. Evaluation and treatment of cryptorchidism. Comparative Effectiveness Review Summary Guides for Clinicians. Rockville: Agency for Healthcare Research and Quality (US); 2013.
2. McCabe MJ, Bancalari RE, Dattani MT. Diagnosis and evaluation of hypogonadism Pediatr Endocrinol Rev. 2014;11(2):214-29.
3. Watson S, Fuqua JS, Lee PA. Treatment of hypogonadism in males Pediatr Endocrinol Rev. 2014;11(2):230-9.

SECTION 9

Infectious Diseases

- Case 65 **Chikungunya**
- Case 66 **Congenital Rubella**
- Case 67 **Congenital Syphilis**
- Case 68 **Dengue Fever**
- Case 69 **Herpes Zoster**
- Case 70 **Human Immunodeficiency Virus**
- Case 71 **Infectious Mononucleosis**
- Case 72 **Malaria**
- Case 73 **Measles**
- Case 74 **Mumps**
- Case 75 **Osteomyelitis**
- Case 76 **Poliomyelitis**
- Case 77 **Septic Arthritis**
- Case 78 **Tetanus Neonatorum**
- Case 79 **Typhoid**
- Case 80 **Varicella**
- Case 81 **Whooping Cough**

CASE 65

Chikungunya

■ PRESENTING COMPLAINTS

An 8-year-old boy was brought with the complaints of:
- Fever since 3 days
- Pain in the joints since 2 days
- Skin rashes since 1 day

History of the Presenting Complaints

Mother gave a history of fever since 3 days. Fever is of moderate to high degree associated with the child and rigor. Fever used to be more in the night. She also gave the history that his son has vomited. Boy also complained of pain in the joints, especially the small joint of the hand. Hence, he was finding difficulty in walking and eating by himself.

His mother noticed the rashes all over his body since 1 day. This led her to bring the child to the hospital. The rash was not pruritic. The boy was receiving treatment for the presenting complaints.

Past History of the Patient

He was the elder sibling of a nonconsanguineous marriage. He was born at term by normal vaginal delivery. There was no significant postnatal event. He was exclusively on breastfeeding for 6 months. Weaning was started as per the advice of the family doctor. The child was on family food by 15 months. He had been completely immunized. All the developmental milestones were normal. The performance at school was good. There was also a history of a similar type of illness in the school.

■ EXAMINATION

The boy was moderately built and moderately nourished. There were signs of moderate dehydration. He was looking toxic and

---

CASE AT A GLANCE

Basic Findings
Height	:	123 cm (50th centile)
Weight	:	25 kg (75th centile)
Temperature	:	38°C
Pulse rate	:	120 beats/min
Respiratory rate	:	26 breaths/min
Blood pressure	:	80/60 mm Hg

Positive Findings

History:
- Fever
- Joint pain
- Skin rash

Examination:
- Dehydrate
- Tender joints
- Swelling of the joints

Investigation:
- ESR: Raised
- IgM antibodies: Raised

(ESR: erythrocyte sedimentation rate; IgM: immunoglobulin M)

dehydrated. The anthropometric measurements included a height was 123 cm (50th centile) and a weight was 25 kg (75th centile).

He was febrile (38°C). The pulse rate was 120 beats/min and the respiratory rate was 26 breaths/min. The blood pressure recorded was 80/60 mm Hg. There were signs of dehydration. There was no pallor, no lymphadenopathy, cyanosis, or icterus.

There was tenderness in the small joints of the hand and leg. There was swelling over the joints. The rashes were present over the body. Macular rashes were present. There was no itching. There was no organomegaly. Bowel sounds were regular. Other systemic examinations were normal.

INVESTIGATION

- *Hemoglobin:* 13 g/dL
- *Total leukocyte count (TLC):* 9.800 cells/mm^3
- *Differential leukocyte count (DLC):* $P_{67}L_{30}E_2M_1$
- *Erythrocyte sedimentation rate (ESR):* 30 mm in the first hour
- *Absolute eosinophil count (AEC):* 320 cells/mm^3
- *X-ray chest:* No abnormality detected (NAD)
- *Immunoglobulin M (IgM) antibodies:* Positive

DISCUSSION

It is an acute disease characterized by fever, arthritis, and skin rash. This is caused by an enveloped virus capable of replicating in mosquitoes.

The chikungunya transmission involves *Aedes Africanus, A. furcifer,* and wild primates. This is seen among the rural population. In urban population, the cycle involves *Aedes aegypti* and humans. Outbreaks typically occur during the rainy season. This is associated with the population density of the mosquito vector. These breed in household containers and puddles with peak activity in midmorning and late afternoon. The disease typically vanishes for years after the epidemics because of the development of immunity among people.

CLINICAL FEATURES (FIG. 1)

The disease has a sudden onset. The incubation period is 2–12 days. The infection is characterized by fever, headache, fatigue, nausea, vomiting, muscle pain, rash, and joint pain. Fever increases abruptly to as high as 103–104°F. It is accompanied by rigors. The acute phase lasts for 2–3 days.

GENERAL FEATURES
• Febrile • Dehydration • Tender joint • Swelling of the joint • Maculopapular rashes

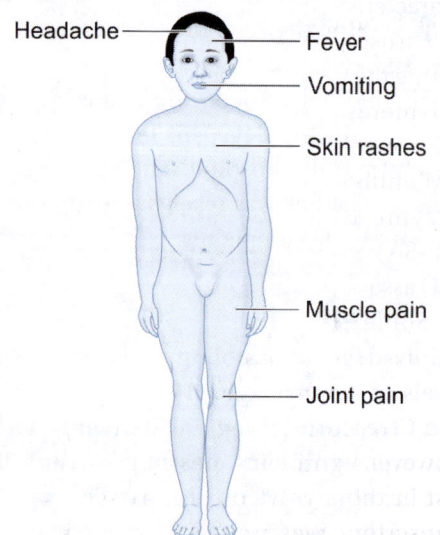

Fig. 1: Clinical features.

Joint pain is often severe in intensity. The arthralgia or arthritis is polyarticular, migrating. It predominantly affects small joints of the hands, wrists, ankles, and feet. There will be less involvement of large joints. Joint pain may continue for months after the illness. Headache is present in 80%. Photophobia and retroorbital pain may also occur.

Maculopapular rashes are seen in 4–8 days later. This affects trunks and limbs. Inguinal lymph nodes may be enlarged. It is associated with young age.

> **ESSENTIAL DIAGNOSTIC POINTS**
> - Out breaks are seen in rainy season
> - Fever, headache, and fatigue
> - *Joint pain:* Polyarticular and migrating
> - Photophobia and retroorbital pain
> - Maculopapular rashes present in trunks and limbs
> - Predominantly affects small joints, joint pain may continue for months

◼ DIAGNOSIS

It should be suspected in patients with a characteristic triad of fever, rash, and arthritis.

Viruses may be isolated in cell cultures during the initial prodromal stage of 2–4 days. Polymerase chain reaction (PCR) can be used to confirm the infection. Virus-related IgM antibodies may be detected by capture enzyme-linked immunosorbent assay (ELISA) and hemagglutination inhibition (HI) assays within 5–7 days of illness.

Some patients show leukopenia with mildly decreased platelet count. Elevated levels of aspartate aminotransferase (AST) and C-reactive protein (CRP) are also seen. However, virus isolation is the most definitive test in the first week. Recently, the reverse transcription PCR (RT-PCR) technique for diagnosis has been developed using nested primer pairs amplifying specific components of three structural gene regions. PCR results can be available within 1–2 days.

Serologic diagnosis can be made by demonstration of a fourfold increase in antibodies in acute and convalescent sera or by demonstrating IgM antibodies specific for chikungunya virus (CHIKV). A commonly used test is the antibody capture enzyme-linked immunosorbent assay (MAC-ELISA), results of MAC-ELISA can be available within 2–3 days. Cross-reaction with other flavivirus antibodies such as O'nyong-nyong and Semliki may occur in MAC-ELBA; however, the latter viruses are relatively rare in Southeast Asia. A positive virus culture supplemented with neutralization is taken as definitive proof of the presence of CHIKV.

Chikungunya should be suspected in patients who present, with the characteristic triad of fever, rash, and arthritis. Viremia is present in most patients during the initial 2–4 days of disease and may be isolated in cell cultures. PCR can be used to confirm the infection. Virus-specific IgM antibodies may be detected by capturing ELISA and HI assays by 5–7 days of illness.

> **LABORATORY SALIENT FINDINGS**
> - Isolation of virus in cell culture
> - Polymerase chain reaction
> - IgM antibodies
> - ELISA and hemagglutination inhibition assays
>
> (ELISA: enzyme-linked immunosorbent assay; IgM: immunoglobulin M)

◼ TREATMENT

No specific treatment is available. Symptomatic treatment includes rest, fluids and ibuprofen, naproxen, acetaminophen, or paracetamol. This may relieve symptoms. Aspirin should be avoided during the acute phase.

BIBLIOGRAPHY

1. Guaraldo L, Wakimoto MD, Ferreira H, Bressan C, Calvet GA, Pinheiro GC, et al. Treatment of Chikungunya musculoskeletal disorders: a systematic review. Expert Rev Anti Infect Ther. 2018;16(4)333-44.
2. Raghavendhar BS, Ray P, Ratagiri VH, Sharma BS, Kabra SK, Lodha R. Evaluation of chikungunya virus infection in children from India during 2009-2010: a cross sectional observational study. J Med Virol. 2016;88(6):923-30.
3. World Health Organization. (2022). Chikungunya. [online] Available from https://www.who.int/news-room/fact-sheets/detail/chikungunya [Last accessed June, 2024].

CASE 66

Congenital Rubella

■ PRESENTING COMPLAINTS

The newborn girl was brought with the complaint of:
- Rashes over the body 4–5 hours after the delivery.

History of Presenting Complaints

A newborn girl was brought to the attention of a pediatrician for the development of petechial rashes all over the body. The rashes appeared about 4–5 hours after the delivery.

She was the first sibling of a consanguineous marriage. She was born at a gestational age of 38 weeks. The delivery was normal. The baby cried immediately after the delivery. Features suggestive of intrauterine growth retardation (IUGR) were present. The birth weight was 1.7 kg.

Antenatal history revealed that the mother had a mild fever at 12 weeks of amenorrhea. There was an associated history of rashes to the mother. This was resolved with symptomatic management.

■ EXAMINATION

The child was a low birth weight (LBW) baby with features of IUGR. Petechial rashes were present all over the body. Anthropometric measurements included, a length of 48 cm (10th centile), a weight of 1.7 kg (LBW), and a head circumference of 33 cm.

The child was afebrile. The pulse rate was 126 beats/min, and the respiratory rate was 36 breaths/min. The blood pressure recorded was 50/40 mm Hg.

CASE AT A GLANCE

Basic Findings
Length	: 48 cm (10th centile)
Weight	: 1.7 kg (LBW)
Temperature	: 37.5°C
Pulse rate	: 126 beats/min
Respiratory rate	: 36 breaths/min
Blood pressure	: 50/40 mm Hg

Positive Findings

History:
- Preterm delivery
- IUGR
- Rashes over the body
- Fever to the mother

Examination:
- Petechial rashes
- Hepatosplenomegaly
- Cataract
- Salt-pepper retinopathy

Investigation:
- *TLC:* Increased
- *IgM level:* Increased
- *BT:* Increased
- *PT:* Increased
- *PTT:* Increased

(BT: bleeding time; IgM: immunoglobulin M; IUGR: intrauterine growth retardation; LBW: low birth weight; TLC: total leukocyte count; PT: prothrombin time; PTT: partial thromboplastin time)

There was no pallor, no cyanosis, and no icterus. Per abdomen examination revealed the presence of hepatosplenomegaly. Eyes were small. There was an absence of red reflex. Fundus could not be visualized probably because of the presence of the cataract in the right eye. In the left eye, the fundus was clotted with fine deposits of pigments, i.e., salt and pepper retinopathy.

■ INVESTIGATION

- *Hemoglobin*: 14.8 g/dL
- *TLC*: 11,000 cells/mm^3
- *ESR*: 24 mm in the first hour
- *Hepatitis B surface antigen (HBsAg)*: Negative
- *Platelet count*: 350,000 cells/mm^3
- *BT*: 7 minutes (normal range: 3–5 minutes)
- *Prothrombin time (PT)*: 25 seconds (normal range: 11–15 seconds)
- *Partial thromboplastin time (PTT)*: 40 seconds (normal range: 60–85 seconds)
- *Liver function test (LFT)*:
  - *Serum glutamic oxaloacetic transaminase (SGOT)*: 45 u/L
  - *Serum glutamic pyruvic transaminase (SGPT)*: 30 u/L
- *Blood IgM*: Increased (normal <20 ng/dL)
- *Throat culture*: Negative

■ DISCUSSION

A child presented with the rashes, i.e., petechial rashes after delivery with a significant history of fever in the first trimester given the suspicion of TORCH (toxoplasmosis, rubella cytomegalovirus, herpes simplex, and human immunodeficiency virus) infection. The associated features such as hepatosplenomegaly, salt and pepper fundal examination, cataract, and thrombocytopenia make the diagnosis of congenital rubella syndrome (CRS).

Congenital infection produces a spectrum of illness known as CRS, a result of multiorgan, noninflammatory vasculitis triggered by persistent viral infection. The first link between rubella virus and fetal damage was made by Gregg, an Australian ophthalmologist, in 1941.

Congenital rubella is a chronic infection, while acquired rubella is an acute infection. The fetus remains infected throughout gestation and for months and sometimes for years thereafter. The gestational age at which maternal infection occurs is a major determinant of the extent of fetal infection as well as its effects on the fetus.

Congenital rubella syndrome refers to infants born with defects secondary to intrauterine infection or who manifest symptoms or signs of intrauterine infection sometime after birth. Congenital infection is considered to have occurred if the infant has IgM rubella antibodies shortly after birth or if immunoglobulin G (IgG) antibodies persist for >6 months by which time maternally derived antibodies would have disappeared.

Rubella (German measles or 3-day measles) is a mild, often exanthematous disease of infants and children that is typically more severe and associated with more complications in adults. Its major clinical significance is transplacental infection and fetal damage as part of the CRS.

Rubella virus is a member of the family *Togaviridae* and is the only species of the genus *Rubivirus*. It is a single-stranded ribonucleic acid (RNA) virus with a lipid envelope and three structural proteins, including a nucleocapsid protein that is associated with the nucleus and two glycoproteins, E1 and E2 that are associated with the envelope.

■ PATHOGENESIS

Rubella demonstrates a vascular endothelial cell tropism directed in large blood vessels at the inner layer of the vascular wall. At the cellular level, the damage is linked to impaired replication, perturbation of cell growth, apoptosis, and postulated interaction between the viral nonstructural protein p90 and host cell regulatory proteins, and the timing of infection is of great importance.

Prospective studies after laboratory-confirmed rubella in pregnancy have documented that the rate of fetal infection is 90% after symptomatic maternal rubella during the first 12 gestational weeks; it drops to 25–30% during the second trimester and rises to 60–100% during the last weeks of gestation. During the second trimester, the fetus develops increasing immunologic competence and no longer seems susceptible to the chronic infection characteristic of intrauterine rubella during the early weeks.

In general, earlier infection produces more extensive damage: Cardiac defects, cataracts, and glaucoma occur predominantly after maternal rubella during the first 2 months of pregnancy. Hearing loss and neurologic manifestations may occur at any time during the first and, less commonly, into the second trimester. Late in pregnancy, infection does not appear to be teratogenic. Maternal infection with rubella during the first trimester of pregnancy frequently results in fetal infection following placental infection during maternal viremia.

Maternal viremia may lead to the seedling of the placenta. The placenta in turn may serve as a source of virus for the fetus. The gestational age of the conceptus at the time of the infection is a critical factor in determining the outcome.

The viral mechanisms for cell injury and death in postnatal or congenital rubella are not well understood. Following infection, the virus replicates in the respiratory epithelium and then spreads to regional lymph nodes. Viremia ensues and is most intense from 10 to 17 days after infection. Viral shedding from the nasopharynx begins approximately 10 days after infection and may be detected up to 2 weeks following the onset of the rash. The period of highest communicability is from 5 days before to 6 days after the appearance of the rash.

The most important risk factor for severe congenital defects is the stage of gestation at the time of infection. Maternal infection during the first 8 weeks of gestation results in the most severe and widespread defects. The risk for congenital defects has been estimated at 90% for maternal infection before 11 weeks of gestation. Defects occurring after 16 weeks of gestation are uncommon, even if fetal infection occurs.

The risk declines with each successive month of the first trimester. However, growth retardation, deafness, microcephaly, and mental retardation occur in infants infected during the fourth month of gestation.

Rubella infection inhibits cell division and is probably the reason for congenital malformation and LBW babies. Necrosis of vascular endothelium is common and may lead to vascular obstruction with secondary damage to organs. Direct lysis of cells by rubella may occur particularly with myocardial, skeletal, muscle cells, and epithelial cells of the lens.

If the infection is serious in the first trimester, spontaneous abortion and stillbirth may occur, or it may develop in multiple defects such as classical triad patent ductus arteriosus (PDA), cataract, or deafness. Infection in the second trimester causes deafness. 50-60% of fetuses are infected prior to the eighth week of gestation. 10–20% of fetuses are infected during the second trimester. Infection during the third trimester is voluminous.

Causes of cellular and tissue damage in the infected fetus may include tissue necrosis due to vascular insufficiency, reduced cellular multiplication time, chromosomal breaks, and production of a protein inhibitor causing mitotic arrests in certain cell types. The most distinctive feature of congenital rubella is chronicity. Once the fetus is infected early in gestation, the virus persists in fetal tissue until well beyond delivery. Persistence suggests the possibility of ongoing tissue damage and reactivation, most notably in the brain.

Blueberry muffins are the skin lesions, hearing loss from sensorineural deafness, and meningoencephalitis. Persistent infection leads to pneumonia, hepatitis, bone lucencies, thrombocytopenia, purpura, and anemia. Later sequelae include motor and mental retardation.

■ CLINICAL FEATURES (FIG. 1)

The consequences of rubella in utero are varied and unpredictable. Spontaneous abortion, stillbirth, live birth with anomalies (single or multiple); and normal infants are represented in this spectrum. Virtually every organ may be involved, transiently or permanently, some with delayed onset.

During the newborn period, congenital rubella may be manifested by several acute conditions that are self-limiting in infants who survive. Neonatal thrombocytopenic purpura, characterized by a variable number of red-purple macular "blueberry muffin" lesions, is the most common and striking of these manifestations. It is usually associated with a high incidence of other transient lesions, such as radiolucencies in the metaphyseal portions of the long bones, hepatosplenomegaly, hepatitis, hemolytic anemia, and bulging anterior fontanelle with or without cerebrospinal fluid (CSF) pleocytosis. This clinical picture (**Figs. 2A to C**) represents the most severe evidence of congenital infection. LBW, cardiac defects, cataracts, deafness, and developmental delay with or without microcephaly frequently accompany these transient lesions.

Signs of congenital heart disease such as cough, tachypnoea, and respiratory distress, LBW are commonly associated with congenital heart disease. Cardiac abnormalities occur in half of the children infected during the first 8 weeks of gestation. PDA is the most frequently reported cardiac defect, followed by lesions of the pulmonary arteries and valvular disease, interstitial pneumonitis leading to death in some cases has been reported. PDA, with or without stenosis of the pulmonary artery or its branches, and atrial and ventricular septal defects are the most common cardiac lesions encountered.

The most characteristic ocular anomaly is a pearly nuclear cataract, unilateral or bilateral, frequently associated with microphthalmia. The lesion may be absent at birth or so small that it may not be detected without careful ophthalmoscopic examination. Congenital glaucoma, which might be present at birth, or which might develop during infancy, is clinically indistinguishable from hereditary infantile glaucoma. The cornea is enlarged and hazy, the anterior chamber is deep, and

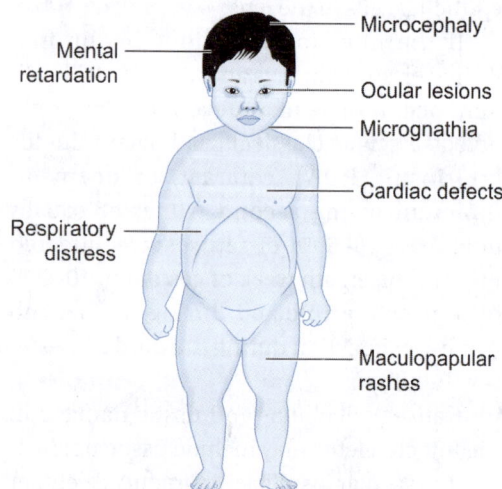

Fig. 1: Clinical features.

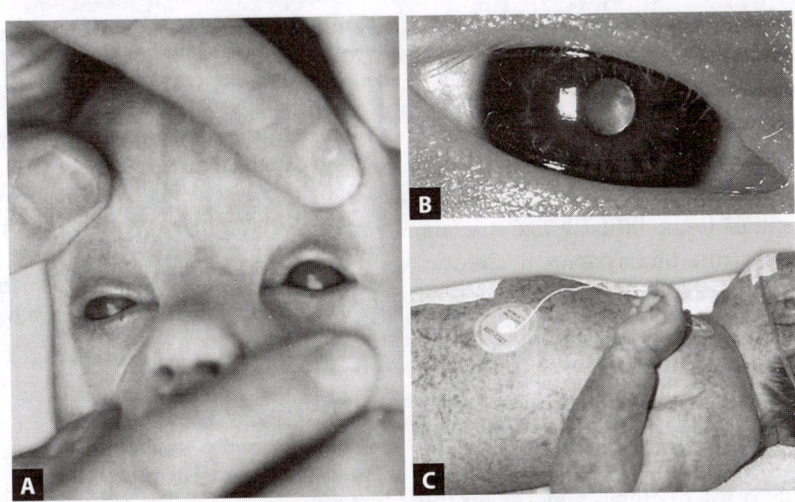

Figs. 2A to C: *(A and B) Cataract and (C) Congenital rubella. (For color version, see Plate 3)*

ocular tension is increased. Retinopathy, characterized by discrete, patchy black pigmentation, quite variable in size and location, is probably the most common ocular manifestation of congenital rubella. There is no evidence that this anomaly of the pigment epithelium of the retina interferes with vision.

Cataract is the most characteristic. Unilateral or bilateral cataracts are the most serious eye finding, occurring in about a third of infants. Ocular lesions may not be recognized until after the neonatal period. The retina may also be involved and lesions may be widespread, mottled with black pigment deposits. These are variable in size and location—the salt and pepper retinitis.

Permanent sensorineural deafness caused by damage to the organ of the corti may be severe or mild and bilateral or unilateral. Defects in the middle ear structures have been reported. Deafness and communication disorders may be the only overt manifestations of congenital rubella, especially if maternal infection occurs after the first 8 weeks of pregnancy. Delayed psychomotor development during infancy is a hallmark of congenital rubella, with the most common consequence of the permanent brain damage being mental retardation, ranging from mild to profound.

Less common are severe spastic diplegia and autism. Progressive rubella panencephalitis, a severe progressive neurologic deterioration beginning during the second decade of life, is a rare complication of congenital rubella. Intellectual deterioration, myoclonus, ataxia, and seizures have progressed to death over the course of several years. High rubella antibody titers in serum and CSF, elevated spinal fluid protein and gamma-globulin levels, histopathologic changes of progressive panencephalitis, and isolation of rubella virus from the brain biopsy specimen add to the obvious parallel between this condition and the subacute sclerosing panencephalitis that is a rare and late sequela of measles.

Neurologic abnormalities are common and may progress following birth. Meningoencephalitis is present in 10–20% of infants with CRS and may persist for up to 12 months. Longitudinal follow-up through 9–12 years of infants without initial retardation revealed progressive development of additional sensory, motor, and behavioral abnormalities, including hearing loss and autism. Lethargy, irritability, bulged anterior fontanelle (AF), and seizures may occur.

Congenital rubella syndrome also poses a risk of type 1 diabetes mellitus. By age 10 years, the risk is at least four times greater in children with CRS than among healthy children, and by adult life, the risk is 10–20-fold greater. In one group of adult survivors, 40% had type 1 diabetes mellitus. The high prevalence of pancreatic islet cell cytotoxic or surface antibodies in congenital rubella patients with and without type 1 diabetes may reflect the in utero infection of pancreatic cells and play a role in the pathogenesis of type 1 diabetes mellitus in genetically susceptible individuals. Thyroiditis also has been described.

Subsequent postnatal growth retardation and ultimate short stature have been reported in a minority of cases. Rare reports of immunologic deficiency syndromes have also been described.

A variety of late-onset manifestations of CRS have been recognized. They include diabetes mellitus (20%), thyroid dysfunction (5%), and glaucoma and visual abnormalities associated with the retinopathy, which had previously been considered benign.

> **ESSENTIAL DIAGNOSTIC POINTS**
> - Adenopathies, bone radiolucencies, and encephalitis
> - *Cardiac defects:* Pulmonary arterial hypoplasia and patent ductus arteriosus
> - Cataracts, retinopathy, and growth retardation
> - Hepatosplenomegaly thrombocytopenia and purpura
> - Late sequalae include diabetes thyroid dysfunction, rubella encephalopathy, and psychomotor problems

■ DIAGNOSIS

The infant with suspected congenital rubella should be evaluated with specimens for viral detection and for rubella-specific IgM. These infants may remain chronically infected for many months after birth and thus are a source of infection for susceptible contacts for a year or more. Virus has been detected in pharyngeal secretions, blood spots, urine, CSF, cataract tissue, and virtually every organ. Reverse transcriptase PCR using dried blood spots, lens aspirates, and oral fluids offers additional evidence for diagnosis in early infancy

Newborn infants with congenital rubella have serum rubella antibody titers comparable to those of their mothers. Much of this antibody is transplacentally acquired IgG, but the presence of rubella-specific IgM reflects in utero antibody production by the fetus and, when present, is diagnostic of congenital rubella. In all but rare infants, by the end of 1 year, IgG is usually the dominant rubella antibody. Detectable levels of antibodies persist for years in most children. Rubella antibody that persists in infancy beyond age 6 months without evidence of postnatal infection essentially confirms the diagnosis of congenital rubella.

Virus can be isolated from the throat and urine from 1 week before to 2 weeks after

> **GENERAL FEATURES**
> - Sensory neural hearing defects
> - *Cardiac defects:* PDA, VSD, and PS
> - *Blood:*
>   – Anemia
>   – Leukopenia
>   – Thrombocytopenia
> - *Ocular:*
>   – Retinopathy
>   – Cataract
>   – Glaucoma
> - Polycystic kidney
>
> (PDA: patent ductus arteriosus; PS: pulmonary stenosis; VSD: ventricular septal defect)

the onset of the rash. Congenital rubella is associated with low platelet counts, abnormal LFTs, hemolytic pleocytosis and very high IgM antibody titer, X-ray shows pneumonitis, and bone metaphyseal longitudinal lucencies in CRS.

> **LABORATORY SALIENT FINDINGS**
> - Leukopenia
> - Low platelet count
> - Abnormal liver function tests
> - Hemolytic anemia and pleocytosis
> - Very high rubella IgM antibody titers
> - Serum IgM elevated
> - Serum IgA and IgG levels may be depressed
>
> (IgA: immunoglobulin A; IgG: immunoglobulin G; IgM: immunoglobulin M)

■ DIFFERENTIAL DIAGNOSIS

- TORCH
- Hepatitis
- Septicemia
- Encephalitis
- Hemolytic anemia
- Immune-mediated thrombocytopenia (ITP)
- Myocarditis

■ TREATMENT

There is no specific treatment. There is no specific antiviral medicine. Acetaminophen and ibuprofen are indicated for the fever.

Prevention is through immunization before puberty. After puberty immunization should be only after the estimation of hemagglutination inhibition (HI) antibody titer and if pregnancy can be avoided for 8 weeks.

If a pregnant mother is suspected to have been exposed to possible rubella during early pregnancy (<16 weeks), HI antibody titer is estimated at 3- and 6-week intervals irrespective of the occurrence of any rash. A fourfold or greater increase in HI antibody indicated rubella infection. If it is confirmed medical termination is advised.

The immunization strategies to prevent congenital rubella infection have been modified.
- To protect the women of childhood-bearing age (15–39 years)
- To prevent the transmission of rubella by vaccinating children ages 1–14 years.

Only 30% of infants with encephalitis appear to escape residual neuromotor defects including autistic syndrome.

■ VACCINATION

Infants with CRS are contagious as long as they are shedding the virus in their pharyngeal secretions. In general, infants who carry rubella for long periods are more severely damaged and delayed in growth and development. There is no specific therapy for congenital rubella. Early detection of auditory and visual impairment and incorporation of adequate educational therapy, including parent education and counseling, are important.

Ideally, postpubertal females should know their immune status before conception and be vaccinated only after assurance that they are not pregnant and can avoid pregnancy for at least 1 month after vaccination. Pregnant women should not be immunized but should be tested for rubella susceptibility. The immediate postpartum period is an excellent time to vaccinate susceptible women, although barriers to postpartum or postabortal vaccination remain challenging. Vaccine virus has been isolated in human breast milk but poses no hazard to the infant. The use of γ-globulin (commercially available human immunoglobulin) in prophylaxis of rubella during pregnancy does not prevent rubella or congenital rubella in a predictable or reliable fashion.

Following a single dose of RA 27/3 vaccine 95% of person 12 months of age and older develop serologic immunity, and after two doses 99% have detectable antibodies. Rubella RA 27/3 vaccine is highly protective as 97% of those vaccinated are protected from clinical disease after one dose. Detectable antibodies remain for 15 years in most individuals vaccinated following one dose, and 91–100% had antibodies after 12–15 years after two doses. Although antibody levels may wane, especially after one dose of vaccine, increased susceptibility to rubella disease does not occur.

Adverse reactions to rubella vaccination are uncommon in children. Measles–mumps–rubella (MMR) vaccine administration is associated with fever in 5–15% of vaccinees and with rash in approximately 5% of vaccinees. Arthralgia and arthritis are more common following rubella vaccination in adults. Approximately 25% of postpubertal women experience arthralgia and 10% experience arthritis. Peripheral neuropathies and transient thrombocytopenia may also occur.

PROGNOSIS

Reinfection with wild virus occurs postnatally in both individuals who were previously infected with wild-virus rubella and vaccinated individuals. Reinfection is defined serologically as a significant increase in IgG antibody level and/or an IgM response in an individual who has a documented preexisting rubella-specific IgG above an accepted cutoff. Reinfection may result in an anamnestic IgG response, an IgM and IgG response, or clinical rubella. There are 29 reports in the literature on CRS following maternal reinfection. Reinfection with serious adverse outcomes to adults or children is rare and of unknown significance.

BIBLIOGRAPHY

1. Centers for Disease Control and Prevention. Rubella and congenital rubella syndrome control and elimination - global progress, 2000-2012. MMWR Morb Mortal Wkly Rep. 2013;62(48):983-6.
2. Gao Z, Wood JG, Burgess MA, Menzies RI, McIntyre PB, MacIntyre CR. Models of strategies for control of rubella and congenital rubella syndrome-a 40 year experience from Australia. Vaccine. 2013;31(4):691-7.
3. Lambert N, Strebel P, Orenstein W, Icenogle J, Poland GA. Lancet. 2015;385(9985):2297-307.
4. Reef SE, Strebel P, Dabbagh A, Gacic-Dobo M, Cochi S. Progress towards control of rubella and prevention of congenital rubella syndrome–worldwide, 2009. J Infect Dis. 2011;204(Suppl 1):S24-7.

CASE 67

Congenital Syphilis

■ PRESENTING COMPLAINTS

A 2-month-old baby was brought with the complaint of:
- Swelling in the right leg since 15 days
- Excessive crying since 2–3 days

History of Presenting Complaints

A 2-month-old boy was brought to the hospital with a history of swelling in his right leg. His mother complained that she noticed a small hard swelling at the lower end of his leg. She also complained, the swelling was painful, his son was crying when it was touched. She also said that her child was crying excessively for 2–3 days. She found it very difficult to console her child. The child used to cry a lot when he was being fed. There was also a history of cough and cold. For the same, the child had received a course of antibiotics.

Past History of the Patient

The boy was the only child of a nonconsanguineous marriage. The child was born at full term by normal delivery. He cried immediately after the delivery. The cry of the baby was good. The birth weight of the child was 2.5 kg. The child was on breast milk after the delivery. There was no significant postnatal event. The child was discharged from the hospital on the third day.

CASE AT A GLANCE

Basic Findings
Length	: 55 cm (25th centile)
Weight	: 4.5 kg (40th centile)
Temperature	: 37°C
Pulse rate	: 126 beats/min
Respiratory rate	: 24 breaths/min
Blood pressure	: 50/40 mm Hg

Positive Findings

History:
- Excessive crying
- Swelling at the right leg
- Snuffles
- Cold
- Prior abortions

Examination:
- Tender swelling
- Snuffles

Investigation:
- Venereal disease research laboratory (VDRL): Positive
- Blood smear: Microcytic hypochromic anemia

■ EXAMINATION

The boy was moderately built and nourished. He was crying excessively and was irritable. He was crying a lot when his limb was touched. Anthropometric measurements included, a length of 55 cm (25th centile), a weight of 4.5 kg (40th centile), and a head circumference of 37 cm.

The child was afebrile, the heart rate was 126 beats/min, and the respiratory rate was 24 breaths/min. The blood pressure recorded was 50/40 mm Hg. There was no pallor, swelling was present on both the lower limbs. There was no lymphadenopathy and no icterus. A small significant swelling was present on the right ankle joint. The swelling was firm in consistency. General signs of rhinitis were present. Other systemic examinations were normal.

INVESTIGATION

- *Hemoglobin:* 12 g/dL
- *TLC:* 7,600 cells/mm^3
- *DLC:* P$_{77}$L$_{20}$E$_1$M$_2$
- *ESR:* 30 mm in the first hour
- *AEC:* 440 cells/mm^3
- *Peripheral blood smear:* Microcytic hypochromic anemia
- *VDRL:* Positive

DISCUSSION

It results from the transplacental transfer of the causative agent, *Treponema pallidum*. Clinical findings may be seen at birth or after several months. These include mucocutaneous manifestations. It is characterized by a bullous rash. The denuded area is left after the rupture leading to crust formation. There will be pink to reddish maculopapular rash.

Congenital syphilis results from the transplacental infection of the developing fetus. An infected pregnant woman has a high probability of transmitting the infection to the fetus. Women with primary and secondary syphilis and spirochetemia are more likely to transmit infection to the fetus than are women with latent infection. Treponemal organisms can cross the placenta at any stage of pregnancy but appear to elicit little tissue response before the 15th week of gestation. The rate of vertical transmission is 70-100% for primary syphilis, 40% for early latent syphilis, and 10% for latent disease.

Transmission can occur at any stage of pregnancy, resulting in early fetal loss, preterm or LBW infants, stillbirths, neonatal deaths, or infants born with congenital disease. Adequate treatment of the mother with penicillin protects the fetus, but the mother may become reinfected. The signs and symptoms are varied and may appear at any time between birth and 3 months of life, with 5 weeks as the median time of onset for those infants appearing normal at birth.

The incidence of congenital infection in the offspring of untreated or inadequately treated infected women remains highest during the first 4 years after acquisition of primary infection, secondary infection, and early latent disease. Maternal factors associated with congenital syphilis include limited access to healthcare, late or no prenatal care, drug use, multiple sex partners, unprotected sexual contact, incarceration, work in the sex trade, and inadequate treatment of syphilis during pregnancy. Congenital syphilis may be seen in the context of untreated, inadequately treated, or undocumented treatment prior to or during pregnancy. In addition, the mother may have been treated appropriately but did not have an adequate serologic response to therapy and the infant was inadequately evaluated or the infant had documented congenital syphilis.

Congenital neurosyphilis is often asymptomatic in the neonatal period, although CSF abnormalities can occur even in asymptomatic infants. Failure to thrive, chorioretinitis, nephritis, and nephrotic syndrome can also be seen. Manifestations of renal involvement include hypertension, hematuria, proteinuria, hypoproteinemia, hypercholesterolemia, and hypocomplementemia, probably related to glomerular deposition of circulating immune complexes. Less-common clinical manifestations of early congenital syphilis include gastroenteritis, peritonitis, pancreatitis, pneumonia, eye involvement (glaucoma and chorioretinitis), nonimmune hydrops, and testicular masses.

■ CLINICAL FEATURES (FIG. 1)

Early Congenital (Prenatal) Syphilis

Untreated syphilis in the pregnant woman can result in stillbirth, spontaneous abortion, nonimmune hydrops, premature delivery, perinatal death, and early or late congenital syphilis. Women with primary or secondary syphilis are more likely to have infants with adverse outcomes compared to women with early- or late-latent syphilis.

Most infants with congenital syphilis are asymptomatic at birth. Infants who develop clinical manifestations during the first 2 years of life are considered to have early congenital syphilis, whereas features that appear later, usually near puberty, compromise late congenital syphilis.

Clinical signs of congenital syphilis appear in approximately two-thirds of affected infants during the third to eighth week of life and in most by 3 months of age. Symptoms may be generalized and nonspecific (e.g., fever, lymphadenopathy, irritability, and failure to thrive).

Alternatively, the highly suggestive triad of snuffles, palmar and plantar bullae, and splenomegaly may be apparent. The severity of clinical illness can vary from mild to fulminant, life-threatening disease. Premature infants are more likely to have hepatomegaly, respiratory distress, and skin lesions than similarly infected term neonates.

Rhinitis (i.e., snuffles) is encountered in 10–50% of infected infants and usually precedes the appearance of cutaneous eruptions by 1–2 weeks. The extremely contagious discharge initially is watery, but it later becomes thicker, purulent, and even hemorrhagic. Without treatment, the nasal cartilage ulcerates with ensuing chondritis, necrosis, and septal perforation (i.e., saddle-nose deformity of late congenital syphilis).

Most live-born syphilitic infants have no visible lesions at birth. When lesions are present, they are most commonly on the skin and in the bones. In the first week of life, syphilis may produce bullous lesions of the skin on the palms and soles. The more usual pattern of skin involvement is a diffuse, symmetric, copper-colored maculopapular rash that is most intense on the face, palms, and soles. It is an infiltrative lesion that when gently scraped with a scalpel yields serum teeming with treponemes. Thus, either dark-field microscopy or direct fluorescent antibody examination may result in a rapid and definitive diagnosis. If left untreated, most syphilitic infants will eventually have some kind of skin lesion.

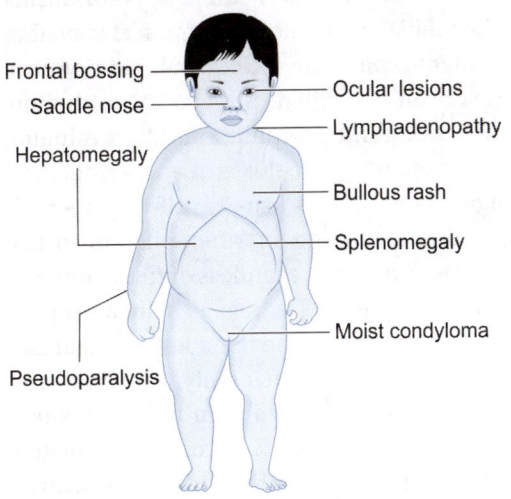

Fig. 1: Clinical features.

A characteristic mucous membrane lesion of infants that has no counterpart in adults is snuffles, rhinitis producing a serous discharge that frequently becomes secondarily infected. Postinflammatory scarring beneath the nose is called rhagades. The lesion may extend to the nasal cartilage and cause sufficient damage to result in saddle nose deformity.

Rhagades are linear scars that extend in a spoke-like pattern from previous mucocutaneous fissures of the mouth. Rhagades are linear scars that radiate from sites of earlier mucocutaneous lesions of the mouth, nares, and anus. Skeletal manifestations are caused by persistent or recurrent periostitis and its associated bone thickening. Throat involvement can produce hoarseness or aphonia.

The mucocutaneous lesions **(Fig. 2)** of congenital syphilis are varied and occur in 30–60% of infants. The most common characteristics are vesiculobullous eruptions that are more pronounced on the palms and soles. The commonly encountered rash consists of oval, red, maculopapular lesions that are most prominent on the buttocks, back, thighs, and soles; they later change to a copper-brown color with superficial desquamation.

Other lesions may be annular, circinate, petechial, or purpuric or have a blueberry muffin appearance. Mucous patches involving the nares, palate, tongue, lips, and anus can occur; these lesions become deeply fissured and hemorrhagic and subsequently result in rhagades (i.e., parrot radial scars of late congenital syphilis).

Condyloma lata usually are encountered later in infancy in untreated patients. These raised, flat, moist, and wart-like lesions most commonly affect perioral (i.e., nares and angles of mouth) and perianal areas.

Congenital syphilis produces widespread lesions in the skeleton resulting in osteochondritis at metaphyseal plates, a generalized symmetric periosteal elevation, and symmetrically occurring osteomyelitic lesions on radiographs. The humerus is the most commonly involved bone, with the tibia next, which often has a highly characteristic pattern with a bilateral moth-eaten appearance; indeed, if other bones are involved these two bones are almost sure to be involved as well.

A bilateral moth-eaten appearance of the medial aspects of the proximal tibia that is highly characteristic of congenital syphilis has been described. About >90% of infants with congenital syphilis manifest skeletal lesions that begin between 1 and 3 months of age; the process is usually self-limited, with healing occurring spontaneously over the next few months, regardless of treatment.

Radiographic findings usually disappear by age 5 months. The bone lesions are often asymptomatic Occasionally, there is pain, often manifested by a pseudoparalysis that may be unilateral, involving either an arm or a leg (parrot paralysis) Later in infancy, there may be recurring isolated bone lesions;

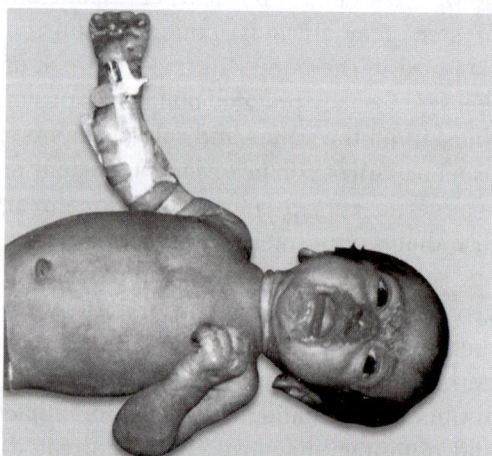

Fig. 2: Mucocutaneous manifestation of an infant.
(For color version, see Plate 4)

dactylitis, frequently asymmetric, is a typical example.

Central nervous system (CNS) involvement with abnormal CSF findings is present in 40-60% of infants with syphilis. Jaundice as a manifestation of syphilitic hepatitis sometimes appears early in congenital syphilis and is resolved with treatment. Syphilitic pneumonitis, or pneumonia alba, is uncommon and usually is only present in fatal cases.

Splenomegaly and generalized lymphadenopathy are found in 20-50% of infants with congenital syphilis. The enlarged nodes are firm and nontender. These are frequent manifestations of early systemic illness. The epitrochlear nodes commonly enlarge. Involvement of the kidney, when present, takes the form of a glomerulonephritis that presents as nephrotic syndrome. Syphilis is responsible for almost half of all nephrotic syndromes in patients <6 months of age.

Hepatosplenomegaly occurs in 50-90% of infants with early congenital syphilis. The enlargement is caused mainly by abundant extramedullary hematopoiesis and by subacute hepatic and splenic inflammation. Jaundice with direct and indirect hyperbilirubinemia, occurs in about one-third of infants and may be contributed to by hepatitis or hemolysis.

Late Congenital Syphilis

Late congenital syphilis may be suspected from the stigmata, from the presence of continued active disease, or from persistently positive tests in an otherwise asymptomatic child. Hutchinson triad includes Hutchinson teeth, interstitial keratitis, and eighth nerve deafness. The most common stigmata are Hutchinson teeth, a screwdriver, or peg-shaped deformity of the upper central incisors of the second dentition. Molars may have extra cusps and are referred to as "Mulberry molars." They are poorly formed and crumble under normal use. All syphilitic teeth demonstrate deficient enamel and decay more readily than normal teeth. Hutchinson incisors are visible by radiography in its site from about age year.

Interstitial keratitis begins between ages 5 and 16 years. Keratitis is an intense inflammatory vascular infiltration of the cornea that may be accompanied by an iritis, which may be followed by a dense cicatricial scar that produces blindness. Although usually bilateral, it may appear in one eye before it appears in the other eye. The lesion is not prevented by treatment given after the first year of disease. Early stages are characterized by marked photophobia, lacrimation, and a hazy appearance of the cornea. Later, scarring occurs.

Other active forms of late disease are gummas and osteitis, which are among the late benign syphilitic lesions. The palate and nasal septum are predilectional sites for destructive gummas, with saddle nose and perforated palatal deformities as possible end results. The saddle nose is the depression of the nasal root. Saddle-nose deformity, high arched palate, and poor maxillary growth are late consequences of syphilitic rhinitis. It occurs as a result of syphilitic rhinitis that destroys the adjacent bone and cartilage. The perforated nasal septum is present.

Persistent periostitis gives rise to thickened clavicles and to a usually asymmetric saber shin. Clutton joints are symmetric synovial effusions, usually of the knees, that are sometimes painless, but which are more often warm and painful.

An important form of active late congenital syphilis involves the CNS, most commonly meningovascular. Paresis, a potentially more dangerous form of CNS syphilis, occurs in juveniles and may be detected in a preparetic state by examination of CSF. The examination shows complement-fixing antibody, pleocytosis, and elevation of protein concentration. If untreated, parenchymal involvement may be severe and eventually irreversible. Juvenile tabes dorsalis rarely occur.

Clinically silent CNS involvement occurs in as many as 60% of infants with congenital syphilis. Acute syphilitic meningitis may present with neck stiffness, vomiting, bulging anterior fontanelle, and a positive Kernig's sign. CSF examination reveals a normal glucose concentration, modestly elevated protein content, and mononuclear pleocytosis (usually <200 cells/mL) a pattern consistent with aseptic meningitis.

Chronic meningovascular syphilis develops in untreated infants and manifests in late infancy with progressive, communicating hydrocephalus, cranial nerve palsies, optic atrophy, and cerebral infarctions leading to hemiplegia or seizure disorders.

ESSENTIAL DIAGNOSTIC POINTS

- Fetal infection results in still birth premature infant
- Mucocutaneous lesions and lymphadenopathy
- Hepatosplenomegaly
- Bony changes and hydrops
- Hutchinson teeth and mulberry molars
- Keratitis and chorioretinitis glaucoma
- Hearing loss saddle nose
- Saber shins and mental retardation

Nephrosis and nephritis may be present at birth. Osteochondritis and syphilitic metaphysitis occur within a few months of life. Upper limbs are more often affected than lower limbs. The condition is generally unilateral. The long bones are painful. The infant may be unable to move the limb, i.e., pseudoparalysis. There may be acute syphilitic leptomeningitis, progressive hydrocephalus and cranial nerve palsies. Congenital glaucoma and chorioretinitis may also be seen.

GENERAL FEATURES

- Early:
  - Bullous rash
  - Moist condyloma
  - Hepatosplenomegaly
  - Generalized lymphadenopathy
  - Hemolytic anemia
  - Nephrosis
  - Nephritis
  - Pseudoparalysis
  - Congenital glaucoma
  - Chorioretinitis
  - Failure to thrive
- Late (after 2–3 years):
  - Hutchinson's teeth
  - Frontal bossing
  - Saddle nose
  - High-arched palate
  - Saber tibia
  - Mulberry molars

■ DIAGNOSIS

Diagnosis of congenital syphilis requires a thorough review of maternal history of syphilis treatment preconception and testing, treatment, and the dynamics of response during the current pregnancy. Regardless of maternal treatment and the presence/absence of symptoms in the infant, proactive evaluation and treatment of exposed neonates is critical.

At birth, diagnosis of congenital syphilis is best established by demonstrating the spirochete or its deoxyribonucleic acid (DNA) in tissues or body fluids as previously alluded to. Serologic data obtained from cord blood or neonatal sera are helpful if interpreted with their limitations in mind.

If the infant's rapid plasma reagin (RPR) or venereal disease research laboratory (VDRL) titer is at least fourfold higher than a concomitantly obtained maternal titer, the diagnosis of congenital syphilis is likely. RPR may be negative in infants whose mother had acquired syphilis shortly before delivery. The fluorescent treponemal antibody absorption IgM (FTA-ABS-IgM) test yields false positive and false negative results in 35 and 10% of cases, respectively.

The diagnosis of congenital neurosyphilis is difficult to ascertain. CSF abnormalities such as mononuclear pleocytosis (≥25 cells/mL), elevated protein concentration (>170 mg/dL) and reactive CSF VDRL are widely used criteria. However, the CSF VDRL can be positive in the absence of neurosyphilis because of passive diffusion of nontreponemal IgG antibodies from serum to CSF and in infants with traumatic lumbar punctures.

Diagnosis of neurosyphilis in the newborn with syphilitic infection is confounded by poor sensitivity of the CSF VDRL test in this age group and lack of CSF abnormalities. A positive CSF VIDRL test in a newborn warrants treatment for neurosyphilis, even though it might reflect passive transfer of antibodies from serum to CSF.

The most useful tests in diagnosis and confirmation include VDRL and FTA-ABS tests. Positive serological tests in mothers may be associated with possible tests in newborns. Passively acquired VDRL from the mother resulting in positive test usually becomes negative within 3 months. A fourfold high titer of VDRL in the fetus as compared to mother is considered diagnostic.

Radiologic changes include osteochondritis, periostitis, and osteitis. The earliest changes occur in the metaphysis and consist of transverse, serrated radiopaque bands (i.e., Wegner sign) alternating the zones of radiolucent osteoporotic bone. Osteochondritis becomes evident radiographically 5 weeks after fetal infection. The metaphysis may become fragmented. Periosteal reactions may consist of a single layer of new bone formation, multiple layers (onion peel periosteum) or a severe lamellar form (periostitis is radiologically apparent after at least 16 weeks) of fetal infection.

Hematologic abnormalities are common and include anemia, leukocytosis, leukopenia, and thrombocytopenia. Anemia may be due to Coombs negative hemolysis, replacement of bone marrow by syphilitic granulation tissue or maturation arrest in the erythroblastoid cell line. Thrombocytopenia is due to shortened peripheral platelet survival.

> **LABORATORY SALIENT FINDINGS**
> - VDRL test
> - FTA-ABS test
> - *CSF analysis:* Mononuclear pleocytosis, elevated proteins, and reactive CSF VDRL
> - FTA-IgM test
> - Demonstration of spirochetes or its DNA in tissue and body fluids
>
> (CSF: cerebrospinal fluid; DNA: deoxyribonucleic acid; FTA-ABS: fluorescent treponemal antibody absorption; IgM: immunoglobulin M; VDRL: venereal disease research laboratory)

■ DIFFERENTIAL DIAGNOSIS

Differential diagnoses include cytomegalovirus (CMV) infection, toxoplasmosis, rubella, and herpes simplex.

■ TREATMENT

Successful treatment also depends upon the integrity of the host's immune response. A transient acute systemic febrile reaction called the Jarisch–Herxheimer reaction (caused by a massive release of endotoxin-like antigens at bacterial lysis) occurs in 15–20% of patients with acquired or congenital syphilis treated with penicillin. It is not an indication for discontinuation of penicillin therapy.

The regimens of choice in proven or highly probable congenital syphilis in infants 4 weeks or younger are as follows:
- Aqueous crystalline penicillin G 100,000–150,000 IU/kg/day (administered as 50,000 U/kg intravenously every 12 hours during the first 7 days of life and every, 8 hours thereafter) for a total of 10 days
Or,
- Procaine penicillin G 50,000 U/kg intramuscularly daily in a single dose for 10 days; adequate CSF concentrations may not be achieved with this regimen.

The VDRL titers should be monitored every 2–3 months until they become nonreactive, or the titer declines by at least fourfold. Untreated infants should have FTA-ABS tests. Passively acquired maternal antibodies usually disappear by 6–12 months of age in uninfected infants.

Treated infants should be followed every 2–3 months to confirm at least a fourfold decrease in nontreponemal titers. Treated infants with congenital neurosyphilis should undergo clinical and CSF evaluation at 6-month intervals until CSF is normal. At the age of 2 years, these infants should receive a full developmental assessment. In a very-low-risk neonate who is asymptomatic and whose mother was treated appropriately, without evidence of relapse or reinfection, but with a low and stable VDRL titer (serofast), no evaluation is necessary. Some specialists would treat such an infant with a single dose of benzathine penicillin G 50,000 units/kg intramuscular (IM).

The penicillin G treatment regimen for children >4 weeks of age is 200,000–300,000 IU/kg/day administered as 50,000 IU/kg intravenously every 4–6 hours for 10 days. If one or more days of therapy are missed, the entire course needs to be restarted.

Follow-up is particularly important for these infants. They should be seen frequently with a careful developmental evaluation, including vision and hearing testing. Nontreponemal tests should be repeated 3, 6, and 12 months after therapy. Titers are expected to decline and become nonreactive or stabilize at very low levels. In infants with congenital neurosyphilis or in those children not evaluated for neurosyphilis, the CSF should also be examined toward the end of therapy. Repeat treatment should be considered if the titer increases or fails to decrease fourfold within 1 year.

Infants with CSF abnormalities should be retested at 6 months of age. If the CSF VDRL is positive at that time, a second course of penicillin is indicated. Follow-up examinations should emphasize developmental assessment and a careful search for stigmata of congenital syphilis.

The following infants are to be treated: (1) Born to a mother who had untreated syphilis at delivery, (2) evidence of maternal relapse of reinfection, (3) physical evidence of active disease, (4) radiological evidence of syphilis, and (5) reactive CSF VDRL.

If CSF is normal 100,000–150,000 IU of penicillin/kg/day in divided dose is given for 10–14 days. If the CSF is abnormal, the infant must be treated with 150,000 IU of penicillin per kilogram body weight per day in two divided doses given IM or intravenous (IV) for a minimum of 21 days.
- *Interstitial keratitis:* Corticosteroids locally
- *Nerve deafness:* Oral steroids and penicillin
- Child should be kept under surveillance for 1 year
- Serological tests are repeated after 4–6 weeks.

PREVENTION

Serologic tests for syphilis should be performed in all pregnant women before delivery and are required by law in many states. No infant should leave the hospital without the serologic status of the infant's mother having been documented at least once during pregnancy. Serologic testing also should be performed at delivery in communities and populations at risk for congenital syphilis. Serologic tests can be nonreactive among infants infected late during their mother's pregnancy.

Penicillin is the only drug that, when given during pregnancy, reliably protects the fetus. If other drugs such as erythromycin are used, the infant should be treated again after birth. The infected pregnant woman's sexual partners must also be treated because the mother could become reinfected and could also reinfect her infant after penicillin therapy. Because most open lesions and possibly blood are contagious, standard precautions are recommended for all patients with suspected or proven syphilis until therapy has been administered for at least 24 hours.

Routine prenatal screening for syphilis remains the most important factor in identifying infants at risk for developing congenital syphilis. Screening all women at the beginning of prenatal care is an evidence-based standard of care and is legally required in all states. In pregnant women without optimal prenatal care, serologic screening for syphilis should be performed at the time pregnancy is diagnosed. Any woman who is delivered of a stillborn infant at 20 weeks or fewer of gestation should be tested for syphilis.

BIBLIOGRAPHY

1. Patten ME, Su JR, Nelson R, Weinstock H; Centers for Disease Control and Prevention (CDC). Primary and secondary syphilis—United States, 2005-2013. MMWR Morb Mortl Wkly Rep. 2014;63(18):402-6.
2. Toltzis P. 50 years ago in the Journal of Pediatrics: congenital syphilis: a laid ghost walks. J Pediatr. 2014;164(1):66.

CASE 68

Dengue Fever

■ PRESENTING COMPLAINTS

A 9-year-old boy was brought with the complaint of:
- Fever since 4 days
- Headache since 4 days
- Vomiting since 3 days
- Abdominal pain since 2 days
- Rashes since 2 days

History of Presenting Complaints

A 9-year-old boy came to the pediatric outpatient department with a history of fever, headache, vomiting, and abdominal pain. The mother said that his son had a high degree of fever associated with chills for about 4 days. For which she took him to her family doctor and got the treatment. The boy was comfortable with treatment for 2–3 days. Later again he developed a fever. This time it was associated with severe headaches not relieved with analgesics. The mother also gave a history of vomiting about three to four times since yesterday. She even said that his son was not tolerating any food. Boy also said that he was having abdominal pain, especially in the upper abdomen. Mother also revealed the presence of some rashes over the body.

Past History of the Patient

He was the elder sibling of a nonconsanguineous marriage. He was born at full term with normal delivery. There were no significant postnatal events. He was on breastfeeding from the delivery and was exclusively on breast milk for

---

CASE AT A GLANCE

Basic Findings
Height	:	128 cm (50th centile)
Weight	:	26 kg (75th centile)
Temperature	:	38°C
Heart rate	:	126 beats/min
Respiratory rate	:	28 breaths/min
Blood pressure	:	70/50 mm Hg

Positive Findings

History:
- High degree of fever
- Headache
- Vomiting
- Abdominal pain
- Rashes

Examination:
- Toxic look
- Moderate dehydration
- Pallor
- Petechiae and ecchymosis
- Congested throat
- Tenderness in right hypochondrium
- Hepatomegaly
- Decreased breath sounds

Investigation:
- Anemia
- Thrombolytopenia
- *Ultrasonography (USG):* Ascites
- *Chest X-ray:* Pleural effusion
- *Tourniquet test:* Positive

3 months. Later weaning was started and was on family food for 1 year. He was completely immunized. His developmental milestones were normal. His scholastic performance was normal. His sister was 5 years old and was maintaining good health.

■ EXAMINATION

The boy was moderately built and moderately nourished. The boy was looking sick, and signs of moderate dehydration were present. He was in agony with pain in his head and in his abdomen. The anthropometric measurement included his weight being 26 kg (75th centile) and his height being 128 cm (50th centile).

The boy was febrile. Signs of moderate dehydration were present. The heart rate was 126 beats/min, respiratory rate was 28 breaths/min, and blood pressure was 70–50 mm Hg.

There was pallor, no lymphadenopathy, no edema, and no clubbing. Petechiae and ecchymotic rashes were present over the face and legs. The throat was congested. Per abdomen examination revealed tenderness at the right hypochondrium and epigastrium. The liver was palpable about 2–3 cm in the midclavicular line and tender.

The respiratory system revealed the presence of decreased breath sounds on the right to basal region. Crepitations were present. The cardiovascular system was normal except for tachycardia. The CNS was normal. The tourniquet test was positive with the appearance of more rashes.

■ INVESTIGATION

- *Hemoglobin:* 8 g/dL
- *TLC:* 14,200 cells/mm^3
- *DLC:* $P_{68}L_{28}E_2M_2$
- *ESR:* 40 mm in the first hour
- *Platelet count:* 35,000 cells/mm^3
- *PCV:* 60 per cent
- *PT:* 12 seconds
- *SGPT:* 750 U/L (normal range 6–50 U/L)
- *Chest X-ray:* Pleural effusion
- *Ultrasound abdomen:* Mild ascites hepatomegaly
- *Stool occult blood:* Positive

■ DISCUSSION

Dengue fever, a benign syndrome caused by several arthropod viruses is characterized by biphasic fever, myalgia or arthralgia, rash, leukopenia, and lymphadenopathy. Dengue hemorrhagic fever (DHF) is an acute infectious thrombocytopenic purpura and is a severe often fatal, febrile disease caused by the dengue virus. It is characterized by capillary permeability, abnormalities of hemostasis, and in severe cases, protein-losing shock syndrome (dengue shock syndrome). It is currently thought to have an immunopathologic basis.

Dengue fever is a benign syndrome caused by several arthropod-borne viruses and is characterized by biphasic fever, myalgia or arthralgia, rash, leukopenia, and lymphadenopathy. DHF is a severe, often fatal, febrile disease caused by 1 of 4 dengue viruses. It is characterized by capillary permeability, abnormalities of hemostasis, and, in severe cases, a protein-losing shock syndrome (dengue shock syndrome), which is thought to have an immunopathologic basis. It occurs when multiple types of dengue virus are simultaneously or sequentially transmitted. It occurs in an endemic where warm temperatures and the practice of water storage at home, harboring the permanent population of *Aedes aegypti*.

■ PATHOGENESIS

Early in the acute stage of secondary dengue infections, there are 15 rapid activations of the complement system. Shortly before or during shock, blood levels of soluble tumor necrosis factor receptor, interferon-γ, and interleukin-2 are elevated. Clq, C3, C4, C5–C8, and C3 proactivators are depressed, and C3 catabolic rates are elevated. Circulating viral nonstructural protein 1 (NS1) is a viral toxin that activates myeloid cells to release cytokines by attaching to toll receptor 4. It also contributes to increased vascular permeability by activating complement, interacting with and damaging endothelial cells, and interacting with blood clotting factors and platelets.

There are at least four distinct antigenic types of dengue virus (dengue 1, 2, 3, and 4), members of the family *Flaviviridae*. In addition, three other arthropod-borne viruses (arboviruses) cause similar or identical febrile diseases with rash.

Two main pathophysiological changes occur. There is increased vascular permeability that gives rise to loss of plasma from the vascular compartment leading to hemoconcentration, low pulse pressure, and other signs of shock. There is a disorder in hemostasis involving thrombocytopenia, vascular changes, and coagulopathy. Platelet defects are both qualitative and quantitative. Maculopapular and peticheal rashes are present.

There is evidence that non-neutralizing antibodies promote cellular infection and enhance the severity of the disease. Dengue viruses demonstrate enhanced growth in cultures of human mononuclear phagocytes. There will be rapid activation of the complement system. Shortly before the shock, blood levels of soluble tumor necrosis factor receptor interferon-γ and interleukin 2 are elevated. These factors may interact with endothelial cells to produce increased vascular permeability through the nitric oxide final pathway.

The mechanism of bleeding in DHF is not known, but a mild degree of disseminated intravascular coagulopathy, liver damage, and thrombocytopenia may operate synergistically. Capillary damage allows fluid, electrolytes, small proteins, and, in some instances, red blood cells to leak into extravascular spaces. This internal redistribution of fluid, together with deficits caused by fasting, thirsting, and vomiting, results in hemoconcentration, hypovolemia, increased cardiac work, tissue hypoxia, metabolic acidosis, and hyponatremia.

The blood clotting and fibrinolytic systems are activated, and levels of factor XII are depressed. The mechanism of bleeding in DHF is not known. However, a mild degree of disseminated intravascular coagulation (DIC), liver damage, and thrombocytopenia may operate synergistically. Capillary damage allows fluid, electrolytes, small proteins, and red cells to lead into extravascular space. This results in hemoconcentration, hypovolemia, increased cardiac work, tissue hypoxia, metabolic acidosis, and hyponatremia.

Early in the acute stage of secondary dengue infections, there is rapid activation of the complement system. Shortly before or during shock, blood levels of soluble tumor necrosis factor receptor, interferon-γ, and interleukin 2 are elevated. Clq, C3, C4, C5–C8, and C3 proactivators are depressed, and C3 catabolic rates are elevated. These factors, the virus itself, or viral NS1 may interact with endothelial cells, blood clotting factors, and platelets to produce increased vascular permeability. The blood clotting and fibrinolytic systems are activated, and levels of factor XII (Hageman factor) are depressed.

Usually, deaths may be due to gastrointestinal or intracranial hemorrhage. Minimal to moderate hemorrhages are seen in the upper gastrointestinal tract (GIT). Petechial hemorrhages are common in the interventricular septum of the heart. Focal hemorrhages are occasionally seen in the lungs, liver, adrenals, and subarachnoid space. The liver is usually enlarged often with changes.

Microscopically there is perivascular edema in the soft tissues and widespread diapedesis of red cells. There may be maturational arrest of megakaryocytes in bone marrow and an increased number of them are seen in capillaries of the lungs, in renal glomeruli, and in sinusoids of the liver and spleen.

Criteria for clinical diagnosis of DHF:
- Clinical criteria
  - *Fever:* Acute onset, high continuous, and lasting for 2–7 days
  - *Hemorrhagic manifestation:* This includes at least a positive tourniquet test. The standard method using the blood pressure cuff is recommended. In DHF, the test usually gives a definite positive result, i.e., >20 petechiae/2.5 cm^2.
  - Enlargement of liver
- *Grading of severity of DHF:*
  - *Grade I:* Fever accompanied by nonspecific constitutional symptoms. The only hemorrhagic manifestation is a positive tourniquet test.
  - *Grade II:* The patient is characterized by spontaneous bleeding usually in the form of skin and other hemorrhagics in addition to the manifestation of grade I.
  - *Grade III:* Circulatory failure characterized by rapid and weak pulse narrowing the pulse pressure (20 mm Hg or less) or hypertension with the presence of cold clammy skin and rashes.
  - *Grade IV:* Profound shock and undetectable blood pressure and pulse.

In dengue shock syndrome, shock supervenes after a fever of 2–7 days. Skin becomes cool, bloately congested, and the pulse becomes rapid. The patient may be lethargic. There will be acute abdominal pain before the onset of shock. It is characterized by a rapid, weak pulse with the narrowing of pulse pressure or hypotension. Untreated shock ends fatally in 12–24 hours. If shock is overcome, complete recovery occurs within 2–3 days.

■ CLINICAL FEATURES (FIG. 1)

The incubation period is 1–7 days. The clinical manifestations are variable and are influenced by the age of the patient. In infants and young children, the disease may be undifferentiated or characterized by fever for 1–5 days, pharyngeal inflammation, rhinitis, and mild cough. A majority of infected older children and adults experience a sudden onset of fever, with temperature rapidly increasing to 39.4–41.1°C (103–106°F), usually accompanied by frontal or retroorbital pain, particularly when pressure is applied to the eyes. Occasionally, severe back pain precedes the fever (back-break fever).

A transient, macular, generalized rash that blanches under pressure may be seen during the first 24–48 hours of fever. The pulse rate

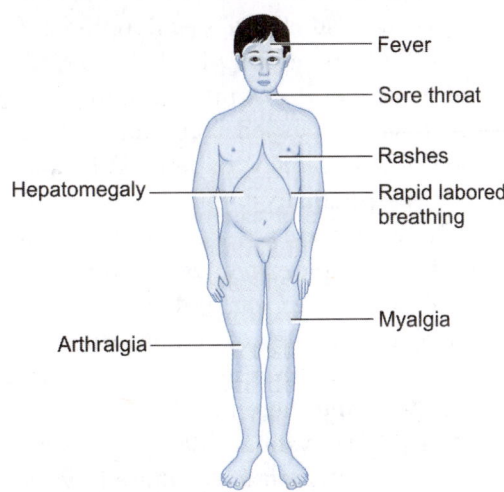

Fig. 1: Clinical features.

may be slow relative to the degree of fever. Myalgia and arthralgia occur soon after the onset of fevers and increase in severity over time. Joint symptoms may be particularly severe in patients with chikungunya infection. From the second to the sixth day of fever, nausea and vomiting are apt to occur, and generalized lymphadenopathy, cutaneous hyperesthesia or hyperalgesia, taste aberrations, and pronounced anorexia may develop.

Approximately 1–2 days after defervescence, a generalized, morbilliform, maculopapular rash appears that spares the palms and soles. It disappears in 1–5 days, desquamation may occur. Rarely there is edema of the palms and soles. About the time this second rash appears, the body temperature, which has previously decreased to normal, may become slightly elevated and demonstrate the characteristic biphasic temperature pattern.

Dengue Hemorrhagic Fever

Differentiation between dengue fever and DHF is difficult early in the course of illness. A relatively mild first phase with abrupt onset of fever, malaise, vomiting, headache, anorexia, and cough may be followed after 2–5 days by rapid clinical deterioration and collapse. In this second phase, the patient usually has cold, clammy extremities, a warm trunk, a flushed face, diaphoresis, restlessness, irritability, midepigastric pain, and decreased urinary output.

Frequently there are scattered petechiae on the forehead and extremities; spontaneous ecchymoses may appear, and easy bruising and bleeding at sites of venipuncture are common. A macular or maculopapular rash may appear, and there may be circumoral and peripheral cyanosis. Respirations are rapid and often labored. The pulse is weak, rapid, and thready and the heart sounds are faint. The liver may enlarge to 4–6 cm below the costal margin and is usually firm and somewhat tender.

Approximately 20–30% of cases of DHF are complicated by shock (dengue shock syndrome). Dengue shock can be subtle, arising in patients who are fully alert, and is accompanied by increased peripheral vascular resistance and raised diastolic blood pressure. Shock is not from congestive heart failure but from venous pooling. With increasing cardiovascular compromise, diastolic pressure rises toward the systolic level and the pulse pressure narrows. Fewer than 10% of patients have gross ecchymosis or gastrointestinal bleeding, usually after a period of uncorrected shock. After a 24–36 hours period of crisis, convalescence is fairly rapid in the children who recover. The temperature may return to normal before or during the stage of shock. Bradycardia and ventricular extrasystoles are common during convalescence.

Criteria for clinical diagnosis of DHF:
- Clinical criteria
- *Fever:* Acute onset, high continuous, and lasting for 2–7 days
- *Hemorrhagic manifestation:* This includes at least a positive tourniquet test. The standard method using the blood pressure cuff is recommended. In DHF, the test usually gives a definite positive result, i.e., >20 petechiae/2.5 cm^2.
- Enlargement of liver

GENERAL FEATURES
- Frontal and retroorbital pain
- Severe back pain
- Transient macular generalized rash
- Relative bradycardia
- Petechial and maculopapular rash
- Circumoral and peripheral cyanosis
- Gastrointestinal bleeding

Criteria for Discharge

- Afebrile for at least 24 hours
- Passing urine normally
- Improved appetite
- No respiratory distress
- Stable Hematocrit
- Platelet count >50,000/mm^3

ESSENTIAL DIAGNOSTIC POINTS

- Fever, sore throat, and retroorbital headache
- Myalgia arthralgia petechial maculopapular rashes
- Hepatomegaly
- Gastrointestinal bleeding
- Thrombocytopenia
- Disseminated intravascular coagulation (DIC)
- Low pulse pressure and circulatory failure
- Intracranial hemorrhage
- Respiratory distress

■ DIAGNOSIS

The World Health Organization criteria for DHF are fever (2–7 days in duration or biphasic), minor or major hemorrhagic manifestations, thrombocytopenia (100,000/μL), and objective evidence of increased capillary permeability (hematocrit increased by 20%), pleural effusion or ascites [by chest radiography or ultrasonography (USG)], or hypoalbuminemia. Dengue shock syndrome criteria include those for DHF as well as hypotension, tachycardia, narrow pulse pressure (<20 mm Hg), and signs of poor perfusion (cold extremities).

Virologic diagnosis can be established by serologic tests, by detection of viral proteins or viral RNA, or by the isolation of the virus from blood leukocytes or acute-phase serum. Following primary and secondary dengue infections, there is a relatively transient appearance of antidengue (immunoglobulin IgM) antibodies. These disappear after 6–12 weeks, a feature that can be used to time a dengue infection. In secondary dengue infections, most antibodies are of the IgG class.

Serologic diagnosis depends on a fourfold or greater increase in IgG antibody titer paired sera by HI, complement fixation, enzyme immunoassay (EIA), or neutralization test. Viral RNA can be detected in blood or tissues by specific complementary RNA probes or amplified first by PCR or by real-time PCR. A viral nonstructural protein, NS1, is released by infected cells into the circulation and can be detected in acute-stage blood samples using monoclonal or polyclonal antibodies. The detection of NS1 is the basis of commercial tests, including rapid lateral flow tests. These tests offer reliable point-of-care diagnosis of acute dengue infection.

Pancytopenia may occur after 3–4 days of illness. Hemoconcentration with an increase in hematocrit by 30% is present. There will be thrombocytopenia, prolonged bleeding time, and decreased prothrombin level. There is a moderate increase in transaminase level, raised blood urea nitrogen (BUN), and hypoalbuminemia. Neutropenia may persist or reappear during the latter stage of the disease and may continue into convalescence, with white blood cell counts < 2,000/mL. Platelet counts rarely fall below 100,000/mL. Venous clotting, bleeding and prothrombin times, and plasma fibrinogen values are within normal ranges. The tourniquet test result may be positive.

Mild acidosis, hemoconcentration, increased transaminase values, and hypoproteinemia may occur during some primary dengue virus infections. The electrocardiogram (ECG) may show sinus bradycardia, ectopic ventricular foci flattened T waves, and prolongation of the P-R interval.

The most common hematologic abnormalities during DHF and dengue shock syndrome are hemoconcentration with an increase of >20% in hematocrit, thrombocytopenia, prolonged bleeding time, and a moderately decreased prothrombin level that is seldom <40% of control. Fibrinogen levels may be subnormal, and fibrin split-product values are elevated.

Other abnormalities include moderate elevations of serum transaminase levels, consumption of complement, mild metabolic acidosis with hyponatremia, occasionally hypochloremia, slight elevation of serum urea nitrogen, and hypoalbuminemia.

Radiographs of the chest reveal pleural effusions (right > left) in nearly all patients with dengue shock syndrome. USG can be used to detect serosal effusions of the thorax or abdomen. Thickening of the gallbladder wall and the presence of perivascular fluid are characteristic signs of increased vascular permeability.

Laboratory Diagnosis

> **LABORATORY SALIENT FINDINGS**
> - Thrombocytopenia
> - Hemoconcentration or raising hematocrit
> - Serological tests
> - Isolation of virus from blood leukocytes or serum
> - Presence of antidengue immunoglobulin; IgM
> - Pancytopenia
> - Abdominal ultrasonography reveals ascites
> - Chest X-ray shows pleural effusion

Confirmation of diagnosis of dengue may be established by following: Direct methods; including (1) virus isolation by culture, (2) genome detection by PCR, and (3) NS1 antigen detection and indirect methods; including (1) IgM detection and (2) IgG detection.

Virus isolation or PCR requires the sample to be obtained within the first 5 days of fever, is technically demanding, not universally available, expensive, and hence of limited practical use. NS1 antigen is a highly conserved glycoprotein of dengue virus and secreted during the initial phase of illness. It disappears as the antibodies appear and hence declines as the illness advances and in secondary dengue infections. The specificity is near 100% and sensitivity in the first 4 days of illness is 90% in primary dengue and 70% in secondary dengue infection.

Antibody determination needs careful interpretation. Following primary dengue infection, 80% of patients will have detectable IgM antibodies by day 5 and 99% by day 10. IgM antibodies peak by day 14 and are undetectable by 2–3 months. IgG antibodies rise later, peak to levels lower than IgM, decline slowly, and remain detectable at low levels for life. Therefore, the diagnosis of primary dengue infection is based on the elevation of IgM.

■ DIFFERENTIAL DIAGNOSIS

- Upper respiratory tract infection
- Influenza
- Malaria
- Yellow fever
- Leptospirosis
- Viral hepatitis

■ COMPLICATIONS

- Dyselectrolytemia
- Hyperpyrexia
- Febrile convulsion
- Epistaxis
- Gastrointestinal bleeding

■ TREATMENT

Treatment of uncomplicated dengue fever is supportive. Bed rest is advised during the febrile period. Antipyretics should be used to keep the body temperature <40°C. Analgesic and mild radiation may be required. Fluid and electrolyte replacement is required for the deficits caused by sweating, fasting, vomiting, and diarrhea.

In the case of DHF, immediate evaluation of the vital signs and degree of hemoconcentration, dehydration, and electrolyte imbalance should be done. Close monitoring is essential for at least 48 hours because shock may occur or recur. Patients who are cyanotic and labored breathing should be given oxygen. When elevation of hematocrit persists after the replacement of fluid, plasma or plasma colloids are indicated. Care must be taken to avoid overhydration. Fresh blood and platelet transfusion should not be given at the time of hemoconcentration.

Bed rest is advised. Antipyretic is advised. Aspirin is avoided because of gastritis, bleeding, and acidosis. A rise in hematocrit indicates significant plasma loss and a need for parenteral fluid therapy. For grades I and II—volume replacement should be done for 12-24 hours. The required fluid volume should be charted on a 2-3 hours basis. The rate of administration is adjusted throughout for 24-48 hours. Serial hematocrit every 4-6 hours and frequent recording of vital signs should be done to avoid fluid overload. The type of fluid are:
- *Crystalloid*:
    - 5% dextrose in Ringer's lactate (RL)
    - 5% dextrose in normal saline (NS)
- *Colloids:* Dextrose 40 and plasma

Paraldehyde may be required for agitated children. DIC should be managed accordingly. Hypovolemia during the fluid reabsorption phase may be life-threatening and is heralded by a fall in hematocrit with a wide pulse presence. Diuretics and digitalization may be necessary.

Severe dengue should be hospitalized and treated with NS or RL; 10-20 mL/kg is infused over 1 hour or as a bolus if blood pressure is not recordable. In critically sick children it is preferable to use two IV lines. One is for NS and the other is for infusing 5% dextrose. If there is no improvement in vital parameters, PCV rises, and colloids 10 mL/kg are given rapidly. If PCV is falling without improvement in vital parameters, blood transfusion is indicated. When massive bleeding cannot be managed with fresh whole blood/fresh packed cells and there is the possibility of DIC, a combination of fresh frozen plasma and platelet concentrates should be considered.

Dextran sulfate sodium (DSS) indicates significant dehydration. Immediate rapid volume replacement is required. Rapid IV 10-20 mL/kg over 20 minutes is recommended. They may be followed by another bolus. If hematocrit is rising plasma or 5% albumin (10-20 mL/kg) as rapid bolus in 20 minutes, is repeated if necessary.

If shock still persists, hematocrit is checked. Declining hematocrit suggests internal bleeding. Fresh whole blood 10 mL/kg is advised if hematocrit is >35%, concentrated platelet transfusion or fresh frozen plasma is indicated in cases of coagulopathy producing massive bleeding.

Dengue Hemorrhagic Fever and Dengue Shock Syndrome

Dengue shock syndrome is a medical emergency that may occur in any child with a recent travel history to a tropical destination. Management begins with diagnostic suspicion and the understanding that shock often occurs during defervescence.

Management of DHF and dengue shock syndrome includes immediate evaluation of vital signs and degrees of hemoconcentration, dehydration, and electrolyte imbalance. Close monitoring is essential for at least 48 hours, because shock may occur or recur precipitously early in the disease. Patients who are cyanotic or have labored breathing should be given oxygen.

Rapid IV replacement of fluids and electrolytes can frequently sustain patients until spontaneous recovery occurs. NS is more effective than the more expensive RL saline in treating shock. When pulse pressure is >30 mm Hg or when the elevation of the hematocrit persists after replacement of fluids, plasma, or colloid preparations are indicated.

Transfusions of fresh blood or platelets suspended in plasma may be required to control bleeding; they should not be given during hemoconcentration but only after the evaluation of hemoglobin or hematocrit values. Salicylates are contraindicated because of their effect on blood clotting.

COMPLICATIONS

Fluid overload should be managed by oral frusemide 0.1–0.5mg/kg/dose once or twice daily or continuous infusion of frusemide 0.1 mg/kg/hour may be administered judiciously.

Hypervolemia during the fluid resorptive phase may be life-threatening and is heralded by a decrease in hematocrit with wide pulse pressure. Diuretics and digitalization may be necessary.

Primary infections with dengue fever and dengue-like diseases are usually self-limited and benign. Fluid and electrolyte losses, hyperpyrexia, and febrile convulsions are the most frequent complications in infants and young children. Epistaxis, petechiae, and purpuric lesions are uncommon but may occur at any stage. Blood from epistaxis that is swallowed, vomited, or passed by the rectum may be erroneously interpreted as gastrointestinal bleeding. In adults and possibly in children, underlying conditions may lead to clinically significant bleeding. Convulsions may occur during high temperatures, especially with chikungunya fever. Infrequently, after the febrile stage, prolonged asthenia, mental depression, bradycardia, and ventricular extrasystoles may occur in children.

PROGNOSIS

Dengue Fever

The prognosis is good. Care should be taken to avoid the use of drugs that suppress platelet activity.

Dengue Hemorrhagic Fever

The prognosis of DHF is adversely affected by late diagnosis and delayed or improper treatment. Death has occurred in 40–50% of patients with shock, but with adequate intensive care, deaths should occur in <1% of cases. Infrequently, there is residual brain damage as a consequence of prolonged shock or occasionally of PBMl hemorrhage. Many fatalities are caused by overhydration.

BIBLIOGRAPHY

1. Cleton N, Koopmans M, Reimerink J, Godeke GJ, Reusken C. Come fly with me: review of clinically important arboviruses for global travelers. J Clin Virol 2012;55(3):191-203.
2. Guzman MG, Harris E. Dengue. Lancet. 2015;385(9966)453-65.
3. Simmons CP, Farrar JJ, Nguyen vV, Wills B. Dengue. N Engl J Med. 2012;366(15):1423-32.
4. Lodha R, Kabra SK. Dengue infection: Challenges and the way forward. Indian J Peditr. 2015;82(12):1077-9.
5. Royal College Physicians of Thailand (RCPT). Practical guidelines for the management of dengue in adults: 2014. Southeast Asian J Trop Med Public Health. 2015;46(Suppl 1): 169-85.

CASE 69

Herpes Zoster

■ PRESENTING COMPLAINTS

An 8-year-old boy was brought with the complaints of:
- Chest pain since 5 days
- Skin lesion since 2 days

History of Presenting Complaints

An 8-year-old boy was brought to pediatric outpatient department with the history of onset of chest pain on the right side. The chest pain was not associated with any respiratory symptoms. It was not related to intake of food. Child had been taken to nearby clinic and he was prescribed some analgesics. But pain was not relieved. After two days boy noticed some skin lesions at the site of chest pain. Skin lesion includes small vesicles. Itching was present along the lesion. Gradually, the skin lesions increased in number along with one plane. Then again, he was taken to pediatric outpatient department, where it was diagnosed.

Past History of the Patient

The patient was the first child of nonconsanguineous marriage. He was born at full term by normal delivery. There was no significant postnatal event. He was on exclusive breast milk for 4 months. Later, weaning was started, and he was on family food by 18 months. His developmental milestones were normal. He had been completely immunized.

CASE AT A GLANCE

Basic Findings
Height	: 130 cm (90th centile)
Weight	: 26 kg (80th centile)
Temperature	: 37°C
Pulse rate	: 96 beats/min
Respiratory rate	: 20 breaths/min
Blood pressure	: 90/60 mm Hg

Positive Findings

History:
- Chest pain
- Vesicular lesion

Examination:
- Vesicular lesion on the dermatome

Investigation:
- *Tzanck preparation:* Showed multinucleated giant cells

■ EXAMINATION

On examination, the boy looked very well built and nourished. He was in agony with pain. Anthropometric measurements included the height of 130 cm (90th centile) and the weight of 26 kg (80th centile).

He was afebrile, the pulse rate was 96 beats per minute, and the respiratory rate was 20 breaths per minute. Blood pressure recorded was 90/60 mm Hg. There was no pallor, no lymphadenopathy, no cyanosis, and no edema. Small vesicular skin lesions were present at the infrascapular and inframammary region on the right side. Other systemic examinations were normal.

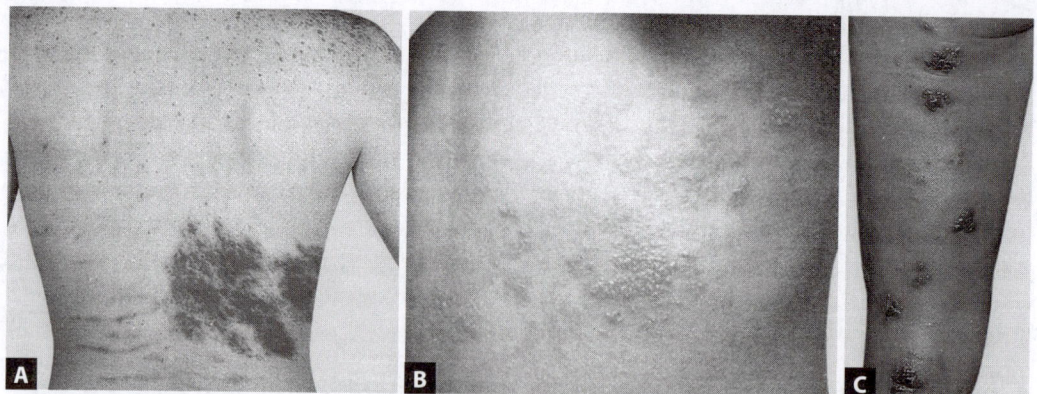

Figs. 1A to C: (A) Herpes zoster rash; (B) Vesicular rash; (C) S1 Dermatome. *(For color version, see Plate 4)*

■ INVESTIGATION

- *Hemoglobin:* 13 g/dL
- *TLC:* 7,600 cells/mm^3
- *ESR:* 22 mm in the 1st hour
- *X-ray chest:* Normal
- *Tzanck preparation:* Showed multinucleated giant cells

■ DISCUSSION

The boy presented with vesicular skin lesion at the right infrascapular region and inframammary region along with the dermatome is characteristic of herpes zoster. It is caused by varicella zoster virus (VZV). The reaction occurs many months or years after the attack of chickenpox. It occurs in dorsal spinal or cranial nerve ganglion. This spreads to appropriate cutaneous dermatome **(Figs. 1A to C)**.

Varicella zoster virus is one of the nine human herpesviruses, which include herpes simplex virus (HSV) types 1 and 2 **(Fig. 2)**, CMV, Epstein–Barr virus (EBV), and human herpesviruses 6A, 6B, 7, and 8. As with HSV-1 and HSV-2, VZV establishes latency in sensory or autonomic ganglia following primary infection, with the ability for subsequent reactivation.

The incidence of herpes zoster is highest in elderly individuals and in immunosuppressed patients. Spread from a contact with varicella is by respiratory secretions or fomites from vesicles or pustules, with a >95% infection rate in susceptible persons.

Herpes zoster is caused by the reactivation of latent VZV. It is not common in childhood and shows no seasonal variation in incidence. Herpes zoster is unusual in healthy children younger than 10 years of age, with the exception of those infected with VZV in utero, or in the 1st year of life, who have an increased risk for development of zoster in the 1st few years of life. Herpes zoster in otherwise healthy children tends to be milder than herpes zoster in adults, is less frequently associated with acute pain, and is generally not associated with postherpetic neuralgia.

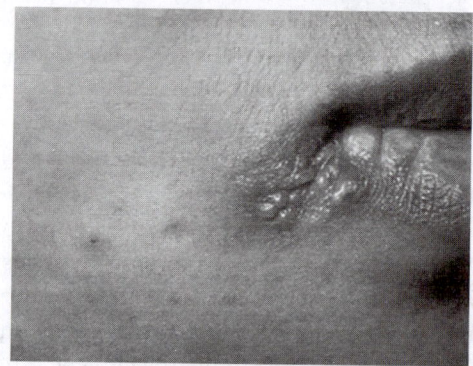

Fig. 2: Herpes simplex vesicles. *(For color version, see Plate 4)*

Varicella zoster virus causes primary, latent, and recurrent infections. The primary infection is manifested as varicella (chickenpox) and results in establishment of a lifelong latent infection of sensory ganglion neurons. Reactivation of the latent infection causes herpes zoster (shingles). Although often a mild illness of childhood, varicella can cause substantial morbidity and mortality in otherwise healthy children. Morbidity and mortality are higher in immunocompetent infants, adolescents, and adults as well as in immunocompromised persons. Varicella predisposes to severe group A *Streptococcus* and *Staphylococcus aureus* infections. A clinically modified disease can occur among vaccinated persons (breakthrough varicella), usually with milder presentation. Varicella and herpes zoster can be treated with antiviral drugs.

PATHOGENESIS

Humans are the only source of infection of VZV. Transmission occurs when aerosolized virus from skin lesions comes into contact with the mucosa of the upper respiratory tract or conjunctivae of susceptible people. Although it was long thought that the source of infection was the respiratory tract of infected individuals, very limited virus has been recovered from an infected person's airways and probably represents a much more limited source of infection than aerosolization from skin lesions.

The infectious period extends from up to 48 hours before the appearance of rash until all skin lesions are crusted over, usually about 5 days in normal hosts. Following infectious contact, the incubation period for varicella is 10–21 days and up to 28 days following a dose of varicella-zoster immunoglobin (VARIZIG).

Infection of cells within the respiratory tract or conjunctivae by inhaled virions is followed by cell-associated spread to local lymph nodes, viremia, and then the development of the vesicular rash approximately 5 days later. Virus can be detected in circulating lymphocytes and monocytes. Cell-to-cell spread of virus within the skin creates infected syncytia with a striking disruption of normal cellular architecture, and VZV-infected keratinocytes that appear to elicit a vigorous type-1 interferon response in neighboring, uninfected cells that restrains horizontal spread of virus, and thus may contribute to the topology of the rash.

Immunocompromised children may have more severe herpes zoster, similar to the situation in adults, including postherpetic neuralgia. Immunocompromised patients may also experience disseminated cutaneous disease that mimics varicella, with or without initial dermatomal rash, as well as visceral dissemination with pneumonia, hepatitis, encephalitis, and disseminated intravascular coagulopathy. Severely immunocompromised children, particularly those with advanced human immunodeficiency virus (HIV) infection, may have unusual, chronic, or relapsing cutaneous disease, retinitis, or CNS disease without rash.

In the immunocompetent host, VZV viremia and the appearance of new skin lesions are curtailed within a few days by a vigorous cellular immune response comprising both natural killer (NK) and antigen-specific (T-cell) components. Conversely, the failure to mount antigen-specific cellular responses is associated with progressive viral replication and dissemination and a potentially fatal outcome.

Individuals with disorders purely of humoral immunity do not suffer unusually severe or repeated episodes of varicella, indicating that cellular immunity affords sufficient protection against primary infection. However, a host humoral response is detectable within 4 days of the onset of the rash and can confer passive immunity; thus, pooled immunoglobulin derived from VZV-immune donors, known as VARIZIG, can be used to protect VZV-exposed subjects at high risk of severe varicella. The presence of VZV-specific antibodies is also the best available correlate of protection against primary infection but is irrelevant to the risk of secondary (reactivation) disease.

Along with measles, varicella is one of the most highly communicable infections in humans, with household attack rates approaching 90%. In the absence of widespread vaccination, outbreaks of varicella occur readily within groups of susceptible children. In unvaccinated populations in temperate climates, seasonal peaks of varicella occur in the spring. These epidemics occur on a background of endemic disease, and 84% of children acquire infection by age 15 years. In contrast, the incidence of varicella in the tropics does not vary by season and tends to be delayed until adolescence or adult life.

Virus also reaches the ganglia by the hematogenous route and subsequent reactivation of latent virus causes herpes zoster, a vesicular rash that usually is dermatomal in distribution. During herpes zoster, necrotic changes may be produced in the neurons and surrounding satellite cells and associated ganglia.

The skin lesions of varicella and herpes zoster have identical histopathology, and infectious VZV is present in both. Varicella elicits humoral and cell-mediated immunity that is highly protective against symptomatic reinfection. Suppression of cell-mediated immunity to VZV correlates with an increased risk for VZV reactivation as herpes zoster.

■ CLINICAL FEATURES (FIG. 3)

Exposure to varicella or herpes zoster in the child has usually occurred 14-16 days previously (range 10-21 days). Contact may not have been recognized, since the index case is infectious 1-2 days before rash appears. Although varicella is the most distinctive childhood exanthema, inexperienced observers may mistake other diseases for varicella.

1-3 days prodrome of fever, respiratory symptoms, and headache may occur, especially in older children. The preeruptive pain of herpes zoster may last several days and be mistaken for other illnesses.

Herpes zoster manifests as vesicular lesions clustered within one or, less commonly, two adjacent dermatomes. In the elderly, herpes zoster typically begins with burning pain followed by clusters of skin lesions in a dermatomal pattern.

The eruption of shingles involves a single dermatome, usually truncal or cranial. The rash does not cross the midline. Ophthalmic zoster may be associated with corneal involvement. The closely grouped vesicles,

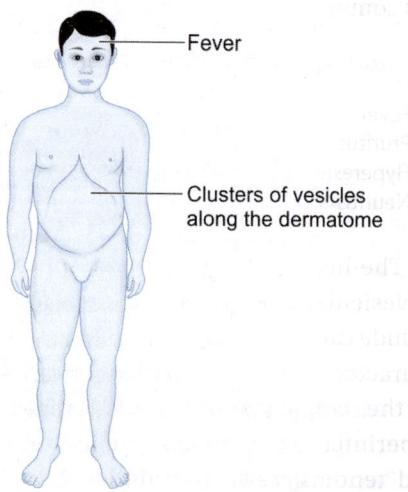

Fig. 3: Clinical features.

which resemble a localized version of varicella or herpes simplex, often coalesce. The duration is 7–10 days before crusting.

Postherpetic neuralgia is rare in children. A few vesicles are occasionally seen outside the involved dermatome. Herpes zoster is a common problem in HIV-infected or other immunocompromised children. Herpes zoster is also common in children who had varicella in early infancy or whose mothers had varicella during pregnancy.

Unlike herpes zoster in adults, zoster in children is infrequently associated with localized pain, hyperesthesia, pruritus, low-grade fever, or complications. In children, the rash is mild, with new lesions appearing for a few days; symptoms of acute neuritis are minimal; and complete resolution usually occurs within 1–2 weeks. An increased risk for herpes zoster early in childhood has been described in children who acquire infection with VZV in utero or in the 1st year of life.

The finding of a lower risk for herpes zoster among vaccinated children with leukemia than in those who have had varicella suggested that the vaccine virus reactivates less commonly than wild-type VZV.

GENERAL FEATURES
- Fever
- Pruritus
- Hyperesthesia
- Neuritis

The history should exclude other cases of vesicular disease. Examination should include careful inspection of the number and character of the vesicles, and the evidence of the complications such as bacterial superinfection, cutaneous dissemination, and tenderness in the abdomen or liver. Fifth cranial nerve involvement produces the possibility of keratoconjunctivitis, uveitis, or both.

ESSENTIAL DIAGNOSTIC POINTS
- History of varicella
- Local paresthesia and pain to eruption
- Dermatomal distribution of grouped vesicles on erythematous base
- *Distribution of rash:* 50% thoracic, 20% cervical, 20% lumbosacral, and 10% cranial nerve

■ COMPLICATIONS

Complications of herpes zoster include secondary bacterial infection, motor or cranial nerve paralysis (1 per 200 cases in adults), encephalitis, keratitis, and dissemination in immunosuppressed patients. These complications are rare in immunocompetent children, and they do not develop prolonged pain. Postherpetic neuralgia does occur in immunocompromised children.

■ DIAGNOSIS

The diagnosis of VZV infection is usually made clinically. VZV is difficult to culture and requires fluid to be obtained from vesicles in the first few days of eruption. When successful, cytopathic effects in cell culture take many days. Detection of VZV DNA using a PCR test, currently, is the diagnostic method of choice. This testing may be used to distinguish between wild-type and vaccine-strain VZV, using genotyping, as well as to predict susceptibility to antiviral drugs.

During the acute phase of illness, the highest diagnostic yield is to test skin lesions by vesicular fluid aspiration or by swabbing or scraping the scab from crusted skin lesions. Early in the infection, VZV may be detected by PCR testing of saliva or buccal mucosal swabs. Tissue biopsy samples, blood, and CSF also can be tested by PCR to confirm the diagnosis. Direct fluorescent antibody (DFA) assay can detect VZV using scrapings of a vesicle base in the first 3–4 days of the eruption and can provide a result quickly; however, the test is not as sensitive as PCR.

A number of sensitive serologic tests are available to measure antibodies to VZV. These include the fluorescent antibody to membrane antigen (FAMA) method, latex agglutination, and enzyme-linked immunosorbent assay. Antibody to VZV develops within a few days after onset of varicella, persists for many years, and is present before the onset of zoster. VZV infections may be documented by a 2–4-fold rise in VZV antibody titer in acute and convalescent-phase serum specimens. Persistence of VZV antibody in infants beyond 8 months of age is highly suggestive of intrauterine varicella. Immunity to varicella is highly likely to be present if a positive titer of antibody (measured by a reliable assay) to VZV is demonstrated with a single serum sample from a child or an adult with no history of disease.

Leukocyte counts are normal or low. Leukocytosis suggests secondary bacterial infection. Multinucleated giant cells in a stained cytologic scraping from a vesicle base (Tzanck test) will indicate the presence of either a VZV or herpes simplex infection. Further distinction is usually made on clinical grounds.

> **LABORATORY SALIENT FINDINGS**
> - *Tzanck preparation:* Multinucleated giant cell
> - Fluorescent antibody staining of lesion smear
> - Serology
> - Elevated serum aminotransferase

■ DIFFERENTIAL DIAGNOSIS

Herpes zoster is sometimes confused with a linear eruption of herpes simplex or a contact dermatitis. Differential diagnoses include the following:
- Atopic dermatitis
- Contact dermatitis
- Seborrheic dermatitis
- Impetigo contagiosa

■ TREATMENT

Treatment with antiviral therapy is dependent on host factors. Antiviral therapy is not recommended for otherwise healthy children with varicella if they are <12 years of age, although some would recommend the use of oral acyclovir or valacyclovir for the treatment of secondary household cases as they tend to experience more severe disease. In these children, benefit is only derived if therapy is started promptly as viral replication only occurs in the first 72 hours of illness.

Oral acyclovir or valacyclovir should be considered for persons who are at an increased risk for severe varicella such as unvaccinated persons older than 12 years, people with chronic cutaneous or pulmonary disorders, people receiving long-term salicylate therapy, and people receiving short, intermittent, or inhaled courses of corticosteroids. Oral acyclovir or valacyclovir should be considered for pregnant women with varicella, with IV acyclovir being administered for more severe disease.

Acyclovir is used especially in immunocompromised person with increasing number of new vesicles, failure of vesicle maturation, abnormal LFTs, and onset of respiratory and CNS symptoms. The dose is 30 mg/kg/day in 3 divided doses for 7 days.

Antiviral drugs are effective for treatment of herpes zoster. In healthy adults, acyclovir (800 mg 5 times a day orally, for 5–7 days), famciclovir (500 mg tid orally, for 7 days), and valacyclovir (1,000 mg tid orally, for 7 days) reduce the duration of the illness and the risk for development of postherpetic neuralgia. In otherwise healthy children, herpes zoster is a less-severe disease, and postherpetic neuralgia usually does not occur. Therefore, treatment of uncomplicated herpes zoster in a child with an antiviral agent may not always be necessary, although some experts would treat with oral acyclovir (20 mg/kg/dose; maximum; 800 mg/dose)4 times a day for 5 days, to shorten the duration of the illness. It is important to start antiviral therapy as soon as possible. Delay beyond 72 hours from onset of rash limits its effectiveness.

Intravenous acyclovir (10 mg/kg every 8 hours) therapy is recommended for all immunocompromised patients, including patients receiving high-dose corticosteroids for 14 days or more. Therapy should be initiated as soon as possible and should continue until no new lesions develop and all lesions have crusted over.

In contrast, herpes zoster in immunocompromised children can be severe, and disseminated disease may be life-threatening. Patients at high risk for disseminated disease should receive IV acyclovir (500 mg/m or 10 mg/kg every 8 hours). Oral acyclovir, famciclovir, and valacyclovir are options for immunocompromised patients with uncomplicated herpes zoster, who are considered at low risk for visceral dissemination. Neuritis with herpes zoster should be managed with appropriate analgesics.

Valacyclovir, which has improved oral bioavailability over oral acyclovir and has been shown to achieve serum levels comparable to IV acyclovir, can be considered in selected circumstances. IV acyclovir also is indicated for both term and preterm neonates who develop varicella from their mothers, and it should be considered for neonates who develop varicella following household exposure. Oral acyclovir is generally not indicated for treatment of young infants because of limited bioavailability and unreliable absorption in infants.

Wet-to-dry soaks are applied to the involved dermatome. Superficial infection is treated with penicillinase-resistant oral penicillin and topical antibiotics.

Analgesics are used to treat the pain. There is no indication for systemic steroids. Scopolamine eyedrops are used to produce mydriasis and cycloplegia. Corticosteroid drops are indicated when interstitial keratitis or uveitis is present and disseminated skin vesicles are seen.

■ BIBLIOGRAPHY

1. American Academy of Pediatrics Committee on Infectious Diseases. Varicella-zoster infections. Red book, 2015 Report of the Committee on Infectious Diseases, 30th edition. Elk Grove Village, IL: AAP publications; 2015. pp. 846-60. [online] Available from https://publications.aap.org/aapbooks/book/498/Red-Book-2015-2015-Report-of-the-Committee-on [Last accessed June, 2024].
2. Chen JJ, Gershon AA, Li Z, Cowles RA, Gershon MD. Varicella zoster virus (VZV) infects and establishes latency in enteric neurons. J Neurovirol. 2011;17(6):578-89.
3. Shapiro ED, Vazquez M, Esposito D, Holabird N, Steinberg SP, Dziura J, et al. Effectiveness of 2 doses of varicella vaccine in children. J Infect Dis. 2011;203(3):312-5.

CASE 70

Human Immunodeficiency Virus

■ PRESENTING COMPLAINTS

A 3-month-old boy was brought with the complaints of:
- Not gaining weight since birth
- Loose motion since 2 months
- Cold and cough since 1 month

History of Presenting Complaints

A 3-month-old boy was brought with the history of not gaining sufficient weight. Mother told that her son's birth weight was 3 kg. It has come down to 2.6 kg when she had checked 2 days back. The child was on exclusive breast milk. Mother also gave the history of loose motion 5–6 times a day since 2 months. She had shown the boy to the nearby practitioner. Mother also revealed the history of repeated attack of cold and cough for which she was showing him to the doctor. As the child was not gaining weight, and because of repeated health problems, it was referred to hospital for the further management.

Past History of the Patient

The patient is the first child of the consanguineous marriage. He was born at full term by vaginal normal delivery. He cried immediately after the delivery. Cry of the child was good. He was on breastfeeds immediately after the delivery. His postnatal period was uneventful. He has received all basic immunization till date.

CASE AT A GLANCE

Basic Findings
Length	:	53 cm (48th centile)
Weight	:	2.6 kg (40th centile)
Temperature	:	39°C
Pulse rate	:	120 beats/min
Respiratory rate	:	28 breaths/min
Blood Pressure	:	50/70 mm Hg

Positive Findings
- Not gaining weight
- Loose motion
- Cold and cough

Examination:
- Poorly built
- Emaciated
- Febrile
- Tachypnea
- Cervical lymphadenopathy
- Hepatosplenomegaly
- Crepitation and rhonchi at lungs

Investigations:
- *Hemoglobin:* Decreased
- *ESR:* Raised
- *Chest X-ray:* Bronchopneumonia
- *USG:* Hepatosplenomegaly
- *CRP:* Positive
- *IgG:* Positive
- *Virology:* Positive

There was a significant history of blood transfusion to the mother for the correction of hemoglobin in the antenatal period.

■ EXAMINATION

On examination, the baby was poorly built and emaciated. These was a loss of pad of fat over the buttocks. The anthropometric measurements included that the height was 53 cm (48th centile) and weight was 2.6 kg (40th centile). The head circumference was 36 cm.

Baby was febrile (39°C). The pulse rate was 120 beats per minute and respiratory rate was 28 breaths per minute. Mild costal retraction was present. Signs of moderate dehydration were present. Blood pressure recorded was 50/70 mm Hg. Cervical lymphadenopathy was present. Per abdomen examination revealed the presence of the hepatosplenomegaly. Respiratory system revealed the presence of crepitation and rhonchi. Cardiovascular system was normal.

■ INVESTIGATION

- *Hemoglobin:* 9.8 g/dL
- *TLC:* 2,800 cells/dL
- *DLC:* $P_{76}L_{20}M_2E_2$
- *ESR:* 50 mm in the 1st hour
- *AEC:* 700 cells/mm^3
- *Chest X-ray:* Suggestive of bronchopneumonia
- *USG AG:* Hepatosplenomegaly
- *CRP:* Positive
- *IgG antibody:* Positive
- *Mantoux test:* Negative
- *Virology:*
  - HIV DNA: Positive
  - HIV PCR: Positive

■ DISCUSSION

Human immunodeficiency virus has become an important cause of childhood morbidity and mortality, especially in developing countries.

The human immunodeficiency virus (HIV-1) and HIV-2 are members of the Retroviridae family. They belong to the *lentivirus* genus. HIV-1 genome has three major regions: Gag region, Pol region, and Env region. The major external protein of HIV-1 is a heavily glycosylated gp120 protein. This contains the binding site for cluster of differentiation-4 (CD_4) molecules. This is the most common T-lymphocyte surface receptor for HIV. Most HIV strains have a specific tropism for one of the chemokines, fusion-inducing molecule, and C-X-C chemokine receptor 4 (CXCR-4).

Conformational changes occur in gp120 and CD4 molecules following the viral attachment. This allows gp41 to interact with the fusion receptor on the cell surface. This results in the entry of viral ribonucleic acid (RNA) into the cell cytoplasm. Viral reverse transcriptase enzyme will transcribe the viral deoxyribonucleic acid (DNA) copies from the virus. RNA duplication of DNA produces double-stranded circular DNA. The circular DNA is transported into the cell nucleus. Here, it is integrated into the chromosomal DNA. This is called provirus. The proviruses can remain dominant for a long period.

Human immunodeficiency virus-1 transcription is followed by translation. This results in a capsid polyprotein. This is cleaved to produce the virus-specific protease. This is a critical enzyme for HIV-1. The RNA genome is then incorporated into the newly formed viral capsid. As the new virus is formed, it buds through the cell membrane and is released.

Human immunodeficiency virus-1 is transmitted via sexual contact, parental exposure to blood, and/or vertical transmission from mother to child. The primary route of infection in the pediatric population is vertical transmission.

Vertical transmission of HIV can occur during the intrauterine, intrapartum period, or through the breast feeding. 30% of infected newborns are infected in utero. The highest percentages of HIV-infected children require the virus intrapartum. Breastfeeding is an important route of transmission. Transfusion of the infected blood or blood products have been accounted for all pediatric acquired immunodeficiency syndrome (AIDS) cases.

The risk factors for vertical transmission include preterm delivery (<34-week gestation), a low maternal antenatal CD4 count, >4-hour duration of ruptured membrane, and birth weight <2,500 g.

■ PATHOGENESIS

If the intrauterine infection coincides with the period of rapid expansion of CD4 cells in the fetus, this could effectively infect the majority of the body's immunocompetent cells.

The mechanisms by which HIV infection causes this CD4+ cell decline are not completely established, although possibilities include ongoing lytic infection, destruction of infected cells by host antiviral immune mechanisms, and death or dysfunction of lymphocyte precursors or accessory cells in the thymus and lymph nodes.

Once established, HIV-1 infection invariably persists. In the absence of antiretroviral therapy (ART), HIV continuously replicates and infects newly activated CD4+ T lymphocytes. Ongoing generation of viral variants bearing escape mutations in immune epitopes contributes to evasion of host-neutralizing antibodies and cytotoxic T cells. Additionally, HIV-I genomes integrate into the host chromosomal DNA to establish latent infection. Resting memory CD4+ T lymphocytes appear to be the most important reservoir of latent HIV-1 infection. These cells stably harbor HIV-1 genomes even after years of viral suppression with ART, allowing viral rebound when ART is stopped. Early initiation of combination antiretroviral therapy (cART) may limit the extent of the latent viral reservoir.

In addition to CD4+ T lymphocytes, other cell types such as tissue-resident macrophages can also be infected by HIV-1. These cells may also function as long-term viral reservoirs and contribute to organ-specific pathology, although some controversy remains. Even in individuals well controlled on cART, HIV-1 DNA may be recovered from brain, lung, liver, kidney, testes, and other tissues. HIV-1-related pathology involves many organs, although it is often difficult to know whether injury is primarily a consequence of local virus infection, immune-mediated cytotoxic effects, or associated infectious complications.

A majority of the prenatally-infected newborns will show much slower progression of disease with a median survival time of 6 years.

CD4 cell depletion may be less dramatic because infants normally have a relative lymphocytosis. Lymphopenia is relatively rare.

B-cell activation occurs in most children. This occurs early in infection as evidenced by hypergammaglobulinemia associated with the high levels of anti-HIV-1 antibody. This response may reflect both dysregulation of T-cell suppression of B-cell antibody synthesis and active CD4 enhancement of B-lymphocyte humoral responses.

■ CLINICAL FEATURES (FIG. 1)

Human immunodeficiency virus-1 infection stage is determined by age-based CD4+ T-cell count criteria. CD4+ T-cell percentage is used for staging when absolute CD4+ T-cell counts are not available. Patients with specific AIDS-defining clinical illnesses indicative of severe immunosuppression are classified as stage 3 regardless of CD4+ T-cell count.

Infant Infection

Perinatal HIV-I infection is most often clinically silent at birth. In some instances,

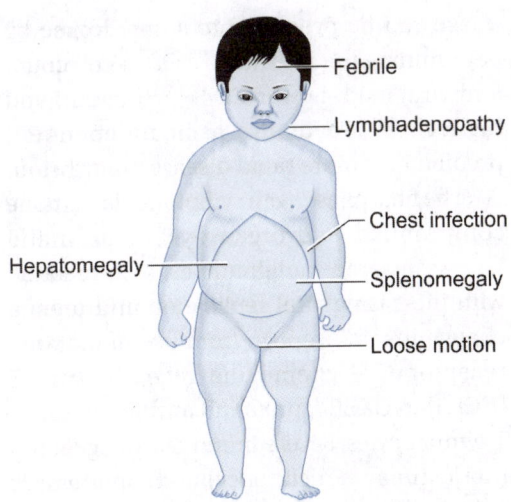

Fig. 1: Clinical features

adenopathy may be detected in the 1st month of life. The incubation period, or interval before symptoms of HIV-1 infection become manifest, is generally shorter following perinatal infection than in adult HIV-1 infection. Viral load [determined by HIV-1 RNA polymerase chain reaction (PCR) quantification] in infants is typically high (>10 copies/mL) and often does not decline to a stable set point for several years. This protracted high-level viremia is likely due to immune immaturity, but it may also reflect the high thymic output of CD4+ T lymphocytes in early childhood that essentially provides fuel for viral replication.

Clinically silent abnormalities of immune function often precede HIV-1 related symptoms. Hypergammaglobulinemia with production of nonfunctional antibodies (polyclonal B-cell stimulation) is more common among HIV-1-infected infants than among adults, typically noted as early as 3–6 months of age. Despite the abundance of immunoglobulins, there is an inability to respond to new antigens with appropriate specific immunoglobulin production. This critically affects infants without prior antigen exposure, contributing to the greater frequency and severity of invasive bacterial infections seen in pediatric HIV-1 infection.

Frequencies of circulating CD4+ T lymphocytes often drop by 1–2 months of age in vertically infected children, but this may not be readily apparent because of the higher baseline percentage and absolute numbers of lymphocytes in infants and young children than adults. The absolute CD4+ count is not as predictive of the risk for opportunistic infections in infants as it is for older children and adults.

The first abnormalities detected include fever, failure to thrive, hepatosplenomegaly, generalized lymphadenopathy, parotitis, and diarrhea. Prior to the early use of cART, approximately 90% of perinatally HIV-1-infected infants would manifest 1 or more of these symptoms in the 1st year of life. In one study, the conditions that best discriminated between untreated HIV-1-infected and uninfected infants were chronic candidiasis, parotitis, persistent lymphadenopathy, and hepatosplenomegaly.

Approximately 20% of untreated HIV-1-infected infants present with rapidly progressive immune compromise and/or an AIDS-defining condition, such as *Pneumocystis jirovecii* pneumonia/*Pneumocystis carinii* Pneumonia (PCP), or serious bacterial or fungal infections within the first 3–6 months of life. These infants have a high rate of mortality in the 1st year of life.

Beyond infancy, common symptoms of untreated HIV-1 infection in childhood include persistent adenopathy, hepatosplenomegaly, recurrent or chronic infections, growth failure, and developmental delay. With the exception of linear growth abnormalities, most of these symptoms are significantly less common and/or less severe with aggressive cART. With successful ART (good adherence and undetectable viral load), opportunistic infections are extremely rare. The development or worsening of HIV-1-related symptoms while receiving effective ART suggests clinical failure and possible resistance to one or more of the medications in the treatment regimen.

The central nervous system is involved in more than 50% of infants infected perinatally. The most common presentation is progressive encephalopathy affecting the developmental milestones drastically. There will be cognitive deterioration and impaired brain growth resulting in acquired microcephaly and motor dysfunction. CNS infection can also occur.

GENERAL FEATURES
• Failure to thrive
• Cold and cough
• Nephritis
• Cardiac involvement
• Hepatitis
• Central nervous system (CNS) involvement

Childhood and Adult Infection

Hallmark stages of HIV-1 infection acquired in childhood or adulthood include an acute infection phase (seroconversion syndrome), often with flu-like symptoms and high-grade viremia; followed by period of immune containment of viral replication, during which the individual is usually free of symptoms; and a final period of progressive symptomatic immune compromise, with increasing viral replication.

During the asymptomatic phase, gradual and progressive abnormalities of immune function appear on testing. Viral load is usually lower than during the acute infection phase and may remain relatively stable at a set point for months to years.

The rapidity with which an infected adult or child progresses through the asymptomatic phase can be predicted to some degree by determining the individual's CD4+ cell count and viral load. Lower CD4+ cell count, and higher viral loads are each independent predictors of more rapid disease progression.

The final phase, with symptomatic immune compromise, end-organ dysfunction, and HIV-associated malignancies, is correlated with increasing viral replication and often a change in viral tropism from use of cytokine receptor C-C chemokine receptor type 5 (CCR5) to CXCR4, profound attrition of CD4+ T lymphocytes, severe immune dysregulation (not just immune deficiency), and opportunistic infections.

Children with HIV infection having severe immunosuppression are susceptible to develop various kinds of infections. The important pathogens are *Pneumocystis jirovecii, Cryptosporidium, Cryptococcus, Isospora,* and CMV. PCP is an opportunistic infection. The infection is more common between 3rd and 6th months of life. Recurrent bacterial infections produce recurrent pneumonia. The common pathogens include *Streptococcus. pneumonia, Haemophilus. Influenzae,* and *Staphylococcus aureus.* Tuberculosis is an important infection associated with HIV. These infected children are likely to have extrapulmonary disseminated tuberculosis. The disease course is likely to be more rapid. The risk of tuberculosis is 5–10 fold higher in HIV patients.

Viral infections due to respiratory syncytial virus (RSV), influenza, and parainfluenza virus result in asymptomatic disease. Adenovirus and measles produce more severe sequelae.

Fungal infections usually present as a part of disseminated disease in immunocompromised children. Pulmonary candidiasis should be suspected in any sick HIV-infected child with lower respiratory tract infection.

A variety of microbes can cause gastrointestinal disease. These include *Salmonella, Campylobacter, Giardia*, CMV, rotavirus, and *Candida*. AIDS enteropathy is a syndrome of malabsorption with partial villus atrophy not associated with a specific pathogen. It is probably the result of direct HIV infection of gut.

The inflammation of liver is caused via hepatitis by CMV, Hepatitis B or C virus, or mycobacteria.

Cardiovascular involvements are commonly persistent and often progressive. The left ventricular (LV) structure and function progressively may deteriorate in the first 3 years of life. This results in subsequent persistent mild LV dysfunction and increased LV mass in HIV-infected children. ECG and echocardiogram are helpful in assessing cardiac function.

Nephritic syndrome is the most common manifestation. Polyuria, oliguria, and hematuria have been observed.

> **ESSENTIAL DIAGNOSTIC POINTS**
> - Multiple serious bacterial infections
> - Encephalopathy, recurrent *Salmonella* septicemia
> - HIV wasting syndrome
> - Disseminated fungal infection
> - Mycobacterial infections
> - Should have positive results for one or more of the HIV-detection tests: HIV culture, HIV polymerase chain rection (PCR), and HIV antigen (p24).
> - HIV-seropositive by repeatedly reactive enzyme immunosorbent assay and confirmatory test

■ DIAGNOSIS

Early diagnosis of the infected infant is critically important, but early (prenatal) identification of the infant at risk for HIV-1 infection is equally vital. Only when HIV-1 infection in the pregnant woman is recognized is there an opportunity to implement strategies to prevent transmission and screen exposed infants. HIV-1 screening and counseling should be a routine part of pregnancy care. Initial testing of the mother should be performed in the first trimester (or first visit later than first trimester) using current HIV-1/2 combination antibody/antigen assays. Repeat HIV testing in the third trimester (prior to 36 weeks of gestation) is recommended for pregnant women at increased risk for infection. Rapid HIV-1 antibody testing is advised for women who present to labor and delivery with unknown HIV status or ongoing high risk of infection.

The persistence of transplacentally-acquired maternal antibody to HIV-1 in the infant complicates the use of conventional IgG antibody tests in diagnosing HIV-1 infection in infancy. Because such HIV-1 antibodies may remain in uninfected infants' blood for up to 24 months, diagnosis of HIV-1 infection in the infant at risk requires the demonstration of HIV-I nucleic acid in the peripheral blood by nucleic acid tests (NAT), namely HIV-1 DNA PCR or HIV-I RNA PCR. Although the HIV-1 RNA PCR could be rendered falsely negative in an infected infant who is on antiretroviral prophylaxis; in practice, the current highly sensitive HIV-1 RNA PCR assays function as well as HIV-1 DNA PCR for screening vertically exposed infants. Serial virologic testing with either HIV-1 DNA PCR or HIV-1 RNA PCR can be expected to establish or exclude the diagnosis of HIV infection in an infant by 4 months of age.

Infants born to HIV-infected mother have antibody positive because of passive transfer of maternal HIV antibody across the placenta. A positive IgG antibody under the age of 18 months cannot be considered as diagnostic because of persistence of maternal antibodies.

After the age of 18 months, IgG antibody to HIV can be detected by reactive enzyme immunoassay (EIA) and confirmatory Western blot test.

The optimal schedule for testing HIV-exposed infant includes HIV-1 NAT at 14–21 days, 4–6 weeks, and 4–6 months of age. Some experts also advise a test in the first 2–3 days after birth to identify infants who are viremic at birth from infection presumably acquired in utero. Because zidovudine (AZT) monotherapy is used commonly in HIV-1-exposed newborns, this early test can help avoid prolonged monotherapy, which could foster development of resistance. Presumptive noninfection with HIV-1 can be determined with negative tests at >2 and >4 weeks of age (or 1 negative test at >8 weeks of age).

Special tests: Specific viral diagnostic assays include HIV DNA or RNA PCR, HIV culture, or immune complex-dissociated p24 antigen assay (ICD-p24). These are essential for the diagnosis of young infants born to HIV-infected mother. HIV DNA PCR is the preferred virologic assay in developed countries. The p24 antigen assay is less sensitive than the other virologic tests.

All infants born to HIV-infected mothers test antibody-positive at birth because of passive transfer of maternal HIV antibody across the placenta. Most uninfected infants lose maternal antibody between 6 and 12 months of age. As a small proportion of uninfected infants continue to have maternal HIV antibody in the blood up to 18 months of age, positive IgG antibody tests cannot be used to make a definitive diagnosis of HIV infection in infants younger than this age. In a child older than 18 months of age, demonstration of IgG antibody to HIV by a repeatedly reactive EIA and confirmatory test (e.g., Western blot or immunofluorescence assay) can/establish the diagnosis of HIV infection.

Although serologic diagnostic tests were most commonly used in the past, tests that allow for earlier definitive diagnosis in children have replaced antibody assays as the tests of choice for the diagnosis of HIV infection in infants.

Specific viral diagnostic assays, such as HIV DNA or RNA PCR, HIV culture, or ICD-p24, are essential for diagnosis of young infants born to H1V-infected mothers. By 6 months of age, the HIV culture and/or PCR identifies all infected infants, who are not having any continued exposure due to breastfeeding. Plasma HIV RNA assays may be more sensitive than DNA PCR for early diagnosis, but data are limited. HIV culture has similar sensitivity to HIV DNA PCR; however, it is more technically complex and expensive, and results are often not available for 2–4 weeks compared to 2–3 days with PCR. The ICD-p24 is less sensitive than the other virologic tests.

The national program (Early Infant Diagnosis) now uses HIV DNA PCR test on dried blood spot samples; the positive tests need confirmation using an HIV DNA PCR on a whole blood sample.

> **LABORATORY SALIENT FINDINGS**
> - Measurement of HIV antibody by enzyme-linked immunosorbent assay (ELISA)
> - *Confirmatory test:* Western bolt
> - *Tests:* HIV culture or nucleic acid tests (NAT)
> - *Special tests:* HIV RNA and DNA PCR at birth, HIV culture, or HIV P24 antigen immune dissociated p24 (1CD-p24)

TREATMENT

Once a decision is made to treat, it should be expected that ART will continue for the remainder of the child's life. Factors to be considered in decisions about initiation of therapy include the risk of disease progression as determined by CD4+ cell count and viral load, the potential benefits and risks of therapy, and the ability of the child and caregiver to adhere to administration of the therapeutic regimen. Issues associated with adherence should be fully assessed, discussed, and addressed with the child, if age-appropriate, and caregiver before the decision to initiate therapy is made.

Clinical and laboratory parameters need to be monitored carefully to detect any evidence of medication toxicity or treatment failure. ART adverse events vary by medication, but some of the more common include neuropsychiatric symptoms (e.g., abnormal dreams and expression), gastrointestinal symptoms (e.g., nausea/vomiting, and diarrhea), rash (rarely severe), lipodystrophy, low bone mineral density, dyslipidemia, hyperglycemia, hematologic abnormalities (e.g., anemia and neutropenia), lactic acidosis, nephrotoxicity, and hepatotoxicity.

To monitor for treatment failure, CD4+ cell count, and viral load should be monitored routinely every 3–4 months for at least the first 2 years of therapy. In children who are adherent to therapy, have CD4+ cell counts well above the threshold for opportunistic infection risk, and have stable clinical status and viral suppression for >2 years, less frequent CD4+ cell count monitoring (every 6–12 months) may be considered.

Effective treatment should result in maximal viral load reduction by 12–16 weeks after initiation of therapy. Virologic failure, defined as a repeated viral load >200 copies/mL after 6 months of therapy, suggests either a lack of adherence to the prescribed regimen or the presence or development of resistant virus.

Decisions concerning change in ART should be guided primarily by the child's prior medication history and antiretroviral resistance testing, including both past and current resistance test results. The initial antiretroviral regimen that a child receives is the one most likely to achieve a sustained antiviral effect. In cases of virologic failure due to resistance, subsequent regimens are likely to be less effective because of the impact of cross-resistance to prior medications.

Clinical status at the time of initial presentation appears to correlate with prognosis in perinatally infected children. Perinatally HIV-1-infected infants appear to follow two basic patterns of disease progression. Approximately 20% of perinatally-infected infants progress rapidly and develop severe immune suppression and stage 3 disease in the 1st year of life if not treated appropriately. The majority of infants, however, have slower disease progression. Approximately 75% develop severe immune suppression by 6–10 years of age.

Assessment of the HIV-1-infected child should include a thorough physical examination and laboratory evaluation. To test for HIV-associated conditions (e.g., cytopenia, kidney disease, and hepatitis) and to set the baseline for monitoring of antiretroviral toxicity, complete blood count with differential, comprehensive metabolic panel, urinalysis, and serum lipids should be measured in newly diagnosed children prior to initiation of ART.

Immunologic testing (CD4+ cell count and quantitative immunoglobulins) will aid in decisions regarding PCP prophylaxis, intravenous immunoglobulin (IVIG) therapy, and initiation of ART. Quantitative HIV-1 RNA PCR (viral load) and antiretroviral drug-resistance testing should also be obtained at the time of diagnosis. Viral load and CD4+

cell counts are independent predictors for the risk of disease progression and should be monitored every 3–4 months whether or not the child is started on ART.

Clinical well-being in HIV-1-infected children can be estimated by assessment of growth rate (weight, length, and head circumference), developmental achievement, and experience with bacterial and viral infections. Following these clinical and laboratory parameters should assist in decisions concerning initiation and switching ART, prophylaxis for opportunistic infections, nutritional interventions, and psychosocial support efforts.

Antiretroviral Therapy

The currently available antiretroviral agents (ART) can be divided into 5 distinct categories:
1. Nucleoside/nucleotide reverse transcriptase inhibitors (NRTIs)
2. Nonnucleoside reverse transcriptase inhibitors (NNRTIs)
3. Protease inhibitors (PIs)
4. Integrase strand transfer inhibitors (INSTIs)
5. Entry and fusion inhibitors

For the treatment of children, cART should usually be initiated with a combination of three drugs. The most effective regimens have included two NRTIs in combination with either an NNRTI, PI, or INSTI. Considerations when choosing a regimen include patient age, results of antiretroviral resistance testing, barriers to adherence, drug toxicities, and differing drug formulations, among others.

Based on pediatric and adult studies of immediate versus deferred therapy, cART is recommended for all HV-1-infected children regardless of clinical symptoms, immune status, or viral load, although the urgency and strength of the recommendation vary by age and level of immune suppression. Because approximately one-sixth of HIV-1-infected children experience rapid progression beginning in the 1st year of life, initiation of treatment is urgent in every child younger than 1 year as soon as the diagnosis is established.

Therapy is also considered urgent in children >1 year of age with an opportunistic illness (infection, HIV-associated malignancy, encephalopathy, or progressive multifocal leukoencephalopathy), as well as for children 1–5 years of age with CD4+ cell count <500 cells/μL and children >6 years of age with CD4+ cell count <200 cells/μL.

The National Program for Management of HIV-infected Children recommends combination of AZT or abacavir + lamivudine + efavirenz as first line of therapy; for children <3 years of age, a PI is used instead of NNRTI.

Cotrimoxazole Therapy: Human Immunodeficiency Virus Exposed

Cotrimoxazole therapy is recommended for all infants starting at 4–6 weeks of age and should be continued till HIV infection is excluded.

All children younger than 1 year of age documented to be living with HIV should receive cotrimoxazole prophylaxis regardless of symptoms or CD4 percentage.

After the age of 1 year, cotrimoxazole prophylaxis is recommended for symptomatic children. All children who begin cotrimoxazole prophylaxis should continue until the age of 5 years, when they can be reassessed.

Immunization

The vaccine as per the schedule should be administered to HIV-infected children. Symptomatic HIV-infected children should not be given oral polio vaccine (OPV) and Bacillus Calmette–Guérin (BCG).

Prevention of Mother-to-Child Transmission

These include antiviral prophylaxis for women during pregnancy and labor and to the infant in the 1st week of the life. Obstetric intervention includes elective caesarian delivery and complete avoidance of breastfeeding.

Treatment of pregnant women includes a combination of AZT (zidovudine), lamivudine (3TC), and nevirapine (NVP). The recommended regimen for pregnant women to prevent mother-to-child transmission is as follows:
- *Antepartum:* AZT starting at 28 weeks of pregnancy
- *Intrapartum:* Combination of single dose of NVP, AZT and 3TC
- *Postpartum:* Combination of AZT and 3TC for 7 days

Antiretroviral therapy for infants born to HIV-positive mothers includes single dose of NVP and AZT for 1 week. When the delivery occurs within 2 hours of a woman taking a single dose NVP, the infant should receive a single dose of NVP immediately after the delivery and AZT for 4 weeks.

■ BIBLIOGRAPHY

1. INSIGHT START Study Group; Lundgren JD, Babiker AG, Gordin F, Emery S, Grund B, Sharma S, et al. Initiation of antiretroviral therapy in early asymptomatic HIV infection. N Engl J Med. 2015;373(9):795-807.
2. Luzuriaga K, Mofenson LM. Challenges in elimination of pediatric HIV-1 infection. N Engl J Med. 2016;374(8):761-70.
3. Tobin NH, Aldrovandi GM. Immunology of pediatric HIV infection. Immunol Rev. 2013;254(1):143-69.

71 CASE

Infectious Mononucleosis

■ PRESENTING COMPLAINTS

A 3-year-old girl was brought with the complaints of:
- Fever since 1 week
- Throat pain since 5 days
- Rashes since 3 days

History of Presenting Complaints

A 3-year-old girl was brought to the pediatric outpatient department with a history of fever, throat pain, and rashes over the body. According to the mother, fever was of moderate-to-high degree, intermittent type, not associated with chills and rigors. Fever used to reduce with paracetamol. Mother also told that her daughter was complaining of the throat pain and difficulty in swallowing food, associated with occasional vomiting. Mother had noticed the maculopapular rashes over the body, which were itching. She also revealed the appetite of her daughter has come down drastically. There was neither loose motion nor cough and cold.

Past History of the Patient

The patient was the only sibling of nonconsanguineous marriage. She was born at full term by normal delivery. Her birth weight was 3 kg. She started taking breast milk immediately after delivery. There was no significant postnatal event. Weaning was started in the 4th month and completed by 1 year. She was immunized completely and all the developmental milestones were normal.

■ EXAMINATION

The girl was moderately built and nourished. She was looking tired and dehydrated. She was carried by her mother. She was irritable and not allowing to examine.

CASE AT A GLANCE

Basic Findings
- Height : 95 cm (75th centile)
- Weight : 13 kg
- Temperature : 39°C
- Pulse rate : 124 beats/min
- Respiratory rate : 22 breaths/min
- Blood pressure : 70/50 mm Hg

Positive Findings

History:
- Fever
- Throat pain
- Maculopapular rashes

Examination:
- Febrile
- Lymphadenopathy
- Dehydration
- Hepatomegaly

Investigation:
- SGOT: Increased
- SGPT: Raised
- Paul–Bunnell test is positive
- USG: Hepatomegaly

Anthropometric measurements included a height of 95 cm (75th centile) and a weight of 13 kg (50th centile). There were signs of moderate dehydration.

The child was febrile (39°C). The pulse rate was 124 beats per minute. The respiratory rate was 22 breaths per minute. Blood pressure recorded was 70/50 mm Hg. There was no pallor. There was generalized lymphadenopathy involving cervical group. There was no cyanosis and no clubbing. There were maculopapular rashes present over the body.

Per abdomen examination revealed the presence of hepatomegaly. Liver was palpable 2 cm below the costal margin and nontender. Throat congestion was present. Bowel sounds were normal. Cardiovascular and respiratory system was normal.

■ INVESTIGATION

- *Hemoglobin:* 11 g/dL
- *TLC:* 12,000 cells/mm^3
- *DLC:* $P_{68}\ L_{28}\ E_2\ M_2$
- *ESR:* 30 mm in the 1st hour
- *LFT:* SGOT—increased; SGPT—increased
- *Paul-Bunnell test:* Positive
- *Chest X-ray:* NAD
- *Ultrasound abdomen:* Hepatomegaly is present

■ DISCUSSION

The child was presented with a history of fever, throat pain, and also maculopapular rashes. This along with lymphadenopathy and hepatomegaly associated with abnormal LFT and positive Paul-Bunnell test indicates infectious mononucleosis (IM).

Epstein-Barr virus was implicated as the etiological agent for IM. Most of the cases are observed in older children but no age is exempted. EBV infections are much more common in pediatric population than commonly believed, for they are by and large subclinical.

Epstein-Barr virus is recognized as the major cause of IM. Most EBV infections are thought to be spread through saliva. Manifestations of EBV infection are varied and range from asymptomatic infection to fulminant lymphoproliferative disease. EBV is also associated with a number of malignancies, including endemic Burkitt lymphoma, nasopharyngeal carcinoma, Hodgkin disease, and a spectrum of post-transplant lymphoproliferative diseases.

Mononucleosis is the most characteristic syndrome produced by EBV infection. Young children infected with EBV have either no symptoms or a mild nonspecific febrile illness. As the age of the host increases, EBV infections are more likely to produce the typical features of the mononucleosis syndrome in 20-25% of infected adolescents. EBV is acquired readily from asymptomatic carriers (15-20% of whom excrete the virus on any given day) and from recently ill patients, who excrete virus for many months. Young children are infected by the saliva of playmates and family members. Adolescents may be infected through sexual activity. EBV can also be transmitted by blood transfusion and organ transplantation.

Epstein-Barr virus can also be associated with Gianotti-Crosti syndrome, a symmetric rash on the cheeks with multiple erythematous papules, which may coalesce into plaques and persist for 15-50 days. The rash has the appearance of atopic dermatitis and may appear on the extremities and buttocks.

Transmission occurs by intimate contact between susceptible individual and asymptomatic shedders of EBV. Blood transfusion is another possible way of transmission.

PATHOGENESIS

Epstein-Barr virus is a member of the family *Herpesviridae* (gammaherpesvirus), which contains linear double-stranded DNA surrounded by a protein capsid. EBV causes lytic infection of human oropharyngeal and salivary cells and latent infection of human and primate B lymphocytes as well as epithelium of the nasopharynx. It has long been recognized to be lymphotropic for B lymphocytes and to infect both oropharyngeal epithelial cells and myocytes, but it is also true that it infects T lymphocytes and natural killer cells.

Infection of lymphocytes with linear EBV DNA can transform them into continuously growing lymphoblastoid cell lines containing a circular DNA episome. Once infected, transformed lymphoblastoid cells rarely continue to produce infectious virus in vitro, although EB antigens can be detected in the cells. The appearance of new antigens on the cell surface of EBV-infected cells is believed to be responsible for the cellular immune response to the virus and for pathogenesis of the resulting disease. The EBV receptor on epithelial cells and B lymphocytes is the CD21 molecule (formerly CR2), which is also the receptor for the C3d fragment of the third component of complement. The virus elicits both humoral and cellular immune responses.

The EBV acquired by ingestion appears to first infect either oropharyngeal resting B cells or epithelial cells and then B cells. Subsequently, the virus infects other susceptible B lymphocytes within the lymphoid tissue of the pharynx. During a 30-50-day incubation period, the virus actively replicates and disseminates throughout the entire lymphoreticular system.

Epstein-Barr virus is excreted in oropharyngeal secretions and is transmitted by contact with saliva via either kissing or other mucosal contact with contaminated objects. Healthy seropositive individuals intermittently shed EBV in their oropharynx. Mucosal contact with the saliva of these individuals is the likely mechanism of infection in preadolescent and adolescent individuals.

Epstein-Barr virus (a DNA virus of herpesvirus group) infects susceptible B lymphocytes by attaching to its specific C3d receptor on the cell surface where it undergoes multiplication. Later, it disseminates throughout the lymphoreticular system. The virus elicits both humoral and cell-mediated immunity. The antibodies are produced against the EBV virus.

The cell-mediated immunity is provided by the T lymphocytes, which proliferate extensively in response to B-lymphocyte infection. In the peripheral blood, this is reflected by the appearance of many atypical T lymphocytes. These cytotoxic/suppressor cells prevent the proliferation of EBV-infected lymphoid cells. Children with defects in their cell-mediated immunity are prone to develop fatal diseases or lymphoproliferative disorders including B-cell lymphomas.

CLINICAL FEATURES (FIG. 1)

The incubation period of EBV-IM is 30-50 days. The clinical syndrome of EBV-IM is usually preceded by a 5-day prodrome of malaise, fatigue, headache, nausea, abdominal pain, or some combination of these symptoms. Over the next 7-20 days, sore throat and fever gradually increase.

The triad of fever, sore throat, and posterior cervical adenopathy occurs in >80% of symptomatic patients. Sore throat is often accompanied by evidence of moderate-to-severe pharyngitis, with marked tonsillar enlargement that may be covered with shaggy gray or white exudate.

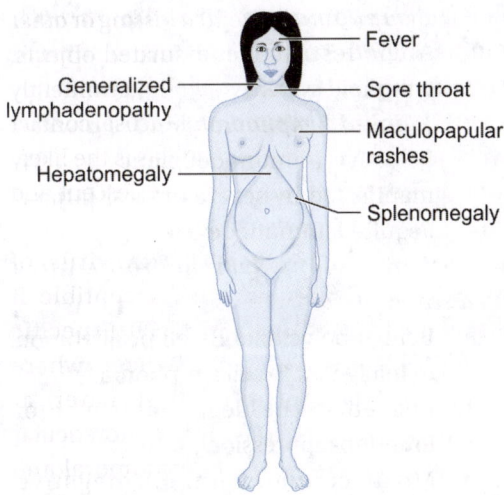

Fig. 1: Clinical features.

Fever is present in 85–95% of patients, from 39°C (102°F) up to 40.5C (105°F), and on average lasts 10 days but may persist for weeks. Fatigue and lymphadenopathy may persist longer.

Adenopathy most often involves only the bilateral posterior cervical nodes but may involve any node, including anterior cervical, epitrochlear, or even generalized lymph nodes. Nodes may be affected singly or in groups (not necessarily symmetrical) and may be very large or small. They are most often firm, discrete, and moderately tender to palpation.

In most cases, a maculopapular rash develops. Patients have a rash, which can be macular, scarlatiniform, or urticarial. Rashes are almost universal in patients taking penicillin or ampicillin. Soft-palate petechiae and eyelid edema are also observed.

Massive splenomegaly may occur, usually defined operationally as a spleen extending well into the left lower quadrant or pelvis or that has crossed the midline of the abdomen and that weighs at least 500–1,000 g. Rupture is rare but can be a potentially fatal complication. Hepatomegaly occurs.

Serum AST and serum lactate dehydrogenase (LDH) are mildly elevated in the majority of patients and may persist for weeks to months. Chronic liver disease, however, does not typically result.

Other clinical findings include bilateral supraorbital edema and rashes. A blanching, erythematous, maculopapular exanthema occurs in about 15–59% of patients, but as many as 80% develop this rash if treated with ampicillin or other B-lactam antibiotics. The same rash may occur with CMV-associated mononucleosis and so does not differentiate CMV from EBV-associated mononucleosis. Urticarial, bullous, hemorrhagic, and scarlatiniform rashes, as well as the Gianotti-Crosti syndrome, are also associated with IM.

Neurologic complications include aseptic meningitis, encephalitis optic neuritis, Guillain–Barré syndrome, transverse myelitis, Bell's palsy, and, in numerous more recent epidemiologic studies, multiple sclerosis following EBV-IM.

GENERAL FEATURES
• Malaise • Loss of appetite • Periorbital edema

There may be ulceration in the oral cavity with enanthems at the junction of hard and soft palate. Spleen is enlarged in more than half of the patients. Periorbital edema is reported in 33% patients. Hepatomegaly is common (30%), and the liver is frequently tender.

COMPLICATIONS

Acute Complications

- *Rash:* Morbilliform rashes, may happen post ampicillin and, to a lesser extent, post penicillin or other antibiotics.

- *Airway obstruction:*
  - Due to massive lymphoid hyperplasia and mucosal edema
  - Steroids may be indicated in impending obstruction
  - Severe obstruction may need tracheostomy or endotracheal intubation
- *Splenic rupture:* One to two cases per thousand cases of IM
- *Lemierre's disease:* Some case series report coinfection with *Fusobacterium*.

Delayed Complications

- *Chronic active EBV infection:*
  - Life-threatening lymphoproliferative disorder that may involve B or T lymphocytes or natural killer (NK) cells
  - Persistent IM-like syndrome and EBV viremia
  - Swelling of lymph nodes and hepatosplenomegaly along with LFT abnormalities and cytopenia
  - If untreated leads to T-cell infiltration of tissues, the curative option being hematopoietic stem cell transplantation (HSCT).
- *Oral hairy leukoplakia:*
  - Corrugated painless plaques on lingual tissue that, unlike *Candida*, cannot be scraped from the surface to which they adhere.
  - Occurs mostly in immunocompromised hosts.
- Lymphoproliferative disorders:
  - *Hemophagocytic lymphohistiocytosis (HLH):* Present with fever, generalized lymphadenopathy, hepatosplenomegaly, hepatitis, pancytopenia, and coagulopathy. One of the most common causes of infectious triggers of HLH.
  - *Lymphomatoid granulomatosis:* Angiodestructive disorder of the lymphoid system
  - *X-linked lymphoproliferative disease:* Selective immunodeficiency to EBV, manifested by severe or fatal IM and acquired immunodeficiency
- *Post-transplant lymphoproliferative disease:*
  - Benign polyclonal B-cell proliferation to malignant B-cell lymphoma
  - Related to the degree and type of immunosuppression
  - Most common in EB-negative recipients who develop primary EBV infection, usually from a graft from an EBV-positive donor.
- *Malignancy:*
  - EBV is a transforming virus and has been causally linked to a variety of malignancies, including lymphomas in transplant recipients.
  - Malignancies include Burkitt lymphoma, tumors in patients with HIV, Hodgkin lymphoma, nasopharyngeal and other head and neck carcinomas, gastric carcinoma, and T cell lymphoma.

Various other complications associated with IM are given in **Box 1**.

> **BOX 1:** Complications of infectious mononucleosis (IM).
>
> - *Respiratory:* Pneumonia and severe airway obstruction
> - *Neurological:* Convulsions, aseptic meningitis, transverse myelitis, and Guillain–Barré syndrome
> - *Hematological:* Immune hemolytic anemia of cold antibody type, thrombocytopenia, aplastic anemia, and hemorrhage
> - *Splenic rupture:* Rupture of rapidly enlarging spleen may follow minor trauma
> - *Others:* Myocarditis, hepatitis, glomerulonephritis, and orchitis

Infection with EBV, the first human virus to be associated with malignancy, accounts for up to 2% of cancers worldwide. Manipulation of infected cells by EBV to establish and maintain latency can lead to transformation and oncogenesis. EBV is associated with lymphoid malignancies, such as Burkitt lymphoma, Hodgkin lymphoma, aggressive NK-cell leukemia, T- and NK-cell lymphoproliferative disorder, and epithelial cell malignancies such as nasopharyngeal carcinoma and gastric carcinoma.

> **ESSENTIAL DIAGNOSTIC POINTS**
> - Prolonged fever
> - Exudative pharyngitis
> - Generalized lymphadenopathy
> - Hepatosplenomegaly
> - Heterophile antibodies
> - Atypical lymphocytes

LABORATORY INVESTIGATIONS

- *Peripheral blood:* Leukopenia may occur early, but an atypical lymphocytosis is most notable. Hematologic changes may not be seen until the 3rd week of illness and may be entirely absent in some EBV syndromes. There is usually an absolute increase in the lymphocytes in the peripheral blood. Most lymphocytes are large and atypical, with pale-blue vacuolated cytoplasm and an eccentric nucleus. SGOT and SGPT levels are elevated in three-fourths of the patients.
- *Heterophile antibodies*: These nonspecific antibodies appear in over 90% of older patients with mononucleosis but in fewer than 50% of children under age 5 years. They may not be detectable until the 2nd week of illness and may persist for up to 12 months after recovery.
- *Paul-Bunnel-Davidsohn test* is positive. The test is often negative in children under 4 years of age. Heterophile antibodies that agglutinate the sheep red cells in a titer of 1 in 56 or more are present. The high titer persists for about 3 weeks. Heterophile antibodies are IgM antibodies, and their titer does not correlate well with the severity of the illness. Rapid screening tests (slide agglutination) are usually positive, they strongly suggest but do not prove EBV infection.
- *Anti-EBV antibodies*: It may be necessary to measure specific antibody titers when heterophile antibodies fail to appear, as in young children. Acute EBV infection is established by detecting IgM antibody to the viral capsid antigen (VCA) or by detecting a fall over several weeks of IgG anti-VCA titers (IgG antibody peaks by the time symptoms appear).
- *EBV PCR:* This assay detects EBV DNA. It is the method of choice for the diagnosis of CNS and ocular infections. Quantitative EBV PCR in peripheral blood mononuclear cells (PBMC) has been studied for the diagnosis of proliferation disorders in transplant patients.
- *Detection of EBV-specific antibodies:* If the heterophile test result is negative and an EBV infection is suspected, EBV-specific antibody testing is indicated. Measurement of antibodies to EBV proteins including VCA, Epstein–Barr nuclear antigen (EBNA), and early antigen (EA) are used most frequently. The acute phase of IM is characterized by rapid IgM and IgG antibody responses to VCA in all cases and an IgG response to EA in most cases. The IgM response to VCA is transient but can be detected for at least 4 weeks and occasionally up to 3 months. The IgG response to VCA usually peaks late in the acute phase, declines slightly over the next several weeks to months,

and then persists at a relatively stable level for life.
- *Detection of viral DNA:* EBV DNA can be detected and viral genome copy number is quantified in whole blood, PBMC, and plasma using real-time PCR. EBV DNA can be detected in PBMC and plasma of patients with IM for a brief period of time after the onset of symptoms and in PBMC for an extended period of time. Virus can be cultivated from the oropharynx for up to 1 year following the acute infection.

Heterophile antibody-negative IM-like syndrome is seen in many conditions such as:
- CMV infection
- *Toxoplasma gondii*
- HIV
- Adenoviral illness
- Group A streptococcal pharyngitis
- HSV
- Human herpes virus-6 (HHV-6)
- Atopic dermatitis, especially Gianotti–Crosti syndrome in which symmetrical cheek rash with multiple erythematous papules coalesce into plaques

---

LABORATORY SALIENT FINDINGS

- Atypical lymphocytosis
- Heterophile antibodies
- Anti-EBV antibodies
- EBV PCR

(EBV: Epstein–Barr virus; PCR: polymerase chain reaction)

■ DIFFERENTIAL DIAGNOSIS

The differential diagnoses of IM include *Toxoplasma*, CMV, adenovirus, rubella, and hepatitis.

■ TREATMENT

Bed rest may be necessary in severe cases. Acetaminophen controls high fever. Potential airway obstruction due to swollen pharyngeal lymphoid tissue responds rapidly to systemic corticosteroids.

Corticosteroids may also be given for hematologic and neurologic complications, although no controlled trials have proved their efficacy in these conditions. Fever and pharyngitis disappear by 10–14 days. Adenopathy and splenomegaly can persist for several weeks longer. Some patients complain of fatigue, malaise, or lack of well-being for several months. Although steroids may shorten the duration of fatigue and malaise, their long-term effects on this potentially oncogenic viral infection are unknown, and indiscriminate use is discouraged. Patients with splenic enlargement should avoid contact sports for 6–8 weeks.

Specific antiviral therapy has generally not been beneficial in treating EBV infections, although treatment of a suspected acute *Streptococcus pyogenes* infection with a non-B-lactam antibiotic such as clindamycin is reasonable. Regarding EBV, several nucleotide analogs have in vitro activity but have little clinical effect. Acyclovir treatment of patients with IM results in interruption of viral shedding in the throat, but clinical progression remains unaffected. However, valacyclovir has been shown to decrease the severity and number of symptoms in several studies. Prophylactic interferon-alpha decreases the incidence of EBV shedding by kidney transplant recipients but is not widely used for prophylaxis or treatment.

Lesions of oral hairy leukoplakia respond to oral or IV acyclovir, but they frequently recur in patients with HIV infection after treatment is discontinued. Aggressive, successful ART frequently results in remission of lesions of oral hairy leukoplakia without specific treatment of EBV.

Treatment with prednisolone (1 mg/kg/day for 7 days) is advised for complications such as hemolytic anemia, airway obstruction, meningitis, and thrombocytopenia with bleeding. Intranasal steroids may be used to relieve nasal obstruction caused by enlarged adenoids.

Acyclovir, valacyclovir, penciclovir, ganciclovir, and foscarnet are active against EBV and are indicated in the treatment of chronic active EBV.

■ PREVENTION

Ganciclovir and valganciclovir have been used to prevent posttransplant EBV disease. Two prophylactic EBV vaccines, gp350 subunit, and CD8 T-cell peptide epitope, have been evaluated in clinical trials.

■ BIBLIOGRAPHY

1. Cohen JI. Epstein-Barr virus infection. N Engl J Med. 2000;343(7):481-92.
2. Dunmire SK, Hogquist KA, Balfour HH. Infectious Mononucleosis. Curr Top Microbiol Immunol. 2015;390:211-40.
3. Rickinson AB. Coinfections, inflammation and oncogenesis: Future directions for EBV research. Semin Cancer Biol. 2014;26:99-115.
4. Stanfield BA, Luftig MA. Recent advances in understanding Epstein-Barr virus. F1000Res. 2017;6:386.

CASE 72

Malaria

PRESENTING COMPLAINTS

A 5-year-old boy was brought with the complaints of:
- Fever since 3 days
- Headache since 2 days
- Vomiting since 1 day

History of Presenting Complaints

A 5-year-old boy came to the hospital with a history of fever, headache, and vomiting.

The child had a high temperature. Moderate-to-high, intermittent fever was associated with chills and rigors. After the chills and rigor, the boy used to sweat a lot. Later, he was taken to the doctor nearby, where he was given antipyretics and antibiotics. He was afebrile for 1 day. Again at midnight, he developed a high temperature followed by chills and rigors. The temperature recorded by the mother was 103°F. Later, child started complaining of headaches. It was associated with vomiting. The next day, child was brought to the hospital.

Past History of the Patient

The patient was the second child of nonconsanguineous marriage. He was born at full term by normal delivery. There was no significant postnatal event. Child was taking breastfeeds as soon as possible. He was exclusively on breastfeeds for the first 4 months. Later, weaning was started. He was on family food by 18 months. He had been completely immunized. His developmental milestones were normal.

CASE AT A GLANCE

Basic Findings
Height	: 107 cm (60th centile)
Weight	: 18 kg (75th centile)
Temperature	: 39°C
Pulse rate	: 110 beats/min
Respiratory rate	: 20 breaths/min
Blood pressure	: 90/70 mm Hg

Positive Findings

History:
- Fever
- Chills and rigors
- Headache
- Vomiting

Examination:
- Febrile
- Splenomegaly

Investigation:
- *TLC:* Increased
- *Malarial parasite (MP) smear:* Positive

EXAMINATION

On examination, the child was moderately built and moderately nourished. His height was 107 cm (60th centile) and weight was 18 kg (75th centile). He was febrile, i.e., 39°C. The pulse rate was 110 beats per minute and respiratory rate was 20 breaths per minute.

Blood pressure recorded was 90/70 mm Hg. There was no pallor, no lymphadenopathy, no icterus, and no edema. Per abdomen examination revealed the presence of spleen measuring about 3 cm below the costal margin. It was firm and nontender. There was no other organomegaly. Other systemic examinations were normal

INVESTIGATION

- *Hemoglobin:* 11 g/dL
- *TLC:* 16,000 cells/mm^3
- *DLC:* P_{72} L_{26} M_2
- *Blood culture and sensitivity:* Negative
- *Malarial parasite (MP) smear:* Plasmodium vivax ring and gametocyte
- *X-ray chest:* Normal
- *Urine culture and sensitivity:* Normal
- *Widal test:* Negative

DISCUSSION

The boy has come with a history of high temperature associated with chills, rigors, and headaches. The fever used to be intermittent and present on alternate days. The child used to be absolutely normal in between the attacks. The history is suggestive of malaria. The MP smear that was taken during the attack at the time of chills proved MP positive.

Malaria occurs when erythrocytes are invaded by any of four species of the plasmodium. It is characterized by high fever, which is often intermittent, anemia, and splenic enlargement.

Life cycle of the Malarial Parasite

Pre-erythrocytic schizogony: As soon as the mosquito bites, within 30 minutes, the sporozoites disappear from the blood. These will invade the liver and reticuloendothelial tissues. The parasites go through asexual reproduction in hepatic cells. Sporozoites divide and form thousands of merozoites. Merozoites will invade red cells but cannot infect hepatocytes. There are no apparent clinical symptoms during this pre-erythrocytic cycle. This phase thus constitutes the incubation period of malaria. This will be generally not <10 days. The process of liver schizogony lasts from 7-10 days for *Plasmodium falciparum, P. ovale,* and *P. vivax,* and 10-14 days for *P. malariae. P. vivax* and *P. ovale* can also produce dormant liver stages (hypnozoites) that can reactivate weeks or months after the initial infection and can cause clinical relapse.

Erythrocytic schizogomy: Merozoites invade erythrocytes. In red blood cells, they become trophozoites. The dividing stage is called erythrocytic schizont. The infected erythrocytes then rupture releasing merozoites into the circulation. The merozoites infect new erythrocytes and start the cycle all over again.

After several stages of schizogony, some merozoites develop into sexual stages, i.e., micro (male) or macro (female) gametes. When a female *Anopheles* mosquito bites a patient, it sucks his/her blood. Only gametocytes form survive in the stomach of the mosquito. The fertilized macrogamete is called a zygote. The zygote enters the wall of the midgut of mosquito and during the migratory stage, it is called ookinete. As it lays below the outer cell layer of the stomach, it is known as an oocyst. Oocyst ruptures and releases sporozoites into the body cavity of the mosquito from where they migrate to salivary glands. When a mosquito bites human beings, it releases sporozoites into their blood.

Malaria can also be acquired by direct blood exposure through blood transfusions. Congenital malaria, with passage of infection from mother to newborn, can also occur, although it is relatively infrequent in endemic areas. It is seen more frequently in nonimmune women and in women who have an overt attack of clinical malaria during pregnancy. In areas where malaria is endemic, infection during pregnancy, even among semi-immune women, can lead to low birth weight and an increased risk of perinatal mortality.

In malaria, many organs are involved. The spleen is enlarged, dark and shows reticular hyperplasia. It returns to normal size as the infection is controlled. In liver, there is Kupffer hyperplasia, sinusoidal and sequestration of the RBCs. Kidneys have ischemic tubular damage resulting in acute transient nephritis. Chronic nephrotic syndrome occurs as a result of *P. malariae*.

In cerebral malaria, there will be plugging of cerebral capillaries with infected erythrocytes, causing hemorrhages and deposition of fibrin in vessels. Brain capillaries, predominantly in white matter, are loaded with parasite RBCs (Fig. 1).

Disease from malaria is caused by the blood stages of the parasite. Rupture of red cells and release of merozoites into the blood lead to the fever, chills, and malaise seen in all forms of malaria. *Plasmodium*-infected erythrocytes, opsonized with antibodies or complement, are less deformable than uninfected erythrocytes and are consequently trapped in the spleen, leading to splenomegaly.

Anemia and thrombocytopenia are due primarily to splenic consumption of erythrocytes and platelets, but autoimmune hemolysis plays a role in the continued destruction of erythrocytes that can occur for weeks after appropriate treatment. In addition, bone marrow suppression occurs in severe malarial anemia, so the anemia seen is due to both erythrocyte destruction (by autoimmune hemolysis and spleen removal of infected erythrocytes) and impaired erythropoiesis. Anemia occurs as a result of the destruction of parasites containing RBCs, bone marrow dysfunction, and hemolysis due to black water fever.

■ CLINICAL FEATURES (FIG. 2)

The incubation period of MP varies between 9 and 30 days. The onset of the disease is sudden with fever, headache, loss of appetite, lassitude, and pain in the limbs. The fever may be continuous. The illness is characterized by chills and rigors, headache, nausea, malaria, and anorexia; the fever occurs on alternate days.

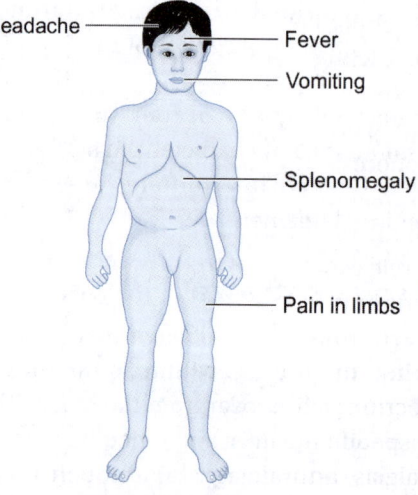

Fig. 2: Clinical features.

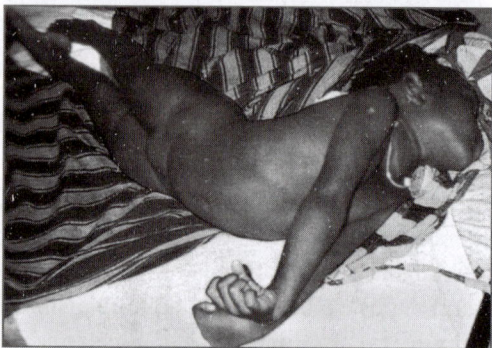

Fig. 1: Cerebral malaria.

The relapse is defined as the recurrence of fever after a period that is greater than normal periodicity. Relapses are more common with *P. falciparum*.

The malaria caused by *P. vivax* is a benign tertian malaria. Malaria is usually acquired from the bites of previously infected female *Anopheles* mosquitoes. Congenital malaria is caused by the transfer of causative agents across the placental barrier. It is rare. Neonatal malaria, on the other hand, is less uncommon and may result from the mingling of infected maternal blood with that of infant during the birth process.

For clinical and diagnostic purposes, malaria may be regarded as having two disease entities. The more dangerous one is caused by *P. falciparum*. It can produce a variety of acute clinical symptoms and signs, and if untreated, it proves fatal.

Children with *P. falciparum*, in particular, may exhibit very irregular fever patterns. Fever is present at some point in the illness in almost all nonimmune children with malaria. Seizures are common in severe malaria. Nonimmune adults frequently exhibit the classic febrile paroxysm, which consists of three phases: A brief "cold" phase, with chills and sometimes rigors; a "hot" phase, with high fever, dry and flushed skin, tachypnea, and thirst; and a "sweating" stage, with defervescence accompanied by diaphoresis and a feeling of great relief but also great weakness. The paroxysms coincide with the rupture of infected erythrocytes and the release of merozoites, pigment, and cell debris into the circulation.

Prodromal, flu-like symptoms occur during the early cycles of erythrocytic infection and may include fever (with no specific pattern), headache, malaise, myalgias, arthralgias, abdominal pain, and diarrhea. The febrile paroxysm may be extremely short or may last for 2–12 hours. Its characteristic pattern is usually observed in children <5 years of age. Fever may be absent or increase gradually for 1–2 days or onset may be sudden with temperature up to 40.6°C with or without prodromal chill.

Children, especially infants, may not exhibit the classic febrile paroxysm seen in adults. In infants, more nonspecific symptoms such as fever, lethargy, decreased appetite, and listlessness may continue to predominate. Vomiting, loose stools, and abdominal pain are very common complaints in both infants and children. Many infants and older children will also have intermittent fevers without a clear pattern, rather than the 48-hour (*P. vivax*, *P. ovale*, *P. falciparum*) or 72-hour (*P. malariae*) fever patterns classically described with these infections.

The physical signs most frequently seen in malaria are hepatomegaly and splenomegaly, which occur in about half of all children with acute malarial disease. In areas where malaria is highly endemic, a large percentage of children develop palpable splenomegaly over time, and the prevalence of splenomegaly in children aged 2–9 years has been used to define an area's malaria-endemicity pattern. In areas of unstable transmission and nonimmune individuals, it is less common.

Although malaria often leads to some degree of anemia, particularly when not treated immediately, pallor is seen in only 25% of children with malaria in endemic areas and jaundice in only 10–15% of children. Scleral icterus may be seen in children. Jaundice is more common in nonimmune adults. Other physical exam findings that relate to complications of malaria include coma or posturing in children with cerebral malaria or chest indrawing and respiratory distress in children with metabolic acidosis.

Nonimmune children with *P. falciparum* malaria often develop complications from the disease. The most common of these complications in children are severe malarial anemia, respiratory distress, and impaired consciousness. Each of these complications can contribute to and exacerbate the others, and mortality increases as the number of malarial complications increases.

Cerebral Malaria

By the definition, cerebral malaria is present in a patient who (i) cannot localize a painful stimulus, (ii) has peripheral asexual *P. falciparum* parasitemia, and (iii) has no other causes of encephalopathy. The pathophysiology of impaired consciousness in a child with severe malaria is likely the same as that of coma.

Cerebral malaria often develops rapidly. Parents typically give a history of 2-5 days of fever, followed by abrupt onset of convulsions or severely impaired consciousness. Children with cerebral malaria may progress from a normal sensorium to coma within hours. Focal seizures are occasionally seen, but focal neurologic deficits are rare. Meningeal signs are usually absent, although abnormal posturing, papillary changes, absent corneal reflexes, Cheyne-Stokes or Kussmaul respirations, and gaze abnormalities may be seen.

Malaria retinopathy consists of four main components: Retinal whitening, vessel changes, retinal hemorrhages, and papilledema. Retinal whitening and vessel color changes are specific to malaria and are not seen in other ocular or systemic conditions. Papilledema is an independent indicator of poor outcomes. Malaria retinopathy appears to distinguish children with cerebral malaria from those with coma due to other causes but is impractical as a standard diagnostic tool because it must be assessed with indirect ophthalmoscopy.

In addition, children who meet the World Health Organization (WHO) criteria for cerebral malaria but do not have retinopathy may still have *P. falciparum* as the primary cause of coma. For this reason, retinopathy is not a requirement for diagnosis of cerebral malaria. Increased intracranial pressure (ICP), generally not seen in adults with cerebral malaria, is a feature of cerebral malaria in children. Studies of interventions that decrease ICP in children with cerebral malaria, including steroids and mannitol, have not shown improved outcomes to date, so understanding and addressing the root cause of increased brain swelling in children with cerebral malaria are key to better outcomes in these children.

Nonimmune adults can develop neurologic sequelae after severe malaria, even without cerebral malaria. Neurologic sequelae seen in nonimmune adults may also be seen in nonimmune older children and may include cranial nerve defects, mononeuritis multiplex, polyneuropathy, and cerebellar dysfunction.

> **ESSENTIAL DIAGNOSTIC POINTS**
> - Fever in endemic area
> - Paroxysms of chills, fever, and sweating
> - Splenomegaly and anemia
> - Headache, vomiting, and diarrhea
> - Backache, cough, and abdominal pain
> - Seizures and coma
> - Malarial parasite in peripheral blood smear

Severe complicated malaria is caused by *P. falciparum*. It is attributed to the high parasitemia, cytoadherence, and sequestration. The manifestation includes:
- Cerebral malaria
- Severe anemia

- Acute renal failure
- Pulmonary edema or acute respiratory distress syndrome (ARDS)
- Hypoglycemia
- Shock
- DIC and repeated generalized convulsions

Blackwater fever is characterized by sudden massive intravascular hemolysis and passage of high-colored urine due to hemoglobinuria. Renal failure may develop. It occurs in glucose-6-phosphate dehydrogenase-(G6PD)-deficiency anemia.

Congenital Malaria

It occurs in nonimmune mothers. Congenital malaria is caused by the transfer of causative agent across the placental barrier. It is probably due to the transplacental transfer of protective maternal IgG antibodies. The incubation period ranges from 2–8 weeks. Clinical manifestation include fever irritability, failure to thrive, pallor, jaundice, and hepatosplenomegaly.

Congenital malaria is acquired from the mother prenatally or perinatally. Congenital malaria usually occurs in the spring from a nonimmune mother with *P. vivax* or *P. malariae* infection, although it can be observed with any of the human malaria species. The first sign or symptom typically occurs between 10 and 30 days of age (range: 14 hours to several months of age). Signs and symptoms include fever, restlessness, drowsiness, pallor, jaundice, poor feeding, vomiting, diarrhea, cyanosis, and hepatosplenomegaly.

Malaria in Pregnancy

Malaria in pregnancy is a major health problem in malaria-endemic countries. It can be severe and is associated with adverse outcomes in the fetus or neonate, including intrauterine growth restriction and low birth weight, even in the absence of transmission from mother to child.

Chronic complications include tropical splenomegaly, nephritic syndrome, endemic Burkitt's lymphoma, and endomyocardial fibrosis. Relapses are not seen with *P. falciparum* and *P. malaria* as there are no persistent exoerythrocytic cycles.

Recrudescence after a primary attack may occur from the survival of erythrocyte forms in the bloodstream. Long-term relapse is caused by the release of merozoites from an exoerythrocytic source in the liver, which occurs with *P. vivax* and *P. ovale*, or from persistence within the erythrocyte, which occurs with *P. malariae* and rarely with *P. falciparum*. A history of typical symptoms in a person >4 weeks after return from an endemic area is, therefore, more likely to be *P. vivax, P. ovale,* or *P. malariae* infection than *P. falciparum* infection.

GENERAL FEATURES
• Sudden onset
• Loss of appetite
• Chills with rigors
• Sweating
• Convulsions

■ DIAGNOSIS

Microscopic Diagnosis

Peripheral smear: The gold standard for diagnosis of malaria is a careful examination of a properly prepared thick film. Thick smears have a sensitivity of detecting 5–10 parasites/µL. Thin smears have a lower sensitivity of 200 parasites/µL but enable species identification. Microscopy also provides information about the parasite load (number of infected RBC/total RBC), prognosis (mature schizonts and pigmented neutrophils indicating a poor prognosis), and tracks response to therapy. The main drawback is the need for expertise, and that they are time consuming (a careful examination of 100 fields needs 20 min). Sometimes, peripheral smears may be negative due to partial antimalarial treatment or sequestration of parasitized cells in deep vascular beds. Repeating smears every 6–8 hours at least 3 times is recommended if the clinical suspicion for malaria is high and the initial smear is negative **(Fig. 3)**.

Sample collection should be done as soon as malaria is suspected. It can be collected any time irrespective of fever and not necessarily only at the height of fever. Collection should be before administration of antimalarials, which makes detection of parasites difficult due to their morphologic alteration.

Examination of Giemsa-stained thick and thin blood smears remains the primary method for diagnosis of malaria. Thick smears are more sensitive in detecting parasites, but thin smears are necessary for identifying *Plasmodium* species and allow estimation of the degree of peripheral blood parasitemia.

It is most important to distinguish *P. falciparum* from the other four human malaria species. *P. falciparum* malaria is suggested by parasitemia that exceeds 2% of red cells, red cells that contain multiple parasites, the almost exclusive presence of ring forms of the parasite, ring forms with a double chromatin dot, and the presence of parasites in all ages of red cells. The banana-shaped gametocyte is pathognomonic for *P. falciparum* malaria. *P. malariae* is characterized by low-level parasitemia and a characteristic band trophozoite. Schüffner's stippling is characteristic of *P. vivax* and *P. ovale*, although it may be more subtle in *P. ovale* infections. *P. ovale*-infected cells often have an oval shape in addition to the stippling.

Quantitative buff coat (QBC) test is a new method for identifying the malarial parasite in the peripheral blood. It involves staining of the centrifuged and compressed red cell layer with acridine orange and its examination under an ultraviolet (UV) light source. It is fast, easy, and claimed to be more sensitive than the traditional thick smear examination. The disadvantages include need for special equipment, cost, false positives due to staining artefacts, and inability to specify the parasite. QBC has been largely supplanted by the rapid diagnostic tests detailed as follows.

Rapid diagnosis tests (RDT): These are immunochromatographic tests (ICTs) to detect *Plasmodium*-specific antigens in blood samples. They employ monoclonal antibodies directed against targeted parasite antigens. In our country, where *P. falciparum* and *P. vivax* malaria parasites cocirculate, typically occurring as a single species infection, an RDT which can detect both *P. falciparum* and *P. vivax* malaria and distinguish between them is warranted.

Other methods of diagnosis: Other diagnostic methods namely microscopy using fluorochromes on centrifuged blood specimens, molecular probes, PCR, and

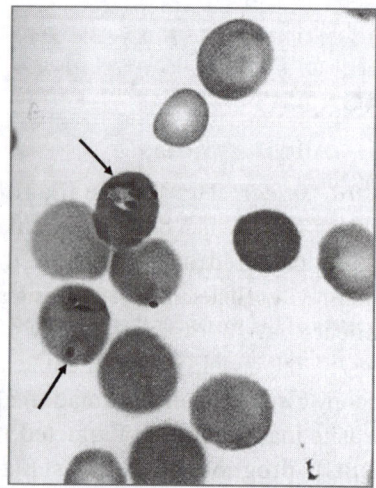

Fig. 3: Peripheral blood smear.
(For color version, see Plate 4)

serology are available. Unfortunately, they are not suitable for routine disease management and do not have wide-field applications. Their use is currently for only research and epidemiological purposes.

Polymerase chain reaction has been found to be highly sensitive and specific for detecting all species of malaria, particularly in cases of low-level parasitemia but is not available commercially, and hence of limited practical utility.

Sensitivity for *P. falciparum* decreases at lower levels of parasitemia, so microscopy is still advised in areas where expert microscopy is available. The test is simple to perform and can be done in the field or laboratory in 10 minutes. PCR is more sensitive than microscopy but is technically more complex. It is available in some reference laboratories and can be useful for confirmation and diagnosis of multiple species of malaria, but the time delay in availability of results generally precludes its use for acute diagnosis of malaria. PCR detection may detect asymptomatic parasitemia in children with very-low-level parasitemia (e.g., internationally adopted children from malaria-endemic areas), with greater sensitivity than microscopy, and may be the preferred method of detection in these children, who, since asymptomatic, do not require immediate treatment.

LABORATORY SALIENT FINDINGS

- Giemsa-stained thick smears
- ELISA
- DNA hybridization.
- Polymerase chain reaction
- *Reflection of severity:* Decreased hematocrit, hemoglobin, haptoglobin levels, increased reticulocyte count, increased LDH levels
- Thrombocytopenia

DNA: deoxyribonucleic acid; ELISA: enzyme-linked immunosorbent assay; LDH: lactate dehydrogenase

---

DIFFERENTIAL DIAGNOSIS

The differential diagnosis of malaria includes the following.
- Typhoid
- Hepatitis
- Septicemia
- Urinary tract infection
- Meningitis
- Encephalitis

TREATMENT

Management includes symptomatic treatment and specific treatment. Fluids and electrolytes are given intravenously to maintain hydration.

All ill-appearing children should be considered nonimmune. Children <5 years old, children traveling to or from malaria endemic areas but originally from a non-endemic area, and children who have been away from an endemic area for >6 months should be considered nonimmune. In many malaria-endemic countries, there are large cities where little or no malaria transmission occurs, and individuals from these cities are essentially nonimmune. A well-appearing child over 5 years of age who has arrived within 6 months from a malaria-endemic area but has *Plasmodium* species infection on a blood smear may be considered semi-immune.

P. falciparum malaria can be a life-threatening emergency, especially in nonimmune individuals. Any child from a malaria-endemic area with signs and symptoms of severe malaria should be treated for *P. falciparum* malaria while awaiting blood smear confirmation. Nonimmune children with documented *P. falciparum* malaria should be hospitalized, because clinical decompensation can occur rapidly, even in children with a relatively benign initial presentation. Nonimmune children with *P. vivax, P. ovale,* or *P malariae* infection can appear quite ill with the initial paroxysm and also typically require hospitalization

Supportive therapy includes fluid and electrolyte balance. Dehydration and shock are corrected. Packed red cells are transfused. Renal failure and seizures are managed accordingly.

Uncomplicated Malaria

Chloroquine 10 mg of base/kg is given stat. This is followed by 5 mg of the base/kg at 12, 24, and 36-hour intervals. Patients with *P. vivax* and *P. ovale* malaria should be given 0.25 mg/kg daily for 14 days to prevent relapse.

Malaria due to P. vivax, P. ovale, P. malariae, and P. knowlesi: Complications due to *P. vivax, P. ovale,* or *P. malariae* are less common than with *P. falciparum*, and severe disease is consequently less common as well, but all malaria species can cause significant illness in a nonimmune child, and in some areas. *P. vivax* is a more common cause of severe illness than *P. falciparum*. Coinfection with *P. falciparum* may be missed on blood smear if the slide reader is inexperienced or if the infection inoculum is low. Children hospitalized with non-*P. falciparum* malaria should be given the same drug treatment regimen as children hospitalized for falciparum malaria.

The guidelines recommend chloroquine or hydroxychloroquine treatment for malaria due to *P. vivax, P. ovale, P. knowlesi,* and *P. malariae*. Prior to treatment with primaquine, all patients should be screened for G6PD deficiency. Individuals with the severe form of G6PD deficiency may experience oxidant hemolysis and methemoglobinemia with primaquine administration and hence should not receive primaquine. There are currently no effective alternatives to primaquine for liver-stage parasite eradication.

Although scattered reports of *P. ovale* and *P. malariae* chloroquine resistance exist, resistance is not widespread and chloroquine remains first-line therapy for these parasites.

Chloroquine-resistant Malaria

The following are used in the case of chloroquine-resistant malaria.

- Quinine 7 mg/kg IV infusion is done over 4 hours followed by 10 mg/kg infusion over 2–8 hours at 8 hours interval until the patient can swallow. The 7-day course should be completed with quinine tablets and syrup 10 mg/kg 3 times a day.
- Artemether 3.2 mg/kg IM stat followed by 1.6 mg/kg at 24-hour interval for 6 days.
- Artesunate 2.4 mg/kg stat by IV injection followed by 1.2 mg/kg after 12 hours and then 1.2 mg/kg daily for 6 days

Treatment of *P. falciparum* Malaria

Intravenous quinidine remains the drug of choice for all children with *P. falciparum*-malaria who require hospitalization. Artesunate is recommended by the WHO in preference to quinidine for the treatment of severe malaria based on studies showing lower mortality in children with severe malaria treated with artesunate. Artesunate has been used worldwide for many years. Treating *P. falciparum* infection with quinine, quinidine, artesunate, or artemether alone has been associated with significant recrudescence rates, which are decreased with the addition of doxycycline, tetracycline, or clindamycin. High-level quinine resistance, although reported, remains uncommon.

The potential cardiac toxicity of quinidine necessitates that patients receive it as an IV infusion, never as a bolus, while on continuous electrocardiographic monitoring. Infusion rates should be reduced if the QT interval is prolonged by >25% of the base-line value. Both quinine and quinidine can induce hyperinsulinemic hypoglycemia, which may cause lethargy or unresponsiveness that is confused with cerebral malaria; therefore, glucose levels should be followed in severely ill patients who are on these medications. Long-term side effects from either medication are uncommon, and the cinchonism (nausea, dysphoria, tinnitus, and high-tone deafness) seen with quinine resolves with cessation of quinine therapy

When children are ready for oral therapy, guidelines suggest completion of the course with oral quinine plus doxycycline, tetracycline, or clindamycin. However, many children do not tolerate oral quinine well, and in practice, a full course of artemether-lumefantrine is often given instead of quinine.

Adjunctive treatment for severe malaria includes blood transfusion for children with severe malarial anemia, seizure medication for children with repeated seizures, and IV antibiotics for children with hypotension or other signs of sepsis. Exchange transfusion for hyperparasitemia is controversial. Some guidelines still recommend exchange transfusion for parasitemia >10%, but a recent review concluded that there was little evidence to suggest benefit to patients from exchange transfusion.

Uncomplicated P. falciparum Malaria

Chloroquine resistant: Artemether-lumefantrine and atovaquone-proguanil are the preferred alternatives to quinine treatment for uncomplicated chloroquine-resistant *P. falciparum* malaria. It has few side effects, and the side effects of atovaquone-proguanil (abdominal pain, vomiting, nausea, and headache) are usually mild and self-limited. In some studies, an elevation of transaminases was seen with atovaquone-proguanil treatment, but transaminase elevations have not been associated with untoward clinical events. Atovaquone-proguanil should be taken with food or a milky drink. Vomiting occurs within 1 hour of dosing of artemether-lumefantrine, a repeat dose should be given. Because atovaquone-proguanil is also used for prophylaxis, it is typically more easily available than artemether-lumefantrine. Children who took atovaquone-proguanil for malaria prophylaxis should not receive it for the treatment of malaria. Instead, artemether-lumefantrine, or, if artemether-lumefantrine is not immediately available, quinine or mefloquine, should be used in children who have received atovaquone-proguanil prophylaxis.

Oral quinine plus doxycycline, tetracycline, or clindamycin can also be used for the treatment of uncomplicated chloroquine-resistant *P. falciparum* infection but has significantly more side effects than artemether-lumefantrine or atovaquone-proguanil.

Children frequently vomit after receiving quinine, especially if they are febrile when receiving the drug. Acetaminophen and sponging prior to administration of oral quinine may decrease the likelihood of vomiting. If vomiting occurs within an hour, the full dose of quinine should be repeated, but it vomiting occurs after 1 hour, no repeat quinine dosing is necessary. Other side effects of quinine have been mentioned earlier. In situations, where urgent treatment is required and IV medications cannot be given, intrarectal or IM quinine has been used successfully.

Mefloquine can be used to treat chloroquine-resistant malaria, but increasing mefloquine resistance and significant CNS side effects with treatment dosages make it an inferior choice, to be used only when artemether–lumefantrine, atovaquone–proguanil, or quinine treatment is not an option. Mefloquine should not be used if the child took mefloquine as prophylaxis, and it should not be used in conjunction with quinine or quinidine, as it may potentiate the cardiac side effects of these medications.

Mefloquine is used in the dose of 15 mg base/kg orally stat and repeated 8–24 hours after, in the dose of 10 mg/kg, i.e., two doses only.

Halofantrine is used in mefloquine-resistant cases. It is used in the dose of 8 mg/kg given 3 times at 6–8 hours intervals for 3 days.

Chloroquine sensitive: Chloroquine remains the drug of choice for chloroquine-susceptible *P. falciparum* malaria. It is inexpensive, generally well tolerated, and easy to administer. Side effects include pruritus in dark-skinned patients (which is fairly common) and, in treatment doses, nausea, dysphoria, and rarely a transient neuropsychiatric syndrome or cerebellar dysfunction. Hydroxychloroquine may be used if chloroquine is not available. If there is any doubt as to whether chloroquine resistance is present in the area malaria was acquired, quinine should be used. Quinidine is the preferred drug in the United States for parenteral treatment of chloroquine-sensitive malaria.

Cerebral Malaria

Chloroquine is used at the dose of 10 mg/kg IV infusion in 0.9% saline and as IV fluid such as 5% or 10% dextrose 10 mg/kg as a maintenance dose.

Treatment of Relapse

Treatment of relapse requires a specific therapy with a combination of chloroquine followed by primaquine for 10–14 days. Treatment of relapsing malaria (*P. vivax* and *P. ovale*) is treated with a standard course of chloroquine followed by primaquine 0.25 mg/kg orally per day for 14 days.

P. Vivax malaria:
- Recurrence within 28 days is due to inadequate treatment or drug resistance.
- Retreatment with different class/regimen is indicated.
- Recurrence after 28 days is due to relapse or reinfection. Weekly suppressive therapy with 10 mg/kg of primaquine for 3–6 months is indicated.

P. falciparum malaria:
- Recurrence within 28 days is due to recrudescence. It is treated with an alternate regimen. If the original regimen was artemisinin-based combination therapies (ACT) regimen, that patient should be treated with quinine plus doxycycline/clindamycin regimen.
- Recurrence after 28 days is due to reinfection and same initial regimen may be restarted.

Prophylaxis

Chloroquine is given (5 mg/kg) orally every week. In prophylaxis, in chloroquine-resistant areas, mefloquine (3.5 mg base/kg weekly) or doxycycline 2 mg/kg daily is given.

Short-term chemoprophylaxis:
- It is indicated in people who plan to stay up to 6 weeks in high-endemic areas of *P. falciparum* malaria.
- Doxycycline 1.5 mg/kg, once daily, maximum dose 100 mg in children above 8 years
- To start 2 days before arrival and continue 4 weeks after leaving an endemic area

Long-term chemoprophylaxis:
- It is indicated in people who plan to stay for >6 weeks in high-endemic areas of *P. falciparum* malaria.
- Mefloquine 5 mg/kg, maximum dose 250 mg, weekly
- Start 2 weeks before and continue for 4 weeks after leaving endemic areas.

■ BIBLIOGRAPHY

1. Crawly J, Chu C, Mtove G, Nosten F. Malaria in children. Lancet. 2010;375:1468-81.
2. Esu EB, Effa EE, Opie ON, Meremikwu MM. Artemether for severe malaria. Cochrane Database Syst Rev. 2019;6(6):CD010678.
3. Griffith KS, Lewis LS, Mali S, Parise ME. Treatment of malaria in the United States: a systematic review. JAMA. 2007;297(20): 2264-77.
4. World Health Organization. (2015). Guidelines for the treatment of malaria, 3rd edition. [online] Available from https://iris.who.int/handle/10665/162441 [Last accessed June 2024].

CASE 73

Measles

■ PRESENTING COMPLAINTS

A 10-month-old girl was brought with the complaint of:
- Cold and cough since 5 days
- Fever since 5 days
- Rashes since 1 day

History of Presenting Complaints

A 10-month-old girl was brought to the pediatric outpatient department with history of rashes all over the body. Her mother told that the child had cough, cold, and fever 3 days back. She was on symptomatic and antibiotic treatment. Fever was of mild-to-moderate degree. Her mother had also told the temperature was not decreasing in spite of antipyretics. In addition, the cold was associated with nasal block and she had feeding problems. Cough used to be more in night, hence child had disturbed sleep. On the fourth day, her mother noticed the small red-colored rashes over the trunk, abdomen, and back. Rashes were not elevated over the skin. There was no itching.

Past History of the Patient

The girl was the first sibling of nonconsanguineous marriage. She was born at term by normal vaginal delivery and cried immediately after the delivery. The birth weight was 3 kg. She started taking the breast milk immediately. There was no significant postnatal event. She was exclusively on breastfeeds for 3 months. Developmental milestones were normal.

CASE AT A GLANCE	
Basic Findings	
Length	: 70 cm (50th centile)
Weight	: 7.5 kg (50th centile)
Temperature	: 39°C
Pulse rate	: 126 beats/min
Respiratory rate	: 28 breaths/min
Blood pressure	: 60/46 mm Hg
Positive Findings	
History:	
• Fever	
• Cough and cold	
• Rashes	
Examination:	
• Febrile	
• Signs of dehydration	
• Sick look	
• Rashes	
Investigation:	
• *X-ray chest:* Signs of bronchopneumonia	

■ EXAMINATION

The child was moderately built and moderately nourished. She was looking sick and was irritable. Signs of mild dehydration were present. Anthropometric measurements included the length 70 cm (50th centile) and the weight 7.5 kg (50th centile). The head circumference was 43 cm.

The child was febrile, i.e., 39°C. The heart rate was 126 beats/min and the respiratory rate was 28 breaths/min. Blood pressure recorded was 60/46 mm Hg. There was no pallor, no lymphadenopathy, no edema, and cyanosis. There were signs of rhinitis.

Respiratory system revealed presence of crepitation at the base. Other systemic examinations were normal.

■ INVESTIGATION

- *Hemoglobin:* 12 g/dL
- *TLC:* 7,600 cells/cumm
- *DLC:* $P_{73}L_{25}E_2$
- *ESR:* 26 mm in the first hour
- *AEC:* 430 cells/cumm
- *X-ray chest:* Signs of bronchopneumonia

■ DISCUSSION

It is a communicable disease characterized by fever, cough, coryza, and Koplik's spots in the preeruptive phase. Maculopapular rashes appear on fourth and fifth day of the illness.

Measles virus is a spherical, nonsegmented, single-stranded, negative-sense RNA virus and a member of the *Morbillivirus* genus in the family of Paramyxoviridae. Measles was originally a zoonotic infection, arising from cross-species transmission from animals to humans by an ancestral *Morbillivirus*. Although RNA viruses typically have high mutation rates, measles virus is considered to be an antigenically monotypic virus, meaning that the surface proteins responsible for inducing protective immunity have retained their antigenic structure across time and space.

Measles virus is transmitted primarily by respiratory droplets over short distances and, less commonly, by small-particle aerosols that remain suspended in the air for long periods of time. Airborne transmission appears to be important in certain settings, including schools, pediatrician offices, hospitals, and enclosed public places, and infectious droplets may persist for several hours after an infected child has left a pediatrician's office. Direct contact with infected secretions can transmit measles virus, but the virus does not survive long on fomites. The disease is more common in preschool children and occurs in all seasons. It is more in winter and spring months.

Infection is initiated when measles virus reaches epithelial cells in the respiratory tract, oropharynx, or conjunctivae. Wild-type measles virus strains preferentially bind to signaling lymphocytic activating molecule (SLAM) (CDI50), expressed on activated T cells, B cells, and antigen-presenting cells. Whereas laboratory-adapted strains can also bind CD46, which is expressed on all nucleated cells.

Measles virus, thus, infects lymphocytes and dendritic cells, as well as respiratory epithelial cells, which contributes to systemic spread. During the first 2–4 days after infection, measles virus proliferates locally in the respiratory mucosa and spreads to draining lymph nodes where further replication occurs. The virus then enters the bloodstream in infected leukocytes, primarily monocytes, producing the primary viremia that disseminates infection throughout the reticuloendothelial system.

Further replication results in a secondary viremia that begins 5–7 days after infection and disseminates measles virus to tissues throughout the body. Replication of measles virus in these target organs, together with the host immune response, is responsible for the signs and symptoms that occur 8–12 days after infection and mark the end of the incubation period.

The incubation period for measles, the time from infection to clinical disease, is approximately 10 days to the onset of fever and 14 days to the onset of rash. The incubation period may be shorter in infants or following a large inoculum of virus and may be longer (up to 3 weeks) in adults.

PATHOLOGY

Measles is caused by RNA paramyxovirus. There is only one serotype. The virus cannot survive outside the human body, for any length or time but retains the infectivity when stored at subzero temperature. The only source of infection is measles case. Carriers are not known to occur. The infective material includes secretion of the nose, throat, and respiratory tract during the prodromal period and early stages of rash.

Measles is highly infectious during the prodromal period and at the time eruption. Communicability declines rapidly after the appearance of rash. The period of communicability is approximately 4 days before and 5 days after the appearance of rash. Isolation of the patient for a week from the onset of rash covers the period of communicability. As there is one antigenic type of measles virus infection, confers lifelong immunity. Hence so-called secondary attacks represent the error in diagnosis.

Cells are killed by cell-to-cell plasma membrane fusion associated with viral replication that occurs in many body tissues, including cells of the CNS. Virus shedding begins in the prodromal phase. With onset of the rash, antibody production begins, and viral replication and symptoms begin to subside.

Diseases other than measles that have been associated with measles virus include subacute sclerosing panencephalitis (SSPE), multiple sclerosis, cirrhosis disease, Paget's disease, and systemic lupus erythematosus (SLE).

There is generalized hyperplasia of the lymphoid tissue. Lesions include superficial vessels of corium of skin and in capillary bed of the mucosa. There is perivascular infiltration with mononuclear and polymorphonuclear leukocytosis. Frank vesicles are formed. Multinucleated giant cells infiltrate into the lymphoid tissue. Multinucleated giant cells are found. They are two types: Warthin-Finkeledy cells of reticuloendothelial system and epithelioid giant cells of respiratory system. Inclusion bodies may be seen in brain cells, CSF examination shows pleocytosis. Lungs may show peribronchial inflammatory reaction with mononuclear cells, giant cell, pneumonia, and secondary bacterial pneumonia.

Measles tend to be more severe in malnourished child. This may be related to poor cell-mediated immunity response secondary to malnutrition. They excrete measles virus for longer periods indicated prolonged risk for themselves and of intensity of spread to others. Local multiplication in respiratory epithelium leads to viremia (day 2–3) and subsequently spread to reticuloendothelial system cells of reticuloendothelial system necrose causing secondary viremia (day 5–7). This is responsible for systemic symptoms.

CLINICAL FEATURES (FIG. 1)

Actually everyone in infancy or childhood between 6 months to 3 years of age in developing countries are vulnerable for disease. No age is immune if there was no previous immunity. Infants are protected by maternal antibodies up to 6 months of age and on some cases the maternal immunity may persist beyond 9 months. Immunity after the vaccination is solid and long-lasting.

In individuals with passively acquired antibody, such as infants and recipients of blood products, a subclinical form of measles may occur. The rash may be indistinct, brief, or rarely, entirely absent. Likewise, some individuals who have received vaccine, when exposed to measles, may have developed a rash but few other symptoms. Persons with inapparent or subclinical measles do not shed measles virus and do not transmit infection to household contacts.

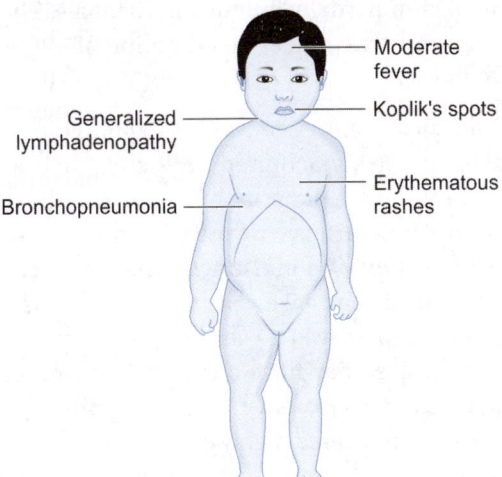

Fig. 1: Clinical features.

There are three stages in the clinical features, which are described in the following text.

Prodromal Stage

Measles is a serious infection characterized by high fever, an enanthem, cough, coryza, conjunctivitis, and a prominent exanthem. After an incubation period of 8–12 days, the prodromal phase begins with a mild fever followed by the onset of conjunctivitis with photophobia, coryza, a prominent cough, and increasing fever. Koplik's spots represent the enanthem and are the pathognomonic sign of measles, appearing 1–4 days prior to the onset of the rash. They first appear as discrete, red lesions with bluish-white spots in the center on the inner aspects of the cheeks at the level of the premolars. They may spread to involve the lips, hard palate, and gingiva. They also may occur in conjunctival folds and in the vaginal mucosa. Koplik's spots **(Figs. 2A and B)** have been reported in 50–70% of measles cases but probably occur in the great majority.

Anorexia and malaise are often accompanied. Moderate generalized lymphadenopathy is also seen. Bleeding occurs from

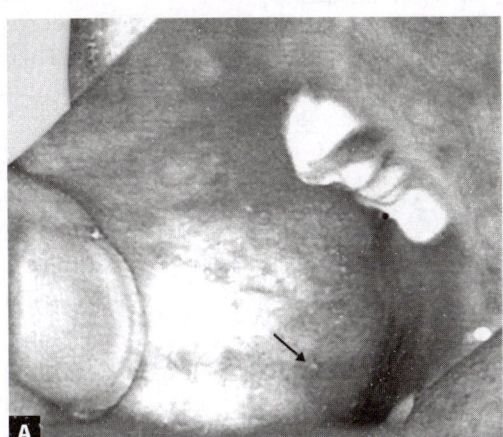
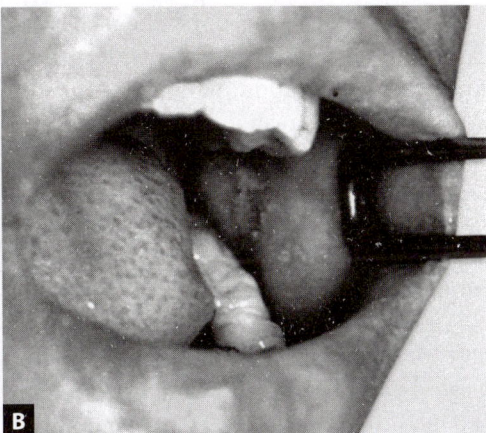

Figs. 2A and B: Koplik spots. *(For color version, see Plate 5)*

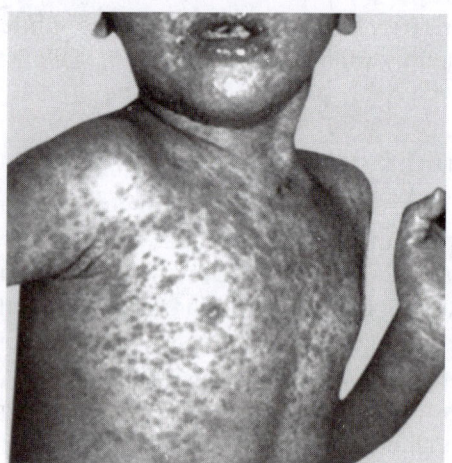

Fig. 3: Maculopapular rashes.
(For color version, see Plate 5)

the mouth, nose and bowel and many result in death.

Eruptive Phase

Symptoms increase in intensity for 2–4 days until the first day of the rash. Typically the rash appears on the fourth day of the fever. This is characterized by typical, macular or maculopapular rashes **(Fig. 3)**. The rash first appears behind the ear, then trunk and extremities. Later, it extends down the body and lower limbs within 2–3 days. The rash may become discrete. In the absence of complication, the rash and fever will disappear in another 4–5 days. The rash fades in the same order of appearance leaving a brownish discoloration, which may persist for 2 months. The rash is erythematous and blanches on pressure. Fever and rash may remain for about a week in uncomplicated cases. Rash may be atypical in few cases. It may be modified to hemorrhagic type. Hemorrhagic measles is characterized by high-fever convulsion, delirium, stupor, and even coma. Of the major symptoms of measles, the cough lasts the longest, often up to 10 days. In more severe cases, generalized lymphadenopathy may be present, with cervical and occipital lymph nodes especially prominent.

Post-measles Stage

There will be loss of weight. Child may fail to recover and there will be gradual deterioration into chronic illness due to increased susceptibility to other bacterial and viral infection. There may be growth retardation and diarrhea, cancrum oris, pyogenic infection, candidosis, and reactivation of pulmonary tuberculosis. Modified measles is seen in partially immune individuals. The symptoms are milder and duration of illness is shorter.

Modified measles infection: In individuals with passively acquired antibody, such as infants and recipients of blood products, a subclinical form of measles may occur The rash may be indistinct, brief, or, rarely, entirely absent. Likewise, some individuals who have received a vaccine, when exposed to measles, may have a rash but few other symptoms. Persons with modified measles are not considered highly contagious.

GENERAL FEATURES
• Dry hacking cough
• Cold and sneezing
• Anorexia, malaise
• Bronchopneumonia
• Encephalitis
• Subacute sclerosing panencephalitis
• Malnutrition

ESSENTIAL DIAGNOSTIC POINTS
• Contact with measles 10–14 days back
• Fever, cough, conjunctivitis, and coryza
• Koplik's spots 1–2 days prior to and after onset of rash
• Maculopapular rash spreading down from the face and hairline to the trunk over 3 days and later becoming confluent
• Leukopenia

DIAGNOSIS

Measles is readily diagnosed on clinical grounds by clinicians familiar with the disease. Koplik's spots are especially helpful because they appear early and are pathognomonic of measles. The case definition for measles requires (1) a generalized maculopapular rash of at least 3 days in duration; (2) fever of at least 38.3°C (101°F); and (3) cough, coryza, or conjunctivitis.

Serology is the most common method of laboratory diagnosis. A positive IgM on a single serum specimen or a significant increase in serum IgG antibody concentration in paired acute and convalescent serum specimens (collected at least 10 days apart) in a patient with clinical manifestations consistent with measles is considered diagnostic of acute infection. Measles virus-specific IgM antibodies may not be detectable until 4–5 days or more after rash onset and usually fall to undetectable levels within 4–8 weeks of rash onset.

Commercially available EIAs can detect either IgM or IgG antibodies to measles virus and are the most frequently used diagnostic methods. Measles can also be diagnosed by isolation of measles virus or identification of measles RNA by RT-PCR amplification of RNA extracted from clinical specimens, such as urine, blood, or throat or nasopharyngeal secretions.

Serologic confirmation is most conveniently made by identification of IgM antibody in serum. IgM antibody appears 1–2 days after the onset of the rash and remains detectable for about 1 month. If a serum specimen is collected <72 hours after onset of rash and is negative for measles antibody, a second specimen should be obtained. Serologic confirmation may also be made by demonstration of a fourfold rise in IgG antibodies in acute and convalescent specimens collected 2–4 weeks apart. Viral isolation from blood, urine, or respiratory secretions can be accomplished by culture at the Centers for Disease Control and Prevention (CDC) or local or state laboratories.

LABORATORY SALIENT FINDINGS

- ELISA
- Hemagglutination tests
- IgM antibodies
- Lymphopenia

(ELISA: enzyme-linked immunosorbent assay; IgM: immunoglobulin M)

DIFFERENTIAL DIAGNOSIS

Differential diagnosis includes rubella, infectious mononucleosis, meningococcemia, and typhoid.

COMPLICATIONS

A wide variety of complications may be observed during the acute stage of measles or shortly thereafter.

A benign asymptomatic keratoconjunctivitis that accompanies measles may persist for as long as 4 months. More severe corneal lesions occur in malnourished children. Transient electrocardiographic abnormalities are common, but true myocarditis is rare. The diffuse lymphadenopathy that accompanies measles involves the mesenteric nodes and is believed to cause the abdominal pain that commonly occurs. Symptoms and signs identical to those of acute appendicitis may result in surgical intervention during the prodromal period.

Complications of bacterial origin result principally from invasion of the respiratory tract by pyogenic organisms. Otitis media and bronchopneumonia are most common. Peribronchitis and interstitial pneumonitis are seen in nearly all children with measles and resolve rapidly after the development of rash and the subsidence of fever. The respiratory tract is involved most often, but severe gastroenteritis also occurs. Acute laryngotracheobronchitis (croup) may cause sufficient airway obstruction to require tracheostomy, especially in children younger than 3 years.

A second fever spike, or failure of the initial spike to drop after the eruption has reached its peak, suggests a secondary bacterial infection. A chest radiograph may disclose bronchopneumonia or a pattern of segmental or lobar involvement.

During the early viremic phase of measles, there is a thrombocytopenia of insufficient magnitude to cause spontaneous bleeding. Another rare and unexplained postinfectious complication, thrombocytopenic purpura, appears 4-14 days after the rash and may produce marked skin purpura, genitourinary and gastrointestinal bleeding, and epistaxis.

Acute postinfectious measles encephalomyelitis is the most common neurologic complication of measles. It is rare in children younger than 2 years, but has occurrence of 1 in 1,000 cases of measles in older children and somewhat more frequently in adults. The onset is usually during the first week after the start of the rash and is typically abrupt, with irritability, headache, vomiting, and confusion, and progressing rapidly to obtundation and coma. These manifestations are frequently accompanied by seizures and recurrence or accentuation of fever.

Subacute Sclerosing Panencephalitis

Subacute sclerosing panencephalitis is a chronic complication of measles with a delayed onset and an outcome that is nearly always fatal. It appears to result from a persistent infection with an altered measles virus that is harbored intracellularly in the CNS for several years. After 7-10 years the virus apparently regains virulence and attacks the cells in the CNS that offered the virus protection. This "slow virus infection" results in inflammation and cell death, leading to an inexorable neurodegenerative process.

The pathogenesis of SSPE remains enigmatic. Factors that seem to be involved include defective measles virus and interaction with a defective or immature immune system. The virus isolated from brain tissue of patients with SSPE is missing 1 of the 6 structural proteins, the matrix or M protein. This protein is responsible for assembly, orientation, and alignment of the virus in preparation for budding during viral replication. Immature virus may be able to reside, and possibly propagate, within neuronal cells for long periods. The fact that most patients with SSPE were exposed at a young age suggests that immune immaturity is involved in pathogenesis.

Clinical manifestations of SSPE begin insidiously 7-13 years after primary measles infection. Subtle changes in behavior or school performance appear, including irritability, reduced attention span, and temper outbursts. This initial phase (first stage) may at times be missed because of brevity or mildness of the symptoms. Fever, headache, and other signs of encephalitis are absent. The hallmark of the second stage is massive myoclonus, which coincides with extension of the inflammatory process site to deeper structures in the brain, including the basal ganglia. Involuntary movements and repetitive myoclonic jerks begin in single muscle groups but give way to massive spasms and jerks involving both axial and appendicular muscles. Consciousness is maintained. In the third stage, involuntary movements disappear and are replaced by choreoathetosis, immobility, dystonia, and lead pipe rigidity that result from destruction of deeper centers in the basal ganglia. The sensorium deteriorates into dementia, stupor, and then coma. The fourth stage is characterized by loss of critical centers that support breathing, heart rate, and blood pressure. Death soon ensues. Progression through the clinical stages may follow courses characterized as acute, subacute, or chronic progressive.

Convalescence is prolonged with respiratory complication. Death may occur. The cause of death may be measles encephalopathy and may be left with severe neurological deficiency.

The diagnosis of SSPE can be established through documentation of a compatible clinical course and at least one of the following supporting findings: (1) Measles antibody detected in CSF, (2) characteristic electroencephalographic findings, and (3) typical histologic findings in and/or isolation of virus or viral antigen from brain tissue obtained by biopsy or postmortem examination.

Cerebrospinal fluid analysis reveals normal cells but elevated IgG and IgM antibody titers in dilutions >1:8. Electroencephalographic patterns are normal in first stage, but in the myoclonic phase, suppression–burst episodes are seen that are characteristic of, but not pathognomonic for, SSPE. Brain biopsy is no longer routinely indicated for diagnosis of SSPE.

Management of SSPE is primarily supportive and similar to care provided to patients with other neurodegenerative diseases. Clinical trials using isoprinosine with or without interferon suggest significant benefit (30–34% remission rate) compared with patients without treatment (5–10% with spontaneous remissions).

It is recognized that carbamazepine is of significant benefit in the control of myoclonic jerks in the early stages of the illness. Virtually all patients eventually succumb to SSPE. Most die within 1–3 years of onset from infection or loss of autonomic control mechanisms. Prevention of SSPE depends on prevention of primary measles infection through vaccination.

■ TREATMENT

Treatment is essentially symptomatic and supportive. Antiviral therapy is not effective in the treatment of measles in otherwise normal patients. Maintenance of hydration, oxygenation, and comfort are goals of therapy. Child should be given adequate amount of fluids orally. Nutrition of the patient should be maintained. If there is vomiting, IV fluid should be given. Fever is controlled by paracetamol and hydrotherapy. Cough may be treated by humidification and saline nebulization. Treatment of the respiratory complications includes antibiotics, oxygen, and supportive measures. Convulsions are managed by injections of diazepam and phenobarbitone.

Secondary bacterial infections are a major cause of morbidity and mortality following measles, and effective case management involves prompt treatment with antibiotics. Antibiotics are indicated tor children with measles, who have clinical evidence of bacterial infection, including pneumonia and otitis media. *Streptococcus pneumoniae* and *Haemophilus influenzae* type B were the most common causes of bacterial pneumonia following measles, and vaccines against these pathogens have lowered the incidence of secondary bacterial infections following measles.

Prophylactic antimicrobial therapy to prevent bacterial infection is not indicated. Measles infection in immunocompromised patients is highly lethal. Ribavirin is active in vitro against measles virus.

Vitamin A treatment results in marked reductions in morbidity and mortality. The WHO currently recommends vitamin A for all children with acute measles, regardless of their country of residence. Vitamin A for treatment of measles is administered once daily for 2 days, at the following doses: 200,000 IU for children 12 months or older; 100,000 IU for infants 6 through 11 months of age; and 50,000 IU for infants younger than 6 months. An additional (i.e., a third) age-specific dose should be given 2–4 weeks later to children with clinical signs and symptoms of vitamin A deficiency.

PREVENTION

Measles vaccine should not be used in patients with leukemia, lymphopenia, steroid therapy, and antimetabolic therapy. Passive immunization is done in exposed infants and younger siblings. Gamma globulin is injected intramuscularly. The doses 0.25 mL/kg and 0.5 mL/kg are recommended for children <1 year and >1 year, respectively.

BIBLIOGRAPHY

1. American Academy of Pediatrics. Measles. 2015 Report of the Committee on Infectious Disease, 30th edition. Elk Grove Village: American Academy of Pediatrics; 2015. pp. 535-47.
2. Fiebelkorn AP, Redd SB, Gastañaduy PA, Clemmons N, Rota PA, Rota JS, et al. A Comparison of Postelimination Measles Epidemiology in the United States, 2009–2014 Versus 2001–2008. J Pediatric Infect Dis Soc. 2017;6(1):40-8.
3. Moss WJ, Griffin DE. Measles. Lancet. 2012;379:153-64.
4. Rota PA, Moss WJ, Takeda M, de Swart RL, Thompson KM, Goodson JL. Measles. Nat Rev Dis Primers. 2016;2:16049.

CASE 74

Mumps

■ PRESENTING COMPLAINTS

An 8-year-old boy was brought with the complaint of:
- Fever since 3 days
- Swelling on both the cheeks since 3 days

History of Presenting Complaints

An 8-year-old boy was brought by his mother with history of swelling on both the cheeks. She told her son developed swelling first on the right side below the ear lobe and later on the left side. There was also associated history of fever. The fever was of moderate-to-high degree and intermittent in nature and used to more in the evening. The child was on treatment for the fever.

Past History of the Patient

He was the elder sibling of nonconsanguineous marriage. He was born at term by normal vaginal delivery. There was no significant postnatal event. He was exclusively on breast milk for 4 months. Weaning was started later as per the advice of family doctor. Child was on family food by 18 months. He had been completely immunized and all the developmental milestones were normal. His performance at school was good. There was also history of similar type of illness in his class. There was no history of rashes over the body.

CASE AT A GLANCE

Basic Findings
Height	:	123 cm (50th centile)
Weight	:	25 kg (75th centile)
Temperature	:	38.6°C
Pulse rate	:	110 beats/min
Respiratory rate	:	26 breaths/min
Blood pressure	:	80/60 mm Hg

Positive Findings

History:
- Fever
- Swelling at cheeks
- Similar complaints in school

Examination:
- Febrile
- Parotid gland swelling

Investigation:
- Normal

■ EXAMINATION

The boy was moderately built and nourished. He was sitting comfortably on examination table. Anthropometric measurements included the height 123 cm (50th centile) and the weight 25 kg (75th centile). He was febrile, i.e., 38.6°C. The heart rate was 110 beats/min, the respiratory rate was 26 breaths/min, and blood pressure recorded was 80/60 mm Hg. There was no pallor, no lymphadenopathy, no cyanosis, and no icterus.

There was diffuse swelling at angle of mandible involving parotid glands on both sides. It was tender. Other systemic examinations were normal.

INVESTIGATION

- *Hemoglobin:* 13 g/dL
- *TLC:* 9,900 cells/cumm
- *DLC:* $P_{67}L_{30}E_2M_1$
- *ESR:* 26 mm in the first hour
- *AEC:* 330 cells/cumm
- *Mantoux test:* Negative
- *X-ray chest:* NAD

DISCUSSION

Mumps is an acute viral infection characterized for painful enlargement of the salivary gland especially parotid gland. Mumps virus is an RNA virus. It spreads from the human reservoir by direct contact or air-borne droplets. The causative agent is myovirus parotiditis. There is only one serotype.

Infants are rarely involved due to the presence of transplacentally acquired maternal mumps antibodies. Carrier state does not exist. Lifelong immunity follows the clinical attack.

Mumps virus is in the family Paramyxoviridae and the genus *Rubulavirus*. It is a single-stranded pleomorphic RNA virus encapsulated in a lipoprotein envelope and possessing seven structural proteins. Surface glycoproteins called HN (hemagglutinin-neuraminidase) and F (fusion) mediate absorption of the virus to host cells and penetration of the virus into cells, respectively. Both of these proteins stimulate production of protective antibodies. Mumps virus exists as a single immunotype, and humans are the only natural host.

PATHOLOGY AND PATHOGENESIS

Mumps is a communicable, systemic viral illness most often characterized by parotitis. Mumps virus is a paramyxovirus closely related to parainfluenza viruses. Mumps is spread by respiratory droplet or through direct contact with saliva. The virus can be isolated from saliva up to 7 days before and through 8 days after parotid swelling.

It commonly occurs between the age of 5 and 15 years. Man is the reservoir of the infection. Saliva is highly infective. Inoculation is by direct contact in infants below the age of 6 months, who are immune because of maternal antibodies.

The virus enters through the nose and mouth and proliferates in parotid gland and respiratory mucosa. This is followed by viremia. Following infection, initial viral replication occurs in the epithelium of the upper respiratory tract. Infection spreads to the adjacent lymph nodes by the lymphatic drainage, and viremia ensues, spreading the virus to targeted tissues. Mumps virus targets the salivary glands, CNS pancreas, testes, and, to a lesser extent, thyroid, ovaries, heart, kidney liver, and joint synovia.

Mumps virus causes necrosis of infected cells and is associated with a lymphocytic inflammatory infiltrate. Salivary gland ducts are lined with necrotic epithelium, and the interstitium is infiltrated with lymphocytes. Swelling of tissue within the testes may result in focal ischemic infarcts. The CSF frequently contains a mononuclear pleocytosis, even in individual without clinical signs of meningitis.

The virus can be isolated from saliva, blood, urine, and CSF. It can be isolated from saliva 6 days before and up to 9 days appearance of the parotid or salivary gland swelling. This is the period of infectivity. It has been isolated from urine from first to 14th day after the onset of salivary gland swelling. Secondary attack rate is 80%. First trimester mumps is associated with increased fetal mortality.

CLINICAL FEATURES (FIG. 1)

The incubation period ranges from 14 to 24 days with the peak at 17–18 days. The

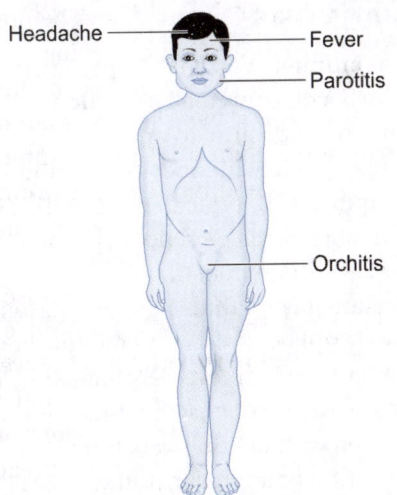

Fig. 1: Clinical features.

ESSENTIAL DIAGNOSTIC POINTS
- No prior mumps immunization
- Parotid gland swelling
- Aseptic meningitis with or without parotitis
- Orchitis

prodromal symptoms may be manifested by fever, muscular pain, headache, and malaise.

A patient with mumps rarely has severe systemic manifestations. Body temperature is typically only moderately elevated for 3–4 days. Symptoms such as abdominal discomfort, anorexia, and headache may precede parotid gland involvement by 1–2 days.

The onset is usually characterized by pain and swelling in one or both parotid glands. Edema of skin and soft tissue extend further and obscure the limit of the glandular swelling. Parotid swelling, however, may be the first sign of illness. It is better seen than felt. It reaches the maximum size by 1–3 days. Swollen tissues push the earlobe upward and outward. Angle of the mandible is not visible. Swelling usually subsides by 3–7 days. Swelling may last 7–10 days and be observed on one or both sides of the face. The submandibular glands may also swell either in addition to the parotid or sometimes in the absence of parotid involvement. Presternal edema is sometimes present. There will be redness and swelling at the orifice of the Wharton's duct. The orifice of the Stensen's duct may show signs of inflammation.

Some patients with mumps complain of abdominal pain, which could represent involvement of the pancreas or, in the female, the ovaries. Serum amylase is usually elevated during mumps infection, and vomiting can occur.

Complications from mumps disease are more common among adults than children. The most feared complication of mumps in males is orchitis. Although orchitis has been reported to occur in persons as young as 3 years of age, it is seen most frequently in postpubertal males, with the highest incidence in those 15–29 years of age. Orchitis is estimated to occur in 14–35% of males with mumps disease. The onset of orchitis is usually heralded by fever toward the first week of illness. Severe pain, swelling, and tenderness, which may persist for weeks, are common. Involvement is most often unilateral, but bilateral involvement has been reported. Testicular atrophy may occur after mumps orchitis unilateral atrophy does not result in sterility, but sterility may occur if the patient has bilateral orchitis. The development of malignancy in mumps-affected testes has been reported.

Other glands may also be occasionally involved with mumps disease. Mastitis is estimated to occur in 31% of females older than 15 years, who are infected with mumps virus. Findings of oophoritis include emesis, fever, and lower abdominal pain. Involvement of the thyroid gland and the development of diabetes mellitus have both been reported to occur after the onset of mumps.

Mumps virus is neurotropic, and >50% of patients with mumps disease have CSF pleocytosis. However, <10% have findings typical of aseptic meningitis. Mumps meningitis can occur in the absence of parotid involvement. CSF findings show predominantly lymphocytic cells, with counts usually <500 cells/μL; CSF glucose is typically normal to slightly low, with CSF protein normal to slightly high. Evidence of encephalitis occurs rarely in mumps disease.

Other manifestations include aseptic meningitis, encephalitis, auditory nerve damage, leading to deafness, cerebellar ataxia-facial neuritis, transverse myelitis, and Guillain–Barre syndrome.

An association has been reported between mumps virus infection in the first trimester of pregnancy and an increased rate of fetal demise/spontaneous abortion. There is no convincing evidence, however, that mumps virus, which can cross the placenta, produces congenital malformations. Mumps virus has been isolated from breast milk. Deafness is a known complication associated with mumps disease, occurring in 1 in 20,000 reported cases. Permanent hearing impairment is most often unilateral, with higher tone frequency loss the most severe. Onset of hearing loss is typically sudden and is not related to CNS involvement. Mumps infected mothers also prone to have low-birth-weight babies. Recently, intrauterine mumps is associated with endocardial fibroelastosis.

GENERAL FEATURES
• Nausea
• Malaise
• Loss of appetite
• Submaxillary and sublingual glands are enlarged
• Encephalitis

DIAGNOSIS

When mumps was highly prevalent, the diagnosis could be made on the basis of a history of exposure to mumps infection, an appropriate incubation period, and development of typical clinical findings. Confirmation of the presence of parotitis could be made with demonstration of an elevated serum amylase value. Leukopenia with a relative lymphocytosis was a common finding. EIA of IgG and IgM levels is commonly used. Mumps virus can be isolated in cell culture inoculated with buccal swab, throat washing, saliva or CSF, or urine during the acute illness.

Serologic testing is usually a more convenient and available mode of diagnosis. A significant increase in serum mumps IgG antibody between acute and convalescent serum specimens as detected by complement fixation, neutralization, hemagglutination, or EIA tests establishes the diagnosis. These are rarely done, but it is possible to identify infection acutely by detecting antibodies to the "S" antigen by complement fixation antibody titers, which rise in first week of illness, and "V" antigen by complement fixation antibody titers that follow with a rise several weeks later, and may persist at low levels for years. Neutralizing and hemagglutination inhibiting antibodies appear during convalescence.

Confirmation of the diagnosis of mumps infection is accomplished by: (1) Isolation of the virus in culture; (2) detection of mumps virus nucleic acid by RT-PCR from either saliva or CSF; (3) detection of mumps-specific IgM antibody's; or (4) demonstration of a significant mumps serum IgG antibody titer rise, quantitatively or semiquantitatively, between acute and convalescent (2 or more weeks apart) serologic assays.

Reverse transcriptase polymerase chain reaction is becoming increasingly more available, and consequently, culture is now performed less frequently. A negative IgM test in a previously immunized individual does not eliminate the diagnosis of mumps, because an IgM response may be absent. In addition, again in a previously immunized patient, an IgG titer rise may be blunted by the presence of preexisting antibody. Viral excretion in saliva from a previously immunized person with possible mumps may also be shortened in duration.

DIFFERENTIAL DIAGNOSIS

Differential diagnosis includes HIV, influenza, CMV, coxsackie virus, suppurative parotitis, recurrent parotitis, lymphadenitis, calculus in stenosis duct.

Parotid swelling may be caused by many other infectious and noninfectious conditions, especially in sporadic cases. Viruses that cause parotitis include parainfluenza 1 and parainfluenza 3 viruses, influenza A virus, CMV, EBV, enteroviruses, lymphocytic choriomeningitis virus, and HIV. Purulent parotitis, usually caused by *Staphylococcus aureus*, is unilateral, extremely tender, associated with an elevated white blood cell count, and may involve purulent drainage from the Stensen's duct. Submandibular or anterior cervical adenitis from a variety of pathogens may also be confused with parotitis. Other noninfectious causes of parotid swelling include obstruction of the Stensen's duct, collagen vascular diseases such as Sjögren syndrome, SLE, immunologic diseases, tumor, and drugs.

LABORATORY SALIENT FINDINGS
- CSF analysis shows lymphocytosis
- Viral culture of saliva throat, urine, spinal fluid
- ELISA
- Compliment fixing antibody to the antigen

(CSF: cerebrospinal fluid; ELISA: enzyme-linked immunosorbent assay)

COMPLICATIONS
- Orchitis, thyroiditis
- Epididymitis
- Pancreatitis
- Oophoritis
- Nephritis
- Meningoencephalomyelitis

TREATMENT

There is no specific treatment. Antipyretics, bed rest, and diet are recommended. Paracetamol and aspirin are given to relieve pain. Warm saline mouthwash is advised. Orchitis is treated with local support and steroids. Steroids relieve pain and swelling of orchitis and arthritis quickly.

PREVENTION

The control of mumps is difficult, because the disease is infectious before a diagnosis can be made. The long and variable incubation period and occurrence of subclinical cases make the control of the spread difficult. However, the cases should be isolated till the clinical manifestations subside. Contacts should be kept under surveillance.

It is given as part of the MMR two-dose vaccine schedule, at 12-15 months of age for the first dose and 4-6 years of age for the second dose. If not given at 4-6 years, the second dose should be given before children enter puberty. Antibody develops in 94% (range: 89-97%) of vaccines after 1 dose. Antibody levels achieved following vaccination are lower than following natural infection.

PROGNOSIS

The outcome of mumps is nearly always excellent, even when the disease is complicated by encephalitis, although fatal cases from CNS involvement or myocarditis have been reported.

BIBLIOGRAPHY

1. Centers for Disease Control and Prevention. (2024). About Mumps. [online] Available from https://www.cdc.gov/mumps/about/index.html [Last accessed June, 2024].
2. Kutty PK, Kyaw MH, Dayan GH, Brady MT, Bocchini JA, Reef SE, et al. Guidance for isolation precautions for mumps in the United States: a review of scientific basis. Clin Infect Dis. 2010;50:1619-28.
3. Livingston KA, Rosen JB, Zucker JR, Zimmerman CM. Mumps vaccine effectiveness and risk factors for disease in households during an outbreak in New York City. Vaccine. 2014;32:369-74.
4. Ogbuanu IU, Kutty PK, Hudson JM, Blog D, Abedi GR, Goodell S, et al. Impact of a third dose of measles–mumps–rubella vaccine on mumps outbreak. Pediatrics. 2012;30:1567-74.

CASE 75

Osteomyelitis

■ PRESENTING COMPLAINTS

A 4-year-old boy was presented with the complaint of:
- Fever since 5 days
- Limping of the right leg since 3 days

History of Presenting Complaints

A 4-year-old boy came to the pediatric outpatient department with a history of fever and limping. The boy was doing well apparently. He developed pain in the right leg at the ankle joint. This was there since last 3 days. There was so much pain that he started to limp while walking. His mother noticed that there was swelling and localized area was more warmer. There was decreased movement of the involved leg. This was associated with the fever. Fever was of moderate-to-high degree and was present since 3 days. The fever was sometimes associated with chills and rigor.

Past History of the Patient

The boy was the second sibling of non-consanguineous marriage. He was born at full term by normal delivery. There was no significant postnatal event. He started taking breast milk. He was on exclusively breast milk for the first 4 months; later weaning was started and the child was on family food by 16 months. His developmental milestones were normal. He was immunized completely apart from regular respiratory tract infection, there was no major health problem. His elder sibling was his sister, who was doing well with the health.

■ EXAMINATION

On examination, the child was moderately built and nourished. He was looking toxic. He was not keeping down his right leg. His anthropometric measurements included

CASE AT A GLANCE	
Basic Findings	
Height	: 99 cm (50th centile)
Weight	: 16 kg (80th centile)
Temperature	: 39°C
Pulse rate	: 120 beats/min
Respiratory rate	: 30 breaths/min
Blood pressure	: 70/50 mm Hg
Positive Findings	
History:	
• Limping	
• Fever	
• Swelling at the right leg	
Examination:	
• Toxic	
• Febrile	
• Right inguinal lymphadenitis	
• Tenderness at the right leg	
Investigation:	
• **TLC:** Raised	
• **ESR:** Raised	
• **X-ray:** Moth-eaten destruction	
(ESR: erythrocyte sedimentation rate; TLC: total leukocyte count)	

the height 99 cm (50th centile) and the weight 16 kg (80th centile). He was febrile, i.e., 39°C. His pulse rate was 120 beats/min. The respiratory rate was 30 breaths/min. The blood pressure recorded was 70/50 mm Hg. There was no pallor and no edema. Right-sided inguinal lymphadenitis was present. There was tenderness at the lower end of the leg. There was swelling over the lower end of the tibia. All the systemic examinations were normal.

■ INVESTIGATION

- *Hemoglobin:* 12 g/dL
- *TLC:* 15,000 cells/cumm
- *DLC:* $P_{78} L_{22}$
- *ESR:* 58 mm in the first hour
- *CRP:* 1,260 µg/L (normal range: 67–1,000 µg/L)
- *Blood culture and sensitivity:* Sterile
- *Mantoux test:* Negative
- *X-ray chest:* Normal
- *Magnetic resonance imaging (MRI):* Normal
- *X-ray of the long bone:* Moth-eaten destruction, cortex is thickened and lamellated

■ DISCUSSION

Osteomyelitis is an infectious process that usually starts in the spongy or medullary bone and then extends to involve compact or cortical bone. The lower extremities are most often affected, and there is commonly a history of trauma.

Osteomyelitis may occur as a result of direct invasion from the outside through a penetrating wound or open fracture, but hematogenous spread of infection (e.g., pyoderma or upper respiratory tract infection) from other infected areas is much more common.

There is frequently a history of some type of minor blunt trauma illness such as an upper respiratory tract infection. Other risk factors include immunodeficiency states, sickle cell anemia, and indwelling vascular catheters.

The most common infecting organism is *Staphylococcus aureus*, which has a tendency to infect the metaphyses of growing bones. Anatomically, circulation in the long bones is such that the arterial supply to the metaphysis just below the growth plate is by end arteries, which turn sharply to end in venous sinusoids, causing a relative stasis.

In the infant under age of 1 year, there is direct vascular communication with the epiphysis across the growth plate, so that direct spread may occur from the metaphysis to the epiphysis and subsequently into the joint.

In the older child, the growth plate provides an effective barrier and the epiphysis is usually not involved, although the infection spreads retrograde from the metaphysis into the diaphysis and, by rupture through the cortical bone, down along the diaphysis beneath the periosteum.

Early recognition of osteomyelitis in young patients is of critical importance. Prompt institution of appropriate medical and surgical therapy before extensive infection develops will minimize permanent damage. The risk is greatest if the physis (the growth plate of bone) is damaged.

Kingella kingae is the second most common cause of osteomyelitis in children younger than 4 years of age. The organism is established as a cause of osteomyelitis, spondylodiskitis, and septic arthritis in this age-group, especially when there is a subacute presentation. *K. kingae* can be difficult to detect unless PCR testing is used.

EXOGENOUS OSTEOMYELITIS

To avoid osteomyelitis by direct extension, all wounds must be carefully examined and cleaned. Osteomyelitis is a common occurrence from pressure sores in anesthetic areas, such as in patients with spina bifida.

Cultures of the wound made at the time of exploration and debridement may be useful if signs of infection develop subsequently. Copious irrigation is necessary, and all nonviable skin, subcutaneous tissue, fascia, and muscle must be excised. In extensive or contaminated wounds, antibiotic coverage is indicated.

Contaminated wounds should be left open and secondary closure performed 3-5 days later. If at the time of delayed closure further necrotic tissue is present, it should be excised. Leaving the wound open allows the infection to stay at the surface rather than extend inward to the bone.

Puncture wounds are especially liable to lead to osteomyelitis and should be carefully debrided if there is suspicion that they are deeper than the subcutaneous fat. The risk is greatest if the physis or growth plate of the bone is involved or synovium is damaged.

Bacteria are the most common pathogens in acute skeletal infections. *S. aureus* is the most common infecting organism in osteomyelitis among all age-groups, including newborns.

Group B *Streptococcus* (GBS) and Gram-negative enteric bacilli (*Escherichia coli*) are also prominent pathogens in neonates; group A *Streptococcus* constitutes <10% of all cases. After 6 years of age, most cases of osteomyelitis are caused by *S. aureus*, *Streptococcus*, or *Pseudomonas aeruginosa*. *P. aeruginosa* from the foam padding of the shoe into bone or cartilage, which develops as osteachondritis. *Salmonella* species and *S. aureus* are the two most common causes of osteomyelitis in children with sickle cell anemia. *Streptococcus pneumoniae* most commonly causes osteomyelitis in children younger than 24 months of age and in children with sickle cell anemia, but its frequency has declined because of pneumococcal conjugate vaccines. *Bartonella henselae* can cause osteomyelitis of any bone, but especially in pelvic and vertebral bones.

Streptococcus agalactiae (GBS) and enteric Gram-negative organisms occur almost exclusively in neonates. *Salmonella* is most commonly isolated in patients with acute hematogenous osteomyelitis (AHO), who have sickle cell anemia, although it can occasionally occur in normal hosts.

Haemophilus influenzae type B, an important pathogen in older series, is now rarely seen in countries that routinely use the *H. influenzae* type B conjugate vaccine. Less common organisms causing osteomyelitis include *B. henselae* (the cause of cat scratch disease), *Brucella*, and *Mycobacterium tuberculosis*.

Causes of nonhematogenous osteomyelitis in children include *Pseudomonas* osteochondritis, usually resulting from puncture wounds to the feet through sneakers, and anaerobic, Gram-negative, and polymicrobial infections that occur after puncture wounds or open fractures.

Infections and other conditions which may predispose may include impetigo, furunculosis, infected lesion of the varicella, infected burns, and direct trauma.

The fungal infection is caused by *Candida*. Infection with atypical mycobacteria can occur with the penetrating injury.

HEMATOGENOUS OSTEOMYELITIS

Hematogenous osteomyelitis is usually caused by pyogenic bacteria; 85% of cases are due to staphylococci. Streptococci are a less common cause of osteomyelitis. *Pseudomonas* organisms are common in cases of nail puncture wounds. Children with sickle cell anemia are especially prone to osteomyelitis caused by salmonellae.

It generally begins as a hematogenous abscess at metaphyses. Abscess ruptures subperiosteally, spreading along the shaft of the bone penetrating the marrow cavity. The periosteum may separate and form shell of the new bones. The pieces of the dead bone is called sequestrum. The new bone formed is called involucrum.

■ PATHOGENESIS

The unique anatomy and circulation of the ends of long bones results in the predilection for localization of blood-borne bacteria. In the metaphysis, nutrient arteries branch into nonanastomosing capillaries under the physis, which make a sharp loop before entering venous sinusoids draining into the marrow. Blood flow in this area is thought to be "sluggish", predisposing to bacterial invasion.

Once a bacterial focus is established, phagocytes migrate to the site and produce an inflammatory exudate (metaphyseal abscess). The generation of proteolytic enzymes, toxic oxygen radicals, and cytokines results in decreased oxygen tension, decreased pH, osteolysis, and tissue destruction. As the inflammatory exudate progresses, pressure increases the spread through the porous metaphyseal space via the Haversian system and Volkmann canals into the subperiosteal space. Purulence beneath the periosteum may lift the periosteal membrane of the bony surface, further impairing blood supply to the cortex and metaphysis.

In newborns and young infants, transphyseal blood vessels connect the metaphysis and epiphysis, so it is common for pus from the metaphysis to enter the joint space. This extension through the physis has the potential to result in abnormal growth and bone or joint deformity. During the latter part of the first year of life, the physis forms, obliterating the transphyseal blood vessels. Joint involvement, once the physis forms, can occur in joints where the metaphysis is intra-articular (hip ankle, shoulder, and elbow), and subperiosteal pus ruptures into of joint space.

In later childhood, the periosteum becomes more adherent, favoring pus to decompress through the periosteum. Once the growth plate closes in late adolescence, hematogenous osteomyelitis more often begins in the diaphysis and can spread to the entire intramedullary canal. Septic arthritis contiguous with a site of osteomyelitis is also seen in older children with *S. aureus* osteomyelitis, which may be related to simultaneous hematogenous inoculation of bone and joint space.

In the metaphysis, there are tiny vascular loops in which blood flow is sluggish. Oral oxygen tension is low. Rupture of sinus of the vessels occurs as a result of trauma. It provides favorable environment for the multiplication of the bacteria.

■ CLINICAL FEATURES (FIG. 1)

Osteomyelitis may occur at any age. But it occurs more commonly between 3 and 12 years. It is more common among boys.

The earliest signs of osteomyelitis in infants may be failure to move the affected extremity (pseudoparalysis), pain on passive movement, or both. Older children typically present with fever, pain at the site of infection, and refusal to use the affected extremity, which usually translates to limping or refusal to bear weight because lower extremity bones are affected more frequently. There can be intense tenderness over the metaphysis of

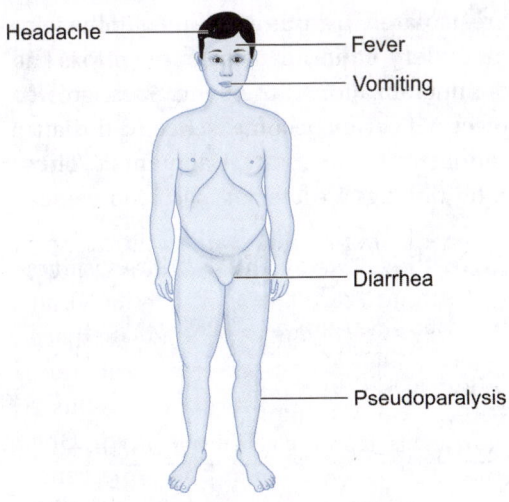

Fig. 1: Clinical features.

the bone on palpation, and muscles of the adjacent joint are frequently in spasm.

In infants, the manifestations of osteomyelitis may be subtle, presenting as irritability, diarrhea, or failure to feed properly; the temperature may be normal or slightly low; and the white blood count may be normal or only slightly elevated.

In older children, the manifestations are more striking, with severe local tenderness and pain, often high fever, rapid plus, and elevated white blood count and sedimentation rate. Osteomyelitis of a lower extremity often occurs around the knee joint in children aged 7–10 years. Tenderness is most marked over the metaphysis of the bone where the process has its origin. The child may limp or refuse to bear weight.

Usually only a single site of bone or joint is involved, although multiple sites of osteomyelitis may be noted in up to 20% of children with *S. aureus* infections. In neonates, two or more bones are involved in almost half of the cases. Children with subacute symptoms and focal findings in the metaphyseal area (usually of tibia) might have a Brodie abscess, with radiographic lucency and surrounding reactive bone. Typically the contents of Brodie abscesses are sterile.

The joint is held in a position of comfort, usually mild flexion, but to a lesser degree than with septic arthritis. Soft-tissue changes of swelling, erythema, and heat are generally late findings in osteomyelitis. After several days, a sympathetic sterile effusion may form in a nearby joint, presenting a problem in differentiation from septic arthritis. It is imperative for the evaluating physician to remember that any infant or child with fever and failure to bear weight or use an extremity needs to be carefully evaluated for potential musculoskeletal infection.

Although essentially any bone can be involved, long bones are most often involved in AHO in children. As noted, the majority of infections occur in the lower extremities, and the most common sites of involvement are the distal femoral and proximal femoral metaphyses. Next in frequency are the proximal femoral metaphysis and distal metaphyses of the radius and humerus. The femur and tibia are equally affected. There will be abrupt illness, fever, and systemic sign of toxicity. There may be associated swelling erythema, tenderness of the involved part. There will be marked tenderness over the involved bone. Hematogenous osteomyelitis of the cervical vertebrae may be manifested as torticollis. Infection in flat bones occurs most often in the pelvis and calcaneus, both of which can present challenges in diagnosis.

GENERAL FEATURES
• Fever
• Pain
• Redness and swelling of the skin and soft tissue
• Nausea

DIAGNOSIS

The diagnosis of osteomyelitis is clinical, blood cultures should be performed in all suspected cases.

There are no specific laboratory tests for osteomyelitis. The white blood cell count and differential, ESR, or CRP are generally elevated in children with bone infections but are nonspecific and not helpful in distinguishing between skeletal infection and other inflammatory processes. Monitoring elevated ESR and CRP may be of value in assessing response to therapy or identifying complications.

Blood cultures are often positive early. The most significant test in infancy is the aspiration of pus when suspicion arises because of lack of movement in a painful extremity. It is useful to needle the bone in the area of suspected infection and aspirate any fluid present. This fluid should be stained for organisms and cultured. Even edema fluid may be useful for determining the causative organism. The white blood cell count is usually elevated, as is the sedimentation rate.

> **LABORATORY SALIENT FINDINGS**
> - Positive blood culture
> - Elevated WBCs, raised ESR
> - *X-ray:* Nonspecific local swelling, elevation of periosteum, formation of new bone, dead bone fragments
> - MRI; edema in early, soft tissue thickening
>
> (ESR: erythrocyte sedimentation rate; MRI: magnetic resonance imaging; WBCs: white blood cells)

Radiograph

Nonspecific local swelling is the first X-ray finding. This is followed by elevation of the periosteum, with formation of new bone from the cambium layer of the periosteum occurring after 3–6 days. As the infection becomes chronic, areas of cortical bone are isolated by pus spreading down the medullary canal, causing rarefaction and demineralization of the bone. Such isolated pieces of cortex become ischemic and form sequestra (dead bone fragments). These X-ray findings are late but specific.

> **ESSENTIAL DIAGNOSTIC POINTS**
> - It is an infectious process
> - It affects metaphysis
> - Pseudoparalysis
> - Toxic look
> - Leukocytosis
> - Focus of infection in hematogenous type

Computed Tomography/Magnetic Resonance Imaging

Computed tomography (CT) can demonstrate osseous and soft-tissue abnormalities and is ideal for detecting gas in soft tissues. CT is a valuable imaging modality. MRI is more sensitive than CT or radionuclide imaging in acute osteomyelitis and is the best radiographic imaging technique for identifying abscesses and for differentiating between bone and soft-tissue infection. MRI provides precise anatomic detail of subperiosteal pus and accumulation of purulent debris in the bone marrow and metaphyses for possible surgical intervention. In acute osteomyelitis, purulent debris and edema appear dark, with decreased signal intensity. MRI can also demonstrate a contiguous or isolated septic arthritis, pyomyositis, or venous thrombosis.

Radiographic Evaluation

Magnetic resonance imaging provides precise anatomic detail of subperiosteal pus and accumulation of purulent debris in the bone marrow and metaphyses for possible surgical intervention. In acute osteomyelitis, purulent debris and edema appear dark, with decreased signal intensity on T1-weighted images, with fat appearing bright.

Magnetic resonance imaging has emerged as an effective alternative to radionuclide imaging where multiple sites of infection are suspected or the site of infection cannot be clearly localized. CT can demonstrate osseous and soft-tissue abnormalities and is ideal for detecting gas in soft tissues but has poor sensitivity for detecting the presence of osteomyelitis.

Radionuclide Studies

Radionuclide imaging can be valuable in suspected bone infections, especially early in the course of infection and/or if multiple foci are suspected or an unusual site is suspected, as in the pelvis. Technetium-99m (99mTc) methylene diphosphonate, which accumulates in areas of increased bone turnover, is the preferred agent for radionuclide bone imaging (three-phase bone scan).

Radionuclide imaging, an alternative to MRI, may be useful if multiple foci are suspected. Three-phase imaging with 99mTc has excellent sensitivity (84–100%) and specificity (70–96%) in hematogenous osteomyelitis and can detect osteomyelitis within 24–48 hours after onset of symptoms.

Bone Aspiration and Biopsy

Bone cultures are positive in 38–91% of cases and confirm the diagnosis. Blood cultures are also very useful, demonstrating, the organism in 30–76% of cases. The highest diagnostic yield occurs when both blood and bone specimens are submitted for culture. Recovery of organisms is enhanced by inoculating bone aspirates into blood culture bottles. This is particularly important when fastidious organisms (e.g., *Kingella*) are suspected, which may require up to a week of incubation before growth is evident. Alternatively, bone aspirates can be submitted for PCR testing when trying to establish a diagnosis in culture-negative osteomyelitis. In multiple studies, PCR testing has been shown to be particularly useful for the diagnosis of *Kingella* AHO, but when available, can also be used to identify other organisms in cases where conventional cultures are negative.

■ DIFFERENTIAL DIAGNOSIS

The differential diagnosis of osteomyelitis includes cellulitis, septic arthritis, pyomyositis, malignancy, collagen vascular disease, and trauma. In differentiating cellulitis from bone infection, tenderness disproportionate to physical findings suggests osteomyelitis. Septic arthritis may be differentiated from osteomyelitis by its more discrete joint findings and its greater degree of joint immobility, in addition to a lack of metaphyseal tenderness. History, physical examination, clinical scenario, and radiologic studies are helpful in differentiating skeletal infection from other diagnoses. Recovery of the causative organism is best obtained by biopsy or aspiration, which not only establishes the diagnosis but also facilitates susceptibility testing and rules out other pathologic processes.

■ TREATMENT

Specific Measures

Optimal treatment of skeletal infections requires collaborative efforts of pediatricians, orthopedic surgeons, and radiologists. Obtaining material for culture (blood, periosteal abscess, bone) before antibiotics are given is essential.

Antibiotic Therapy

The empiric antibiotic therapy is based on the knowledge of likely organism with particular age-group.

In the young infant, GBS and *S. aureus* are the major pathogens, but coverage of enteric Gram-negatives must be included. An appropriate initial therapeutic regimen includes an antistaphylococcal agent plus a third-generation cephalosporin, such as cefotaxime.

In neonates, an antistaphylococcal penicillin, such as nafcillin or oxacillin (150–200 mg/kg/24 h divided q 12 h IV), and a broad-spectrum cephalosporin, such as cefotaxime (150–225 mg/kg/24 h divided q 8 hours IV), provide coverage for the methicillin-susceptible *S. aureus* (MSSA), GBS, and Gram-negative bacilli. If methicillin-resistant *Staphylococcus* is suspected, vancomycin is substituted for nafcillin.

If the neonate is a small premature infant or has a central vascular catheter, the possibility of nosocomial bacteria (Gram-negative enteric, *Pseudomonas*, or *S. aureus*) or fungi (*Candida*) should be considered. In older infants and children, the principal pathogens are *S. aureus* and *Streptococcus*.

In children <4 years of age, a regimen providing coverage for *S. aureus*, *Streptococcus pyogenes*, *S. pneumoniae*, and *Kingella* should be used. An antistaphylococcal agent plus a third-generation cephalosporin may provide appropriate coverage.

In infants and children, about 4–5 years, the main pathogen may be *S. aureus*, *Streptococcus*, and *H. influenzae*. Then the third-generation cephalosporins are used. Cefuroxime (100–150 mg/kg/24 h) in three divided doses, cefotaxime 150 mg/kg/day in three divided doses and ceftriaxone (50 mg/kg/24 h) given once daily. Antistaphylococcal antibiotics such as nafcillin (15 mg/kg/day) in four divided doses, or cephalothin 100–150 mg/kg/24 h in four divided doses.

A major factor influencing the selection of empirical therapy is the rate of methicillin resistance among community *S. aureus* isolates. If methicillin-resistant *S. aureus* (MRSA) accounts for >10% of community *S. aureus* isolates, including an antibiotic effective against MRSA in the initial empirical antibiotic regimen is suggested, vancomycin (60 mg/kg/24 h divided q 6 hours IV) is the gold standard agent for treating invasive MRSA infections, especially when the child is critically ill. Clindamycin (40 mg/kg/24 h q 8 hours) is also recommended when the rate of clindamycin resistance is 5–10% among community *S. aureus* isolates, the child is not severely ill and bacteremia is not a concern or blood cultures are known to be negative. Cefazolin (100 mg/kg/24 h divided q 8 hours IV) or nafcillin (150–200 mg/kg/24 h divided q 6 hours) is the agent of choice for parenteral treatment of osteomyelitis caused by MSSA. Penicillin is first-line therapy for treating osteomyelitis caused by susceptible strains of *S. pneumoniae* as well as all group A streptococci. Cefotaxime or ceftriaxone is recommended for pneumococcal isolates with resistance to penicillin and for most *Salmonella* spp.

In immunocompromised children or those with underlying medical conditions, broader-spectrum coverage may be appropriate. *Pseudomonas* is a consideration, and antipseudomonal agent may be part of the regimen.

For immunocompromised patients, combination therapy is usually initiated, such as with vancomycin and ceftazidime, or with piperacillin–tazobactam and aminoglycoside. *K. kingae* usually responds to beta-lactam antibiotics including cefotaxime.

If possible, initiating treatment with a single agent is preferred. If cultures remain sterile, treatment should be continued based on the most common organism for the age-group, usually *S. aureus*. If there is no response to treatment, less common organisms may be suspected, although there may be other causes as well (e.g., the common etiologic agent is resistant to the chosen antibiotic regimen or there are complications of the infection). In children under 1 years of age with negative cultures, *K. Kingae* should strongly be considered.

After the initial period of IV antibiotic therapy for 5-7 days, patient should be treated adequately with oral antibiotics. Inadequate antibiotic therapy often leads to chronic disease and orthopedic deformity. Changing antibiotics from the IV route to oral administration when a patient's condition clearly has improved and the child is afebrile for 48-72 hours may be considered. For the oral antibiotic regimen with beta-lactam drugs for susceptible staphylococcal or streptococcal infection, cephalexin (80-100 mg/kg/24 h q 8 hours) or oral clindamycin (30-40 mg/kg/24 h q 8 hours) can be used to complete therapy for children with clindamycin-susceptible MRSA or for patients who are seriously allergic or cannot tolerate beta-lactam antibiotics. Surgical treatment involves surgical removal of sinus and debridement of sequestrum.

The usual recommended duration is 4-6 weeks, but depends on the cause and extent of infection as well as clinical and laboratory response. However, some newer studies have shown successful outcomes with 3 weeks of therapy. Each patient must be evaluated individually, taking into account the speed of clinical response, whether surgical debridement was done, normalization of CRP or ESR, and radiologic findings.

General Measures

Splinting of the limb minimizes pain and decreases spread of the infection by lymphatic channels through the soft tissue. The splint should be removed periodically to allow active use of adjacent joints and prevent stiffening and muscle atrophy. In chronic osteomyelitis, splinting may be necessary to guard against fracture of the weakened bone.

Surgical Measures

Treatment of chronic osteomyelitis consists of surgical removal of sinus tracts and sequestrum, if present. Antimicrobial therapy is continued for several months or longer until clinical and radiographic findings suggest that healing has occurred. Normalization of ESR and CRP is expected in successful treatment of chronic osteomyelitis but does not by itself indicate clearance of the underlying infection. Many patients with chronic osteomyelitis have a normal CRP and ESR even at the onset of illness.

The need for open surgery in osteomyelitis depends on the extent of the pathologic process in individual patients and likely somewhat on the virulence of the specific pathogen. In children who present early in the "cellulitic phase", antibiotic therapy alone is usually sufficient for treatment. If pus is encountered during diagnostic aspiration, if a subperiosteal or intramedullary abscess is detected by ultrasound or MRI, or if a bone lesion is evident on plain films, surgical intervention may be warranted. Patients initiated on medical therapy who do not promptly improve should also be evaluated for surgical intervention.

Surgical drainage and debridement removes inflammatory products more rapidly than do host defense mechanisms, providing a more effective environment for antibiotic penetration and preventing further bone necrosis. Drainage of an abscess also reduces the inoculum of bacteria present. Any patient with a lytic lesion on plain films should have, in addition to cultures, the bone biopsy sent to pathology for histology and special stains to rule out other pathologic processes such as malignancy and to evaluate for unusual organisms such as fungi or acid-fast bacilli (AFB).

It is important that all devitalized soft tissue be removed and adequate exposure of the bone obtained to permit free drainage. Excessive amounts of bone should not be removed when draining acute osteomyelitis, because they may not be completely replaced by the normal healing process. Little damage is done by surgical drainage, but failure to drain the pus in acute cases may lead to more severe damage.

Treatment of chronic osteomyelitis consists of surgical removal of sinus tracts and sequestrum, if present. Antibiotic therapy is continued for several months or longer until clinical and radiographic findings suggest that healing has occurred. Monitoring the CRP or ESR is not helpful in most cases of chronic osteomyelitis.

Aspiration of the metaphysis for culture and Gram stain is the most useful diagnostic measure in any case of suspected osteomyelitis. In the first 24–72 hours, it may be possible to treat osteomyelitis by antibiotics alone. If frank pus is aspirated from the bone, however, surgical drainage is indicated. If the infection has not shown a dramatic response within 24 hours, surgical drainage is also indicated.

■ COMPLICATIONS

Chronic Osteomyelitis

The most common complication of AHO is chronic or recurrent osteomyelitis, which occurs in fewer than 5% of cases. Symptoms may include chronic or recurrent pain, swelling, erythema, or purulent discharge, and in some cases, sinus tract formation. Development of chronic osteomyelitis is more common following nonhematogenous osteomyelitis (e.g., following penetrating trauma). The hallmark of chronic osteomyelitis is bone necrosis. Therapy is primarily surgical with adjunctive long-term antibiotics. A bone biopsy should be obtained in chronic osteomyelitis for culture and for histopathology to exclude Langerhans cell histiocytosis, malignancy, and other causes.

Other Complications and Outcomes

Pathologic fractures can occur but are rare. If the bone growth plate is involved, there is a risk of abnormal length of the affected bone. In general, the outcome of well-managed cases of cute osteomyelitis in pediatric patients is favorable.

■ PHYSIOTHERAPY

The major role of physical medicine is a preventive one. If a child is allowed to lie in bed with an extremity in flexion, limitation of extension can develop within a few days. The affected extremity should be kept in extension with sandbags, splints, or, if necessary, a temporary cast. Casts are also indicated when there is a potential for pathologic fracture. After 2–3 days, when pain is easing, passive range of motion exercises are started and continued until the child resumes normal activity. In neglected cases with flexion contractures, prolonged physical therapy is required.

■ PROGNOSIS

When osteomyelitis is diagnosed in the early clinical stages and prompt antibiotic therapy is begun, the prognosis is excellent. If the process has been unattended for a week to 10 days, there is almost always some permanent loss of bone structure, as well as the possibility of growth abnormality.

BIBLIOGRAPHY

1. Bouchoucha S, Drissi G, Trifa M, Saied W, Ammar C, Smida M, et al. Epidemiology of acute hematogenous osteomyelitis in children: a prospective study over a 32 months period. Tunis Med. 2012;90(6):473-8.
2. Dartnell J, Ramachandran M, Katchburian M. Hematogenous acute and subacute paediatric osteomyelitis: a systemic review of literature. J Bone Joint Surg Br. 2012;94(5):584-95.
3. Keren R, Shah SS, Srivastava R, Rangel S, Bendel-Stenzel M, Harik N, et al.; Pediatric Research in Inpatient Settings Network. Comparitive effectiveness of intravenous vs oral antibiotics for postdischarge treatment of acute in children. JAMA Pediatr. 2015;169:120-8.
4. Peltola H, Pääkkönen M, Kallio P, Kallio MJ; Osteomyelitis-Septic Arthritis Study Group. Short- versus long-term antimicrobial for acute osteomyelitis of childhood: prospective, randomized trial on 131 culture-positive cases. Pediatr Infect Dis J. 2009;29:1123-7.

76 CASE

Poliomyelitis

■ PRESENTING COMPLAINTS

An 18-month-old boy was brought with the complaint of:
- Loose motion since 2 days
- Vomiting since 2 days
- Fever since 2 days
- Sudden onset of weakness in the left leg since 1 day

History of Presenting Complaints

An 18-month-old boy was brought to pediatric outpatient department with history of sudden onset of weakness in left leg. The child was not able to stand as he was not able to put his left leg to the ground. His mother gave the history that her son was suffering from loose motion, vomiting, and fever since last 2 days. He was receiving treatment from general practitioner. As child had persistent vomiting, the doctor had given an injection to control the vomiting. His mother noticed the development of weakness in the left leg after the injection. Coincidentally, the injection was given on the left gluteal region. Again she rushed back to the doctor and informed about the weakness. Later after examination, he referred to pediatrician.

Past History of the Patient

The boy was the only child of nonconsanguineous marriage. He was delivered at term by normal vaginal delivery. His mother never had any antenatal health checkup. There were no significant postnatal events. The child was given breast milk immediately. He was on exclusively breast milk for 6 months. Later, the child was given family food. He was not given any immunization. His developmental milestones were normal.

■ EXAMINATION

The child was moderately built and nourished. He was irritable and was not allowing anybody to touch his left leg.

CASE AT A GLANCE

Basic Findings
Length	: 80 cm (50th centile)
Weight	: 10 kg (75th centile)
Temperature	: 38°C
Pulse rate	: 120 beats/min
Respiratory rate	: 24 breaths/min
Blood pressure	: 60/40 mm Hg

Positive Findings

History:
- Weakness in left leg
- Intramuscular weakness
- Crying
- Not immunized

Examination:
- Febrile
- Weakness in left leg
- Paresthesia
- Moderate dehydration

Investigation:
- *Lumbar puncture:* Pleocytosis, increased protein

He was not able to stand. The anthropometric measurements included weight 10 kg (75th centile) and length 80 cm (50th centile). He was febrile, heart rate was 120 beats/min, respiratory rate was 24 breaths/min, and the blood pressure recorded was 60/40 mm Hg.

Child was pale, there was no edema, no lymphadenopathy, no cyanosis, and icterus.

There were signs of moderate dehydration. CNS revealed higher mental functions were normal. Anterior fontanelle is closed. No cranial nerve is involved. There were no meningeal signs. There was weakness and hypotonia in the left leg. Deep tendon reflexes were exaggerated. The child was not allowing anybody to touch his left leg. Other systemic examinations were normal.

■ INVESTIGATION

- *Hemoglobin:* 12 g/dL
- *TLC:* 9,600 cells/cumm
- *DLC:* $P_{78} L_{18} E_2 M_2$
- *ESR:* 21 mm in first hour
- *Chest X-ray:* NAD
- *Lumbar puncture:* Pleocytosis cells 300 cells/cumm; proteins raised 100 mg/dL

■ DISCUSSION

The combination of fever, asymmetric fluid paralysis, without sensory loss and pleocytosis in CSF fluid helps to arrive at diagnosis of poliomyelitis.

The polioviruses are nonenveloped, positive-stranded RNA viruses belonging to the Picornaviridae family, in the genus *Enterovirus* and consist of three antigenically distinct serotypes (types 1, 2, and 3). Polioviruses spread from the intestinal tract to the CNS, where they cause aseptic meningitis and poliomyelitis, or polio. The polioviruses are extremely hardy and can retain infectivity for several days at room temperature. Poliovirus can survive for long periods for external environments. It can live in water for 4 months and in feces for 6 months. It is therefore well adapted for fecal-oral transmission.

Man is the only reservoir and natural host of virus. Most infections are subclinical. It is the mild and subclinical infections that play a dominant role in the spread of infection. There are no chronic carriers. Poliovirus is excreted in the stools of the patient for 2 weeks before and 6–8 weeks after the onset of illness, sometimes as long as 3–4 months. Fecal contamination of the edible substance may occur either due to human association or through the flies. The virus is found in fecal and oropharyngeal secretion of the infected person.

The vulnerable age is between 6 months to 3 years. Several predisposing risk factors include fatigue, trauma, IM infection, open procedure such as tonsillectomy done during the epidemics of polio and administration of alum containing DPT (diphtheria, tetanus, and pertussis).

Poliomyelitis virus multiplies in the intestine. If there is no local immunity it travels to the required lymph nodes and reticuloendothelial structure. As a result, specific antibodies are produced in the blood and the gut. Antibodies act mainly at the site of extraneural proliferation of the virus.

Infants acquire immunity transplacentally from the mother. This immunity will last for 4–6 months of life and disappear at a variable rate. Active immunity after the natural infection lasts for life. Neutralizing antibodies develop within several days after the exposure often before the onset of illness. The early production of IgG antibodies is a result of replication of the virus in the intestinal tract and deep lymphatic tissue. This occurs before the CNS is invaded. Local mucosal immunity, conferred mainly by IgA is an important defense against poliovirus.

PATHOGENESIS

Polioviruses infect cells by adsorbing to the genetically determined poliovirus receptor. The virus penetrates the cell, is uncoated, and releases viral RNA. The RNA is translated to produce proteins responsible for replication of the RNA, shut of host cell protein synthesis, and synthesis of structural elements that compose the capsid. Mature virus particles are produced in 6-8 hours and are released into the environment by disruption of the cell.

The exact mechanism of entry into the CNS is not known. However, once entry is gained the virus may traverse neural pathways, and multiple sites within the CNS are often affected. The effect on motor and vegetative neurons is most striking and correlates with the clinical manifestations. Perineuronal inflammation, a mixed inflammatory reaction with both polymorphonuclear leukocytes and lymphocytes, is associated with extensive neuronal destruction. Petechial hemorrhages and considerable inflammatory edema also occur in areas of poliovirus infection.

Poliovirus selectively damages the motor and autonomic nervous system. Most commonly affected areas are the anterior horn cells of the spinal cord, vestibular and cranial nerve nuclei, vital centers in medulla and vermis, and nuclei in the roof of cerebellum.

The poliovirus primarily infects motor neuron cells in the spinal cord (the anterior horn cells) and the medulla oblongata (the cranial nerve nuclei). Because of the overlap in muscle innervation by 2-3 adjacent segments of the spinal cord, clinical signs of weakness in the limbs develop when >50% of motor neurons are destroyed. In the medulla, less-extensive lesions cause paralysis, and involvement of the reticular formation that contains the vital centers controlling respiration and circulation may have a catastrophic outcome. Involvement of the intermediate and dorsal areas of the horn and the dorsal root ganglia in the spinal cord results in hyperesthesia and myalgias that are typical of acute poliomyelitis.

Other neurons affected are the nuclei in the roof and vermis of the cerebellum, the substantia nigra, and, occasionally, the red nucleus in the pons; there may be variable involvement of thalamic, hypothalamic, and pallidal nuclei and the motor cortex.

The neuropathy of poliomyelitis is due to direct cellular destruction. Neurological damage may include chromatolysis of Nissl substance in the cytoplasm. This is followed by changes in the nuclei and pericellular infiltration. The process is reversible till this stage. If neurons undergo necrosis, the process becomes irreversible.

In the contact host, wild-type and vaccine strains of polioviruses gain host entry via the GIT. Recent studies in nonhuman primates demonstrate that the primary sites of replication are in the CD155 epithelial cells lining the mucosa of the tonsil follicle and small intestine, as well as see the macrophages/dendritic cells in the tonsil follicle and Peyer's patches. Regional lymph nodes are infected, and primary viremia occurs after 2-3 days. The virus seeds multiple sites, including the reticuloendothelial system, brown fat deposits, and skeletal muscle. Wild-type poliovirus probably accesses the CNS along peripheral nerves. Reversion occurs in the small intestine and probably accesses the CNS via the peripheral nerves. Poliovirus has almost never been cultured from the CSF of patients with paralytic disease, and patients with aseptic meningitis caused by poliovirus never have paralytic disease.

With the first appearance of non-CNS symptoms, a secondary viremia probably occurs as a result of enormous viral replication in the reticuloendothelial system.

Secondary damage may be due to immunological mechanism. In poliomyelitis, the neural lesions occur in the roof and vermis of the cerebellum, the substantia nigra, and, occasionally, the red nucleus in the pons; there may be variable involvement of thalamic, hypothalamic, and pallidal nuclei and the motor cortex.

Apart from the histopathology of the CNS, inflammatory changes occur generally in the reticuloendothelial system. Inflammatory edema and sparse lymphocytic infiltration are prominently associated with hyperplastic-lymphocytic follicles.

Infants acquire immunity transplacentally from their mothers. Transplacental immunity disappears at a variable rate during the first 4–6 months of life. Active immunity after natural infection is probably lifelong but protects against the infecting serotype only; infections with other serotypes are possible. Poliovirus neutralizing antibodies develop within several days after exposure as a result of replication of the virus in the M cells in the intestinal tract and deep lymphatic tissues. This early production of circulating IgG antibodies protects against CNS invasion. Local (mucosal) immunity, conferred mainly by secretory IgA, is an important defense against subsequent reinfection of the GIT.

ESSENTIAL DIAGNOSTIC POINTS
• Headache, fever, muscle weakness • Asymmetric flaccid paralysis • Muscle tenderness and hyperesthesia late atrophy • Aseptic meningitis • Inadequate immunization • Underlying immune deficiency

■ CLINICAL FEATURES (FIG. 1)

Inapparent Infections

Inapparent infections include approximately 91–96% of cases. There will not be presenting complaints. Diagnosis is done by isolation of virus and rising antibody titers.

Abortive Poliomyelitis

In approximately 5% of patients, a nonspecific influenza-like syndrome occurs 1–2 weeks after infection, which is termed abortive poliomyelitis. Fever, malaise, anorexia, and headache are prominent features, and there may be sore throat and abdominal or muscular pain. Vomiting occurs irregularly. The illness is short-lived, lasting up to 2–3 days. The physical examination may be normal or may reveal nonspecific pharyngitis, abdominal or muscular tenderness, and weakness. Recovery is complete, and no neurologic signs or sequelae develop. The features of abortive poliomyelitis are as follows:
- Fever
- Anorexia, nausea
- Abdominal pain
- Constipation
- Loose motion
- Sore throat

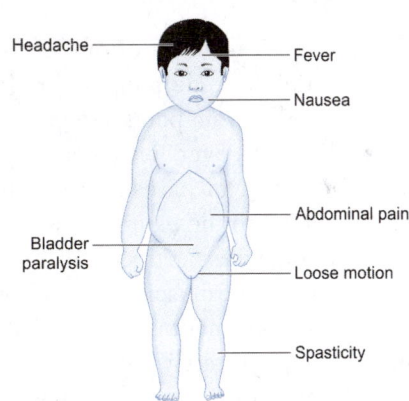

Fig. 1: Clinical features.

Nonparalytic Poliomyelitis

In approximately 19% of patients infected with wild-type poliovirus, signs of abortive poliomyelitis are present, as are more intense headache, nausea, and vomiting, as well as soreness and stiffness of the posterior muscles of the neck, trunk, and limbs. Fleeting paralysis of the bladder and constipation are frequent. Approximately two-thirds of these children have a short symptom-free interlude between the first phase (minor illness) and the second phase (CNS disease or major illness). Nuchal rigidity and spinal rigidity are the basis for the diagnosis of nonparalytic poliomyelitis during the second phase.

The features of nonparalytic poliomyelitis are as follows:
- Headache
- Fleeting paralysis of the bladder
- First phase—minor
- Second phase—CNS
- Nuchal rigidity
- Spinal rigidity
- Tripod sign
- Kiss-knee sign
- Head drop
- Reflexes are active

Paralytic Poliomyelitis

The paralytic phase of poliomyelitis is extremely variable; some patients progress during observation from paresis to paralysis, whereas others recover, either slowly or rapidly. The extent of paresis or paralysis is directly related to the extent of neuronal involvement; paralysis occurs if >50% of the neurons supplying the muscles are destroyed. The extent of involvement is usually obvious within 2–3 days; only rarely does progression occur beyond this interval. Bowel and bladder dysfunction ranging from transient incontinence to paralysis with constipation and urinary retention often accompany paralysis of the lower limbs.

The onset and course of paralysis are variable in developing countries. The biphasic course is rare; typically the disease manifests in a single phase in which prodromal symptoms and paralysis occur in a continuous fashion.

Impaired ventilation must be recognized early; mounting anxiety, restlessness, and fatigue are early indications for preemptive intervention. Tracheostomy is indicated for some patients with pure bulbar poliomyelitis, spinal respiratory muscle paralysis, or bulbospinal paralysis, because such patients are generally unable to cough, sometimes for many months. Mechanical respirators are often needed. The features of paralytic poliomyelitis are as follows:
- Bladder paralysis
- Bowel atony
- Pain, flaccid paralysis
- Spasticity
- Nuchal and spinal rigidity
- Respiratory and cardiac arrhythmias
- Blood pressure and vasomotor changes
- Spotty paralysis
- Spinal form—muscles of neck, abdomen, trunk, diaphragm
- Bulbar form—cranial nerves, vital centers
- Encephalitic—irritability, disorientation, drowsiness, coarse tremors

Postpolio Syndrome

After an interval of 30–40 years, as many as 30–40% of persons who survived paralytic poliomyelitis in childhood may experience muscle pain and exacerbation of existing weakness or development of new weakness or paralysis. This entity, referred to as postpolio syndrome, has been reported only in persons who were infected in the era of wild-type poliovirus circulation. Risk factors for postpolio syndrome include increasing length of time since acute poliovirus infection, presence of permanent residual impairment after recovery from acute illness, and female sex.

GENERAL FEATURES
• Nuchal rigidity • Spinal rigidity • Tripod sign • Head drop • Kiss-knee sign • Spotty paralysis

■ DIAGNOSIS

The combination of fever, headache, neck and back pain, asymmetric flaccid paralysis without sensory loss, and pleocytosis gives diagnosis of poliomyelitis. CSF fluid during minor illness shows pleocytosis. Protein is normal, usually rises to between 50 and 100 mg/dL by the second week of illness.

Characteristic clinical presentation of acute lower motor neuron type of asymmetrical paralysis of proximal limb muscles without any sensory involvement is highly suggestive of poliomyelitis. However, cases of acute flaccid paralysis (AFP) cases should be investigated by sending a stool sample for isolation of virus.

Stool Virus Isolation

Stool examination is recommended in every case of AFP. Virus can be detected from onset to 8 or more weeks after paralysis; the highest probability of detection is during the first 2 weeks after onset of paralysis. Examination of the CSF (cell count, Gram stain, protein, and glucose) is useful in eliminating other conditions that cause AFP. Isolation of wild poliovirus from stool is the recommended method for laboratory confirmation of paralytic poliomyelitis. Two stool specimens are collected from each case for laboratory confirmation.

LABORATORY SALIENT FINDINGS
• *CSF analysis:* Lymphocytosis, mild elevated protein, normal protein • Cell culture • ELISA test (CSF: cerebrospinal fluid; ELISA: enzyme-linked immunosorbent assay)

The WHO recommends that the laboratory diagnosis of poliomyelitis be confirmed by isolation and identification of poliovirus in the stool, with specific identification of wild-type and vaccine-type strains.

In suspected cases of AFP, two stool specimens should be collected 24-48 hour apart as soon as possible after the diagnosis of poliomyelitis is suspected. Poliovirus concentrations are high in the stool in the first week after the onset of paralysis, which is the optimal time for collection of stool specimens. Polioviruses may be isolated from 80-90% of specimens from acutely ill patients, whereas <20% of specimens from such patients may yield virus within 3-4 weeks after onset of paralysis. Because most children with spinal or bulbospinal poliomyelitis have constipation, rectal straws may be used to obtain specimens; ideally a minimum of 8-10 g of stool should be collected.

The CSF is often normal during the minor illness and typically contains a pleocytosis with 20-300 cells/dL, with CNS involvement. The cells in the CSF may be polymorphonuclear early during the course of the disease but shift to mononuclear cells occurs soon afterward. By the second week of major illness, the CSF cell count falls to near-normal values. In contrast, the CSF protein content is normal or only slightly elevated at the outset of CNS disease but usually rises to

50-100 mg/dL by the second week of illness. In polioencephalitis, the CSF may remain normal or show minor changes. Serologic testing demonstrates seroconversion or a fourfold or greater increase in antibody titers from the acute phase of illness to 3-6 weeks later.

DIFFERENTIAL DIAGNOSIS

- Guillain-Barre syndrome
- Aseptic meningitis
- Viral encephalitis
- Peripheral neuritis
- Encephalomyelitis

TREATMENT

There is no specific antiviral treatment for poliomyelitis. The management is supportive and aimed at limiting progression of disease, preventing ensuing skeletal deformities, and preparing the child and family for the prolonged treatment required and for permanent disability if this seems likely. Patients with the nonparalytic and mildly paralytic forms of poliomyelitis may be treated at home. All IM injections and surgical procedures are contraindicated during the acute phase of the illness, especially in the first week of illness, because they might result in progression of disease.

The broad principles of management are to allay the fear, to minimize skeletal deformities, to anticipate and meet the complications. Patients with nonparalytic and mildly paralytic forms may be treated at home.

Abortive Poliomyelitis

Supportive treatment with analgesics, sedatives, an attractive diet, and bed rest until the child's temperature is normal for several days is usually sufficient. Avoidance of exertion for the ensuing 2 weeks is desirable, and careful neurologic and musculoskeletal examinations should be performed 2 months later to detect any minor involvement.

Nonparalytic Poliomyelitis

Treatment for the nonparalytic form is similar to that for the abortive form; in particular, relief is indicated for the discomfort of muscle tightness and spasm of the neck, trunk, and extremities. Analgesics are more effective when they are combined with the application of hot packs for 15-30 minutes every 2-4 hours. Hot tub baths are sometimes useful. A firm bed is desirable and can be improvised at home by placing table leaves or a sheet of plywood beneath the mattress. A footboard or splint should be used to keep the feet at a right angle to the legs. Because muscular discomfort and spasm may continue for some weeks, even in the nonparalytic form, hot packs and gentle physical therapy may be necessary. Patients with nonparalytic poliomyelitis should also be carefully examined 2 months after apparent recovery to detect minor residual effects that might cause postural problems in later years.

Paralytic Poliomyelitis

Most patients with the paralytic form of poliomyelitis require hospitalization with complete physical rest in a calm atmosphere for the first 2-3 weeks. Suitable body alignment is necessary for comfort and to avoid excessive skeletal deformity. A neutral position with the feet at right angles to the legs, the knees slightly flexed, and the hips and spine straight is achieved by use of boards, sandbags, and, occasionally, light splint shells. The position should be changed every 3-6 hours.

Active and passive movements are indicated as soon as the pain has disappeared.

Moist hot packs may relieve muscle pain and spasm. Opiates and sedatives are permissible only if no impairment of ventilation is present or impending. Constipation is common, and fecal impaction should be prevented.

When bladder paralysis occurs, a parasympathetic stimulant such as bethanechol may induce voiding in 15–30 minutes; some patients show no response to this agent, and others respond with nausea, vomiting, and palpitations. Bladder paresis rarely lasts more than a few days. If bethanechol fails, manual compression of the bladder and the psychologic effect of running water should be tried. If catheterization must be performed, care must be taken to prevent urinary tract infections.

A proper diet and a relatively high fluid intake should be started at once unless the patient is vomiting. Additional salt should be provided if the environmental temperature is high or if the application of hot packs induces sweating. Anorexia is common initially. Adequate dietary and fluid intake can be maintained by placement of a central venous catheter. An orthopedist and a physiotherapist should see patients as early in the course of the illness as possible and should assume responsibility for their care before fixed deformities develop.

The management of pure bulbar poliomyelitis consists of maintaining the airway and avoiding all risks of inhalation of saliva, food, and vomitus. Gravity drainage of accumulated secretions is favored by using the head low (foot of bed elevated 20°–25°) prone position with the face to one side. Patients may require tracheostomy because of vocal cord paralysis or constriction of the hypopharynx; most patients who recover have little residual impairment, although some exhibit mild dysphagia and occasional vocal fatigue with slurring of speech.

Patients with weakness of the muscles of respiration or swallowing should be nursed in a lateral or semi-prone position. Aspirators with rigid or semirigid tips are preferred for direct oral and pharyngeal aspiration, and soft, flexible catheters may be used for nasopharyngeal aspiration.

Fluid and electrolyte equilibrium is best maintained by IV infusion because of tube or oral feeding in the first few days may incite vomiting. In addition to close observation for respiratory insufficiency, the blood pressure should be measure at least twice daily, because hypertension is not uncommon and occasionally leads to hypertensive encephalopathy.

Impaired ventilation must be recognized early; mounting anxiety, restlessness, and fatigue are early indications for presumptive intervention. Tracheostomy is indicated for some patients with pure bulbar poliomyelitis, spinal respiratory muscle paralysis, or bulbospinal spinal paralysis, because such patients are generally unable to cough, sometimes for many months. Mechanical respirators are often needed.

■ COMPLICATIONS

Paralytic poliomyelitis may be associated with numerous complications. Acute gastric dilation may occur abruptly during the acute or convalescent stage, causing further respiratory embarrassment; immediate gastric aspiration and external application of ice bags are indicated. Melena severe enough to require transfusion may result from single or multiple superficial intestinal erosions; perforation is rare. Mild hypertension for days or weeks is common in the acute stage and probably related to lesions of the vasoregulatory centers in the medulla and especially to underventilation.

Dimness of vision, headache, and a light-headed feeling associated with hypertension should be regarded as premonitory of a frank convulsion. Acute pulmonary edema occurs occasionally, particularly in patients with arterial hypertension. Hypercalcemia occurs because of skeletal decalcification that begins soon after immobilization and results in hypercalciuria.

PROGNOSIS

In general, the more extensive the paralysis in the first 10 days of illness, the more severe the ultimate disability. Unexpected improvement may appear soon after defervescence and again about 6 weeks after the onset. This time that corresponds to functional restoration of temporarily inactive neurons. The degree of functional recovery depends upon adequacy and promptness of the supportive treatment, proper body positioning, active motion, use of assertive devices, and psychological motivation of the patient.

BIBLIOGRAPHY

1. Poh CL, Tan EL. Detection of the enteroviruses from the clinical specimens. Methods Mol Biol. 2001;665:65-77.
2. Polio Global Eradication Initiative. [online] Available from www.polioeradication.org [Last accessed June, 2024].
3. Rhoades RE, Tabor-Godwin JM, Tsueng G, Feuer R. Enterovirus infections of the central nervous system. Virology. 2011;411(2):288-305.

CASE 77

Septic Arthritis

PRESENTING COMPLAINTS

A 9-month-old boy was brought with the complaint of:
- Fever since 2 days
- Swelling in the right knee since 1 day
- Decreased movements since 1 day

History of Presenting Complaints

A 9-month-old boy was brought to the pediatric outpatient department with history of sudden onset of fever. The child was crying when his leg was touched. He was apparently normal about 2 days back. His mother told that all of a sudden, her son became much irritable and started crying excessively. On careful observation, his mother found that there was swelling around right knee joint. He was not allowing anyone to touch his leg. His mother had noticed that there was little warmth over the knee joint compared to the surrounding region. There was history of fever, moderate to high degree. Fever used to be more in the evening and night and used to be relieved by antipyretics to little extent.

Past History of the Patient

The boy was the only and first sibling of non-consanguineous marriage. He was born at full term by normal vaginal delivery. The baby cried immediately after delivery. The birth weight of child was 3 kg. Child was on breast milk immediately after the delivery, weaning of food was started at the age of 4 months. His developmental milestones were normal. Before the development of this problem, he had upper respiratory tract infection (URTI) about 1 week back, for which he had received treatment. He had been completely immunized.

CASE AT A GLANCE

Basic Findings
Length	: 70 cm (50th centile)
Weight	: 7.75 kg (40th centile)
Temperature	: 39°C
Pulse rate	: 116 beats/min
Respiratory rate	: 28 breaths/min
Blood pressure	: 70/50 mm Hg

Positive Findings

History:
- Sudden onset of fever
- Redness and pain in the right knee
- Limping
- Past history of upper respiratory tract infection (URTI)

Examination:
- Arthritis at right knee
- Tenderness
- Crepitation at right base chest

Investigation:
- TLC: Raised
- ESR: Raised
- CRP: Raised

(CRP: c-reactive protein; ESR: erythrocyte sedimentation rate; TLC: total leukocyte count; URTI: upper respiratory tract infection)

EXAMINATION

On examination the child was moderately built and nourished. He was looking toxic, irritable, and crying excessively. Anthropometric measurements included the length 70 cm (50th centile) and the weight 7.75 kg (40th centile). The head circumference was 40 cm. The child was febrile 39°C, and toxic signs of mild dehydration were present. The pulse rate was 116 beats/min. The respiratory rate was 28 breaths/min. The blood pressure recorded was 70/50 mm Hg.

He was looking pale, no edema, and no icterus. The right inguinal lymph nodes were enlarged. There was swelling in and around the knee joint. There was limitation of the movements at knee joint. Erythema, tenderness, and warmth were present. Respiratory system revealed the presence of the basal crepitation on both lungs. Other systemic examinations were normal.

INVESTIGATION

- *Hemoglobin:* 12 g/dL
- *TLC:* 22,000 cells/cumm
- *DLC:* $P_{72} L_{25} E_3$
- *ESR:* 56 mm in the first hour
- *Antistreptolysin O (ASLO):* 200 Todd units
- *CRP:* 2,200 µg/L (normal range: 70–1,800 µg/L)
- *X-ray chest:* Normal
- *X-ray of the right knee:* Normal

DISCUSSION

The boy presented with sudden onset of pain in knee joint, which was associated with raised ESR. Leukocytosis and raised CRP point to the diagnosis of septic arthritis. It most commonly occurs during the first year of life. It frequently follows the infection of the skin and upper respiratory tract.

Septic arthritis is more common in young children. Half of all cases occur by 2 years of age and three-fourths of all cases occur by 5 years of age. Adolescents and neonates are at risk of gonococcal septic arthritis.

Hemophilus influenzae type B accounted for more than half of all cases of bacterial arthritis in infants and young children. Since the development of the conjugate vaccine, it is now a rare cause; *S. aureus* is now the most common infection in all age-groups.

In sexually active adolescents, gonococcus is a common cause of septic arthritis and tenosynovitis, usually of small joints or as a monoarticular infection of a large joint (knee). *Neisseria meningitidis* can cause either a septic arthritis that occurs in the first few days of illness or a reactive arthritis that is typically seen several days after antibiotics have been initiated. Group B *Streptococcus* is an important cause of septic arthritis in neonates.

Fungal infections usually occur as part of multisystem disseminated disease; *Candida* arthritis can complicate systemic infection in neonates with or without indwelling vascular catheters. Primary viral infections of joints are rare, but arthritis accompanies many viral (parvovirus, mumps, rubella live vaccines) syndromes, suggesting an immune-mediated pathogenesis.

PATHOGENESIS

Predisposing factors for the development of septic arthritis vary with age. For example, in neonates, the presence of indwelling catheters including those in the umbilical vessels increases the risk, whereas in older children, risk factors include underlying medical conditions such as immunodeficiencies, diabetes, juvenile idiopathic in arthritis (JIA), and hemoglobinopathies.

The source of pyogenic arthritis varies according to the child's age. In the infant, pyogenic arthritis often develops by spread from adjacent osteomyelitis. In the older child, it presents an isolated infection, usually without bony involvement. In teenagers with pyogenic arthritis, an underlying systemic disease is usually the cause, such as an obvious generalized infection or an organism (e.g., the *Gonococcus*) that has an affinity for joints.

The anatomy of the synovial joint provides an environment conducive to bacterial infection. The synovial tissue lining the joint lacks a basement membrane and therefore secretes a transudate of serum. The rest of the joint surface is composed of a vascular cartilage. Bacteria enter the joint by hematogenous seeding, direct extension from an adjacent focus, or direct inoculation during a joint aspiration, arthrotomy, or trauma.

Initially, after bacterial invasion occurs, the synovial membrane swells and produces increased amounts of fluid, distending the joint. It infection persists without treatment, pus accumulates in the area and destruction of cartilage follows. Subluxation or dislocation of the joint may result from increased intra-articular pressure occurring when the joint capsule is distended by purulent fluid. This increased pressure may compromise blood supply in certain areas. In the hip, this may lead to a vascular necrosis of the femoral head.

Bacteria are deposited in the subsynovial capillary vessel network, with the migration of the bacteria and blood products into the joint space. If the host's immune system is well prepared, the arthritis does not progress and process is aborted.

Septic arthritis primarily occurs as a result of hematogenous seeding of the synovial space. Less often, organisms enter the joint space by direct inoculation or extension from a contiguous focus. The synovial membrane has a rich vascular supply and lacks a basement membrane, providing an ideal environment for hematogenous seeding.

The presence of bacterial products (endotoxin or other toxins) within the joint space stimulates cytokine production (tumor necrosis factor alpha, interleukin-1) within the joint, triggering an inflammatory cascade. The cytokines stimulate chemotaxis of neutrophils into the joint space, where proteolytic enzymes and elastases are released by neutrophils, damaging the cartilage.

Proteolytic enzymes released from the synovial cells and chondrocytes also contribute to destruction of cartilage and synovium. Bacterial hyaluronidase breaks down the hyaluronic acid in the synovial fluid, making the fluid less viscous and diminishing its ability to lubricate and protect the joint cartilage.

Damage to the cartilage can occur through increased friction, especially for weight-bearing joints. The increased pressure within the joint space from accumulation of purulent material can compromise the vascular supply and induce pressure necrosis of the cartilage. Synovial and cartilage destruction results from a combination of proteolytic enzymes and mechanical factors.

Articular cortical degradation occurs because of depletion of collagen and proteoglycan. Pus in the joint space increases intracapsular pressure with the resulting decrease in blood flow to the epiphyses. This can lead to irreversible ischemic damage if the pressure is nor relieved promptly.

The initial effusion of the joint rapidly becomes purulent. An effusion of the joint may accompany osteomyelitis in the adjacent bone. A white cell count exceeding 100,000/mL in the joint fluid indicates a definite purulent infection. Generally, spread of infection is from the bone into the joint, but unattended pyogenic arthritis may also affect adjacent bone. The sedimentation rate is often above 50 mm/h.

Delayed or inadequate treatment of a septic joint can result in permanent joint damage with subsequent disability. Septic arthritis is most common in children <3 years of age. In most cases, a single, large joint is involved, usually in the lower extremity. As in osteomyelitis, males are affected more frequently. There may be a history of trauma or recent infection of the skin or upper respiratory tract.

■ CAUSATIVE AGENTS

As in osteomyelitis, etiologic agents of septic arthritis vary by age. *Staphylococcus aureus* (MSSA and MIRSA) is the leading organism in all age-groups neonates, and enteric Gram-negative organisms are also important to consider and may be isolated from an affected joint as a consequence of an adjacent osteomyelitis. *S. aureus*, *Streptococcus pyogenes*, and *Kingella kingae* are the most prominent causative pathogens in children <4 years of age. *H. influenzae* type B, the most common organism in this age-group in the past, is rarely seen now in countries that routinely vaccinate against this agent. In children older than 4 years, *S. aureus* and *S. pyogenes* are the chief pathogens. *Klebsiella* is a Gram-negative bacterium that occasionally causes pyarthrosis.

Fungal infections usually occur as part of multisystem disseminated disease. Candida arthritis can complicate systemic infection in neonates with or without indwelling vascular catheters. Primary viral infections of joints are rare, but arthritis accompanies many viral (parvovirus, mumps, rubella live vaccines) syndromes, suggesting an immune-mediated pathogenesis.

■ CLINICAL FEATURES (FIG. 1)

The onset may be sudden with systemic symptoms and fever. Local swelling may appear with pain and muscular rigidity, erythema, tenderness, and warmth.

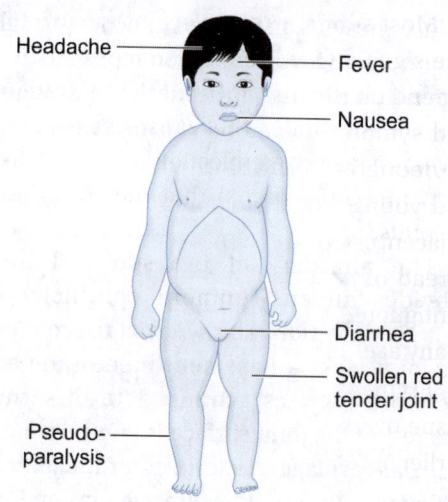

Fig. 1: Clinical features.

Joints of the lower extremity constitute 75% of all cases of septic arthritis. The elbow, wrist, and shoulder joints are involved in approximately 25% of cases, and small joints are uncommonly infected.

Children generally present acutely with a painful, erythematous, warm joint, and refusal to move or bear weight on the affected extremity. Fever, toxicity, and irritability are often accompanying features.

The joint is held in the position of most comfort, usually mild flexion when the hip is involved, erythema or joint swelling is generally not obvious, but the affected hip is held in a position of flexion abduction, and external rotation. Young children may exhibit the phenomenon of "referred pain", in which symptoms from an infected hip joint are referred to the ipsilateral knee. The differential diagnosis of septic arthritis includes cellulitis, bursitis, osteomyelitis (including patellar) with or without a sympathetic effusion, reactive arthritis, transient synovitis, and arthritis associated with systemic disease, such as juvenile idiopathic arthritis (JIA), or malignancy.

Most septic arthritis are monoarticular. The signs and symptoms of septic arthritis depend on the age of the patient. Early signs and symptoms may be subtle, particularly in neonates. Septic arthritis in neonates and young infants is often associated with adjacent osteomyelitis caused by transphyseal spread of infection, although osteomyelitis contiguous with an infected joint can be seen at any age.

Erythema and edema of the skin and soft tissue overlying the site of infection are seen earlier in septic arthritis than in osteomyelitis, because the bulging infected synovium is usually more superficial, whereas the metaphysis is located more deeply. Septic arthritis of the hip is an exception because of the deep location of the hip joint.

Joints of the lower extremity constitute 75% of all cases of septic arthritis. The elbow, wrist, and shoulder joints are involved in approximately 25% of cases, and small joints are uncommonly infected. Suppurative infections of the hip, shoulder, elbow, and ankle in older infants and children may be associated with an adjacent osteomyelitis of the proximal femur, proximal humerus, proximal radius, and distal tibia because the metaphysis extends intra-articularly.

In older children, the signs may be striking, with fever, malaise, vomiting and restriction of motion. In infants, paralysis of the limb due to inflammatory neuritis may be evident. Infection of the hip joint in infants should be suspected if decreased abduction of the hip is present in an infant who is irritable or feeding poorly. A history of umbilical catheter treatment in the newborn nursery should alert the physician to the possibility of pyogenic arthritis of the hip.

> **ESSENTIAL DIAGNOSTIC POINTS**
> - Fever, malaise vomiting
> - *Pseudoparalysis:* Paralysis of limb due to inflammatory neuritis
> - Redness and swelling of the skin soft tissue
> - *Leukocytosis:* >100,000/dL, indicate sepsis

Infants may have only pseudoparalyses of the extremity or apparent pain on movement of the joint. Most older infants and children have fever and localizing signs. Redness and swelling of the skin and soft tissue tend to be seen. The bulging, infected synovium is near the surface. Nonspecific systemic signs of infection such as nausea, vomiting, diarrhea, and headache are present in disseminated infection syndrome with multiple foci of infection or disease.

■ DIAGNOSIS

Because of the risk of long-term orthopedic complications, septic arthritis is an orthopedic emergency. Joint aspiration is the most important component of the diagnostic evaluation. Other laboratory tests and radiologic studies are generally nonspecific, but findings may be useful to direct the evaluation.

Blood cultures should be performed in all cases of suspected septic arthritis. Aspiration of the joint fluid for Gram stain and culture when the history and physical findings indicate septic arthritis remains the definitive diagnostic technique and provides the optimal specimen for culture to confirm the diagnosis. Most large joint spaces are easy to aspirate, but the hip can pose technical problems; ultrasound guidance facilitates aspiration. Aspiration of joint pus provides the best specimen for bacteriologic culture of infection. If *Gonococcus* is suspected, cervical, anal, and throat cultures should also be obtained.

Multiplex bacterial PCR panels appear to have a yield around 50% from joint fluid specimens, but this increase over culture is almost entirely due to their enhanced ability to detect *K. kingae*. Other strategies to increase detection of *K. kingae* include prompt inoculation onto solid media and inoculation of the joint fluid in blood culture bottles. A diagnosis of Lyme arthritis is made through via a two-step test of an ELISA or IEA followed by a reflex Western blot for samples that are positive or equivocal by the first methodology Patients with Lyme arthritis are seropositive because arthritis is a late manifestation of infection.

The white blood cell count and differential, ESR, and CRP are generally elevated in children with joint infections but are nonspecific and might not be helpful in distinguishing between infection and other inflammatory processes. Monitoring elevated ESR and CRP may be of value in assessing response to therapy or identifying complications. In one study of *S. aureus* septic arthritis, risk features for a site of osteomyelitis contiguous with septic arthritis included a CRP >10 mg/dL at the time of admission, positive blood cultures or >2 days of fever following admission.

Ultrasonography

Ultrasonography is particularly helpful in detecting joint effusion and fluid collection in the soft-tissue and subperiosteal regions. USG is highly sensitive in detecting joint effusion, particularly for the hip joint, where plain radiographs are normal in >50% of cases of septic arthritis of the hip. USG can serve as an aid in performing hip aspiration.

Radionuclide Imaging

Radionuclide imaging compared to radiographs is more sensitive in providing supportive evidence of the diagnosis of septic arthritis; a scan may be positive within 2 days of the onset of symptoms.

Radiography

Early distension of the joint capsule is nonspecific and difficult to measure by X-ray. In the infant with unrecognized pyogenic arthritis, dislocation of the joint may follow within a few days as a result of distension of the capsule by pus. Later changes include destruction of the joint space, resorption of epiphysial cartilage, and erosion of the adjacent bone of the metaphysis. The bone scan shows increased flow and increased uptake about the joint.

Magnetic resonance imaging and CT can confirm the presence of joint fluid in patients with suspected osteoarthritis infections but are not routinely indicated. MRI is useful in evaluating for adjacent osteomyelitis or pyomyositis but is typically reserved for cases when the index of suspicion for these conditions is high.

LABORATORY SALIENT FINDINGS
• Increased leukocyte count • Elevated ESR • *Arthrocentesis:* Gram stain, antinuclear antibodies, elevated WBCs in joint fluid • Blood culture and sensitivity • Lactic acid concentration in joint fluid
(ESR: erythrocyte sedimentation rate; WBCs: white blood cells)

Joint Fluid Analysis

For patients in whom the diagnosis of septic arthritis is suspected, aspirating the affected joint can be both diagnostic and, in many cases, therapeutic. Synovial fluid should be sent for Gram stain, aerobic cultures, and cell count with a leukocyte differential. Anaerobic, fungal, and acid-fast bacilli (AFB) cultures may be considered in some instances (e.g., immune compromised patients, penetrating injuries to the joint, postprocedure septic arthritis).

Joint fluid cultures are positive in 30–60% of cases. Inoculation of joint fluid into blood culture bottles increases the yield of cultures, particularly when the etiologic agent is fastidious such as in the case of *K. kingae*. Leukocyte counts greater than 50,000 cells/μL, with a predominance of segmented neutrophils, are suggestive of bacterial arthritis, even in the absence of a positive culture. However, it should be recognized that white blood cells in infected joint fluid can vary widely, ranging from 2,000 to 300,000/μL. Synovial fluid glucose and protein may be measured but are nonspecific.

Lactic acid concentration within the joint fluid is a reliable method for establishing a diagnosis of septic arthritis. In patients with septic arthritis, the mean lactic acid concentration in synovial fluid is 11.6 mmol/L (normal level is 2.3 mmol/L).

GENERAL FEATURES
• Toxic
• Fever
• Dehydration

■ DIFFERENTIAL DIAGNOSIS

Differential diagnosis includes deep cellulitis, fungal arthritis, acute rheumatic fever, rheumatoid arthritis, toxic synovitis, traumatic arthritis, and Henoch–Schönlein purpura (HSP).

■ TREATMENT

The goals of therapy are as follows: Decompression or the joint space and removal of inflammatory debris by adequate drainages sterilization of the joint through the use of appropriate antimicrobial agents; relief of pain; and prevention of joint deformity. It includes the choice of antibiotics. It is based on the microscopic examination of Gram-stained smear. Surgical drainage should be performed especially if hip and shoulder are involved.

Antibiotic Therapy

Antimicrobial therapy should be instituted immediately after blood cultures and joint fluid samples are obtained. Empiric, initial antibiotic choice is based on the likely pathogens at various ages, the results of Gram stain of the joint aspirate, and any special considerations dictated by the patient's underlying medical problems or clinical situation.

Empiric choice of antimicrobials is similar to that recommended for osteomyelitis, and regimens for all age-groups should include an antistaphylococcal agent with coverage for methicillin-resistant *Staphylococcus* aureus (MRSA) as dictated by local prevalence.

If *Neisseria gonorrhoeae* is a consideration, ceftriaxone, or cefotaxime should be used. Parenteral antibiotics are used initially and continued until there is no further need for surgical intervention and the child is afebrile with clinical improvement and improvement of laboratory parameters. The exact length of therapy is dependent on the clinical situation, the patient's response, and the particular organism. Traditionally, therapy is continued for at least 2 weeks after the patient is afebrile, joint fluid accumulation has resolved, and laboratory parameters have normalized.

Antibiotics can be selected based on the child's age, results of the Gram stain, and culture of the aspirated pus. Reasonable empiric therapy in infants is nafcillin or oxacillin plus a third-generation cephalosporin. An antistaphylococcal agent alone is usually adequate for children over age 5 years.

For staphylococcal infections, 3 weeks of therapy is recommended; for other organisms, 2 weeks is usually sufficient.

Oral therapy may began when clinical signs have improved markedly. It is not necessary to give intra-articular antibiotics, because good levels are achieved in the synovial fluid.

In neonates, an antistaphylococcal penicillin, such as nafcillin or oxacillin (150–200 mg/kg/24 h divided q 6 hours IV), and a broad-spectrum cephalosporin, such as cefotaxime (150–225 mg/kg/24 h divided q 8 hours IV), provide coverage for the *S. aureus*, group B *Streptococcus*, and gram-negative bacilli. If MRSA is a concern, vancomycin is selected instead of nafcillin or oxacillin.

In older infants and children with septic arthritis, empirical therapy to cover for *S. aureus*, streptococci, and *K. kingae* includes cefazolin (100–150 mg/kg/24 h divided q 8 hours) or nafcillin (150–200 mg/kg/24 h divided q 6 hours).

In areas where methicillin resistance is noted in 10% of community-acquired methicillin-resistant *S. aureus* strains (CA-MRSA), including an antibiotic that is effective against CA-MRSA isolates is suggested. Clindamycin (40 mg/kg divided q 8 hours) and vancomycin (15 mg/kg q 6 hours IV) are alternatives when treating CA-MRSA infections. For immunocompromised patients, combination therapy is usually initiated, such as with vancomycin and ceftazidime or with extended-spectrum penicillin's and beta(β)-lactamase inhibitors with an aminoglycoside.

When the pathogen is identified, appropriate changes in antibiotics are made, if necessary. If a pathogen is not identified and a patient's condition is improving, therapy is continued with the antibiotic selected initially. If a pathogen is not identified and a patient's condition is not improving, reaspiration or the possibility of a noninfectious condition should be considered.

Duration of antibiotic therapy is individualized depending on the organism isolated and the clinical course. 10–14 days is usually adequate for streptococci, *S. pneumoniae*, and *K. kingae*; longer therapy may be needed for *S. aureus* and Gram-negative infections (3 weeks), concomitant osteomyelitis (4 weeks), extensive disease, or slow response to treatment.

Intravenous antibiotics for 14–21 days must be used. Chloramphenicol in the dose of 100 mg/kg/24 hour in 4 divided IV doses. Ampicillin in the dose of 200 mg/kg/24 h in six divided doses, or cefotaxime in the dose of 150 mg/kg/24 h in four divided doses is recommended. If there is no clinical improvement within 48 hours, then the surgical drainage of the infected joint should be undertaken immediately.

Normalization of ESR and CRP in addition to a normal examination supports discontinuing antibiotic therapy. Oral antibiotics can be used to complete therapy once the patient is afebrile for 48–72 hours and is clearly improving.

In the hip joint, pyogenic arthritis is most easily treated by surgical drainage, because the joint is deep and difficult to aspirate and is also inaccessible to thorough cleaning through needle aspiration.

Arthroscopic irrigation and debridement have been successful in treating pyogenic arthritis of the knee. If fever and clinical symptoms do not subside within 24 hours after the treatment is begun, open surgical drainage is indicated.

Surgical Therapy

Drainage of the infected joint may require repeated aspiration, arthroscopic lavage, or open drainage with lavage. Repeated aspiration may be appropriate in a setting where no surgeon is readily available to perform arthroscopic or open drainage, but drainage with lavage, either via an arthroscopic or an open procedure, is superior because it allows thorough cleansing and removal of inflammatory debris that cannot be evacuated by aspiration. Arthrotomy may not be necessary for infection of all joints, but is indicated for patients who fail to respond to repeated joint aspirations and in those with infections of the hip (and perhaps the shoulder). Recently, arthroscopic techniques have become more popular and cause less morbidity, with similar results.

Infection of the hip is generally considered a surgical emergency because of the vulnerability of the blood supply to the head of the femur. For joints other than the hip, daily aspirations of synovial fluid may be required. Generally, one or two subsequent aspirations suffice. If fluid continues to accumulate after 4–5 days, arthrotomy or video-assisted arthroscopy is needed. At the time of surgery, the joint is flushed with sterile saline solution. Antibiotics are not instilled, because they are irritating to synovial tissue, and adequate amounts of antibiotic are achieved in joint fluid with systemic administration.

■ PROGNOSIS

The prognosis for the patient with pyogenic arthritis is excellent if the joint is drained early, before damage to the articular cartilage has occurred. If infection is present for >24 hours, there is dissolution of the proteoglycans in the articular cartilage, with subsequent arthrosis and fibrosis of the joint. Damage to the growth plate may also occur, especially within the hip joint, where the epiphysial plate is intracapsular.

Sequelae of septic arthritis include joint deformity and residual dysfunction, abnormal bone growth, and in the hip, avascular necrosis of the femoral head. Risk factors for subsequent complications include delay in drainage, age <1 year, involvement of the hip or shoulder, adjacent osteomyelitis, and infection with *S. aureus*.

■ BIBLIOGRAPHY

1. Arnold JC, Bradley JS. Osteoarticular Infections in Children. Infect Dis Clin North Am. 2015;29:557-74.
2. Peltola H, Pääkkönen M, Kallio P, Kallio MJ; Osteomyelitis-Septic Arthritis (OM-SA) Study Group. Prospective, randomized trial of 10 days versus 30 days of antimicrobial treatment, including a short-term course of parenteral therapy, of childhood septic arthritis. Clin Infect Dis. 2009;48:1201-10.
3. Sukswai P, Kovitvanitcha D, Thumkunanon V, Chotpitayasunondh T, Sangtawesin V, Jeerathanyasakun Y. Acute hematogenous osteomyelitis and septic arthritis in children: clinical characteristics and outcome study. J Med Assoc Thai. 2011;94Suppl 3:S209-16.
4. Tanwar YS, Jaiswal A, Singh S, Arya RK, Lal H. Acute pediatric septic arthritis: a systematic review of literature and current controversies. Pol Orthop Traumatol. 2014;79:23-9.

CASE 78

Tetanus Neonatorum

■ PRESENTING COMPLAINTS

A 6-day-old newborn was brought with the complaint of:
- General rigidity of the body since 2 days
- Breathlessness since 2 days
- Not taking feeds since 1 day
- Excessive crying since 1 day

History of Presenting Complaints

A 6-day-old boy was brought to the hospital with history of excessive crying and not taking feeds since 2 days. His mother had noticed that he was apparently normal till the third day and was crying excessively. She was trying to feed him and thinking that he might be hungry. But her efforts used to be in vain.

She had also noted that he had generalized rigidity and bending of the body in extension since 2 days. There was also history of fever, moderate to high degree. This was not associated with chills and rigors. There was also history of respiratory distress.

Past History of the Patient

The infant was the only sibling of nonconsanguineous marriage. He was born at home at full term by normal delivery. Delivery was conducted by untrained personnel. The baby cried immediately after the delivery. His mother was doubtful whether she had been received tetanus toxoid antenatally.

CASE AT A GLANCE

Basic Findings
Length	: 51 cm (50th centile)
Weight	: 3 kg (50th centile)
Temperature	: 38°C
Pulse rate	: 120 beats/min
Respiratory rate	: 38 breaths/min
Blood pressure	: 50/30 mm Hg

Positive Findings

History:
- Excessive crying
- Not taking feeds
- Muscular rigidity
- Cyanosis
- Home delivery

Examination:
- Excessive crying
- Not taking feeds
- Cyanosis
- Tachycardia
- Tachypnea
- Infected umbilical stump

Investigation:
- Normal

■ EXAMINATION

On examination, the child was moderately built and nourished. He was crying excessively and was not taking feeds. The mouth of the child was kept slightly opened. There was generalized rigidity. At the time of the examination, the child was cyanosed as a result of the spasm of the larynx and respiratory muscles.

Anthropometric measurements included the length of the infant 51 cm (50th centile) and the weight 3 kg (50th centile). The head circumference was 34 cm. He was febrile, 38°C. Heart rate was 120 beats/min and the respiratory rate was 38 breaths/min. Blood pressure recorded was 50/30 mm Hg.

There was no pallor, no lymphadenopathy, and no edema. Cyanosis was evident. Umbilical stump was infected. Other systemic examinations were normal.

■ INVESTIGATION

- *Hemoglobin:* 12 g/dL
- *TLC:* 10,200 cells/cumm
- *ESR:* 20 mm in the first hour
- *CRP:* 1,900 µg/L
- *Blood culture and sensitivity:* No growth
- *X-ray chest:* Normal
- *CSF examination:* Normal

■ DISCUSSION

Tetanus neonatorum is caused by Gram-positive motile, anaerobic spore-bearing bacillus called *Clostridium tetani*. The organism enters the body through the open wounds by the soil containing clostridial spores from animal manure. The toxin reaches the CNS by retrograde axon transport, is bound to cerebral gangliosides, and is thought to increase reflex excitability in neurons of the spinal cord by blocking function of inhibitory synapses. Intense muscle spasms result. It produces powerful neurotoxin, i.e., tetanospasmin enters into the circulation. It enters into the motor end plates. It spreads to the nervous system along with the axon cylinders of the motor nerves.

■ ETIOLOGY

Tetanus is an acute, spastic paralytic illness historically called lockjaw that is caused by the neurotoxin produced by *C. tetani*, a motile, Gram-positive, spore-forming obligate anaerobe whose natural habitat worldwide is soil, dust, and the alimentary tracts of various animals. *C. tetani* forms spores terminally, producing a drumstick or tennis racket appearance microscopically. Tetanus spores can survive boiling but not autoclaving, whereas the vegetative cells are killed by antibiotics, heat, and standard disinfectants. Unlike many clostridia, *C. tetani* is not a tissue-invasive organism and instead causes illness through the effects of a single toxin, tetanospasmin, more commonly referred to as tetanus toxin. Tetanospasmin in the second most poisonous substance known, surpassed in potency only by botulinum toxin. The human lethal dose of tetanus toxin is estimated to be 10^{-5} mg/kg.

■ PATHOGENESIS

Tetanus occurs after introduced spores germinate, multiply, and produce tetanus toxin in the low oxidation–reduction potential of an infected injury site. A plasmid carries the toxin gene. Toxin is released after vegetative bacterial cell death and lysis.

Tetanus toxin (and the botulinum toxins) is a 150 kDa simple protein consisting of a heavy chain (100 kDa) and a light (50 kDa) chain joined by a single disulfide bond. Tetanus toxin binds at the neuromuscular junction and enters the motor nerve by endocytosis, after which it undergoes retrograde axonal transport to the cytoplasm of the alpha motor neuron. In the sciatic nerve, the transport rate was found to be 3.4 mm/h.

The toxin exits the motoneuron in the spinal cord and next enters adjacent spinal inhibitory interneurons, where it prevents release of the neurotransmitters glycine and gamma-aminobutyric acid (GABA). Tetanus toxin thus blocks the normal inhibition of antagonistic muscles on which voluntary coordinated movement depends; as a consequence, affected muscles sustain maximal contraction and cannot relax. The autonomic nervous system is also rendered unstable in tetanus. Because C. *tetani* is not an invasive organism, its toxin-producing vegetative cells remain where introduced into the wound, which may display local inflammatory changes and a mixed bacterial flora.

The phenomenal potency of tetanus toxin is enzymatic. The light chain of tetanus toxin (and of several botulinum toxins) is a zinc-containing endoprotease whose substrate is synaptobrevin, a constituent protein of the docking complex that enables the synaptic vesicle to fuse with the terminal neuronal cell membrane. The heavy chain of the toxin contains its binding and internalization domains.

In many cases, no history of a wound can be obtained. In the newborn, usually in underdeveloped countries, infection generally results from contamination of the umbilical cord. The incubation period typically is 4–14 days but may be longer.

Tetanus spores can survive boiling but not autoclaving, whereas vegetative cells are killed by antibiotics, heat and disinfectant. The toxin is produced by vegetative form.

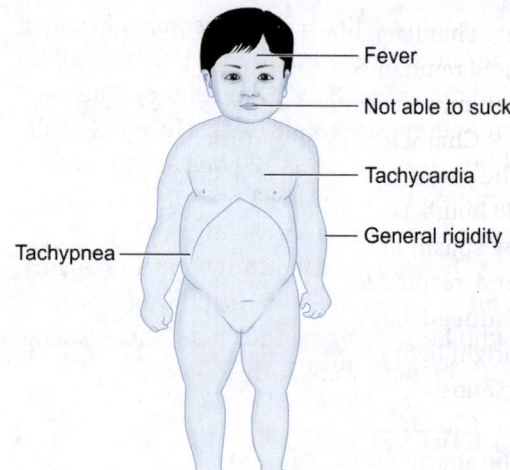

Fig. 1: Clinical features.

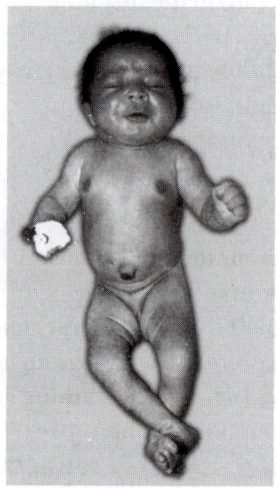

Fig. 2: Neonatal tetanus.

■ CLINICAL FEATURES (FIG. 1)

The symptom is often mild pain at the site of inoculation, followed by hypertonicity and spasm of the regional muscles. The most common age at the onset of the symptoms is 3–15 days. Excessive unexplained crying followed by the refusal of the feeds is seen. The mouth is kept slightly opened due to pull and spasm of the neck muscles.

Neonatal tetanus, the first signs are irritability and inability to feed. The infant may then develop stiffness of the jaw and neck, increasing dysphagia, and generalized hyperreflexia with rigidity and spasms of all muscles of the abdomen and back (opisthotonos)**(Fig. 2)**. The facial distortion resembles a grimace (risus sardonicus) The sardonic smile, i.e., risus sardonicus, results from intractable spasm of facial and buccal muscles. Paralysis or diminished movement, stiffness and rigidity to the touch, and spasms with or without opisthotonos are characteristic. The umbilical stump may hold remnants of dirt, dung, clotted blood, or serum, or it may appear relatively benign.

Characteristically, difficulty in opening the mouth (trismus) is evident within 48 hours. Lockjaw or reflex spasm is followed by spasm of limbs and spasm of the larynx and respiratory muscles characteristically induced by stimuli of touch, noise, and bright light results in episodes of apnea and cyanosis.

Choking and dysphagia occur due to the spasm of the pharyngeal muscles. There is generalized rigidity and opisthotonus in extension. Difficulty in swallowing and convulsions triggered by minimal stimuli such as sound, light, or movement may occur. There will be episodes of apnea and cyanosis due to the spasm of the larynx and respiratory muscle. Spasms are characteristically induced by the touch, noise, and light. Spasms are less marked in preterm babies. Individual spasms may last for seconds or minutes. Recurrent spasms are seen several times each hour, or they may be almost continuous. Fever, tachycardia, and tachypnea are present. Umbilical stump may show the evidence of sepsis.

The convulsions are characterized by sudden, severe tonic contractions of the muscle. There is first clinching, flexion, adduction of arms, and hyperextension of the legs. But there are no changes in sensorium.

In most cases, the temperature is normal or only mildly elevated. A high or subnormal temperature is bad prognostic sign. Patients are fully conscious and lucid.

A profound circulatory disturbance associated with sympathetic over activity may occur on the second to fourth day, which may contribute to the mortality rate. This is characterized by elevated blood pressure, increased cardiac output, tachycardia (>20 beats/min), and arrhythmias.

Constipation persists until the spasms are relieved. Intercurrent infections, dehydration, and acidosis may complicate the clinical picture.

Cephalic tetanus follows head injury and otitis media. Sometimes it may follow the generalized tetanus. Cranial nerve involvement is present.

ESSENTIAL DIAGNOSTIC POINTS

- History of skin wound
- Not immunized child
- *Trismus:* Spasms jaw muscles
- Stiffness of neck, back, and abdominal muscles
- Hyperirritability and hyperreflexia
- Generalized, episodic muscle contraction
- No altered sensorium

GENERAL FEATURES

- Lockjaw
- Risus sardonicus
- Convulsions
- No altered sensorium
- Choking
- Opisthotonus

■ DIAGNOSIS

The picture of tetanus is one of the most dramatic in medicine, and the diagnosis may be established clinically. The typical setting is an unimmunized patient (and/or mother), who was injured or born within preceding 2 weeks, who presents with trismus, other rigid muscles, and with clear sensorium.

There may be a mild polymorphonuclear leukocytosis. The CSF is normal with the exception of mild elevation of opening pressure.

Serum muscle enzymes may be elevated. Transient electrocardiographic and electroencephalographic abnormalities may occur. Anerobic culture and microscopic examination of pus form the wound can be helpful, but *C. tetani* is difficult to grow, and the drumstick-shaped Gram-positive bacilli often cannot be found.

> **LABORATORY SALIENT FINDINGS**
> - Polymorphonuclear leukocytosis
> - Serum muscle enzymes may be elevated
> - ECG and EEG abnormalities
> - Anerobic culture examination of pus: Drumstick gram positive bacilli
>
> (ECG: electrocardiogram; EEG: electroencephalogram)

■ DIFFERENTIAL DIAGNOSIS

The differential diagnosis includes retropharyngeal abscess, trauma, meningitis and poliomyelitis. Poliomyelitis is characterized by asymmetric paralysis in an incompletely immunized child. The history of an animal bite, absence of trismus, and CSF pleocytosis suggests rabies. Local infections of the throat and jaw should be easily recognized. Bacterial meningitis, phenothiazine reactions, decerebrate posturing, narcotic withdrawal, spondylitis, and hypocalcemic tetany may be confused with tetanus.

■ MANAGEMENT

The aims of treatment are airway maintenance, prevention of further toxin absorption, relieving clinical features, controlling automatic instability and antibiotics.

Airway management may require intubation and mechanical ventilation, especially in severe cases.

Management of tetanus requires eradication of *C. tetani* and the wound environment conducive to its anerobic multiplication, neutralization of all accessible tetanus toxin, control of seizures and respiration, palliation, provision of meticulous supportive care, and, finally, prevention of recurrences.

Surgical wound excision and debridement are often needed to remove the foreign body or devitalized tissue that created anerobic growth conditions. Surgery should be performed promptly after administration of *human tetanus immunoglobulin (TIG)* and anti serum. Excision of the umbilical stump in the neonate with tetanus is no longer recommended.

Tetanus toxin cannot be neutralized by TIG after it has begun its axonal ascent to the spinal cord. TIG should be given as soon as possible to neutralize toxin that diffuses from the wound into the circulation before the toxin can bind at distant muscle groups. The optimal dose of TIG has not been determined. A single IM injection of 500–1,000 IU of TIG is sufficient to neutralize systemic tetanus toxin, but total doses as high as 3,000–6,000 IU are also recommended. Infiltration of TIG into the wound is now considered unnecessary.

If TIG is unavailable, use of human IVIG may be necessary. IVIG contains 4–90 units/mL of TIG; the optimal dosage of IVIG for treating tetanus is not known, and its use is not approved for this indication.

Another alternative is equine- or bovine-derived tetanus antitoxin (TAT). The usual dose of TAT is 50,000–100,000 units, with half given intramuscularly and half intravenously, but as little as 10,000 units may be sufficient. Approximately 15% of patients are given the usual dose of TAT experience serum sickness. When TAT is used, it is essential to check for possible sensitivity to horse serum; desensitization may be needed. The human-derived immunoglobulins are much preferred because of their longer half-lives (30 days) and the virtual absence of allergic and serum sickness adverse effects. Intrathecal TIG, given to neutralize tetanus toxin in the spinal cord, is not effective.

Penicillin G (100,000 units/kg/day divided every 4–6 hours IV for 10–14 days remains the antibiotic of choice because of its effective clostridiocidal action and its diffusibility, which is an important consideration because blood flow to injured tissue may be compromised. Metronidazole (500 mg every 8 hours IV for adults) appears to be equally effective. Erythromycin and tetracycline (for persons >8 years of age) are alternatives for penicillin-allergic patients.

All patients with generalized tetanus need muscle relaxants. Diazepam provides both relaxation and seizure control. The initial dose of 0.1–0.2 mg/kg every 3–6 hours given intravenously is subsequently titrated to control the tetanic spasms, after which the effective dose is sustained for 2–6 weeks before a tapered withdrawal. Magnesium sulfate, other benzodiazepines (midazolam), chlorpromazine, dantrolene, and baclofen are also used. Diazepam prevents by GABA-mediated central inhibition. Intrathecal baclofen produces such complete muscle relaxation that apnea often ensues; like most other agents listed, baclofen should be used only in an intensive care unit setting. Oral drugs used for severe spasms include pancuronium bromide. Autonomic instability is controlled with the use of alpha- and beta-adrenergic blockers and IV magnesium.

The highest survival rates in generalized tetanus are achieved with neuromuscular blocking agents, such as vancuronium and pancuronium, which produce a general flaccid paralysis that is then managed by mechanical ventilation. Autonomic instability is regulated with standard alpha- or beta- (or both) blocking agents; morphine has also proved useful.

■ SUPPORTIVE CARE

Meticulous supportive care in a quiet, dark, secluded setting is most desirable. Because tetanic spasms may be triggered by minor stimuli, the patient should be sedated and protected from all unnecessary sounds, sights, and touch. All therapeutic and other manipulations must be carefully scheduled and coordinated.

Cardiorespiratory monitoring, frequent suctioning, and maintenance of the patient's substantial fluid, electrolyte, and caloric needs are fundamental. Careful nursing attention to mouth, skin, bladder, and bowel function is needed to avoid ulceration, infection, and obstipation. Prophylactic subcutaneous heparin may be of value but must be balanced with the risk for hemorrhage.

Endotracheal intubation may not be required, but it should be done to prevent aspiration of secretions before laryngospasm develops. A tracheostomy kit should be immediately available at hand for unintubated patients. Endotracheal intubation and suctioning easily provoke reflex tetanic seizures and spasms, so early tracheostomy should be considered in severe cases not managed by pharmacologically induced flaccid paralysis. Therapeutic botulinum toxin has been used for this purpose, that is, to overcome trismus.

■ COMPLICATIONS

The seizures and the severe, sustained rigid paralysis of tetanus predispose the patient to many complications. Aspiration of secretions and pneumonia may have begun before the first medical attention was received. Maintaining airway patency often mandates endotracheal intubation and mechanical ventilation with their attendant hazards, including pneumothorax and mediastinal emphysema.

The seizures may result in lacerations of the mouth or tongue, in IM hematomas or rhabdomyolysis with myoglobinuria and renal failure, or in long bone or spinal fractures. Venous thrombosis, pulmonary embolism, gastric ulceration with or without hemorrhage, paralytic ileus, and decubitus ulceration are constant hazards. Excessive use of muscle relaxants, which are an integral part of care, may produce iatrogenic apnea. Cardiac arrhythmias, including asystole, unstable blood pressure, and labile temperature regulation reflect disordered autonomic nervous system control that may be aggravated by inattention to maintenance of intravascular volume needs.

PROGNOSIS

The most important factor that influences outcome is the quality of supportive care. Mortality is highest in the very young and the very old. A favorable prognosis is associated with a long incubation period, absence of fever, and localized disease.

An unfavorable prognosis is associated with onset of trismus <7 days after injury and with onset of generalized tetanic spasms <3 days after onset of trismus. Sequelae of hypoxic brain injury, especially in infants, include cerebral palsy, diminished mental abilities, and behavioral difficulties. Most fatalities occur within the first weeks of illness. Reported case fatality rates for generalized tetanus are 5–35%, and for neonatal tetanus they extend from <10% with intensive care treatment to >75% without it. Cephalic tetanus has an especially poor prognosis because of breathing and feeding difficulties.

Prognosis is worse if onset of symptoms occur within the first week of life, if the interval between lockjaw and the onset of the spasm is <48 hours, if high fever and tachycardia are present. Laryngeal spasm resulting in apnea are frequent. Many deaths are due to pneumonia or respiratory failure. If the patient survives 1 week, recovery is likely.

PREVENTION

Tetanus is an entirely preventable disease. A serum antibody titer of >0.01 units/mL is considered protective.

Active immunization should begin in early infancy with combined diphtheria toxoid–tetanus toxoid–acellular pertussis (DTaP) vaccine at 2, 4, 6 and 15–18 months of age, with boosters at 4–6 years (DTaP) and 11–12 years [tetanus–diphtheria–pertussis (Tdap)] of age and at 10-year intervals thereafter throughout adult life with tetanus and reduced diphtheria toxoid (Td).

Immunization of women with tetanus toxoid prevents neonatal tetanus, and pregnant women should receive one dose of reduced diphtheria and pertussis toxoids (Tdap) during each pregnancy, preferably at 27–36 weeks gestation.

Arthus reactions (type III hypersensitivity reactions), a localized vasculitis associated with deposition of immune complexes and activation of complement, are reported rarely after tetanus vaccination. Mass immunization campaigns in developing countries have occasionally provoked a widespread hysterical reaction.

BIBLIOGRAPHY

1. American Academy of Pediatrics. Tetanus. In: Kimberlin DW, Brady MT, Jackson MA (Eds). Red Book:2015 Report of Committee on Infectious Diseases, 30th edition. Elk Grove Village: American Academy of Pediatrics; 2015; pp. 773-8.
2. Centre for Disease Control and Prevention. Tetanus. [online] Available from https://www.cdc.gov/tetanus/ [Last accessed June, 2024].
3. Ergonul O, Egeli D, Kahyaoglu B, Bahar M, Etienne M, Bleck T. An unexpected tetanus case. Lancet Infect Dis. 2016;16:746-52.
4. Okoromah CN, Lesi FE. Diazepam for treating tetanus. Cochrane Database Syst Rev. 2004;2004(1):CD003954.

CASE 79

Typhoid

■ PRESENTING COMPLAINTS

A 10-year-old boy was brought with the complaint of:
- Fever since 10 days
- Headache since 10 days
- Tiredness since 5 days
- Loose motion since 3 days

History of Presenting Complaints

A 10-year-old boy was brought to the hospital with history of fever, lethargy, and headache for 10 days. Fever was of moderate to high degree, intermittent, and more in the evening and night. It was associated with chills and rigors. Headache was diffuse in nature and was severe, throbbing type. It used to be relieved by taking analgesics. There was no history of vomiting.

A week back, he had been to an endemic area where malaria was more common. His mother told that he had been treated with intravenous (IV) antibiotics, and the temperature was present with spikes. Later he developed loose motion.

Past History of the Patient

The child was the eldest sibling of nonconsanguineous marriage. He was born at full term by normal delivery. There were no significant postnatal events. His developmental milestones were normal. He had been completely immunized. His performance at school was good.

■ EXAMINATION

The boy was moderately built and nourished. He was looking sick and moderately dehydrated. The anthropometric measurements included the height 135 (50th centile) and the weight 29 kg (75th centile). He was

---

CASE AT A GLANCE

Basic Findings
Height	: 135 cm (50th centile)
Weight	: 29 kg (75th centile)
Temperature	: 39°C
Pulse rate	: 116 beats/min
Respiratory rate	: 22 breaths/min
Blood pressure	: 100/70 mm Hg

Positive Findings

History:
- Fever with rigors
- Headache
- IV antibiotics did not control temperature
- Loose motions

Examination:
- Febrile
- Cervical lymphadenopathy
- Splenomegaly

Investigation:
- *Hb:* Anemia
- *TLC:* Leukopenia
- *Widal:* Positive

(Hb: hemoglobin; TLC: total leukocyte count)

febrile, i.e., 39°C. The pulse rate was 116 beats/min and the respiratory rate was 22 breaths/min. The blood pressure recorded was 100/70 mm Hg. There was pallor, no icterus, and no edema. There was cervical lymphadenopathy.

Per abdomen examination revealed the enlargement of the spleen. Splenomegaly was present about 2 cm below the costal margin. It was nontender. Other systemic examinations were normal.

■ INVESTIGATION

- *Hemoglobin:* 8 g/dL
- *TLC:* 5,200 cells/cumm
- *DLC:* P_{65} L_{30} M_2 E_1
- *Platelet count:* 6,50,000 cells/cumm
- *Blood culture and sensitivity:* No growth
- *Widal test:* O 1:320; H 1:320

■ DISCUSSION

Fever, headache, associated splenomegaly, and loose motion lead to the provisional diagnosis of enteric fever and malaria. The diagnosis of typhoid is favored because of the presence of leukopenia especially neutropenia. Diagnosis of typhoid is mainly made by blood culture and sensitivity in the first week.

■ ETIOLOGY

Typhoid fever is caused by *Salmonella enterica* serovariant Typhi (*Salmonella* Typhi), a Gram-negative bacterium. A very similar but often less-severe disease is caused by *Salmonella* Paratyphi A and rarely by *Salmonella* Paratyphi B and *Salmonella* Paratyphi C.

■ PATHOGENESIS

Typhoid fever is caused by the Gram-negative bacillus *S.* Typhi. Parathyroid fevers, which are usually milder but may be clinically indistinguishable, are caused by *S.* Paratyphi A, *Salmonella schottmuelleri*, or *Salmonella hirschfeldii* (formerly Salmonella Paratyphi A, B, and C); children have a shorter incubation period than do adults (usually 5–8 days instead of 8–14 days).

Enteric fever occurs through the ingestion of the organism, and a variety of sources of fecal contamination have been reported, including street foods and contamination of water reservoirs. With an incubation period ranging from 4 to 14 days, depending on the inoculating dose of viable bacteria.

Typhoid fever is transmitted by the fecal-oral route and by contamination of food and water. Unlike other *Salmonella* species, there are no animal reservoirs of *S.* Typhi; each case is the result of direct or indirect contact with the organism or with an individual who is actively infected or a chronic carrier.

The infected persons excrete the bacilli in stools and urine. Food and water may be contaminated by hands of carrier of patients. It is transmitted by ingestion of the infected food, milk, or water. The period of infectivity or communicability lasts as long as bacteria are present in excreta.

After ingestion, *S.* Typhi organisms are thought to invade the body through the gut mucosa in the terminal ileum, possibly through specialized antigen-sampling cells known as M-cells that overlie gut-associated lymphoid tissues, through enterocytes, or via a paracellular route. *S.* Typhi crosses the intestinal mucosal barrier after attachment to microvilli by an intricate mechanism involving membrane ruffling actin rearrangement and internalization in an intracellular vacuole.

Salmonella Typhi has three main antigens O, H, and Vi and a number of phage types. It survives intracellularly in the tissue of various organs. The factors which influence the onset of typhoid fever in man are the infecting dose and virulence of organism.

Salmonella Typhi expresses virulence factors that allow it to downregulate the pathogen recognition receptor-mediated host inflammatory response. Within the Peyer's patches in the terminal ileum, *S.* Typhi can traverse the intestinal barrier through several mechanisms, including the M-cells in the follicle-associated epithelium, epithelial cells, and dendritic cells. At the villi, *Salmonella* can enter through the M-cells or by passage through or between compromised epithelial cells.

After passing through the intestinal mucosa, *S.* Typhi organisms enter the mesenteric lymphoid system and then pass into the bloodstream via the lymphatics. This primary bacteremia is usually asymptomatic, and blood culture results are frequently negative at this stage of the disease. The bloodborne bacteria are disseminated throughout the body and are thought to colonize the organs of the reticuloendothelial system, where they may replicate within macrophages. After a period of bacterial replication, *S.* Typhi organisms are shed back into the blood, causing a secondary bacteremia that coincides with the onset of clinical symptoms and marks the end of the incubation period.

On contact with the epithelial cell, *S.* Typhi assembles type III secretion system encoded on *Salmonella* pathogenicity *i*slands-1 (SPI-1) and translocates effectors into the cytoplasm. These effectors activate host Rho guanosine triphosphatases, resulting in the rearrangement of the actin cytoskeleton into membrane ruffles, induction of mitogen-activated protein kinase (MAPK) pathways, and destabilization of tight junctions. Changes in the action cytoskeleton are further modulated by the actin-binding proteins SipA and SipC and lead to bacterial uptake. MAPK signaling activates the transcription factors activator protein 1 (AP-1) and nuclear factor (NF)-κB, which lead to production of interleukin 8.

The destabilization of tight junctions allows the transmigration of polymorphonuclear leukocytes (PMNs) from the basolateral surface to the apical surface, paracellular fluid leakage, and access of bacteria to the basolateral surface. Shortly after internalization of *S.* Typhi by macropinocytosis, salmonellae are enclosed in a spacious phagosome formed by membrane ruffles.

Later, the phagosome fuses with lysosomes, acid's, and shrinks to become adherent around the bacterium, forming the *Salmonella*-containing vacuole. A second type II secretion system encoded on SPI-2 is induced within the *Salmonella*-containing vacuole and translocates effector proteins SifA and PipB2, which contribute to *Salmonella*-induced filament formation along microtubules. After passing through the intestinal mucosa, *S.* Typhi organisms enter the mesenteric lymphoid system and then pass into the bloodstream via the lymphatics. This primary bacteremia is usually asymptomatic, and blood culture results are frequently negative at this stage of the disease. The bloodborne bacteria are disseminated throughout the body and are thought to colonize the organs of the reticuloendothelial system (RES), where they may replicate within macrophages. After a period of bacterial replication, *S.* Typhi organisms are shed back into the blood, causing a secondary bacteremia that coincides with the onset of clinical symptoms and marks the end of the incubation period.

The organism enters the body through the walls of the intestinal tract, and following a transient bacteremia multiplies in the reticuloendothelial cells of the liver and spleen. Persistent bacteremia and symptoms then follow. The organism does not invade the mucosa. But it goes into the submucosal tissue where they proliferate in the lymphoid tissue of the ileum. Peyer's patches are swollen and show marked round cell infiltration. Macrophages engulf the bacteria, and they carry them to distant site.

The mesenteric lymph nodes, liver and spleen are hyperemic and generally reveal the area of focal necrosis. Reinfection of the intestine occurs as organisms are excreted in the bile. Bacterial emboli produce the characteristic skin lesions (rose spots). Hyperplasia of the reticuloendothelial system with proliferation of mononuclear cell is predominant finding. Symptoms in children may be mild or severe, but children under age of 5 years rarely have severe typhoid fever.

Importantly, *S.* Typhi and *S.* Paratyphi both express typhoid toxin, whereas "nontyphoidal" *Salmonella* spp. do not express. Not only does this offer the prospect that typhoid toxin may help explain important clinical distinctions between typhoidal and nontyphoidal *Salmonella* infections, it raises hopes for new approaches to disease treatment and diagnostics.

■ CLINICAL FEATURES (FIG. 1)

The primary sources of infection are feces and urine of the carrier cases. The secondary sources are contaminated finger and food.

The incubation period of typhoid fever is usually 7–14 days but depends on the infecting dose and ranges between 3 and 30 days. Many factors influence the severity and overall clinical outcome of the infection. They include the duration of illness before the initiation of appropriate therapy, choice

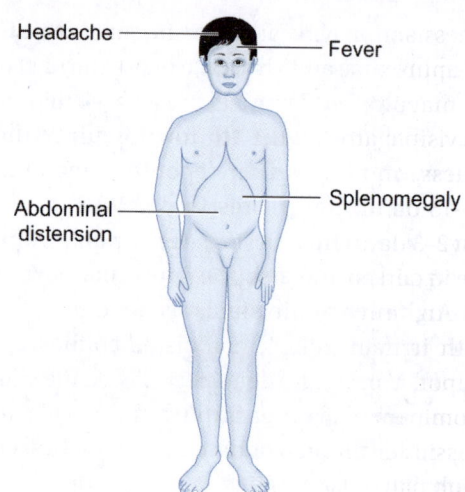

Fig. 1: Clinical features.

of antimicrobial treatment, age, previous exposure, or vaccination history, virulence of the bacterial strain, quantity of inoculum ingested, and several host factors affecting immune status.

In children, the onset of typhoid fever is sudden rather than insidious, with malaise, headache, crampy abdominal pains and distension and sometimes constipation followed within 48 hours by diarrhea, high fever, and toxemia.

The presentation of typhoid fever may also differ according to age. Diarrhea, toxicity, and complications such as disseminated intravascular coagulopathy are also more common in infancy, resulting in higher case fatality rates. However, some of the other features and complications of typhoid fever seen in adults, such as relative bradycardia, neurologic manifestations, and gastrointestinal bleeding, are rare in children.

Typhoid fever usually manifests as high-grade fever with a wide variety of associated features, such as generalized myalgia, abdominal pain, hepatosplenomegaly, abdominal pain, and anorexia. In children, diarrhea may occur in the earlier stages of the illness and may be followed by constipation. In approximately 25% of cases, a macular or maculopapular rash (rose spots) may be visible around the 7th to 10th day of the illness, and lesions may appear in crops of 10–15 on the lower chest and abdomen and last 2–3 days. These lesions may be difficult to see in dark-skinned children.

An encephalopathy may be seen with irritability, confusion, delirium, and stupor. Vomiting and meningismus may be prominent in infants and young children. The classic lengthy three-stage disease seen in adult patients is often shortened in children. The prodrome may last only 2–4 days, the toxic stage only 2–3 days, and the defervescence stage 1–2 weeks.

During the prodromal stage, physical findings may be absent, or there may merely be some abdominal distension and tenderness, meningismus, mild hepatomegaly, and minimal splenomegaly.

The typical typhoidal rash (rose spots) is present in 10–15% of children. It appears during the second week of the disease and may erupt in crops for the succeeding 10–14 days. Rose spots are erythematous maculopapular lesions 2–3 mm in diameter that fade on pressure. They are found principally on the trunk and chest, and they generally disappear within 3–4 days. The lesions usually number fewer than 20.

If no complications occur, the symptoms and physical findings gradually resolve within 2–4 weeks; however, the illness may be associated with malnutrition in a number of affected children. Although enteric fever caused by *S. Paratyphi* organisms has been classically regarded as milder illness, there have been several outbreaks of infection with drug-resistant *S. Paratyphi* A, suggesting that paratyphoid fever may also be severe, with significant morbidity and complications.

> **ESSENTIAL DIAGNOSTIC POINTS**
> - Insidious or acute onset headache vomiting, anorexia, constipation or diarrhea, ileus, and high fever
> - Meningismus, splenomegaly
> - Leukopenia
> - Positive stool, blood, bone marrow, and urine culture

In severe toxic state, there is altered sensorium. The child may be in apathy and stuperous and may be muttering in delirium. This peculiar state is called typhoid state.

Convalescent carriers excrete *Salmonella* for 3 months after the illness. Few of them may become permanent carriers. Permanent carriers excrete *Salmonella* in their stool for more than a year after an episode of enteric fever. This occurs in 1–4% of cases. Carrier state is more common under 5 years of age. Few may continue to excrete the organism in urine.

> **GENERAL FEATURES**
> - Fever
> - Chills and rigors
> - Loose motion
> - Rashes

■ DIAGNOSIS

Complete Blood Count

Change in complete blood count is nonspecific. Leukopenia is found in 20–25% cases, whereas leukocytosis makes the diagnosis less probable. White blood cell (WBC) count remains low mostly. In differential count, absolute eosinopenia and thrombocytopenia may be seen. Presence of severe anemia is unlikely, if present, points toward complications like perforation, hemolysis, or an alternative diagnosis like malaria.

Biochemical

Mild elevation of bilirubin and SGOT, SGPT may occur.

Culture

Definitive diagnosis is by isolation of organism by culture of different specimen.

Blood culture: It is gold standard investigation with overall sensitivity of 50% and specificity of 100%. Sensitivity is maximum in first week and reduces with time.

BACTEC, an automated blood culture, system certainly increases isolation rate. Blood culture should be done in all suspected cases as positive culture riot not only unequivocally establishes the diagnosis but also gives the sensitivity pattern, which is important in this era of multidrug-resistant typhoid fever (MDRTF).

Stool, urine, and other cultures: These are not done routinely. Bacilli can be isolated in third week if untreated. Stool specimen of adequate amount should be processed within 2 hours or should be kept in 4°C. For the detection of carrier, several samples should be examined because of irregular shedding of organism. Sensitivity of urine culture is very poor. Duodenal string and skin snip culture of rose spots is of academic interest only.

Serological Tests

No tests are enough sensitive or specific to replace culture-based diagnosis.

Widal Test

It detects agglutinating antibodies against the somatic O and flagellar H antigen of *S.* Typhi, *S.* Paratyphi A and B. "O" antigen is also shared by other *Salmonella* species and other members of Enterobacteriaceae family. Anti-O titer is mainly IgM type, rises and falls sharply early in the illness, whereas anti-H titer is both IgM and IgG type, rises late in the illness and persists for longer time.

Conventionally, positive Widal implies rising titer in paired samples done at a gap of weeks, but use of antibiotics dampens the immune response and may prevent rise in titer. In endemic area, baseline antibodies are present due to repeated subclinical infections with *Salmonella* and other Enterobacteriaceae. This antibody titer varies with age, socioeconomic condition, urban or rural area, and prior immunization status. For optimal result, Widal test should be done by tube method after 5–7 days of fever and single result of 1:160 against both O and H antigen should be taken as cutoff value for diagnosis.

It is most widely used diagnostic tool, but the sensitivity and specificity is suboptimal. It may be negative in up to 30% culture positive enteric fever.

Enzyme immunoassay test or Typhidot test: This is a simple, rapid test for early diagnosis and has high positive and negative predictive values. It detects IgM and IgG antibodies against outer membrane protein of Typhi and is commercially available as Typhidot. Detection of IgM indicates acute infection in early stage. Whereas IgG antibodies can persist till 2 years following an infection. So, the test cannot distinguish between acute infection and convalescence phase.

This test has been improved in modified Typhidot M test which detects only IgM antibodies.

TUBEX test: Positive test detect only IgM antibodies against O9 antigens, specifically found in group-D *Salmonella*. It is not positive with other groups of *Salmonella*-like paratyphoid.

Antigen detection tests: To detect serum or urinary O, H, or Vi, antigens have suboptimal with variable sensitivity and specificity.

LABORATORY SALIENT FINDINGS

- Positive blood culture in the first week
- Positive stool culture after first week
- Leukopenia
- *Serological test:* Widal test, Typhidot
- Proteinuria
- Thrombocytopenia
- Mild elevation of liver enzymes

COMPLICATIONS

Complications occur in about 30% of unattended patients. These include bronchitis, pneumonia, myocarditis, liver abscess, diarrhea, and encephalitis. There may be perforation of the intestine, peritonitis, and chronic osteomyelitis.

The most serious complications of typhoid fever are gastrointestinal hemorrhage (2–10%) and perforation (1–3%). They occur toward the end of the second week or during the third week of the disease.

Intestinal perforation is one of the principal causes of death. The site of perforation generally is the terminal ileum or cecum. The clinical manifestations are indistinguishable from those of acute appendicitis, with pain, tenderness, and rigidity in the right lower quadrant. The X-ray finding of the free air in the peritoneal cavity is diagnostic.

Bacterial pneumonia, meningitis, septic arthritis, abscesses, and osteomyelitis are uncommon complications, particularly if specific treatment is given promptly. Shock and electrolyte disturbances may lead to death.

About 1–3% of patients become chronic carriers of *S.* Typhi. chronic carriage is defined as excretion of typhoid bacilli for more than a year, but carriage is often lifelong. Adults with underlying biliary or urinary tract disease are much more likely than children to become chronic carriers.

Relapse may occur up to 2 weeks after the termination of therapy. Complication occur in about 30% of untreated patients.

DIFFERENTIAL DIAGNOSIS

The differential diagnosis includes malaria, kala-azar, brucellosis, infectious mononucleosis, and leptospirosis.

TREATMENT

An early diagnosis of typhoid fever and institution of appropriate treatment are essential. The vast majority of children with typhoid fever can be managed at home with oral antibiotics and close medical follow-up for complications or failure of response to therapy. Patients with persistent vomiting, severe diarrhea, and abdominal distention may require hospitalization and parenteral antibiotic therapy.

There are general principles of typhoid fever management. Adequate rest, hydration, and attention are important to correct fluid and electrolyte imbalance. Antipyretic therapy (acetaminophen 10-15 mg/kg every 4-6 hours PO) should be provided as required. A soft, easily digestible diet should be continued unless the patient has abdominal distention or ileus.

Antibiotic therapy is critical to minimize complications. It has been suggested that traditional therapy with either chloramphenicol or amoxicillin is associated with relapse rates of 5–15% and 4–8%, respectively, whereas use of the quinolones and third-generation cephalosporins is associated with higher cure rates.

The antibiotic treatment of typhoid fever in children is also influenced by the prevalence of antimicrobial resistance. Over the past two decades, emergence of multidrug-resistant strains of *S.* Typhi (i.e., isolates fully resistant to amoxicillin, trimethoprim-sulfamethoxazole, and chloramphenicol) has necessitated treatment with fluoroquinolones, which are the antimicrobial drug of choice for treatment of salmonellosis in adults, with cephalosporins as an alternative. The emergence of resistance to quinolones places tremendous pressure on public health systems, because alternative therapeutic options are limited.

In addition to antibiotics, the importance of supportive treatment and maintenance of appropriate fluid and electrolyte balance must be underscored. Although additional treatment with dexamethasone (3 mg/kg for the initial dose, followed by 1 mg/kg every 6 hours for 48 hours) is recommended for severely ill patients with shock, obtundation stupor, or coma; corticosteroids should be administered only under strictly controlled conditions and supervision, because their use may mask signs of abdominal complications.

Antimicrobial susceptibility testing and local experience are used to guide therapy. Equally effective regimens for susceptible strains include the following: Oral cefixime at the dose of 20 mg/kg/day (ceiling dose of 1,200 mg) is the drug of choice. Azithromycin 10–20 mg/kg/day is a good second choice. Trimethoprim–sulfamethoxazole (10 mg/kg trimethoprim and 50 mg/kg sulfamethoxazole per day orally in two or three divided doses), amoxicillin (100 mg/kg/day in four divided doses), and ampicillin (100–200 mg/kg/day intravenously in four divided doses) can be used **(Table 1)**.

Treat for at least 7 days after defervescence or a total of 14 days, whichever is later. Azithromycin is used for a total of 7 days.

Steroids are indicated only in severe illness. If the patient presents with shock, coma, or in altered sensorium, dexamethasone in the dose of 3 mg/kg followed by 1 mg/kg every 6 hours for 2 days may be given. Prolonged use of steroids can increase the relapse rate and cause adverse effects, hence should be used judiciously.

Treatment of carrier is ampicillin 200 mg/kg/day orally. Other drugs used are ceftriaxone and ciprofloxacin.

Third-generation cephalosporins are used for resistant strains. Ceftriaxone and cefotaxime may be used parenterally. Cefixime is efficacious orally. Ciprofloxacin or other fluoroquinolones are efficacious but not approved in children but may be used for multiple resistant strains.

Occasionally the presence of multiple resistant strains requires the use of chloramphenicol (50–100 mg/kg/day orally or intravenously in four doses). Treatment duration is 14–21 days. Patients remain febrile for 3–5 days even with appropriate therapy.

For severe illness and complications, IV ceftriaxone and cefotaxime are used in doses of 100 mg/kg/day and 200 mg/kg/day, respectively. Parenteral treatment is continued until defervescence has occurred, oral intake has improved, and complications resolved. Therapy may be switched to oral cefixime to total duration of 14 days of treatment. Other oral drugs can be used are azithromycin, cotrimoxazole, and amoxicillin.

Relapse

Even after adequate treatment, enteric fever has a relapse rate of 5–20%. Recurrence of fever 2–3 weeks after its initial resolution is

TABLE 1: Drug dosage guideline.

Drug	Dose (mg/kg/day)	Maximum dose (per day)
Ceftriaxone	100	4 g
Cefotaxime	150–200	8 g
Cefixime	20	1,200 mg
Azithromycin	20	1 g
Aztreonam	50–100	8 g

called relapse. It is usually milder. Treatment of relapse is with the same drug used for initial therapy. Relapse can be differentiated from reinfection only by molecular typing.

Carrier State

Carrier state is defined as an asymptomatic person who sheds *Salmonella* in stool or urine beyond 3 months of an episode of enteric fever. It is uncommon in pediatric age-group hence post-illness screening for *S.* Typhi carriage is not recommended. If detected treat with trimethoprim–sulfamethoxazole (10 mg/kg/day for 6–12 weeks) or high-dose amoxicillin (75–100 mg/kg/day for 4–6 weeks) to decrease the risk to close contacts.

Treatment of Relapse

Relapses may be treated with the same drug as used for primary therapy; azithromycin is the preferred drug since it is associated with very low relapse rate.

■ PREVENTION

Three types of vaccine are available:
1. Heat-killed, phenol-preserved whole cell *S.* Typhi vaccine
2. Purified and adjuvenated Vi polysaccharide vaccine
3. Oral live-attenuated Ty21a typhoid vaccine.
   Globally, two vaccines are currently able for potential use in children. An oral, live-attenuated preparation of the Ty21a strain of *S.* Typhi has good efficacy (67–82%) for up to 5 years. Significant adverse effects are rare. The Vi capsular polysaccharide can be used in people 2 years of age and older. It is given as a single intramuscular (IM) dose, with a booster every 2 years and has a protective efficacy of 70–80%. The vaccines are currently recommended, for anyone traveling into endemic areas, but a few countries have introduced large-scale vaccination strategies. Several large-scale demonstration projects using the Vi polysaccharide vaccine have demonstrated protective efficacy against typhoid fever across all age-groups. Recent Vi-conjugate vaccine has a protective efficacy exceeding in younger children and may offer protection of preschool children, who are at risk for the case of enteric or typhoid fever.

■ PROGNOSIS

A prolonged convalescent carrier stage may occur in children. Three negative cultures after all antibiotics have been stopped are required before contact precautions are stopped. With early antibiotic therapy, the prognosis is excellent. With early treatment, the mortality rate is <1%. Relapse occurs 1–3 weeks later in 10–20% of patients despite appropriate antibiotic treatment.

■ BIBLIOGRAPHY

1. Crump JA, Sjölund-Karlsson M, Gordon MA, Parry CM. Epidemiology, Clinical Presentation, Laboratory Diagnosis, Antimicrobial Resistance, and Antimicrobial Management of Invasive Salmonella Infections. Clin Microbial Rev. 2015;28: 901-37.
2. Date KA, Newton AE, Medalla F, Blackstock A, Richardson L, McCullough A, et al. Changing Patterns in Enteric Fever Incidence and Increasing Antibiotic Resistance of Enteric Fever Isolates in the United States, 2008-2012. Clin Infect Dis. 2016;63:322-9.
3. Date KA, Bentsi-Enchill AD, Fox KK, Abeysinghe N, Mintz ED, Khan MI, et al.; Centers for Disease Control and Prevention (CDC). Typhoid Fever surveillance and vaccine use – South-East Asia and Western Pacific regions, 2009–2013. MMWR Morb Mort Wkly Rep. 2014;63(39):855-60.
4. Kumar P, Kumar R. Enteric Fever. Indian J Pediatr. 2017;84:227-30.

CASE 80

Varicella

■ PRESENTING COMPLAINTS

A 6-year-old boy was brought with the complaint of:
- Fever since 2 days
- Headache since 2 days
- Anorexia since 1 day
- Skin lesion since 1 day

History of Presenting Complaints

A 6-year-old boy was brought to the pediatric outpatient department with history of skin lesions all over the body. His mother complained that he was absolutely normal previous day. It started suddenly and spread all over the body within 24 hours. Skin lesions included vesicles containing clear water, while lesions were opened. These lesions first appeared on scalp and on face and later over chest and back. She had noticed that he was having a mild degree of fever before development of skin rashes. The symptoms of headache and anorexia were recollected and considered as significant. There was history of itching.

Past History of the Patient

The boy was the only child of consanguineous marriage. He was born at full term by normal vaginal delivery. There was no significant postnatal event. He was breastfed for 3 months and weaning of the food was started at third month according to advice of family doctor. His developmental milestones were normal. He had been completely immunized. His performance at school was good. There was history of similar type of skin lesions at school.

■ EXAMINATION

The child was moderately built and moderately nourished. He looked and signs of moderate dehydration were present. He was lying on the examination table with anxious look. Anthropometric measurements included his height 118 cm (75th centile) and weight 19 kg (50th centile).

CASE AT A GLANCE	
Basic Findings	
Height	: 118 cm (75th centile)
Weight	: 19 kg (50th centile)
Temperature	: 39°C
Pulse rate	: 120 beats/min
Respiratory rate	: 24 breaths/min
Blood pressure	: 70/50 mm Hg
Positive Findings	
History:	
• Fever	
• Skin lesions	
• Similar attack in school	
Examination:	
• Febrile	
• Pleomorphic skin lesions	
Investigation:	
• Normal	

He was febrile, i.e., 39°C. The heart rate was 120 beats/min and the respiratory rate was 24 breaths/min. Blood pressure recorded was 70/50 mm Hg. There was no icterus, no cyanosis, no lymphadenopathy, and no pallor. There were skin rashes of varying morphology. These included vesicle, pustule, and crusted lesions. Itching marks were present. Other systemic examinations were normal.

INVESTIGATION

- *Hemoglobin:* 12 g/dL
- *TLC:* 8,600 cells/cumm
- *DLC:* $P_{72} L_{18} E_5 M_2 B_3$
- *ESR:* 24 mm in first hour
- *AEC:* 440 cells/cumm
- *X-ray chest:* Normal

DISCUSSION

It is a highly contagious disease presenting with sudden onset of mild fever, with mild constitutional symptoms. The rash is centripetal, pleomorphic (**Fig. 1**) appearing on the first day and has relative short course of illness.

Varicella virus produces primary, latent, and recurrent infections. The primary infection is manifested as chickenpox. It results in establishment of lifelong latent infection of sensory ganglion neurons. Gestational chickenpox can be severe in mother and can cause distinct intrauterine syndrome.

Man is the only reservoir. Children of all ages including the neonates are susceptible with the peak incidence between 5 and 9 years.

Varicella virus is a neurotropic human herpes virus. The patients with varicella are contagious from 24 to 48 hours before appearance of rash till the vesicles are crusted, i.e., usually 3–7 days of the onset of rash. Scab formation occurs and fall by 5–20 days.

Varicella is transmitted by contact with oropharyngeal secretions and the fluid of skin lesions of infected individuals, either by airborne spread or through direct contact. Primary infection (varicella) results from inoculation of the virus onto the mucosa of the upper respiratory tract and tonsillar lymphoid tissue. During the early part of the 10–21 day incubation period, virus replicates in the local lymphoid tissue, and then a brief subclinical viremia spreads the virus to the reticuloendothelial system. Widespread cutaneous lesions occur during a second viremic phase that lasts 3–7 days. Peripheral blood mononuclear cell (PBMC) carry infectious virus, generating new crops of vesicles during this period of viremia.

Varicella is also transported back to the mucosa of the upper respiratory tract and oropharynx during the late incubation period, permitting spread to susceptible contacts 1–2 days before the appearance of rash. Host immune responses limit viral replication and facilitate recovery from infection.

Widespread cutaneous lesions occur during viremic phase. Mononuclear cells carry

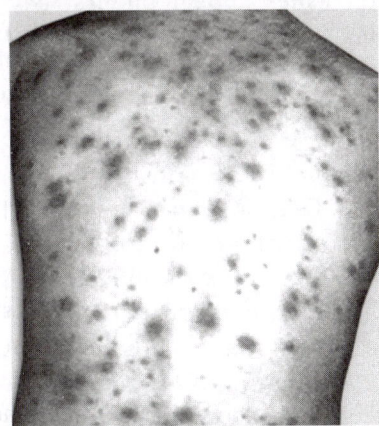

Fig. 1: Pleomorphic rashes.
(For color version, see Plate 5)

the infection. This results in generation of new crops of vesicles for 3–7 days. The lesions begin as macules and quickly develop into papules and vesicles with scab and crest formation. The skin lesions are concentrating on trunk, back, and shoulder.

Later, the viruses are transported back to respiratory mucosal sites during late incubation period. In immunocompromised state, it results in continued viral replication. This may cause injury to lungs, liver, and brain.

Ballooning degeneration of cells in viscera results in giant cells (cowdry type A) eosinophilic intranuclear acidophilic inclusion bodies. Foci of necrosis may be present in esophagus, pancrease, liver, genitourinary tract, adrenal, etc. In post-varicella encephalitis, perivascular demyelination may be seen in the white matter in brain.

It establishes latent infection of sensory ganglia cells in all individuals, who have primary infection. Subsequent reactivation of the latent virus results in herpes zoster. There is vesicular rash in dermatomal distribution. It elicits humeral and cell-mediated immunity.

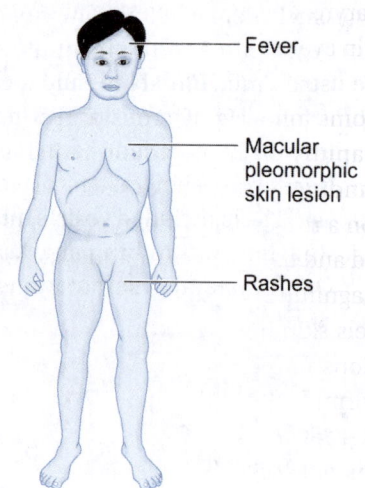

Fig. 2: Clinical features.

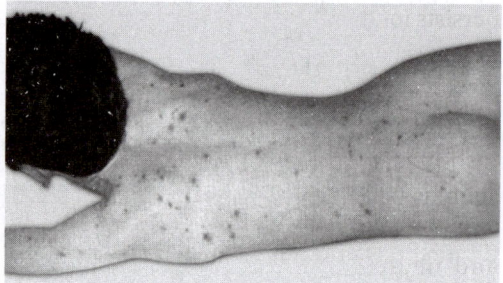

Fig. 3: Rashes. *(For color version, see Plate 5)*

■ CLINICAL FEATURES (FIG. 2)

The illness usually begins 14–16 days after exposure. The incubation period can range from 10 to 21 days. Prodromal symptoms include fever, malaise, anorexia, headache, and mild abdominal pain. These symptoms may occur between 24 and 48 hours before the appearance of rash. They may persist 2–4 days after onset of rash **(Figs. 3 and 4)**.

> **ESSENTIAL DIAGNOSTIC POINTS**
> - Contact with varicella or herpes zoster
> - Widely spread red macules and papules
> - Concentrated on the face and trunk
> - Vesicles, pustules, and then crusting in 5–6 days
> - Variable fever nonspecific symptoms

The rashes appear on first day. The macules quickly develop into papules and vesicles on an erythematous base or areola. New lesions appear for 1–7 days.

It has a characteristic centripetal distribution. The lesions appear first on the scalp, face, or trunk. The lesions being mainly concentrated on trunk, back, and shoulders with fewer lesions on face, scalp, extremities, nose, mouth, conjunctiva, and vagina. The initial exanthem consists of pruritic erythematous macules. These later form clear fluid-filled vesicles. Clouding and umbilication begin in 24–48 hours. The initial lesions are crusted. Ulcerative lesions involve oropharynx and vagina. Vesicular lesions are found in eyelids and conjunctiva.

The usual case consists of mild systemic symptoms followed by crops of red macules that rapidly become small vesicles with surrounding erythema (described as a dew drop on a rose petal), form pustules, become crusted and then scab over and leave no scar. The magnitude of systemic symptoms usually parallels skin involvement. Up to five crops of lesions may be seen. New crops usually stop forming after 5–7 days. Pruritis is often intense. If varicella occurs in the first few months of life, it is often mild as a result of persisting maternal antibody. Once crusting begins, the patient is no longer contagious. Hypopigmentation and hyperpigmentation persists for days to weeks. Scarring is unusual unless secondarily infected.

Severity of the disease is indicated by high temperature 40°C and hemorrhagic rash in child on immunosuppressive drugs such as cortisone. Fetal infection produces embryopathy with limb atrophy, skin scarring, and neurological and eye manifestation. Zoster or shingles activate the latent primary infection.

VARICELLIFORM RASHES IN VACCINATED INDIVIDUALS

Varicelliform rashes that occur after vaccination could be a result of wild-type varicella-zoster virus (VZV), vaccine strain VZV, or other etiologies (e.g., insect bites, coxsackievirus). During days 0–42 after vaccination, the likelihood of rash from wild-type or vaccine strain VZV varies depending on the stage of a country's vaccination program. In the early stages of a vaccine program, rash within 1–2 weeks is still most commonly caused by wild-type VZV, reflecting exposure to varicella before vaccination could provide protection. Rash occurring 14–42 days after vaccination is a result of either wild-type or vaccine strains, reflecting exposure and infection before protection from vaccination or an adverse event of vaccination (vaccine-associated rash), respectively.

Breakthrough varicella is disease that occurs in a person vaccinated >42 days before rash onset and is caused by wild-type virus. One dose of varicella vaccine is 98% effective in preventing moderate and severe varicella and is 82% [95% confidence interval (CI):79–85%; range: 44–100%] effective in preventing all diseases after exposure to wild-type VZV. This means that after close exposure to VZV, as may occur in a household or an outbreak setting in a school or daycare center, about one of every five children, who received one dose of vaccine may experience breakthrough varicella. Exposure to VZV may also result in asymptomatic infection in the previously immunized child. The rash in breakthrough disease is frequently atypical and predominantly maculopapular, and vesicles are seen less commonly. The illness is most commonly mild with <50 lesions, shorter duration of rash, fewer complications, and little or no fever.

Breakthrough cases are overall less contagious than wild-type infections within household settings, but contagiousness varies proportionally with the number of lesions; typical breakthrough cases (<50 lesions) are about one-third as contagious as disease in unvaccinated cases, whereas breakthrough cases with 250 lesions are as contagious as wild-type cases. Consequently, children with breakthrough disease should be considered potentially infectious and excluded from school until lesions have crusted or, if there are no vesicles present, until no new lesions are occurring.

NEONATAL VARICELLA

Mortality is particularly high in neonates born to susceptible mothers, who contract varicella around the time of delivery. Infants whose mothers demonstrate varicella in the period from 5 days prior to delivery to 2 days afterward are at high risk for severe varicella. These infants acquire the infection transplacentally as a result of maternal viremia, which may occur up to 48 hours prior to onset of maternal rash. The infant's rash usually occurs toward the end of the first week to the early part of the second week of life (although it may be as soon as 2 days). Because the mother has not yet developed a significant antibody response, the infant receives a large dose of virus without the moderating effect of maternal anti-VZV antibody.

If the mother demonstrates varicella >5 days prior to delivery, she still may pass virus to the soon-to-be-born child, but infection is attenuated because of transmission of maternal VZV-specific antibody across the placenta. This moderating effect of maternal antibody is present it delivery occurs after about 30 weeks of gestation, when maternal IgG is able to cross the placenta in significant amounts.

CONGENITAL VARICELLA SYNDROME

In utero transmission of VZV can occur; however, because most adults in temperate climates are immune, pregnancy complicated by varicella is unusual in these settings. When pregnant women do contract varicella in early pregnancy, experts estimate that as many as 25% of the fetuses may become infected. Fortunately, clinically apparent disease in the infant is uncommon: The congenital varicella syndrome occurs in approximately

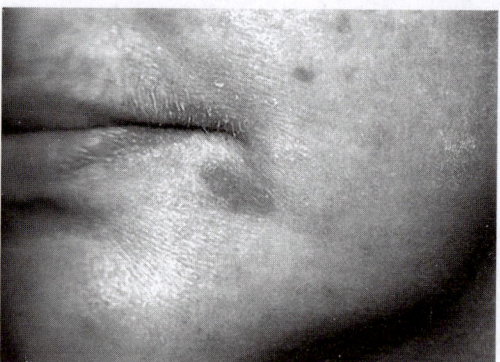

Fig. 4: Herpes simplex. *(For color version, see Plate 5)*

0.4% of infants born to women who have varicella during pregnancy before 13 weeks of gestation and in approximately 2% of infants born to women with varicella between 13 and 20 weeks of gestation. Rarely, cases of congenital varicella syndrome have been reported in infants of women infected after 20 weeks of pregnancy, the latest occurring at 28 weeks of gestation.

GENERAL FEATURES
• Mild fever
• Dehydration
• Decreased appetite
• Centripetal distribution
• Papules, vesicles and erythematous rashes

DIAGNOSIS

The diagnosis of VZV fetopathy is based mainly on the history of gestational varicella combined with the presence of characteristic abnormalities in the newborn infant. Virus cannot be cultured from the affected newborn, but viral DNA may be detected in tissue samples by PCR. Since many infants with congenital varicella syndrome develop zoster before a year of age, it may be possible to isolate VZV from that rash. Alternatively, use of PCR to identify VZV DNA in vesicular fluid or scabs from zoster lesions in such an infant may be diagnostic. Chorionic villus sampling and fetal blood collection for the detection of viral DNA, virus, or antibody have been used in an attempt to diagnose fetal infection and embryopathy.

Diagnosis is clinical and not usually difficult in a typical case. Often a history of exposure to the disease is helpful in reaching the diagnosis. Chickenpox should be differentiated from other exanthemata such as herpes simplex, enteroviral infections, insect bites, and drug reactions.

Leukopenia is typical during the first 72 hours. This is followed by relative or absolute lymphocytosis. LFTs are usually mildly elevated.

Cerebrospinal fluid examination shows mild lymphocytic pleocytosis and moderate increase in protein.

Varicella pneumonia classically produces numerous bilateral nodular densities and hyperinflation. This is very rare in immunocompetent children. Abnormal chest X-rays are seen more frequently in adults.

LABORATORY SALIENT FINDINGS
• Leukopenia • Mildly elevated LFT • *CSF analysis:* Mild lymphocytic pleocytosis, moderate increase in protein • Isolation of virus from vesicles • ELISA and compliment fixation
(CSF: cerebrospinal fluid; ELISA: enzyme-linked immunosorbent assay; LFT: liver function test)

■ DIFFERENTIAL DIAGNOSIS

Differential diagnosis includes vesicular rashes by herpes simplex, *Enterovirus*, *Staphylococcus*, and drug reactions.

■ COMPLICATIONS

The rate of severe or complicated varicella is low among immunocompetent children, but such cases are numerically common in unvaccinated populations. The most frequent complication in the young is secondary bacterial infection of the skin. The other complications of varicella reflect overwhelming viral infection and are more likely to occur in the context of defective cell-mediated immunity.

Secondary Bacterial Infections

Scratching of the intensely itchy skin lesions of varicella often leads to the introduction of bacteria, typically *S. aureus* or *S. pyogenes*. Local skin infection in a well child can be treated with an oral antibiotic, with close clinical follow-up. Progression of erythema around lesions, formation of bullae, or development of regional lymphadenitis should prompt consideration of IV antibiotic therapy. Recent varicella confers a significantly increased risk of invasive bacterial disease, particularly group A streptococcal (GAS) infections; these include necrotizing fasciitis, bacteremia, pneumonia, empyema, and toxic shock syndrome. It has been estimated that varicella directly precedes approximately 15% of invasive GAS infections.

Varicella Pneumonia

Although rates are lower among immunocompetent children, pneumonia commonly accompanies varicella in immunocompromised hosts. Respiratory symptoms (e.g., dyspnea, tachypnea, chest tightness, cough) develop in the context of acute varicella, usually 1 to 6 days after the onset of the rash, and may progress rapidly to respiratory failure. The severity of clinical signs is a poor guide to prognosis, therefore, the patient with new respiratory symptoms in the context of varicella should be urgently evaluated.

IV antiviral therapy and improved intensive care have markedly improved survival of these patients over recent years, but deaths continue to occur.

Varicella may be life-threatening in immunosuppressed patients (especially those with leukemia or lymphoma or those receiving high doses of steroids). Their disease is complicated by severe pneumonitis, hepatitis, and encephalitis.

Hemorrhagic varicella lesions may be seen without other complications. This is most often caused by autoimmune thrombocytopenia, but hemorrhagic lesions can occasionally represent idiopathic disseminated intravascular coagulation (purpura fulminans).

Neonates born to mothers who develop varicella from 5 days before to 2 days after delivery are at high risk for severe or fatal (5%) disease and must be given varicella-zoster immune globulin (VZIG) and followed closely.

Varicella occurring during the first 20 weeks of pregnancy may cause (2% incidence) congenital infection associated with cicatricial skin lesions, associated limb abnormalities, and cortical atrophy.

The complications of VZV infection occur with varicella or wither activation of infection, more commonly in immunocompromised patients. Mild thrombocytopenia occurs in 1-2% of children with varicella and may be associated with transient petechiae. Purpura, hemorrhagic vesicles, hematuria, and gastrointestinal bleeding are rare complications that may have serious consequences.

Neurologic Complications

Varicella is classically associated with three neurologic pictures: (1) Cerebellar ataxia, (2) encephalitis, and (3) Reye's syndrome. Rarely, it has been associated with Guillain-Barre syndrome, stroke, transverse myelitis, and aseptic meningitis. Cerebellar ataxia complicates approximately 1 in 4,000 cases of varicella and usually follows the onset of rash, making the diagnosis clear. Vomiting and headache often accompany the ataxia, whereas only one-fourth of patients experience neck stiffness or nystagmus. It is not known whether this syndrome results from VZV replication within the CNS or instead reflects a parainfectious autoimmune process, but the typical timing of onset in the second week following the onset of illness suggests the latter.

Encephalitis occurs in <0.1% of cases, usually in the first week of illness. It is usually limited to cerebellitis with ataxia, which resolves completely. Diffuse encephalitis can be severe.

Protracted vomiting or a change in sensorium suggests Reye syndrome or encephalitis. Because Reye syndrome usually occurs in patients who are also using salicylates, these should be avoided in patients with varicella.

■ TREATMENT

The only antiviral drug available in liquid formulation that is available for treatment of varicella for pediatric use is acyclovir. Given the safety profile of acyclovir and its demonstrated efficacy in the treatment of varicella, treatment of all children, adolescents, and adults with varicella is acceptable. Oral therapy with acyclovir (20 mg/kg/dose maximum: 800 mg/dose) given as 4 doses/day for 5 days can be used to treat uncomplicated varicella in individuals at increased risk for moderate-to-severe varicella: Nonpregnant individuals older than

12 years of age and individuals older than 12 months of age with chronic cutaneous or pulmonary disorders; individuals receiving short-term, intermittent, or aerosolized corticosteroid therapy; individuals receiving long-term salicylate therapy; and possibly secondary cases among household contacts.

Immunocompromised individual needs IV antiviral (even if 72 hours of exanthema have crossed) for 7–10 days or till no new lesions for 48 hours.

Acyclovir-resistant varicella (primarily in children infected with HIV) may be treated with foscarnet or cidofovir.

Children <2 years: Acyclovir in dose of 10 mg/kg (maximum 800 mg) four times daily for 7 days beginning 7–10 days after exposure.

Children 2 to <18 years: Oral acyclovir in dose of 10 mg/kg (maximum 800 mg) four times daily or valacyclovir in dose of 20 mg/kg (maximum 1,000 mg) three times daily for 7 days.

To be most effective, treatment should be initiated as early as possible, preferably within 24 hours of the onset of the exanthem. Valacyclovir (20 mg/kg/dose; maximum: 1,000 mg/dose administered three times daily for 5 days) is licensed for treatment of varicella in children 2 to <18 years of age, and both valacyclovir and famciclovir are approved for treatment of herpes zoster in adults.

Intravenous therapy is indicated for severe disease and for varicella in immunocompromised patients (even if begun >72 hours after the onset of rash). Any patient who has signs of disseminated VZV, including pneumonia, severe hepatitis, thrombocytopenia, or encephalitis should receive immediate treatment. IV acyclovir therapy (500 mg/m^2 every 8 hours) initiated within 72 hours of development of initial symptoms decreases the likelihood of progressive varicella and visceral dissemination in high-risk patients.

Treatment is continued for 7–10 days or until no new lesions have appeared for 48 hours. Delaying antiviral treatment in high-risk individuals until it is obvious that prolonged new lesion formation is occurring is not advisable, because visceral dissemination occurs during the same period.

Acyclovir-resistant VZV has been identified primarily in children infected with HIV. These children may be treated with IV foscarnet (120 mg/kg/day divided every 8 hours for up to 3 weeks). The dose should be modified in the presence of renal insufficiency. Resistance to foscarnet has been reported with prolonged use. Cidofovir is also useful in this situation. Because of the increased toxicity profile of foscarnet and cidofovir, these two drugs should be initiated in collaboration with an infectious disease specialist.

■ PREVENTION

The recommendations for use of human VZIG differ based on when the infant is exposed to varicella. Newborns whose mothers develop varicella during the period of 5 days before to 2 days after delivery should receive VZIG as soon as possible after birth. Although neonatal varicella may occur in about half of these infants despite administration of VZIG, it is milder than in the absence of VZIG administration.

Varicella-zoster immune gammaglobulin 125 U/kg (maximum 625 U) may prevent in contact if administered IM within 96 hours of exposure. The group who require protection are children under the age of 1 month, pregnant women, patients with leukemia and those on steroid therapy. Use of acyclovir as chemoprophylaxis is not recommended.

VZIG is available for postexposure prevention of varicella in high-risk susceptible persons. Postexposure prophylaxis with acyclovir is effective when it is started at 8 or 9 days after exposure and is continued for 7 days.

The live attenuated vaccine should be given as part of routine childhood immunization and "catch-up" immunization is recommended for all other susceptible children and adults.

Varicella vaccine is also useful for postexposure prophylaxis when given within 3–5 days of the exposure.

PROGNOSIS

Except for secondary bacterial infection, serious complications are rare and recovery complete in immunocompetent hosts. A live vaccine prepared with Oka strain is now available. The vaccine is given within 3 days of exposure, may prevent disease in >80% of individuals.

BIBLIOGRAPHY

1. Bialek SR, Perella D, Zhang J, Mascola L, Viner K, Jackson C, et al. Impact of a routine two-dose varicella vaccination program on varicella epidemiology. Pediatrics. 2013;132:1134-40.
2. Chen JJ, Gershon AA, Li Z, Cowles RA, Gershon MD. Varicella zoster virus (VZV) infects and establishes latency in enteric neurons. J Neuroviral. 2011;17:578-89.
3. English R. Varicella. Pediatr Rev. 2003;24:372-9.
4. Marin M, Marti M, Kambhampati A, Jeram SM, Seward JF. Global Varicella Vaccine Effectiveness: A Meta-analysis. Pediatrics. 2016;137(3):e20153741.
5. Shapiro ED, Vazquez M, Esposito D, Holabird N, Steinberg SP, Dziura J, et al. Effectiveness of 2 doses of varicella vaccine in children. J Infect Dis. 2011;203(3):312-5.

CASE 81

Whooping Cough

■ PRESENTING COMPLAINTS

An 8-month old girl was brought with the complaint of:
- Cough since 1½ months
- Congestion of face since 15 days
- Vomiting since 15 days
- Noisy respiration since 15 days

History of Presenting Complaints

An 8-month-old girl was brought with history of episodes of paroxysm of the cough since 1 month. Her mother complained that the child was having repeated episodes of cough. Each paroxysm of cough was followed by vomiting. She further told that her child used to vomit ingested food material. It was associated with intense congestion of face and sometimes bluish coloration of face. Usually the cough was associated with inspiratory sound.

Past History of the Patient

The child was the second child of nonconsanguineous marriage. She was born at full term by normal vaginal delivery. She did not have any postnatal significant event, was discharged on the fourth day, and was exclusively on breastfeeds for first 4 months. Later weaning started gradually with cereals and fruits. There was no feeding problems. She was not immunized with pertussis component because of apprehension. Her elder sister was 3 years old and had intermittent cough for 3 weeks.

■ EXAMINATION

The girl was moderately built and nourished. She was looking ill and mildly dehydrated. Anthropometric measurements included the length 70 cm (75th centile) and the weight 7 kg (50th centile). The head circumference was 42 cm.

CASE AT A GLANCE

Basic Findings
Length	: 70 cm (75th centile)
Weight	: 7 kg (50th centile)
Temperature	: 37°C
Pulse rate	: 120 beats/min
Respiratory rate	: 32 breaths/min
Blood pressure	: 60/40 mm Hg

Positive Findings

History:
- Paroxysm of cough
- Whoop
- Vomiting
- Congestion

Examination:
- Sick look
- Mild dehydration

Investigation:
- Erythrocyte sedimentation rate (ESR): Decreased
- Lymphocytosis

She was afebrile, the pulse rate was 120 beats/min, and the respiratory rate was 32 breaths/min. Blood pressure recorded was 60/40 mm Hg. There was no pallor, no lymphadenopathy, and no cyanosis.

Respiratory system revealed the presence of occasional crepitation on the right lung base. Other systemic examinations were normal.

INVESTIGATION

- *Hemoglobin:* 10.8 g/dL
- *TLC:* 18,200 cells/cumm
- *DLC:* $P_{40} L_{56} E_3 M_1$
- *ESR:* 8 mm in the first hour
- *AEC:* 334 cells/cumm
- *Mantoux test:* Negative
- *X-ray chest:* Normal

DISCUSSION

Pertussis is an acute, highly communicable infection of the respiratory tract caused by *Bordetella pertussis*. Children usually acquire the disease from symptomatic family contacts. The risk of the disease is highest under the age of 5 years. Regular immunization reduces the incidence and mortality of the pertussis.

A suspected case of pertussis is defined as follows: A patient with a cough lasting for 2 weeks or more, with at least one of the following:
- Paroxysms of coughing
- Inspiratory whooping
- Post-tussive vomiting
- Apneic spells and cyanosis with cough of any duration, in infants, without any obvious systemic cause
- High index of suspicion for cough of any duration in unvaccinated children

Adults who have mild respiratory illness, not recognized as pertussis, frequently are the source of infection. Asymptomatic carriage of *B. pertussis* is not recognized. Infectivity is greatest during the catarrhal and early paroxysmal cough stage (for about 4 weeks after onset).

Neither natural disease nor vaccination provides complete or lifelong immunity against pertussis reinfection or disease. Subclinical reinfection undoubtedly contributed significantly to immunity against disease ascribed previously to both vaccine and prior infection. The resurgence of pertussis has been attributed to a variety of factors, including partial control of pertussis leading to less continuous exposure, increased awareness, improved diagnostics, suboptimal vaccines, waning vaccine-induced immunity, and pathogen adaptation.

Protracted coughing (which in some cases is paroxysmal) can be caused by *Mycoplasma*, parainfluenza viruses, influenza viruses, enteroviruses, respiratory syncytial virus (RSV), or adenoviruses.

Pertussis-like illness is caused by adenovirus, *Bordetella parapertussis*, *Bordetella bronchie septicum*, and *Chlamydia*.

Active immunity follows natural pertussis. Reinfections occur years to decades later but are usually milder. Immunity following vaccinations wanes in 5–10 years.

Although the DTaP series is protective, short-term, vaccine effectiveness wanes rapidly, with estimates of only 10% protection 8.5 years after the fifth dose. Tdap protection also is short-lived, with efficacy falling from >70% initially to 34% within 2–4 years. Divergence of circulating strains from vaccine strains began with the introduction of DTP, but with the exclusive use of acellular pertussis vaccines, *pertactin-deficient strains* emerged and have become dominant in countries where these vaccines are used.

PATHOGENESIS

Bordetella organisms are small, fastidious, Gram-negative coccobacilli that colonize only ciliated epithelium. The exact mechanism of disease symptomatology remains unknown. *Bordetella* species share a high degree of DNA homology among virulence genes. *B. pertussis* produces numerous virulence factors, including toxins and attachment agents, many of which are antigenic and included in the acellular vaccine. The bacteria attach to ciliated epithelial cells of the respiratory tract, induce ciliary paralysis and local inflammation, and thicken and decrease clearance of secretions. Only *B. pertussis* expresses pertussis toxin, the major virulence protein. Pertussis toxin has numerous proven biologic activities (e.g., histamine sensitivity, insulin secretion, leukocyte dysfunction).

Pertussis is extremely contagious, with attack rates as high as 100% in susceptible individuals exposed to aerosol droplets at close range. High airborne transmission rates were shown in a baboon model of pertussis despite vaccination with the acellular vaccine.

These bacteria will multiply only in association with ciliated epithelium. They produce various active substances or virulent factors. These inflammatory debris accumulate in lumen of the bronchi. Bronchiolar obstruction and atelectasis result due to accumulation of mucus secretion. Pathological changes are also seen in brain and liver. Fatty infiltration of liver may be noted and cortical atrophy has been documented.

Bordetella pertussis is not invasive. Pertussis toxin, necessary but not sufficient to cause clinical pertussis, is secreted by the bacteria-and affects G-protein function, which prevents migration of lymphocytes to the area of infection, and inhibits the function of neutrophils, macrophages, monocytes, and lymphocytes. Adenylate cyclase toxin invades phagocytes and induces high levels of cyclic adenosine monophosphate (AMP), which impairs immune cell function and induces apoptosis.

Other cell-surface proteins, including filamentous hemagglutinin, pertactin, and fimbrial agglutinogens, are involved in bacterial attachment to ciliated respiratory epithelium. The function of additional factors, including tracheal cytotoxin, surface lipooligosaccharide, and cytoplasmic heat-labile toxin, is less well characterized. Communicability is highest early in the disease (catarrhal phase), but may persist for weeks in some individuals. Unrecognized disease serves as a reservoir tor spread of infection.

Tracheal cytotoxin, adenylate cyclase, and pertussis toxin appear to inhibit clearance of organisms. Tracheal cytotoxin, dermo-necrotic factor, and adenylate cyclase are postulated to be predominantly responsible for the local epithelial damage that produces respiratory symptoms and facilitates absorption of pertussis toxin. Both antibody and cellular immune responses follow infection and immunization.

■ CLINICAL FEATURES (FIG. 1)

It is more infectious during catarrhal stage. The period may be considered to extend from the week after exposure to about 3 weeks after the onset of paroxysmal stage. It is spread mainly by droplet infection and direct cataract.

Pertussis is extremely contagious, with attack rates as high as 100% in susceptible individuals exposed to aerosol droplets at close range. High airborne transmission rates were shown in pertussis despite vaccinated with the acellular vaccine. *B. pertussis* does not survive for prolonged periods in the environment.

Chronic carriage by human is not documented. After intense exposure as in

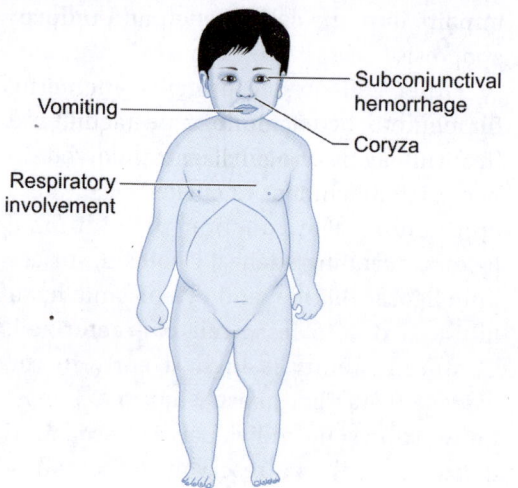

Fig. 1: Clinical features.

households, the rate of subclinical infection is as high as 80% in fully immunized or previously infected individuals. When carefully sought a symptomatic source case can be found for most patients.

Infants <3 months old do not display the classic stages. The catarrhal phase lasts only a few days or is unnoticed, and then, after the most insignificant startle from a draft, light, sound, sucking, or stretching, a well-appearing young infant begins to choke, gasp, gag, and flail the extremities, with face reddened. Cough may not be prominent, especially in the early phase, and whoop is infrequent. Apnea and cyanosis can follow a coughing paroxysm, or apnea can occur as the only symptom (without cough). Both are more common with pertussis than with neonatal viral infections. The paroxysmal and convalescent stages in young infants are lengthy.

The incubation period is 7–14 days but not >3 weeks. Clinically whooping cough has got three stages:

1. *Catarrhal stage:* This stage lasts for 10–14 days. The onset of pertussis is insidious, with catarrhal upper respiratory tract symptoms (rhinitis, sneezing, and an irritating cough). Slight fever may be present; temperature greater than 38.3°C suggests bacterial superinfection or another cause of respiratory tract infection. The child has cough and coryza with nasopharyngeal (NP) secretion. The paroxysmal nature of cough can be suspected toward the latter part of this phase. The rapid succession of cough may be in an explosive manner. The child may appear choked, unable to breath.

2. *Paroxysmal stage:* This stage lasts for 2–4 weeks. After about 2 weeks, the cough becomes paroxysmal, characterized by 10–30 forceful coughs terminate with a long drawn-out inspiratory crowing sound or whoop. The paroxysm of cough terminates into vomiting. Whoop is produced by the air rushing during inspiration through the half open glottis. The whoop may not be present in a neonate, where it is manifested with apnea and cyanotic spells. Paroxysms of cough are precipitated by food, cold air, and liquid. Paroxysmal stage is considerably prolonged in young infants <3 months. Coughing is accompanied by cyanosis, sweating, prostration, and exhaustion. This stage lasts for 2–4 weeks, with gradual improvement. Clinical pertussis is milder in immunized children. The bout of cough petechial and conjunctival hemorrhages are seen.

3. *Convalescent stage:* Vomiting becomes less severe. Appetite and general condition improve. This stage lasts for 2–4 weeks. The interval between the paroxysm of cough is prolonged. Severity of episodes decreases gradually. It is prolonged because of atelectasia, pneumonia, and bronchiectasis. During the convalescent

period, coughing in the young infant may actually become louder, although generally less distressing. Overall, the paroxysmal coughing gradually lessens in severity and frequency during convalescence. Paroxysms may disappear, only to reappear in a milder form during a subsequent respiratory illness over the ensuing year. Persons with pertussis are considered infectious from onset of the catarrhal stage through the third week of the paroxysmal stage or until 5 days after starting treatment.

Uncomplicated pertussis is usually an afebrile disease, so fever should prompt evaluation for a secondary bacterial infection. Otitis media and pneumonia are the most common secondary infections. Other pulmonary complications include atelectasis, emphysema, pneumothorax, and pulmonary hypertension.

Coughing and vomiting may result in esophageal tears with hematemesis and melena. Neurologic complications include hypoxic encephalopathy, seizures, and intracranial bleeds. Nutritional compromise and resultant failure to thrive are common in young infants recovering from pertussis.

Classic pertussis in the nonimmune host is difficult to confuse with other illnesses. In the immunized individual symptoms are less likely to be characteristic, A coughing illness for >2 weeks and/or post-tussive emesis should arouse suspicion. In infants presenting with apnea, RSV or other viral infection, and serious bacterial illness need to be excluded.

Bordetella pertussis is the cause of epidemic pertussis as well as of most sporadic pertussis. *B. parapertussis* may cause a similar syndrome that is less severe and of shorter duration. Protracted coughing illness mimicking pertussis may also be seen with adenovirus, *Mycoplasma*, and *Chlamydia*. Ancillary features of the illness such as sore throat, headache, or swollen lymph nodes, as well as knowledge of epidemiologically significant local pathogens, will aid diagnostically.

> **ESSENTIAL DIAGNOSTIC POINTS**
> - Cough, coryza, and fever
> - Persistent staccato, paroxysmal cough ending with high pitched inspiratory "whoop"
> - Leukocytosis with absolute lymphocytosis
> - Diagnosis is confirmed by fluorescent stain or culture of nasopharyngeal secretion

> **GENERAL FEATURES**
> - Cough
> - Coryza
> - Choking
> - Whoop
> - Decreased appetite
> - Malnutrition
> - Convulsions
> - Hernia
> - Rectal prolapse

Apnea and respiratory distress were the most frequent complications, followed by pneumonias. The frequency of complications declines with increasing age; however, post-tussive emesis, protracted cough (>3 months), sleep disturbances, and weight loss are common in adults with pertussis; subcutaneous emphysema, pulled muscles and even broken ribs may occur in adults following paroxysmal coughing. The characteristic "whoop" is often absent in older individuals.

■ DIAGNOSIS

Classical pertussis should be readily diagnosed based on clinical features. The presence of absolute peripheral lymphocytosis (>10,000 lymphocytes/μL) is supportive evidence for systemically active pertussis toxin. Absolute lymphocyte counts of >20,000 cells/μL are not uncommon, and total white blood cell counts >100,000 cells/µL have been reported.

Leukocytosis (15,000–100,000 cells/µL) caused by absolute lymphocytosis is characteristic in the catarrhal stage. Lymphocytes are normal small cells, rather than the large, atypical lymphocytes seen with viral infections. Adults, partially immune children, and occasionally infants may have less impressive lymphocytosis.

Methods for confirmation of infection by *B. pertussis* [culture, polymerase chain reaction (PCR), serology] have limitations in sensitivity, specificity, or practicality, and tests relative values depend on the setting, phase of disease, and purpose of use (e.g., as clinical diagnostic versus epidemiologic tools). PCR testing on NP wash specimens is the laboratory test of choice for *B. pertussis* identification.

A confirmed case is defined as one with any cough illness in which *B. pertussis* is isolated and cultured, or a case with symptoms confirmed by PCR or epidemiologic linkage to a laboratory-confirmed case.

Culture is considered the gold standard as it is the only 100% specific method for identification, specimen for culture is obtained by deep NP aspiration, and inoculation in Bordet-Gengou agar, Regan-Lowe or modified Stainer-Scholte media causes growth in 3–4 days. Recovery of organisms is highest during catarrhal and early paroxysmal stages. Previously immunized or antibiotic treated patients may produce a negative culture; however, this does not exclude the diagnosis of pertussis.

Blood and laryngeal swab cultures are incubated at 35–37°C in a humid environment and examined daily for 7 days for slow-growing, tiny, glistening colonies. Direct fluorescent antibody testing of potential isolates using specific antibody for *B. pertussis* and *B. parapertussis* maximizes recovery rates.

Identification of *B. pertussis* by culture or PCR from NP swabs or nasal wash specimens proves the diagnosis. PCR detection is replacing culture in some hospitals because of improved sensitivity and decreased time to diagnosis and cost. The organism may be found in the respiratory tract in diminishing numbers beginning in the catarrhal stage and ending about 2 weeks after the beginning of the paroxysmal stage.

Polymerase chain reaction should be tested from NP specimens taken at 0–3 weeks following cough onset, but may provide accurate results for up to 4 weeks. The optimal timing for specimen collection is 2–8 weeks following cough onset, when the antibody titers are at their highest; however, serology may be performed on specimens collected up to 12 weeks following cough onset.

After 4–5 weeks of symptoms, cultures and fluorescent antibody tests are almost always negative. Charcoal agar containing an antimicrobial should be inoculated as soon as possible. *B. pertussis* does not tolerate drying or prolonged transport.

Currently, the most generally accepted serologic criterion for diagnosis of pertussis is the use of an enzyme-linked immunosorbent assay to demonstrate a significant increase in IgG serum antibody concentrations against pertussis toxin between acute and convalescent specimens or a single point test collected 2–8 weeks following cough onset. Results may not correlate with clinical disease and can be difficult to interpret in a highly immunized population.

Enzyme-linked immunosorbent assays for detection of antibody to pertussis toxin or filamentous hemagglutinin may be useful for diagnosis but are currently not widely available and interpretation of antibody titers may be difficult in previously immunized patients.

The blood picture may resemble lymphocytic leukemia or leukemoid reactions. Fluorescent antibody staining of the laryngeal swab is a quick diagnostic test. ESR is reduced.

The chest X-ray reveals thickened bronchi and sometimes shows a shaggy heart border, indicating bronchopneumonia and patchy atelectasis.

Following natural infection, antibodies develop to several *B. pertussis* antigens. These responses do not confer lifetime immunity but rather wane in 7–20 years. Immunization with whole-cell vaccine likewise results in response to multiple antigens, but responses last only 6–12 years. The acellular pertussis vaccines are well tolerated, offer very targeted responses, but do not have durability of response. Recent outbreaks and increases in disease incidence suggest the protection afforded by acellular vaccines may be as short as 4–5 years.

LABORATORY SALIENT FINDINGS

- Lymphocytosis
- Culture
- PCR reaction from nasopharyngeal swabs
- ELISA test
- *Chest X-ray:* Bronchopneumonia and patchy atelectasis

(ELISA: enzyme-linked immunosorbent assay; PCR: polymerase chain reaction)

■ DIFFERENTIAL DIAGNOSIS

The differential diagnosis of pertussis includes bacterial tuberculosis, chlamydial, and viral pneumonia. Cystic fibrosis and foreign body aspiration may be considerations. Adenovirus and RSV may cause paroxysmal coughing with an associated elevation of lymphocytes in the peripheral blood, mimicking pertussis.

- Foreign body
- Tuberculous lymph node
- Bronchiolitis
- Tracheitis
- Bronchiectasis

■ COMPLICATIONS

Infants >6 months old have excessive mortality and morbidity; infants <2 months old have the highest reported rates of pertussis-associated hospitalization (82%), pneumonia (25%), seizures (4%), encephalopathy (19%), and death (19%). Infants <4 months old account for 90% of cases of fatal pertussis.

The principal complications of pertussis are *apnea*, *secondary infections* (e.g., otitis media, pneumonia), and *physical sequelae* of forceful coughing. Fever, tachypnea or respiratory distress between paroxysms and absolute neutrophilia are clues to pneumonia.

Respiratory failure from apnea may mandate intubation and ventilation through the days when disease peaks; prognosis is good. Progressive *pulmonary hypertension* in very young infants and secondary *bacterial pneumonia* are severe complications of pertussis and are the usual causes of death.

Acute neurologic events during pertussis almost always are the result of *hypoxemia* or *hemorrhage* associated with coughing or apnea in young infants.

The infants below 6 months have high maturity:
- *Respiratory:*
  - Patchy atelectasis
  - Pneumonia
  - Interstitial pneumonia
  - Bronchiectasis
  - Subcutaneous emphysema
  - Pneumothorax
  - Flaring of tuberculosis
- *Neurological:*
  - Resistant seizers
  - Ataxia

- Intracranial hemorrhage
- Aphasia
- Hemiplegia
- Paraplegia
- *Gastrointestinal:*
  - Hernia
  - Rectal prolapse
  - Malnutrition

Bronchopneumonia due to superinfection is the most common serious complication. It is characterized by abrupt clinical deterioration during the paroxysmal stage, accompanied by high fever and sometimes a striking leukemoid reaction with a shift to predominantly polymorphonuclear neutrophils.

Atelectasis is a second common pulmonary complication. Atelectasis may be patchy or extensive and may shift rapidly to involve different areas of lung. Intercurrent viral respiratory infection is also a common complication and may provoke worsening or recurrence of paroxysmal coughing.

Otitis media is common residual chronic bronchiectasis is infrequent despite the severity of the illness.

Apnea and sudden death may occur during a particularly severe paroxysm. Seizures complicate 1.5% of cases and encephalopathy occurs in 0.1%. the encephalopathy frequently is fatal.

Anoxic brain damage, cerebral hemorrhage, or pertussis neurotoxins are hypothesized, but anoxia is most likely the cause. Epistaxis and subconjunctival hemorrhages are common.

TREATMENT

Specific Measures

Limited goals of hospitalization are to (1) assess progression disease and likelihood of life-threatening events at peak of disease; (2) maximize nutrition; (3) prevent or treat complications; and (4) educate parents in the natural history of the disease and in care that will be given at home. Heart rate, respiratory rate, and pulse oximetry are monitored continuously with alarm settings so that paroxysms can be witnessed and recorded by healthcare personnel.

Treatment for clinical pertussis is primarily supportive. Hospitalization is indicated for all infants with severe paroxysms associated with cyanosis or apnea. Infants with potentially fatal pertussis may appear to be amazingly well between paroxysms. Caution should be exercised when suctioning these young, exhausted infants because it may precipitate a paroxysm.

Admission to an intensive care setting is indicated if emergent response to paroxysms cannot be managed on the ward. Supplemental oxygen, IV fluids, and nutritional support are frequently required in severe and protracted disease. Some have suggested that early extracorporeal membrane oxygenation with leukodepletion in the most severe cases may decrease mortality. Young infants should remain hospitalized until nutrition is adequate, no supportive intervention is required during paroxysms, disease is unchanged or improved for at least 48 hours, and the infant's care can be safely managed at home.

Antibiotic therapy has no discernible effect on the course of the illness once the paroxysms are well established; however, treatment may ameliorate disease expression for those who are treated in the catarrhal phase. Clinicians should strongly consider treating prior to test results if clinical history is strongly suggestive or patient is at risk for severe or complicated disease (e.g., infants).

All suspected and confirmed cases of pertussis should be treated in order to minimize secondary spread. The CDC recommends treating patients >1 year of age within 3 weeks of cough onset and those 1 year of age and pregnant women within 6 weeks of cough onset. Treatment and postexposure prophylaxis dosing is based on age and weight.

Infants younger than 3 months of age with suspected pertussis usually are admitted to hospital, as are many between 3 and 6 months of age unless witnessed paroxysms are not severe, as well as are patients of any age if significant complications occur.

Macrolides are the drugs of choice for the treatment of pertussis and may improve infant survival. Studies have demonstrated that both azithromycin and clarithromycin are as effective as erythromycin is in eliminating *B. pertussis* from the nasopharynx, although there are no data of infants younger than 1 month of age. Because of the known association of erythromycin and infantile hypertrophic stenosis, it is not a preferred agent for use in neonates and should be used only if azithromycin is not available. There are data demonstrating that 7 days of erythromycin estolate are as effective as 14 days, which may reflect the improved penetration of this erythromycin formulation over others. Stomach upset is the most commonly reported side effect of erythromycin and frequently is a reason for patient noncompliance.

Azithromycin is the drug of choice in all age-groups, for treatment or postexposure prophylaxis. Infantile hypertrophic pyloric stenosis (IHPS) is associated with macrolide use in young infants, especially in those <14 days old, with highest risk in those receiving erythromycin versus azithromycin. Benefits of postexposure prophylaxis or treatment of infants far outweigh risk of IHPS. Trimethoprim–sulfamethoxazole (TMP-SMX) is an alternative to azithromycin for infants >2 months old and children unable to receive azithromycin. Because of limited effectiveness, treatment of *B. parapertussis* is based on clinical judgment and is considered in high-risk populations.

Antibiotics may ameliorate early infections but have no effect on clinical symptoms in the paroxysmal stage. Erythromycin is the drug of choice because it promptly terminates respiratory tract carriage of *B. pertussis*. A single resistant strain has been reported. Patients should be given erythromycin estolate (40–50 mg/kg/24 h in four divided doses for 14 days). Erythromycin ethylsuccinate is efficacious, but the higher dose recommended causes considerable gastrointestinal intolerance. A recent study suggests that 7 days and 14 days of treatment are equally effective. Clarithromycin for 7 days and azithromycin for 5 days were equal to erythromycin for 14 days in one small study.

Ampicillin (100 mg/kg/day in four divided doses) may also be used for erythromycin-intolerant patients. Household or other close contacts (e.g., in day care centers) should be given erythromycin to reduce secondary transmission. This prophylaxis should be used regardless of age or immunization status.

Corticosteroids reduce the severity of disease but may mask signs of bacterial superinfection. Albuterol (0.3–0.5 mg/kg/day in four doses) has reduced the severity of illness, but tachycardia is common when the drug is given orally and aerosol administration may precipitate paroxysms.

General Measures

Nutritional support during the paroxysmal phase is important. Frequent small feedings, tube feeding, or parenteral fluid supplementation may be needed. Minimizing stimuli that trigger paroxysms is probably the best way of controlling cough. In general, cough suppressants are of little benefit.

Treatment of Complications

Respiratory insufficiency due to pneumonia or other pulmonary complications should be treated with oxygen and assisted ventilation if necessary. Convulsions are treated with oxygen and anticonvulsants. Bacterial pneumonia or otitis media requires additional antibiotics.

Antibiotics are given to shorten the coarse during catarrhal phase. Erythromycin is given in the dose of 40–50 mg/kg/day for 14 days. Small dose of bronchodilator may be helpful to relieve the spasms. Betamethasone 0.75 mg/kg/day may be helpful. Humidification of the air diminishes the viscosity of the mucus and child can bring it out more easily.

Pertussis vaccine should not be given to an infant with the history of convulsions associated with progressive neurological manifestation. This is to minimize the risk of encephalopathy following pertussis vaccine.

■ PREVENTION

Active immunization with DTP vaccine should be given in early infancy. Acellular pertussis (DTaP) vaccines cause less fever and fewer local and febrile systemic reactions and have replaced the former whole cell vaccines. The recent increase in incidence of pertussis is primarily due to increased recognition of disease in adolescents and adults.

Chemoprophylaxis with erythromycin should be given to exposed family and hospital contacts, particularly those under age 2 years. Hospitalized children with pertussis should be isolated because of the great risk of transmission to patients and staff.

■ PROGNOSIS

The prognosis for patients with pertussis has improved in recent years because of excellent nursing care, treatment of complications, attention to nutrition, and modern intensive care. However, the disease is still very serious in infants under age of 1 year; most deaths occur in this age-group. Children with encephalopathy have a poor prognosis.

■ BIBLIOGRAPHY

1. Atwell JE, Salmon DA. Pertussis resurgence and vaccine uptake: implications for reducing vaccine hesitancy. Pediatrics. 2014; 134(3):602-4.
2. McGirr A, Fisman DN. Duration of pertussis immunity after DTaP immunization: a meta analysis. Pediatrics. 2015;135(2):331-43.
3. Quinn HE, Snelling TL, Habig A, Chiu C, Spokes PJ, McIntyre PB. Parental Tdap boosters and infant pertussis: a case-control study. Pediatrics. 2014;134(4):713-20.
4. Thampi N, Gurol-Urganci I, Crowcroft NS, Sander B. Pertussis post-exposure prophylaxis among household contacts: a cost-utility analysis. PLoS One. 2015;10(3): e1119271.
5. Yeung KHT, Duclos P, Nelson EAS, Hutubessy RCW. An update of the global burden of pertussis in children younger than 5 years: a modelling study. Lancet Infect Dis. 2017; 17(9):974-80.

SECTION 10

Newborn

- Case 82 **Birth Asphyxia**
- Case 83 **Neonatal Seizures**
- Case 84 **Neonatal Hypoglycemia**
- Case 85 **Neonatal Pathological Jaundice**
- Case 86 **Normal Newborn**
- Case 87 **Premature Infant**
- Case 88 **Respiratory Distress Syndrome**

CASE 82

Birth Asphyxia

■ PRESENTING COMPLAINTS

A newborn child was brought with the complaint of:
- Did not cry
- Flabby
- Noot breathing

History of Presenting Complaints

A multigravida mother aged about 28 years came to the labor room with delivery pain. This was her fourth pregnancy. There was a history of delivery pain once in every 3 minutes. There was a history of rupture of the membrane about 1 hour back. Amniotic fluid was clear. Over the next 4 hours, she delivered spontaneously by vertex presentation. The duration of the second stage of delivery was 10 minutes.

A female child was born. The child did not cry immediately after the delivery. The child was in a state of limp and apneic. Apgar score at 1 minute was 2/10. The head was positioned, and the airway was cleared. Respiration is assessed. The child was dried, and suctioning was done. Oxygen was given. The child started having spontaneous breathing. Oxygen was on flow at the rate of 4 L to maintain satisfactory oxygen saturation. The child became pink, her tone became hypertonic, and started to cry. The heart rate came to normal. Apgar score at 5 minutes was 8/10. The child was later shifted to the neonatal intensive care unit (NICU) for further management.

CASE AT A GLANCE

Basic Findings
Length	: 48 cm (10th centile)
Weight	: 2.5 kg (third centile)
Temperature	: 37°C
Pulse rate	: 86 beats/min
Respiratory rate	: No spontaneous breathing
Blood pressure	: 50/30 mm Hg

Positive Findings

History:
- Multigravida
- Fast delivery
- No spontaneous breathing
- Apneic and limp

Examination:
- Limp and apneic
- No spontaneous breathing
- Cyanosis
- Bradycardia
- Bilateral basal crepitation

Investigation:
- *Arterial blood gas (ABG):* Acidotic feature

■ EXAMINATION

The newborn baby was moderately built and nourished. The child was limp and apneic. The child was not breathing spontaneously. The child was flabby. The child was not crying even to the little stimulation on the back and sole. The child was completely cyanosed.

The anthropometric measurements included the weight was 2.5 kg (3rd centile) the length of the baby was 48 cm (10th centile). The head circumference recorded was 33 cm. The gestational age corresponds to 36 weeks.

Newborn was afebrile. The heart rate was 66 beats/min. The child was not spontaneously breathing. The blood pressure recorded was 50/30 mm Hg. The baby looked pale, cyanosis was present. There was no edema, no lymphadenopathy. The respiratory system revealed no breath sounds in the beginning. Later after suctioning and oxygen, breath sounds were heard at both bases. Crepitations were present. The cardiovascular system revealed bradycardia in the beginning and later it became normal. Per abdomen examination was normal.

INVESTIGATION

- *Hemoglobin:* 12 g/dL
- *Total leukocyte count (TLC):* 13,600 cells/mm^3
- *Differential count (DLC):* $P_{78}L_{18}E_2B_2$
- *Blood glucose:* 56 g/dL
- *Packed cell volume (PCV):* 45%
- *Blood group and Rh typing:* A positive
- *Blood urea nitrogen (BUN):* 20 mg/dL
- *Serum creatinine:* 1 mg/dL
- *Serum electrolyte:*
  - *Na:* 107 mEq/L
  - *K:* 4 mEq/L
  - *Cl:* 80 mEq/L
- *ABG:*
  - pH <7 mm Hg
  - Partial pressure of arterial carbon dioxide (PaCO$_2$) 60 mm Hg
  - Partial pressure of arterial oxygen (PaO$_2$): 40 mm Hg CO$_3$
- *Chest X-ray:* No abnormality detected.
- *Blood culture:* Sterile
- *Swab culture—ear and throat:* Sterile

DISCUSSION

Birth asphyxia is a clinical condition, wherein the cell is deprived of oxygen, and carbon dioxide accumulates in the tissue. It is the most common medical emergency in newborn infants. It is the leading cause of neonatal mortality and morbidity. To prevent this, adequate ventilation and proper circulation should be established.

After the birth, the lungs expand as they are filled with air. The fetal lung fluid gradually leaves the alveoli. One-third of the fetal lung fluid is removed during vaginal delivery as the chest is squeezed, and the lung fluid comes through the nose and mouth. The first few breaths are very powerful. This helps in expanding alveoli and replaces the lung fluid with air. The first breath is usually followed by a cry. This enables the infant to breathe out against the closed glottis. This produces positive intrathoracic pressure up to 40 cmH$_2$O. Functional residual capacity (FRC) reaches about 75% of the final aeration.

The first functional breath is stimulated by many factors:
- *Physiological hypoxia:* This is present at birth. The average volume of oxygen saturation of arterial blood is 22%. Partial pressure of carbon dioxide (pCO$_2$) level 60 torr, pH is 7.28. This stimulates carotid and aortic receptors.
- *Clamping of the cord:* This increases arterial pressure. This in turn stimulates aortic baroreceptors and the sympathetic nervous system.
- *Sudden cooling of the body:* This acts through the trigeminal cold receptors.

An infant should breathe spontaneously after delivery. In about 6% of delivery cases, infants require some intervention, immediately after birth. This intervention is more common among very low-birth-weight (LBW) babies. 70% of the infants requiring resuscitation come under high-risk pregnancy. Hence, high-risk pregnancy should always be attended by a pediatrician.

Full-term mature infants delivered normally, will breathe within a few seconds. The time interval between the delivery of the nose and the first breath is about 20–30 seconds. The child will have rhythmic respiration within 90 seconds.

Fetal lungs contain fluid. They do not contain oxygen. Blood flow through the lungs is markedly diminished following birth. This is due to the partial closing of arteries in the lungs. This results in a large amount of blood being directed away from the lungs to the ductus arteriosus.

High-risk pregnancies are anticipated with certain problems. For the development of spontaneous breathing, these pregnancies should be attended by a pediatrician. These include meconium-stained liquor, breech delivery, assisted delivery, abnormal fetus, postdated pregnancy, maternal hypertension, Rh incompatibility, maternal diabetes, preterm delivery, and young or elderly primi.

PATHOPHYSIOLOGY OF ASPHYXIA

A rational approach to resuscitation must be based on the physiologic changes in the circulatory and respiratory systems that occur normally as the newborn infant adapts to extrauterine life.

The human infant is particularly vulnerable to asphyxia in the perinatal period. During normal labor, transient hypoxemia occurs with uterine contractions, but the healthy fetus tolerates this well. There are five basic causes of asphyxia during labor and delivery:
1. Interruption of the umbilical blood flow (e.g., cord compression)
2. Failure of gas exchange across the placenta (e.g., placental abruption)
3. Inadequate perfusion of the maternal side of the placenta (e.g., severe maternal hypotension)
4. An otherwise compromised fetus who cannot further tolerate the transient, intermittent hypoxia of normal labor, (e.g., the anemic or growth retarded fetus)
5. Failure to inflate the lungs and complete the change in ventilation and lung perfusion that must occur at birth.

Asphyxia in the fetus or newborn infant is a progressive and reversible process. The speed and extent of progression are highly variable. Sudden, severe asphyxia can be lethal in <10 minutes. Mild asphyxia may progressively worsen over 30 minutes or more. Repeated episodes of brief, mild asphyxia may reverse spontaneously but produce a cumulative effect of progressive asphyxia. In the early stages, asphyxia usually reverses spontaneously if its cause is removed. Once asphyxia is severe, spontaneous reversal is unlikely because of the circulatory and neurologic changes that accompany it (Fig. 1).

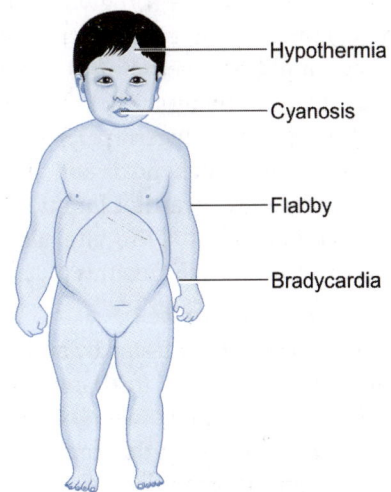

Fig. 1: Clinical features.

Cardiac output is maintained early in asphyxia, but its distribution changes radically. Selective regional vasoconstriction reduces blood flow to less vital organs and tissues, such as the gut, kidneys, muscles, and skin. Blood flow to the brain and myocardium increases, thereby maintaining adequate oxygen delivery despite the reduced oxygen content of the arterial blood. Other organs and tissues must depend on increased oxygen extraction to maintain oxygen consumption. Pulmonary blood flow is low in the fetus. It is decreased further by hypoxia and acidosis. As a consequence of these adaptations, fetal oxygen consumption decreases.

Early in asphyxia, newborns make vigorous attempts to inflate their lungs. If successful, the lungs become adequately ventilated and perfused, but the mere presence of gasping does not ensure that this will happen. As asphyxia becomes more severe, the respiratory center is depressed, and the chances of an infant spontaneously establishing effective ventilation and pulmonary perfusion diminish.

If asphyxia progresses to the severe stage, oxygen delivery to the brain and heart decreases. The myocardium then uses its stored reserve of glycogen for energy. Eventually, the glycogen reserve is consumed, and the myocardium is exposed simultaneously to progressively lower values of partial pressure of oxygen (pO_2) and pH. The combined effects of hypoxia and acidosis lead to decreased myocardial function and decreased blood flow to the vital organs. Brain injury begins late during this phase.

Hypoxia in newborns can be:
- *Intrauterine:* It is manifested by abnormal fetal heart rate pattern, fresh meconium, and reduced fetal movements. It may be acute, chronic, or acute-on-chronic.
- *Intrapartum:* It may be acute, acute-on-chronic due to placental insufficiency.

This may be also the cause of prolonged labor due to oxytocin infusion or cord compression. It implies fetal bradycardia and hypoxemia. This may lead to metabolic acidosis.

GENERAL FEATURES
• No breathing
• Apnea
• Mottling

CAUSES OF ASPHYXIA

Maternal
- Sedation
- Hypertension
- Eclampsia
- Acute hypotension
- Maternal diabetes
- Age <15 years and >35 years

Fetal
- Malpresentation
- Cephalopelvic disproportion
- Multiple births
- Premature
- Postmature
- Hydrops

Placental
- Abruptio placenta
- Placenta previa
- Cord prolapses
- Twin-to-twin transfusion
- Bleeding into the mother.

There are many situations that cause the delayed onset of respiration other than asphyxia. These include:
- Drugs
  - Depressing the central nervous system (CNS)
  - Pethidine 4 hours before delivery
- Trauma to CNS
- Prematurity

- Anemia
- Congenital malformation

Delivery

Delivery room resuscitation of the newborn infant: The presence of certain antepartum, intrapartum, or postpartum risk factors predicts many but certainly not all infants who require help in the delivery room. Premature infants, when compared to term infants, are at particular risk for a difficult transition following birth. The most common contributing factor for infants in need of resuscitation is asphyxia. Asphyxia results in concomitant hypoxia and hypercapnia and causes mixed metabolic and respiratory acidosis. The asphyxia can result from either failure of placental gas exchange before birth or deficient pulmonary gas exchange once the newborn is delivered.

The following equipment should always be immediately available:
- A functional positive-pressure ventilation (PPV) device capable of delivering oxygen, suction devices (bulb syringe as well as wall suction and suction catheters), a functional laryngoscope with appropriate-sized blades, and appropriate endotracheal tubes and end-tidal CO_2 detectors. Pulse oximetry monitoring should be available for every delivery. Cardiac monitoring may help to monitor infants receiving PPV and is recommended if cardiac compressions are initiated. In certain potentially dire circumstances, an umbilical venous line should be prepared, and resuscitation medications drawn up and labeled for potential use.

Resuscitation of the child requires a rapid and systematic response that is well rehearsed. A team approach works better, in which each member should take the responsibilities. The leader should identify the problem and direct the personnel. The intervention should begin instantly.

The main principle of resuscitation is to assist the infant in establishing adequate ventilation, pulmonary perfusion, and adequate cardiac output. Other supportive and important care includes adequate peripheral circulation, maintaining blood sugar level, electrolyte balance, and prevention of heat loss. The cause of the cardiorespiratory problem should be corrected.

Immediately after delivery of the head, but prior to first breaths, the infant's nose and mouth should be gently suctioned. The infant is then delivered, and the umbilical cord is clamped and cut. Neonates should be kept on their sides with necks in a neutral position. Care should be taken to prevent hyperextension or underextension of the neck, since either of these may decrease air entry.

- Delayed cord clamping (DCC) after birth provides a transfusion of placental blood to the newly born infant. In full-term infants, the placental blood volume at birth is approximately 35 mL/kg of birth weight. If the infant is held at the level of the introitus after birth, 40% of this blood volume will be transferred to the infant within 1 minute after birth. In full-term infants, DCC improves hemoglobin levels at birth and iron stores throughout infancy. The only known negative outcome of DCC is hyperbilirubinemia, leading to an increased need for phototherapy. In preterm infants, DCC improves short-term outcomes. For example, it reduces the need for blood transfusion and reduces intraventricular hemorrhage (IVH) (all grades) and necrotizing enterocolitis (NEC). Based on the available data, DCC should be performed in preterm and term infants who do not require resuscitation at birth.

An infant is transferred to a prewarmed towel or blanket. It is very important to keep the baby warm. Baby should be quickly dried and wrapped in a warm blanket to prevent heat loss from evaporation. Hypothermia increases the metabolic rate and oxygen consumption. This causes acidosis, and hypoglycemia and predisposes coagulation abnormalities. If the infant is preterm, place the infant on a portable, chemically activated heating pad under a layer of warm blankets. If the baby is <32 weeks estimated gestational age, place the trunk and extremities into a food-grade resealable polyethylene bag or plastic wrap.

Next, clear the airway. Gently suction the oropharynx and nose. If the infant's respiration is vigorous, nothing more may be necessary. Attach electrocardiogram (ECG) electrodes and pulse oximeter and monitor the heart rate and oxygen saturation. The infant should be placed with the neck in mild extension so that the airway is maximally patent. Sometimes shoulder roll helps to maintain the correct position of the head. If the airway is obstructed or PPV is required secretions should be gently suctioned from the mouth and then nose with a bulb syringe or suction catheter. Take care to avoid vigorous or deep suction because it can cause vagal stimulation with apnea and bradycardia.

Both drying and suctioning are forms of tactile stimulation. These are sufficient to initiate and support respiration. An infant with primary apnea will respond to almost any form of stimulation; however, if the baby remains apneic, gasping, or with an inadequate heart rate, the infant is in secondary apnea, and effective PPV must be initiated without delay. If the infant is not breathing or has inadequate respiratory effort, brief tactile stimulation either by rubbing the back or by slapping/flicking the soles of the feet. If the infant does not respond within a few seconds, PPV should be initiated promptly. Gentle rubbing of the trunk or extremities may help the rate and depth of respiration once the breathing has been established.

The process of evaluation and resuscitation begins as soon as the child is born. The mouth, oropharynx, and nose are thoroughly suctioned. This helps to keep the airway patent. If the thick meconium is present, aspiration is done directly from the trachea, after intubation. In the meanwhile, Apgar scoring is done to assess the status of the baby.

Apgar Scoring

Virginia Apgar was an anesthetist, who tabulated scoring to assess the infant's response to stress of the labor and delivery. It consists of total points assigned to the five objective signs in the newborn. The signs are evaluated, and scoring is done. Unusually the scoring is done at 1 and 5 minutes and updated every 5 minutes until it is normal.

Sign	0	1	2
Appearance	Pale or blue	Peripheral cyanosis	Pink
Pulse rate	No	<100	>100
Grimace	No	Examine	Cry
Activity	Flaccid	In between	Flexed
Respiration	No	Slow and gasping	Crying

Inference

Apgar score	Inference
8–10	No asphyxia
5–7	Mild asphyxia
3–4	Moderate asphyxia
0–3	Severe asphyxia

Because of the practical limitations of Apgar scoring, an action-oriented assessment is done. This offers an immediate therapeutic guide for the management.

Action-oriented assessment:

- *Fetal distress:* Yes/No
- *Medication:* Yes/No
- *First cry:* Minutes after the births
- *Respiration:* Absent/slow/irregular/crying
- *Heart rate:* Absent/up to 100/>100

Steps in Resuscitation

- If the 1-minute Apgar score is 5–7, i.e., mild asphyxia, a baby requires to be administered oxygen with a bag and mask.
- If 1 minute Apgar score is 3–4—moderate asphyxia, oxygen is administered by bag and mask. If spontaneous breathing is not established and if there is history of pethidine administration, naloxone is given in the dose of 0.1 mg/kg. Simultaneously heart rate is evaluated.
- If 1 minute Apgar score is 0–2—severe asphyxia. Here failure of the bag and mask requires prompt intubation to establish respiration. The size of the endotracheal tube is decided depending upon the weight of the child.

1 minute Apgar: It correlates with umbilical cord pH. It is an index of intrapartum asphyxia. In very LBW babies, Apgar may not indicate the severity of asphyxia.

Apgar score beyond 1 minute: This reflects the child's changing conditions and response to resuscitation efforts. A low Apgar score indicates further therapeutic effects. Apgar score of 3 or less is likely to be associated with long-term neurological regulation. By this time a child can be clinically classified, and action can be started promptly. The clinical classification can be done as:

- Vigorous crying
- Pale apneic and bradycardia
- Gasping and bradycardia
- Asystole but potentially revivable
- Stillborn or macerated.

However, some infants with severe acidosis have normal Apgar scores, and with some normal blood gases and pH have very low scores. Maternal anesthetics, sedatives, maternal drugs, fetal sepsis, and CNS pathologic conditions can lower the Apgar score; extremely premature infants often have low scores without any other evidence of asphyxia. Regardless of the cause, an Apgar score that remains low calls for action. The clinical significance of the Apgar score increases with time. Scoring should continue every 5 minutes until the score increases to 7 or above. The length of time it takes to reach a score of 7 is a rough indication of the severity of asphyxia.

Indications for Resuscitation

Infants with poor, gasping, or absent respiratory effort—with inadequate heart rate below 100 beats/min; or who are born preterm should be taken to the radiant warmer for further assessment and possible resuscitation interventions. Heart rate may initially be assessed by listening to the precordium with a stethoscope, but cardiac monitoring can be used at any time as well. Palpation of the base of the cord should not be performed as this is not accurate. Gasping, apnea, and a heart rate below 100 beats/min are signs that indicate the need to clear the airway and provide PPV.

Infant weight (grams)	Size of the tube (internal diameter)
<1,000	2 mm
1,000–2,000	2.5 mm
2,000–3,000	3 mm
>3000	3.5 mm

Modalities of Intervention

Once the neonate is assessed, the mode of intervention should be clear. There are a few modes of intervention as given below:

Modalities of intervention:
- No further action
- Suctioning
- Oxygen
- Bag and mask
- Intubation
- Intubation
- External cardiac massage

No Further Action

Here the baby is crying lustily. The heart rate and respiratory rate are good. No resuscitation is required, a cord is clamped, and vitamin K is given. The baby is given to the mother.

Suctioning

This should be gentle suction. A large amount of secretion is found in the mouth and pharynx. Gentle oropharynx and nasal nares suctioning is done. This will also act as a stimulus but should be done carefully. Catheter size numbers 8F or 10F should be used. Suctioning should not be continued for more than 5 seconds. This should be accompanied by monitoring heart rate. Deep and longer-duration suctioning at the oropharynx produces bradycardia and apnea.

If there is evidence of meconium staining, thorough suctioning of the mouth, nose, and posterior pharynx should be performed soon after the delivery of the head. If the meconium is thick and the child is depressed, direct endotracheal tube suction should be done. Tracheal suctioning should be repeated until no further meconium can be aspirated.

An infant is positioned in supine. A small roll of towel is kept under the shoulders in order to extend the neck and open the airways. Suctioning of the oral cavity, hypopharynx, and nose is done. The mask should be tightly fit on the face enclosing the nose and mouth of the baby. This should not injure the eye and other facial structures. The oxygen reservoir should be attached to the bag to increase the concentration of oxygen delivered to the baby.

Facial Oxygen

In utero, the oxygen tension of the fetus is relatively low compared to adult levels. Healthy-term newborns take 5–10 minutes for preductal oxygen saturations to reach 90% without intervention. In term infants, resuscitation should be initiated with a 2% fraction of inspired oxygen (FiO_2), and the oxygen subsequently be adjusted to meet normal oxygen saturation goals per minute of life for healthy term infants.

Oxygen use during the resuscitation of preterm infants remains controversial. Preterm infants are often hypoxemic due to lung immaturity and impaired gas exchange. However, they are also deficient in antioxidant protection and thus face potential adverse effects from exposing developing organs to high concentrations of inspired oxygen or high blood oxygen tension.

For all infants who require respiratory support or supplemental oxygen during resuscitation, pulse oximetry should target oxygen saturations based on published nomograms of preductal oxygen saturations during the first 10 minutes of life.

This is indicated when there is cyanosis. Here a child may be breathing spontaneously with a normal heart rate, but the child may be slightly cyanotic. Oxygen is given at the rate of 5 L/min. It is quite safe to administer 80% oxygen.

Bag and Mask (Table 1)

About 100% oxygen is provided during bag and mask ventilation. The left hand is used to hold the mask to the baby's face while the right-hand squeezes the bag. Little or ring fingers of the left hand are placed under the baby's chin and the neck is slightly extended. This prevents the head from moving around and maintains an open airway. With other fingers and thumbs, a mask is firmly placed to ensure a tight seal. A tight seal is confirmed by the characteristic rasping noise when the bag is squeezed only the thumb, and two fingers are used to squeeze the bag. A bag should be squeezed gently to depress a few centimeters. The rate should be maintained at 40–60/min.

If the child is gasping and taking shallow breathing and is bradycardiac, then ventilation is achieved by using a bag and mask. The indications are listed in the box.

Indications for bag and mask:
- Apnea unresponsive to suctioning and gentle stimulation
- Heart rate <100 beats/min
- Persistent central cyanosis with 100% oxygen
- Gasping respiration.

The primary mechanism is the initiation of spontaneous breathing due to the head's paradoxical reflex. The rapid inflation of the lungs causes the baby to take inspiration, which is followed by gasps and then normal breathing.

Effective ventilation of the lungs is the most critical step in the stabilization of the newborn infant who is not transitioning well at birth.

Three different devices (self-inflating bag, flow-inflating bag, and T-piece resuscitator) are currently available for ventilation of the

TABLE 1: Types of positive ventilation devices for the newborn.

Characteristic	Self-inflating bag	Flow-inflating	T-piece resuscitator
• Appropriate-sized masks	• Available	• Available	• Available
• Oxygen concentration • 90–100% capability • Variable concentration	• Only with reservoir • Only with blender plus reservoir • 40% O_2 delivered with no reservoir attached	• Yes • Only with blender	• Yes • Only with blender
• Peak inspiratory pressure	• Amount of squeeze measured by pressure gauge	• Amount of squeeze measured by pressure gauge	• Peak inspiratory pressure determined by adjustable mechanical setting
• Positive end-expiratory pressure (PEEP)	• No direct control (unless optional PEEP valve is attached)	• Flow control valve adjustment	• PEEP control
• Inspiratory time	• Duration of squeeze	• Duration of squeeze	• The duration that the PEEP cap is occluded
• Appropriately sized bag • Safety features	• Available • Pop off valve • Optional pressure gauge	• Available • Pressure gauge	• Available • Maximum pressure relief valve pressure gauge

newborn in the delivery room, each with its particular positive and negative features.

Ventilation can be provided via an appropriately sized face mask, laryngeal mask, or endotracheal tube. In order to provide effective ventilation via face mask, the first step is to make sure the infant is maintained in the open airway position. The mask must be appropriately sized to achieve a good seal. It should fit snugly around the mouth, supported by the chin and bridge of the nose. The mask should not rest on the eyes because adequate pressure to achieve an adequate seal often elicits an adverse vagal reflex. Lack of appropriate airway position and poor seal are common causes of inadequate ventilation and resultant poor response to PPV in the delivery room. The best sign that effective ventilation is underway is a rapid rise in heart rate, followed by improvement in oxygen saturation and tone. If there is no rapid improvement, then look for the presence of chest rise with each ventilation and listen for breath sounds.

Ventilation rates of 40–60 breaths/min are recommended. It is easy for an inexperienced provider to deliver much higher rates than are beneficial, so counting out loud, and maintaining a steady rhythm of 1 breath per second can be helpful. Initial inflation pressures may be high to inflate the lungs, but having done so, adjust the inspiratory pressure to maintain a heart rate greater than 100° bpm avoiding overdistending the lungs. The optimum inspiratory pressure, inflation time, and flow rate required to maintain effective ventilation vary. If the heart rate (>100 beats/min), oxygen saturation, and tone improve, and the baby begins to breathe spontaneously, then the bagging rate can be gradually reduced. The stomach should be decompressed to prevent gas distention and aspiration of stomach contents (which can further impede effective ventilation) via placement of an orogastric tube if prolonged bagging is needed.

If the chest expansion is inadequate the following steps are to be taken: (1) Reapply the mask, (2) reposition the head, (3) remove the secretion from the mouth, (4) open the infant's mouth slightly, and (5) ventilate with larger pressures.

The inflation pressure should be around 30–40 cmH_2O for 1 second. This should be adequate enough to expand the lung. This should be given at the rate of 40/min. In an apneic child, the pressure should be around 40 cmH_2O. The inspiration and expiration ratio should be around 1:1. To maintain the maximum residual capacity, the lungs should be kept inflated for 3 seconds. In an apnea, gradual inflation of the lungs to a peak pressure of 40 cmH_2O over 3.5 seconds once or twice is best.

Bag and mask ventilation may produce gastric distension. This will compromise diaphragmatic movements. It may be necessary to decompress the stomach with a nasogastric tube.

Bag and mask ventilation can be stopped if the neonate resumes normal respiration and heart rate remains above 100 beats/min. Otherwise, it should be continued, and cardiac compression should be provided.

Three signs that indicate improvement include (1) increasing heart rate, (2) spontaneous respiration, and (3) improving color.

Intubation

Intubation may be performed for a variety of indications during resuscitation. These include suctioning an obstructed airway, inadequate response and/or poor chest rise during bag-mask ventilation, need for PPV beyond a few minutes, need for external chest compressions, endotracheal delivery of epinephrine if the intravenous (IV) route is inaccessible, surfactant administration, and suspected diaphragmatic hernia.

Laryngoscope blade size, endotracheal tube size, and insertion depth for babies of various estimated gestational ages.

Blade size	ETT size (mm)	EGA (weeks)	Depth of insertion (cm)
No. 0 or No. 00	2.5	23–24	5.5
No. 0 or No. 00	2.5	25–26	6.0
No. 0	2.5–3.0	27–29	6.5
No. 0	3.0	30–34	7.0–75
No. 1	3.5	34–38	8.0–8.5
No. 1	3.5–40	>38	9.0–10.0

(EGA: estimated gestational age; ETT: endotracheal tube)

This is indicated in terminal apnea. The state is diagnosed in a child who is pale or even white. The child is completely limp and makes no effort at all to breathe. The child is bradycardiac, i.e., 80 beats/min and asystole. The child who is under 32 weeks of gestation and who is not breathing well should be intubated quickly. Elective intubation should be given to those who are under 28 weeks of gestational maturity.

For endotracheal tube size, laryngoscope blade size, and depth of insertion. Use of a stylet is an option as long as care is taken that the tip does not protrude beyond the tube, and it is secured so that accidental trauma does not occur. Intubation is a skill that takes practice. An increasing heat rate and end-tidal carbon dioxide detection after several breaths are the primary methods of confirming ventilation.

The infant is positioned with the neck slightly extended. Free flow oxygen is provided during the procedure. The laryngoscope is held with the left hand, the mouth is opened with the right index finger, and the blade is inserted under the tongue. The laryngoscope blade is lifted upward and forward so that the blade is parallel to the infant's body. Epiglottis, vocal cords, and glottis are visualized. If the esophagus is seen, the laryngoscope is withdrawn until epiglottis is seen. If the tongue is seen, the laryngoscope is advanced until it enters the vallecula or passes under the epiglottis. Gentle pressure is provided over the cricoid cartilage of the trachea. A slightly curved endotracheal tube is inserted through a C-shaped arch. The tube is passed into the mouth at the right corner. The visualization of the glottis is maintained. The tip of the tube passes through the vocal cord. The best location for an endotracheal tube is mid way between the glottis and carina.

Intubation attempt should be limited to 20 seconds. Bag and mask ventilation should be done if the attempt is unsuccessful. Endotracheal tube position is confirmed by auscultation and chest wall movements.

The key point in the intubation is the correct position of the laryngoscope and the position of the baby. The baby's chin sternum and genitalia are lined up in a single plane. A laryngoscope and blade are placed in that angel. Then intubator can see the anatomical landmarks, such as the posterior tongue, epiglottis, larynx, and esophagus. Then intubator can make adjustments in the position of the blade and can locate the vocal cords.

The most common sign that ETT is not in the trachea is that the child is not becoming pink and remains bradycardiac. Additional indications are a lack of any chest movements, unequal chest movements, and abdominal distension. Listening with the stethoscope can be misleading especially in a small child as the breath sounds are easily transmitted to the lungs even though the tube is in the esophagus.

Either measure the distance from the septum of the nose to the tragus of the ear and add 1 cm for tube insertion depth or use the gestational age-based depth of insertion table. Secondary confirmation includes seeing the chest rise after beginning positive pressure breaths through the tube, listening for equal breath sounds, and seeing condensation within the tube. Subsequent radiographic confirmation of proper placement is needed. Prolonged or repetitive intubation attempts should be interrupted for the reapplication of bag-mask ventilation to avoid exacerbation of hypoxia and hypoventilation.

External Cardiac Massage

Chest compression consists of rhythmic compression of the sternum pressing the heart against the spine. It results in the rise of intrathoracic pressure and circulation of blood to the vital body organs.

The heart circulates blood throughout the body and delivers oxygen to the vital organs. When the infant becomes hypoxic, heart rate slows and myocardial contractility decreases. That compression is used to increase circulation and oxygen delivery. It should be accompanied by ventilation with 100% oxygen.

If even after intubation for 15–30 seconds and with 100% oxygen the heart rate remains low, i.e., 60 beats/min, cardiac massage should be done.

Current resuscitation guidelines recommend cardiac compressions for a newborn infant with a heart rate below 60 beats/min despite adequate ventilation with supplementary oxygen for 30 seconds. Because ventilation is the most effective action in newborn resuscitation and because chest compressions are likely to interfere with effective ventilation. Resuscitation providers are strongly encouraged to optimize assisted ventilation via an endotracheal tube before initiating chest compressions. Once compressions are initiated, the oxygen concentration should be increased to 100%.

Chest compression should be given to a depth of approximately one-third the anteroposterior diameter of the chest. Back support should be provided by the tips of the encircling finger in the two-thumb method or by the second hand being placed in the two-finger method compression coordinated, with the ventilation should be continued until the heart rate is >60 beats/min.

The best technique is to stand at the foot end of the infant. Both the thumbs are placed one above the other at the junction of the middle and lower third of the sternum. The remaining fingers of both hands are wrapped around the chest supporting the back.

In the other technique, the sternum is compressed by using two fingers, a ring, and a middle finger. The fingers are placed about 2 cm below the nipple line. Despite all these maneuvers, if the child is not reviving then the following condition should be thought of.

Compression is done at the rate of 90/min. One ventilation should follow every third chest compression. Thus in 1 minute 90 chest compressions and 30 positive pressure breaths should be given in the ratio of 3:1. Carotid and femoral pulse are checked to know the effectiveness of compression. If the heart rate is >60 beats/min, chest compression is stopped, but the ventilation should be continued till the heart rate reaches 100 beats/min and the infant is breathing spontaneously.

If the heart rate is <60 beats/min, the chest compression bag and mask ventilation are continued, and medication is started.

The goal of cardiac compressions is to perfuse the heart and the brain. If severe asphyxia results in asystole or agonal bradycardia, the newborn myocardium is depleted of energy substrate. Adequate coronary perfusion must be re-established with oxygenated blood in order to regenerate sufficient adenosine 5'-triphosphate required for effective myocardial function and return of spontaneous circulation.

Coronary perfusion pressure is the difference between the aortic diastolic blood pressure and the right atrial end-diastolic blood pressure. Thus, cardiac compressions and adequate systemic vascular resistance are needed to generate adequate diastolic blood pressure in order to achieve a return of spontaneous circulation. Given the profound vasodilation that typically results from the significant acidemia induced by asphyxia, a vasopressor agent, such as epinephrine will frequently be required to achieve an adequate aortic diastolic pressure for sufficient coronary perfusion.

Conditions not responding to resuscitation procedure:
- Tension pneumothorax
- Prematurity
- Cardiac anomalies
- Pulmonary hypoplasia
- Diaphragmatic hernia

Use of Drugs

If the baby is apneic despite intubation and ventilation and requires external cardiac massage for asystole or severe bradycardia then the drugs are necessary.

Routes of Administration

Intratracheal: This route is excellent for the administration of adrenaline and atropine. It can be used immediately, and the lungs absorb it immediately. The dose is double the IV dose. Drugs should be diluted with 2 mL of normal saline and then injected along the endotracheal tube. Ventilation is then reconnected, which ensures the drug reaches the lung.

Intravenous
A central venous line is used.

Intracardiac
This is extremely hazardous as it is easy to puncture the lungs or rupture the coronary artery. The drugs do not work any better just because they are in the heart.

The umbilical vein provides ready venous access. A loose tie of the umbilical tape is tied around the base of the cord. French catheter of 3.5–5 size is flushed with normal saline. The umbilical cord is cut with a sterile scalpel about 1–2 cm from the base. A large thin-walled umbilical vein is identified. An umbilical catheter is inserted into the vein until the free flow of the blood is aspirated. This should be only a few centimeters into the vein. The catheter is then connected to the stop clock. This helps to administer the medicine and normal saline flush.

Drugs and Dosages

Epinephrine
Although based primarily on adult and animal studies, epinephrine has long been the preferred vasopressor agent for the treatment of ventilation-resistant neonatal cardiac arrest. The most important action of epinephrine is to stimulate α-adrenergic receptor-mediated vasoconstriction in order to elevate the diastolic blood pressure and thus the coronary perfusion pressure. Consequently, during neonatal cardiac arrest, if effective ventilation and cardiac compressions have failed to re-establish perfusion, epinephrine should be given rapidly.

Current guidelines recommend that if agonal bradycardia (heart rate <60 beats/min) or asystole persists despite 30 seconds of effective PPV, followed by 30 seconds of co-ordinated cardiac compressions and ventilation, then 0.1–0.3 mL/kg of 1:10,000 epinephrine solution should be given rapidly via the IV route followed by 0.5–1.0 mL of normal saline flush. The emphasis on IV delivery of epinephrine rather than the previously acceptable endotracheal route mandates that delivery room resuscitation providers be well-trained in the rapid placement of umbilical venous catheters. The endotracheal route is not efficacious or reliable, but it must be used due to persistent lack of IV access, a higher dose (0.5–1.0 mL/kg) of epinephrine should be used, in hopes of improving efficacy. The higher endotracheal dose should always be drawn up in a larger 3–5 mL. Syringe to help alert the resuscitation team of the route for which the dose is intended because high doses of epinephrine should not be given intravenously.

Volume Infusion

Volume infusion should be given only if there is a high suspicion for rounding the delivery (cord avulsion, velamentous insertion of the cord, traumatic abruption, etc.); or if the baby appears to be in shock and unresponsive to apparently adequate resuscitation. If there is a suspicion of significant blood loss, then the best replacement fluid is an emergency supply of O-negative blood, but normal saline is acceptable until blood is available. It should be given in 10-mL/kg aliquots slowly over 5–10 minutes with assessment for response.

It is important to remember, though, that the majority of severely depressed infants have suffered an asphyxial injury and are not hypovolemic. In an asphyxia-induced hypotension and bradycardia model (without hypovolemia), volume infusion during resuscitation increased pulmonary edema, decreased pulmonary dynamic compliance, and did not improve blood pressure either during or after the resuscitation. Thus, volume infusions during delivery room resuscitation may be detrimental and exacerbate poor cardiac output when hypovolemia is not present.

Sodium Bicarbonate

There is no evidence to support the use of sodium bicarbonate during the resuscitation of the newborn. Its use in the newborn should be moved to postresuscitation care that can be guided by assessment of acid–base balance. Bicarbonate should never be given unless the lungs are being adequately ventilated. Otherwise, acidemia will be increased due to increased respiratory acidosis.

Glucose

Hypoglycemia causes derangement in the myocardium. If the baby is hypoglycemic and venous access is not available, then intramuscular injection is given.

Albumin

This is the plasma expander. It helps to correct metabolic academia.

Atropine

It may be used for prolonged bradycardia if it is vagally stimulated. In asphyxia, it can be given intravenously or intratracheally.

Postresuscitation Care

If the 5-minute Apgar score is >7 and no other complication, the baby is transferred to the mother and kept under observation.

If the 5-minute Apgar score is <7 and the baby has other complications such as suspected meconium aspiration and LBW, the baby is transferred to NICU. The temperature of the infant is to be monitored to avoid hypothermia. Fluids are restricted to two to third of a normal requirement to avoid the syndrome of inappropriate antidiuretic hormone (SIADH) and to maintain fluid and electrolyte balance. Ventilators should be monitored depending on blood gas reports. Metabolic complications should be monitored and treated. These include metabolic acidosis, hypoglycemia, hypocalcemia, and hyperbilirubinemia.

The next step is to treat complications such as convulsion by phenobarbitone 20 mg/kg and or phenytoin sodium 20 mg/kg loading dose and 3–4 mg/kg maintenance dose. Lumbar puncture is done to reduce intracranial tension in IVH. Infections are treated with appropriate antibodies.

Subsequent Care

Most of them survive if they are breathing by 24 hours of age. Once the infant does not have convulsions for 4–8 hours and does not show any neurological abnormality, anticonvulsions may be stopped. Long-term anticonvulsions should be given if the convulsions persist and if there are persisting electroencephalogram (EEG) changes associated with abnormal neurological signs.

The prognosis is guarded if the following features persist:
- Persisting fits and apnea attacks
- Prolonged hypotonia
- Prolonged hyperirritability
- Persistent vomiting
- Persistent failure to suck adequately.

■ BIBLIOGRAPHY

1. Bry K. Newborn resuscitation and the lung. NeoReviews. 2008;9:e306.
2. Datta V. Therapeutic hypothermia for birth asphyxia in neonates. Indian J Pediatr. 2017; 84(3):219-26.
3. Deorari AK. Newer guidelines for birth asphyxia in neonates Indian J Pediatrics. 2001;38:496-99.
4. International guidelines for neonatal Resuscitation. Pediatrics. 2000;106:1-16.
5. Kattwinkel J. Textbook of Neonatal Resuscitation. American Heart Association; 2000.
6. Neonatal Resuscitation: National Neonatology Forum of India, 2nd edition. 2014.
7. Thoreson M. Cooling the newborn after asphyxia—physiological and experimental background and its clinical use. Semin Neonatal. 2000;5(1):61-73.

CASE 83

Neonatal Seizures

PRESENTING COMPLAINTS

A 2-day-old girl was brought with the complaint of:
- Weak cry since 1 day
- Not taking feeds since 1 day
- Fever since 6 hours
- Uprolling of eyeballs since 20 minutes

History of Presenting Complaints

A 2-day-old female newborn was referred to the pediatric outpatient department with a history of weak crying, and not taking feeds regularly. Mother told the history of uprolling of the eyeballs. The mother felt that her daughter was warm. When the mother brought these changes in her child to the notice of the ward sister, she referred to the pediatric outpatient.

Past History of the Patient

The newborn baby was the second sibling of a nonconsanguineous marriage. The baby was born at term by normal vaginal delivery. There was no postnatal problem at the time of delivery. The baby cried immediately after the delivery. The cry of the baby was good. The child started breastfeeding immediately. Mother was having vaginal discharge for a long time for which she had treatment.

CASE AT A GLANCE

Basic Findings
Length	: 49 cm (50th centile)
Weight	: 3 kg (25th centile)
Temperature	: 38.5°C
Pulse rate	: 140 beats/min
Respiratory rate	: 28/min
Blood pressure	: 50/40 mm Hg

Positive Findings

History:
- Weak cry
- Not taking feeds
- Uprolling of eyeballs
- Fever

Examination:
- Febrile
- Depressed Moro reflex
- Weak cry
- AF full

Investigation:
- TLC: More
- CRP: Positive
- CSF:
  – Turbid, leukocyte 102
  – Glucose—10 mg/dL

(CRP: C-reactive protein; CSF: cerebrospinal fluid; TLC: total leukocyte count)

EXAMINATION

The newborn was lying on the examination table. It appeared to be appropriate for gestation. The child was lying without much movement. It was responding to the flickering of the sole by a weak cry. Cry was very weak. The anterior fontanelle was full and tense. Neonatal reflexes (NNR) were sluggish.

His anthropometric measurements included a weight of 3 kg (25th centile), a length of 49 cm (50th centile), and a head circumference of 33 cm.

The baby was febrile at 38.5°C. The heart rate was 140 beats/min and the respiratory rate was 287 breaths/min. The blood pressure recorded was 50/40 mm Hg.

There was hypotonia, depressed Moro reflex, and a weak cry. Deep tendon reflexes are normal. The anterior fontanelle was full and bulging. The fundoscopic examination was normal.

INVESTIGATION

- *Hemoglobin:* 12 g/dL
- *TLC:* 16,200 cell/mm^3
- *DC:* $P_{75}L_{20}M_2E_3$
- *C-reactive protein (CRP):* Positive
- *Random blood sugar (RBS):* 38 mg/dL
- *Calcium:* 3.6 mg/dL
- *Sodium:* 132 mmol/L
- *Potassium:* 4.9 mmol/L
- *pH:* 7.37
- *pCO$_2$:* 38 mm Hg
- *pO$_2$:* 95 mm Hg
- *Chest X-ray:* NAD
- *Cerebrospinal fluid (CSF):*
  - Turbid
  - *Leukocyte*: 102
  - 60% polymorphs
  - *Glucose:* 10 mg/dL
  - *Protein:* 300 mg/dL
  - *CSF gram stain:* Negative

DISCUSSION

Seizures are a common manifestation of serious CNS disease in the newborn. Prompt diagnosis and intervention are indicated because seizures indicate serious underlying disease and may interfere with supportive care, e.g., ventilation and alimentation.

PATHOPHYSIOLOGY

The immature brain has many differences from the mature brain that render it more excitable and more likely to develop seizures. In addition, the specific types of these receptors that are increased are those that are permeable to calcium [glutamate receptor 2 (GLUR2) α-amino-3-hydroxy-5-methyl-4-isoxazolepropionic acid (AMPA) receptors]. This contributes to increased excitability and the long-term consequences associated with seizures, particularly those resulting from perinatal hypoxia. Medications that block AMPA receptors, such as topiramate, may thus prove useful in this clinical setup.

Another difference is the delay in the development of inhibitory gamma-aminobutyric acid (GABA)-ergic transmission. In fact, GABAergic in the immature brain has an excitatory function as the chloride gradient is reversed relative to the mature brain, with higher concentrations of chloride being present intracellularly than extracellularly. Thus, opening of the chloride channels in the immature brain results in depolarizing the cell and not in hyperpolarizing it. This phenomenon appears to be more prominent in male neonates, perhaps explaining their greater predisposition to seizures.

Although it is susceptible to developing seizures, the immature brain appears to be more resistant to the deleterious effects of seizures than the mature brain, as a result of increases in calcium-binding proteins that buffer injury-related increases in calcium, increased extracellular space, decreased levels of the second messenger inositol triphosphate, and the immature brain's ability to tolerate hypoxic conditions by resorting to anaerobic energy metabolism.

ETIOLOGY

When neonatal seizures occur, immediate attention must be directed toward the identification of an underlying etiology in order to permit rapid and appropriate intervention (when available) as well as meaningful prediction of outcome. Although neonatal seizures may be due to numerous underlying causes, most result from relatively few causes, e.g., hypoxic-ischemic cerebral injury, intracranial hemorrhage, or metabolic derangements.

Seizures are distinctly uncommon manifestations of withdrawal from passive addiction to narcotics, e.g., heroin, methadone, or barbiturates. In contrast, maternal cocaine abuse may be associated more commonly with epileptiform EEG abnormalities or seizures in newborns exposed in utero or by breastfeeding. This may relate to direct neuronal excitotoxicity, teratogenic effects, or destructive ischemic and hemorrhagic lesions.

Characteristically, severe, tonic seizures begin during the first hours of life, associated with apnea and severe hypoventilation, bradycardia, hypotonia, fixed and dilated pupils, and absence of extraocular movements in response to the doll's head maneuver. The later features are useful for distinguishing anesthetic intoxication from hypoxic-ischemic encephalopathy.

Early myoclonic encephalopathy presents within hours of birth with severe, fragmentary, refractory myoclonus, which often is worsened by handling or stimulation. Infants often have a high-arched palate. The initial neuroimaging is normal, but diffuse cerebral atrophy develops, and affected infants frequently die in the first 2 years of life.

Perinatal Complications

These include neonatal encephalopathy, cerebral contusion, and intracranial Hemorrhage. This will account for 40% of seizures. A posthypoxic ischemic state is suspected when there is an abnormal fetal heart rate pattern, low Apgar score, jitteriness, lethargy, and seizures.

Neonatal Encephalopathy

These children are apneic at birth, i.e., within 12 hours of life. The types of seizures may be subtle, tonic seizures, and multifocal. This is associated with metabolic disorders, such as hypocalcemia, hypoglycemia, inappropriate secretion of antidiuretic hormone (ADH), hyponatremia, and diabetes insipidus.

Intracranial Hemorrhage and Central Nervous System Trauma

The main cause is breech delivery and forceps delivery. Trauma may produce cerebral contusion or Hemorrhage, subdural Hematoma, and subarachnoid bleeding. Seizures are seen on the first day of life. It is usually associated with prematurity and signs of encephalopathy.

Primary Subarachnoid Hemorrhage

This is mainly seen among premature babies. Seizures occur on the second day. Children will be normal in between the seizures. 90% will have normal development.

Periventricular Hemorrhage

This occurs within 3 days of life. These are mainly seen in premature children. Tonic seizures are presenting complaints. This is associated with rapid deterioration, respiratory arrest, and death.

Subdural Hemorrhage

This results during the tearing of falx tentorium, superficial cortical veins. These are commonly seen with large babies and breech deliveries. Seizures occur on the first day. These are associated with cerebral contusion and Hemorrhage.

Metabolic Disorders

- Hypoglycemia
- Hypocalcemia
- Hypomagnesemia
- Hyponatremia
- Hypernatremia
- Pyridoxine dependency
- *Amino acid metabolism disorder:*
  - Maple syrup urine disorder
  - Phenylketonuria
  - Urea cycle disorder
- *Organic acidemia:*
  - Methyl melanic acidemia
  - Propionic acidemia
  - Congenital lactic acidosis
- Biotin-response disorder
- Fructose intolerance

Infections

- *Bacterial:*
  - Meningitis
  - Brain abscess
- *Viral:*
  - Coxsackie
  - ECHO
  - *Cytomegalovirus* (CMV)
- Toxoplasmosis
- Syphilis

Developmental Problems

- Cerebral dysgenesis
- Neurocutaneous syndrome

Drugs

- Narcotic and sedative withdrawal
- Inadvertent use of local anesthesia
- Theophylline

Polycythemia Hyperviscosity

Focal Infarcts

Familial Neonatal Seizures

Hypertensive Encephalopathy

Coarctation of aorta

Unknown Cause

Associated events causing CNS damage are increased cerebral blood flow, and accompanying seizures may result in infarction of the vascular bed. This is a germinal matrix in preterm. Changes in the concentration of critical high-energy phosphate bonds, such as adenosine triphosphate (ATP) and phosphocreatinine are the contributing factors. Depletion of the brain substrate such as cerebral glucose despite of increased cerebral blood flow and excessive release of synaptic excitatory amino acids such as glutamate, exerts a toxic effect. The incidence of etiology of newborn seizures is depicted in **Table 1**.

Causes of seizures can be classified depending on the day of the appearance of seizures. These are placed as follows:

TABLE 1: Incidence of etiology.

• Perinatal hypoxia	• 50%
• Infection	• 12%
• Hypoglycemia	• 12%
• Hypocalcemia	• 12%

Day 1:
- Birth asphyxia
- Birth injury
- Hypoglycemia
- Subarachnoid hemorrhage
- Congenital infection

Day 2:
- Intracerebral bleed
- Hypoxia
- Hypoglycemia

Day 3:
- Hypocalcemia
- Inborn errors

Day 4:
- Hypocalcemia
- Drug withdrawal
- Meningitis

CLINICAL FEATURES (FIG. 1)

Neonatal seizures differ considerably from seizures observed in older children, principally because the immature brain is less capable of propagating generalized or organized electrical discharges. The principal types of neonatal seizures are summarized below. Focal clonic seizures may be associated with focal cerebral infarction or traumatic cerebral contusion.

Benign neonatal sleep myoclonus occurs during active sleep in healthy premature and term newborns. Myoclonus may be florid and consists of either bilateral synchronous or asynchronous or asymmetric movements that are not stimulus sensitive, but which cease on arousal from sleep.

GENERAL FEATURES
• Convulsions • Fever • Not taking feeds • Flabby

Infants with severe dysfunction of the CNS may have stimulus-sensitive myoclonus, which may be associated with spike or sharp wave discharges on the EEG.

Subtle clinical phenomena correlate more frequently with simultaneous abnormal EEG discharges in premature than in term newborns.

The brain of the newborn is immature. Therefore, well-organized tonic-clonic type of convulsion is not seen in newborns. Hence, convulsions in newborns will have different presentations.

Presentations of Convulsions

- Jerking of eyes
- Repetitive blinking of fluttering of eyelids
- Oral or buccal movements—drooling, sucking, yawning
- Tonic postures of limb
- Apnea

These are associated with hypocalcemia, hypoglycemia, neonatal encephalopathy, and drug withdrawal. These are seen in premature children. It is also seen in children of diabetic mothers with normal blood sugar and calcium levels.

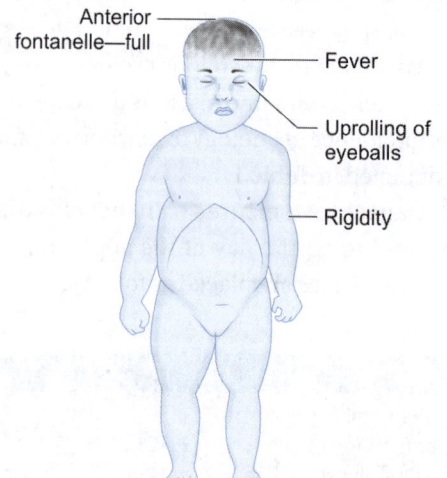

Fig. 1: Clinical features.

TYPES OF NEONATAL SEIZURES

There are five main neonatal seizure types: (1) Subtle, (2) clonic, (3) tonic, (4) spasms, and (5) myoclonic. Spasms, focal clonic, focal tonic, and generalized myoclonic seizures are, as a rule, associated with electrographic discharges (epileptic seizures), whereas motor automatisms, the subtle, generalized tonic, and multifocal myoclonic episodes are frequently not associated with discharges and thus are thought to often represent release phenomena with abnormal movements secondary to brain injury rather than true epileptic seizures. To determine clinically whether such manifestations are seizures or release phenomena is often difficult, but precipitation of such manifestations by stimulation and aborting them by restraint or manipulation would suggest that they are not seizures.

Thus, in many cases, specifically in sick neonates with a history of neurologic insults, continuous bedside EEG monitoring helps make this distinction. Such monitoring has become the standard of care in most intensive care nurseries.

Subtle Seizures

This accounts for 50% of convulsions in newborns. It may be subcortical in origin. This may not be associated with an epileptic form or hypersynchronous EEG. Subtle seizures include transient eye deviations, nystagmus, blinking, mouthing, abnormal extremity movements (rowing, swimming, bicycling, pedaling, and stepping), fluctuations in heart rate, hypertension episodes, and apnea. Subtle seizures occur more commonly in premature than in full-term infants.

Clonic Seizures

Here movements are localized, clonic jerking type. There will not be a loss of consciousness. Clonic seizures can be focal or multifocal. Multifocal clonic seizures incorporate several body parts and are migratory in nature. The migration follows a non-Jacksonian trend; for example, jerking of the left arm can be associated with jerking of the right leg. Generalized clonic seizures that are bilateral, symmetric, and synchronous are uncommon in the neonatal period presumably due to decreased connectivity associated with incomplete myelination at this age. This is associated with or precipitated by metabolic disturbances and trauma. Trauma may be cerebral contusion, subarachnoid hemorrhage, or focal infarct. Unifocal abnormal EEG is reported. The prognosis is good.

Tonic Seizures

Movements may be focal or localized type. These may resemble decerebrate or decorticate rigidity. These are associated with eye movements or apnea. This is more often seen with premature children. Focal tonic seizures include persistent posturing of a limb or posturing of the trunk or neck in an asymmetric way often with persistent horizontal eye deviation. Generalized tonic seizures are bilateral tonic limb extension or tonic flexion of upper extremities often associated with a tonic extension of lower extremities and trunk. This is associated with CNS disease, IVH, multifocal, abnormal EEG with burst suppression pattern, with extremely attenuated amplitude. The prognosis is poor.

Spasms Seizures

Spasms are sudden generalized jerks lasting 1–2 seconds that are distinguished from generalized tonic spells by their shorter duration and by the fact that spasms are usually associated with a single, very brief, generalized discharge.

Myoclonic Seizures

Movements are single or multiple with slow jerks. Movements are synchronous. This involves upper and lower limbs with CNS pathology. Burst suppression pattern EEG with focal sharp transient waves is seen. These will evolve into hypsarrhythmia. The prognosis is poor.

Myoclonic seizures are divided into focal, multifocal, and generalized types. Myoclonic seizures can be distinguished from clonic seizures by the rapidity of the jerks (<50 milliseconds) and by their lack of rhythmicity. Focal myoclonic seizures characteristically affect the flexor muscles of the upper extremities and are sometimes associated with seizure activity on EEG. Multifocal myoclonic movements involve asynchronous twitching of several parts of the body and are not commonly associated with seizure discharges on EEG. Generalized myoclonic seizures involve bilateral jerking associated with flexion of the upper and occasionally lower extremities. The latter type of myoclonic jerks is more commonly correlated with EEG abnormalities than the other types.

■ SEIZURES VERSUS JITTERINESS

Jitteriness can be defined as rapid motor activities, such as a tremor and shake, which can be ended by flexion or holding the limb. Seizures, on the other hand, generally do not end with tactile or motor suppression. Jitteriness, unlike most seizures, is usually induced by a stimulus.

Jitteriness and Clonus

These are characterized by the absence of abnormal gaze or eye movements. These can be provoked by stimulation or by stretching of the joint. Passive flexion or gentle restrain can stop the movements. These are accompanied by increased blood pressure or bradycardia. There is no associated EEG abnormality. Tremors are a prominent type of movement.
- Jitteriness is not accompanied by abnormal eye movements.
- Jitteriness may be spontaneous or stimulus sensitive
- The flexion and extension phases of the tremor are equal in amplitude compared to the unequal phases observed with clonic seizure movements.
- Jitteriness may be stopped by passive flexion or repositioning of the affected body part.

Causes of Jitteriness
- Normal infants
- Hypocalcemia
- Cerebral hyperexcitability
- Infants of diabetic mother (IDM)
- Hypoglycemia
- Congenital thyrotoxicosis
- Drug toxicity
  - Atropine
  - Ephedrine

■ HYPOXIC-ISCHEMIC ENCEPHALOPATHY

This is the most common cause of neonatal seizures, accounting for 50–60% of patients. Seizures secondary to this encephalopathy occur within 12 hours of birth.

■ VASCULAR EVENTS

These include intracranial bleeds and ischemic strokes and account for 10–20% of patients. Three types of hemorrhage can be distinguished primary subarachnoid hemorrhage, germinal matrix- IVH, and subdural hemorrhage. Patients with arterial strokes or venous sinus thrombosis can present with seizures and these can be diagnosed by neuroimaging. Venous sinus thrombosis could be missed unless magnetic resonance (MR) or computed tomography (CT) venography studies are requested.

■ INTRACRANIAL INFECTIONS

Bacterial and nonbacterial infections account for 5-10% of the cases of neonatal seizures and include bacterial meningitis, TORCH (toxoplasmosis, other infections, rubella, CMV, herpes simplex virus) infections, particularly herpes simplex encephalitis.

Hypoglycemia can cause neurologic disturbances and is very common in small neonates and neonates whose mothers are diabetic or prediabetic. The duration of hypoglycemia is very critical in determining the incidence of neurologic symptoms.

Hypoglycemia occurs at two peaks. The first peak corresponds to low birthweight infants and is evident in the first 2-3 days of life. The second peak occurs later in neonatal life and often involves large, full-term babies who consume milk that has an unfavorable ratio of phosphorus to calcium and phosphorus to magnesium. Hypomagnesemia is often associated with hypocalcemia. Hyponatremia can cause seizures and is often secondary to inappropriate antidiuretic hormone secretion.

Local anesthetic intoxication seizures can result from neonatal intoxication with local anesthetics administered to the infant's scalp.

Neonatal seizures can also result from disturbances in amino acid or organic acid metabolism. These are usually associated with acidosis and/or hyperammonemia. However, even in the absence of these findings, if the cause of the seizures is not immediately evident, then ruling out metabolic causes requires a full metabolic work-up.

Pyridoxine and pyridoxal dependency disorders can cause severe seizures. These seizures, which are often multifocal clonic, usually start during the first few hours of life.

■ DRUG WITHDRAWAL

Seizures can rarely be caused by the neonate's passive addiction and then drug withdrawal. Such drugs include narcotic analgesics, sedative-hypnotics, and others. The associated seizures appear during the first 3 days of life.

■ NEONATAL SEIZURE SYNDROMES

Seizure syndromes include benign idiopathic neonatal seizures (fifth-day fits), which are usually apneic and focal motor seizures that start around the fifth day of life. Patients have a good response to medications and a good prognosis. Autosomal dominant benign familial neonatal seizures have onset at 2-4 days of age and usually remit at 2-15 weeks of age. The seizures consist of ocular deviation, tonic posturing, clonic jerks, and, at times, motor automatisms. Interictal EEG is usually normal.

> **ESSENTIAL DIAGNOSTIC POINTS**
> - Varying clinical presentation
> - Results from underlying central nervous system (CNS) dysfunction or can cause CNS damage
> - Intravenous anticonvulsants in correct doses is essential.
> - Abnormal eye movements, limb movements, orobuccal-lingual movements, and apnea may be the presentation
> - Treatment of underlying cause

■ DIAGNOSIS

Some cases can be correctly diagnosed by simply taking the prenatal and postnatal history and performing an adequate physical examination. Depending on the case, additional tests or procedures can be performed. EEG is considered the main tool for diagnosis. It can show paroxysmal activity (e.g., sharp waves) in between the seizures and electrographic seizure activity if a seizure is captured. However, some neonatal seizures might not be associated with EEG abnormalities.

Continuously monitoring the EEG at the bedside in the NICU for neonates at risk for neonatal seizures and brain injury is part of routine clinical practice in most centers, providing real-time measurements of the brain's electrical activity and identifying seizure activity.

Careful neurologic examination of the infant might uncover the cause of the seizure disorder. Examination of the retina might show the presence of chorioretinitis, suggesting a congenital TORCH infection in which case titers of mother and infant are indicated. Inspection of the skin might show hypopigmented lesions characteristic of tuberous sclerosis [seen best on ultraviolet (UV) light examination] or the typical crusted vesicular lesions of incontinentia pigmenti; both neurocutaneous syndromes are often associated with generalized myoclonic seizures beginning early in life. An unusual body or urine odor suggests an inborn error of metabolism.

Blood should be obtained for determinations of glucose, calcium, magnesium, electrolytes, and BUN. If hypoglycemia is a possibility, serum glucose testing is indicated so that treatment can be initiated immediately. Hypocalcemia can occur in isolation or in association with hypomagnesemia. A lowered serum calcium level is often associated with birth trauma or a CNS insult in the perinatal period.

A lumbar puncture is indicated in virtually all neonates with seizures unless the cause is obviously related to a metabolic disorder, such as hypoglycemia and hypocalcemia. The CSF findings can indicate bacterial meningitis or aseptic encephalitis. Prompt diagnosis and appropriate therapy improve the outcome for these infants. Bloody CSF indicates a traumatic tap or a subarachnoid or intraventricular bleed. Immediate centrifugation of the specimen can assist in differentiating the two disorders. A clear supernatant suggests a traumatic tap and a xanthochromic color suggests a subarachnoid bleed. Mildly jaundiced normal infants can have a yellowish discoloration of the CSF that makes inspection of the supernatant less reliable in the newborn period.

Additional causes include maternal diabetes, prematurity, DiGeorge syndrome, and high phosphate feedings. Hypomagnesemia (<1.5 mg/dL) is often associated with hypocalcemia and occurs particularly in infants of malnourished mothers. In this situation, the seizures are resistant to calcium therapy but respond to intramuscular magnesium, 0.2 mL/kg of a 50% solution of $MgSO_4$. Serum electrolyte measurement can indicate significant hyponatremia (serum sodium <115 mEq/L) or hypernatremia (serum sodium >160 mEq/L) as a cause of the seizure disorder.

Many inborn errors of metabolism cause generalized convulsions in the newborn period. Because these conditions are often inherited in an autosomal recessive or X-linked recessive fashion, it is imperative that a careful family history be obtained to determine if there is consanguinity or whether siblings or close relatives developed seizures or died at an early age. Serum ammonia determination is useful for screening for hypoglycemic hyperammonemia syndrome and for suspected urea cycle abnormalities.

Maple syrup urine disease should be suspected when a metabolic acidosis occurs in association with generalized clonic seizures, vomiting, bulging fontanel, and muscle rigidity during the first week of life. The result of a rapid screening test using 2,4-dinitrophenylhydrazine that identifies keto derivatives in the urine is positive for maple syrup urine disease.

Pyridoxine dependency must be considered when seizures begin shortly after birth with signs of fetal distress in utero and are resistant to conventional anticonvulsants, such as phenobarbital and phenytoin. The history may suggest that similar seizures occurred in utero. When pyridoxine-dependent seizures are suspected, 100–200 mg of pyridoxine or pyridoxal phosphate should be administered intravenously during the EEG, which should be promptly performed once the diagnosis is considered. The seizures abruptly cease, and the EEG often normalizes in the next few hours or longer.

■ INVESTIGATION

Investigations of neonatal convulsions can be categorized as:
- *Immediate:* These are done at the time of convulsions, as the investigations done will help in the immediate management.
  - Blood glucose
  - Serum electrolytes—sodium and potassium
  - Serum calcium
  - PCV
  - Acid–base gas analysis
- *Early:* This is done once the baby has stopped convulsing. This will help to find out the cause.
  - Complete blood count (CBC)
  - Blood culture
  - Lumbar puncture
  - CT scan
- *Late:* These are not always necessary. This is indicated when the convulsions are recurrent. Etiology has not been established by routine investigations:
  - Serum magnesium
  - Amino acid chromatography
  - Urine for drug screening
  - CT scan
  - Magnetic resonance imaging (MRI)
  - EEG

> **LABORATORY SALIENT FINDINGS**
> - Blood sugar
> - Serum electrolytes, calcium, magnesium
> - Hematocrit
> - Lumbar puncture
> - CT scan
> - EEG
> - Septic profile
> - Screening for inborn error of metabolism
>
> (CT: computed tomography; EEG: electroencephalogram)

■ TREATMENT

The mainstay in the therapy of neonatal seizures is the diagnosis and treatment of the underlying etiology (e.g., hypoglycemia, hypocalcemia, meningitis, drug withdrawal, and trauma), whenever one can be identified.

Lorazepam

The initial drug used to control acute seizures is usually lorazepam. Lorazepam is distributed to the brain very quickly and exerts its anticonvulsant effect in <5 minutes. It is not very lipophilic and does not clear out from the brain very rapidly. Its action can last 6–24 hours. Usually, it does not cause hypotension or respiratory depression. The dose is 0.05 mg/kg (range: 0.02–0.10 mg/kg) every 4–8 hours intravenously. It is useful in acute situations. This is given for about 2–5 minutes.

Diazepam

Diazepam can be used as an alternative initial drug. It is highly lipophilic, so it distributes very rapidly into the brain and then is cleared very quickly out, carrying the risk of recurrence of seizures. Like other IV benzodiazepines, it carries a risk of apnea and hypotension, particularly if the patient is also on a barbiturate, so patients need to be observed for 3–8 hours after administration. The usual dose is 0.1–0.3 mg/kg IV over 3–5 minutes, given every 15–30 minutes to a maximum total dose of 2 mg. However, because of the respiratory and blood pressure limitations and because the IV preparation contains sodium benzoate and benzoic acid, it is currently not recommended as a first-line agent. The initial dose is 0.1–0.3 mg/kg. This acts synergistically with phenobarbitone hence, there is a high risk of respiratory arrest.

Midazolam

Midazolam can be used as an initial drug as a bolus or as a second- or third-line drug as a continuous drip for patients who did not respond to phenobarbital and/or to phenytoin. The doses used have been in the range of 0.05–0.1 mg/kg IV initial bolus, with a continuous infusion of 0.5–1 µg/kg/min IV that can then be gradually titrated upward, if tolerated, every 5 minutes or longer, to a maximum of approximately 33 µg/kg/min (2 mg/kg/h).

Phenobarbital

It is given in a dose of 10–20 mg/kg to control seizures for several minutes. If the seizure persists, even after 1 hour, a second dose of 10 mg/kg can be repeated. If the seizure still persists, another dose of 10 mg/kg can be repeated after 2–4 hours. The maximum loading dose is 30–40 mg/kg. Cumulating loading dose >20 mg/kg requires careful monitoring of blood pressure and respiratory status. Apnea and hypertension are rarely encountered. Respiratory support may be needed after phenobarbital loading. 24 hours after starting the loading dose, maintenance dosing can be started at 3–6 mg/kg/day usually administered in two separate doses.

In seizure-free periods phenobarbitone is given at the dose of 15–20 mg/kg intravenously. This will help to attain therapeutic plasma levels. The maintenance dose of phenobarbitone is 3.5–4.5 mg/kg/day. This can be given as a single dose or divided into two doses.

The therapeutic plasma level range is from 15 to 45 mg/dL. This should be measured at least 1 hour after the IV dose or 2–4 hours oral dose. The lowest therapeutic dose is 15–30 mg/dL.

Phenytoin and Fosphenytoin

The dose of 15–25 mg/kg IV in normal saline at a rate not faster than 1 mg/kg/min is given. The rate at which the dose should be given must not exceed 0.5–1.0 mg/kg/min so as to prevent cardiac problems, and the medication needs to be avoided in patients with significant heart disease. Heart rate should be monitored while administrating the drug. The maintenance dose is 4–8 mg/kg/day. This is divided into two to three doses. The therapeutic plasma level is 10–20 mg/dL.

Fosphenytoin, which is a phosphate ester prodrug, is preferable. It is highly soluble in water and can be administered very safely intravenously and intramuscularly, without causing injury to tissues. Fosphenytoin is administered in phenytoin equivalents (PEs). The usual loading dose of fosphenytoin is 15–20 PE/kg administered over 30 minutes. Maintenance doses of 4–8 PE/kg/day can be given.

If required, as well as correction of hypoglycemia, hypocalcemia, or other metabolic derangements. If seizures persist, a single loading dose of phenobarbitone (20 mg/kg) should be administered intravenously, which may be followed by additional doses of 5 mg/kg to a total of 40 mg/kg (including loading dose) as required, if there is no cardiac decompensation. If seizures are still uncontrolled, a single loading dose of phenytoin (20 mg/kg) may be administered slowly with concomitant careful monitoring of cardiac function. If seizures remain refractory to therapy, the use of benzodiazepine, lorazepam, or midazolam is recommended.

Seizures in the neonatal period are often life-threatening. It may lead to incredible brain damage. Vital parameters should be maintained. Serum electrolytes and pH should be monitored. The underlying cause should be treated. IV therapy and glucose therapy are included.

Serum glucose level should be maintained around 70–120 mg/dL, and 2–4 mL/kg of 25% dextrose is given over 3–4 minutes. This should be followed by 4–8 mg/kg/min as a maintenance dose.

Pyridoxine Dependency

This is diagnosed by giving pyridoxine 50 mg IV as a therapeutic trial. The diagnosis is confirmed if the seizure stops within a minute. A maintenance dose of 10–100 mg of pyridoxine orally four times a day is advised. In case of deficiency, the dose is 5 mg orally.

Duration of Therapy

Duration of therapy is related to the risk of developing later epilepsy in infants suffering from neonatal seizures, which ranges from 10 to 30% and depends on the individual neurologic examination, the etiology of the seizures, and the EEG at the time of discharge from the hospital. In general, if the EEG at the time of discharge does not show evidence of epileptiform activity, then medications are usually tapered at that time. If the EEG remains paroxysmal, then the decision is usually delayed for several months after discharge.

Other Anticonvulsants

Pyrimidine, carbamazepine, and valproic acid are used.

Treatment for Refractory Seizures

If the seizures are refractory, 40 mg/kg of an initial dose of phenobarbitone, then phenytoin at the dose of 20 mg/kg is administered. Then if the seizures remain unresponsive, benzodiazepine (diazepam and lorazepam) or paraldehyde is used. Simultaneous EEG should be performed to document the cessation of seizure activity. Magnesium sulfate at the dose of 0.2 mL/kg/dose of 50% solution can be used. Pyridoxine is also tried at the dose of 50–100 mg IV.

If the convulsions are intractable and the baby is in state convulsions, clonazepam 50 µg/kg IV slowly for 2–5 minutes is given. Alternatively, clonazepam 100–200 µg/kg can be given intravenously over 30 seconds. Benzodiazepam can be repeated as and when needed. Midazolam can be repeated as and when needed. Midazolam 0.05–0.15 mg/kg/dose is effective when given intramuscularly.

Follow-up of Anticonvulsant Therapy

All the medications that are used to control the seizures can be stopped. The only maintenance dose of phenobarbitone is continued. Indications for stopping anticonvulsants are normal examination findings and the absence of recurrent and nonepileptic forms of seizures.

The duration of the therapy is guided by the neurological status of the infant, the cause of the seizures, and EEG findings. The infant is evaluated at 6–8 weeks. If there is no recurrence of seizures, CNS examination and EEG are normal, the phenobarbitone is stopped. When the phenobarbitone is continued, the child is evaluated at the age of 6 months. The infant is treated like a case of epilepsy if the seizures are recurrent or if there is any evidence of neuronal disabilities or if these are EEG normalities at 6 months.

PROGNOSIS

The most important determinant of outcome is the underlying neurologic disease. In addition, the early onset of seizures, frequent or prolonged seizures, and seizures that are refractory to multiple anticonvulsants often are associated with poor prognosis. However, in a significant proportion of newborns, the EEG is borderline, equivocal, or contains less marked abnormalities that are associated with an uncertain prognosis.

Normal outcome	56%
Neurological sequelae	30%
Death	15%

Seizures are more common with the gestational age <30 weeks. Neonatal mortality is higher with lesser gestational age. Seizures of different Etiology will have different prognoses. The outcome will reflect the seriousness of the disease. The prognosis depends upon the type of the seizure.

10% of the seizure children will have normal EEG. 90% of the seizure children will burst the suppression pattern with electrical silence with marked voltage suppression. 50% of seizures with immaturity and voltage asymmetry will have neurological deficits.

Bad Prognostic Factors

- *Apgar score:* <6 at 5 minutes
- 5 minutes of intermittent positive-pressure ventilation (IPPV) following birth
- Early onset of seizure
- Seizures lasting > 30 minutes
- Hypotonia at 5 minutes following birth
- Uncontrolled seizures for 3 or more days
- Presence of tonic or myoclonic seizures

BIBLIOGRAPHY

1. Boylan GB, Stevenson NJ, Vanhatalo S. Monitoring Neonatal seizures. Semin Fetal Neonatal Med. 2013;18(4):202-8.
2. Clancy RR. The contribution of EEG to the understanding of neonatal seizures. Epilepsia. 1996;37(1):S52-9.
3. Dulac O, Milh M. Brain maturation and epilepsy. Handb Clin Neurol. 2013;111:441-6.
4. Glass HC. Neonatal seizures: advances in mechanisms and management. Clin Perinatol. 2014;41(1):177-90.
5. Hill A. Neonatal seizures. Pediatr Rev. 2000; 21(4):117-21.
6. www.newbornwhocc.org. WHO Guidelines on neonatal seizures. (2012). [online] Available from https://iris.who.int/bitstream/handle/10665/77756/9789241548304_eng.pdf;sequence=1 [Last accessed June, 2024].

CASE 84

Neonatal Hypoglycemia

■ PRESENTING COMPLAINTS

A newborn baby was brought with the complaint of:
- Not active since 4 hours
- Apathy since 4 hours
- Not taking feeds since 2 hours

History of Presenting Complaints

The newborn baby was brought to the pediatric outpatient department with a history of apathy, not active since 4 hours, and not taking feeds since 2 hours. The child was delivered about 12 hours back to the hospital. This was a normal full-term delivery. Newborn was delivered by vertex presentation. The baby cried immediately after the delivery. The cry of the baby was good. The Apgar score was 8 and 10 at 1 and 5 minutes respectively. The mother was advised to feed her baby after some time. The mother said that his son was sucking at her breast in the beginning. But now he was not at all getting up even after the tactic stimulus. That worried her and she came to show her son to the pediatrician.

Antenatal history and check-up showed the development of diabetes in the mother after the first trimester. She was advised GTT and diagnosed to have gestational diabetes. However, her diabetes status was under control with medicines. All the antenatal scanning to rule out congenital anomalies was normal.

CASE AT A GLANCE

Basic Findings
Length	: 53 cm (97th centile)
Weight	: 4 kg (97th centile)
Temperature	: 37°C
Pulse rate	: 146 beats/min
Respiratory rate	: 24/min
Blood pressure	: 50/40 mm Hg

Positive Findings

History:
- Diabetic mother
- Not active
- Not taking feeds

Examination:
- Big baby
- *BBR:* Neonatal reflexes- not satisfactory

Investigation:
- *Random blood sugar (RBS):* 40 mg/day

■ EXAMINATION

The newborn was big in size. The newborn baby was lying on the examination table, without any movements. The child was not active. Hypotonia was present. His cry was feeble after tactile stimulation. Neonatal reflexes (NNR) were not satisfactory. The anthropometric measurements included a weight was 4 kg (97th centile), a length was 53 cm (97th centile), and a head circumference of 35 cm. The child was afebrile, heart rate was 146 beats/min, and respiratory rate was 24 breaths/min. The blood pressure recorded was 50/40 mm Hg. All systemic examinations were normal. There was no clinical evidence of congenital anomalies.

■ INVESTIGATION

- *Hemoglobin:* 4 g/dL
- *TLC:* 12,400 cells/mm^3
- *DC:* $P_{68}L_{28}E_2M_2$
- *RBS:* 40 mg/dL
- *Blood urea:* 20 mg/dL
- *Creatinine:* 1 mg/dL
- *Serum calcium:* 8 mg/dL
- *CRP:* Negative
- *Blood culture and sensitivity:* Sterile
- *Chest X-ray:* No abnormality detected (NAD).
- *Echocardiogram (ECHO):* NAD

■ DISCUSSION

Hypoglycemia is a metabolic disorder, where the blood glucose level is <45 mg/dL. During gestation, the glucose is freely transferred across the placenta by the process of facilitated diffusion. After the birth infant must adjust with sudden withdrawal of transplacental supply. There will be a decrease in blood sugar levels between 1 and 3 hours of life. This fall is accentuated in preterm infant IDMs, birth asphyxia, and intrauterine growth restriction (IUGR) babies.

Neonatal Hypoglycemia

Hypoglycemia is a low level of plasma or blood glucose in a neonate.

In healthy-term neonates, there is a transient, physiological fall in the blood glucose concentration with a nadir at 60–90 minutes after birth, without any symptoms later rising to levels above 60 mg/dL by 4 hours.

Breastfed infants may tolerate lower blood sugar levels because of bioavailable alternate fuels such as ketone bodies, thus facilitating adaptation during transition.

Definition

- *Symptomatic:* Blood sugar < 40 mg/dL
- *Asymptomatic:*
  - <4 hours of age—25 mg/dL
  - 4–24 hours of age—35 mg/dL
  - 24–48 hours—45 mg/dL
  - >48 hours—60 mg/dL

It is a metabolic disorder, where the blood glucose level is <45 mg/dL. Any child with blood glucose <40 mg/dL should be evaluated. The incidence is 0.4%.

During gestation, glucose is freely transferred across the placenta by the process of facilitated diffusion. However, after birth, an infant must adjust with the sudden withdrawal of this transplacental supply. In all infants, there is a nadir in blood sugar between 1 and 3 hours of life. This fall is accentuated in preterm infants, IDM, infants with erythroblastosis fetalis, asphyxiated infants, and in small-for-gestational-age (SGA) infants. Brain dysfunction occurs at 45 mg/dL at any age or gestation.

All conditions associated with the development of hypoglycemia in the neonate result from one or a combination of two basic mechanisms: Inadequate production or excessive tissue use. Inadequate glucose production results from a lack of glycogen stores, an inability to synthesize glucose, or both. Excessive tissue uses results from increased insulin secretion.

■ CLINICAL FEATURES (FIG. 1)

Clinical manifestations of hypoglycemia in neonates are discussed in **Table 1**.

The clinical features of hypoglycemia are many. These are listed further.

Clinical Features of Hypoglycemia

- Lethargy, apathy, weak or high-pitched cry, poor feeding

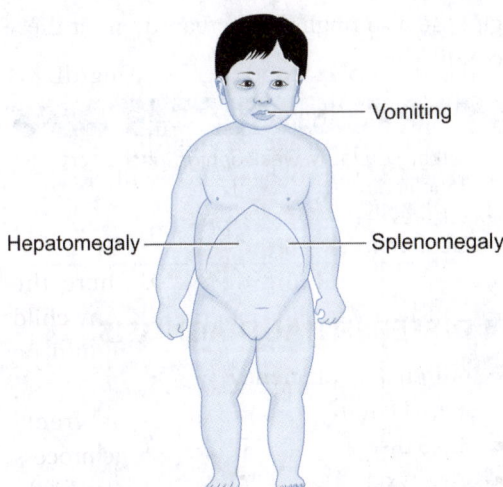

Fig. 1: Clinical features.

TABLE 1: Clinical manifestations of hypoglycemia in the neonate.	
Adrenergic	**Neuroglycopenic**
• Tachypnea • Tachycardia • Poor suck • Poor feeding • Pallor • Temperature instability • Sweating	• Lethargy and hypotonia • Apnea or irregular breathing efforts • Cyanosis • Seizures

- Tremors, jitteriness, apnea, and cyanosis
- Seizures
- Vomiting
- Macrosomia favors hyperinsulinism
- *Jaundice:*
  - Galactosemia
  - Sepsis
- *Hepatomegaly:* Glycogen storage disorder
- *Splenomegaly:* Rh immunization

Causes

Causes of Hypoglycemia

- Infants of diabetic mother
- Erythroblastosis fetalis
- Prematurity
- IUGR
- Birth asphyxia
- Hypothermia
- Galactosemia
- Adrenal insufficiency
- Congenital hypopituitarism
- Polycythemia

The third trimester of pregnancy is an important period for hepatic glycogen deposition. An infant delivered prematurely without having had the benefit of part of or the entire third trimester will have limited hepatic glycogen stores. The greater the degree of prematurity, the less glycogen will be present. SGA premature infants are at extremely high risk for the development of hypoglycemia because available nutrients life is channeled toward growth, with little set aside for glycogen storage. For this reason, SGA premature infants have extremely limited glycogen stores.

Hypoxia, acidosis, and alterations in fetal blood pressure and flow can stimulate catecholamine secretion in utero, which in turn will mobilize hepatic glycogen stores. In addition, hypoxia increases the rate of anaerobic glycolysis, therapy accelerating glucose use. These events deplete fetal glycogen stores and place the infant at risk for hypoglycemia after delivery.

Full-term and premature SGA neonates are at great risk for the development of hypoglycemia as a result of inadequate hepatic glycogen stores. A delay in the induction of gluconeogenic capability probably is responsible for this prolonged hypoglycemia. These SGA neonates have elevated plasma concentrations of gluconeogenic precursors, suggesting an inability to convert exogenous gluconeogenic precursors such as alanine to glucose.

Infants of diabetic mothers are at great risk for the development of hypoglycemia as a result of the carry-over of the fetal hyperinsulinemic state into neonatal life. They have elevated plasma insulin concentrations and release insulin briskly in response to glucose challenges. The problems of the infant of diabetic mother (IDM) are presented in the following sections.

Infants with Beckwith–Wiedemann syndrome, erythroblastosis fetalis and those whose mothers have taken chlorpropamide or benzothiazides are at risk for the development of hypoglycemia as a result of hyperinsulinism. Infants with erythroblastosis fetalis caused by Rh compatibility were reported in the past to be at risk for hypoglycemia from hyperinsulinism secondary to β-cell hyperplasia.

Maternal use of chlorpropamide and benzothiazide can directly increase insulin secretion in the neonate. β-sympathomimetic agents used to stop premature labor have been reported to cause neonatal hypoglycemia. These drugs stimulate glycogen breakdown and gluconeogenesis in the mother and fetus. Large-for-gestational-age (LGA) infants whose mothers do not have diabetes mellitus are at risk for transient hypoglycemia. This is particularly true for LGA infants of obese women. Sepsis in a neonate often is heralded by hypoglycemia or hyperglycemia. Hypoglycemia is a well-acknowledged complication of neonatal polycythemia-hyperviscosity syndrome.

Although polycythemia is more likely to occur in SGA and LGS infants who are at risk for hypoglycemia for other reasons, hypoglycemia occurs at an increased rate in polycythemic approximately grown infants. Infants who have suffered hypothermia are at increased risk for development of hypoglycemia. This may result from increased availability of catecholamines, which would deplete glycogen reserves. Tissue use of glucose also might be increased under these conditions.

GENERAL FEATURES
• Lethargy, apathy, weak or high-pitched cry • Poor feeding • Seizures • Jaundice

DIFFERENTIAL DIAGNOSIS

- Adrenal insufficiency
- Renal failure
- CNS disease
- Asphyxia
- Liver failure
- Cardiac failure
- Sepsis

DIAGNOSIS AND TREATMENT HYPOGLYCEMIA

Prevention of Hypoglycemia

High babies should receive adequate breastfeeding and should be assessed. Small babies not able to suck effectively on the breast should receive expressed breast milk by alternate methods.

If the blood sugar level is >20 mg/dL in an asymptomatic baby, a trail of oral feeds is given, and blood sugar is tested after 30–45 minutes. If the sugar values are above 40 mg/dL, frequent feeding is advised, and blood sugar level is monitored every 6 hours for 48 hours. If the blood sugar level persists below 40 mg/dL, a baby should receive an IV glucose infusion. If the initial blood sugar level is <20 mg/Dl, an IV glucose infusion is started.

In infants with the risk of hypoglycemia, blood glucose levels should be checked at 3, 6, 12, and 24 hours of age. These children should be given 10% glucose and water every 2–4 hours until the glucose level is stable.

The blood glucose should be maintained above 2.0 mmol/dL.

In symptomatic hypoglycemia, blood glucose levels should be monitored every 1-4 hours. Milk feeds are better than glucose feeds.

ESSENTIAL DIAGNOSTIC POINTS

- Blood sugar <40 mg/dL in term and preterm infants
- Often asymptomatic detected on screening
- Manifestations; lethargy, poor cry, poor activity, refusal of feeds, apnea, cyanosis, tremors, and rarely seizures
- Should be treated quickly and promptly as it produces brain damage

Glucose in the dose of 2-4 mL/kg (0.5-1.0 mg/kg) of 25% dextrose is given by rapid IV infusion. The rate of administration should be 1 mL/min. This should be followed by continuous infusion of glucose in the dose of 4-8 mg/kg/minute.

Some infants with hyperinsulinism and infants with IUGR will require a glucose dose of 12-15 mg/kg/min. Glucose is tapered to 4-6 mg/kg/minute after monitoring the glucose level. Glucagon 0.1 mg/kg intramuscularly is given with a maximum dose of 1 mg/kg in infants with good glycogen storage.

Small for the date babies should be started with milk feeds within 2 hours of the birth and can be fed every third hourly for the first 24 hours. Premature babies should have an IV line started without delay. 10% glucose infusion is started with maintenance sodium.

If hypoglycemia is found in children born to a diabetic mother, feeding should be started as early as possible. Feeding should be given a third hour for the first 24 hours. Breastfed babies should be put to the breast. They may require a complimentary milk formula if the glucose level falls below 1.5 mmol/L.

LABORATORY SALIENT FINDINGS

- Hematocrit
- Sepsis screen
- Blood grouping for Rh incompatibility
- Investigate maternal diabetes

In comatose children or in babies with convulsions, 25% dextrose intravenously for 1 mL/min and 10% glucose infusion at the rate of 60-90 mL/kg/day is given. Then it should be tapered to avoid the rebound phenomenon. This is seen especially with hyperinsulinemia.

If the glucose level remains low, then a 15-20% dextrose infusion is started. Then hydrocortisone is started in the dose of 2.5 mg/kg 12th hourly. If the blood glucose level is still less than 46 mg/dL, then glucagon's in the dose of 0.1 mg/kg is used. This should be given intramuscularly.

Treatment of Refractory Hypoglycemia

- *Corticosteroids:* This reduces peripheral glucose utilization and promotes gluconeogenesis. Hydrocortisone is given at the dose of 5 mg/kg.
- *Glucagon:* This releases glycogen from hepatic stores and promote gluconeogenesis. The dose of glucagon's is 0.25 mg/kg.
- *Epinephrine:* This promotes gluconeogenesis and glycogenolysis and augments glycogen secretion. It inhibits insulin secretion.
- *Diazoxide therapy:* This is used only in extreme cases after other therapies have failed.

All infants at risk for the development of hypoglycemia should undergo frequent plasma glucose determinations. Infants at risk for hypoglycemia should be checked frequently during the first 4 hours of life and then at 4-hour intervals until the risk period has passed. If an infant is feeding, blood sampling should be done before feeding. For IDMs and SGA infants, the screening should continue for at least 24 hours.

Intravenous administration of glucose in a quantity sufficient to meet tissue requirements is the treatment of choice for hypoglycemia. The administration of 10 or 15% dextrose solution at 5–10 mL/kg body weight, followed by a continuous infusion at 5–6 mg/kg body weight/min of glucose, will increase plasma glucose concentrations to 40 mg/dL or greater and acutely meet tissue requirements. The maintenance rates may require adjustment depending on the Etiology of hypoglycemia.

Glucagon and epinephrine increase glucose production. Because both mobilize hepatic glycogen stores, their efficacy in treating hypoglycemia is variable, particularly in infants with limited hepatic stores. The numerous cardiovascular effects of epinephrine also limit its usefulness in infants.

Infants who are hypoglycemic for prolonged periods as a result of an inability to produce glucose can be treated with corticosteroids (hydrocortisone 5 mg/kg/day every 12 hours; prednisone 2 mg/kg/day orally). Steroids exert some of their effects by inducing gluconeogenic enzyme activity.

■ BIBLIOGRAPHY

1. Rozance PJ, Hay WW Jr. Neonatal hypoglycemia. NeoReviews. 2010;11:e681.
2. Sweet CB, Grayson S, Polak M. Management strategies for neonatal hypoglycemia. J Pediatr Pharmacol Ther. 2013;18(3):199-208.

Neonatal Pathological Jaundice

■ PRESENTING COMPLAINTS

A 2-day-old newborn was brought with the complaint of:
- Yellowish discoloration of skin since 2 days
- Not taking feeds since 1 day

History of Presenting Complaints

A 2-day-old newborn baby was brought to the pediatric outpatient department with a history of yellowish discoloration of skin. The mother said that she had noticed yellowish discoloration 5–6 hours after the delivery. She also revealed that her baby was not taking feed or sucking at breasts since morning, i.e., on the second day. She brought this to the notice of the resident working in the ward. Later boy was referred to the pediatric outpatient department for further management.

Past History of the Patient

This newborn boy was the second sibling of a nonconsanguineous marriage. The baby was born at term by normal vaginal delivery. There was no postnatal problem at the time of delivery. The baby cried immediately after the delivery. The cry of the baby was good. The child started breastfeeding immediately. The mother did not have any antenatal health records. On the leading question, there was one abortion before the delivery of the present baby. The first child was the girl's baby, and she never had any problem at the time of delivery.

■ EXAMINATION

Child was lying on the examination table. It appeared to be appropriate for gestation. The child was lying without much movement. It was responding to the flickering of the sole by crying. But the cry was very weak. Anterior fontanelle was depressed. NNR were sluggish. The anthropometric measurements included, weight was 3 kg (25th centile), and

---

CASE AT A GLANCE

Basic Findings
Length	: 49 cm (50th centile)
Weight	: 3 kg (25th centile)
Temperature	: 37°C
Pulse rate	: 140 beats/min
Respiratory rate	: 28 breaths/min
Blood pressure	: 50/40 mm Hg

Positive Findings

History:
- Yellowish discoloration
- Not taking feeds

Examination:
- **Hb:** 8.8 g/dL
- **Blood group of child:** O positive
- **Packed cell volume (PCV):** 58%
- Raised serum bilirubin
- Increased reticulocyte count
- *Coombs test:* Positive

length was 49 cm (50th centile). The head circumference was 33 cm.

Baby was afebrile, the heart rate was 140 beats/min and respiratory rate was 28 breaths/min, blood pressure recorded was 50/40 mm Hg.

Baby was pale. Icterus was present even on the palm and sole. There was no edema, no lymphadenopathy. All the systemic examinations were normal.

■ INVESTIGATION

- *Hemoglobin:* 8.8 g/dL
- *Total leukocyte count (TLC):* 12,300 cells/mm^3
- *DLC:* $P_{72}L_{18}E_6M_2B_2$
- *Blood group of mother:* O negative
- *Blood group of the newborn:* O positive
- *PCV:* 58%
- *Peripheral blood smear:* Immature red blood cells (RBCs) were present
- *Reticulocyte count:* 5%
- *Coombs test:* Positive
- *Serum bilirubin:* 28 mg/dL
  - *Direct:* 2 mg/dL
  - *Indirect:* 26 mg/dL

■ DISCUSSION

Introduction

Jaundice, a yellow discoloration of the skin and sclerae resulting from bilirubin deposition in tissues arises when the rate of bilirubin production exceeds the rate of its elimination. Although jaundice can result from an increase in either unconjugated (indirect) or conjugated (direct) bilirubin, a rise in the indirect fraction is the most common cause of newborn jaundice and is the focus of this chapter.

Pathological Hyperbilirubinemia

The diagnosis of physiologic jaundice in term or preterm infants can be established only by excluding known causes of jaundice based on history, clinical findings, and laboratory data. In general, a search to determine the cause of jaundice should be made if (1) it appears in the first 24–36 hours after birth, (2) serum bilirubin is rising at a rate faster than 5 mg/dL 24 hours, (3) serum bilirubin is >12 mg dL in a full-term infant (especially in the absence of risk factors) or 10–14 mg/dL in a preterm infant, (4) jaundice persists after 10–14 days after birth, or (5) direct bilirubin fraction is >2 mg/dL at any time.

Other factors suggesting a pathologic cause of jaundice are family history of hemolytic disease, pallor, hepatomegaly, splenomegaly, failure of phototherapy to lower the bilirubin level, vomiting, lethargy, poor feeding excessive weight loss, apnea, bradycardia, abnormal vital signs (including hypothermia), light-colored stools, dark urine positive for bilirubin, bleeding disorder, and signs of kernicterus.

Delayed physiologic processes or pathologic conditions can result in severe hyperbilirubinemia requiring treatment. Jaundice occurring in the first 24 hours of life or persisting beyond 2 weeks of age in a term infant, a rapid rate of rise of bilirubin >0.2 mg/dL/h, a serum bilirubin level greater than the 95th percentile for age in hours, or a direct bilirubin level greater than 1 mg/dL are all suggestive of pathologic jaundice.

Pathologic jaundice is due to an imbalance between bilirubin production and elimination. Increased production can result from hemolysis arising from blood group incompatibilities, erythrocyte enzyme deficiencies, or structural defects of the erythrocytes. Increased bilirubin production is also seen in premature infants because of the shortened red cell lifespan; in infants of diabetic mothers due to polycythemia or ineffective erythropoiesis; in infants with dosed-space bleeding, such as bruising and hemorrhage into internal organs due to the breakdown of extruded blood; in infants with polycythemia; and in infants with sepsis. Decreased elimination of bilirubin can result from either a genetic defect in hepatic uptake, as seen in newborn infants with a polymorphic variant of the organic anion transporter polypeptide-2 (OATP-2) gene, or impaired conjugation of bilirubin from inherited defects in uridine diphosphate-glucuronosyltransferase (UGT) as seen in Gilbert syndrome and Crigler–Najjar syndrome types I (severe deficiency) and II (less severe form). In Gilbert syndrome, the mildly decreased UGT activity is related to an increased number of thymine-adenine repeats in the promoter region.

Severe Jaundice—Hyperbilirubinemia

Any jaundice visible in the first 24 hours of life

Yellow staining of palms and soles or deep yellow appearance (measure bilirubin values using transcutaneous bilirubinometer or laboratory testing of serum sample, when in doubt)

Bilirubin values >95 centiles for gestation/weight/age in hours.

Warning signs of encephalopathy, such as poor feeding and lethargy.

Kramer's Criteria (**Table 1**) is helpful in clinical assessment of the severity of jaundice. The clinical assessment requires natural light (which can be faulty in hospital lighting). It also depends on the experience of personnel and the subjectivity of assessment.

All babies were reviewed within 48 hours and babies with higher risk within 24 hours of discharge for yellow staining of palms and soles or deep yellow appearance (measure values using transcutaneous bilirubinometer or laboratory testing of serum sample).

Look for lactation problems (excess weight loss and delayed transition of stool to yellow color), infrequent stool, and urine.

Exclude early signs of encephalopathy (poor feeding and lethargy)

Risk Groups: Need Close Attention

- Mother Rh-negative or O group
- Gestation of baby < 38 completed weeks
- Lactation not established
- Predischarge bilirubin in a high-risk zone [transcutaneous bilirubin (TcB) >13 mg/dL]
- Cephalohematoma
- Previous baby with jaundice
- Glucose-6-phosphate dehydrogenase (G6PD) deficiency.

Increased enterohepatic circulation of bilirubin (and decreased elimination) occurs if there is a failure to establish breastfeeding or with conditions that result in decreased intestinal motility such as ileus, pyloric stenosis, and intestinal obstruction. In breastfeeding failure characterized by a decreased feeding frequency, weight loss, and dehydration, there is not only increased enterohepatic circulation but also caloric deprivation.

True breast milk jaundice syndrome develops more gradually, presents typically in the second week of life, and requires the exclusion of other causes of unconjugated hyperbilirubinemia, and generally resolves between 1 and 3 months of age. The etiology

TABLE 1: Visual assessment by *Kramer Criteria*.	
Face	4–8 mg/dL
Upper trunk	5–12 mg/dL
Lower trunk and things	8–16 mg/dL
Arms and lower legs	11–18 mg/dL
Palms and soles	>15 mg/dL

of breast milk jaundice is unclear but probably multifactorial. Exaggerated enterohepatic circulation, variations in the *Glucuronidase* gene, and variations in the breast milk microbiome have been implicated as factors contributing to the development of breast milk jaundice.

PATHOGENESIS

Bilirubin Metabolism

Bilirubin is derived from the catabolism of heme. Approximately 75% of bilirubin is derived from the breakdown of hemoglobin from senescent RBCs and the rest from ineffective erythropoiesis and the breakdown of hemoproteins, such as cytochromes, myoglobin, nitric oxide synthase, glutathione peroxidase, and catalase.

Heme is degraded in a two-step process by the enzyme heme oxygenase resulting in the formation of biliverdin and carbon monoxide in equimolar amounts. Carbon monoxide, which diffuses from the cell, binds to hemoglobin in circulating red blood cells to form carboxyhemoglobin (COHb) and is eventually excreted during exhalation (measurable as end-tidal carbon monoxide). Bilirubin is produced from biliverdin by the action of biliverdin reductase, and on entering the circulation, bilirubin binds to albumin and is transported to the liver. Fat-soluble, nonpolar bilirubin crosses the plasma membrane of the hepatocyte and binds to cytoplasmic ligandin, for transport to the endoplasmic reticulum.

Conjugation with glucuronic acid in a reaction catalyzed by UGT transforms bilirubin into a water-soluble form, bilirubin glucuronide, which is easily excretable. The distribution of bilirubin into tissues depends on its binding to albumin and the serum pH. The greater the binding to albumin is and the more alkaline the pH is, the more likely it is that bilirubin will remain in circulation until it enters the liver.

Conjugated bilirubin is excreted into the intestine via the bile, where it is either deconjugated by the enzyme—glucuronidase and reabsorbed into the circulation (enterohepatic circulation) or converted by bacteria to nonabsorbable breakdown products. Because the newborn infant has few intestinal bacteria, the enterohepatic circulation of bilirubin is active in the newborn and contributes to the increased propensity for jaundice.

Although not all full-term infants become visibly jaundiced, nearly all have a higher total serum bilirubin (TSB) concentration (hyperbilirubinemia 1 mg/dL) compared to adults. The range of normal TSB levels in a population depends on race, ethnicity, genetic factors, and rates of breastfeeding. In terms of healthy infants, jaundice resolves by 2 weeks of age but may take longer in late preterm infants (35–37 weeks of gestation).

CLINICAL FEATURES (FIGS. 1 AND 2)

The baby developed jaundice, i.e., indirect type on the first day. The baby blood group was O-positive to O-negative mother indicates

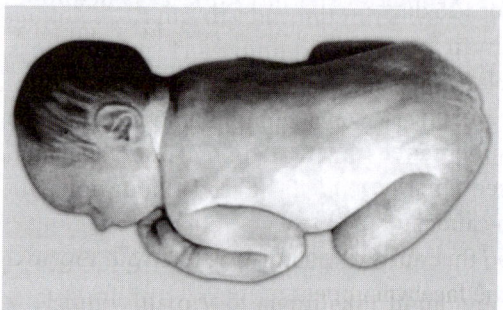

Fig. 1: A child with pathological jaundice.

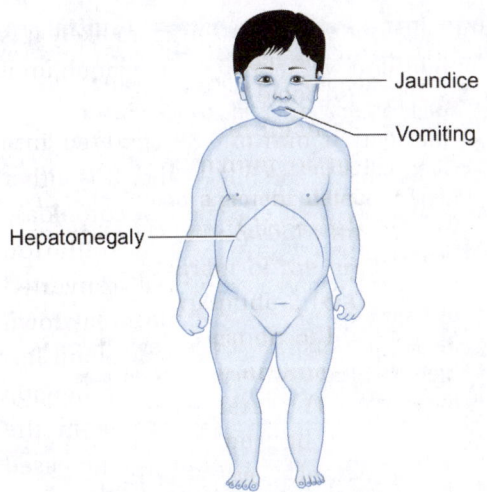

Fig. 2: Clinical features.

GENERAL FEATURES
• Jaundice • Not taking feeds • Convulsion

hemolytic. It is very difficult to differentiate it from the physiological type. Damage can occur even with the physiological range of bilirubin levels in sick preterm infants. Hence, it is a collective diagnosis.

Pathological jaundice appears before 36 hours of age. The rate of increase in bilirubin levels will be 5 mg/dL/kg/day. Total bilirubin may rise up to 15–20 mg/dL. This may persist for >10 days in term babies and for >15 days in preterm babies.

In newborns, jaundice is detected by blanching the skin with digital pressure, thus revealing the underlying color of the skin and subcutaneous tissue. This dermal icterus is seen first in the face and then progresses in a caudal manner to the trunk and extremities so that, for a given bilirubin level, the skin of the face will appear more yellow than that of the foot.

The cephalocaudal color difference in newborns is best explained by a conformational change in the bilirubin–albumin complex. Following its formation, bilirubin is bound tightly to albumin and the initial binding process is extremely rapid (within 10 months). This is followed by a train of slow, relaxing changes in the conformation of the bilirubin albumin complex commencing within 1–30 seconds, final conformation being reached 8 minutes after the initial binding. This time course suggests that, initially there is a lower bilirubin-binding affinity to albumin (until the final stage of conformation has occurred) and thus less effective bilirubin–albumin binding in the blood immediately after it has left the reticuloendothelial system. The affinity increases after the blood reaches the distal portions of the body and the conformational changes in the bilirubin–albumin complex are completed.

All pregnant women should be tested for ABO and Rh (D) typing and a serum screen performed for unusual isoimmune antibodies. If such prenatal testing has not been performed, then a direct Coombs test, blood type, and an Rh (D) type on the infant's (cord) blood should be done, and this should always be done if the mother is Rh-negative. In addition to the identification of potentially Rh-sensitized infants, this testing is obligatory because it identifies Rh-negative mothers who require anti-D globulin to prevent Rh (D) sensitization.

Although, there is certainly a wide spectrum of hemolysis in ABO hemolytic disease, this diagnosis generally should not be made unless there is a positive direct agglutination test and clinical jaundice within the first 12–24 hours. Reticulocytosis and the presence of microspherocytes on the smear help to confirm the diagnosis.

It depends upon the nature of the individual immune response. The severity of the illness ranges from mild hemolysis to severe anemia with compensatory hyperplasia of erythropoietic tissue, leading to enlargement of the spleen and liver.

Child will be many a time premature. Any evidence of IUGR should be looked for. Associated features of polycythemia and in utero infection should be looked for. Microcephaly may be present with toxoplasmosis, other (congenital syphilis and viruses), [toxoplasmosis, others (syphilis, hepatitis B) rubella, CMV, and herpes simplex virus (TORCH)] infection. The presence of pallor suggests a hemolytic type of anemia. This diagnosis is supported by hepatosplenomegaly. Features of omphalitis and hypothyroidism should be looked for.

Profound anemia results in pallor, signs of cardiac decompensation, i.e., cardiomegaly and respiratory distress, massive anemia, and circulatory collapse. This leads to excessive abnormal fluid in two or more fetal compartments, i.e. skin, pleura, and pericardium, termed hydrops fetalis. It frequently results in death in utero or shortly after birth.

The severity of hydrops is related to the level of anemia and the degree of reduction in serum albumin. This is due to hepatic dysfunction. Petechiae, purpura, and thrombocytopenia may also be present in severe cases.

Icterus is generally evident on the first day of life. This is because the infant bilirubin conjugating and the excretory system are unable to cope with the load resulting from massive Hemolysis. Indirect bilirubin accumulates postnatally. It may rapidly reach extremely high levels. This represents a significant risk of bilirubin encephalopathy. Hypoglycemia occurs more frequently in infants with severe hemolytic disease.

> **ESSENTIAL DIAGNOSTIC POINTS**
> - Clinical jaundice in the first 24 hours of life
> - Total bilirubin increasing by >5 mg%/day
> - Total serum bilirubin of >12.9 mg% in full term
> - Direct bilirubin >2 mg%
> - Clinical jaundice persisting for more than one week in full term and >2 weeks in preterm infants
> - It is clinically appreciated with bilirubin values of 7 mg%
> - Babies with asphyxia, acidosis, hypoglycemia, preterm infant are at higher risk bilirubin encephalopathy

Infants with Severe Jaundice

In those infants with severe jaundice (TBS levels >18 mg/dL), it is worth looking for ABO immunization and other causes of hemolysis. If ABO or some other type of hemolytic disease is strongly suspected, these infants generally require more aggressive therapy than those with non-hemolytic jaundice. In the absence of Hemolysis and any abnormal historical or physical findings, jaundice by itself is rarely a sign of serious illness and although, some reports have suggested that unexplained indirect hyperbilirubinemia may be the only manifestation of sepsis in otherwise healthy-appearing newborns.

Prolonged Jaundice (Beyond 3 Weeks)

This is the persistence of significant jaundice (10 mg/dL) beyond three weeks in a term baby. The common causes include inadequate feeding, breast milk jaundice, cephalhematoma hemolytic disease, (G6PD) deficiency, and hypothyroidism. Urinary tract infection should be considered.

Danger Signs in Jaundiced Infants

- Family history of significant hemolytic disease

- Onset of jaundice in first 24 hours of life
- Onset of jaundice after 3 days of life
- Vomiting
- Lethargy
- Poor feeding
- Fever
- High-pitched cry
- Dark urine
- Light stools

Every infant who is jaundiced beyond 3 weeks of age must have a measurement of direct bilirubin performed. If the level is elevated, the urine should be tested for bile and the stool color evaluated. This approach is essential for the early identification of infants with biliary atresia. If these infants are to benefit from the operation of portoenterostomy, surgery should be performed before 60 days of age. If an elevated direct bilirubin measurement is obtained while the infant is in the nursery, it must be repeated; if it remains elevated, the infant must be investigated for possible causes of cholestatic jaundice.

■ DIAGNOSIS

Evaluation of a jaundiced infant should try to identify the type of hyperbilirubinemia (indirect or direct), its severity, the risks of bilirubin encephalopathy, and the cause of the hyperbilirubinemia.

A review of the maternal, family, and infant history should aim to identify blood group incompatibilities, congenital infections, maternal diabetes, maternal drugs, birth trauma, closed space bleeding in the newborn, familial causes such as hereditary spherocytosis, G6PD deficiency, family history of liver disease, and siblings with jaundice (which may suggest blood group incompatibilities, breast milk jaundice, or Lucey–Driscoll syndrome). The newborn should be assessed for poor feeding, decreased stooling or urination, excessive weight loss, and poor breastfeeding or poor milk intake.

Physical examination of the infant should try to identify whether the infant is preterm, SGA, or LGA. The infant should be assessed for ruddiness (suggestive of polycythemia), pallor, presence of extravasated blood (e.g., cephalohematoma), petechiae, hepatosplenomegaly, chorioretinitis, omphalitis, evidence of sepsis, and features of congenital hypothyroidism. Finally, careful examination and documentation should be made of features of bilirubin encephalopathy.

Visual inspection of the degree of yellow discoloration of the skin is unreliable, and a TSB level should be obtained. Other common laboratory tests to identify the presence of hemolysis and its etiology and severity may be indicated. These include maternal and infant ABO and Rh blood types, indirect and direct antiglobulin tests, complete blood count, reticulocyte count, peripheral blood smear, a G6PD level, and if necessary, specific tests suck as an osmotic fragility test. Finally, assessment of serum albumin, and if the infant appears ill, the blood pH may be helpful in assessing the risk of bilirubin encephalopathy **(Table 2)**.

Evaluation for infection may be warranted depending on the history and physical examination. ABO hemolytic disease is the most common form of hemolysis diagnosed in the newborn. Only half of those infants with a positive direct antibody (Coombs) test are likely to have significant hemolysis. On the other hand, some infants with a negative direct Coombs test have increased rates of hemolysis. Reticulocytosis and the presence of microspherocytes on a peripheral blood smear may help confirm the diagnosis but are not pathognomonic.

TABLE 2: Guidelines for initial evaluation and follow-up of jaundice in apparently healthy term and near-term infants.

Clinical observation	Initial actions	Other evaluations	Follow-up
Onset of jaundice in first 24 hours	• Clinical evaluation • Measure TSB and TcB	• Blood group (ABO, Rh) • Direct Coombs test • CBC, smear for red cell morphology, reticulocyte count	Repeat TSB in 4–24 hours
The onset of jaundice is 24–72 hours	• Clinical evaluation • Assess cephalocaudal distribution TcB	TSB if indicated by TcB or clinical evaluation	Clinical evaluation and/or TcB or TSB within 24–72 hours and repeat as necessary

(CBC: complete blood count; TcB: transcutaneous bilirubin; TSB: total serum bilirubin)

Routine testing for G6PD deficiency is indicated when family history or ethnic or geographic origin suggests the likelihood of G6PD deficiency. However, not all infants with G6PD deficiency have hemolysis, and G6PD levels can be high in the presence of hemolysis. Also, such testing is not available currently in all institutions, and, when done, the results are usually not timely enough for immediate decision-making careful follow-up is required for all discharged newborn infants who have hemolysis.

Transcutaneous bilirubinometry has been investigated as a substitute for serum bilirubin assessment. Noninvasive transcutaneous bilirubin (TcB) measurements have been shown to underestimate TSB measurements, especially with advancing chronological age.

If an infant is significantly jaundiced clinically, it is prudent to immediately institute phototherapy while waiting for the laboratory test results. If the serum bilirubin exceeds thresholds described in published guidelines, then phototherapy should be continued, and periodic serum bilirubin assessments performed until the bilirubin drops below the phototherapy threshold **(Table 3)**.

TABLE 3: Phototherapy maximum indirect levels.

Suggested maximal indirect serum bilirubin-concentrations (mg/dL) in preterm infants

Birthweight (g)	Uncomplicated	Complicated
<1,000	12–13	10–12
1,000–1,250	12–14	10–12
1,251–1,499	14–16	12–14
1,500–1,999	16–20	15–17
2,000–2,500	20–22	18–20

All the neonates with icterus warrant the investigation. The clinical and biochemical jaundice asks for a detailed investigation. This is enlightened as follows:
- *Clinical jaundice:*
  - Early onset, i.e., within 24 hours
  - Sick infant
  - Persistent jaundice of more than a week at term and >2 weeks at preterm babies
- *Biochemical jaundice:*
  - Rising bilirubin, i.e., >5 mg/dL/day
  - Conjugated serum bilirubin >1.5 mg/dL
  - Conjugated hyperbilirubin >2 mg/dL
  - To the serum bilirubin level of >18 mg/dL in a term at the 3–5 days in premature infants 12–15 mg/dL.

These help to know the severity of the icterus and help in the management. These are classified and investigations are again dependent on the time of onset of jaundice. These are depicted below.

- *Onset within 24 hours:*
  - Serum bilirubin:
    - Conjugated
    - Unconjugated
  - Total count and differential count
  - Blood group and typing
  - Coombs test
- *Onset after 24 hours:*
  - Serum bilirubin
  - Blood group and typing
  - Coombs test
  - Urine culture and sensitivity
  - Total count and differential count
  - Blood culture and sensitivity
  - G6PD
- *Prolonged jaundice:*
  - Serum bilirubin
  - Thyroid function test
  - Liver function test
  - Urine culture and sensitivity
  - Total count and differential count
  - G6PD
  - Blood culture and sensitivity
  - *Others:* sepsis screen; thyroid function test; urine for reducing substances to rule out galactosemia; specific enzyme/genetic studies for Crigler–Najjar, Gilbert, and other genetic enzyme deficiencies.

LABORATORY SALIENT FINDINGS

- Serum bilirubin direct and indirect
- Blood grouping of the mother and child ABO and Rh
- Direct Coombs in infant
- Hematocrit
- Peripheral blood smear red blood cell (RBC) morphology and reticulocyte count

---

Rh Isoimmunization

Hemolytic disease of newborns results from transplacental passage of the maternal antibody active against red blood cell (RBC) antigens of the infant. This leads to an increased rate of RBC destruction. It is an important cause of pathological jaundice in newborns.

The Rh antigenic determinants are genetically transmitted from each parent and determine the Rh type. This will direct the production of the number of blood group factors.

When Rh-positive blood is infused into Rh-negative women, or Rh-positive fetal blood containing D antigen inherited from a Rh-positive father enters the maternal circulation during pregnancy, with spontaneous or induced abortion or at delivery, this leads to antibody formation against the D may be induced in inseminated Rh-negative recipient mother. Hemolytic disease rarely occurs during the first pregnancy. This is because transfusion of Rh-positive fetal blood into a Rh-negative mother tends to occur near the time of delivery.

Hemolytic Disease

The combination of antepartum and postpartum prophylaxis with Rh immunoglobulin has dramatically reduced the incidence of erythroblastosis fetalis and the contribution of ABO hemolytic disease to neonatal jaundice was discussed in the section on laboratory evaluation. Other hemolytic processes to be considered include spherocytosis and other morphologic abnormalities of the erythrocyte, in addition to the erythrocyte enzyme deficiencies.

Infants with G6PD deficiency have an increased rate of red cell breakdown and bilirubin production, in those who develop significant hyperbilirubinemia, the major problem appears to be abnormal bilirubin elimination.

The risk of kernicterus in G6PD deficient infants with TSB levels above 20 mg/dL (342 mmol/L) appears to be comparable to that associated with Rh disease. Thus, in the presence of G6PD deficiency, more aggressive treatment of these infants probably is indicated.

Antenatal Diagnosis

The presence of a measurable antibody titer of 1:64 or greater suggests significant hemolytic disease. Although exact titer correlates poorly with the severity of the disease. If the mother is found to have antibodies against D at a titer of 1:16 or greater at any time during subsequent pregnancy, the severity of the fetal disease should be monitored by amniocentesis, percutaneous umbilical blood sampling (PUBS), and ultrasonography. Real-time ultrasonography is used to detect the progression of the disease.

Amniocentesis is used to assess fetal hemolysis. Hemolysis of the fetal RBCs produces hyperbilirubinemia before the onset of severe anemia. Bilirubin is cleared by the placenta. However, a significant proportion enters the amniotic fluid. This can be measured by spectrophotometry. Amniocentesis is performed if there is evidence of maternal sensitization (titer >1:16). Spectrophotometric scanning of amniotic fluid wavelengths demonstrates a positive optical density, and deviation of absorption for bilirubin from normal at 450 mm. The optical density of 1,450 is a reflection of the fetal bilirubin level and thus hemolysis and indicates the severity of anemia and risk of intrauterine deaths.

Postnatal Diagnosis

Immediately after the birth of any infant to a Rh-negative mother, blood from the umbilical cord or from the infant should be examined for ABO blood group, Rh type, hematocrit, and hemoglobin. The Coombs test should be done. If the Coombs test is positive, baseline serum bilirubin should be measured. Direct Coombs test will result in strongly positive in clinically affected infants. It may remain there for a month.

Kernicterus

Kernicterus, or bilirubin encephalopathy, is a neurologic syndrome resulting from the deposition of unconjugated (indirect) bilirubin in the basal ganglia and brainstem nuclei. The pathogenesis of kernicterus is multifactorial and involves an interaction between unconjugated bilirubin levels, albumin binding and unbound bilirubin levels, passage across the blood–brain barrier (BBB), and neuronal susceptibility to injury. Disruption of the BBB by disease, asphyxia, and other factors and maturational changes in BBB permeability affect risk.

Signs and symptoms of kernicterus usually appear 2–5 days after birth in term infants and as late as the seventh day in preterm infants, but hyperbilirubinemia may lead to encephalopathy at any time during the neonatal period. The early signs may be subtle and indistinguishable from those of sepsis, asphyxia, hypoglycemia, intracranial hemorrhage, and other acute systemic illnesses in a neonate. Lethargy, poor feeding, and loss of the Moro reflex are common initial signs. Subsequently, the infant may appear gravely ill and prostrate, with diminished tendon reflexes and respiratory distress. Opisthotonos with a bulging fontanel, twitching of the face or limbs, and a shrill, high-pitched cry may follow. In advanced cases, convulsions and spasms occur, with affected infants stiffly extending their arms in an inward rotation with their fists clenched. Rigidity is rare at this late stage.

> **CLINICAL FEATURES OF KERNICTERUS**
>
> - Acute form:
>   - *Phase 1 (first 1–2 days):* Poor suck, stupor, hypotonia, seizures
>   - *Phase 2 (middle of first week):* Hypertonia of extensor muscles, opisthotonos, retrocollis, and fever
>   - *Phase 3 (after the first week):* Hypertonia
> - Chronic form:
>   - *First year:* Hypotonia, active deep tendon reflexes, obligatory tonic neck reflexes, and delayed motor skills
>   - *After the first year:* Movement disorders (choreoathetosis, ballismus, and tremor), upward gaze, and sensorineural hearing loss

Acute bilirubin encephalopathy caused by unconjugated bilirubin in the infant presents with a poor suck, lethargy, hypotonia in the first 2 days of age followed by hypertonia of extensor muscles, opisthotonus, retrocollis, and fever in the middle of the first week and hypertonia after the first week. Surviving infants may have exaggerated deep tendon reflexes, obligatory tonic neck reflexes, delayed motor skills, and after the first year, movement disorder (choreoathetosis, ballismus, and tremor), upward gaze, paralytic palsies, intellectual deficits, and sensorineural hearing loss.

Kernicterus is characterized pathologically by staining and necrosis of neurons in the basal ganglia, hippocampus, and subthalamic nuclei of the brain. Those regions most commonly affected are the basal ganglia, particularly the subthalamic nucleus and the globus pallidus; the hippocampus, the geniculate bodies, various brainstem nuclei, including the inferior colliculus, oculomotor, vestibular, cochlear, and inferior olivary nuclei; and the cerebellum, especially the dentate nucleus and the vermis. MR imaging of infants with kernicterus has shown abnormalities in these regions. Bilirubin may also cause changes in brain-stem-evoked responses and abnormal infant cries in the acute phase, and sensorineural hearing loss long term.

Neuronal necrosis is the dominant histopathologic feature after 7–10 days of postnatal life. For the most part, its distribution corresponds with the distribution of bilirubin staining, although there are some exceptions to this rule. Intense staining develops in the olivary and dentate nuclei, but there is little neuronal necrosis in these regions. The important areas of neuronal injury (as opposed to staining) include the basal ganglia, brainstem oculomotor nuclei, and brainstem auditory pathways, especially (cochlear) nuclei.

Pathogenesis is a complex process, it is related to the interaction between the level of bilirubin, gestational maturity, and integrity of BBB.

Serum bilirubin and protein ratio >3.5 will be associated with brain damage.

The classical neurological signs are not seen at prematurity. Here bilirubin staining is limited to cranial nerves, subthalamus, and thalamus.

The inhibition of protein phosphorylation is probably an important mechanism in bilirubin toxicity and lysine binding may have an important role in the mediation of this toxicity.

It is not known why bilirubin is deposited preferentially in the basal ganglia, but it is possible that it may first attach to nerve terminals, thus lowering membrane potentials and decreasing nerve conduction and after further exposure, may penetrate nerve terminals or axons with retrograde uptake of bilirubin in the cell body.

Albumin has a primary binding site with the capacity for binding up to 1 molecule of bilirubin per molecule of albumin and one or more binding sites with much lower affinities. When the bilirubin–albumin ratio exceeds 1, the concentration of free or unbound bilirubin increases, but binding at the lower affinity sites continues up to a molar bilirubin–albumin ratio of 3:1. It has been widely accepted that bilirubin toxicity occurs when free bilirubin enters the brain and binds to cell membranes.

No association can be made between a specific serum bilirubin level duration of exposure to high bilirubin levels and the risk of neurotoxicity, although the risk is higher with a serum bilirubin level of >25 mg/dL. Low serum albumin levels and the use of agents that displace bilirubin from albumin such as sulfisoxazole, benzyl alcohol, and ceftriaxone, can increase the risk of bilirubin encephalopathy. A decrease in blood pH may render unbound (free) bilirubin lipophilic, thereby enhancing tissue uptake.

Premature infants are particularly at risk of encephalopathy because of low serum albumin concentrations and frequency of acidosis. Albumin-bound bilirubin and conjugated bilirubin do not cross the BBB but when the barrier is disrupted, as in prematurity, asphyxia, meningitis, sepsis, and intracranial hemorrhage, bilirubin may access vulnerable areas of the developing brain.

Blood–Brain Barrier

A BBB exists that limits the entry of certain substances into the CNS. This barrier, at the cerebral blood vessels, is due to a continuous lining of endothelial cells connected by tight junctions that restrict intercellular diffusion. The BBB normally excludes most water-soluble substances and proteins but is permeable to lipid-soluble substances that are not protein-bound. Large molecules, such as albumin, are excluded from the brain but may enter when the brain is made permeable by the infusion of a hypertonic solution.

Opening of a BBB allows albumin-bound bilirubin to bathe the neurons, but whether or not free bilirubin binds to albumin or to cellular membranes may be determined by the binding of bilirubin to albumin.

In the first few days, the infant becomes lethargic and hypotonic and sucks poorly. Later in the first week, the second phase evolves. The infant becomes hypertonic and frequently develops a fever and a high-pitched cry. Hypertonia involves the extensor muscle groups, and most infants exhibit backward arching of the neck (i.e., retrocollis) and trunk (i.e., opisthotonus). The fever may be due to diencephalic involvement. In the third phase, usually after 1 week, hypertonia subsides and is replaced by hypotonia. Infants who manifest hypertonia during the second phase invariably develop the clinical features of chronic bilirubin encephalopathy.

Extrapyramidal Disturbances

Athetosis (i.e., involuntary, sinuous, writhing movements) may develop as early as 18 months but may be delayed as late as 8 or 9 years. If sufficiently severe, athetosis may prevent useful limb function. These movements are described as uncontrollable, purposeless, involuntary, and incoordinate. They may be rapid and jerky (choreiform), slow and worm-like (orthodox athetosis) or so slowed by hypertonicity that the patient may assume momentarily fixed attitudes with a stiffness of the extremities (dystonia). Severely affected children also may have dysarthria, facial grimacing, drooling, and difficulty in chewing and swallowing.

Auditory Abnormalities

Some degree of hearing loss is often found in children with chronic bilirubin encephalopathy. Pathologic studies and studies of hearing tests indicate that injury to the brainstem, specifically the cochlear nuclei, is the principal cause of hearing loss, although occasional studies suggest possible involvement of the peripheral auditory system as well.

Hearing loss is generally most severe in the high frequencies and an association between moderate hyperbilirubinemia and subsequent sensorineural hearing loss has been described in LBW infants.

Gaze Abnormalities

The limitation of upward gaze and other gaze abnormalities occur, and full vertical eye movements during the Doll's eye maneuver are attained in most affected children suggesting that the lesion is above the level of the oculomotor nuclei. Some patients have paralytic gaze palsies. Supranuclear palsies can be explained by bilirubin deposition. Neuronal injury in the rostral midbrain and nuclear palsies can be explained by damage to the oculomotor nuclei.

> **ORGANS STAINED BY BILIRUBIN IN KERNICTERUS**
> - Basal Ganglia
> - Globus pallidus
> - Putamen
> - Caudate nucleus

The serum bilirubin level again varies to produce early symptoms in kernicterus. This can be called symptomatic levels displayed in the **Box 1**.

> **BOX 1:** Symptomatic levels for kernicterus.
> - *Term:* 25–30 mg/dL
> - *Rhesus:* 20–25 mg/dL
> - *Preterm:* 10 mg/dL

> **BOX 2:** Risk factors for kernicterus.
> - <2 weeks old
> - Displacement of bilirubin from albumin
> - Infection
> - Hypothermia
> - Excessive hemolysis
> - Rh incompatibility
> - Congenital spherocytosis
> - Prematurity
> - Acidosis
> - Asphyxia
> - Drugs—diazepam and sulfonamide
> - ABO incompatibility
> - Septicemia

The precise level of bilirubin at which brain damage occurs is uncertain. There are many other factors responsible for kernicterus. These are called risk factors and are placed in the **Box 2**.

Clinical Classification of Kernicterus

Kernicterus can be classified clinically as follows:
- *State I:* Decreased tone, lethargy, poor feeding, vomiting, and poor Moro reflex
- *State II:* Opisthotonus, seizures, fever, rigidity, and oculogyric crisis
- *State III:* Spasticity at about 1 week of age
- *State IV:* Late sequela

Biochemical and Biological Determinants of Bilirubin Encephalopathy

- *Bilirubin level:* In term babies, serum bilirubin should not be allowed to cross 25 mg/dL. There is no safe level in babies. Every attempt should be made to see that serum bilirubin level should not cross 1 mg/dL/100 mg.

- *Bilirubin-protein ratio:* Bilirubin-protein ratio of 3:5 or more may be associated with the development of bilirubin encephalopathy.
- *BBB:* Gestational immaturity, hypoxia, hypoglycemia, acidosis, birth injury, and septicemia.
- *Salicylate saturation index:* It determines the extent to which albumin is saturated with bilirubin. This can be assessed by displacement or addition of salicylate in vitro. A salicylate index of 8 or more is associated with bilirubin encephalopathy.

TREATMENT (TABLE 4)

Mechanisms and Principles

Hyperbilirubinemia can be treated by exchange transfusion, which removes bilirubin mechanically. Phototherapy, which converts bilirubin to products that can bypass the liver's conjugating system and be excreted in the bile or in the urine without further metabolism; and pharmacologic agents that interfere with heme degradation and bilirubin production, accelerate the normal metabolic pathways for bilirubin clearance or inhibit the enterohepatic circulation of bilirubin. Phototherapy is the most common treatment in use for hyperbilirubinemia; exchange transfusions generally are reserved for phototherapy failures. The bilirubin levels at which intervention is necessary are still a contentious issue.

Phototherapy

Phototherapy is thought to modify bilirubin deposited within the first few millimeters of the skin surface. It should not be used with a child with liver disease or obstructive type of jaundice. Because this causes the retention of products of phototherapy, this may cause bronze baby syndrome. In such a situation, the exchange transfusion is the safer method of treatment **(Box 3)**.

Indications for Phototherapy

- Abnormal rise in bilirubin level
- Prophylactic therapy in premature with jaundice
- Hemolytic disease in newborns impending for exchange transfusion
- Serum bilirubin >16–17 mg/dL on day 4
- Non-hemolytic type of jaundice with bilirubin level >15 mg/dL on day 4.

Laboratory investigations such as serum bilirubin can also be considered as a cut-off point for phototherapy.

Weight of the infant	Serum bilirubin level
- <1,500 g	- 5 mg/dL
- 1,500–2,000 g	- 8–12 g/dL
- 2,000–2,500 g	- 13–15 mg/dL
- Full term	- 15–20 mg/dL

TABLE 4: Management of hyperbilirubinemia in the healthy term and near-term newborn.

Age (h)	TSB level [mg/dL(mmol/L)]			
	Consider phototherapy	Phototherapy	Exchange transfusion if intensive phototherapy fails	Exchange transfusion and intensive phototherapy
≤24	—	—	—	—
25–48	≥12 (205)	≥15 (260)	≥20 (340)	≥25 (430)
49–72	≥15 (260)	≥18 (310)	≥25 (430)	≥30 (510)
≥72	≥17 (290)	≥20 (340)	≥25 (430)	≥30 (510)

> **BOX 3:** Factors that determine to dose of phototherapy.
> - Spectrum of light emitted
> - Irradiance of light source
> - Design of phototherapy unit
> - Surface area of an infant exposed to the light
> - Distance of infant from the light source

Mechanism of Action in Phototherapy

It helps to understand how phototherapy works if we consider that light is an infusion of discrete photons of energy that correspond to the individual molecules of a drug in a conventional medication. Absorption of these photons by bilirubin molecules in the skin leads to the therapeutic effect in much the same way as binding of drug molecules to a receptor has a desired effect.

Light Spectrum

The spectrum of light delivered by the phototherapy unit is determined by the type of light source and any filters used. Because of the optical properties of bilirubin and skin, the most effective lights are those with wavelengths that are predominantly in the blue-green spectrum.

Photoisomerization occurs when bilirubin is exposed to light. This occurs in the extravascular space of the skin. This leads to the conversion of bilirubin-to-bilirubin isomer, i.e., lumirubin. This isomer diffuses into the blood and is bound to albumin. Later it is transported to the liver. It is excreted with the bile in the bowel. Here it may be converted back into unconjugated bilirubin.

Intramolecular cyclization of bilirubin to lumirubin: It is rapidly excreted in the bile and urine. It is the most important pathway to lower serum bilirubin levels.

Photooxidation: Bilirubin is converted to pale colored product. They are excreted in urine.

Bilirubin absorbs the light in the 400–500 nm range. Irradiation in this range will be more effective. White lamps with peaks out at 425–475 nm are more effective. White lamps with peaks at 550–600 nm are also effective. The range of 380–700 nm white lamp is adequate for treatment.

Technique of Phototherapy

The source of light is four white lights and four blue lights. The length of the fluorescent lamp is 18 inches. These should be 45 cm above the infant. A shield made of plexiglass may be used. This screens out the wavelength below 300 nm. Hence, less harm to the child. Eyes and external genitalia should be covered by an eye patch and diaper. The posture of an infant should be changed every 2 hourly. The child should be weighed daily, extra fluid should be given. Bilirubin level should be monitored every 12th hourly. Once it begins to fall, the phototherapy can be stopped. Sometimes it may be restarted if the bilirubin level is not low.

Side effects of Phototherapy

Insensible water loss: This is more common among preterm infants. These children should be given extra fluid. The extra amount is 30 mL/kg/day. This may not be required in a full-term baby who is taking feeds well.
- *Hypocalcemia*
- *Loose green stool:* There will be increased fetal water loss. The cause is thought to be increased bile salts and unconjugated bilirubin in guts. This produces changes in the bacterial flora. Hence, these children should be fed with lactose-free until phototherapy is stopped.

- **Skin may be erythematous:** Because of the hyperemia or increased blood circulation
- **Retinal damage:** Occurs if the phototherapy is given without covering the eyes. This leads to visual defects.
- **Bronze baby syndrome:** This occurs if phototherapy is given to infants with obstructive jaundice. In obstructive jaundice, there will be an accumulation of the photoxidized isomerase, and this is called bronze baby syndrome.
- **Cellular damage:** Includes chromatid exchange and deoxyribonucleic acid (DNA) strand breakages. It may be necessary to cover the scrotum.

Phenobarbitone

The dose of phenobarbitone is 5–8 mg/kg/body weight every 24 hours. This induces microsomal enzymes in the liver. This increases bilirubin conjugation and excretion. It takes 3–7 days to become effective and may take much longer time in premature babies. Phenobarbitone can be used in type II Crigler–Najjar syndrome. It cannot be used for prophylactic purposes.

Contradictions of Phototherapy

- Significantly elevated direct bilirubin
- Family history of porphyrias
- Loss of rods and cones in the retina

Discontinue phototherapy once two TSB values 12 hours apart are below current age-specific cut-offs. The infant should be monitored clinically for rebound bilirubin rise within 24 hours for babies with hemolytic disorders.

Intravenous Immunoglobulin

The administration of intravenous immunoglobulin (IVIG) is an adjunctive treatment for hyperbilirubinemia caused by isoimmune hemolytic disease. Its use is recommended when serum bilirubin is approaching exchange levels despite maximal interventions, including phototherapy IVIG (0.5–1.0 g/kg/dose; repeat in 12 hours) reduces the need for exchange transfusion in both ABO and Rh hemolytic disease, presumably by reducing hemolysis.

Metalloporphyrins

A possible adjunct therapy is the use of metalloporphyrins for hyperbilirubinemia. The metalloporphyrin Sn-mesoporphyrin (SnMP) offers promise as a drug candidate. The proposed mechanism of action is competitive enzymatic inhibition of the rate-limiting conversion of hemeprotein to biliverdin (an intermediate metabolite in the production of unconjugated bilirubin) by hemeoxygenase. A single intramuscular dose on the first day of life may reduce the need for subsequent phototherapy. Complications from metalloporphyrins include transient erythema if the infant is receiving phototherapy. Administration of SnMP may reduce bilirubin levels and decrease both the need for phototherapy and the duration of hospital stay.

Exchange Transfusion (Table 5)

It reduces the level of bilirubin effectively. Indications for exchange transfusion are listed in the **Box 4**.

Serum bilirubin for exchange transfusion.

TABLE 5: Serum bilirubin for exchange transfusion.

Birth weight	Serum bilirubin
<1,250 g	13
1,250–1.499 g	15
1,500–1,999 g	17
2,000–2,499 g	18
>2,500 g	20

> **BOX 4:** Indications of exchange transfusion.
>
> - Severe nonhemolytic anemia
> - Septicemia with sclerema
> - Cord bilirubin level >5 mg
> - Chronic anemia
> - Disseminated intravascular coagulation
> - Hypoxemia in respiratory distress syndrome (RDS)
> - Cord hemoglobin level <10 mg/mL
> - Indirect serum bilirubin level 20 mg/100 mL
> - Acute renal hepatic failure

Types of Blood Used for Exchange Transfusion

The blood being used must be crossmatched with the mother's blood.

For Rh-isoimmunization: O-negative packed cells suspended in AB plasma or O-negative whole blood or Rh-negative baby's ABO group after crossmatch.

For ABO isoimmunization: O group (Rh-compatible) packed cell suspended in AB plasma or O group whole blood (Rh-compatible with baby) after crossmatch.

In other situations, the baby's blood group should be used.

The procedure will correct anemia and congestive cardiac failure (CCF) in hydrops. These children would have already received an intrauterine transfusion. The rebound of bilirubin after the exchange is expected because of sequestered sensitized RBCs and Hemolysis of transfused RBCs.

Technique

The sick neonate should be stable before starting an exchange transfusion. This includes control of asphyxia, hypoglycemia, acidosis, and temperature. A cardiac monitor and blood pressure cuff should be placed. An intravenous line is maintained for glucose and medications. Blood glucose, serum potassium, and pH should be measured.

If the umbilical cord is old and dried, it can be softened by soaking it in saline water for half an hour. This makes the insertion of the catheter easier. A catheter is inserted as far as required for free exchange. The position of the venous catheter should be left open for the risk of air embolism.

Purse string silk suture should be placed after the completion of the exchange transfusion. The tie around the cord should be tightened for 1 hour. This is to avoid necrosis of the skin. The venous catheter should be pulled out quickly to check the blood from the distal end.

If umbilical vein catheterization is not possible, exchange transfusion can be carried out by a central vein placed through the anterior cubital fossa.

It is a common practice to administer calcium during exchange transfusion to CPD anticoagulated blood. The citrate present in the blood can bind calcium and magnesium. This produces a decrease in these ions.

Albumin infusion has been proposed 1-2 hours before exchange transfusion. During the process, an attempt will be made to remove the bilirubin in a hastened way. Albumin may draw the tissue-bound bilirubin into the circulation.

Albumin should be administered with caution in infants with respiratory distress and congestive heart failure.

Isovolumetric exchange transfusion: It is done in a small sick and hydropic child. Here blood is pulled out of umbilical arteries and simultaneous blood is pushed in the umbilical vein.

Two-volume exchange: This usually involves double the blood volume of the infant's blood. The blood of an infant is 80 mL/kg; therefore, an exchange transfusion uses 160 mL/kg of the blood.

In the procedure, the blood is removed in aliquots that are tolerated by infants. The amount of blood removed depends upon the weight of the infants.
- 1,500 g: 5 mL
- 1,500–2,500 g: 10 mL
- 2,500–3,500 g: 15 mL
- 3,500 g or more: 20 mL

Blood volume removed by exchange:
- *Volume exchange:* 63%
- *Volume exchange:* 87%
- *Volume exchange:* 95%

Anemic sick children should be given partial exchange transfusion with packed cells, i.e., 25–80 mL/kg. This will raise hematocrit to 40%. The recommended time of exchange transfusion is 1 hour. Blood should be shaken well after every deciliter of exchange. This avoids the sedimentation of RBCs. Phototherapy should be continued after the exchange transfusion.

Complications of Exchange Transfusion
- Electrolyte imbalance
- *Cardiac problem:* Cardiac arrest, arrhythmias, and volume overload
- *Vascular:* Air embolism, thrombosis, infarction
- *Bleeding:* Thrombocytopenia, deficient clotting factor
- *Infection:* Septicemia, hepatitis, CMV, and acquired immunodeficiency syndrome (AIDS)
- *Metabolic:* Hypoglycemia, hypocalcemia, hypercalcemia, and acidosis

Potential complications from exchange transfusion are not trivial and include metabolic acidosis, electrolyte abnormalities, hypoglycemia, hypocalcemia, thrombocytopenia, volume overload, arrhythmias, NEC, infection, graft-versus-host disease, and death.

Various factors may influence the decision to perform a double-volume exchange transfusion in an individual patient. The appearance of clinical signs suggesting kernicterus is an indication for exchange transfusion at any level of serum bilirubin. A healthy full-term infant with physiologic or breast milk jaundice may tolerate a concentration slightly higher than 25 mg/dL with no apparent ill effect; whereas, kernicterus may develop in a sick premature infant at a significantly lower level A level approaching that considered critical for the individual infant may be an indication for exchange transfusion during the first or second day after birth, when a further rise is anticipated, but not typically after the fourth day in a term infant or after the seventh day in a preterm infant, because an imminent fall may be anticipated as the hepatic conjugating mechanism becomes more effective.

Supportive Treatment
- *Adequate feeding:* Hydration should be maintained, and hypoglycemia should be prevented. This is done by early feeding. Early feeding helps in the building up of bacterial flora. This reduces enterohepatic circulation.
- *Aspiration of cephalohematoma:* Cephalohematoma will also cause severe jaundice in newborns. Here aspiration of the cephalohematoma should be done, as it is the root cause of jaundice.
- *Treatment of sepsis and hepatitis:* Septicemia will present with jaundice in newborns. Septicemic work-up and treatment with suitable antibiotics should be done.

BIBLIOGRAPHY
1. American Academy of Pediatrics on Hyperbilirubinemia. Management of

hyperbilirubinemia in newborn infant 35 or more weeks of gestation. Pediatrics. 2004;114(1)297-316.
2. Bhutani VK, Johnson L. The jaundiced newborn in the emergency Department: Prevention of kernicterus. Clin Peditr Emerg Med. 2008,9(3):149-59.
3. Bhutani VK, Johnson L. Kernicterus in late preterm infants cared for as term healthy infants. Semin Perinatol. 2006,30(2): 89-97.
4. Gamaleldin R, Sampson PD, Seoud I, Aboraya H, Aravkin A, Sampson D, et al. Risk factors for neurotoxicity in newborns with severe neonatal hyperbilirubinemia. Pediatrics. 2011;128(4):e925-31.
5. Lauser BJ, Specter NJ. Hyperbilirubinemia in the newborn. Pediatr Rev. 2010;32(8):341-9.
6. Murki S, Kumar P. Blood exchange transfusion for infants with severe neonatal hyperbilirubinemia. Semin Perinatol. 2011;35(3): 175-84.

CASE 86

Normal Newborn

■ PRESENTING COMPLAINTS

A newborn child was brought for a general checkup.

History of Presenting Complaints

A newborn baby was brought to pediatric OPD for a general checkup. Mother had delivered the baby in a primary health center (PHC) in village. This baby was the first sibling of a consanguineous marriage. Mother had an antenatal checkup in the PHC. She was having regular checkups and had received immunization as per the advice. Antenatal health checkup investigations were within normal range.

She went to the PHC with delivery pain and there was drainage of the amniotic fluid, which was clear. She delivered vaginally with vertex presentation. The delivery was conducted by the nurse. Baby cried immediately after the delivery. Cry of the baby was good. Neonatal reflexes were satisfactory. Baby was put to the breast immediately. Baby started to take the feeds regularly. Later, the baby was sent to pediatric OPD the next day for general checkup.

■ EXAMINATION

Newborn child was moderately built and moderately nourished. Baby was active, alert, and crying. The anthropometric measurements included that the weight of the child was 3 kg (50th centile), length was 51 cm (75 centile), and the head circumference was 35 cm.

The child was afebrile, the heart rate was 140 beats per minute the respiratory rate was 24 breaths per minute. Blood pressure was 50/40 mm Hg. There was no pallor and acrocyanosis was present. There was no edema and no lymphadenopathy.

Neonatal reflexes were satisfactory. Anterior fontanelle was normal and skin and

---

CASE AT A GLANCE

Basic Findings
Weight	: 3 kg (50th centile)
Length	: 51 cm (75th centile)
Temperature	: 37°C
Pulse rate	: 140 beats/min
Respiratory rate	: 24 breaths/min
Blood pressure	: 50/40 mm Hg

Positive Findings

History:
- FTND
- Delivered in PHC
- Antenatal care was present

Examination:
- Normal child
- NNR satisfactory
- No evidence of congenital anomaly

Investigation:
- Normal

(FTND: full-term normal delivery; NNR: neonatal reflexes; PHC: primary health center)

spine were normal. There were no clinically evident congenital anomalies. The baby was appropriate for gestational age (AGA).

Cardiovascular system revealed the first and second heart sounds heard. No murmur is suggestive of congenital heart disease (CHD). Respiratory system revealed the presence of crepitation and rhonchi. Per abdomen examination showed mild distension of the abdomen. There was no significant organomegaly. Bowel sounds were normal.

■ INVESTIGATION

- *Hemoglobin:* 14 g/dL
- *TLC:* 12,3000 cells/mm^3
- *DLC:* $P_{72}L_{24}E_2M_2$
- *Blood culture and sensitivity:* Sterile
- *Urine culture sensitivity:* Sterile
- *Blood group and Rh typing:* O+ve
- *Chest X-ray:* No abnormality detected

■ DISCUSSION

It includes history taking and physical examination. History dates from the day of conception till the delivery and also a few days after the delivery. Birth history includes antenatal, natal, and postnatal events. Family history of other siblings should also be ascertained.

Antenatal history includes previous obstetric history and number of gravida and para. History suggestive of abortion and stillbirth should be sought. Chronic diseases of the mother such as cardiac disease, tuberculosis, and hypertension should be ascertained. History of any drug intake and antenatal investigation should be noted.

Natal history includes birth of the child. The mode of delivery, place of the delivery, presentation of the baby, and direction of the labor should be ascertained.

In postnatal history, birth asphyxia should be noted down. Apgar scoring at 1 minute and 5 minutes should be sought. History of passing of urine and meconium should be ascertained. Presence of jaundice and time of onset of jaundice should be noted.

The neonatal examination is best performed in an appropriately equipped, well-lit, warm, draft-free room, with the parents present. Examining the infant under a servo-controlled radiant warmer is an alternative. Thorough hand-washing before and after handling each infant is essential to prevent the spread of pathogenic organisms, and if the infant has not had a first bath, gloves should be worn.

Isolated minor congenital anomalies are quite common, with some studies reporting these in as many as so of the newborn population, but the presence of three or more increases the risk of the infant having a syndrome. Evidence of trauma in a part of the baby should lead to a search for trauma in other areas, particularly in large infants and in infants who underwent difficult deliveries such as breech or forceps delivery. It is also important to be able to distinguish malformations from deformations as the etiology and management differ.

Gestational Age Assessment

The infant's gestational age should be estimated and body size should be compared with appropriate normal standards. There are several ways to estimate gestational age, including reliable maternal history, prenatal ultrasound scan performed before 20 weeks of gestation, and physical examination of the infant's skin, external genitalia, ears, breasts, and neuromuscular behavior **(Table 1)**. Infants are classified as preterm (born at <37 completed weeks of gestation), early term (37–38 weeks), term (39–41 weeks), and post-term (>42 weeks).

TABLE 1: Gestational age assessment.

Score	−1	0	1	2	3	4	5
Skin	Sticky, friable, and transparent	Gelatinous, red, and translucent	Smooth pink and visible veins	Superficial peeling and/or rash, few veins	Cracking pale areas, rare veins	Parchment-deep, cracking, no vessels	Leathery, cracked, and wrinkled
Lanugo	None	Sparse	Abundant	Thinning	Bald areas	Mostly bald	
Plantar surface	Heel–toe 40–50 mm: 1	<50 mm, no crease	Faint red marks	Anterior transverse crease only	Creases anterior 2–3	Creases over the entire sole	
Breast	Imperceptible	Barely perceptible	Flat areola no bud	Stippled areola 1–2 mm bud	Raised areola 3–4 mm bud	Full areola 5–10 mm bud	
Eye/ear	Lids fused: loosely: −1 and Tightly: −2	Lids open, pinna flat, stays folded	Slightly curved pinna, soft slow recoil	Well-curved pinna, soft but ready recoil	Formed and firm, instant recoil	Thick cartilage, ear stiff	
Genitals (male)	Scrotum flat, smooth	Scrotum empty, faint rugae	Testes in upper canal, rare rugae	Testes descending, few rugae	Testes down good rugae	Testes pendulous, deep rugae	
Genitals (female)	Clitoris prominent	Prominent clitoris, small labia minora	Prominent clitoris enlarging minora	Majora and minora equally prominent	Majora large, minora small	Majora covers clitoris and minora	

Birth weight, head circumference, and length should be measured. Length is measured from vertex to heel with the infant's legs fully extended. These measurements are then compared for gestational age against standard population-based growth charts. An infant is considered to be AGA if the birth weight for gestational age falls between the 10th and 90th percentile. 20% of infants with serious congenital malformations are small for gestational age.

Two methods that are commonly used clinically for the assessment of gestational age are: (1) Parkin method and (2) the new Ballard method.

Gestational age assessment again depends on skin texture, skin color, breast size, and breast firmness.

Skin Texture

Skin texture is tested by picking up the fold of abdominal skin between fingers and thumb and inspecting it.
- *Score 0:* Very thin and gelatinous feel
- *Score 1:* Thin and smooth
- *Score 3:* Slight thickening and stiff feeling
- *Score 4:* Thick and parchment-like with superficial or deep cracking

Skin Color

- *Score 0:* Dark red
- *Score 1:* Uniformly pink
- *Score 2:* Pale pink
- *Score 3:* Pale

Breast Size

Breast size is measured by feeling the breast nodule by finger and thumb.
- *Score 0:* No breast tissue palpable
- *Score 1:* Not >0.5 cm in diameter
- *Score 2:* 0.5–1 cm in diameter
- *Score 3:* >1 cm in diameter.

Ear Firmness

Ear firmness is tested by palpation and folding of the upper pinna and notching and recoiling.

Score 0: Pinna feels soft and is easily folded in a bizarre position without springing back into position spontaneously.

Score 1: Pinna feels softer along the edge and easily folded and returns slowly to the correct position spontaneously.

Score 3: Pinna feels firm with definite cartilage extending up to the periphery and springs back immediately into the position after being folded.

The maturity rating is calculated as given in the **Tables 2 and 3**.

GENERAL PHYSICAL EXAMINATION

All the babies should, however, be examined in more detail by a pediatrician preferably within 24 hours. The baby should be at least 6 hours old before the preliminary detailed examination. However, the examination of

TABLE 2: Maturity rating—Parkin method.

Parkin score	Age (in weeks)
1	26
2	30
3	33
4	34
5	35
6	36
7	37
8	38
9	39
10	40
11	41
12	42

TABLE 3: Maturity rating—Ballard method.

Ballard score	Age (in weeks)
–10	20
–5	22
0	24
5	26
10	28
15	30
20	32
25	34
30	36
35	38
40	40
45	42
50	44

BOX 1: Normal vital data of newborn.

- *Core temperature:* 36.5–37°C
- *Respiratory rate:* 40 breaths per minute
- *Heart rate:* 120–140 beats per minute
- *Blood pressure:* 60/40 mm Hg

the child should be conducted usually three times:
1. At birth
2. After 24 hours
3. At the time of discharge

The main objective of the examination is to screen hidden abnormalities of the heart, abdomen, and hips and reassure parents about the minor abnormalities and normal variants. Mother should always be at the bedside so that she is allowed to express her concern. As soon as the baby is delivered, he/she should be taken in a prewarmed baby tray. Cord is clamped and cut. Baby should never be kept naked for >1 minute.

Once the respiratory status of the child is settled, then the routine examination of the child is designed to assess the general status of health and to detect the hidden congenital anomalies.

Much of the time is devoted to inspection of the child. It includes awareness and activity of the child. Peripheral cyanosis is normal in newborns, but central cyanosis will indicate cardiac or respiratory disease. Cyanosis in the mucous membrane is more reliable in dark neonates. Presence of jaundice in the first 24 hours is pathological and should be investigated.

Vernix caseosa, a greasy cheese-like material that disappears after a few hours is present at the folds of the neck and groin. Newborns will have extremely smooth skin. Thin gelatinous skin is seen in preterm babies. Dry and cracked skin which tends to peel is seen in postmature child. An abnormally high-pitched cry indicates central nervous system (CNS) insult. Weak and feeble cry should be investigated.

Next, anthropometric measurements of the neonate should be done. These include length, weight, head circumference, chest circumference, and upper segment and lower segment ratio. These vital parameters indicate the status of the neonate. The normal ranges are given in the **Box 1**.

After glancing through the inspectory findings and recording the vital parameters, any clues regarding congenital anomalies in the baby should be looked for. History suggestive of the amount of the amniotic fluid should be ascertained. Polyhydramnios in the mother is associated with upper intestinal obstruction like esophageal atresia and duodenal atresia. Oligohydramnios is associated with bilateral renal agenesis and obstructive uropathy.

Incidences of congenital anomalies are common among preterm babies. Usually, one congenital anomaly will be associated with other congenital anomalies. Hypoplastic type of small-for-the-date babies are prone to have congenital anomalies.

Single umbilical artery is usually associated with imperforate anus, genitourinary abnormalities, and esophageal atresia. Asymmetry of the face occurs as a result of congenital hypoplasia of depressor anguli oris muscle. Single palmar crease is seen in Down syndrome. Potency of all the orifices and midline abnormalities should be seen.

Heart should be examined when the child is calm. Some systolic murmurs are common during the first 48 hours. Breath sounds are equal and clear on both sides. Faint crepitations heard are due to retained lung fluids. These are absorbed spontaneously. Coarse crepitations are due to loose secretion in the upper airway and throat.

REGIONAL PHYSICAL EXAMINATION

Head

The shape and symmetry of the newborn vary considerably. Many factors are responsible for these variabilities. These include intrauterine position and pressure, presentation at the time of the delivery, and the amount of molding during labor and delivery. The shape returns to normal within 3 days.

Babies born by vertex vaginal delivery will have some overriding or overlapping of the sutures. Caput succedaneum and cephalohematoma may be encountered **(Figs. 1 and 2)**. One should be able to feel all the sutures in the baby's head. Sutural separation should also be examined. Normally, sutural separation will not be >0.5 cm. Plagiocephaly is due to the flattening of the occiput and opposite frontal region. Head is lengthened in mentovertical axis with vertex and fronto-occipital axis in breech presentation.

The head shape of newborns is influenced by their presentation in utero. After vertex presentation and vaginal delivery, infants demonstrate pronounced vertical elongation of the head referred to as molding. Breech infants often have occipital–frontal head elongation, with a prominent occipital shelf.

The cranial sutures should be palpably open and may be separated by up to several millimeters at birth. Temporary overlap of bones, due to molding, should be distinguished from craniosynostosis (premature closure of a suture). If a suture

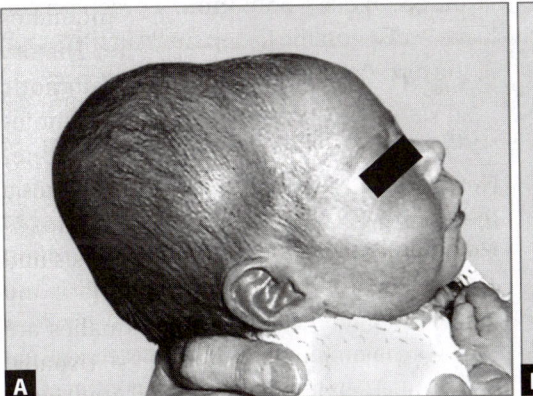
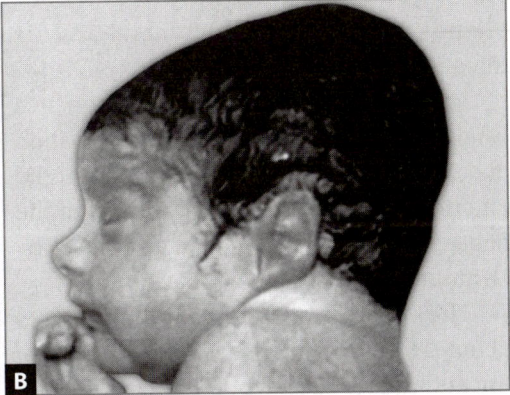

Figs. 1A and B: Caput succedaneum.

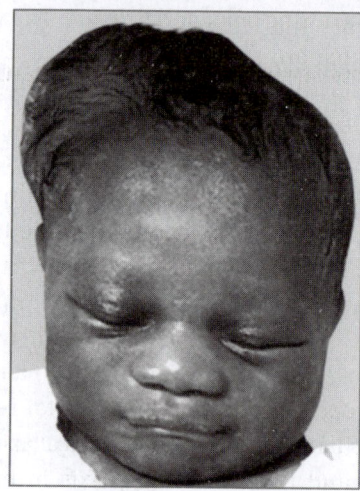

Fig. 2: Cephalohematoma.

Transillumination of the head is performed as a screening test in a baby with an unusually large and asymmetrically shaped head. This is done before performing more accurate forms of intracranial diagnosis.

Transillumination test will be positive when there is increased amount of fluid in subarachnoid, subdural, or ventricular space. The condition includes severe hydrocephalus, chronic subdural hematoma or effusion, and hydranencephaly. A bulging or tense fontanelle, with separation of the bony sutures, indicates increased intracranial pressure. A circular hematoma may be seen at the site of application of a vacuum extractor.

closes in utero, it prevents growth of the skull perpendicular to the fused suture line, resulting in a sustained, abnormal skull configuration. In contrast, after molding occurs, the bones return to their normal positions in a few days, sometimes with a small concomitant decrease in head circumference.

Fontanelle is the depression between the skull bones and is covered by connective tissue. The gap may disappear if there is an overlapping of bones due to molding. This should be differentiated from the craniosynostosis. There will be ridges in craniosynostosis. Usually there are six fontanelle at birth.

Anterior fontanelle is flat or concave when the baby is held in an upright position and when the child is quiet. The size of the anterior fontanelle usually admits tip of the finger. It varies from 3 to 4 cm and closes by 18 months. It is sometimes pulsatile.

The posterior fontanelle measures about 0.5–4 cm and closes by 3–4 months. Encephalocele and depressed fracture are rare findings.

Face

The newborn's face may indicate the presence of a dysmorphic syndrome. There may be obvious malformations, such as cleft lip or a small mandible (micrognathia). Intrauterine position may cause asymmetry in the face. Pressure over the stylomastoid foramen during labor may cause peripheral facial paralysis, which is obvious during crying. The paralysis usually resolves and should be distinguished from congenital absence of the depressor anguli oris muscle, which also results in asymmetric crying facies **(Fig. 3)**. Fracture of the zygomatic arch can occur and is detectable by palpation. Forceps often leave bruises on the face, usually in the shape of the forceps blade.

Eyes

Newborns generally open their eyes when they are awake, held upright, and shaded from bright light. An infant who is quiet and alert will fix on the examiner's face and follow it.

The normal appearance of eyes should be established. Eyelids are usually puffy and swollen at the time of birth. Eyes should

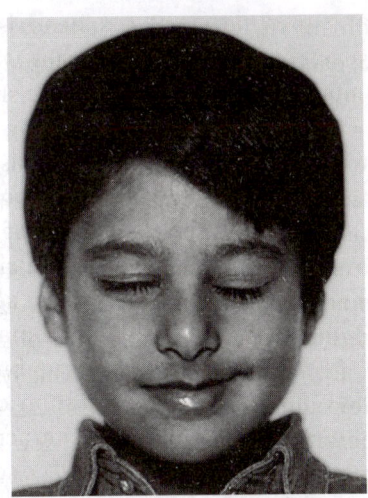

Fig. 3: Bell's palsy.

never be attempted to open. This maneuver will be many a times unsuccessful. The main ingredient in success is patience. If the baby is in a quiet and alert state, it may open its eyes spontaneously. Then baby may fix gaze on the examiner. Baby will follow the examiner through an area of at least 90°. This along with presence of bilateral red reflex gives good first-line assurance about baby's vision. Babies open their eyes when they are being fed. Eye movements are not fully coordinated at birth. Babies may have strabismus because of conjugate movement of the eyes in young infants. This is only intermittent. Fundoscopy is not done routinely in newborns. This is limited to those in whom there is a specific concern of the eyes, such as prematurity, and congenital infections, like rubella or CMV.

It is mandatory to look at the pupil through the fundoscope from a distance to see the red reflex. This is done by looking straight on the pupil from a few feet away. Bright red and orange glow of the pupils is the reflection of the light from the back of the retina. In congenital cataract, pupil will appear dull grey rather than bright orange.

Ophthalmoscopic examination should be performed in newborn infants prior to their discharge. One holds the ophthalmoscope close to the examiner's eye with the lens power set at 0. In a dark room, light is allowed to project simultaneously in both eyes and then individually from 18 inches away. It should begin by focusing on the anterior portion of the eye and then progressing back to the retina. This allows detection of anterior lesions, such as cataracts and colobomas of the iris. In fair babies, a red reflex is transmitted back through the lens, whereas in darker-skinned infants, a pale orange-tan color may be seen. It should be symmetrical in color and intensity. Visualizing retinal vessels verifies focusing on the retina. A diminished or absent red reflex suggests a cataract or other opacities. A white pupillary reflex is abnormal and may occur with a large retinoblastoma or developmental abnormalities such as retinal coloboma, retinopathy of prematurity, and persistent hypoplastic primary vitreous.

Birth trauma may cause subconjunctival hemorrhages or hemorrhages in the anterior chamber, vitreous, and retina. Forceps deliveries can result in lacerations of the lid or globe. A rupture of the Descemet membrane in the cornea may result in corneal clouding.

Ears

At term, the ears are well formed and contain sufficient cartilage to retain a normal shape and resist deformation. Gently pulling the pinna back and down aids examination of the ear canal and tympanic membrane. An alert, normal newborn will turn toward human speech and startle to a loud noise, which is considered a crude estimate of hearing.

Nose

The main aim of examining nose is to assess the patency of both nares. Patency can be established by blocking one nostril and then the other with a finger while the baby's mouth is closed. Air movement in each nostril is heard either directly or by stethoscope. Nasal stuffiness can occur as a result of retained mucus or trauma but could also suggest drug withdrawal.

In a suspected case of choanal atresia or stenosis, a soft catheter is passed through the passage. A baby with bilateral choanal atresia usually presents with respiratory distress and cyanosis. Distress and cyanosis will be relieved when the baby opens the mouth or while crying.

Mouth

Examination of the mouth includes inspection and palpation. A cleft palate **(Fig. 4)** may not be seen but may be detectable by palpation; a cleft uvula should raise suspicion of a palatal defect. Small, shiny white masses on the gums (epithelial pearls) are common. White Epstein pearls are found in the midline on the roof of the mouth, at the junction of the hard and soft palate. A ranula is a small benign mass (i.e., mucocele) that arises from the floor of the mouth. A high-arched or narrow palate is found in many dysmorphic syndromes.

The tongue **(Fig. 5)** may be attached to a short central frenulum (i.e., ankyloglossia). An enlarged or protruding tongue can be seen with hemangiomas, isolated macroglossia, hypothyroidism, or in Down and Beckwith syndromes. A normal, awake newborn will usually suck vigorously on a finger placed in the mouth. Natal teeth, if present, usually erupt in the lower incisor position. These can either be supernumerary teeth or true, deciduous milk teeth. If they are very loose or cause painful breastfeeding, they may be removed.

Some newborns will have some mucus or saliva drooling from their mouth in the first few hours of the birth. This occurs as a result of swallowing amniotic fluid and regurgitating the stomach contents.

Bluish retention cyst is present on the floor of the mouth. Sucking blisters are found on lips. Glossoptosis is the potential cause of airway obstruction.

Neck

The neck of the newborn should have a full range of motion; limitation may indicate an

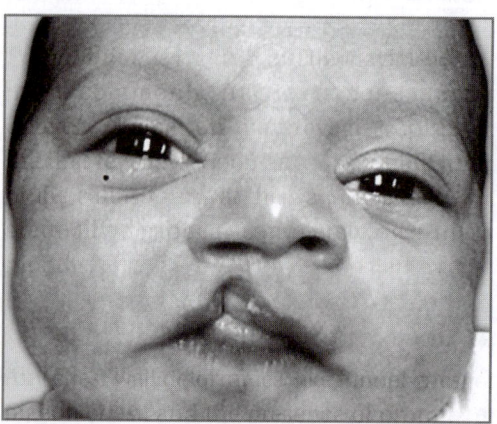

Fig. 4: Cleft lip.

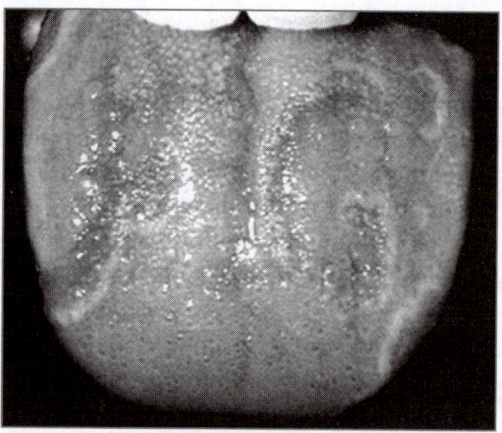

Fig. 5: Geographic tongue.
(For color version, see Plate 6)

abnormality of the cervical spine. Cervical masses, such as a goiter, cavernous hemangioma, or cystic hygroma **(Figs. 6A and B)**, may compress the trachea and cause inspiratory obstruction. Branchial cleft anomalies **(Fig. 6C)** include cysts or sinuses along the anterior edge of the sternocleidomastoid muscle **(Fig. 6D)**. Thyroglossal duct cysts **(Figs. 7A and B)** usually occur in the ventral midline. Torticollis is seen with a tightened sternocleidomastoid muscle on one side and an atretic sternocleidomastoid muscle on the side toward which the head is turned; facial asymmetry is a common accompaniment.

Lateral traction during delivery may damage the upper root of the brachial plexus (C5 or C6 vertebra), resulting in paralysis of the shoulder and arm. The arm is held alongside the body in internal rotation (i.e., Duchenne–Erb paralysis) **(Figs. 8A and B)**. The lower root of the brachial plexus (C8 or T1 vertebra) may be damaged, particularly during breech delivery. When this occurs, the small muscles of the hand are paralyzed, resulting in the absence of a grasp reflex (i.e., Klumpke paralysis). When there is neck trauma, the cervical sympathetic nerves may be damaged (i.e., Horner syndrome), and the phrenic nerve may be injured, causing diaphragmatic paralysis.

Neck will be usually short in the newborn and fibroma of the sternocleidomastoid muscle, thyroglossal cyst, dermoid cyst, and cystic hygroma are differential diagnoses of swelling of the neck.

Thyroid areas should be examined thoroughly to rule out thyroid swelling, especially if the mother is taking iodides

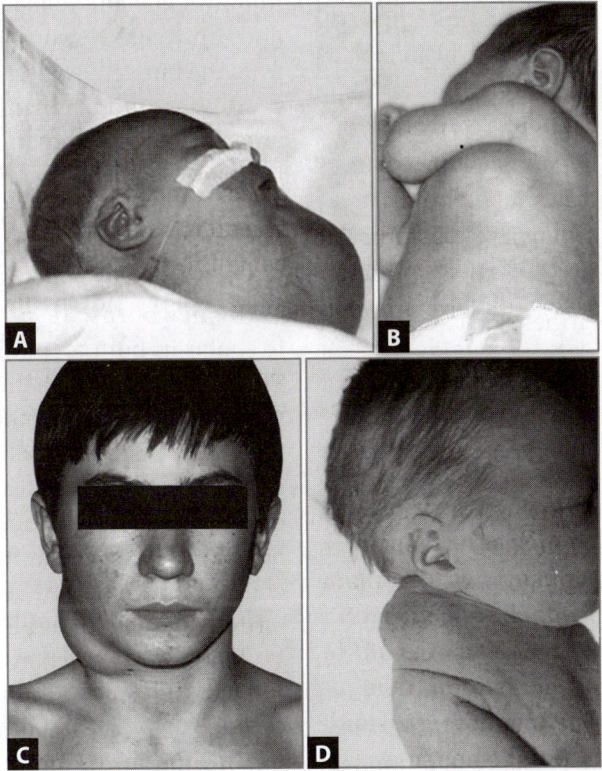

Figs. 6A to D: (A and B) Cystic hygroma; (C) Branchial cyst; (D) Sternocleidomastoid muscle tumor.

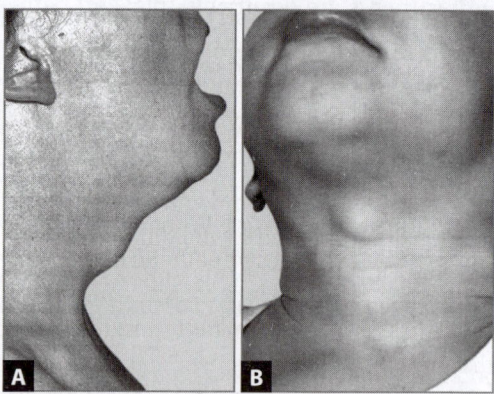

Figs. 7A and B: (A) Thyroglossal cyst on elevation; (B) Thyroglossal cyst.

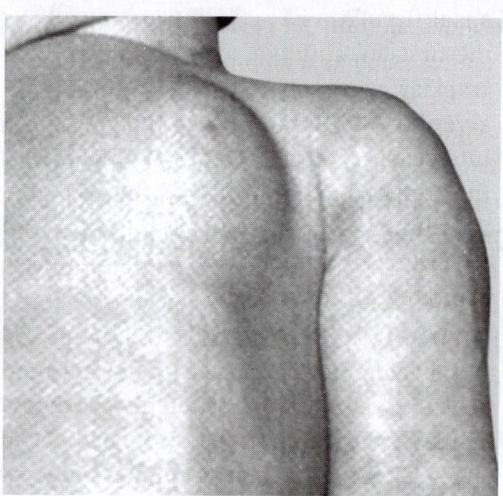

Fig. 9: Breast engorgement—newborn.

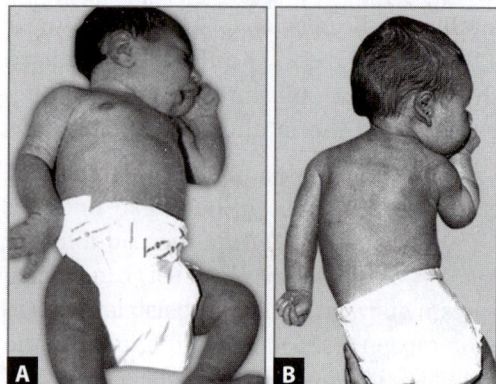

Figs. 8A and B: Erb's palsy.

during pregnancy or if there is a family history of thyroid disease.

Palpation of the clavicle: The clavicle is the most commonly fractured bone during delivery. Palpation may reveal crepitus in the first few days. Soon after, a sizeable lump of the callus forms at the fracture site. It will gradually disappear completely over many months.

Chest

Any chest wall deformities, like funnel chest or pigeon chest, and the presence of prominent xiphisternum are noted. Position, contour, and form of the nipple or the presence of accessory nipple should be looked for. Enlargement of the breast **(Fig. 9)** may occur in both male and female infants during 3rd and 4th week. Newborns may secrete milk from the nipple.

Ribs are more horizontal with increasing anteroposterior diameter of the chest. This limits the movements of the thoracic cage, the descent of the diaphragm, the abdominal controls, and pushes the abdominal wall forward.

In newborns, respiration is normally irregular in both amplitude and frequency. This is associated with the pauses lasting <10 seconds. Irregular breathing pattern is more marked in premature babies. The respiratory rate average is 30–40 breaths per minute in a resting full-term baby. Breath sounds should be heard well in the front and the back, few crackles may be heard immediately after the birth within a few hours.

Intercostal retractions are normal during the first few minutes after birth. Thereafter, they are usually a sign of increased inspiratory effort from noncompliant lungs or airway obstruction. Mild expiratory grunting, nasal flaring, and tachypnea occur during the first few minutes after birth. Scattered crackles caused by residual retained intra-alveolar lung fluid often clear rapidly. Intercostal indrawing is very common among the preterm babies because of the softness of the ribs.

Overinflated chest is seen in meconium-aspirated newborns.

When the airway is obstructed or the lungs are stiff, the abdomen appears to enlarge and the chest cage appears to get smaller with inspiration (i.e., thoracoabdominal asynchrony). Persistence or worsening of respiratory symptoms may indicate more serious problems.

Cardiovascular System

The point of maximal cardiac impulse is at the fourth to fifth intercostal space and medial to the midclavicular line on the left side of the chest. This may be displaced if there is a pneumothorax or space-occupying lesion.

The heart rate may be 160–180 beats per minute during the first few hours after birth. Thereafter, the normal awake heart rate averages 120–130 beats/min. Occasionally, a normal newborn infant may have a heart rate of 80 beats/min, which may tall transiently to 60 beats/min for short periods.

It will vary when the child is crying and taking feeds. Occasional extra systoles are common. The two heart sounds are usually equal in intensity. The normal variation of the width of the split in the second sound with the respiration may be difficult to appreciate because the respiratory or heart rate is rapid.

Despite the rapid heart rate, heart sounds can be clearly distinguished. The pulmonic component of the second sound may be prominent on the 1st day. The splitting of the second sound is audible along the left upper and mid sternum. While postnatal circulatory adjustments are occurring, transient benign murmurs can be heard over the pulmonic area or cardiac apex. Murmurs and other physical signs such as cyanosis, poor perfusion, tachypnea, difficulty in palpating pulses, or brachiofemoral delay require further evaluation.

Sometimes, in the first few days, it is common to hear soft precordial systolic murmurs. This is probably due to flow through ductus arteriosus that remains patent immediately after the birth. This closes gradually over the hours or days. Cardiac murmur heard during the first 48 hours can be transient or a significant murmur.

Criteria for significant murmur.
- Loud grade III murmur—abnormal second heart sound
- Associated ejection click

Cyanosis in neonates indicates hypoxemia. It is due to the shunting of the venous blood from pulmonary to systemic circulation, i.e., right-to-left shunt.

Radial and femoral pulses should be palpated and compared to the other side. Absence of femoral pulse and brachiofemoral delay indicates the coarctation of the aorta.

Abdomen

Infants often have abdomens that are bulging at the sides but they should be soft. History of maternal polyhydramnios should raise concern for possible intestinal obstruction. A gap between the abdominal rectus muscles in the midline (i.e., diastasis recti) **(Fig. 10)**, most noticeable with crying, is quite common. There is also often a small defect in the periumbilical musculature of the anterior abdominal wall, which may allow an umbilical hernia; this usually closes as the muscles develop toward the end of the 1st year.

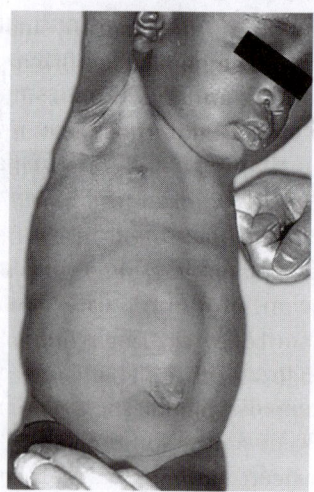

Fig. 10: Diastasis recti.

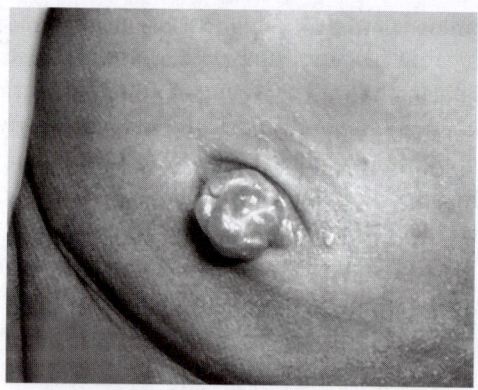

Fig. 11: Umbilical granuloma.
(For color version, see Plate 6)

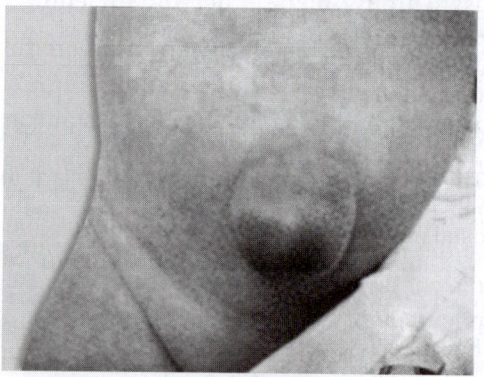

Fig. 12: Umbilical hernia.

The umbilical cord should be inspected for a number of vessels present in it. Shrinkage of the cord with drying occurs rapidly after the birth as a result of the closure of umbilical arteries. This produces deprivation of the blood supply to tissues.

The umbilical cord normally contains two arteries and one vein, with the vein being larger than the arteries. Approximately 1% of newborns have a single umbilical artery, and 15% of these have one or more congenital anomalies, usually involving the nervous, gastrointestinal, genitourinary, pulmonary, or cardiovascular systems.

The umbilical cord usually falls off between 10 and 14 days, releasing a small amount of opaque, yellowish discharge. Delayed separation of the cord, past 3 weeks, often occurs in infants with defective phagocyte function. Application of local antiseptics prevents the delay in separation. A discharge from the cord stump should exclude an infant with persistent urachus. Umbilical granuloma is a firm tissue present at the site of separation **(Fig. 11)**. This has to be distinguished from the polyp in the persistent part of mesenteric duct. This requires surgical removal. Cord granuloma can be treated with copper sulfate granule application.

In an intrauterine growth-retarded baby, the cord is often thin and stingy with little Wharton's jelly. In a baby who has been bathed in meconium in utero for more than a few hours, the cord may be stained green.

Umbilical hernia may be present at birth **(Fig. 12)**. It is more common among preterm and LBW babies. Gastroschisis or omphalocele can occur due to the diversification of recti.

Inguinal hernia **(Fig. 13)** occurs, when tissue such as part of intestine protrudes through weak part of inguinal canal.

Palpation of the abdomen is simple during the feed, but care must be taken not to cause vomiting.

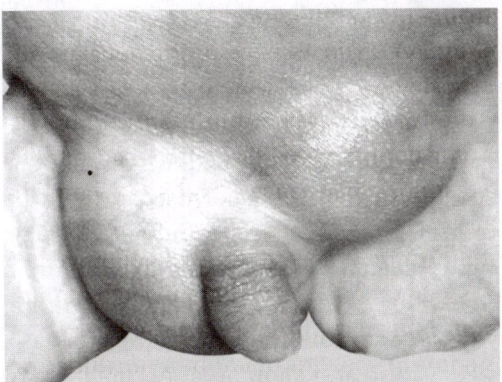

Fig. 13: Bilateral inguinal hernia.

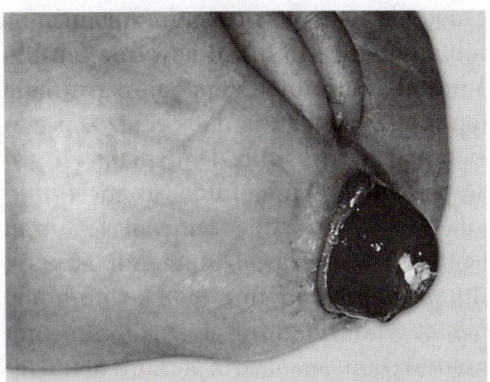

Fig. 14: Rectal prolapse. *(For color version, see Plate 6)*

Liver
Normally, the liver is palpable in epigastrium. Poorly defined liver edge is palpable in the right upper quadrant by applying the thumb or fingers gently to the surface of the skin. The edge is normally felt 1–2 cm below the right costal margin in the mid-axillary line.

Spleen
The spleen may or may not be palpable in a newborn. It is enlarged more laterally than in the older children. Tip points to the left rather than the right loin. The ability to palpate the tip of the spleen on deep inspiration is not always an indication of abnormality. But this should be considered along with other findings. Palpation should also include a search for unusual masses.

Kidneys
The renal examination is easiest on the 1st day before the bowel is filled with gas. The lower portion of each kidney is normally palpable on each side and the lateral and lower edges can be felt above the level of the umbilicus and lateral to the midclavicular line. During the 3rd day, only the lower pole is palpable. The right kidney is situated slightly lower than the left kidney, and the palpable portion of the kidney normally feels about 2 cm wide. Unless they are enlarged and the abdomen is unusually soft, bladder is usually palpable in infancy.

Anus
A thorough examination is required to confirm anal patency, as an imperforate anus is not always obvious on inspection. A normal-appearing anal dimple can exist with no opening. A fistula that opens onto the perineum, ventral to the normal anus, may also accompany the imperforate anus. However, this fistula will not have the radiating skin creases of a normal anus. Presence of meconium on the perineum and perianal area does not rule out imperforate anus; meconium in the anal area may have been passed by way of the skin fistula or, in a girl, a fistula from the rectum to the vagina.

Rectal prolapse (**Fig. 14**) in which rectum starts to push through the anus. This is seen in malnutrition and whooping cough.

Genitalia
Genitalia examination will help to estimate the gestational age. In males, glans penis is normally covered completely by prepuce that should not be fully retracted. Penile foreskin

is adherent. Normally, urine should pass in full stream without ballooning the prepuce.

Identification of the urethral opening is important. Hooded prepuce is present with hypospadias.

Scrotum is best examined with a quiet baby and warm hand. Scrotum is usually large as it is the embryonic analog of the tibia of a female. Scrotum in a full-term boy is pendulous and rugosity is well formed. It may be more pigmented than the rest of the skin.

Both the gonads should be palpable and capable of being brought into the scrotum. The testes should be completely descended. The normal testis is 1–2 cm long and both the testes should be identical in size, neither soft nor hard in consistency.

Hydrocele **(Fig. 15)** *of the tunica vaginalis:* Small collection of fluid disappears within a few days if it is communicating type. A large collection of fluid around the cord leads to hernia.

In preterm female infants, separation of the labia majora may give the illusion that the clitoris is enlarged. In term female infants, the labia majora meet in the midline, covering the rest of the genitalia. It is important to identify the urethra, which is just below the clitoris, and the vagina as distinct orifices; a single orifice or urogenital sinus is abnormal.

In female newborns, genitalia will have relatively large labia majora, that cover and occlude the labia minora and vaginal introitus. Considerable thick vaginal discharge may be present, especially on the 2nd and 3rd day. Minor bleeding is also noted. This is normal unless there is more blood loss in the urine. Mucosal tag from the wall of the vagina is seen. These are common abnormalities. In girls, clitoris is prominent. If the infant is premature, labia minora is also seen covered by labia majora. In case of ambiguous genitalia, a chromosomal analysis should be done.

Ambiguous genitalia is a term that encompasses a wide range of findings such as enlargement of the clitoris and varying degrees of labial fusion in females or micropenis, hypospadias with bifid scrotum, and cryptorchidism in males. As the distinction between a male and female can often be difficult, the assistance of a pediatric endocrinologist is warranted. In such situations, it may be prudent to avoid assigning a sex until further investigation.

Extremities

Upper limb abnormalities of the hands are common features of dysmorphism. Number of the fingers and toes and the presence of syndactyly should be looked and noted. Slight syndactyly of the second and third toes is a common minor congenital anomaly.

Traumatic injuries to the limbs can occur as a consequence of intrauterine positioning and delivery. These include fractures in the shaft of the femur, humerus, or clavicles and injury to the brachial plexus, causing paralysis of the hand and arm.

It is important to be able to distinguish normal variations in joint positions from

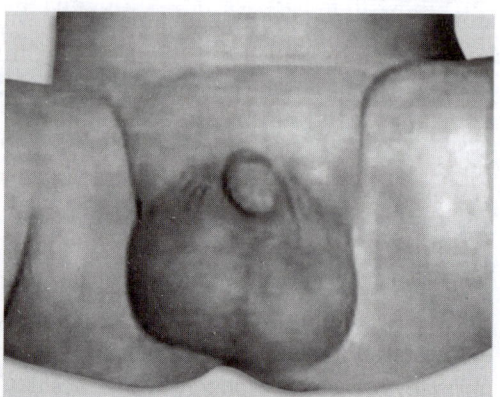

Fig. 15: Congenital hydrocele.

joints that are deformed. As a rule, if simple manual pressure will correct a deformed joint back to its neutral position, then corrective positioning or simple exercise and stretching will correct the deformity. If the deformity cannot be corrected by gentle pressure, orthopedic evaluation is needed.

With the hips flexed to 90° angle, the legs normally can be abducted until the knees and touch the table the infant is lying on. If this cannot be done, there may be developmental dysplasia of the hip. Female infants constrained in a breech position in utero are at a higher risk. In this condition, the head of the femur is displaced posteriorly, out of the acetabular fossa. The affected leg may appear shorter. The examiner will feel a click when abducting and adducting the hips in about 10% of all infants. However, only 10% of infants with hip clicks have developmental dysplasia of the hip. The Ortolani and Barlow maneuvers can test for a dislocatable hip.

Malformations of the limbs are often obvious **(Figs. 16A and B)**. Often, limb abnormalities are indicators of underlying genetic syndromes. The notable exceptions are those associated with traumatic amputation from amniotic band syndrome. These intrauterine constriction bands may amputate the digits or cause localized edema by obstructing lymphatic drainage.

Rudimentary skin tags at the lateral border of either the fifth finger or toe may represent rudimentary supernumerary digits. Extra-long nails are common in post-term infants.

Most normal newborns have slight bowing of legs. This disappears gradually as the child gets older. This reflects intrauterine position.

Postural talipes should be differentiated from true talipes. Postural type can always be straightened. It usually reverts to normal within few weeks.

Back

Spine: The spine of the newborn is quite flexible in both the dorsoventral and lateral axes; restricted movement suggests vertebral anomalies. The entire length of the spine, including the sacrum, should be palpated for bony defects and asymmetries. A midline abnormality of the skin over the spine, such as a small dimple, tufts of hair, or a pilonidal sinus, may indicate an occult spina bifida, or a diastematomyelia (i.e., a division of the spinal cord into two parts, which may become tethered as the child grows). Neural tube defects (i.e., meningocele and myelomeningocele) and tumors of the spine (i.e., teratomas) also may be present at birth.

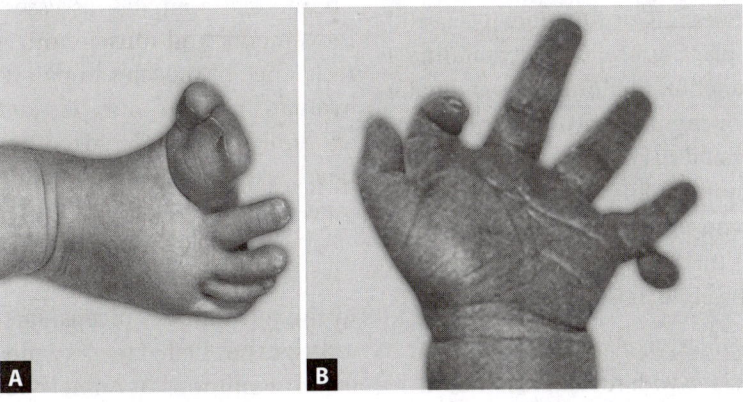

Figs. 16A and B: (A) Polydactyly and syndactyly; (B) Extra digit.

Back is completely examined till the natal cleft. Congenital defects in the dorsal surface may give clues for internal anomalies. Pilonidal sinus is a common finding present. This may disappear gradually and has no special significance.

Any hemangioma, lipoma, or tuft of hair that crosses the midline of the lower back has a high probability of internal structural spinal abnormalities.

Neural tube defects may be small but they are always on the midline. It is the common site for stroke bite, midline hairy nevus, and spina bifida. Any fixed deformity should be ruled out such as kyphosis and scoliosis. Sacrococcygeal teratoma is seen immediately posterior to anus. 4% of them are malignant.

Truncal tone is assessed by supporting the baby with left hand. The right hand is used to steady the back. In case of floppy baby, child remains like ragdoll. The spine and limbs are normally flexed, but there may be a momentary extension of the neck. This is called ventral suspension.

Nervous System

Interpretation of neurologic signs in a newborn infant requires knowledge of normal development because maturational changes parallel an increase in the level and complexity of neurologic function. It is useful to retain the basic approach in evaluating a neurologic function, including a systematic assessment of mental status (i.e., level of alertness), cranial nerve function, the motor and sensory systems, and the evoked reflexes.

The nervous system starts with the sensorium of the child. It is, otherwise, the alertness of the child. It is classified as:

State of wakefulness in a neonate:
State I: Deep sleep with regular respiration
State II: Light sleep with regular respiration
State III: Eyes open with no gross body movements
State IV: Eyes open with gross body movements
State V: Eyes open or closed and crying.

BEHAVIOR OF THE NEWBORN INFANT

Mental status examination consists of observing spontaneous eye opening and movements of the eyes, face, and extremities, as well as the response to stimulation. A preterm infant born before 32 weeks of gestation spends much of the time sleeping but can be aroused by gentle stimulation. After 32 weeks of gestation, there are periods of spontaneous eye opening with roving eye movements and movements of the face and extremities. The irritable and agitated infant cries spontaneously with minimal stimulation and cannot be calmed. Delayed or poorly-maintained response to stimulation suggests lethargy, in coma, and arousal is impossible.

It is determined by internal resources and the response to external environment. Infant's behavior can be judged at rest after stimulation. The mother and child can start with positive attitude.

Motor Functions

The motor examination assesses spontaneous movements and muscle tone. Posture and resistance of muscles to passive movement evaluate passive tone. Evoked changes in extremity tone and evoked postures of the head, trunk, and extremities assess active tone.

Tendon Reflexes

In the term infant, biceps, knee, and ankle jerks can be elicited readily, and ankle clonus is also common. Asymmetry or absence of reflexes may indicate a significant central or peripheral nervous system abnormality. Eliciting a plantar response is of limited value.

Spontaneous movements normally take place when the baby is awake consisting of alternating flexion and extension. Normally, the tone of the newborn is hypertonia and that of preterm is hypotonia. Deep tendon reflexes are usually brisk and variable. Normally ankle clonus may be present with 6–8 jerks uninterrupted.

Examination of the Cranial Nerve

First cranial nerve cannot be tested in the newborn or neonate. Second cranial nerve can be examined by the way the child turns to diffuse light. If both eyes rotate in the same direction, it suggests that the III, IV, and VI cranial nerves are intact. Doll's eyes response in turning of the eye in the opposite direction involves the integrity of III, IV, and VI cranial nerves. Ptosis **(Fig. 17)** and pupillary reaction signify II cranial nerve.

The presence of the rooting reflex indicates that V nerve is intact and crying and grimacing suggest the VII cranial nerve.

Optokinetic nystagmus is elicited by holding the baby on the back with outstretched arms, hands supporting the occiput, and gently turning slowly in a clockwise direction. This suggests the intact vestibular part of the VIII nerve. Startled response indicates auditory part of the VIII nerve. IX and X cranial nerves are judged by gag reflex. Vigorous sucking and striping action by the tongue suggests that XII cranial nerve is intact.

During the last trimester of gestation, changes occur in tone and primitive reflexes. Flexor tone increases in the lower extremities and progresses cephalad between 28 and 40 weeks of gestation. After 40 weeks of gestation, maturation of tone and coordination begins rostrally and progresses caudally. For example, the infant at 28 weeks of gestation lies with both upper and lower extremities fully extended with little or no resistance to passive movement of the extremities. As the infant matures, by 34 weeks, the lower extremities are flexed, and by 36 weeks, the upper extremities are flexed. Term infants demonstrate flexion in both upper and lower extremities. At term, both neck flexors and extensors can maintain the head in the axis of the trunk for more than a few seconds.

Involuntary Movements

The frequency and symmetry of spontaneous movements vary with the infant's level of arousal; normal spontaneous movements of the extremities in the term infant are organized and smooth. The ability to abduct the thumb is particularly meaningful, as persistent adduction suggests a corticospinal tract lesion. Jitteriness and seizures are involuntary movements that require further evaluation. Jitteriness consists of tremor-like movements of extremities that are very sensitive to stimuli and can be stopped with gentle passive flexion. Jitteriness may be found in hypoglycemia, hypocalcemia, and hypoxic–ischemic encephalopathy, but often no specific cause is identified. Seizures are difficult to diagnose clinically

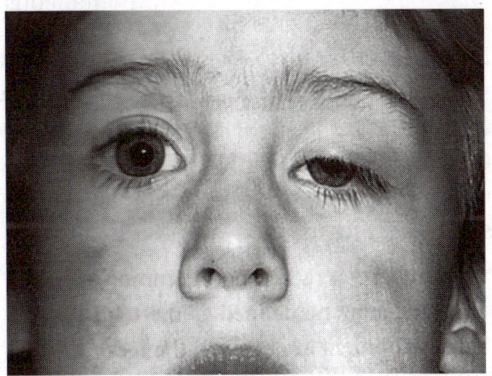

Fig. 17: Ptosis of left upper lid.

and suspicion requires confirmation with electroencephalography. Many infants demonstrate myoclonic jerks during the onset of sleep that are mistaken for seizures.

Posture and Passive Tone

The symmetry and maturity of passive tone are evaluated by observing the resting posture of the infant and by moving the extremities while the infant is awake and quiet. The degree of resistance to slow, gentle movement of the extremities and extremity angles ascertain passive tone. The infant's head must be in the midline position during the motor examination to avoid eliciting asymmetries in tone provoked by the asymmetric tonic neck reflex. In a normal baby, flexion always exceeds extension.

Active Tone and Primitive Reflexes

Active tone refers to the infant's tone during active movement in reaction to certain situations. Active tone and evoked reflexes are evaluated by observing changes in the infant's posture in response to changes in position with respect to gravity or by observing the infant's responses to other stimuli, such as touch and pressure. Of the many primitive reflexes described in neonates, only a few, including the righting reaction and raise-to-sit maneuver, are routinely assessed. These are normally present in term and preterm infants and do not disappear until the infant reaches several months of age. Absence of primitive reflexes in the newborn infant indicates CNS depression.

Maturational Changes in Tone and Reflexes

Maternal menstrual history or early fetal sonography provides the best possible dating before 32 weeks of gestation; from 32 weeks on, it appears reasonable to confirm gestational age by physical criteria and CNS function of the infant according to the normal steps of development. In this assessment, structured evaluation of passive tone, active tone, and primary reflexes are used to determine gestational age within 2-week periods. A definite conclusion on neurologic maturation is reached only if 7 of the 10 responses correspond to the same 2-week gestation period. When >3 responses are out of line, no firm conclusion can be made. Such a result also raises the probability of a neurologic abnormality.

Sensory Examination

Sensory function has limited value in newborns. Anal reflex should be tested for neural tube defects. Vision is very difficult to test. It is told that visual acuity in newborns is 6/45.

Hearing is judged by startle response including blinking of the eye and changes in the heart rate. These changes are seen as a response to 500–1,000 cycles per second.

Hip Joint Examination

Stability of the Joint

The most common screening maneuver combines those described by Ortolani and Barlow. With the baby supine on a firm surface, flex its thighs to right angle to the abdomen and its knees to the right angle to the thighs. Then, the thigh is grasped with the examiner's fingers along the outside of the shaft of the femur, with the middle fingertips on the greater trochanter, and the examiner's thumb medially in the femoral triangle.

With the baby at rest, the first femur is adducted completely and gently abducted from the position of full adduction so that knees come to lie laterally on the mattress. During abduction, the greater trochanter is pushed medially with the fingers. If there is a click either during adduction or abduction, or if there is resistance as the knee approaches full abduction, or if there is a spasm or discomfort of the abductor muscles of the femur, the baby probably has congenitally dislocated or dislocatable hip.

Unstable hips: Many unstable joints following breech delivery become stable within few days. It is prudent to reexamine the hips after 24–48 hours.

Dislocated hips: Here, abduction at the affected hip is limited and difficulty in abducting either hip to 80° angle should arise the suspicion of congenital dislocation.

Pediatricians should be alerted if some of the signs or symptoms listed in the **Box 2** are noticed.

Reflexes

- *Grasp reflex:* This is elicited in hands and feet. This is done by pressing the finger lightly against the palm and sole. The lightness of the grasp is often sufficient. This is enough for traction response. It is generally safer to do this by holding the infant's wrist and pulling him slowly to the sitting posture. The infant flexes his elbows as if he/she is trying to assist the movements. Hence, attempt should be made to hold the head in line with the trunk as it is raised.
- *Moro reflex:* This is elicited by allowing the head to fall back unsupported for a short distance. Sudden extension and abduction of the limbs are followed by slower adduction and flexion to the resting position.
- *Rooting reflex:* This is elicited by touching the infant's cheeks to turn eagerly to the side. This is stimulated in the hope of finding the nipple.
- *Crossed extension response:* This is elicited by extending one leg and tickling the other sole. A positive response is movement of extension possibly with the adduction to the lower leg.
- *Stepping movements:* When the child is held erect with the feet on a firm surface, a full-term infant attempts to straighten trunk and makes a stepping movement with his/her legs.

■ SKIN OF THE NEWBORN

Fine, soft, lanugo hair cover the entire body in very preterm infants and disappears from the face and lower back between 32 and 37 weeks. The term infant has lanugo hair on the upper back and dorsal aspects of the limbs. Vernix caseosa, a thick, white material with the consistency of soft cheese, covers the skin of the entire body until 35–37 weeks. By term, the amount of vernix is limited mainly to the flexor creases.

The subcutaneous tissue is relatively thick, and the fingernails and toenails are fully formed and extend slightly beyond the ends of the digits. If fetal stress occurs at term, meconium may be passed into the amniotic fluid. If meconium has been in the amniotic fluid for several hours, it will also stain the

---

BOX 2: Alarming signs in neonate.

- Bleeding from any site
- Appearance of jaundice within 24 hours
- Poor feeding
- Lethargy
- Excessive crying
- Respiratory distress or cyanosis
- Convulsions
- Not passing urine within 72 hours
- Not passing motion within 24 hours

skin, fingernails, toenails, and umbilical cord, with fetuses at <34 weeks of gestation rarely passing meconium. The postmature infant (beyond 42 weeks) may have a somewhat wasted appearance with dry and peeling skin, a decreased amount of subcutaneous tissue, long fingernails, and an alert appearance.

Skin Abnormalities

Neonates often have skin rashes, some of which indicate a serious systemic issue. Much more common than these serious rashes are many benign skin lesions that are important to recognize and explain to parents **(Figs. 18A to G)**.

Color

There may be cyanosis of the hands and feet (acrocyanosis), which is normal immediately after birth or if the infant has been exposed to a cold environment. Harlequin skin describes a transient change in the skin color with no known pathologic significance: One side of the body turns pale while the other side remains pink with a sharp line of demarcation in the midline.

Ecchymoses or localized petechiae generally result from birth trauma and are often present over the head after vertex delivery or on the feet, lower limbs, and buttocks following breech delivery. More generalized

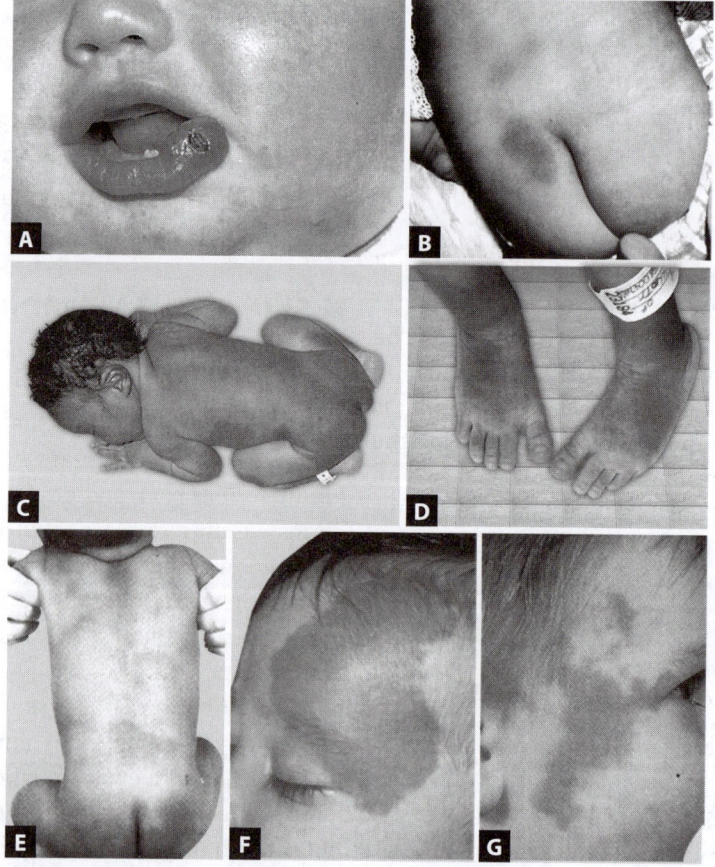

Figs. 18A to G: (A) Strawberry hemangioma; (B) Mongolian spots; (C to E) Mongolian blue spots; (F and G) Port-wine stains. *(For color version, see Plate 7)*

petechiae suggest thrombocytopenia. Subcutaneous fat necrosis appears as red lesions where the subcutaneous tissue is hard and sharply demarcated and is usually seen over the cheeks, buttocks, limbs, or back.

Neonatal jaundice is caused by an elevation in indirect-reacting bilirubin, resulting in a yellow-to-green discoloration of the skin. It is assessed by briefly pressing on the infant's skin with a finger and observing the color in the blanched area. One must be cautious in interpreting the intensity of jaundice based on physical examination as visual assessment of jaundice has been shown to be unreliable. Mild physiologic jaundice usually develops 2–4 days after birth. However, jaundice on the first day warrants prompt investigation; it is usually from sepsis or hemolytic anemia.

Keloid is a raised scar caused by excess of protein (collagen) in skin during healing **(Fig. 19)**.

Vernix Caseosa

At birth, the normal full-term infant is covered by vernix caseosa. It is a greasy substance that protects the skin during the lengthy immersion in amniotic fluid. This is the normal sebaceous secretion of the skin.

The skin of the face and head may exhibit a variety of changes. It is important to reassure the parents.

Angiomatous Lesion (Figs. 20 and 21)

These are small, flame-shaped, flat hemangiomas over the eyelids and the roof of the nose. These should be differentiated from port-wine stains. These are larger, permanent, and may involve areas of the face or head in

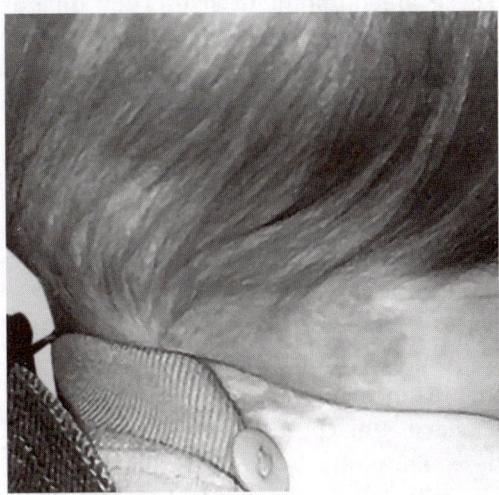

Fig. 20: Salmon patch. *(For color version, see Plate 8)*

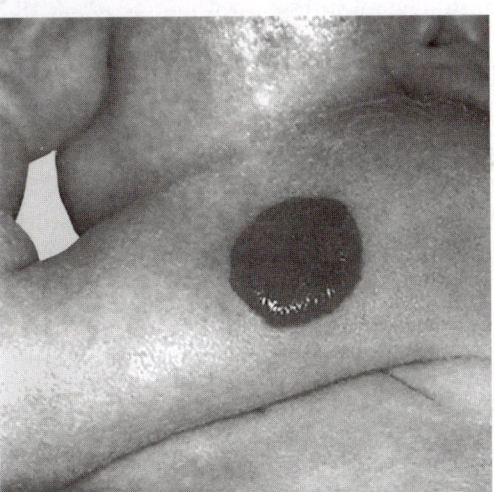

Fig. 21: Strawberry hemangioma. *(For color version, see Plate 8)*

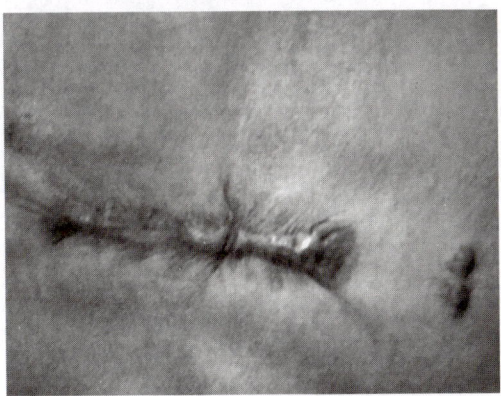

Fig. 19: Keloid.

a particular nerve distribution, especially trigeminal nerve distribution.

Milia

These are small white spots on the face. These represent hyperactive sebaceous glands with visible retained secretion.

Petechiae

Petechiae on the face are quite common. These are pinpoint in size. They do not blanch with pressure. They usually result from an increased presence in the venous system during a vertex vaginal delivery. They may appear on the face-on-face presentation on buttocks after breech delivery. Bruising, i.e., ecchymoses may be related to delivery trauma.

Erythema Toxicum

It is a newborn rash that is extremely common in full-term infants. The lesions usually appear as white pustules on an erythematous base. These are 1–3 mm in diameter and occur singly or in groups. The lesions contain many eosinophils. In the case of pustules, lesions contain gram-positive cocci-like characteristic pustules.

Visceral larva migrans is caused by migratory larvae of certain nematodes such as Toxacara Canis, Toxacara Catis and Ascaris **(Fig. 22)**.

The skin changes seen in post-maturity are dryness, flakiness, or cracking of the skin. The skin lesions that should cause concern and warrant close observation, investigation, and treatment often include

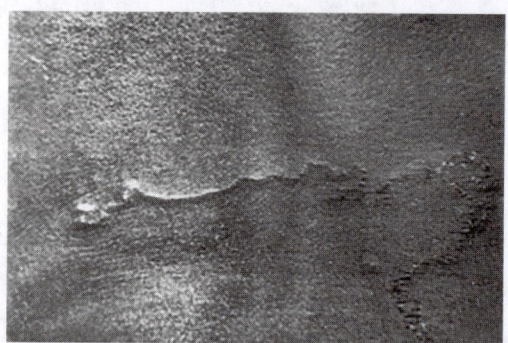

Fig. 22: Visceral larva. *(For color version, see Plate 8)*

vesicles, pustules, areas of absent skin either congenital or acquired, and large bulky subcutaneous hemangioma.

■ BIBLIOGRAPHY

1. Behrman RE, Kliegman RM, Jenson HB. Nelson textbook of pediatrics, 19th edition. Philadelphia: W.B. Saunders Company; 2011.
2. Bhat BV, Neonatal care. In: Bhave S, Parthasarathy A, Borker AS, Nair MKC Partha's Fundamentals of Pediatrics, 2nd edition. New Delhi: Jaypee Brothers Medical Publishers (P) Ltd; 2013.
3. Cloherty JP, Echenwald EC, Hansen AR, Stark AR. Cloherty and Stark Manual of Neonatal Care, 7th edition. Philadelphia, PA; Wolters Kluwer; 2012.
4. Illingworth RS. The normal child, 10th edition. Amsterdam, Netherlands: Elsevier; 1997.
5. Khan OA, Garcia-Sosa R, Hageman JR, Msall M, Kelley KR. Neonatal Neurological Examination. NeoReviews. 2014;15(8): e316-24.
6. Rennie JM, Roberton NRC. Rennie and Roberton's Textbook of Neonatology, 5th edition. Edinburgh: Churchill Livingstone Elsevier; 2012.

CASE 87

Premature Infant

■ PRESENTING COMPLAINTS

A newborn was brought with the complaint of:
- Preterm delivery of the newborn
- LBW baby

History of Presenting Complaints

The newborn delivered by emergency cesarean section was referred to the doctor in charge of the neonatal intensive care unit (NICU). The delivery was attended by the resident doctor working in pediatrics department. The mother was not registered case in antenatal health checkup. She was not aware of duration of the pregnancy.

One day, she came with history of epigastric pain with swelling of the face and lower limbs. On examination, her blood pressure was recorded as 210/160 mm Hg. Her urine albumin was +++. These along with her clinical findings suggested that she was in imminent eclampsia. Hence the obstetrician decided to induce the delivery. As she had first sibling being delivered by cesarean section, the emergency cesarean section was planned. Before the section, emergency ultrasound examination showed approximate age of the fetus was 30 weeks.

The female baby cried immediately, after the delivery. The cry of the baby was good. Apgar score at 1 minute and 5 minutes were 8 and 10, respectively. The birth weight of the female baby was 1.1 kg. Hence, later the baby was shifted to NICU. This was the second sibling of nonconsanguineous marriage. The first child was 2 years old and maintains the good health.

■ EXAMINATION

The girl baby was low-birth-weight (LBW). She was lying on the bed with increased tone. She used to respond to the tactile stimulus

CASE AT A GLANCE

Basic Findings
Length	: 45 cm (<3rd centile)
Weight	: 1.1 kg (<3rd centile)
Temperature	: 37°C
Pulse rate	: 136 beats/min
Respiratory rate	: 42 breaths/min
Blood pressure	: 50/30 mm Hg

Positive Findings

History:
- Unbooked cases
- Maternal blood pressure
- Swelling of the face
- Epigastric pain

Examination:
- Maternal hypertension
- Imminent eclampsia
- Low birth weight
- Respiratory system:
  - Crepitation
  - Preterm baby

by crying. Signs of prematurity were present. Premature edema was present. Acrocyanosis was present. Features of intrauterine growth restriction (IUGR) were present. Labia were separated. Newborn was afebrile. The heart rate was 136 beats/min. The respiratory rate was 42 breaths/min. The blood pressure recorded was 50/30 mm Hg.

The anthropometric measurements included the weight 1.1 kg (<3rd centile), the length 45 cm (<3rd centile), and the head circumference 30 cm.

Respiratory system revealed presence of crepitation. Cardiovascular system showed first and second heart sounds were normal, with no evidence of congenital heart disease (CHD). Her abdomen examination was normal. There was no clinical evidence of congenital anomalies.

■ INVESTIGATION

- *Hemoglobin:* 13 g/dL
- *TLC:* 10,500 cells/cumm
- *DLC:* $P_{78}L_{20}E_2M_0$
- *CRP:* Negative
- *Blood sugar:* 80 mg/dL
- *Serum calcium:* 8 mg/dL
- *Blood group and Rh typing:* AB positive
- *Chest X-ray:* No abnormality detected

■ DISCUSSION

Ten to thirty percent of all the births are of LBW. Majority of them will be small for age, 60% of the LBW babies are AGA.

Extremely and Very Preterm Infants

Infants born before 37 weeks from the first day of the last menstrual period (LMP) are termed premature by World Health Organization (WHO). Infants born before 28 weeks gestation are extremely preterm, also referred to as extremely low-gestational-age newborns (ELGANS); whereas infants born between 28 and 31 weeks are very preterm.

In addition to classification by gestational age, classification is also based on birth weight. Extremely low birth weight (ELBW) is used to describe infants with a birth weight <1,000 g; very low birth weight (VLBW) describes infants <1,500 g at birth; and LBW describes infants <2,500 g at birth.

Birth weight in general is a proxy for gestational age but in the cases of IUGR and small-for-gestational-age (SGA) infants, birth weight can sometimes be misleading for true gestational age.

If the gestational age is <37 weeks, then it is called preterm or premature delivery. 5% of the pregnancies are preterm delivery and 2% of them are before 32 weeks. These children are immature both anatomically and functionally.

■ PROBLEMS OF PREMATURITY

The basic underlying feature of the LBW babies is immaturity of organ system. These basics lack brown fat, which helps to keep themselves warm. Infants born before 34 weeks of gestational age will have uncoordinated neonatal reflex.

Respiratory System

These neonates will have poor alveolar diffusion of gases. This predisposes to resuscitation difficulties. Hence these neonates present with respiratory distress syndrome (RDS) and apnea. These are associated with poor surfactant.

Central Nervous System

Interventricular hemorrhage is more common because of delicate vessels. Immaturity of the system is manifested by inactivity, lethargy, poor cough reflex, uncoordinated sucking and swallowing reflexes. Blood–brain barrier is inefficient and hence the damage may occur at low serum bilirubin levels.

Cardiovascular System

The closure of ductus arteriosus is delayed. Hence patent ductus arteriosus (PDA) may present with CCF. Hypovolemia will result with hypotension. Cardiac dysfunction will also occur.

Gastrointestinal System

Regurgitation and aspiration are common because of uncoordinated sucking, small capacity of the stomach, incompetence of the cardioesophageal junction, and poor cough reflex. Abdominal distension and functional obstruction are due to hypotonic.

Infection

The low levels of IgG antibodies and inefficient cellular immunity predispose them to infections. Humid atmosphere, contaminated instrument will contribute to the incidence of infection.

Metabolic Disorders

The poor hepatic glycogen stores, birth asphyxia, and RDS contribute to the development of hypoglycemia. The BUN is high due to low glomerular filtration rate and acidosis develops early. These infants are prone to develop hypoglycemia, hypocalcemia, and hypoxia. Electrolyte imbalance occurs due to immature kidneys.

Blood Disorder

These infants are prone to develop hemolytic anemia, thrombocytopenia, and edema at 6–10 weeks of age. Hyperbilirubinemia is also a feature.

Eye

Retrolental fibroplasia due to oxygen toxicity is seen particularly in newborn with gestational age <35 weeks.

■ CLINICAL FEATURES (FIG. 1)

- Thin red shiny skin, often covered with lanugo
- Lanugo are specially seen on back and shoulder
- Poor muscle tone, floppy and lie in frog-like posture
- Ears of little cartilage and very soft
- Genitalia are poorly developed
- Small scrotum with scaly rugosity
- Prominent labia minora and an enlarged clitoris
- Testes are present in external ring
- Breast nodule is with 5 mm
- Single deep crease in anterior one-third of the sole

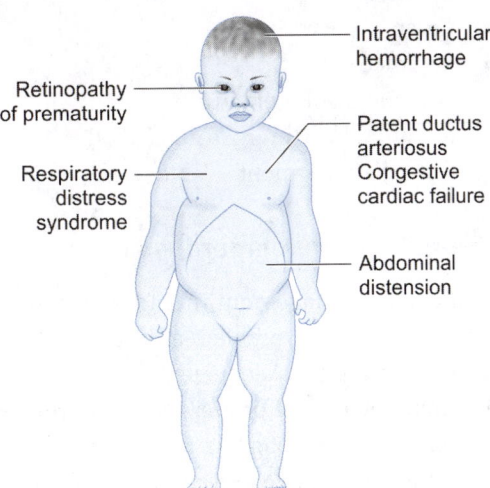

Fig. 1: Clinical features.

GENERAL FEATURES
• Immaturity of organ system • Regurgitation and aspiration • Infection • Hypoglycemia • Hypoxia • Hypocalcemia • Hemolytic anemia • Thrombocytopenia

PROBLEMS OF PREMATURE INFANT

Early

- Hypoxia, apnea
- RDS
- Patent ducts arteriosus
- Septicemia
- Jaundice
- Periventricular bleeding
- Hypoglycemia, hypocalcemia, hypothermia

Late

- Septicemia, NEC
- Bronchopulmonary dysplasia (BPD)
- Anemia
- Cerebral palsy
- Jaundice
- Osteopenia of prematurity
- Retinopathy of prematurity (ROP)
- Growth impairment

Neonatal Management

Immediate management includes management of respiratory problem and stabilization of vital parameters. Adequate oxygen delivery and maintenance of proper temperature are the mainstay of management.

Administering oxygen to reduce the risk of injury from hypoxia and circulatory insufficiency (risk of cerebral palsy, death) must be balanced against the risk of hyperoxia to the eyes (ROP) and oxygen injury to the lungs (BPD). For ELBW infants at birth, guidelines should be followed to determine need for oxygen during resuscitation to maintain goal oxygen saturation limits.

Warm condition of the baby should be given prime importance as hypothermia can lead to hypoglycemia, bleeding diathesis, pulmonary hemorrhage, acidosis, apnea, and respiratory failure. Adequate oxygenation is achieved by oxygen therapy and assisted ventilation. PDA requires conservative management with adequate oxygenation, fluid restriction, and diuretics. Indomethacin may be necessary. Skin leads to marked evaporation. Fluid loss particularly if baby is under radiant warmer in turn leads to hypernatremia. Alternatively immature kidney fails to conserve sodium resulting in hyponatremia.

The management of a patient with impending premature delivery should include the following: Evaluation of gestational age by dates and/or early ultrasound, fetal size and position, condition of the fetal membranes, amount of amniotic fluid volume, and evidence of chorioamnionitis, and other obstetric complications, such as bleeding and toxemia.

For patients between 23 and 34 weeks gestation, administration of two doses of 12 mg of betamethasone, 24 hours apart, and administer a booster dose of 12 mg weekly for those patients who continue to be at risk of delivering prematurely. Beyond 34 weeks, steroids are used only when an amniocentesis is indicated and the lecithin/sphingomyelin (L/S) ratio shows persistent lung immaturity.

■ DELIVERY ROOM MANAGEMENT

The basic principle guiding successful management should be directed toward prevention of any physiologic deviation from normality, such as hypothermia, acidosis, or hypoxia. At the same time, it is important that each intervention during the resuscitation process be adapted carefully to the size and the needs of the tiny infant. Brisk maneuvers, excessive positive pressure with bagging, or inappropriate administration of drugs and fluids can induce permanent CNS or lung injuries.

Neonatal Resuscitation

Failure to initiate or sustain respiratory effort is fairly common at birth, with 5–10% of births requiring some intervention. Infants with primary apnea respond to stimulation by establishing normal breathing. Infants with secondary apnea require some ventilatory assistance in order to establish spontaneous respiratory effort. Secondary apnea usually originates in the CNS as a result of asphyxia or peripherally because of neuromuscular disorders. The lungs in infants affected by conditions such as pulmonary hypoplasia and prematurity may be noncompliant, and initial efforts to begin respirations may be inadequate to initiate sufficient ventilation.

In term infants after stimulation, if no respirations are noted, or if the heart rate is <100 beats/min, positive-pressure ventilation (PPV) should be given through a tightly fitted and appropriately sized bag-mask device. PPV should be initiated at pressures of approximately 20 cm H_2O at a rate of 40–60 breaths/min initially with 21% FiO_2 for full-term infants.

Successful and effective ventilation is signified by adequate chest rise, symmetric breath sounds, improved pink color, heart rate >100 beats/min, increasing oxygen saturation, spontaneous respirations, and improved tone. If after 30 seconds of providing PPV there are no signs of effective ventilation, corrective steps should be performed to improve ventilation.

Delayed cord clamping for 1–3 minutes can be performed in both preterm and term infants but is especially recommended for preterm infants. Benefits to term infants include higher hemoglobin levels at birth with improved iron stores in the first few months of life. Additional benefits for preterm infants include improved hemodynamic stability, decreased need for inotropic support, decreased need for transfusions, and decreased risk of NEC and IVH.

During the initial steps of stabilization, the condition of the infant is assessed rapidly. After drying, positioning on warm blankets, and suctioning, most of the LBW infants require immediate initiation of IPPV with a bag and mask. For the LBW infants, ventilation is more effective if performed at a higher ventilatory rate than for the term infant. We use anesthesia bags and ventilate at a rate of 60–80 breaths/minute, adjusting the pressure to provide adequate bilateral air entry. For extremely premature infants, intubation in the delivery room may follow rapidly. Because NICU is adjacent to the delivery room, if the infant is responding well to manual ventilation (heart rate >100, pink color), he or she is transferred to the NICU for further management.

Even following optimal resuscitation, the Apgar scores of LBW infants rarely exceed 6 or 7 in view of their decreased tone and reactivity, poor respiratory effort, and initially poor peripheral perfusion. The infant's heart rate is thus the best measure of the effectiveness of resuscitation efforts.

ADMISSION TO THE NEONATAL INTENSIVE CARE UNIT

It is well established that the majority of cerebral injuries occur around the time delivery or in the immediate postnatal period. Acute changes in cerebral blood flow may predispose the very fragile network of periventricular vessels to rupture. Hence, it is essential to handle these fragile infants with extreme care, avoiding unnecessary disturbances, and preventing rather than correcting physiologic deviations in acid–base balance, blood gases, blood pressure, or body temperature. During the first hours after admission, the premature infant is placed in an open radiant warmer to allow for easier access.

Blood is analyzed for glucose, electrolytes, blood gases, hemoglobin, and leukocytes; and intravenous 10% dextrose is initiated at a rate varying from 85 to 100 mL/kg/day, according to the degree of immaturity and the type of incubator used (radiant heater vs. closed incubator).

Total parenteral nutrition (TPN) generally is started after the first 48 hours of life, when electrolytes, glucose, urea, and acid–base status are well controlled. When the mother receives intravenous fluids during her labor, a baseline electrolytic profile of the newborn shortly after birth seems to be the proper way to follow up subsequent changes. Electrolytes are repeated between 12 and 18 hours of age. During the first 72 hours, the body weight is recorded every 8 hours, and fluid intake is adjusted accordingly.

In order to establish prognostic criteria, it is important to obtain a cranial ultrasound in the first 24 hours of life. This ultrasound needs to be repeated at least 1 week later, or as often as necessary, depending on the pathology detected on admission or if the infant's condition has deteriorated, suggesting CNS involvement.

RESPIRATORY SUPPORT

The introduction of exogenous surfactant therapy has reduced significantly the mortality of all newborns suffering from respiratory failure secondary to RDS, but its impact has been particularly important among the most premature infants. Administration of surfactant in these very tiny infants requires extra care, as rapid changes in lung compliance may not only damage the lungs by creating overinflation and overdistension, but also may predispose to acute changes in ductal circulation, which, in turn, could lead to both cerebral and or pulmonary hemorrhage. With rapid improvement in oxygenation, persistent hyperoxia also may be detrimental to the eyes. Hence, the administration of surfactant should be performed by an experienced person, under close monitoring of ventilatory parameters and rapid reduction of peak inspiratory pressures (PIP) and oxygen concentrations.

In RDS, there are compartments in the lung with relatively normal ventilation perfusion ratios and others with poor ventilation and adequate perfusion, it seems reasonable to attempt to improve ventilation of the poor ventilation–perfusion (V-Q) compartment without overdistension of the normal V-Q compartment. Raising the ventilatory rate, which raises the mean airway pressure (MAP) without changing the PIP, appears to accomplish this goal.

When the oxygen requirement exceeds 40% or the initial X-ray shows severe RDS, we immediately administer exogenous surfactant and rapidly adjust the ventilatory parameters according to the new lung compliance.

The concept of permissive hypercapnia for patients requiring mechanical ventilation gives priority to the prevention or limitation of severe pulmonary hyperinflation over the maintenance of normal ventilation. The principle consists of allowing the pCO_2 to rise by minimizing ventilator pressures and tidal volume. Potential risks of high pCO_2 values include increased cerebral perfusion, increased retinal perfusion, increased pulmonary vascular resistance (PVR), and reduction of pH. Based on epidemiologic observation, it appears that respiratory acidosis, unlike metabolic acidosis, is not associated with poor neurologic outcomes.

■ CARDIOVASCULAR SUPPORT

By far, the major cardiovascular problem in ELBW infants is the presence of a PDA. More than 50% of infants born weighing <1,000 g will have a PDA diagnosed during the first few days of life. The onset of clinical manifestations of the PDA is related to the timing of improvement of the infant's respiratory status, which is associated with decreasing PVR and predominantly left-to-right shunt. However, the patency of the ductus arteriosus can be documented easily in the first hours of life, with the help of echocardiography. At this early stage of life, the shunt is either right to left or bidirectional, depending on the severity of the infant's respiratory condition.

An active pericardium, with bounding pulses and visible carotid pulse, often will precede auscultation of a murmur. If left untreated, the infant may develop left-sided heart failure and pulmonary edema or hemorrhagic pulmonary edema, with significant deterioration of the respiratory status. Significant left-to-right ductal shunting may cause decreased peripheral perfusion and oxygen delivery. ELBW infants with significant PDA are at risk of IVH, NEC, renal failure, chronic liver disease (CLD), and metabolic acidosis.

Left-to-right shunting along with patent ductus leads to development of BPD. It prolongs the ventilator dependency. The diagnosis is confirmed by contrast echo.

Restriction of fluid therapy and administration of diuretics will help in managing the ductus. If the ductus persists after fluid restriction, indomethacin is given in the dose of 0.2 mg/kg/dose for three doses at 12 hourly interval, which is safe and effective. This will help in >70% of cases.

Contraindications to indomethacin therapy are renal failure, active bleeding, thrombocytopenia, and severe indirect hyperbilirubinemia. The presence of IVH does not appear to be an absolute contraindication to the use of indomethacin. Recent studies indicate that there is no progression of the severity of IVH after administration of indomethacin for PDA closure.

■ FLUID AND ELECTROLYTES

It is important to remember that the body of the ELBW infant is made up of 85–90% water, which is distributed as one-third intracellular water (ICW). Immediately following birth glomerular filtration rate and fractional excretion of sodium (FENa) are low and urine output is minimal. This is followed by the diuretic phase, which results in a decrease in the extracellular compartment.

Once the infant's respiratory status has stabilized and the need for ready access to the infant is not as essential as it is during the hours following admission, the infant is transferred to an incubator maintaining 75–80% humidity for the first week of life. This approach allows limitation of fluid intake to between 80 and 100 mL/kg/day for the first day of life. In addition, we monitor the infant's weight every 8 hours during the first days of life and adjust fluid intake consequently.

Electrolyte abnormalities such as hypernatremia, hyponatremia, and hyperkalemia frequently are seen in LBW infants. Hypernatremia is usually the result of severe insensible water loss, but can be secondary to the treatment of metabolic acidosis with large amounts of sodium bicarbonate. Hyponatremia (<130 mmol/L) more frequently is seen because of the high FENa during the diuretic phase.

On admission, infants receive only a 10% dextrose solution in water. We monitor blood glucose and electrolytes closely and we test all urines for glucose. We subsequently adjust the intravenous dextrose according to the blood glucose values. We start sodium supplementation only when its serum value is <140 mmol/L, which usually happens between the second and third days of life.

■ NUTRITION

The goals of early nutritional support for extremely premature infants include approximating the rate and composition of growth for a normal fetus at the same postmenstrual age. Achieving this goal requires an understanding of the intrauterine growth rate to be targeted as well as the unique nutrient requirements of premature infants. Strategies to prevent growth faltering include a combined approach of early parenteral and enteral nutrition, fortification of human milk, and the use of standardized feeding guidelines. In addition, careful monitoring of not only weight gain but also length and head circumference using appropriate intrauterine growth curves, as well as consultation with an experienced neonatal dietitian, is important to achieve optimal growth outcomes.

Nutrition is an essential part of the care of the ELBW infant. These tiny infants are born with very low reserves of fat and carbohydrates, and they rapidly develop nutritional deficiencies in calcium, phosphorous, iron, trace minerals, and vitamins. Their endocrine and enzymatic capability is limited due to immaturity. Postnatally, they rapidly enter a catabolic state unless sufficient nutrients are given. But reversal of this catabolic state often is difficult because of limited feeding tolerance. The gastrointestinal tract is immature in terms of digestive pathways and motor function, increasing the risk of developing NEC.

Because the first goal of nutrition is to prevent catabolism, usually this will be achieved by providing a minimum of 50 kcal/kg/day growth will require additional caloric intake. Achieving steady growth is essential for the LBW infant, because the growth velocity at 25–30 weeks gestation is relatively higher than at term. If reasonable caloric intake cannot be provided, catch-up growth may never be achieved.

In the early days of life, satisfactory nutrition can never be achieved exclusively with milk. Parenteral nutrition provides the additional calories. In contrast to oral nutrition parenteral administration of 80–85 kcl/kg/day can provide the necessary calories for growth. When the infant no longer is receiving intravenous nutrition, 100–120 kcl/kg/day are needed to maintain growth. Appropriate growth, if one wants to mimic intrauterine growth, should be a 2% daily increase in body weight, slowing to 1% near term.

Both parenteral nutrition and oral nutrition are not without difficulties and complications in the LBW infant, TPN requires intravenous access and this can be associated with a variety of infections. Exclusive intravenous nutrition affects the mucosal lining of the gastrointestinal tract, which is bypassed and eventually may lead to villous atrophy. TPN also requires regular metabolic monitoring for glucose, electrolytes urea, lipids and acid–base balance. Cholestatic jaundice is a frequent complication of TPN.

Early Parenteral Nutrition

In the absence of intravenous amino acids, extremely premature infants lose 1–2% of body protein stores per day. IV amino acids and dextrose should be started immediately after birth. Many units use a starter or stock solution of amino acids and dextrose to accomplish this goal in infants weighing <1,500 g. A minimum of 2 g/kg of amino acids should be given in the first 24 hours after birth, with the goal of supplying at least 3.5 g/kg within 24-48 hours after birth. To meet total energy requirements, IV lipids will also be needed.

Enteral Nutrition

Early enteral feedings are recommended in ELBW and VLBW infants, typically beginning between 6 and 48 hours with some period of trophic/minimal enteral feeding volume. Feedings are typically advanced slowly (15–30 mL/kg/day) with a target goal of delivering approximately 110–135 kcal/kg/day and 3.5–4.5 g protein/kg/day. To accomplish these goals, human milk must be fortified, or a premature formula can be given.

Enteral nutrition may consist of either breast milk or premature formulas. During fetal life, the fetus constantly swallows amniotic fluid, promoting intestinal development.

Enteral feeding, even in small amounts, has been demonstrated to stimulate trophic factors and hormonal maturation of the gastrointestinal tract, thus improving overall intestinal function and potentially improving feeding tolerance and preventing mucosal atrophy. Whether early introduction of feedings and stimulation of the gastrointestinal tract could prevent or decrease the incidence of NEC has not yet been established. Breast milk contains lipase, which improves fat tolerance.

Feeding difficulties are common in babies under 34 weeks of gestation. The babies do not suck. They have poor gag reflex. So, care should be taken to avoid aspiration. If baby is unable to take feeds by mouth, then nasogastric tube feeds are given. Oral iron started after second week.

Neonates weighing <1,200 g or gestational age <30 weeks, IUGR infants should be started with intravenous fluids initially. TPN is administered through the central line.

Ten percent dextrose solution in the initial dose of 60 mL/kg body weight is started. Blood glucose level is checked every 3rd hourly. If it is <7 mm, intravenous fluid is changed to 5% dextrose. Amino acids are added up to 25%, if intravenous fluids are required for >3 days.

Oral feeds are started if the bowel sounds are heard or once the meconium is passed. It usually taken about 2–3 days. But by the end of the first week combined intravenous and enteral feeds should amount about 120–150 mL/kg body weight.

Neonates weighing 1,200–1,800 g or gestational age maturity is 30–34 weeks, should be put on gavage feeds. LBW babies weighing >1,800 g or gestational age maturity of >34 weeks should be given breast milk directly.

Breastfeeding alone contains insufficient nutrients for babies under 1,500 g. Hence, suitable supplements like medium-chain triglyceride, glucose polymer, phosphorus, and sodium should be given. Hyperbilirubinemia is treated by phototherapy and exchange transfusion.

GLUCOSE, CALCIUM, AND PHOSPHORUS HOMEOSTASIS

Early hypoglycemia frequently is seen in this group of infants because of poor glycogen reserves and the immaturity of the postnatal adaptive mechanism of endocrine as well as enzymatic control of glucose. In particular, ketogenesis and lipogenesis, which lead to the production of alternate fuels, are limited in very premature infants, making the infant more dependent on glucose. Hence, an infusion of dextrose at the rate of 5-7 mg/kg/min is necessary to maintain normoglycemia.

Hyperglycemia is a frequent and challenging complication, particularly in extremely immature infants of 23-24 weeks gestation.

The sudden onset of a glycosuria in a previous stable infant may be an early sign of infection. Hyperglycemia also is seen frequently with initiation of dexamethasone therapy for BPD. Because of the slow metabolic adaptation of the LBW infant, rapid and significant changes in glucose intake should be avoided in order to prevent episodes of hypo- or hyperglycemia, which can become difficult to control. Finally, for the treatment of acute and severe hypoglycemia, a bolus of no >200 mg/kg of dextrose can be administered as needed, while at the same time, increasing the concentration of the intravenous glucose infusion.

Because hypocalcemia also can induce apnea, we always verify calcium levels after the first 24 hours of life. It is important of remember that metabolic acidosis can give falsely reassuring values of ionized serum calcium, which decline rapidly with the improvement of acid-base balance. Mechanisms involved in the early manifestations of hypocalcemia include parathyroid dysfunction, renal immaturity, and calcitonin stimulation. Our treatment of hypocalcemia consists of administering 500 mg/kg/day of calcium gluconate. As soon as we introduce TPN 300 mg/kg/day of calcium gluconate is added daily to the solution, together with multivitamins.

It is important to mention at this point that both the classic and hypophosphatemic forms of rickets nowadays are seen only in nutritionally neglected LBW infants.

ACID-BASE BALANCE

Acid-base homeostasis varies in relation to the degree of renal maturity. The renal threshold for loss of bicarbonate can be as low as 15 mEq/L hence, there is often a need for more buffer with sodium bicarbonate in ELBW infants. The need for supplemental sodium bicarbonate also is frequent during the introduction of amino acids in the TPN.

Although acidosis is the main concern in the early days of life, later on, many of these tiny babies may develop a metabolic alkalosis due to the administration of diuretics, in combination with fluid restriction.

JAUNDICE

Hepatic immaturity and reduced erythrocyte lifespan, blood group incompatibilities, extensive extravasation of blood, and increased enterohepatic circulation due to poor bowel motility all contribute to the fact that LBW infants are very prone to develop jaundice.

Because the serum bilirubin binding capacity is decreased in premature infants due to the lower serum albumin, the level at which toxicity for the brain and acoustic nerves may occur is much lower than that of the more mature infant. When the bilirubin level approaches the exchange transfusion level, it is important to void variations in acid–base balance, high levels of lipid infusion, hypothermia, and certain medications which may compete with and displace bilirubin from albumin, thus precipitating kernicterus.

INTERVENTRICULAR HEMORRHAGE

The IVH is a major and unfortunately frequent complication in the LBW infant. Its incidence is correlated with the degree of prematurity. Potential complications of IVH include hemorrhagic periventricular infarction, hydrocephalus, periventricular leukomalacia (PVL), and seizures.

Intraventricular hemorrhage may present acutely, leading to shock and death; it may be clinically silent, or more commonly, it may present with cardiorespiratory instability.

The incidence is indirectly proportional to LBW of the babies. Many of the bleeds are asymptomatic. Hence the routine cranial ultrasound is used for scanning. This should be performed at 24th day, 3rd day, and 7th day. Prevention is the ideal way of management. This includes preventing birth asphyxia and correcting bleeding diathesis, which will help in preventing IVH and PDA.

The immediate management of IVH involves stabilization of the cardiovascular system, correction of any bleeding diathesis, if present and monitoring for hyperbilirubinemia and hyperkalemia. Careful neurologic examination and serial measurement of head circumference and serial cranial ultrasounds must be performed to allow early detection of hydrocephalus. If there is rapidly progressive dilatation of the ventricles, neurosurgical intervention may be necessary for temporary or permanent drainage of the CSF.

PERIVENTRICULAR LEUKOMALACIA

The PVL has been reported in varying incidence from 4% to 15% and is the consequence of hypoxic–ischemic lesions, leading to necrosis of the white matter. Most commonly affected are white matter near the trigone of the lateral ventricles and around the foramen of Monro. PVL may occur in association with IVH, but also may be diagnosed independently as the only CNS lesion.

Cystic PVL among preterm infants is the single best predictor of adverse long-term neurologic outcomes.

The diagnosis of PVL is made by cranial ultrasonography. When the lesions have occurred in utero, it is possible to make the diagnosis soon after birth. However, for postnatally acquired PVL, several weeks may be necessary before the diagnosis can be secured. The characteristic evolution of PVL is the formation of multiple echolucent cysts. Because of the delayed appearance of the cystic lesions, it is important, even for those infants with normal early cranial ultrasonography.

SEIZURES

Compared to full term infants, seizures are more difficult to diagnose clinically, which probably is due to cortical underdevelopment at early gestational age. The etiology of seizures in the LBW infant, as for the term, infant, may be related to CNS pathology, metabolic derangements (i.e., hypoglycemia, hypocalcemia, severe hyponatremia), infectious causes, and drug withdrawal.

The order of preference for medications to control seizures is as follows: Phenobarbital at a loading dose of 20 mg/kg, which, on occasion, can be increased to 30 mg/kg, phenytoin at a loading dose of 15 mg/kg, paraldehyde rectally at 0.3 mL/kg (diluted 1:1 in mineral oil), and occasionally diazepam at 0.1–0.2 mg/kg/dose.

■ HEARING IMPAIRMENT

Early diagnosis of hearing loss and the use of hearing aids as early as 6 months of age, together with speech therapy, are essential in order to reduce the disability of deafness. The most objective tests are the measure of evoked auditory brain stem responses or otoacoustic emissions.

■ HEMATOLOGICAL DISORDERS

Low iron stores, multiple blood tests, blood loss due to either organ hemorrhage or hemolysis and rapid growth are some of the factors that make anemia a practically unavoidable hematologic complication for any LBW infant.

To decrease the risk of infection, one unit of packed red cells from a single, properly screened donor, divided into several small bags (satellite bags), could be used for the same infant.

■ HOMEOSTASIS AND BLEEDING DIATHESIS

Conditions requiring immediate administration of additional vitamin K include hemorrhagic pulmonary edema, pulmonary or gastric hemorrhage, and disseminated intravascular coagulation. The management of these conditions often will require, in addition to vitamin K, administration of fresh frozen plasma, transfusion of platelets, and treatment of the underlying condition.

■ APNEA OF PREMATURITY

Apnea of prematurity is a feature of nearly all infants with a birth weight <1,000 g. Its incidence and frequency decrease with advancing gestational age, but at times it may be seen up to 42 weeks of gestation in the ELBWs population, it is a frequent indication for mechanical ventilation, thus exposing these infants to the potential complications of ventilatory support.

Apnea usually is defined as a cessation of breathing for 20 seconds or more, or of a shorter duration if associated with cyanosis or bradycardia. Different patterns have been observed in premature infants, such as central apnea (absent breathing movements) and obstructive apnea (central and obstructive).

Low-birth-weight infants are particularly prone to obstructive apnea, especially when in the supine position with the neck in the midline because of the weakness of the muscles of the oropharynx. Apnea due to obstruction of the lower airways also have been reported, suggesting of lung mechanics. The cessation of gas exchange during a significant apneic episode is manifested by hypoxemia and/or bradycardia. Recurrent episodes of apnea may affect neurodevelopmental outcome.

Patient management will depend on the severity and frequency of apneic episodes. Methylxanthines, which stimulate the respiratory center, are the most effective pharmacologic treatment for apnea of prematurity.

Another drug that has been used for the treatment of apnea is doxapram. Like methylxanthines, doxapram has been observed to improve minute ventilation and tidal volume, lower pCO_2, and increase blood pressure.

■ NEONATAL INFECTIONS

As the clinical signs of infection often are nonspecific, the index of suspicion and the concern about the possibility of intrauterine infection should be very high in the presence of a premature birth. Hence, screening for infection should be an integral part of the evaluation of the LBW infant.

Diagnosis of neonatal infection sometimes can be difficult, as early neonatal infection often manifests with respiratory symptomatology, which is also the overwhelming pathology of prematurity. Early appearance of recurrent apnea, poor perfusion, hypotension, and significant metabolic acidosis, often in the presence of an abnormal leukocyte count, are very strong elements in favor of infection.

If the infant's condition improves rapidly, the blood culture is negative and the acute phase reactants are normal, we discontinue antibiotics can be discontinued after 3-5 days.

■ FOLLOW-UP

All the danger signs should be explained to parents and informed to report in case of development of any danger sign.
- Difficulty in feeding
- Reduced activity
- Baby is too cold or too warm
- Fast breathing and chest indrawing
- Abnormal movements
- Jaundice

■ BIBLIOGRAPHY

1. Agostoni C, Buonocore G, Carnielli VP, De Curtis M, Darmaun D, Decsi T, et al.; ESPGHAN Committee on Nutrition. Enteral nutrient supply for preterm infants: commentary from the European Society for Paediatric Gastroenterology, Hepatology and Nutrition Committee on Nutrition. J Pediatr Gastroenterol Nutr. 2010;50(1)85-91.
2. Bombell S, McGuire W. Early trophic feeding for very low birth weight infants. Cochrane Database Syst Rev. 2009;(3):CD000504.
3. Engle WA. Infants born preterm: defination, physiologic and metabolic immaturity, and outcomes. NeoReviews. 2009;10:e280-e286.
4. Lucas A, Fewtrell M. Feeding low birth infants. In: Rennie JM (Ed). Roberton's Textbook of Neonatology, 4th edition. Edinburgh: Churchill Livingstone; 2005. pp. 314-24.

CASE 88

Respiratory Distress Syndrome

■ PRESENTING COMPLAINTS

A newborn (6 hours) was brought with the complaint of:
- Breathlessness since birth
- Bluish color since birth
- Indrawing of chest since 1 hour

History of Presenting Complaints

The newborn was referred to NICU from pediatrician who attended the delivery. The boy was born at preterm at 35 weeks. The age of the mother at the time of the delivery was 18 years.

The baby was delivered vaginally at 35 weeks of amenorrhea. He was delivered normally without any intervention. The Apgar score at 1 minute was 4 and at 5 minutes was 8. He required resuscitative intervention such as bag and mask ventilation to establish spontaneous respiration. He was given oxygen at the rate of 4 L to maintain oxygen saturation up to 95. There was tachypnea with respiratory rate of 50 breaths/min. But there was no indrawing subcostal recession. Attending pediatrician discussed the case with senior doctor and then referred to NICU.

His mother was not booked for antenatal health checkups. She was very irregular to antenatal health checkup. She never had any antenatal investigation. In the third trimester, she noticed swelling of the legs. She was diagnosed with having hypertension. She was on antihypertensive medication.

CASE AT A GLANCE	
Basic Findings	
Length	: 48 cm (<10th centile)
Weight	: 1,500 g (<3rd centile)
Temperature	: 37°C
Pulse rate	: 146 beats/min
Respiratory rate	: 80 breaths/min
Blood pressure	: 50/30 mm Hg
Positive Findings	
History:	
• Primi	
• Young mother	
• Difficulty in breathing	
• No antenatal checkup	
• Maternal hypertension	
Examination:	
• Tachypnea	
• Respiratory distress	
• Grunting	
• Low birth weight	
• Preterm delivery	
• Basal crepitation	
• Abdominal distension	
Investigation:	
• Chest X-ray: Reticular granular pattern	

■ EXAMINATION

The newborn was lying in the bed with respiratory distress (RD). Features suggestive of IUGR were present. There were sternal retraction, intercostal indrawing, expiratory grunt, and tachypnea. He was on oxygen at a rate of 4 L to maintain oxygen saturation of 98.

The anthropometric measurements included the weight 1,500 g (<3rd centile), length 48 cm (10th centile), and the head circumference 33 cm.

The baby was afebrile, with heart rate 146 beats/min and respiratory rate 80 breaths/min. The blood pressure recorded was 50/30 mm Hg. There was no pallor, no cyanosis, and no lymphadenopathy. Acrocyanosis and bluish discoloration over the tongue was present.

Respiratory system revealed presence of crepitation at both bases. Per abdomen examination showed mild distension. Cardiovascular system revealed presence of tachycardia, with no features suggestive of CHD.

■ INVESTIGATION

- *Hemoglobin:* 12 g/dL
- *TLC:* 14,000 cells/cumm
- *DLC:* $P_{71}L_{25}E_2B_2$
- *Blood sugar level:* 70 mg/dL
- *Platelet count:* 300,000 cells/dL
- *Electrolyte:*
  - *Na:* 110 mEq/L
  - *K:* 4 mEq/L
  - *Cl:* 80 mEq/L
- *Blood group and Rh typing:* O positive
- *Chest X-ray:* Reticular granular pattern
- *Blood culture and sensitivity:* Sterile
- *Urine culture and sensitivity:* Sterile
- *ABG:* pH—7; $PaCO_2$—55 mm Hg; PaO_2—45 mm Hg; HCO_3—18 mEq/L

■ DISCUSSION

Neonatal RDS is the most common cause of respiratory failure in preterm infants. Its incidence is inversely related to gestational age and increases to as high as 95% in infants born at 22-24 weeks of gestation.

Hyaline membrane disease (HMD) is the important cause of RD in newborns. It occurs as a result of deficiency of surfactant. The name is derived from amorphous material that lines the terminal bronchiole and alveoli in this disease. Pathologically, there will be diffuse alveolar atelectasis, edema, and cell injury. It is the most common cause of death before 30 weeks.

■ INCIDENCE

- *A ratio of L/S less than:*
  - 1.5—70%
  - 1.5-2.0—40%
  - 2—unlikely
- Incidence is more in males, especially in cases with prematurity, perinatal asphyxia, maternal diabetes, and cesarean section, but not in labor.
- Incidence is reduced in stressful pregnancy such as eclampsia and infection, maternal drug addiction, IUGR, and corticosteroid administration prior to the delivery.

■ ETIOLOGY

- *Prematurity:* Surfactant appears in the lung in the third trimester hence, the preterm infant, i.e., delivered before the term will not have sufficiently developed surfactant.
- *Asphyxia:* Acidosis, hypothermia, and hypoxia will inhibit surfactant synthesis. This is more important in premature children.
- *Maternal diabetes:* There is increased incidence of RDS in infants of diabetic mother. The simple rationale is infants are delivered by cesarean section without having been in labor.
- *Cesarean section:* During the process of labor, there will be increased activity of adrenergic system. This will help to

release surfactant. This phenomenon is not available to the infants born with cesarean section.

The main feature of RDS is compromised lung function caused by both structural and biochemical immaturity of the lung.

Structural Immaturity

Lung development during fetal life occurs in different stages. Following organogenesis in the first two stages (embryonic and pseudoglandular) of lung development, the canalicular stage, starting at approximately 16 weeks after conception, is the first step in lung differentiation, involving formation of an actual air–blood barrier. Differentiation continues in both the saccular and alveolar stages of lung development starting at 24 and 36 weeks postconceptional age, respectively. This means that, at the time of birth, lung development of most preterm infants is still at the saccular stage, resulting in a reduced surface area for gas exchange and limited diffusion capacity due to thickened membranes at the air–blood interface.

Surfactant deficiency (decreased production and secretion) is the primary cause of RDS. In the absence of pulmonary surfactant, significantly increased alveolar surface tension leads to atelectasis, and the ability to attain an adequate FRC is impaired. As a consequence of progressive injury to epithelial and endothelial cells from atelectasis (atelectrauma), volutrauma, ischemic injury, and oxygen toxicity, effusion of proteinaceous material and cellular debris into the alveolar spaces (forming the classic hyaline membranes) further impairs oxygenation.

Biochemical Immaturity

The major constituents of surfactant are dipalmitoylphosphatidylcholine (lecithin), phosphatidylglycerol, apoproteins (surfactant proteins SP-A, SP-B, SP-C, and SP-D), and cholesterol. With advancing gestational age, increasing amounts of phospholipids are synthesized and stored in type II alveolar cells. These surface-active agents are released into the alveoli, where they reduce surface tension and help maintain alveolar stability at end expiration. Synthesis of surfactant depends in part on normal pH, temperature, and perfusion. Asphyxia, hypoxemia, and pulmonary ischemia, particularly in association with hypovolemia, hypotension, and cold stress, may suppress surfactant synthesis. The epithelial lining of the lungs may also be injured by high oxygen concentrations and mechanical ventilation, thereby further reducing secretion of surfactant.

The hallmark of RDS is a deficiency of pulmonary surfactant, a complex mixture of lipids (90%) and proteins (10%) that is synthesized in alveolar epithelial type II cells. Type II cells are 1 of the 2 epithelial cell types that line the alveolus. The most important function of surfactant is lowering of the alveolar surface tension, the force directed from the wall to the center of the alveolus at the air–liquid interface. This function is mainly attributed to the surfactant phospholipid dipalmitoylphosphatidylcholine and the surfactant hydrophobic proteins B and C. The hydrophilic surfactant proteins A and D play a role in innate host defense. Synthesis and storage of surfactant begins at about 16 weeks' gestation, and lung homogenates have high concentrations of surfactant by 20 weeks. However, surfactant is not secreted until later, appearing in amniotic fluid at approximately 28 weeks gestation, although this may vary greatly among individuals. This explains why some infants with a gestational age of <30 weeks do not develop neonatal

RDS while other infants, born at a more advanced gestation, do.

The high alveolar surface tension accompanying surfactant deficiency will increase the elastic recoil forces of the lung and decrease compliance of the respiratory system. As a result, preterm infants with RDS need to create large transpulmonary pressures to establish an adequate tidal volume. The absence of surfactant will also compromise lung volume stability, especially at the end of expiration. This makes the lung prone to a low end-expiratory lung volume and atelectasis, partly because the highly compliant chest wall is unable to counteract the increase in elastic recoil forces of the lung. A low end-expiratory lung volume may further compromise lung compliance and increase airway resistance and PVR. Due to the fact that the hypoxic pulmonary vasoconstriction response is often not functional in newborns, perfusion of collapsed sacculi–alveoli, also referred to as intrapulmonary right-to-left shunt, increases and results in (severe) hypoxemia.

Predisposing Factors

As mentioned, the incidence of RDS is inversely related to gestational age. It is twice as common in males than in females at all gestational ages and is more common in white infants. Delivery by cesarean section, particularly if performed before the onset of spontaneous labor, is an independent risk factor as well. Infants of diabetic mothers are five times more likely to develop RDS than infants of nondiabetic mothers with the same gestational age, sex, and mode of delivery. A higher maternal age also predisposes for RDS. Finally, the second-born twin is more likely to be affected, and a family history of RDS increases the risk for any given premature infant.

On the other hand, complications of pregnancy, such as pregnancy-induced hypertension, chronic maternal hypertension, premature rupture of membranes, intrauterine infection, and subacute placental abruption, all decrease the incidence of RDS. Infants born to mothers addicted to narcotics are also at less risk for developing RDS.

Risk Factors for Hyaline Membrane Disease

- Prematurity
- Male sex
- Cesarean section
- Maternal diabetes
- Second born twin
- Perinatal asphyxia

The risk for development of RDS increases with maternal diabetes, multiple births, cesarean delivery, precipitous delivery, asphyxia, cold stress, and a maternal history of previously affected infants. The risk of RDS is reduced in pregnancies with chronic or pregnancy-associated hypertension, maternal heroin use, prolonged rupture of membranes (PROM), and antenatal corticosteroid prophylaxis.

Factors which hasten the lung development include:

- Toxemia in mother
- PROM
- Glucocorticoid

PATHOLOGY

Pathologic findings early in the course of RDS include atelectasis, pulmonary edema, pulmonary vascular congestion, pulmonary hemorrhage, and evidence of direct injury to the respiratory epithelium. Epithelial cell injury is especially evident in the bronchiolar region of the lung. Histologic findings include the presence of hyaline membranes, the characteristic eosinophilic material derived from bronchial and bronchiolar injury to epithelial cells. Pulmonary edema, hemorrhage, and hemorrhagic edema are common pathologic features in RDS, especially if the clinical course is further complicated by PDA and congestive heart failure.

At postmortem examination, the lungs from infants with RDS are firm and airless. Atelectasis is striking on gross inspection, when the lungs are fixed in inflation, only the airways and a few alveolar ducts are air-filled. Diffuse atelectasis and dilated terminal bronchioles and alveolar ducts lined with a homogenous hyaline staining material characterize the microscopic picture. The hyaline membranes are plasma clots containing fibrin, other plasma constituents, and cellular debris. The small pulmonary arterioles appear constricted. There is congestion of pulmonary capillaries and veins and an increase in pulmonary water with dilation of the lymphatics. Because of these histological features, RDS was initially named HMD.

Interstitial air leaks are common, and collections of air are often seen around small airways and vessels. In some cases, the alveoli and hyaline membranes contain red cells. Electron microscopic examination shows degeneration of epithelial and endothelial cells and rupture of the basement membranes. If death occurs after 3 or 4 days of RD, the hyaline membranes are fragmented and numerous macrophages appear in the intra-alveolar spaces. The pulmonary interstitium is widened and filled with round cells and fibroblasts. After the first week, there is a proliferation of alveolar epithelial type II cells and capillaries, In, severe cases, chronic changes occur, including metaplasia of the bronchiolar epithelium and interstitial fibrosis.

■ PATHOPHYSIOLOGY

Normally surfactant begins to reappear in the lungs from 36 to 48 hours of age. Hence the condition worsens during the first 24 hours. Later, once the surfactant appears, it starts improving.

Histologically, there will be interstitial congestion of the alveolar wall. This causes desquamation of alveolar pneumonocytes. Alveolar ducts are dilated. There will be exudation of plasma into the alveoli. This again compromises with surface tension. Hyaline membrane is formed over the respiratory bronchioles and alveoli. This occurs as a result of coagulation of proteins of plasma exudate.

These changes lead to collapse of alveoli and stiffness of the lung. Lung compliance is decreased by 25%. Hence there will be increased work of breathing (WOB). There will also be increased pulmonary shunting producing, hypoxia, hypoventilation, and respiratory acidosis.

Pulmonary artery pressure and right heart pressure remain at the fetal level. This leads to right-to-left shunt across the ductus arteriosus and foramen ovale. Resultant hypoxia will produce alveolar damage.

This causes transudation of fluid and peripheral edema. Hypoxia produces hypotension, low blood volume, and hyperoxemia. This depresses myocardium. Accumulation of lactic acid occurs from anaerobic metabolism secondary to hypoxia.

The diuretic phase of RDS is characterized by 6–8 hours period of increased urine output. This occurs between 24 and 60 hours of life. The urine output is at least 80% of the intake. This phase heralds rapid improvement in lung function and recovery from RDS. Infants with delayed diuretic phase are more likely to develop BPD.

The characteristic clinical features of infants with neonatal RD are an expiratory grunt, tachypnea, intercostal and sternal retractions, and cyanosis. Grunting respiration is caused by a prolonged expiratory effort against a partially closed glottis. It is usually preceded by a strong inspiratory effort during which the intrathoracic pressure drops well below atmospheric pressure. During the prolonged expiration, intrathoracic pressure is maintained above atmospheric pressure. Infants do not grunt with every breath, and those with severe disease grunt most frequently. By maintaining a positive intrapulmonary pressure during most of the respiratory cycle, grunting probably helps to prevent atelectasis, which is one of the hallmarks of RDS.

Due to their decreased lung compliance, infants with RDS need to generate large transpulmonary pressures to establish an adequate tidal volume. The large negative intrathoracic pressures generated as the infant attempts to inflate its lungs cause the soft tissues of the chest cage to retract. These retractions are particularly notable in very small preterm infants as they have highly compliant chest walls. With severe RD, the lower sternum may be pulled in almost to the vertebral column by the forceful contraction of the diaphragm. Infants breathe primarily with the diaphragm and have very compliant chest walls; as a result they often have paradoxical breathing movements. Thus, as the chest caves in, its circumference becomes smaller while the abdominal circumference increases. As a result, breathing becomes less efficient and tidal volumes become smaller. By increasing their respiratory rate, the infants try to maintain an adequate minute volume as much as possible.

The combination of reduced alveolar ventilation and stability explains that breath sounds are often diminished in intensity and have a harsh, tubular quality. Occasionally, there are fine rales, particularly in those infants born by cesarean section, who may have excessive lung liquid.

Cyanosis is an early sign of RDS and, as the disease progresses, may be present even when an infant breathes 100% oxygen. As the lungs become more difficult to ventilate, the WOB increases, the infant tires, and arterial carbon dioxide tension rises. At the same time, the hypoxemia and diminished peripheral blood flow cause metabolic acidosis as lactic acid accumulates. With the development of acidosis, potassium leaves the cells and its concentration in serum rises, in some instances to very high levels.

Urine output is usually diminished early in the course of the disease, and the infants may become progressively edematous. Some infants, especially VLBW infants, have systemic hypotension, peripheral pallor, slow capillary filling, and hypothermia when not treated in time with sufficient respiratory support and exogenous surfactant.

■ POSTNATAL LUNG MATURATION

It takes only 1–2 days following birth for an immature lung to mature as it responds to the surge of glucocorticoids and beta-adrenergic compounds released by the stress of delivery. Glucocorticoids increase surfactant synthesis, and beta-adrenergic stimulation promotes its secretion. At the same time, structural changes occur in the lung. Thin-walled respiratory units develop, and the number of capillaries increases. With these changes, the signs and symptoms of RD usually subside after 48–72 hours of life. Recovery is usually heralded by diuresis. Clinical improvement is accompanied by a rapid fall in PVR and a rise in systemic arterial pressure. In some infants, particularly the least mature with birth weight <1,500 g, this may permit development of a large shunt from the aorta through a PDA to the pulmonary artery. In these infants, recovery may be interrupted by the development of pulmonary edema.

CAUSES OF RESPIRATORY DISTRESS IN PRETERM

The causes of RD in preterm are as follows:
- Subglottic stenosis
- Congenital pneumonia
- *Cardiac:* CHDs and PPHN (persistent pulmonary hypertension of the newborn) (primary/secondary)
- Congenital bilateral vocal cord palsy
- Air leak syndromes
- *Metabolic:* Hypothermia, hypoglycemia, metabolic acidosis, polycythemia, and hyperthermia
- Subglottic hemangioma
- Congenital airway malformation and congenital diaphragmatic hernia
- *CNS causes:* Seizures, perinatal asphyxia, IVH, and maternal medications (anesthetics and $MgSO_4$)
- *Cysts/masses:* Vallecular cyst, cystic hygroma
- Meconium aspiration syndrome (MAS)
- *Others:* Tracheoesophageal fistula (TEF), bilateral pulmonary hypoplasia, and anemia
- Laryngomalacia
- Short neck syndromes causing glossoptosis
- Laryngeal stenosis or atresia

CLINICAL FEATURES (FIG. 1)

Respiratory Distress in the Term Newborn

Respiratory distress in newborn is characterized by increased WOB in the form of tachypnea, grunting, chest retractions, and often associated with reduced air entry and cyanosis.

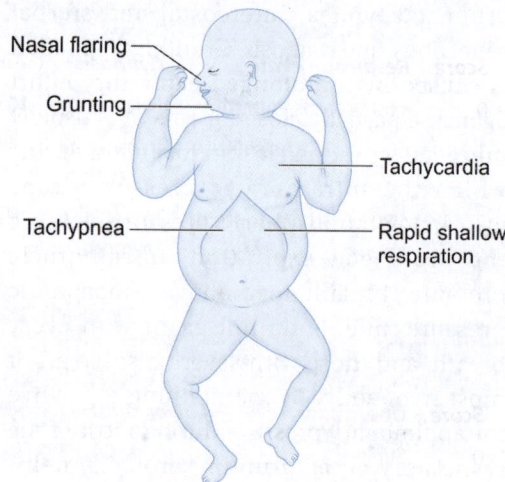

Fig. 1: Clinical features.

There are various clinical scoring systems for assessing the severity of RD objectively, out of which Downes scoring **(Table 1)** and Silverman–Anderson Score (SAS) **(Table 2)** scoring systems are widely used. Downes scoring system is used for term neonates, whereas SAS score is often used in preterm neonates.

Pulse oximetry screening is useful in early detection of critical CHD. All neonates must undergo preductal (right upper limb) and postductal (one of the lower limb) saturation check, around or after 24 hours of life and saturation <95% or saturation difference between preductal and postductal of 3% is considered as screen-positive and should undergo echocardiography.

Blood Gas Analysis

Arterial or capillary blood gas analysis helps in assessing the severity of RD and guiding the management.

Normal range of blood gas values in neonates are: pH 7.35–7.45, $PaCO_2$ 35–45 mm Hg, PaO_2 45–80 mm Hg, bicarbonate 20–24 mEq/L, and base deficit 3–7 mEq/L.

TABLE 1: Downes score.

Score	Respiratory rate	Cyanosis	Air entry	Grunt	Retraction
0	<60 breaths/minute	Nil	Normal	None	Nil
1	60–80 breaths/minute	In room air	Mild decrease	Audible with stethoscope	Mild
2	>80 breaths/minute or apnea	In >40% oxygen	Marked decrease	Audible without stethoscope	Moderate-to-severe

TABLE 2: Silverman–Anderson Score (SAS).

Score	Upper chest	Lower chest	Xiphoid retractions	Nares dilatation	Grunting
0	Synchronized	No retractions	None	None	None
1	Lag on inspiration	Just visible	Just visible	Minimal	Heard with stethoscope
2	Seesaw	Marked	Marked	Marked	Heard without stethoscope

TABLE 3: Grading of the severity of respiratory distress.

	Score	0	1	2
1	Respiratory rate	Less than 60	60–80	>80
2	Cyanosis	No	No cyanosis at 40% O_2	Require >40% O_2
3	Retraction	No	Mild	Moderate to severe
4	Grunting	No	Audible with stethoscope	Audible without Stethoscope
5	Air entry	Good	Decreased	Nonaudible

Characteristically, tachypnea, prominent (often audible) expiratory grunting, intercostal and subcostal retractions, nasal flaring, and cyanosis are noted. Breath sounds may be normal or diminished with a harsh tubular quality, and on deep inspiration, fine crackles may be heard. The natural course of untreated RDS is characterized by progressive worsening of cyanosis and dyspnea. If the condition is inadequately treated, blood pressure may fall; cyanosis and pallor increase, and grunting decreases or disappears, as the condition worsens. Apnea and irregular respirations are ominous signs requiring immediate intervention. Untreated patients may also have a mixed respiratory-metabolic acidosis, edema, ileus, and oliguria. Respiratory failure may occur in infants with rapid progression of the disease. In most cases the signs reach a peak within 3 days, after which improvement is gradual.

■ CLINICAL EXAMINATION

The clinical examination should include the assessment of severity of the disease as well as the cause of the distress **(Table 3)**.

Obstructed breathing occurs due to Pierre Robin anomaly and is relieved by prone position. Child turning pink on crying and cyanosed on nose breathing is seen with choanal atresia. Froth in the mouth and cyanosis during the feed first indicate TEF.

Pneumothorax and lobar emphysema will produce asymmetrical chest movements. Scaphoid abdomen and grossly shifted mediastinum suggests diaphragmatic hernia. Pink frothy tracheal fluid is encountered in pulmonary hemorrhage.

Time of onset of RD. Causes of the RD can be analyzed with the clue of time of onset of distress.

Within 4-6 hours of birth:
- Premature—HMD
- Term—meconium aspiration
- *Any gestational age:*
  - Pneumothorax
  - Asphyxia
  - Transient tachypnea of the newborn (TTN)
- Transposition of great arteries—failure to become pink

After 4 hours:
- Pneumonia
- CHD
- Metabolic acidosis or lung malformation.

The infant attempts to maintain alveolar volume by prolonging and increasing expiratory pressures by breathing against a partially closed glottis, causing the grunting noise characteristic of RDS but is often seen in other respiratory disorders. Increasing oxygen requirements and the need for ventilatory support often occur rapidly in the first 24 hours of life and continue for several days thereafter.

The clinical course depends on the severity of RDS and the size and maturity of the infant at birth. In uncomplicated RDS, typically seen in more mature infants, recovery is rapid and infants generally no longer require oxygen or ventilatory support after the first week of life. The most premature infants are at risk for severe RDS and frequently develop complications, including CNS, hemorrhage, PDA, air leak, and infection, which contribute to prolonged requirements for oxygen and ventilatory support.

Altered lung function test is depicted in the **Table 4**.

TABLE 4: Lung function test in respiratory distress syndrome (RDS).

	Measurement	Normal	RDS
1	Lung compliance (mL/H$_2$)	5–6	0.87–1.5
2	Forced residual capacity (mL/kg)	30	10–20
3	Tidal volume (mL/kg)	6–8	4–7
4	Alveolar volume (mL/kg/min)	200 mL	250–350 mL

The clinical signs to diagnose RDS include respiratory rate >60 beats/min, sternal retraction, intercostals and subcostal recession. To confirm our diagnosis all these signs should appear within 4 hours of birth and should persist for >4 hours.

CAUSES OF CYANOSIS IN RESPIRATORY DISTRESS SYNDROME

- Ventilation-perfusion mismatch due to atelectasis secondary to surfactant deficiency
- Intrapulmonary shunting of the blood due to pulmonary vasoconstriction secondary to hyperoxemia and acidosis
- Shunting across the foramen ovale and ductus arteriosus
- Atelectasis
- Acidosis
- Surfactant deficiency

GENERAL FEATURES
• Preterm baby
• Intercostal and subcostal retractions
• Cyanosis
• Breathlessness
• Apnea

ESSENTIAL DIAGNOSTIC POINTS

- Respiratory rate >60 breaths/min
- Cyanosis
- *Use of accessory muscles of respiration:* Nasal flaring, intercostals, and subcostal retraction
- Expiratory grunt
- Is caused by respiratory and nonrespiratory cause

DIAGNOSIS

The clinical course, radiograph of the chest, blood gas and acid-base values help to establish clinical diagnosis. Chest radiograph shows characteristic reticular granularity of the parenchyma. The laboratory findings are characterized initially by progressive hypoxemia, hypercarbia, and variable metabolic acidosis.

LABORATORY SALIENT FINDINGS

- L/S ratio in amniotic fluid
- Gastric shake test
- *X-ray chest:* Reticular granular pattern
- ABG to confirm hypoxemia, hypercarbia metabolic acidosis

(ABG: arterial blood gas; L/S: lecithin/sphingomyelin)

CHEST X-RAY

Table 5 shows the chest X-ray and ultrasound findings in various conditions.

This is the most useful investigation that can help in the etiological diagnosis of RDS in the newborn. The radiographic appearance of the lungs in infants with RDS is characterized by reduced aeration with a diffuse reticulogranular pattern of increased density, usually uniform in distribution but is occasionally more marked in the bases or on one side. The densities are due to miliary atelectasis and interstitial edema. Lung volumes are small, and even radiographs taken after a maximal inspiration rarely show the diaphragm to be below the eighth or ninth interspace. The heart is usually normal in size, although it often appears large because of the large thymic shadow and decreased lung volume. In RDS, the radiological features include symmetrical fine reticulogranular pattern, reduced lung volume, diffuse haziness (ground-glass appearance), air bronchograms, and complete white-out of lungs in late stages.

In (TTN), the chest X-ray shows normal or increased lung inflation, streaky perihilar infiltrates, and fluid in horizontal fissure. In MAS, chest X-ray shows hyperinflation, coarse irregular opacities, and sometimes pneumothorax air leaks, esophageal atresia, and diaphragmatic hernia.

TABLE 5: Chest X-ray and ultrasound findings in various conditions.

Condition	Chest X-ray	Ultrasound lung
TTN	Sunburst appearance; fluid in minor fissure	Thickened pleural lines, B lines, double lung point
MAS	Hyperinflation with bilateral patchy lung opacities	Disappearance of A lines, scattered B lines
RDS	Reticulogranular opacities/ground-glass appearance	B lines, white lungs
Pneumonia	Asymmetrical parenchymal infiltrates	Nonspecific changes
Pneumothorax	Collapsed lung border with air in pleural space with mediastinal shift	Absence of sliding sign; Barcode sign

(MAS: meconium aspiration syndrome; RDS: respiratory distress syndrome; TTN: transient tachypnea of the newborn)

DIFFERENTIAL DIAGNOSIS

- Group B streptococcal septicemia
- Cyanotic heart disease
- Persistent pulmonary hypertension
- Aspiration syndrome
- Diaphragmatic hernia
- Cystic adenomatoid malformation
- Pulmonary lymphangiectasia
- TTN

TRANSIENT TACHYPNEA OF THE NEWBORN

It may be difficult to distinguish RDS from normal, physiological pulmonary transition after birth. During this transition, fluid needs to be cleared from the lung and an air-filled FRC need to be created. Preterm infants often show signs of RD, including grunting and retractions. Furthermore, some infants may be oxygen dependent. In some infants, pulmonary transition may take several hours, a condition also referred to as TTN, or wet lung. However, in contrast to RDS, these symptoms are usually not progressive but instead resolve within the first 24–48 hours. Furthermore, the chest X-ray shows hyperaeration of the lungs, perihilar streaking and fluid in the interlobar fissures.

CONGENITAL PNEUMONIA

Infants with congenital pneumonia, especially group B streptococcus may also present with signs of RD that can be clinically and radiologically indistinguishable from RDS.

In the differential diagnosis, early-onset sepsis may be indistinguishable from RDS. In neonates with pneumonia, the chest radiograph may be identical to that for RDS. Clinical factors such as maternal group B streptococcal colonization with inadequate intrapartum antibiotic prophylaxis, maternal fever (>38.6°C) or chorioamnionitis, or PROM (>12 hours) are associated with an increased risk of early-onset sepsis. Echocardiography with color-flow imaging should be performed in infants, who show no response to surfactant replacement, to rule out cyanotic CHD as well as ascertain patency of the ductus arteriosus and assess PVR.

TREATMENT

At the time of birth, most of the lung is still fluid-filled, and the infant clears the fluid by creating large expiratory pressures, also referred to as expiratory braking. Clinically, expiratory braking often presents itself as grunting and retractions. Due to the fact that fluid clearance takes time, most infants are cyanotic at birth and it takes them up to 10 minutes to attain an oxygen saturation (SpO_2) of 90% or more. It is clear that normal physiological pulmonary transition may be difficult to distinguish from RDS. For this reason, the initial treatment should be similar and consist of supporting the infant without causing injury to the vulnerable lungs.

The main aim of treatment is to keep the baby alive and in good condition. This should continue until he starts synthesizing his own surfactant. Hence, any condition which inhibits surfactant synthesis should be managed carefully.

If the infant is spontaneously breathing, the expiratory phase of respiration should be supported with continuous positive airway pressure (CPAP). If spontaneous breathing is absent or inadequate, PPV should be initiated. If clinical signs of RD and cyanosis persist after the transitional phase, RDS is very likely and appropriate treatment should be started.

The primary aim in treatment of RDS is to restore lung function and gas exchange while avoiding treatment-induced injury to the vulnerable lungs of preterm infants. As low end-expiratory lung volume is the most prominent feature of RDS, stabilizing end-expiratory lung volume should be the first goal of treatment.

The following parameters should be monitored continuously in all babies.
- PaO_2 level by umbilical artery catheter (UAC) or by transcutaneous every 4-6 hourly
- ABG
- Fractional impaired oxygen concentration
- ECG
- Ventilator
- Electrolyte, calcium, and albumin daily or twice daily
- *Investigation:*
  - PCV
  - Chest radiography
  - Tracheal respiration for culture

Surfactant replacement therapy is provided through the endotracheal tube (ETT) and is often used several times during the early course of RDS to maintain pulmonary function. Exogenous surfactants are given by intratracheal instillation of doses of approximately 100 mg of phospholipids per 1 kg of body weight.

Supportive Treatment

- *Acid–base homeostasis:* It is necessary to keep infant's pH >7.25.
  - *Metabolic acidemia:* It is diagnosed when there is base deficit of >5 mmol/L. It is very important to treat the etiology like anemia, hypoxemia, and sepsis. However, treatment of academia is important, when the base deficit exceeds 5 mmol/L. Spontaneous correction is expected in an infant who is stable, i.e., normally perfused and normotensive. Again after waiting for 2-3 hours, base deficit is measured, if there is no improvement sodium bicarbonate can be used. But the rate of infusion should be slow. It should not exceed 0.5 mmol/min.

    Dose can be calculated as follows:
    Dose = Base deficit (mmol/L) × body weight (kg) × 0.4.

- *Respiratory academia and alkalemia:* Respiratory alkalemia is diagnosed when $PaCO_2$ level is below 30 mm Hg. This in turn produces decreased cardiac output and cerebral blood flow and interventricular hemorrhage.

    Most of the time is can be iatrogenic or over vigorous IPPV. A steady rise in $PaCO_2$ with the help of ventilator is advised. A sudden rise will suggest pneumothorax. Atelectasis misplaces ETT. Plasma expanders can be used at the dose of 10-20 mL/kg if the blood pressure is <30 mm Hg.

- *Feeding:* Oral feedings are withheld for first 2-3 days because of paralytic ileus. Many infants will pass meconium by third day. Bowel sounds will be present. Hence, 1 mL of expressed breast milk (EBM) hourly can be increased and if it is not tolerated, parenteral nutrition should be considered.

Fluid electrolyte balance: The main aim is to take care of excessive fluid administration. Infant with RDS are prone to develop pulmonary edema because of presence of hypoalbuminemia and increased capillary leak. Fluid overload gives rise to NEC, PDA, and chronic lung disease. Fluid intake is calculated or restricted to 60 mL/kg/day. Hypokalemia, hyperkalemia, and calcium hemostasis should be monitored and maintained. Infusion of dopamine (5–10 ug/kg/min) may help maintain the circulation and avoid excessive fluid administration, especially in the VLBW infant.

To avoid opening of the ductus arteriosus by fluid overload, 60 mL/kg fluid should be given the first day, 80 mL/kg in the next 3 days. Glucose is given at the strength of 10–50%. Sodium, calcium, and amino acids are also added. Hypoalbuminemia is seen among premature infants. Peripheral and pulmonary edema will result if the albumin level is below 20 g/L. Hence, infusion of 0.5–1g/kg is advised. Apprehension of the oligemia state in the first 24 hours of RDS can be alleviated by trial of frusemide at dose of 1.5 mg/kg.

Indomethacin is inhibitor of prostaglandin synthetase. This helps in closure of ductus arteriosus. The dose is 0.2 mg/kg orally or intravenously every 12th hourly for total of three doses. This is advised in infants with hypoxemia and CCF secondary to PDA.

Hypotension is the feature in the first few hours of life. Systolic blood pressure should be maintained at 30–40 mm Hg. PCV should be recorded. If it is <40, blood transfusion is advised. If PCV is 45%, albumin is given. If still hypotension persists, dopamine 5–10 mg/kg/min is given intravenously.

Surfactant Replacement Therapy

Surfactant deficiency, one of the main features of RDS, can be treated by exogenous surfactant replacement. Administering exogenous surfactant into the lungs will lower the surface tension, improve lung compliance, and stabilize end-expiratory lung volume.

Timing of Surfactant Therapy

There are two clearly defined treatment strategies tor administration of surfactant: (1) Prophylactic therapy, which requires the surfactant preparation to be instilled in the infant's trachea shortly after birth, preferably in the delivery room and (2) rescue therapy, which is designed to treat infants with established RDS. The latter can be divided into early (<2 hours after birth) or delayed (2 hours after birth) rescue treatment.

More recent studies comparing invasive mechanical ventilation combined with prophylactic surfactant treatment to primary nasal CPAP (nCPAP) and, if indicated, rescue surfactant treatment have shown that prophylactic treatment is associated with an increased risk of death or BPD. For this reason, prophylactic surfactant treatment is no longer recommended when using primary nasal CPAP at birth.

Modes of Surfactant Delivery

Historically, surfactant was administered via an ETT during invasive mechanical ventilation. As the latter has been identified as a major risk factor for ventilator-induced lung injury and subsequent BPD, alternative, less invasive strategies of surfactant administration have been investigated.

During the Intubate, Surfactant, and Extubate (INSURE) protocol, infants are intubated and surfactant is administered followed by immediate extubation to nasal CPAP. Compared with traditional surfactant treatment INSURE reduces the need for mechanical ventilation, but the effect on other clinical outcomes, such as mortality and BPD at 36 weeks postmenstrual age, is limited. With the aim of avoiding intubation altogether, some investigators explored the feasibility of administering surfactant during spontaneous breathing on nasal CPAP. Several studies have now shown that this route of administration, often referred to as less-invasive surfactant application (LISA) or minimally invasive surfactant therapy (MIST), reduces the need for invasive mechanical ventilation and death or BPD at 36 weeks postmenstrual age. Other modes of surfactant delivery, including the use of a laryngeal mask or nebulized surfactant administration, still need further evaluation.

Artificial surfactant, i.e., Exosurf in 67.5 mg phospholipids per kg administered gradually for over 15–40 minutes. Surfactant improves oxygenation by resolving atelectasis and improving lung compliance. Hence, it reduces the duration of ventilatory support and decreases the incidence of air leaks.

Before starting the surfactant therapy, these should be adequate oxygenation and perfusion. The dose of the survertor is 100 mg/kg (4 mL/kg). The route of administration is intratracheal. This is done by 5 Fr end-hole catheter. This tip of the catheter should come just beyond the ETT.

Repeat doses of the medicine may be administered depending upon the severity of the disease. Infant should be given 100% oxygen to aerosolize surfactant into all the lobes of both the lungs as the administration of the medicine. The therapy is followed by improved oxygenation, this requires reduction of MAP and FiO_2 to present development of air leaks, damage to retina and lungs. ETT are used. The frequent adverse effects are bradycardia, desaturation, apnea, and pulmonary hemorrhage. Risk can be decreased by prenatal glucocorticoid therapy. Early postnatal PDA treatment is done by indomethacin or ligation.

Oxygen Therapy

Aim of oxygen therapy is to keep PaO_2 level at 60–90 mm Hg. Higher concentration will cause ROP, pure oxygen administration is not advised. It inactivates surfactant and produces atelectasis and eventually produces pulmonary edema and hemorrhage. Purity of oxygen should limit to 95%.

Frequent checking of infant's PaO_2 is always mandatory. Along with it acid–base status should be monitored. Umbilical artery catheterization is a widely used technique. Problems associated with the catheter block should be looked for. The findings of the catheter blocks are pale, mottled legs, discolored legs, hematuria, and abdominal distension and blood in the stool.

Warmed and humidified oxygen is used. This is very useful for mild-to-moderate RDS. This should be given by head box. If the oxygen concentration required is >60%, alternative form of oxygen is started.

The basic defect requiring treatment in RDS is inadequate pulmonary oxygen–carbon dioxide exchange. Basic supportive care (thermoregulatory, circulatory, fluid, electrolyte, and respiratory) is essential, while FRC is established and maintained. Careful and frequent monitoring of heart and respiratory rates, arterial oxygen saturation (SaO_2), PaO_2, $PaCO_2$, pH, electrolytes, glucose, hematocrit, blood pressure, and temperature are essential. Arterial catheterization is frequently necessary. Because most cases of RDS are self-limited, the goal of treatment is to minimize abnormal physiologic variations and superimposed iatrogenic problems. Treatment of infants with RDS is best carried out in the NICU.

Nasal Continues Positive Airway Pressure

Recognizing the benefits of surfactant replacement therapy, in addition to the potential protective effects of prophylactic nCPAP some experts recommend intubation for prophylactic or early rescue surfactant replacement therapy, followed by extubation back to nCPAP immediately once the infant is stable (usually within minutes to <1 h). The aforementioned method is commonly referred to as *intubate, surfactant, and extubate*. A variation of the INSURE method has evolved known as *minimally invasive surfactant therapy* or *less invasive surfactant administration*, in which a small feeding tube, rather than an ETT, is used to deliver intratracheal surfactant to a spontaneously breathing infant on nCPAP. The combination of early rescue surfactant by the INSURE, MIST, or LISA method with nCPAP has been associated with the reduced need for mechanical ventilation, and emerging evidence suggests modest benefits in terms of preventing BPD. The amount of nCPAP required usually decreases after approximately 72 hours of age, and most infants can be weaned from nCPAP shortly thereafter. Assisted ventilation and surfactant are indicated for infants with RDS who cannot keep oxygen saturation >90% while breathing 40–70% oxygen and receiving nCPAP.

Mechanical Ventilation

The goal of mechanical ventilation is to improve oxygenation and ventilation without causing pulmonary injury or oxygen toxicity. Acceptable ranges of ABG values vary significantly among institutions, but generally range from PaO_2, 50–70 mm Hg, $PaCO_2$, 45–65 mm Hg (and higher after the first few days when risk of IVH is less), and pH 7.20–7.35. During mechanical ventilation, oxygenation is improved by increasing either FiO_2, or the MAP.

Modes of Mechanical Ventilation

Synchronized intermittent mechanical ventilation (SIMV) delivered by time-cycled, pressure-limited, continuous flow ventilators is a common method of conventional ventilation for newborns. With pressure-limited SIMV, a set PIP is delivered in synchrony with the patients' own breaths for a specified rate per minute. For breaths above the set rate, pressure support breaths [8–10 cm H_2O above positive end-expiratory pressure (PEEP)] are provided to help overcome the resistance associated with spontaneous breathing through the ETT.

High-frequency ventilation (HFV) achieves desired alveolar ventilation by using smaller tidal volumes and higher rates (300–1,200 breaths/min or 5–20 Hz). HFV may improve elimination of CO_2, and improve oxygenation in patients, who show no response to conventional ventilators, as well as those who have severe RDS, interstitial emphysema, recurrent pneumothoraces, or meconium aspiration pneumonia.

High-frequency oscillatory ventilation (HFOV) and *high-frequency jet ventilation* (HFJV) are the most frequently used methods. HFOV may reduce BPD, but the effect size is likely small. In severe respiratory failure unresponsive to conventional mechanical ventilation, HFOV strategies that promote lung recruitment, combined with surfactant therapy, may improve gas exchange. HPJV is particularly useful to facilitate resolution of air leaks. Elective use of either HFV method, in comparison with conventional ventilation, generally does not offer advantages when used as the initial ventilation strategy to treat infants with RDS.

Continuous Positive Airway Pressure

Adequacy of ventilation and oxygenation must be established as soon as possible to avoid pulmonary vasoconstriction, further V-Q abnormalities and atelectasis. PPV, CPAP, and oxygen therapy may be required at any time during the course of RDS and must be readily available to the infant. Close monitoring of pH, oxygen saturation, pCO_2 by transcutaneous monitors, and by arterial catheterization or sampling of arterialized capillary blood is critical in guiding mechanical ventilation and ambient oxygen requirements.

This improvement in oxygenation has been linked to a higher end-expiratory lung volume. Recent studies have also shown that primary CPAP is the preferred mode of respiratory support after birth, as it reduces the need for invasive mechanical ventilation, surfactant treatment, and the risk of death or BPD.

Continuous positive airway pressure is usually administered via the nasal route using either a mask or prongs. Although the optimal level of CPAP still needs to be established, a continuous positive pressure of up to 6–10 cmH_2O can be tolerated by the nasal route. Minimal invasive surfactant treatment and nasal IPPV might further enhance the success of CPAP in patients with RDS. However, there is insufficient evidence to support the use of humidified high-flow nasal cannula as an alternative primary mode for CPAP in infants with RDS.

In cases in which nasal noninvasive support is not effective in restoring lung function and gas exchange or if severe apnea occurs, intubation and mechanical ventilation should be started using either conventional modes or HFV. Again, maintaining an optimal lung volume should be the primary ventilation strategy when using these modes.

Here the applied pressure is up to 8–10 cmH_2O. This pressure keeps the alveoli open and preserves the surfactant. Splinting of the alveoli by pressure reduces the shearing forces.

Lung function shows improvement; respiration become regular; FRC increases; airway resistance decreases; CVP is raised by 10–20%; pulse pressure falls slightly.

Continuous positive airway pressure can be 8 L/min. The gas should be warmed and humidified. The level of the CPAP can be adjusted by tightening the gate clip. This should be accompanied by varying the distance between the water surface of the tube in the water bottle. The conventional pressure monitor is used to check the amount of CPAP.

The CPAP is indicated when the $PaCO_2$ is <60 mm Hg in recurrent apnea and during the weaning phase of ventilator. More effective CPAP is seen when it is started early. CPAP is more useful when the child requires oxygen at the concentration of 60–70%. It is useful in infants of <1.5 kg weight who need 30–40% oxygen during the first 24 hours of life. The initial pressure applied is 5–6 cmH_2O of CPAP. Once the condition improves CPAP is reduced to 1–2 cmH_2O. Finally, reduction is 2 cmH_2O.

Partial pressure of arterial oxygen is checked for each change. Once the PaO_2 is satisfactory at the CPAP of 2 cmH_2O, CPAP can be discontinued. If the same thing is maintained minimum for 4 hours and again if it deteriorates, CPAP can be restarted.

As forced inspiratory oxygen requirements decrease during recovery, airway pressure is decreased and the infant is weaned to head hood or nasal cannula oxygen. Apnea, inadequacy of ventilation, atelectasis, mucous plugging, and hyperaeration or air leak may complicate the care of infants with RDS.

Nasogastric tube feeding is well tolerated. Oral feeds can complicate into regurgitation. Intravenous fluid should be carefully monitored for the fear of fluid retention by retarding venous return.

Intermittent Positive Pressure Ventilation

Indications:
- Electively in VLBW, i.e., <1,000 g
- Blood gas analysis is poor
- Severe retraction
- Intractable apnea
- Laboratory indication—respiratory acidosis pH <7.2
- Severe hypoxemia
- Clinical failure to establish effective ventilation, onset of apnea irregular, and exhausted respiration
  - $PaCO_2$ >Torr
  - PaO_2 <50–60 Torr

Principles: Normal lungs require low pressure, i.e., 12–14 cmH_2O to inflate. The inspiratory time is 0.2 seconds and expiratory time is 0.4 seconds [inspiratory to expiratory (I:E)—1:2]. This is the time required for the lungs to inflate to 60% of its minimum. At this level airway resistance and lung compliance coincide with each other, i.e., apnea of premature.

Low compliance of lungs in RDS: It requires relatively more I:E time to inflate lungs. It requires high inspiratory pressure with the PEEP to keep alveoli open. This requires MAP of 12–14 cmH_2O volume by rising the respiratory rate and tidal volume or lowering PEEP. High resistance as in meconium aspiration requires prolonged expiratory time, no PEEP, and slow rate.

The aim of the IPPV is to keep PaO_2 level above 40 mm Hg and $PaCO_2$ level below 60 mm Hg. $PaCO_2$ level more than this produces IVH in an infant weighing <1.5 kg.

Endotracheal tube number 3.0 or 3.5 mm diameter should be used. Oral ETT is used for shorter duration, i.e., for 24 hours. If the longer periods of IPPV is expected, nasal ETT are used. Outer margin of the ETT at the end of the nostril should be marked and fixed to avoid displacement. Immobilization of the tube is very important. Position of the tube is checked radiologically. Baby's head should be placed in slight extension. This will avoid trauma to laryngeal mucosa.

Small dead space should be maintained in the ventilator circuit and in baby. This will help to prevent atelectasis. Good humidifier is required. Suctioning of the ETT is repeated every fourth hourly. Swift and efficient suctioning is accepted. 0.5 mL of normal saline should be instilled before suctioning. Child should be observed during suctioning. Suctioning should stopped immediately if there is cyanosis and if $PaCO_2$ levels falls below 50 mm Hg and if the heart rate is below 80 beats/min.

Initial Ventilator Settings

- *Respiratory rate:* 30–40 breaths/min; inspiratory time: 0.2–0.6 seconds.

  In VLBW 60–40 breaths/min may be more physiological. Baby synchronizes better with ventilator to give improved oxygen and pH. This will lower the incidence of pneumothorax.
- Peak pressure initially 25 mm Hg
  I:E ratio is 1:2
  Gas flow rate—5–10 L/min
- Continuous distending pressure of 4–6 cmH_2O to keep alveoli open.

  Failure to synchronize with a ventilator may be an indicator for transiently raising inspiratory pressure or plasma infusion. If the infant's fighting continues, a high pressure of 30–40 cmH_2O is continued for exceptionally stiff lung. Child may require sedation.

Ventilator setting is done according to the readings given as follows:
- *Rate:* 30–40/minute
- *FiO_2:* 0.8

- *Positive inflation pressure:* 25 cmH$_2$O
- *PEEP:* 5 cmH$_2$O
- *I:E ratio:* 1:1::1.5:1
- *Gas flow per minute:* 5–10 L/minute

Subsequent alteration to ventilator settings: This is in order of adjustment while improving ventilation to minimize atelectasis, BPD, and pneumothorax.
- Oxygen is raised to not >95%.
- Altering I:E ratio can be prolonged, the inspiration raised PaO$_2$ 1:1; 1:2 for ventilating healthy lung
- Respiratory rate is raised to reduce CO$_2$ retention. Sometimes, it is better to accept raised PaCO$_2$ than increasing the peak inflation pressure.
- The inflation pressure is raised to 5 cmH$_2$O.

  Once these improve in the status, peak pressure is reduced. Oxygen and respiratory rate is reduced to minimize barotrauma, pneumothorax, and BPD.

  Mechanical problems associated with the ventilator should also be kept in mind when there is no improvement in the child's condition.
- *No chest wall movements:* Hand ventilation with 100% oxygen by bag and mask. Improvement indicates ventilator leak or stiff lung needing higher pressure. Poor or no response means tube higher pressure. Poor or no response means tube is partially or totally blocked and infant should be reintubated.
- If the chest wall is moving it means ventilator is working, then tube should be checked to know whether it is in right main bronchus. Adequate oxygen concentration rate of inflation pressures are monitored.
- If the child is still fighting nonsynchronized, then oxygen concentration is increased up to 95%. Respiratory rate is increased in steps like 10 breaths/min up to 60–90 per minute. Inflation pressure can be increased. If the child is still fighting then pancuronium is continuously used.
- If still the child is fighting to improve, then pneumothorax, septicemia, hypotension, hypoglycemia should be suspected. Metabolic acidosis, NEC, PDA should also be considered.

Partial pressure of oxygen is directly related to the MAP. MAP is the measure of the average pressure to which the lungs are exposed during the respiratory cycle. This can be calculated by dividing the area under the airway pressure curve by the duration of the cycle. The MAP is affected by the changes in the inspiratory flow, peak respiratory pressure, and the ratio of I:E. MAP can be measured directly from ventilator. Retention of CO$_2$ occurs when there is slow respiratory rate, short expiratory time, and high levels of PEEP. If there is hypercapnia and hypoxia, PIP is increased until satisfactory gas analysis is obtained.

Optimal PEEP is the end-expiratory pressure at which oxygenation is minimum with the minimal effect of cardiovascular function. To determine this, PEEP is maintained at the level equal to 10% of the inspired oxygen concentration.

To improve oxygenation when PaCO$_2$ is normal, i.e., 35–55 mm Hg, MAP is increased. PEEP is also increased. Inspiration should, however, rarely last longer than 1.5 seconds. I:E ratio is of no use.

To improve oxygenation when PaCO$_2$ is <30–35 mm Hg, diagnosis should be rechecked. Other causes to be considered are CHD, persistent fetal circulation, and overventilation. Chest X-ray is helpful. If still the diagnosis is RDS, MAP should be sustained. When PEEP is increased, rate is decreased.

When there is hypercapnia, i.e., >70 mm Hg, it is managed by increasing the rate and decreasing the PEEP. PEEP should not be reduced below 3 cmH_2O as it preserves the surfactant. Infant can be paralyzed by pancuronium.

In spite of all these maneuvers, if the blood gas analysis is not satisfactory, the following possibilities are suspected:
- Blocked or leaking tube
- Noncorrected metabolic and electrolytic imbalance
- Complications of RDS.

For diagnosis in RDS, PIP and MAP are pushed until PaO_2 is 50 mm Hg. This is used in children with CO_2 retention. The disadvantage is air leak syndrome and chronic lung disease. Other method is increasing the fast ventilatory rate and this causes pulmonary vascular dilatation.

If all the procedures fail, the three most common diagnoses to be kept in mind are pneumonia or septicemia, massive IVH and primary pulmonary hypoplasia.

Once the reasonable, satisfactory blood gases are obtained this should be maintained for 3–4 hours. If PIP is >30 cm H_2O, every attempt is made to bring it down. RDS tends to get worse for the first 36–48 hours.

As RDS resolves, the peak pressure is reduced in steps of 2–4 cm H_2O and oxygen steps of 5–10% down to 40–45%.

Antibiotics

As infant is on IPPV, antibiotics should be started. Some antibiotics are maintained until the infant is on IPPV or for 1 week after IPPV.

Vitamin E

Vitamin E is a biological antioxidant. This inhibits peroxidation of membrane lipids by the radical such as superoxide. It is advised in LBW babies receiving 100 per oxygen, which will cause retrolental fibroplasia and BPD. The dose is 100 IU/kg/day intramuscular to maintain blood vitamin E level between 2.0 and 3.0 IU/dL.

Sedation

Pancuronium is the drug for sedation. Indications for sedation are:
- Child fighting with ventilatory breath to avoid risk of pneumothorax
- Child who requires greater than 75% of oxygen and or PIP greater than 30 cmH_2O
- In case of fluctuation in blood pressure, if untreated, infants may have increased IVH.

Position of the infant should be changed every 2–3 hourly. If this is done promptly, secretion is rarely a problem. ETT should be sucked out every 4–6 hourly instilling normal saline. Chest physiotherapy is done if the secretion become a problem.

Weaning of Intermittent Positive-Pressure Ventilation

This process takes several weeks. Sometimes it will be completed within 24 hours. Weaning off is slower in LBW babies. Weaning process is started by reducing high pressure and oxygen concentration. Pressure is reduced at the rate of 2–3 cmH_2O and oxygen concentration by 5–10% at a time. Such reduction step can be done once in 4 hours.

In VLBW, rate is reduced gradually, i.e., 15/min, 10/min, and 5/min. Prolonged apnea is avoided. This will help infants to develop spontaneous respiratory effort. While reducing the rate, the inspiratory time should never exceed 1 second. This is known as intermittent mandatory ventilation.

While changing to CPAP, forced inspiratory oxygen level should be increased to

0.05–0.1. This is because infant may become transiently hypoxia or apneic during or after transfer. After changing there will be immediate surge in PaO_2 because of increased FiO_2. Hence, it is necessary to check $PaCO_2$, 30–60 minutes after the transfer to CPAP.

Extubation

When the child's condition is good, chest X-rays show no pneumothorax, PCV is >40%, and extubation is done. Adequate humidification of inspired air should be ensured. Nasal prone CPAP at the same pressure should be contained. Oral feeding should be stopped for 12–24 hours as feeds decrease PaO_2. Careful aspiration of the mouth and oropharynx is done. Once the infant is extubated and is on nasal CPAP, CPAP can be discontinued gradually, 1–2 cm H_2O at a time for a week or more.

Causes of failure of weaning of IPPV:
- PDA with pulmonary edema
- Secretions
- Laryngeal edema and stenosis
- BPD
- Recurrent apnea

■ COMPLICATIONS

Complications of the RDS
- Pneumothorax
- BPD
- IVH
- PDA
- Fluid overload
- PIF
- Laryngeal stenosis
- Neurological handicap
- Septicemia
- Complication of RDS

Central nervous system hemorrhage, IVH, and PDA represent significant clinical problems affecting the care of infants with RDS. PDA and subsequent congestive heart failure and pulmonary edema further compromise respiratory function, decreasing pulmonary compliance and perhaps inactivating pulmonary surfactant.

Prompt diagnosis and medical or surgical treatment of PDA are indicated during the treatment of RDS.

Acute CNS hemorrhage is often associated with shock, pulmonary compromise, and pulmonary hemorrhage. Fluctuations in respiratory status may contribute to IVH and can be minimized by careful attention to respiratory care and by judicious use of sedation.

Intravenous fluids and administration of oral feedings must be adjusted carefully during acute and convalescent care of infants with RDS. Excessive fluid administration impairs pulmonary function and increases the risk of PDA.

■ PREVENTION

Neonatal RDS is associated with incomplete development of the lung at the time of birth. Thus, premature delivery should be delayed, where possible. If this cannot be avoided, additional efforts should be made to accelerate lung maturation. Animal studies have shown that antenatal administration of glucocorticoids accelerates both structural and biochemical (surfactant) lung maturation.

Administration of betamethasone to women in premature labor at least 2 days before delivery significantly reduced the incidence of RD. Numerous studies following this pivotal publication have confirmed that antenatal glucocorticoids reduce mortality and perinatal morbidities, such as RDS, IVH, and NEC. Treatment consists of two doses of 12 mg of betamethasone given intramuscularly 24 hours apart, or four doses of 6 mg of dexamethasone given intramuscularly 12 hours apart. The benefits of antenatal steroid typically begin at around 24 hours after initiation of therapy and last 7 days. Current guidelines recommend treatment with antenatal glucocorticoids if preterm delivery is imminent between 24 and 34 weeks of gestation.

BIBLIOGRAPHY

1. Bahrami KR, Van Meurs KP. ECMO for neonatal respiratory failure. Semin Perinatol. 2005;29(1):15-23.
2. Donn SM, Sinha SK. Manual of Neonatal Respiratory Care, 4th edition. Germany: Springer International Publishing; 2016.
3. Gelfand SL, Fanaroff JM, Walsh MC. Meconium stained fluid: approach to the mother and baby. Pediatr Clin North Am. 2004;51(3):655-67, ix.
4. Pfister RH, Soll RF. Initial respiratory support of preterm infants: the role of CPAP, the INSURE method and noninvasive ventilation. Clin Perinatal. 2012;39:459-81.
5. Sweet DG, Carnielli V, Greisen G, Hallman M, Ozek E, Plavka R, et al.; European Association of Perinatal Medicine. European consensus guidelines on the management of neonatal respiratory distress syndrome in preterm infant—2010 update. Neonatology. 2010;97:402-17.
6. Warren JB, Anderson JM. Newborn respiratory disorders. Pediatr Rev. 2010;31:487-95; quiz 496.
7. Yeh TF. Core concepts: meconium aspiration syndrome: pathogenesis and current management. NeoReviews. 2010;11:e503-e12.

SECTION

Nutrition

- Case 89 **Obesity**
- Case 90 **Protein–Energy Malnutrition**
- Case 91 **Rickets**
- Case 92 **Scurvy**

CASE 89

Obesity

PRESENTING COMPLAINTS

A 10-year-old boy was brought with the complaint of:
- Obesity since 6 months
- Withdrawal behavior since 6 months
- Pessimistic attitude since 3 months

History of Presenting Complaints

A 10-year-old boy was brought to hospital with problem of obesity, which worried him. That made him to develop withdrawal behavior. His psychosomatic symptoms started worrying his parents. His mother complained that he would remain alone. He was not showing much interest in playing along with his peers. His mother also told that he used to avoid any work which requires physical exercise. He started developing pessimistic attitude.

Past History of the Patient

The boy was the elder sibling of consanguineous marriage. He was delivered at full term by normal vaginal delivery. The birth weight of the child was 3.5 kg. There was no significant postnatal event except normal physiological jaundice. He was bottle-fed since birth and cereals and fruits were started when he was 6 months old. His mother had no records of infancy but she told that he had been always with big body. His developmental milestones were normal. He had been completely immunized. She never thought his son ate excessively and never worried that he was overweight. A dietician assessed and calculated that his daily intake was about 3,500 calories.

CASE AT A GLANCE	
Basic Findings	
Height	: 135 cm (50th centile)
Weight	: 46 kg (>97th centile)
Temperature	: 37°C
Pulse rate	: 100 beats/min
Respiratory rate	: 20 breaths/min
Blood pressure	: 110/80 mm Hg
Positive Findings	
History:	
• Overweight	
• Psychosomatic symptoms	
Examination:	
• Normal	
Investigation:	
• Normal	

EXAMINATION

The child was obese. He was moderately built. His anthropometric measurements included the height 135 cm (50th centile) and the weight 46 kg (>97th centile). He was tall and weight was out of proportion.

He was afebrile. Pulse rate was 100 beats/min and the respiratory rate was 20 breaths/min. The blood pressure recorded was 110/80 mm Hg. There was no pallor, no lymphadenopathy, no cyanosis, and no clubbing. Other systemic examinations were normal.

INVESTIGATION

- *Hemoglobin:* 14 g/dL
- *Total leukocyte count (TLC):* 7,200 cells/cumm
- *Differential leukocyte count (DLC):* $P_{55}L_{40}E_3M_0$
- *Erythrocyte sedimentation rate (ESR):* 26 mm in the first hour
- *Absolute eosinophil count (AEC):* 300 cells/dL
- *Urine examination:* Normal
- *X-ray chest:* Normal

DISCUSSION

Obesity is the most common nutritional disorder of children. Here adipose tissue is enlarged out of proportion to other body organs. It is the term used when the weight exceeds 120% of standard weight. In practice, simple observation of undressed child leaves little doubt about the diagnosis.

The body mass index (BMI) defined as weight/height^2 (in kg/m^2) is most useful index. It correlates significantly with subcutaneous and total fat in adolescents. The term overweight is used when BMI exceeds 95th percentile for that age and gender. Skinfold thickness above 85th percentile for age and gender also suggests obesity. It can be measured at triceps, midabdominal or subscapular sites.

Obesity is defined as BMI at or above the 95th percentile for the child's age and gender. Severe or extreme levels of pediatric obesity have also been defined using several different criteria. Extreme obesity has been reported as BMI at the 97th and 99th percentiles; at the 120th percentile above the 95th percentile; or as excess overweight calculated as 100 × (BMI/50th percentile BMI for child age and gender).

The hypothalamus contains two important sets of neurons: Anorexigenic (appetite suppressing) proopiomelanocortin (POMC) neurons and orexigenic (appetite promoting) neuropeptide Y (NPY) neurons. Hormones that are direct measures of the energy status of an individual (i.e., fasting or fed) can directly activate or suppress these neurons to bring the individual back to equilibrium. Insulin, glucose, leptin, lipids, and the gut-derived peptides cholecystokinin, amylin, peptide YY (PYY), glucagon-like peptide-1 (GLP-1), ghrelin, and gastric inhibitory peptide (GIP) all have actions within the brain to control food intake. For instance, after a meal, glucose levels rise along with insulin levels. Insulin can activate POMC neurons and inhibit NPY neurons, which promotes satiety and the cessation of eating. There is also evidence that the body will defend a higher body weight through decreased energy expenditure and/or increased hunger after weight loss. These pathways are highly complex and contribute to the difficulty in losing weight and maintaining weight loss in the obese individual.

GENETICS

One important example, the *FTO* gene at 16q12, is associated with adiposity in childhood, probably explained by increased energy intake. Monogenic forms of obesity have also been identified, including melanocortin-4 receptor (MC4R) deficiency, associated with early-onset obesity and food-seeking behavior. Mutations in MC4R are a common cause of monogenetic obesity but a rare cause of obesity in general. Deficient activation of MC4R is seen in patients with

POMC deficiency, a prohormone precursor of adrenocorticotropic hormone (ACTH) and melanocyte-stimulating hormone (MSH), resulting in adrenal insufficiency, light skin, hyperphagia, and obesity.

There are genetic conditions associated with obesity, such as Prader–Willi syndrome, which results from absence of paternally expressed imprinted genes in the 15q11.2-q13 region.

ENDOCRINE AND NEURAL PHYSIOLOGY

Gastrointestinal (GI) hormones, including cholecystokinin, GLP-1, PYY, and vagal neuronal feedback promote satiety. Ghrelin stimulates appetite. Adipose tissue provides feedback regarding energy storage levels to the brain through hormonal release of adiponectin and leptin. Adipocytes secrete adiponectin into the blood, with reduced levels in response to obesity and increased levels in response to fasting. Reduced adiponectin levels are associated with lower insulin sensitivity and adverse CV outcomes. Leptin is directly involved in satiety; low leptin levels stimulate food intake, and high leptin levels inhibit hunger in animal models and in healthy human volunteers.

Numerous neuropeptides in the brain, including PYY, agouti-related peptide, and orexin, appear to affect appetite stimulation, whereas melanocortins and d-melanocortin-stimulating hormone are involved in satiety.

The most common method for clinically identifying a child as being overweight or obese relies on the definition for children using the BMI. BMI percentile is used and recommended most frequently because it is easy and inexpensive to obtain. This index is a reflection of weight for height. As a child grows, normal BMI values vary with age and sex, thus, a single absolute cutoff of BMI as a measure of obesity is not available in youth. Overweight for children is defined as a BMI at or above the 85th percentile but below the 95th percentile for the child's age and gender.

CLINICAL FEATURES (FIG. 1)

Many times diagnosis is made from child's appearance. Obesity **(Fig. 2)** or overnutrition is generalized. Excessive accumulation of fat in the subcutaneous and other tissues can be quantitated by measuring skinfold thickness

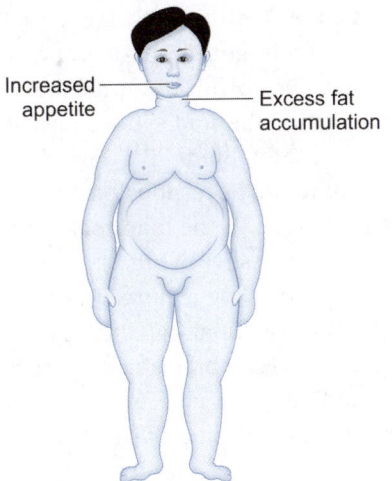

Fig. 1: Clinical features.

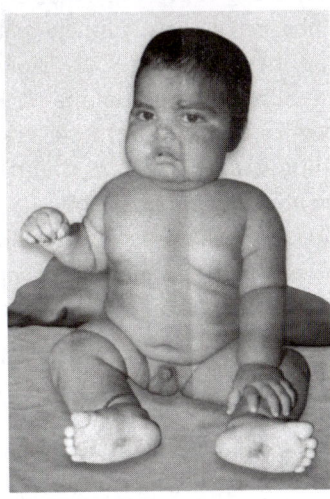

Fig. 2: Obesity.

with skin fold calipers. It is mainly due to excessive intake of the food.

Genetic predisposition may also be present. Lack of activity may be responsible for obesity even though intake of food may not be unusual. It may result from increase in number or size of fat cells, adipocytes. Adipocytes appear to increase in number when caloric intake is increased.

Stocky children may have relatively large skeletal frames and have more than average amount of muscular tissue. Appetite may be influenced by various factors. These include psychogenic disturbances and hypothalamus, pituitary, or other brain lesions. Some inherited syndromes such as Laurence-Moon-Biedl, Prader-Willi, and Cushing may also be responsible.

The adiposity in the mammary region of boy is often suggestive of breast development and an embarrassing feature. The obesity of the extremities is usually greater in the upper arm and thigh. The hands may be relatively small and fingers are tapering. Genu valgum is common. Psychological disturbance is also common.

Obese children carry a large body weight. This tires them more easily and further reduces physical activity. Clinical features of endocrine, hypothalamic, or various cryptogenic syndromes are obvious. Traumatic inflammation and neoplastic lesion of hypothalamus and pituitary gland causes increased appetite and hence obesity.

Leptin is adipose tissue secreted hormone with receptors in hypothalamus. Plasma level of leptin correlates with body fat mass and is regulated by feeding, fasting, insulin, and steroid.

Insulin decreases lipolysis and increases fat syntheses and uptake. Genetic studies have shown the relation between leptin, gene, and obesity.

The obese respond to carbohydrate meal with increased insulin and decreased utilization of free fatty acids. Protein conservation is facilitated as the brain utilizes ketones for energy. If the obesity is initiated early, it is likely to persist. There is good evidence that fatty children will become obese adults.

It can become evident at any age, but most frequently it is seen in the first year, 5-6 years of age, and during adolescence. The facial features often appear disproportionately fine. The abdomen is tender to be pendulus. White and purple striae are often present. The external genitalia of the boy is disproportionately small. Penis is often embedded in pubic fat.

Puberty may occur early, hence ultimate height of the person is less. The development of external genitalia is normal in majority of girls. Menarche is not usually delayed.

The extreme exogenous obesity produces severe cardiorespiratory distress in pulmonary, tidal, and expiratory reserve volume. The manifestations include polycythemia, hypoxemia, cyanosis, cardiac enlargement, and congestive cardiac failure.

Obesity may be exogenous and endogenous.

Exogenous obesity:
- Constitutional
- Excessive food intake
- Decreased energy expenditure
- Fat cell hyperplasia

Endogenous obesity:
- *Genetic:*
  - Prader-Willi syndrome
  - Laurence-Moon-Biedl syndrome
- *Hormonal:*
  - Hypothyroidism
  - Hypogonadism
  - Pseudohypoparathyroidism
  - Cushing's syndrome

- *Hypothalamic:*
  - Obesity

Those with BMI >85 percentile for the age should be investigated, if they have any of the following:
- Family history of cardiovascular complications of type II diabetes
- Rapid increase in obesity
- Hypertension

Blood sugar, serum cholesterol, lipid profile, LFT, skeletal maturity evaluation, hormonal test, i.e., urine free cortisol, free thyroxine (FT4) and thyroid-stimulating hormone (TSH), testosterone, estradiol and gonadotropin assay as suggested by clinical examination.

CLINICAL EVALUATION

Laboratory testing for fasting plasma glucose, triglycerides, low-density lipoprotein and high-density lipoprotein cholesterol, and liver function tests are recommended as part of the initial evaluation for newly identified pediatric obesity. Overweight children (BMI 85-95th percentile) who have a family history of diabetes mellitus or signs of insulin resistance should also be evaluated with a fasting plasma glucose test. Other laboratory testing should be guided by history or physical examination findings.

The evaluation of obesity has three main purposes: (1) To exclude underlying pathology, (2) to evaluate potential comorbidities of obesity, and (3) to identity underlying behavioral and environmental variables that can be targeted to improve the child's weight status.

Possible identifiable causes of obesity include iatrogenic, endocrine, or genetic conditions. Iatrogenic causes include glucocorticoids, appetite stimulants, certain antidepressants, antipsychotics, oral hypoglycemic agents, or surgical injury to the hypothalamus. Endocrine causes, such as hypothyroidism or Cushing syndrome, are almost always accompanied by decreased linear growth. Very early-onset obesity, developmental delays, and/or impaired learning may be signs of a genetic disorder. MC4R mutations are the most common genetic form of obesity and are associated with early-onset obesity and a strong family history of severe obesity. Prader-Willi syndrome (loss of imprinted genes on 15q11-q13) is the most common syndromic form of obesity. Given the rarity of genetic syndromes in causing obesity in the general population, further discussion is outside the scope of this chapter. A good history and physical examination are often sufficient to identify whether there is any concern for an underlying genetic or hormonal etiology of obesity.

GENERAL FEATURES
• Overweight
• Behavioral problems

DIFFERENTIAL DIAGNOSIS

- Overeating
- Endocrine disorders such as hypothyroidism, pseudohypoparathyroidism, and Cushing's syndrome
- Fröhlich's syndrome (adipose genital dysmorphy)
- Prader-Willi syndrome—obesity starts from late infancy, upper slanting of palpable fissure, hypogonadism, mental retardation, strabismus, and short stature.

Initial laboratory screening tests may include fasting blood sugar and/or hemoglobin, alanine aminotransferase (ALT), aspartate aminotransferase (AST), and a fasting lipid panel, to assess for metabolic dysfunction. Further laboratory evaluation tor polycystic ovary syndrome or hypertension should be performed as needed.

Unless the history and physical examination suggest concern for other conditions, such as hypothyroidism, additional laboratory screening is not necessary. Although the initial screening [e.g., thyroid stimulating hormone (TSH)] tests for the evaluation of obesity are consistent across guidelines, there is no clear consensus on when subsequent screening should be performed.

■ TREATMENT

These children should be encouraged to take foods rich with fiber but low caloric content before they take their main meals. A full stomach gives a feeling of satisfaction and therefore the intake is reduced. Greater physical activity should be encouraged. Attempts should be made to reduce the weight gradually rather than promptly. Use of drugs to reduce appetite should be discouraged. Surgical methods are not recommended in children. It is considered only when obesity is life-threatening.

Caloric intake should be reduced. Children should be encouraged to take high-fiber food but low caloric content. General physical activity should be encouraged. Sometimes the child may require psychological support and encouragement. Use of drugs to reduce appetite should be discouraged.

■ PHARMACOTHERAPY

Two medications (orlistat, sibutramine) have been tested in randomized control trials. Orlistat is a GI lipase inhibitor, and sibutramine is a serotonin and norepinephrine reuptake inhibitor. Combined with behavioral interventions, these two drugs resulted in low-to-moderate short-term weight loss in obese adolescents (BMI reduction of 2.6 kg/m^2 more for sibutramine, 0.85 kg/m^2 more for orlistat compared to placebo).

Potential side effects include increase in heart rate and blood pressure with sibutramine and GI side effects with orlistat that can be prohibitive for continued use. There have also been reports of liver injury, cholelithiasis, and pancreatitis with orlistat. Data on weight maintenance after interruption of therapy are not available.

Only orlistat is Food and Drug Administration (FDA) approved for use in children and adolescents 12 years and older. Sibutramine was voluntarily withdrawn in 2010 because of an association with increased incidence of cardiovascular events among adults at high risk for cardiovascular disease. Metformin, an insulin sensitizer, is approved for the treatment of type 2 diabetes in children 10 years of age and older. It can result in modest weight loss among children with type 2 diabetes.

■ SURGERY

Bariatric surgery is a consideration in the setting of severe obesity in adolescents, particularly if associated with comorbidities. However, experts recommend that adolescents should be considered for bariatric surgery only if they are severely obese (BMI >40 kg/m^2) and have serious medical comorbidities associated with their obesity, have reached Tanner stage of 4 or greater to ensure skeletal maturity, have demonstrated commitment to lifestyle change, have tailored at least 6 months to a structured weight loss program, and have a stable psychosocial environment. It may also be appropriate with BMI >35 kg/m^2 if associated with severe comorbidities such as type 2 diabetes mellitus, moderate-to-severe sleep apnea, or pseudotumor cerebri. These factors are best assessed in a pediatric tertiary care center in the context of a multidisciplinary program.

Different surgical modalities, including restrictive or malabsorptive procedures, or a combination, can be employed. They include the Roux-en-Y gastric bypass (RYGB), biliopancreatic diversion, adjustable gastric banding (AGB), and the vertical sleeve gastrectomy (VSG). Bariatric surgery can lead to massive reductions in body weight, BMI, and fat mass, with reports of 50–60% of excess weight loss in the first year, with absolute BMI reduction or about 30%. This reduction is associated with marked improvement or resolution of obesity-related comorbidities and improvement in mental health and quality of life.

Side effects include potential serious surgical complications, including pneumonia, deep venous thrombosis, pulmonary embolus, GI hemorrhage, anastomotic obstruction, wound infections, risk for cholelithiasis, and even death.

Postoperatively, nutritional status should be closely monitored and supplementation provided to avoid macronutrient (mostly protein) and micronutrient (fat-soluble vitamins, iron, and calcium) deficiencies, which are particularly concerning in growing adolescents. Bariatric surgery and continued management of adolescents should be done only by a multidisciplinary team with pediatric expertise.

CONCLUSION

Obesity remains a common pediatric medical condition that most clinicians will have to address among their patients due to the impact that obesity has on many disease processes and conditions. In pediatric primary care, overweight and obesity should be screened for and, depending on the weight status of the child, either obesity prevention or weight management should be addressed during well-child and/or follow-up visits. Clinicians should help advocate for children both in their clinical practice and in their community for healthy eating and physical activity behaviors, along with health-promoting environments for children.

BIBLIOGRAPHY

1. August GP, Caprio S, Fennoy I, Freemark M, Kaufman FR, Lustig RH, et al.; Endocrine Society. Prevention and treatment of obesity: an endocrine society clinical practice guideline based on expert opinion. J Clin Endocrinol Metab. 2008;93(12):4576-99.
2. Dennison BA, Erb TA, Jenkins PL. Television viewing and television in bedroom associated with overweight risk among low-income preschool children. Pediatrics. 2002;109(6):1028-35.
3. Keiss W, Wabitsch M. Metabolic Syndrome and Obesity in children. Pediatric Adolesc Med Basel. 2015;19:166-70.
4. Mathai S, Derraik JG, Cutfield WS, Dalziel SR, Harding JE, Biggs J, et al. Increased adiposity in adults born preterm and their children. PLoS One. 2013;8:e81840.
5. Wu J, Cohen P, Spiegelman BM. Adoptive thermogenesis in adipocytes: is beige the new brown? Genes Dev. 2013;27(3):234-50.

CASE 90

Protein–Energy Malnutrition

■ PRESENTING COMPLAINTS

An 18-month-old boy was brought with the complaint of:
- Irritability since 6 months
- Generalized swelling since 4 months
- Skin lesion since 1 month
- Loose motion since 15 days

History of Presenting Complaints

An 18-month-old boy was brought to the pediatric outpatient department with history of irritability, generalized swelling, and skin changes. His mother complained that her son was more irritable, and he was not taking feeds regularly. His food intake was very low. She told that he used to sit quietly in one place and was not playful. His mother also told that his son was getting repeated episodes of loose motions. She noticed that the child developed the swelling of the limbs and face. The swelling was gradually increasing. She told about the presence of skin lesions at the elbow. Itching and desquamation were present.

Past History of the Patient

He was the third sibling of nonconsanguineous marriage. He was born at full term by normal vaginal delivery. The baby cried immediately after the delivery. The birth weight was 2.5 kg. He started to take breastfeeds regularly. He was on breastfeed for first 3 months. Later weaning started. He was on family food by 1 year. His developmental milestones were delayed. He had been completely immunized.

CASE AT A GLANCE	
Basic Findings	
Height	: 78 cm (25th centile)
Weight	: 8 kg (below 3rd centile)
Temperature	: 37°C
Pulse rate	: 110 beats/min
Respiratory rate	: 26 breaths/min
Blood pressure	: 60/40 mm Hg
Positive Findings	
History:	
• Irritability	
• Generalized swelling	
• Skin changes	
• Poor appetite	
Examination:	
• Irritability	
• Generalized edema	
• Skin changes	
• Hair changes	
Investigation:	
• Anemia	
• Abnormal LFT	
• ESR raise	

(ESR: erythrocyte sedimentation rate; LFT: liver function test)

■ EXAMINATION

On examination, the child was moderately built and poorly nourished. He was irritable and crying. Anthropometric measurements included the height 78 cm (25th centile) and the weight 8 kg (below 3rd centile). The head circumference was 45 cm.

He was afebrile, the heart rate was 110 beats/min, and the respiratory rate was 26 breaths/min. The blood pressure recorded was 60/40 mm Hg.

There was a pallor. Generalized edema was present. There was no cyanosis and no clubbing. Skin changes included the hyperpigmented areas in flexor place on ventral surface. Desquamation was present. The hair changes included, the sparse lusterless, easily pluckable hair. The texture of the hair was coarse. Muscles were thin and weak.

Respiratory system revealed the presence of bilateral coarse crepitation at the base. Per abdomen examination revealed the presence of hepatomegaly measuring about 3 cm. below the costal margin. The cardiovascular system and central nervous system were normal.

■ INVESTIGATION

- *Hemoglobin:* 8 g/dL
- *TLC:* 7,600 cells/cumm
- *ESR:* 40 mm in the first hour
- *Blood glucose:* 60 mg/dL
- *Serum potassium:* 3 mEq/dL
- *Serum magnesium:* 2 mEq/dL
- *Serum bilirubin:* 1.2 mg/dL
- *Alkaline phosphatase:* 600 U/L
- *Serum glutamic oxaloacetic transaminase (SGOT):* 150 IU/L
- *Serum glutamic pyruvic transaminase (SGPT):* 70 IU/L
- *Peripheral blood smear:* Microcytic hypochromic anemia
- *X-ray chest:* Suggestive of pneumonia

■ DISCUSSION

The clinical state is mainly because of insufficient protein. It may also be because of impaired absorption of protein as in chronic diarrhea or chronic liver disorders. The growing child must maintain a positive nitrogen balance. Deficiency of calories and other nutrients will complicate the clinical and chemical patterns.

Acute malnutrition results in wasting (decrease in weight for height) and occurs when food consumption is suddenly severely reduced. Chronic under nutrition occurs when long-term food consumption is insufficient to cover the requirements for daily energy expenditure. It results in stunting (decrease in height-for-age).

■ ETIOLOGY

Large families: Rapid succession of pregnancies adversely affects the nutritional status of mothers. Their fetuses tend to be small and this is reflected in high incidence of low birth weight.

Feeding habits: A child is more likely to have protein–energy malnutrition (PEM) if exclusive breastfeeding is not given for first 4–6 months, lactation fails, breast milk supply is not sufficient, and introduction of solid energy-dense and protein-rich complementary food is delayed.

Infections: Infections such as malaria, whooping cough, tuberculosis, and measles precipitate acute malnutrition and aggravate the existing nutritional deficit. Recurrent attacks of diarrhea in preschool children are a major contributory factor in etiology. Malnutrition may adversely affect the immune status and make the malnourished individuals more vulnerable to infections. This sets up a vicious cycle of malnutrition, infection, malnutrition.

■ PATHOPHYSIOLOGY

When a child's intake is insufficient to meet daily needs, physiologic and metabolic changes take place in an orderly progression to conserve energy and prolong life. This process is called reductive adaptation. Fat stores are mobilized to provide energy. Later protein in muscle, skin, and the GI tract is mobilized. Energy is conserved by reducing physical activity and growth, reducing basal metabolism and the functional reserve of organs and by reducing inflammatory and immune responses. These changes have important consequences:

- The liver makes glucose less readily, making the child more prone to hypoglycemia. It produces less albumin, transferrin, and other transport proteins. It is less able to cope with excess dietary protein and to excrete toxins.
- Heat production is less, making the child more vulnerable to hypothermia.
- The kidneys are less able to excrete excess fluid and sodium, and fluid easily accumulates in the circulation, increasing the risk of fluid overload.
- The heart is smaller and weaker and has a reduced output, and fluid overload readily leads to death from cardiac failure.
- Sodium builds up inside cells due to leaky cell membranes and reduced activity of the sodium/potassium pump, leading to excess body sodium, fluid retention, and edema.
- Potassium leaks out of cells and is excreted in urine, contributing to electrolyte imbalance, fluid retention, edema, and anorexia.
- Loss of muscle protein is accompanied by loss of potassium, magnesium, zinc, and copper.
- The gut produces less gastric acid and enzymes, motility is reduced, and bacteria may colonize the stomach and small intestine, damaging the mucosa and deconjugating bile salts. Digestion and absorption are impaired.
- Cell replication and repair are reduced, increasing the risk of bacterial translocation through the gut mucosa.
- Immune function is impaired, especially cell-mediated immunity. The usual responses to infection may be absent, even in severe illness, increasing the risk of undiagnosed infection.
- Red cell mass is reduced, releasing iron, which requires glucose and amino acids to be converted to ferritin, increasing the risk of hypoglycemia and amino acid imbalances. If conversion to ferritin is incomplete, unbound iron promotes pathogen growth and formation of free radicals.
- Micronutrient deficiencies limit the body's ability to deactivate free radicals, which cause cell damage. Edema and hair/skin changes are outward signs of cell damage.

When prescribing treatment, it is essential to take these into account, otherwise organs and systems will be overwhelmed, and death will rapidly ensue.

CLASSIFICATION OF PROTEIN–ENERGY MALNUTRITION

Protein–energy malnutrition may be classified according to the severity, course, and the relative contributions of energy or protein deficit. Severity classifications are based on anthropometric measurements, mainly weight and height. Accordingly several classifications are suggested:

- *Indian Academy of Pediatrics (IAP) Classification:* More than 80% of expected weight-for-age is taken as normal. Grades of malnutrition are grade I (71–80%), II (61–70%), III (51–60%), and IV (<50%) expected weight for that age.
- *Welcome Trust Classification:* This is based on deficit in body weight for age

and presence or absence of edema. Children weighing between 60% and 80% of their expected weight-for-age with edema are classified as having kwashiorkor. Those weighing between 60% and 80% of expected without edema are known as having undernutrition. Those without edema and weighing <60% of their expected weight-for-age are considered to be having marasmus. Children with edema and body weight <60% of expected are labeled as having marasmic kwashiorkor.
- *World Health Organization (WHO) Classification:* This is based on all four parameters, i.e., weight-for-age, height-for-age, and weight-for-height, and edema. WHO recommends three terms, i.e., stunting, underweight, and wasting for assessing the magnitude of malnutrition in under five children.

■ CLINICAL FEATURES (FIG. 1)

Malnutrition causes a variety of metabolic disturbances. Resistance to infections is decreased, GI functions are disturbed and learning ability is adversely affected.

The growth of children is retarded and there is high morbidity and mortality among malnourished individuals.

Nutritional Marasmus and Kwashiorkor

The two extreme forms of malnutrition account only for a small proportion of malnourished children. A much larger number of subjects suffer from mild-to-moderate nutritional deficit.

If the food deficit persists for a longer period, the malnourished subject conserves his energy by curtailing physical activity. Moderately malnourished children appear slower and less energetic. If the nutrition deficit continues longer, growth of the child is affected. Growth lag is more pronounced in weight than the length. With prolonged deprivation, height is also stunted. Head circumference is not reduced significantly. Chest circumference normally exceeds the head circumference by the age of 1 year, but it may not do so till much later in malnourished children.

The weight of the child is reduced and appears disproportionate with long body, thin limbs, and unduly large head. Buttocks are flattened with wrinkling of skin over the front of thighs. The scapulae look winged. Abdominal wall is thin and therefore abdomen appears distended. As the nutritional deficit exaggerates with the onset of infections, the child may become marasmic or develop kwashiorkor.

Marasmus

A marasmic subject is markedly emaciated. The body weight is <60% of the expected weight for the age. The fat in the adipose tissues is severely depleted, because it is used up for providing energy. The contour of atrophic muscles is evident under the thin

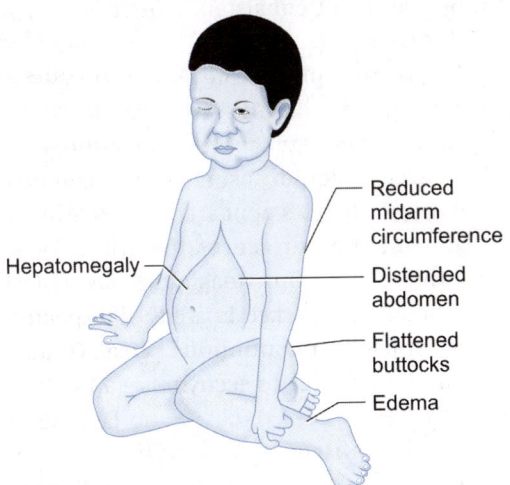

Fig. 1: Clinical features.

and wrinkled skin. Loose folds of skin are prominent over the gluten and the inner side of thigh. The buccal pad of fat is preserved till the malnutrition becomes extreme.

A higher proportion of saturated fatty acids is stored there, and the saturated fat is the last to be depleted. The skin appears dry and inelastic and is prone to be infected. The hair is hypopigmented.

The abdomen is distended due to wasting and hypotonia of abdominal wall muscles. The midarm circumference is reduced. The bony points appear unduly prominent due to emaciation. The baby appears alert but is often irritable. Marasmic children may show voracious appetite.

Kwashiorkor

Markedly retarded growth, psychomotor changes, and edema of dependent parts are three essential clinical features of kwashiorkor. The edema starts in the lower extremities and later involves upper limbs and the face. Muscles of the upper limbs are wasted, but the lower extremities appear swollen. The face appears moon-shaped and puffy. The trunk is affected to a lesser extent. Debilitating illnesses such as measles or diarrhea can precipitate edema. With the onset of kwashiorkor, the previously peevish and irritable undernourished child becomes lethargic, listless, and apathetic. The child takes little interest in the environment and does not play with his toys.

The kwashiorkor patient appears miserable and resents examination by the physician. Appetite is impaired and it is difficult to feed him orally.

The hair is thin, dry, brittle, and devoid of its normal sheen. The length of the hair growing during the period of nutritional deprivation appears reddish brown. During the phases of better nutrition, the growing part of the hair gets appropriately pigmented.

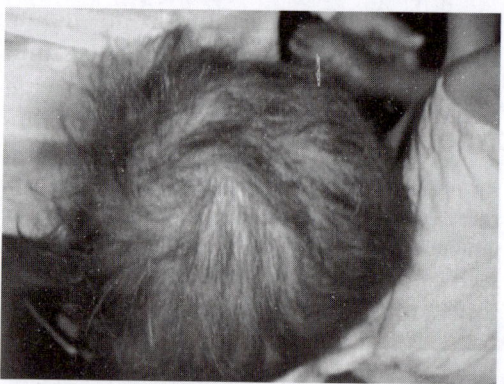

Fig. 2: Flag sign.

This gives appearance of alternate bands of hypopigmented and normally pigmented hair (flag sign) **(Fig. 2)**. These children often suffer from recurrent episodes of diarrhea and respiratory and skin infections.

> **ESSENTIAL DIAGNOSTIC POINTS**
> - Growth retardation
> - Anorexia
> - Generalized edema
> - Skin changes
> - Hepatomegaly
> - Electrolyte disturbances
> - Hair changes

The liver is enlarged with rounded lower margin and soft consistency in about one-third of cases.

Large areas of skin may show erythema or hyperpigmentation. The skin becomes dry and hyperkeratotic. The epidermis peels off in large scales, exposing tender raw area underneath. It gives appearance of old paint flaking off the surface of the wood. The underlying raw skin is easily infected. The skin lesions are marked in areas of the body, most exposed to continuous pressure and irritation. Petechiae or ecchymosis appear in severe cases.

As the nutritional deficiencies are generally multiple, anemia due to iron, protein, vitamin B, or folate deficiency is

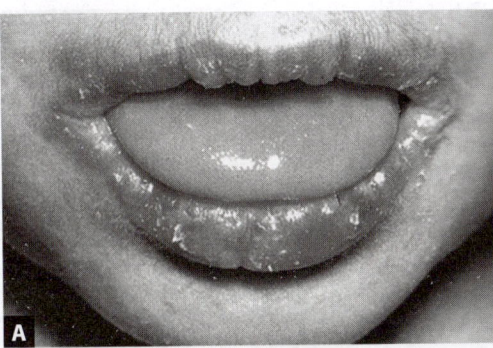

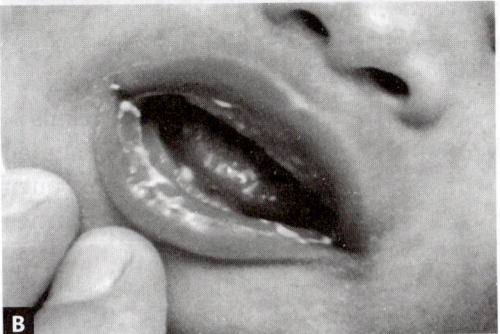

Figs. 3A and B: (A) Glossitis; (B) Oral thrush.
(For color version, see Plate 9)

often associated. Deficiencies of vitamin B complex factors, especially ariboflavinosis are common **(Figs. 3A and B)**. Keratomalacia due to vitamin A deficiency is reported in 10–20% of patients with kwashiorkor. Associated scorbutic changes manifest as bleeding gums, subperiosteal hemorrhage or even ecchymotic spots. Subclinical ascorbic acid deficiency is frequent in malnutrition. Rickets due to vitamin D deficiency is present in only 5% cases, though almost all cases would have subclinical vitamins D and A deficiency.

Severe Acute Malnutrition

Children will mix of marasmus and kwashiorkor. They will have any of the following three criteria:

1. Weight for height below −3 standard deviation
2. Presence of bipedal edema
3. Midarm circumference below 11.5 cm.

Severe wasting is most visible on the thighs, buttocks, and upper arms, as well as over the ribs and scapulae, where loss of fat and skeletal muscle is greatest. Wasting is preceded by failure to gain weight and then by weight loss. The skin loses turgor and becomes loose as subcutaneous tissues are broken down to provide energy. The face may retain a relatively normal appearance, but eventually becomes wasted and wizened. The eyes may be sunken from loss of retroorbital fat, and lacrimal and salivary glands may atrophy, leading to lack of tears and a dry mouth. Weakened abdominal muscles and gas from bacterial overgrowth of the upper gut may lead to a distended abdomen. Severely wasted children are often fretful and irritable.

In *edematous malnutrition* the edema is most likely to appear first in the feet and then in the lower legs. It can quickly develop into generalized edema affecting also the hands, arms, and face. Skin changes typically occur over the swollen limbs and include dark, crackled peeling patches ("flaky paint" dermatosis) with pale skin underneath that is easily infected. The hair is sparse and easily pulled out and may lose its curl. In dark-haired children, the hair may turn pale or reddish. The liver is often enlarged with fat. Children with edema are miserable and apathetic, and often refuse to eat.

GENERAL FEATURES

- Placid, slow, less active
- Wrinkling of the skin over front of thigh
- Irritable
- Edema
- Thin, dry, brittle hair
- Chronic diarrhea
- Hypopigmentation
- Hyperpigmentation

TABLE 1: Clinical signs of malnutrition.

Site	Signs
Face	Moon face (kwashiorkor), simian facies (marasmus)
Eye	Dry eyes, pale conjunctiva, Bitot spots (vitamin A), periorbital edema
Mouth	Angular stomatitis, cheilitis, glossitis, spongy bleeding gums (vitamin C, parotid enlargement
Teeth	Enamel mottling, delayed eruption
Hair	Dull, sparse, brittle hair; hypopigmentation; flag sign (alternating bands of light and normal color; broomstick eyelashes, alopecia
Skin	Loose and wrinkled (marasmus); shiny and edematous (kwashiorkor); dry, follicular hyperkeratosis; patchy hyper- and hypopigmentation ("crazy paving" or flaky paint dermatoses); erosions; poor wound healing
Nails	Koilonychia, thin and soft nail plates, fissures, or ridges
Musculature	Muscle wasting, particularly buttocks and thighs; Chvostek or Trousseau sign (hypocalcemia)
Skeletal	Deformities, usually as a result of calcium, vitamin D, or vitamin C deficiencies
Abdomen	*Distended:* Hepatomegaly with fatty liver, ascites may be present
Cardiovascular	Cardiovascular bradycardia, hypotension, reduced cardiac output, small-vessel vasculopathy
Neurologic	Global developmental delay, loss of knee and ankle reflexes, impaired memory
Hematologic	Pallor, petechiae, bleeding diathesis
Behavior	Lethargic, apathetic, irritable on handling

The clinical signs of malnutrition are given in **Table 1**.

DIFFERENTIAL DIAGNOSIS

- Nephrotic syndrome
- Angioneurotic edema
- Chronic diarrhea
- Malnutrition
- Infestation
- Malabsorption syndrome

TREATMENT

Management

The management of PEM depends on nutritional status, degree of hypermetabolism, expected duration of illness, and associated complications. The goals are to minimize weight loss, maintain body mass, and encourage body mass repletion or growth.

The management consists of three phases:
1. *Resuscitation:* Lasts for 6–24 hours
2. *Acute phase:* 1 day to 1 week/+
3. *Rehabilitation:* Through second and third weeks to 6 weeks; the period of phases especially the first two phases may vary depending on the condition of the child when brought for medical attention.

World Health Organization has suggested guidelines for the inpatient treatment of severely malnourished children, the general principles are as follows:

Dehydration

Assessment of dehydration is difficult due to wasting and edema. However, dry oral mucosa, acidotic breathing, oliguria, absence of tears, and peripheral circulatory failure are most reliable signs.

The amount of fluid and sodium should not exceed 75% of the allowances calculated on the basis of weight and age (because of reduced capacity to excrete water and inability to excrete sodium).

Additional fluid can be given if needed. Fluid deficit and maintenance fluids are calculated. Deficit fluid volume is replaced by 5% dextrose in N/2 saline in 6–8 hours, and maintenance fluid volume is given as isolyte P over 16 hours.

If child has shock, Ringer's lactate 30 mL/kg or 20 mL/kg of 0.45% saline (1/2) in 5% dextrose is given in hour, then 70 mL/kg of Ringer's lactate or 10 mL/kg in 1 hour of glucose saline for 2 hours. If shock does not improve then 10 mL/kg of plasma is infused. Potassium is added in infusion in dosage of 2–3 mEq/kg (maximum dose 40 mEq/L), when a flow of urine is observed.

In mild dehydration, ORS (oral rehydration salt—WHO—sodium chloride 3.5 g, potassium chloride 1.5 g, sodium citrate 2.9 g, glucose 20 g) should be given. Severely malnourished children with dehydration may not tolerate this high-sodium, low-potassium oral rehydration salt (ORS).

Ongoing loss of water in stool is provided at 10 mL/kg/stool. Once the child is stable and he is able to accept oral feeds, milk-based therapeutic nutrition is started.

The indications for hospitalization are hypothermia, infection, fluid and electrolyte imbalance, convulsions, unconsciousness, xerophthalmia, severe dermatosis, extreme weight deficit, bleeding, marked hepatomegaly, jaundice, purpura raised liver enzymes, severe anemia and cardiac failure, persistent vomiting, severe anorexia, distended tender abdomen, and age <1 year.

Correction of Electrolyte Imbalance

All severely malnourished child usually have potassium and magnesium deficiencies, which may take at least 2 weeks to correct. It is corrected by giving extra potassium 2–4 mmol/kg/day, extra magnesium 0.3–0.6 mmol/kg/day and restricting the salt. When rehydrating low-sodium rehydration fluid is given. The extra potassium and magnesium can be prepared in a liquid form and added directly to feeds during preparation.

Hypothermia: It is common in marasmus and is usually a manifestation of infection, hypoglycemia or severe energy deficit. Child is kept in warm room, well covered, close to mother, and is given frequent feeds and antibiotics for infection. If the axillary temperature is <35°C take rectal temperature using a low reading thermometer, if below 35.5°C (95°F) feed straight away (or start rehydration if needed).

Hypoglycemia: It is again more common in Marasmus with hypothermia, septicemia, and coma. It requires 10% glucose 1–2 mL/kg in bolus followed by 10% dextrose in N/5 saline in maintenance dose for 24 hours. Antibiotics are given and continue 2 hourly feeds, day and night. As hypoglycemia and hypothermia usually occur together and are signs of infection, check for hypoglycemia whenever hypothermia is found. Frequent feeding is important in both conditions.

Infection: Diagnosis of fulminant infection is made by high index of suspicion or in the presence of hypothermia, apathy, convulsion, or coma. Antimicrobials (broad spectrum) are started immediately while awaiting culture reports. Gastric aspirate examination and culture, X-ray chest and Mantoux test are done to diagnose pulmonary tuberculosis. Blood film for malaria may be required.

If the child has no complications, *cotrimoxazole* 5 mL orally twice daily for 5 days (2.5 mL if weight <4 kg) (5 mL is equivalent to 40 mg Trimethoprim + 200 mg sulfamethoxazole (SMX)] or if the child is severely ill, has complications give intravenous (IV) ampicillin (50 mg/kg/6 hourly for 2 days) then oral amoxicillin for 5 days or continue ampicillin for 5 days. Add gentamicin 7.5 mg/kg intramuscular (IM)/IV for once.

If no improvement within 48 hours add chloramphenicol 25 mg/kg/IM/IV for 5 days or appropriate antibiotic, if specific infections are identified. If anorexia persists after 5 days course, antibiotics are continued for full 10 days. If no/poor response, reassess the child fully. Some experts routinely give metronidazole 7.5 mg 8 hourly for 7 days to hasten intestinal repair of mucosa and reduce the risk of potential anerobic infection.

Human immunodeficiency virus (HIV)/ acquired immunodeficiency syndrome (AIDS): In children with HIV/AIDS, good recovery from malnutrition is possible though it may take longer and treatment failures may be common. Lactose intolerance occurs in severe HIV-related chronic diarrhea. Treatment should be same as for HIV-negative children.

Anemia: If hemoglobin is <5 g/dL, small packed cells transfusion (5–10 mL/kg) is given. In children with impending cardiac failure, partial exchange transfusion (10–20 mL/kg) may be quite beneficial. Whole blood transfusion (10 mL/kg) has been recommended for severely ill-malnourished children. Iron supplementation for anemia is withheld for first 1–2 weeks to allow transferring regeneration and to permit resolution of infection.

Xeropthalmia: Vitamin A 1 lakh units aqueous preparation should be given to all severely malnourished children on days 1, 2, and 28th in children above 1 year of age or >10 kg weight. In infants below 1 year or weight <10 kg, half of the above dose is given. If the infant is between 0 and 6 months 50,000 units are given.

Congestive heart failure is most common after 3 days of acute phase usually in kwashiorkor. Oxygen inhalation and diuretics are helpful.

Hypocalcemia: Requires correction by calcium gluconate IV 1–2 mL/kg or calcium lactate powder 3 g/day orally.

Zinc deficiency: Role of zinc supplementation is controversial. Dose of zinc is 2 mg/kg/day.

Other vitamins: Appropriate vitamins should be supplied with 10 mL, multivitamin injection (MVI) 1–2 mL daily in drip and later orally plus vitamin K 1–5 mg weekly.

Copper, chromium, and manganese deficiency: Dose of copper is 20 µg/kg/day, that of chromium is 0.2 µg/kg/day, and manganese is 10 µg/kg/day.

Although the phases of resuscitation and acute phases are divided separately, quite often the medical treatment started during the phase of resuscitation continues into acute phase. The acute phase also may be prolonged to 2–3 weeks instead of 1 week as suggested.

> **LABORATORY SALIENT FINDINGS**
> - Anemia
> - Hypoglycemia
> - Hypocalcemia
> - Hypomagnesemia
> - Altered liver function test (LFT)
> - Septic screen

DIETARY MANAGEMENT OF SEVERE PROTEIN–ENERGY MALNUTRITION

Initial Phase

In the initial stabilization phase, a cautious approach is required because of the child's fragile physiological state and reduced homeostatic capacity. Feeding should be started as soon as possible after admission and should be designed to provide just sufficient energy protein to maintain physiological processes.

It is for mild-to-moderate PEM and for those uncomplicated severe PEM who have fairly good appetite, normal body temperature, and who are conscious and active and without evidence of serious infection. These children are managed at home by parents under observation and supervision.

The main goal of treatment is to provide adequate calories for dual purpose, replace losses, and build up nutrition and promote growth. Caution must be taken to gradually build up the calories and proteins. The energy recommended is 120–150 kcal/day and protein 2–3 g/kg/day of high biological value. Both of these should be based on locally available and affordable food sources, commonly consumed by the family.

Frequent small feeds with calories and proteins distributed proportionately are encouraged rather than 1 or 2 major bulky meals. Parents are educated about hygienic way of preparation and handling of food, use of safe and clean drinking water, and importance of personal hygiene.

The regime recommended is one that provides near-maintenance requirement, i.e., approximately 80 cal/kg/day and 0.7 g protein/day with the calculation being based on actual rather than expected weights. The second rule is to offer small amount of feeds of low osmolarity and low lactose at frequent intervals to avoid the incidence of vomiting, hypoglycemia, and hypothermia. The intake can be gradually stepped up so that by the end of first week the child is able to take approximately 100 cal/kg/day and 1 g protein/kg/day. Some authorities suggest 100 kcal/kg/day and 1–1.5 g of proteins/kg/day.

Some basic advice is also given, for management of diarrhea by oral rehydration solution, immediate attention for treatment of common infestations, and infections and appropriate management of anemia by oral iron and folic acid supplements and associated vitamin deficiencies.

To promote growth, zinc supplements are given when positive nutrition balance starts occurring and child manifests with an increase in weight gain.

If the child is breastfed, continue to breastfeed but give starter formula (milk-based formulas containing 75 kcal/100 mL (0.9 g protein/100 mL), which will be satisfactory for most children. Very weak children may be fed by spoon, dropper, or syringe. A recommended schedule in which volume is gradually increased and feeding frequency gradually decreased is:

Days	Frequency	Vol/kg/feed	Vol/kg/day
1–2	2 hourly	11 mL	130 mL
3–5	3 hourly	16 mL	130 mL
6–7+	4 hourly	22 mL	130 mL

For children with a good appetite and no edema this schedule can be completed in 2–3 days (e.g., 24 hours at each level).

Severely malnourished children often have refusal to feed and hence "forced feeding" by intragastric tube has to be done. Milk is the most common and nutritional liquid food and is also well tolerated except by children with secondary disaccharide (lactose) intolerance. Fluid volume is usually calculated approximately 130 mL/kg/day. This may be divided into 2 hourly feeds in the first week and 3 hourly thereafter, the calorie content of milk can be increased by adding oil as follows:

COMPOSITION OF ENRICHED MILK		
Component	Energy (cal)	Protein (g)
Cow's milk (300 mL)	198	9.6
Sugar (85 g)	340	–
Vegetable oil (30 g)	270	–
Total	808	9.6

The amount of water added to this formulation would depend on the desired concentration of calories and proteins required and state of hydration of the individual patient since milk is the only fluid offered to the child. If the volume is of 1,000 mL then 120 mL/kg/day and 1.1 g protein/kg/day. Coconut oil is the recommended oil as it is supposed to provide medium-chain triglyceride (MCT); other oils are equally effective besides coconut oil is not culturally used by all communities for feeding. Dietary LC-PUFA (long-chain polyunsaturated fatty acids) have been known to improve intestinal repair in severe PEM, therefore its quantitative and qualitative supply should be considered.

World Health Organization has recommended milk-based formulas containing 75 cal/100 mL and 0.9 g protein/100 mL in the initial feeding schedule and then gradually increasing to supply 100 and 135 cal/100 mL of feed, respectively, for catchup growth. These formulas are mainly based on the use of dried skimmed milk or dried whole milk and the use of these formulas is limited because of the economic constraints of the less advantaged communities of India where the problem of PEM is most common.

Phase of High-energy Feeding

After the child passes through the initial phase and shows signs of improvement and tolerates the prescribed diet, one can then gradually increase the calorie intake to approximately 150–180 cal/kg/day. The amount of milk could be gradually decreased and the intake of semisolid/solids increased. The protein intake recommended during phase is in the range of 1.5–2 g/kg/day.

Therapeutic Diet

Therapeutic diet should provide 150 kcal/kg/day for moderately undernourished and about 200 kcal/kg/day for severely malnourished children. About 10–15% of total calories should be obtained from proteins. A protein intake of 3 g/kg/day is sufficient. Milk is most frequent source of protein used in therapeutic diets.

As a general rule, the diet prescribed for the child should be such, which the family can afford to provide for the baby within its limited income, can be easily cooked at home, does not perish easily, and is culturally acceptable and easily available in the local market. Expensive prestige foods may not necessarily be the most nutritious foods. Routine advice for giving fruit and eggs should be made only after due consideration of the family's economic constraints.

Milk-based diets may not be tolerated by some malnourished infants in the first few days due to transient lactose intolerance. If tolerated, milk-based diets are most suitable at the beginning of the treatment. If dried skimmed milk powder is used for reconstituting the milk, sugar and oil should be added to provide extra calories.

It is necessary to introduce semisolid diet with high calories and protein content, a week or fortnight after the start of the therapy. Extreme apathy and disinclination to eat make the treatment of kwashiorkor a trying experience. Feeding through a nasogastric tube for a few days results in a dramatic change in the behavior of the patient, who then starts accepting oral feeds after a few days.

Every child should receive following intervention:
- Antibiotic therapy
- Dose of vitamin A—100,000 units (xerophthalmia, Bitot spots or keratomalacia)
- Albendazole single dose

ASSESSMENT OF RECOVERY AND FOLLOW-UP

Recovery can be assessed by:
- Improvement of general condition, alertness, and smile.
- Return of appetite.
- Gain in weight 50–70 g/day.
- Disappearance of edema (7–10 days) and hepatomegaly.
- Rise in serum albumin over the first 2 weeks of therapy.

The measure of efficacy of treatment of mild-to-moderate malnutrition is weight gain. Recovery is complete when the child reaches his or her standard weight, which usually takes 6–8 weeks. Follow-up of such children is essential because, mortality rates of 10–30% have been reported after discharge from hospital. Continued supervision is necessary, till the expected weight for height has been achieved.

PROGNOSIS

Mortality rates in severe PEM vary between 10% and 30%. The causes of deaths are same which determine hospitalization. Long-term sequelae of PEM are irreversible stunting and mental impairment.

BIBLIOGRAPHY

1. Bhatnagar S, Lodha R, Choudhary P, Sachdev HPS, Shah N, Narayan S, et al. IAP guidelines 2006 on hospital based management of severely malnourished children (adapted from the WHO Guidelines). Indian Pediatr. 2007;44(6)443-61.
2. Indian Academy of Pediatrics; Dalwai S, Choudhury P, Bavadekar SB, Dalal R, Kapil U, Dubey AP, et al. Consensus statement of Indian Academy of Pediatrics on integrated management of severe acute malnutrition. Indian Pediatr. 2013;50:399-404.
3. Morris SS, Cogill B, Uauy R; Maternal and Child Undernutrition Study Group. Effective international action against undernutrition: why has it proven so difficult and what can be done to accelerate progress? Lancet. 2008;371(9612):608-21.
4. Wikipedia. (2019). Malnutrition in children. [online] Available from https://en.wikipedia.org/wiki/Malnutrition_in_children [Last accessed June, 2024].

CASE 91

Rickets

■ PRESENTING COMPLAINTS

An 18-month-old boy was brought with the complaint of:
- Bow legs since 1 week
- Vomiting and loose motion since 15 days
- Abnormal walking since 1 week

History of Presenting Complaints

A 18-month-old boy was brought to the pediatric outpatient department with history of abnormal walking. His mother told that his son's walking stature was different from other. She describes that it was just like waddling gait. She had also expressed the bow legs in his son. Change in walking style had changed or worsened after the recent acute gastroenteritis.

Past History of the Patient

The child was the only sibling of nonconsanguineous marriage. He was born at full term by vaginal delivery. He cried immediately after the delivery. There was no significant postnatal event. He was exclusively on breast milk for 4 months. Weaning started later with cereals and fruits. He was on family food by 15 months. His motor developmental milestones were slightly delayed. He had been completely immunized.

CASE AT A GLANCE

Basic Findings
Height	: 80 cm (50th centile)
Weight	: 11 kg (60th centile)
Temperature	: 38°C
Pulse rate	: 106 beats/min
Respiratory rate	: 26 breaths/min
Blood pressure	: 70/50 mm Hg

Positive Findings

History:
- Abnormal walking
- Bow legs
- Delayed motor milestones

Examination:
- Febrile
- Moderate dehydration
- Bow legs
- Double malleoli
- Abdominal distension

Investigation:
- Microcytic hypochromic anemia
- Anemia
- Hypocalcemia
- Hypophosphatemia
- Increased alkaline phosphatase

■ EXAMINATION

On examination, he was looking pale, and signs of moderate dehydration were present. He was moderately built and moderately nourished. Anthropometric measurements included the height 80 cm (50th centile) and the weight 11 kg (60th centile).

He was febrile, the pulse rate was 106 beats/min, and the respiratory rate was 26 breaths/min. The blood pressure recorded was 70/50 mm Hg. There was pallor, no lymphadenopathy, and no edema.

Anterior fontanelle was large and not closed. The wrist and knees were swollen. Bow legs were evident. Power in the lower limbs was less and finding very difficult to stand for a long time. Double medial malleoli were present.

Respiratory system revealed presence of crepitations. Per abdomen examination showed the abdominal distension. There was no organomegaly.

INVESTIGATION

- *Hemoglobin:* 8 g/dL
- *TLC:* 13,600 cells/cumm
- *Platelet count:* 5,00,000 cells/cumm
- *Serum calcium:* 2.5 mmol/L (Normal range: 2.2–2.7 mmol/L)
- *Serum phosphorus range:* 0.8 mmol/L (normal 1.25–2.1 mmol/L)
- *Alkaline phosphatase range:* 500 U/L (Normal 30–120 U/L)
- *Peripheral blood smear:* Microcytic hypochromic anemia
- *X-ray of long bone:* Showed the cupping and flaring of the ends of the bone

DISCUSSION

In general, the child had slightly delayed gross motor milestones. He managed to walk without support by the age of 16 months. But later he refused to walk and to bear weight on his lower limbs. Preceding history of gastroenteritis, swollen wrists and knee, bow legs, microcytic hypochromic anemia, mild hypocalcemia, and marked hypophosphatemia is seen in severe form of the rickets. Raised alkaline phosphatase level is also seen.

Rickets occurs as a result of dietary deficiency of vitamin D. The diet of infants contains only small amount of vitamin D. Several factors predispose to vitamin D deficiency. Rickets particularly develops during rapid growth in low birth weight (LBW) and adolescents.

Bone consists of a protein matrix called osteoid and a mineral phase, principally composed of calcium and phosphate, mostly in the form of hydroxyapatite. Osteomalacia is present when there is inadequate mineralization of bone osteoid and occurs in children and adults.

Rickets is a disease of growing bone that is caused by unmineralized matrix at the growth plates and occurs in children only before fusion of the epiphyses. Because growth plate cartilage and osteoid continue to expand but mineralization is inadequate, the growth plate thickens. There is also an increase in the circumference of the growth plate and the metaphysis, increasing bone width at the location of the growth plates and causing some of the classic clinical manifestations, such as widening of the wrists and ankles.

There is a general softening of the bones that causes them to bend easily when subject to forces such as weight-bearing or muscle pull. This softening leads to a variety of bone deformities. There is an increase in overall bone turnover and concomitant rise in alkaline phosphatase.

Subsequent bone deformities result in craniotabes, greenstick fracture, impairment of the linear growth, rickety rosary, bowed legs, and swollen wrist and knee. New bone formation is initiated by osteoblast. This is responsible for matrix deposits and its subsequent mineralization.

ETIOLOGY

Vitamin D deficiency most commonly occurs in infancy because of a combination of poor intake and inadequate cutaneous synthesis. Transplacental transport of vitamin D, mostly 25-D, typically provides enough vitamin D for the first 2 months of life unless there is severe maternal vitamin D deficiency. Infants who receive formula receive adequate vitamin D, even without cutaneous synthesis.

Because of the low vitamin D content of breast milk, breastfed infants rely on cutaneous synthesis or vitamin supplements. Cutaneous synthesis can be limited because of the ineffectiveness of the winter sun in stimulating vitamin D synthesis; avoidance of sunlight because of concerns about cancer, neighborhood safety, or cultural practices; and decreased cutaneous synthesis because of increased skin pigmentation.

The causes of rickets are given in **Box 1**.

Valgus or varus deformities of the legs are common; windswept deformity occurs when one leg is in extreme valgus and the other is in extreme varus.

Cutaneous synthesis mediated by sunlight exposure is an important source of vitamin D. It is important to ask about time spent outside, sunscreen use, and clothing, especially if there may be a cultural reason for increased covering of the skin. Because winter sunlight is ineffective at stimulating cutaneous synthesis of vitamin D, the season is an additional consideration. Children with increased skin pigmentation are at increased risk for vitamin D deficiency because of decreased cutaneous synthesis.

PATHOPHYSIOLOGY

Vitamin D deficiency causes decreased absorption of calcium from gut. The resulting hypocalcemia leads to increase in parathormone secretion. This helps in the release of calcium from bone. Parathormone also reduces the excretion of calcium by kidneys and renal tubular absorption of phosphate. As a result, the serum calcium level tends to become normal, while the serum phosphate level falls.

BOX 1: Causes of rickets.

Vitamin D disorders:
- Nutritional vitamin D deficiency
- Congenital vitamin D deficiency
- Secondary vitamin D deficiency
  - Malabsorption
  - Increased degradation
  - Decreased liver 25-hydroxylase
- Vitamin D-dependent rickets types 1A and 1B
- Vitamin D-dependent rickets types 2A and 2B
- Chronic kidney, disease

Calcium deficiency:
- Low intake
  - Diet
  - Premature infants (rickets of prematurity)
- Malabsorption
  - Primary disease
  - Dietary inhibitors of calcium absorption

Phosphorus deficiency:
- Inadequate intake
  - Premature infants (rickets of prematurity)
  - Aluminum-containing antacids

Renal losses:
- X-linked hypophosphatemic rickets
- Autosomal dominant hypophosphatemic rickets
- Autosomal recessive hypophosphatemic rickets types 1 and 2
- Hereditary hypophosphatemic rickets with hypercalciuria
- Overproduction of fibroblast growth factor-23
  - Tumor-induced rickets
  - McCune-Albright syndrome
  - Epidermal nevus syndrome
  - Neurofibromatosis
  - Fanconi syndrome
- Dent disease
- Distal renal tubular acidosis

After sometime, this compensatory mechanism fails and both calcium and phosphorous levels fall. Since calcium phosphate is necessary for deposition of calcium of growing bones, decrease in blood levels of calcium, phosphorous, or both interferes with the calcification of the osteoid tissue. Serum alkaline phosphatase level also gets increased due to increase in osteoblastic activity.

Children with the disorder of the absorption such as celiac disease, steatorrhea, pancreatitis, cystic fibrosis may acquire rickets, because of deficient absorption of the vitamin D and calcium or both. This leads to lower serum calcium level. This in turn releases parathyroid hormone (PTH), restoring calcium to normal or near normal. This occurs at expense of the loss of phosphate in urine resulting in hypophosphatemia. The inorganic serum phosphate level is usually reduced to 0.5 mmol/L.

The other conditions which interfere with metabolic conversion and activation of vitamin D such as hepatic and renal lesions are also implicated in rickets.

■ PATHOLOGY OF RICKETS

The epiphyseal plate is a narrow well-defined strip from where cartilage cells grow in parallel column toward the metaphysis. After initial proliferation, the old cartilage cells degenerate and disappear, leaving spaces into which the blood vessels and osteoblasts of the shaft can penetrate. Calcium is deposited in the zone of degenerating cartilage, which is then called "zone of preparatory calcification".

In rickets, the cartilage cells go on multiplying giving rise to a broad irregular cartilaginous zone. The process of degeneration and calcification becomes incomplete, leading to softness of the bone. Rapidly growing cartilage cells particularly affect the costochondral junctions and end of long bones. There is also defective mineralization in the subperiosteal bone. In long-standing cases, the bones under stress may become deformed or even have pathological fractures.

Supplementation of vitamin D restores the normal development of the bone with calcification starting at the zone of preparatory calcification, which in a radiography would be seen as a thin dense line near the epiphysis.

■ CLINICAL FEATURES (FIG. 1)

Rickets is a disease of growing bones, and its incidence is particularly high between 4 and 18 months. Skeletal deformities are the most striking feature of rickets.

Most manifestations of rickets are a result of skeletal changes. One of the early signs of rickets is craniotabes. Craniotabes is a softening of the cranial bones and can be detected by applying pressure at the occiput or over the parietal bones. The sensation is similar to the feel of pressing into a ping-pong ball and then releasing. It results from the thinning out of the inner table of the skull

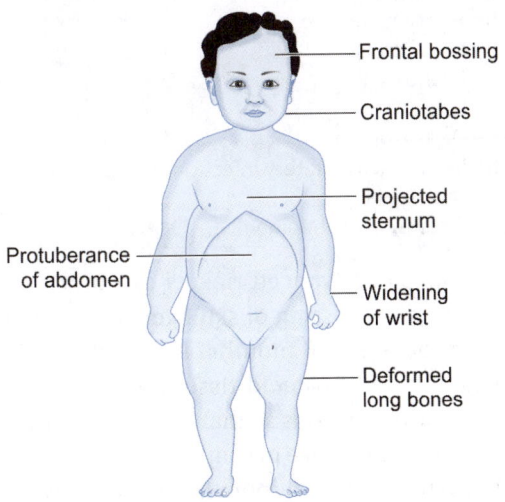

Fig. 1: Clinical features.

due to absorption of noncalcified osteoid tissue. Craniotabes may also be secondary to osteogenesis imperfecta, hydrocephalus, and syphilis. It is a normal finding in many newborns, especially near the suture lines, but it typically disappears within a few months of birth.

Other early evidences of osseous changes are palpable enlargement of costochondral junctions, i.e., rachitic rosary and widening of the wrists and ankles **(Figs. 2 to 4)**. Widening of the costochondral junctions results in a rachitic rosary, which feels like the heads of a rosary as the examiner's fingers move along the costochondral junctions from rib to rib. Growth plate widening is also responsible for the enlargement at the wrists and ankles.

The horizontal depression along the lower anterior chest known as Harrison's groove occurs from pulling of the softened ribs by the diaphragm during inspiration. Softening of the ribs also impairs air movement and predisposes patients to atelectasis and pneumonia.

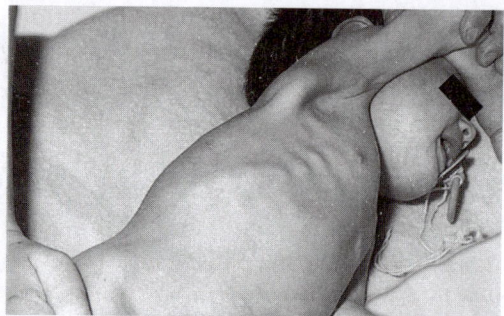

Fig. 2: Ricket rosary.

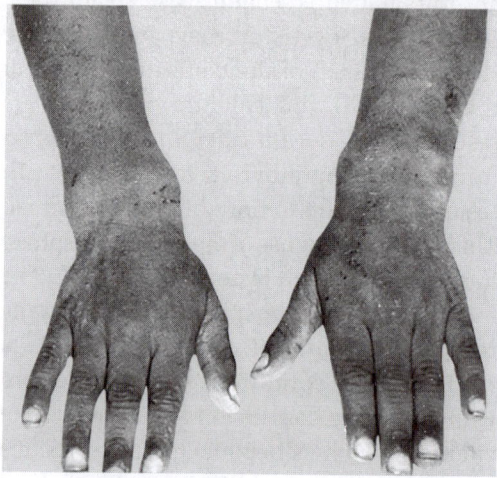

Fig. 3: Widened wrist.

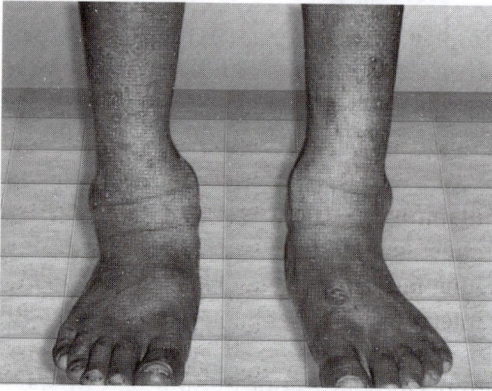

Fig. 4: Widened ankle.

ESSENTIAL DIAGNOSTIC POINTS
• Bossing of skull • Pigeon chest • Harrison's groove • Craniotabes • Kyphosis • Scoliosis • Dwarfism • Recurrent respiratory infection • Hypotonia • Distension of abdomen

Signs of advanced rickets can be easily recognized. Bossing of skull generally starts after the age of 6 months. It occurs due to heaping up of osteoid tissue in the frontal and parietal regions so that the skull appears squarish or box-like in shape.

In thorax, the sternum is pushed forward, producing a "pigeon chest". A horizontal depression known as Harrison's groove, corresponding to costal insertion of the

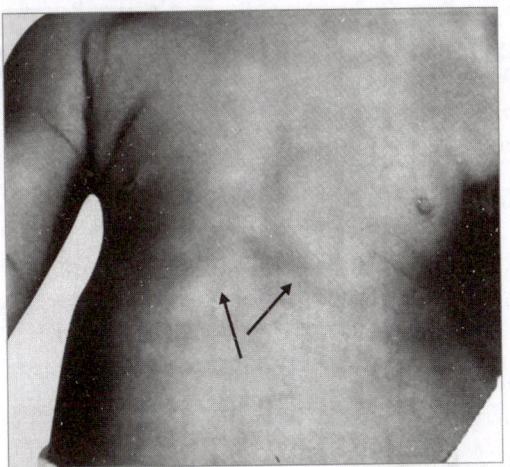

Fig. 5: Harrison sulcus.
(For color version, see Plate 9)

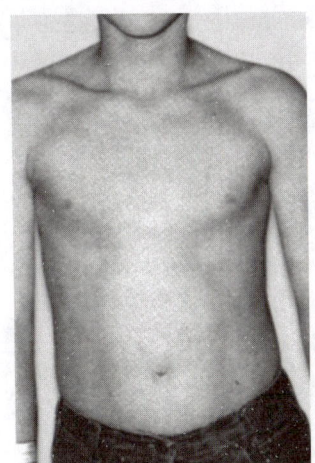

Fig. 7: Hyperexpand chest.

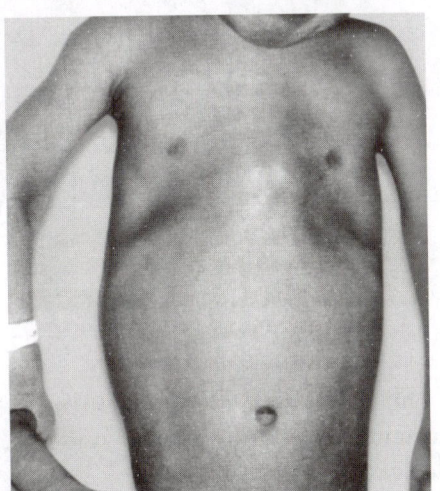

Fig. 6: Pectus carinatum.
(For color version, see Plate 10)

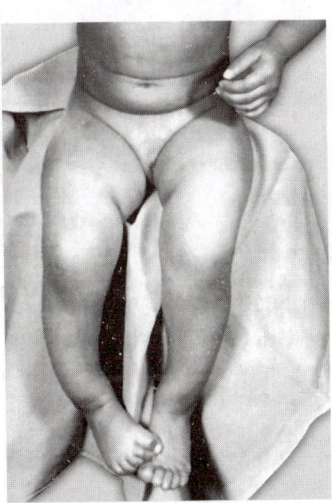

Fig. 8: Broad ankles—rickets.

diaphragm develops **(Figs. 5 and 6)**. The chest deformities **(Fig. 7)** decrease the lung resilience and predispose the child to intercurrent infections.

Bending of the spine backward (kyphosis) and laterally (scoliosis) may occur. Pelvis may become softened, and the promontory of the sacrum is pushed anteriorly and the acetabulae inward, resulting in a narrowed pelvic inlet. This is helped by lax ligaments. Deformity of a pelvis in a female, results in difficulty during labor at a later stage.

Long bones of the legs get deformed when the child starts bearing weight and is thus, usually seen after the age of 1 year. Bending of the femur, tibia, and fibula, result in bow legs or knock knees **(Figs. 8 to 15)**. Coxa vara and green stick fractures may also occur. All deformities of bones result in rachitic dwarfism.

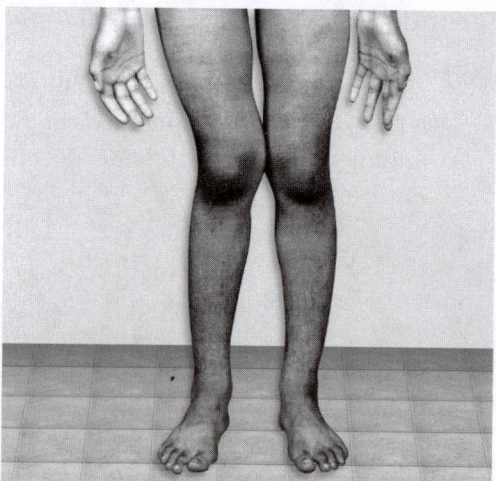

Fig. 9: Genu valgum.

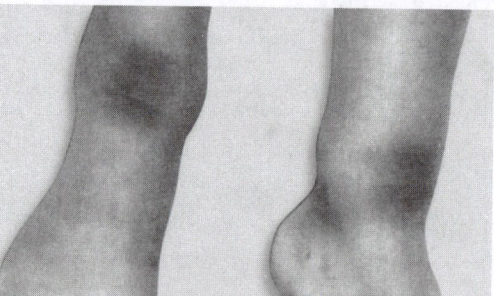

Fig. 12: Broad ankles.

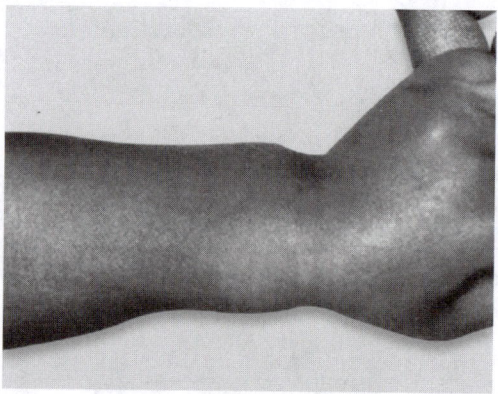

Fig. 10: Widening of the wrist.

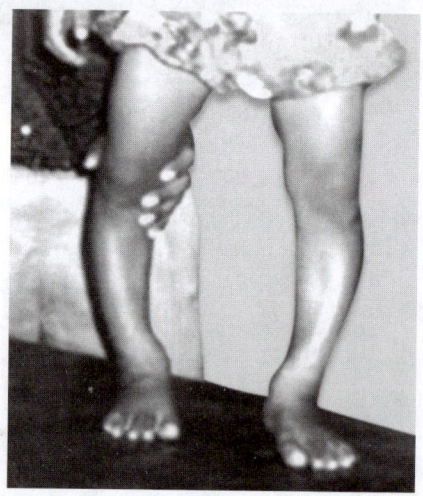

Fig. 13: Bow legs.

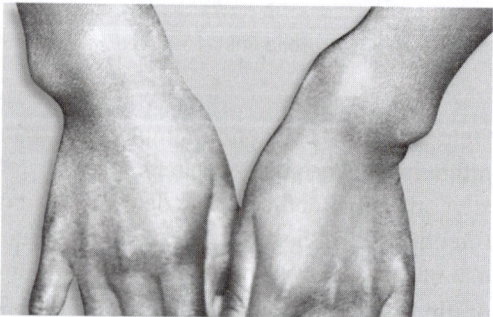

Fig. 11: Broad wrists.

Dentition may be delayed and disordered eruption of temporary teeth occurs. In children between 8 and 18 months, permanent teeth, which are undergoing calcification, may be affected.

Besides skeletal deformities, there is generalized hypotonia with delay in motor development. The abdomen is protuberant, and generalized flabbiness of muscles may result into visceroptosis with downward displacement of spleen and liver.

Deficiency of vitamin D in early infancy results in bilateral lamellar cataracts. They may even be seen in neonatal period.

Clinical variants of rickets include type I calcium deficient, type II phosphate deficient and type III end organ resistance to 1,25 $(OH)_2D_3$.

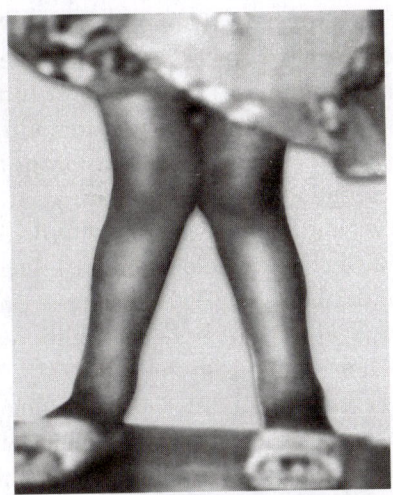

Fig. 14: Knock knees.

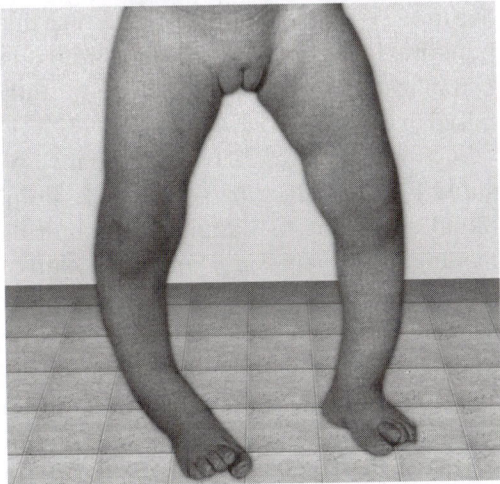

Fig. 15: Genu varum.

■ BIOCHEMICAL INVESTIGATIONS

First line:
- Serum calcium (no tourniquet), phosphorus, alkaline phosphatase, creatinine, and albumin—all fasting samples
- Liver and kidney functions (if clinically indicated)
- In nonnutritional cases:
  - Venous blood gas
  - Serum PTH, 25(OH)D, and 1,25 (OH)$_2$D
- Urinary calcium/creatinine ratio (spot or 24 hours urine sample)
- Thymolphthalein monophosphate (TmP) (morning spot urinary sample and simultaneous fasting serum sample)

GENERAL FEATURES
• Rachitic rosary
• Harrison's groove
• Delayed dentition
• Lumbar lordosis

■ DIAGNOSIS

The diagnosis of rickets is based on the clinical features, biochemical findings, and characteristic radiological picture. The serum calcium level may be normal or low, the serum phosphorous level is below 4 mg/dL, and the serum alkaline phosphatase is usually elevated.

Radiology

Radiological changes are best seen on posteroanterior radiographs of the wrist, although characteristic rachitic changes can be seen at other growth plates. Decreased calcification leads to thickening of the growth plate. The edge of the metaphysis loses its sharp border, which is described as *fraying*. The edge of the metaphysis changes from a convex or flat surface to a more concave surface. This change to a concave surface is termed *cupping* and is most easily seen at the distal ends of the radius, ulna, and fibula **(Fig. 16)**. There is widening of the distal end of the metaphysis, corresponding to the clinical observation of thickened wrists and ankles as well as the rachitic rosary. Other radiologic features include coarse trabeculation of the diaphysis and generalized rarefaction.

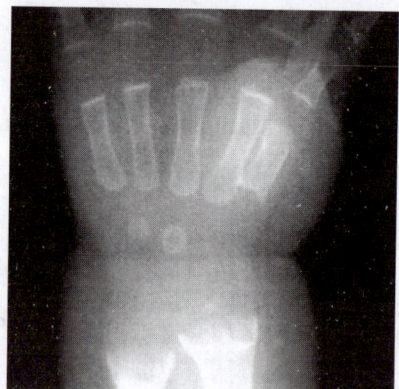

Fig. 16: Cup-shaped rarefied radius and ulna.

Skiagram of the wrist shows widening, cupping, and fraying of the epiphyses, in contrast to the normally sharply demarcated and slightly convex epiphyseal line. The density of shafts decreases with prominent trabeculae. There is an increase in distance between concave epiphyseal line and the ends of metacarpals. Greenstick fractures, expansion of bone ends, and bending of bones may be evident on radiographs. Some raising of the periosteum is due to excess of osteoid lying under the periosteum.

The initial laboratory tests in a child with rickets should include serum calcium, phosphorus, alkaline phosphatase, PTH, 25-hydroxyvitamin D, 1,25-dihydroxyvitamin D (1,25-D), creatinine, and electrolytes. The diagnosis of vitamin D deficiency is based on low circulating levels of $25(OH)D_3$. Values above 20 ng/mL are normal, between 10 and 20 ng/mL are insufficient and below 10 ng/mL are indicative of deficiency.

Urinalysis is useful for detecting the glycosuria and aminoaciduria (positive dipstick for protein) seen with Fanconi syndrome. Evaluation of urinary excretion of calcium (24-hour collection for calcium or calcium–creatinine ratio) is helpful if hereditary hypophosphatemic rickets with hypercalciuria or Fanconi syndrome is suspected. Direct measurement of other fat-soluble vitamins (A, E, and K) or indirect assessment of deficiency (prothrombin time for vitamin K deficiency) is appropriate if malabsorption is a consideration.

If a good clinical examination does not provide a clue to etiology, then PTH should guide further workup. Primary and secondary hyperparathyroidism result in increased phosphorus leak from the proximal tubule. Thus, a child with any cause of calcipenic rickets, such as malabsorption or distal renal tubular acidosis (RTA), due to concomitant secondary hyperparathyroidism, may appear to have hypophosphatemic rickets. Serum PTH is a useful investigation at this juncture, being only marginally elevated in hypophosphatemic rickets, and significantly raised in calcipenic rickets.

Cases with high PTH should be investigated for distal RTA by serum potassium, blood and urine pH, ammonium chloride loading test if necessary, and ultrasound of kidneys for nephrocalcinosis. Malabsorption tests include ESR, antiendomysial or tissue transglutaminase antibodies, D-xylose test, and endoscopic duodenal biopsy. If these are negative, serum 25-OHD and $1,25(OH)_2D$ can throw light on 1 alpha-hydroxylase defect and calcitriol receptor defect [vitamin D-resistant rickets, (VDRR)] 1 and 21. Low PTH type of resistant rickets should be worked tip for phosphate clearance (phosphate clearance/creatinine clearance) and TmP/GFR (glomerular filtration rate) measurement. Proximal RTA is tested by bicarbonate loading test and documenting aminoaciduria, glycosuria, and uric aciduria in addition to phosphaturia. Plain radiology reveals coarse trabecular pattern in RTA and renal failure, and dense bone in hypophosphatemic rickets.

LABORATORY SALIENT FINDINGS
• Low serum phosphorus level • High serum alkaline phosphatase level • High parathyroid hormone (PTH) levels • Low-level serum calcifedoil

Vitamin D Levels in Serum

	25-dydroxyvitamin D level (ng/mL)
▪ Deficient:	<10
▪ Insufficient:	10–20
▪ Optimal:	20–60
▪ High:	60–90
▪ Toxic:	Greater than 90

Changes of active rickets in spine and pelvis are rarely seen even in advanced stages. The level of serum calcium is normal or slightly low (9–9.5 mg/dL) and that of phosphate decreased (1.5–3 mg/dL). Serum alkaline phosphatase level is raised. PTH levels are normal. Blood levels of $1,25(OH)_2D_3$ are inappropriately low for the level of serum phosphate. Urinary phosphate excretion is increased with decreased TmP.

■ DIFFERENTIAL DIAGNOSIS

- Hypophosphatemia
- Metaphyseal dysostosis
- Fanconi's syndrome
- Cystinosis

Nutritional rickets should be differentiated from other types of rickets and chondrodystrophy. Other conditions producing bony deformities may, sometimes, need consideration. Craniotabes and a large head apart from rickets, occurs in hydrocephalus, congenital syphilis, and osteogenesis imperfecta. Enlargement of costochondral junctions may also be seen in scurvy and chondrodystrophy.

■ TREATMENT

Children with nutritional vitamin D deficiency should receive vitamin D and adequate nutritional intake of calcium and phosphorus. There are two strategies for administration of vitamin D. With stoss therapy, 300,000–600,000 IU of vitamin D are administered orally or intramuscularly as 2–4 doses over 1 day. Because the doses are observed, stoss therapy is ideal in situations where adherence to therapy is questionable.

The alternative is daily, high-dose vitamin D, with doses ranging from 2,000 to 5,000 IU/day over 4–6 weeks. Either strategy should be followed by daily vitamin D intake of 400 IU/day if <1 year old or 600 IU/day if >1 year old. It is important to ensure that children receive adequate dietary calcium and phosphorus; this dietary intake is usually provided by milk, formula, and other dairy products.

It is now advised to use lower daily doses of 2,000 IU, 3,000–6,000 IU, and 6,000 IU for infants below 12 months, 1–12 years, and >12 years, respectively, for the duration of 12 weeks followed by maintenance dose of 400–600 IU/day.

Children who have symptomatic hypocalcemia might need IV calcium acutely, followed by oral calcium (30–75 mg/kg/day) supplements, which typically can be tapered over 2–6 weeks in children who receive adequate dietary calcium. Transient use of IV or oral 1,25-D (calcitriol) is often helpful in reversing hypocalcemia in the acute phase by providing active vitamin D during the delay as supplemental vitamin D is converted to active vitamin D.

Calcitriol doses are typically 0.05 ug/kg/day. IV calcium is initially given as an acute bolus for symptomatic hypocalcemia (20 mg/kg of calcium chloride or 100 mg/kg of calcium gluconate. Some patients require continuous IV calcium drip, titrated to maintain the desired serum calcium level. These patients should transition to enteral calcium, and most infants require approximately 1,000 mg of elemental calcium.

Management of Nonnutritional Rickets

- *Hypophosphatemic rickets:* Oral phosphorous 35–75 mg/kg/day and oral calcitriol 20–40 ng/kg/day
- *Vitamin D-dependent rickets type 1 (VDDR 1):* Calcitriol 150–200 ng/kg/day and oral calcium (30–75 mg/kg/day)
- *Vitamin D-dependent rickets type 2 (VDDR 2):* Very high doses of calcitriol (1–6 µg/day) and IV calcium or high-dose calcium (150–200 mg/kg/day)

Orthopedic corrective surgery, i.e., osteotomy is indicated for deformities. This is done only after active rickets is brought under control. Diet should be supplemented with adequate dose of vitamin D_3. Steatorrhea or malabsorption of fat should be treated. If there is no response even to the second dose other variants of rickets should be looked for.

■ BIBLIOGRAPHY

1. Elder CJ, Bishop NJ, Rickets. Lancet. 2014;383:1665-76.
2. National Institute of Nutrition. (2011). Dietary Guidelines for Indians. [online] Available from https://www.nin.res.in/downloads/DietaryGuidelinesforNINwebsite.pdf [Last accessed June, 2024].
3. Wagner CL, Greer FR; American Academy of Pediatrics Section on Breastfeeding; American Academy of Pediatrics Committee on Nutrition. Prevention of rickets and vitamin D deficiency in infants, children, and adolescents. 2008;122:1142-52.

CASE 92

Scurvy

■ PRESENTING COMPLAINTS

An 18-month-old boy was brought with the complaint of:
- Decreased appetite since 2 months
- Irritability since one month
- Loose motion since 3–4 days
- Rashes since 2 days

History of Presenting Complaints

An 18-month-old boy was brought to the hospital with history of irritability, digestive disturbance, and loss of appetite. His mother had noticed that he was more irritable for last 2 months. She had even noticed that he was becoming more irritable recently. She also complained that her son had on and off attack of loose motions, which were semisolid. She also complained that her son's appetite has come down drastically and made a note of development of small rashes over the recently. There was no history suggestive of hematuria.

Past History of the Patient

He is the only child of nonconsanguineous marriage. He was born at full term by normal vaginal delivery. His birth weight was 2.5 kg. He started to take the breast milk immediately. Weaning started at fourth month. His developmental milestones were normal. He had been completely immunized. He was suffering from repeated respiratory tract infections.

CASE AT A GLANCE

Basic Findings
Height	: 83 cm (90th centile)
Weight	: 10 kg (75th centile)
Temperature	: 37°C
Pulse rate	: 110 beats/min
Respiratory rate	: 22 breaths/min
Blood pressure	: 60/40 mm Hg

Positive Findings

History:
- Irritability
- Bowel disturbance
- Loss of appetite

Examination:
- Frog-leg posture
- Hypertrophy of gums
- Subperiosteal hemorrhage
- Petechial hemorrhage
- Pallor
- Scorbutic rosary

Investigation:
- *Hemoglobin:* Decreased
- *X-ray of long bone:* Showed periosteal hematoma

■ EXAMINATION

The boy was moderately built and nourished. He was irritable. There was evidence of generalized tenderness. He had assumed frog-leg posture. Hips and knees were semiflexed. Hypertrophy of the gums was present. There was prominent costochondral junction. Subperiosteal hemorrhages were palpated at the end of femur. Petechial hemorrhages were seen in skin and mucous membrane.

Anthropometric measurements included the height 83 cm (90th centile), the weight 10 kg (75th centile), and the head circumference 47 cm.

The child was afebrile. Heart rate was 110 beats/min and respiratory rate was 22 breaths/min. Blood pressure recorded was 60/40 mm Hg. Pallor was present. Cervical lymphadenopathy was present. There was no cyanosis and clubbing. Other systemic examinations were normal.

■ INVESTIGATION

- *Hemoglobin:* 9.3 g/dL
- *TLC:* 10,800 cells/cumm
- *ESR:* 16 mm in the first hour
- *Platelet count:* 4,40,000 cells/cumm
- *Bleeding time:* 6 minutes
- *Clotting time:* 10 minutes
- *X-ray of the long bone:* Showed periosteal hematoma

■ DISCUSSION

In scurvy, there is defective formation of connective tissues and collagen in skin, cartilage, dentine, bone, and blood vessels, leading to their fragility. In the long bones, osteoid is not deposited by osteoblasts, cortex is thin, and the trabeculae become brittle and fracture easily.

Vitamin C is important for synthesis of collagen at the level of hydroxylation of lysine and proline in precollagen. It is also involved in neurotransmitter metabolism (conversion of dopamine to norepinephrine and tryptophan to serotonin), cholesterol metabolism (conversion of cholesterol to steroid hormones and bile acids), and the biosynthesis of carnitine. Vitamin C functions to maintain the iron and copper atoms, cofactors of the metalloenzymes, in a reduced (active) state. Vitamin C is an important antioxidant (electron donor) in the aqueous milieu of the body. Vitamin C enhances nonheme iron absorption, the transfer of iron from transferrin to ferritin, and the formation of tetrahydrofolic acid and thus can affect the cellular and immunologic functions of the hematopoietic system.

Vitamin C is potent reducing agent. The adrenals and lens have particularly high content of vitamin C. When a mother's intake of vitamin C during pregnancy and lactation is adequate, the newborn will have adequate tissue levels of vitamin C related to active placental transfer, subsequently maintained by the vitamin C in breast milk or commercial infant formulas. Breast milk contains sufficient vitamin C to prevent deficiency throughout infancy.

Absorption of vitamin C occurs in the upper small intestine by an active process or by simple diffusion when large amounts are ingested. Vitamin C is not stored in the body but is taken up by all tissues; the highest levels are found in the pituitary and adrenal glands.

Humans depend on dietary sources for vitamin C. An adequate intake is 40 mg for age 0–6 months and 50 mg for age 6–12 months. For older children, the recommended dietary allowance is 15 mg for age 1–3 years, 25 mg for age 4–8 years, 45 mg for age 9–13 years, and 65–75 mg for age 14–18 years. The requirement for vitamin C is increased during infectious and diarrheal diseases. The best food sources of vitamin C are citrus fruits and fruit juices, peppers, berries, melons, tomatoes, cauliflower, and green leafy vegetables.

The need for vitamin C is increased by febrile illness, diarrheal disease, iron deficiency, and exposure to cold. It is essential for the formation collagen and intracellular matrix in teeth, bones and capillaries. It is also involved in tyrosin metabolism, adrenal cortical functioning, and electron transport. It is a cofactor in activation of hydroxylating enzymes in oxidation process. It helps in the transfer of iron from the plasma transferring into tissue ferritin and thus helps in storage of iron in the bone marrow, spleen, and liver. It provides protection to eyes and lungs against oxidizing agents. Hence reduces oxidation of low-density lipoprotein and prevents the deposition of atheromatous plaque. It helps in maintenance of vascular integrity through the prostacyclin, i.e., anti-platelet and vasodilating effect.

Ascorbic acid is essential for normal formation of collagen. Alteration in collagen formation is partly due to failure to incorporate hydroxyproline and proline. Formation of collagen and chondroitin sulfate is impaired. The periosteum becomes loosened. Subperiosteal hemorrhages occur especially at ends of femur and tibia. In severe scurvy, there may be degeneration in the skeletal muscles, cardiac hypertrophy, bone marrow depression, and adrenal atrophy.

A deficiency of vitamin C results in the clinical presentation of *scurvy*. Children fed predominantly heat-treated (ultra-high temperature or pasteurized) milk or unfortified formulas and not receiving fruits and fruit juices are at significant risk for symptomatic disease.

Infants and children on highly restrictive diets, devoid of most fruits and vegetables, are at risk of acquiring severe vitamin C deficiency. Such diets are occasionally promoted with unsubstantiated claims of benefit in autism and other developmental disorders.

In scurvy, there is defective formation of connective tissues and collagen in skin, cartilage, dentin, bone, and blood vessels, leading to their fragility. In the long bones, osteoid is not deposited by osteoblasts, cortex is thin, and the trabeculae become brittle and fracture easily.

■ CLINICAL FEATURES (FIG. 1)

Scurvy may occur at any age. The usual age of onset is 6–18 months. Breastfed infants are well protected in breast milk contains adequate amount of vitamin C. Clinical manifestations require time to develop. The symptoms may include irritability, tachypnea, digestive disturbances, and loss of appetite.

Irritability becomes progressive. There is evidence of generalized tenderness. Pain results in pseudoparalysis. Child will assume frog-leg position. Hips and knees are semiflexed with feet rotated outward. Subperiosteal swelling can be palpated at the end of femur. Hypertrophy of gums **(Figs. 2 and 3)** is present. There may be scorbutic rosary at the costochondral junction.

Subperiosteal hemorrhages in the lower limb bones sometimes acutely increase the swelling and pain, and the condition might mimic acute osteomyelitis or arthritis. Costochondral junction becomes prominent and appear as a sharp and angular, scorbutic rosary is attributed to the separation of epiphyses of ribs and backward displacement of sternum. A "rosary" at the costochondral

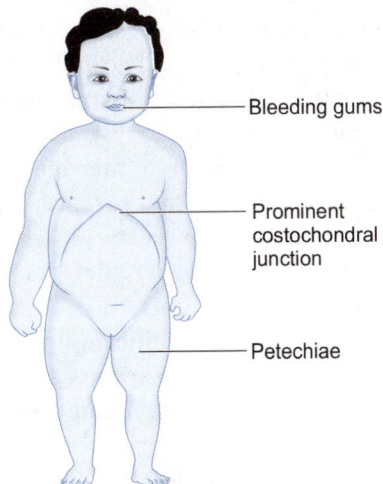

Fig. 1: Clinical features.

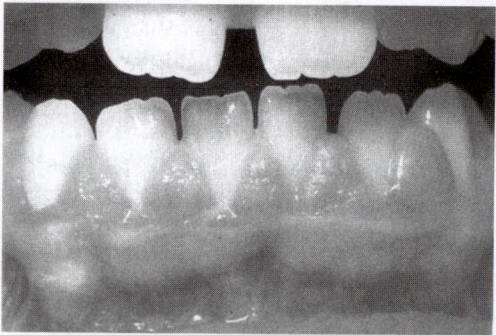

Fig. 2: Gingival hypertrophy. *(For color version, see Plate 10)*

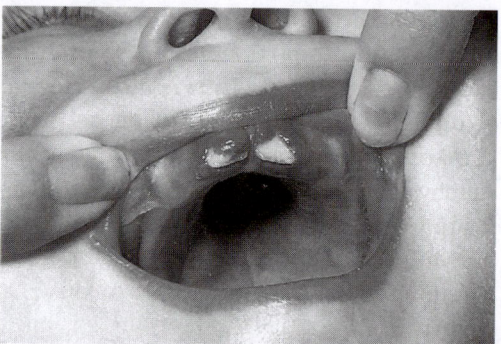

Fig. 4: Bleeding gum. *(For color version, see Plate 11)*

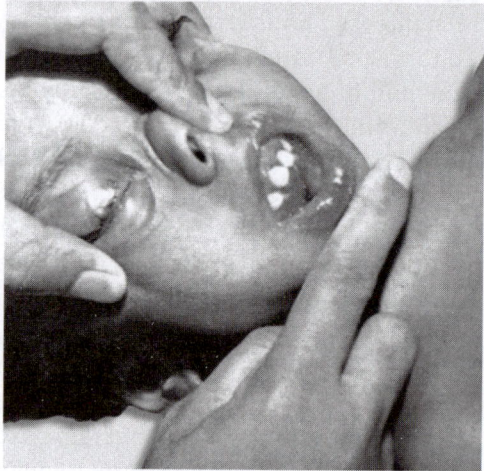

Fig. 3: Gum hypertrophy. *(For color version, see Plate 10)*

junctions and depression of the sternum are other typical features. The angulation of scorbutic beads is usually sharper than the angulation of a rachitic rosary. Gum changes are seen in older children after teeth have erupted and are manifested as bluish purple, spongy swellings of the mucous membrane, especially over the upper incisors. Gum bleeds are common **(Fig. 4)**.

Anemia, a common finding in infants and young children with scurvy, is related to impaired iron absorption and coexistent hematopoietic nutrient deficiencies including iron, vitamin B_{12}, and folate. Hemorrhagic manifestations of scurvy include petechiae, purpura, and ecchymoses at pressure points; epistaxis; gum bleeding; and the characteristic perifollicular hemorrhages. Other manifestations are poor wound and fracture healing, hyperkeratosis of hair follicles, arthralgia, and muscle weakness.

Petechial hemorrhages occur in skin and mucous membrane. Hematuria, melena or orbital, conjunctival, and subdural hemorrhage may be found. The anemia is associated with that of scurvy. These are sickle cell anemia, iron deficiency anemia, and sometimes dimorphic anemia.

ESSENTIAL DIAGNOSTIC POINTS
- Irritability, generalized tenderness
- Pseudoparalysis, frog-leg position
- Bleeding and hypertrophy of gums
- Prominent costochondral junction
- Petechial hemorrhage in skin mucous membrane
- Orbital and conjunctival hemorrhage

GENERAL FEATURES
- Child is listless
- Anorexia
- Paradoxical cry
- Frog-like posture
- Hemorrhages

■ DIAGNOSIS

The typical radiographic changes occur at the distal ends of the long bones and are particularly common at the knees. The shafts of the long bones have a ground-glass appearance because of trabecular atrophy. The cortex is thin and dense, giving the appearance of pencil outlining of the diaphysis and epiphysis. Epiphyseal ends are sharply outlined.

The white line of Frankel, an irregular but thickened white line at the metaphysis, represents the zone of well-calcified cartilage. White line may also be seen with healing rickets, severe protein-energy malnutrition (PEM), plumbism, acute leukemia, and congenital syphilis. Epiphyseal centers of ossification are surrounded by white ring—Wimberger sign.

The epiphyseal centers of ossification also have a ground-glass appearance and are surrounded by a sclerotic ring. The more specific but late radiologic feature of scurvy is a zone of rarefaction under the white line at the metaphysis. This zone of rarefaction (Trümmerfeld zone), a linear break in the bone that is proximal and parallel to the white line, represents area of debris of broken-down bone trabeculae and connective tissue.

A Pelkan spur is a lateral prolongation of the white line and may be present at cortical ends. Epiphyseal separation can occur along the line of destruction, with either linear displacement or compression of the epiphysis against the shaft. Subperiosteal hemorrhage produces periosteal elevation.

Magnetic resonance imaging (MRI) can demonstrate acute as well as healing subperiosteal hematomas along with periostitis, metaphyseal changes, and heterogeneous bone marrow signal intensity even in absence of changes in plain radiographs. Gelatinous transformation of bone marrow, on aspiration, has been reported in children with suspected malignancy.

Evidence of vitamin C deficiency is better furnished by ascorbic acid concentration in white cells, platelet layer (buffy layer) of centrifuged oxalated blood. A level of zero in this layer indicates latent scurvy.

■ DIFFERENTIAL DIAGNOSIS

Differential diagnosis includes arthritis, acrodynia, osteomyelitis, pseudoparalysis, syphilis, poliomyelitis, and leukemia.

■ TREATMENT

Administration of ascorbic acid is preferred. The only therapeutic dose is 100–200 mg or more orally or parenterally. Three to four ounces of orange or tomato juice will be of help.

Vitamin C supplements of 100–200 mg/day orally or parenterally ensure rapid and complete cure. The clinical improvement is seen within a week in most cases, but the treatment should be continued for up to 3 months for complete recovery.

■ BIBLIOGRAPHY

1. Indian Council of Medical Research, National Institute of Nutrition. (2024). Dietary Guidelines for INDIANS. [online] Available from https://main.icmr.nic.in/sites/default/files/upload_documents/DGI_07th_May_2024_fin.pdf [Last accessed June, 2024].
2. Sethuraman U. Vitamins. Pediatr Rev. 2006; 27:44-55.
3. Shah D, Sachdev HPS. Vitamin C (ascorbic acid). In: Kliegman RM, Stanton BF, St Geme III JW, Schor NF, Behrman RE. Nelson Textbook of Pediatrics, 19th edition. United Kingdom: Elsevier Health Sciences; 2011.
4. Suskind DL. Nutritional deficiencies during normal growth. Pediatric Clin North Am. 2009;56:1035-53.

SECTION 12

Neoplastic Diseases

- Case 93 **Ewing's Sarcoma**
- Case 94 **Hodgkin's Disease**
- Case 95 **Leukemia**
- Case 96 **Neuroblastoma**
- Case 97 **Osteosarcoma**
- Case 98 **Retinoblastoma**
- Case 99 **Wilms' Tumor**

CASE 93

Ewing's Sarcoma

■ PRESENTING COMPLAINTS

A 3-year-old boy was brought with the complaint of:
- Swelling in the right leg since 2 months
- Pain in the leg since 15 days
- Fever since 7 days
- Not able to walk since 2 days

History of Presenting Complaints

A 3-year-old boy was brought to the hospital with a history of pain in the right leg. His mother said that he had been complaining of pain in his right leg for the last 2 weeks. The mother also said that the child had a fever since the last 1 week. The fever was moderate to a high degree, intermittent. It was not associated with chills and rigors. It used to be more in the evening. The child was not able to walk because of pain in the leg. He was limping. The mother had also noted that there was a small swelling in the leg.

Past History of the Patient

He was the only sibling of a consanguineous marriage. He was born at full term by normal vaginal delivery. He cried immediately after the delivery. He started taking feeds as early as possible. There was no significant postnatal event. He was sent home on the third day. Weaning started from the fourth month as per advice from a family doctor. He was on family food for 1 year. All the developmental milestones were normal. He had been completely immunized.

■ EXAMINATION

The child was moderately built and nourished. He was not allowing anybody to touch his right leg. Anthropometric measurements included, his height was 93 cm (50th centile), and his weight was 13 kg (75th centile).

CASE AT A GLANCE

Basic Findings
Height	: 93 cm (50th centile)
Weight	: 13 kg (75th centile)
Temperature	: 38°C
Pulse rate	: 120 beats/min
Respiratory rate	: 20 breaths/min
Blood pressure	: 70/50 mm Hg

Positive Findings

History:
- Pain
- Fever
- Swelling

Examination:
- Tenderness
- Limping
- Swelling
- Febrile

Investigation:
- *X-ray of leg:* Irregularly thickened cortical wall
- *Fine-needle aspiration cytology (FNAC):* Small uniform round cells

He was febrile, the heart rate was 120 beats/min, and the respiratory rate was 20 breaths/min. The blood pressure recorded was 70/50 mm Hg. There was no pallor. The right inguinal lymph nodes were enlarged and tender. There was erythema and tenderness in the upper part of the right leg.

INVESTIGATION

- *Hemoglobin:* 12 g/dL
- *Total leukocyte count (TLC):* 7,800 cells/mm^3
- *Erythrocyte sedimentation rate (ESR):* 32 mm in the first hour
- *Absolute eosinophil count (AEC):* 330 cells/mm^3
- *X-ray chest:* No abnormalities detected (NAD)
- *X-ray of the leg:* Irregularly thickened cortical wall of the proximal half of the tibia.
- *Bone marrow biopsy:* NAD
- *Computed tomography (CT) scan chest:* NAD
- *Fine-needle aspiration cytology (FNAC):* Small uniform round cells

DISCUSSION

It is a small round blue cell tumor of the bone. It is more common in males. The primary symptom is pain. This may be accompanied by fever and tenderness. The soft tissue involvement varies but may be massive.

Other conditions that may be confused are osteomyelitis and eosinophilic granuloma. Ewing's sarcoma (EWS) and primitive neuroectodermal tumor (PNET) are the second most common malignant bone tumors, after osteogenic sarcoma in children and adolescents.

Ewing's sarcoma may arise in the bone or soft tissues throughout the body. They may be undifferentiated (pathologically termed EWS) or show evidence of neural differentiation (pathologically termed primitive neuroectodermal tumor). Moreover, a subset of these tumors that arise in the chest wall have historically been referred to as Askin tumors. As EWS, PNET, and Askin tumors are now understood to share the same fundamental biology, the principles that drive the management of patients with these tumors are largely identical.

It is an uncommon type of highly malignant small round cell undifferentiated bone tumor occurring in children. Ewing's tumor forms about 20% of all malignant bone tumors. It occurs in the age group of 10–20 years and is more common in males. It can also be seen below the age of 10 years. It arises from the primitive mesenchymal cells of the medullary cavity. The sites affected are the diaphyseal regions of long bones, such as the femur, tibia, and humerus. It also occurs in flat bones like pelvic bones.

PATHOGENESIS

Additionally, microneme protein 2 (MIC-2) [cluster of differentiation 99 (CD99)] staining is usually positive. A specific chromosomal translocation, t (11;22), or a variant thereof is found in most of the EWS family of tumors. The feature of EWS is the presence of one of several recurrent chromosomal translocations involving members of the *TET* transcription factor family and *ETS* transcription factor gene family members. The translocation results in a novel chimeric transcription factor that brings the activation domain of the TET family with the deoxyribonucleic acid (DNA) binding domain of the ETS family member. Analysis for the chain reaction translocation by fluorescence in situ hybridization (FISH) or polymerase analysis for the chimeric fusion gene products EWS/friend leukemia integration 1 transcription (FLI1) or EWS/ERG (for other variants) is utilized routinely in diagnosis. The most common translocation involves EWSR1 on chromosome 22 with FLI1 on chromosome 11, leading to the classic t(11;22) translocation. These fusions are believed to be the inciting event in the development of these tumors.

Immunohistochemical staining assists in the diagnosis of EWS to differentiate it from small, round, blue cell tumors, such as lymphoma, rhabdomyosarcoma, and neuroblastoma. Histochemical stains may react positively with certain neural markers on tumor cells (neuron-specific enolase and S-100), especially in peripheral PNETs. Reactivity with muscle markers (e.g., desmin and actin) is absent.

■ PATHOLOGY

These tumors can arise in any bone. But the most common sites are flat bones, such as the pelvis, chest wall, head, vertebrae, and the diaphyseal region of long bones. The most commonly involved bone is the femur. The most common sites of metastasis are the lungs, bone marrow, central nervous system (CNS), and other bones

Macroscopically the tumor is a pale soft mass with minimal bone tissue. There are areas of degeneration and hemorrhage. There is further simulation of osteomyelitis by the presence of milky pus-like fluid in the tumor tissue due to degeneration.

Microscopically the tumor is very cellular with minimal stromal tissue. The characteristic cell is the small polyhedral cell with scanty cytoplasm and a large nucleus. The appearance is monotonously uniform with cells arranged in compact sheets with loose and vacuolated formation by the tumor cells. This stimulates the rosette formation of neuroblastoma. The presence of glycogen helps in differentiating this condition from neuroblastoma. This is indicated by periodic acid–Schiff (PAS) reaction. The tumor must be differentiated from lymphoma (reticulum cell sarcoma).

> **ESSENTIAL DIAGNOSTIC POINTS**
> - Small, round blue cell malignancy
> - Pain and swelling
> - Fever, anemia, and leukocytosis
> - Weight loss

■ CLINICAL FEATURES (FIG. 1)

The patient presents with pain which gradually increases and is followed by swelling. The swelling is firm to soft in consistency with indefinite margins. The duration of the symptoms may vary from a few weeks to a few months and sometimes >1 year. The most common presenting symptom is pain, and occasionally swelling will occur, depending on the location and size of the primary tumor. As patients with EWS tend to be otherwise healthy, active adolescents, it is not unusual for initial musculoskeletal complaints to be attributed to injury, often responsive to nonsteroidal anti-inflammatory drugs, and for there to be repeated visits for persistent pain before diagnosis. Some patients have a palpable mass at initial presentation, and some may have functional consequences related to the location of the tumor.

Ewing's sarcoma often is associated with systemic manifestations, such as fever and weight loss; patients may have undergone treatment for a presumptive diagnosis of osteomyelitis fever of unknown origin. Patients also may have a delay in diagnosis when their pain or swelling is attributed to a sports injury.

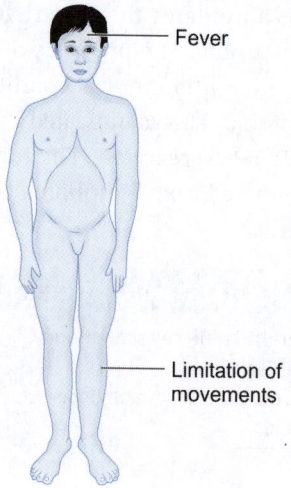

Fig. 1: Clinical features.

The swelling rapidly increases in size with the involvement of soft tissues and the general condition deteriorates. The peculiar feature of Ewing's tumor is that metastasis occurs in other bones such as the skull, vertebrae, and ribs, in addition to the lungs by spreading through the bloodstream.

Approximately 80% of patients have a primary tumor arising from a bone, while the other 20% have soft tissue primary tumors. Among patients with bone tumors, approximately half of the cases will arise in the long bones of the extremities while the other half will arise in flat bones such as the pelvis and ribs, a distribution that is markedly different from pediatric osteosarcoma, which is predominantly a disease of the long bones. Metastatic disease is present at initial diagnosis in a quarter of cases, with lung, bone, and bone marrow being the most common metastatic sites.

GENERAL FEATURES
• Pain • Swelling • Weight loss

DIAGNOSIS

Once a diagnosis of EWS is established, staging studies are performed to assess for the presence of disseminated disease. Patients require CT of the chest and staging for bone metastases, either with a bone scan or whole-body positron emission tomography (PET) scan. PET scanning has become more prevalent in recent years and appears to be more sensitive than bone scans in detecting metastatic disease. For bone marrow staging, bilateral bone marrow aspirates and biopsies are commonly performed, though recent evidence indicates that PET imaging results may guide the need for whether or not bone marrow biopsies should be performed. Some centers do not perform staging bone marrow biopsies in patients who: have no evidence of metastatic disease by PET scans, as there is a low likelihood of isolated metastatic disease to the bone marrow.

Ewing's sarcoma occurs primarily between 10 and 20 years. It is suspected of clinical history and radiographic features. It should be confirmed by surgical biopsy. Once the diagnosis is made the patients should be screened for metastasis in the lung.

The radiograph shows areas of mottled rarefaction in the affected diaphysis of the bone. There will be marked destruction of the bone cortex and involvement of the soft tissues. There is also reactive new bone formation in layers under the raised periosteum producing the characteristic "onion-peel" appearance. A large, associated, soft tissue mass often is visualized on magnetic resonance imaging (MRI) or CT. the differential diagnosis includes osteosarcoma, osteomyelitis, Langerhans cell histiocytosis, primary lymphoma of bone, metastatic neuroblastoma, or rhabdomyosarcoma in the case of a pure soft tissue lesion.

To avoid compromising the ultimate potential for limb salvage by a poorly planned biopsy incision, the same surgeon should perform the biopsy and the surgical procedure. CT-guided surgical biopsy of the lesion often provides diagnostic tissue. It is important to obtain adequate tissue for special stains and molecular studies. CT scans of bone and marrow biopsy are advised. Pathological fracture may occur through the bone as a result of tumor destruction or at a biopsy site. They may heal poorly during radiotherapy (RT) and chemotherapy. This may cause pain.

Special histochemical staining should be done to distinguish EWS from another metastatic round-cell tumors, such as rhabdomyosarcoma, neuroblastoma, and non-Hodgkin's lymphoma (NHL).

Thorough evaluation for the metastatic disease includes CT of the chest, radionuclide bone scan, and bone marrow aspiration, and biopsy specimens from at least two sites. MRI of the tumor and the entire length of the involved bone should be performed to determine the exact extension of the soft tissue and bony mass and the proximity of the tumor to neurovascular structures.

Ewing sarcoma is a classic small round blue cell tumor, characterized pathologically by sheets of monomorphic cells with a high nuclear-to-cytoplasmic ratio. Immunohistochemistry and cytogenetic/molecular studies are critical to differentiate EWS from other childhood small round blue cell tumors. CD99, while not specific to EWS, is the most useful stain, with a strong membranous pattern classically described. Additional testing to confirm a diagnosis will include cytogenetic studies such as FISH that reveal a break at the EWSRI locus and polymerase chain reaction (PCR) to assess and detect a specific EWS-ETS translocation.

> **LABORATORY SALIENT FINDINGS**
> - CT scan, and MRI of the primary lesion
> - CT scan of the chest
> - Bone scanning, bilateral bone marrow aspirates, and biopsy
> - Special histochemical staining
> - *Radiograph:* Onion-peel appearance
>
> (CT: computed tomography; MRI: magnetic resonance imaging)

■ DIFFERENTIAL DIAGNOSIS

Differential diagnoses include osteosarcoma, osteomyelitis, eosinophilic granuloma, lymphoma, rhabdomyosarcoma, and neuroblastoma.

■ TREATMENT

Ewing's sarcoma is considered a radiosensitive tumor, and local control may be achieved with irradiation or surgery. Radiation therapy is associated with risks of radiation-induced second malignancies, failures of bone growth, and fibrosis. It is the traditional treatment for Ewing's tumor. This tumor is radiosensitive and regression following therapy is remarkable. Surgical resection is indicated to achieve local control. Chemotherapy should be resumed as soon as possible after surgery.

However, with this type of treatment, the local recurrence rate is high. Hence, currently after preoperative chemotherapy, surgical resection of the tumor-bearing bone is done with skeletal reconstruction followed by postoperative chemotherapy. This regimen has increased the survival rate from 5 to 50%. Chemotherapy should be resumed as soon as possible after surgery. It is important to provide the patient with crutches if the tumor is in a weight-bearing bone, to avoid a pathologic fracture before definitive local control. Tumor control with RT requires moderately high doses ranging from 5.500 to 6.000 cGy.

Multiagent chemotherapy is important because it can shrink the tumor rapidly and is usually given before local control is attempted. Standard chemotherapy for nonmetastatic EWS includes vincristine, doxorubicin, cyclophosphamide, etoposide, and ifosfamide. Chemotherapy usually causes dramatic shrinkage of the soft tissue mass and rapid, significant pain relief.

■ PROGNOSIS

The stage at initial diagnosis is the strongest clinical prognostic factor for EWS. Approximately 70% of patients with localized disease can be expected to survive at least 5 years without relapse or progression with contemporary therapy, compared to only 30% or less for patients with metastatic disease. Among patients with metastatic disease, the location of metastases appears to have important prognostic value, as those with bone and/or bone marrow metastasis have dismal outcomes compared to those with isolated pulmonary metastatic disease. Other adverse prognostic factors at the initial presentation include older age, larger tumor size, and primary pelvic site. Poor response to initial chemotherapy, based upon imaging and/or histopathology, is also associated with inferior outcomes.

Long-term follow-up of patients with EWS is important because of the potential for late effects of treatment, such as anthracycline cardiotoxicity; second malignancies, especially in the radiation field; and late relapses, even as long as 10 years after initial diagnosis.

■ BIBLIOGRAPHY

1. Meyer JS, Nadel HR, Marina N, Womer RB, Brown KL, Eary JF, et al. Imaging guidelines for children with Ewing sarcoma and osteosarcoma: a report from the Children's Oncology Group Bone Tumor Committee. Pediatr Blood Cancer. 2008;51(2):163-70.
2. Moore DD, Haydon RC. Ewing's sarcoma of the bone. Cancer Treat Res. 2014;162:93-115.
3. Womer R, West DC, Krailo MD, Dickman PS, Pawel BR, Grier HE, et al. Randomized Controlled Trial of Interval-Compressed Chemotherapy for the Treatment of Localized Ewing Sarcoma: A Report From the Children's Oncology Group. J Clin Oncol. 2012;30(33):4148-54.

CASE 94

Hodgkin's Disease

■ PRESENTING COMPLAINTS

A 7-year-old girl was brought with the complaint of:
- Swelling in the neck since 6 months
- Fever since 15 days
- Tiredness since 1 week

History of Presenting Complaints

A 7-year-old girl came to the pediatric outpatient department, referred by a general practitioner for evaluation of swelling of the neck. The girl's mother had noticed a small swelling on the left side of her daughter's neck about 6 months back. Then she was taken to their family doctor. The doctor told her that it could be because of the respiratory tract infection and a course of antibiotics was given. But the increasing swelling still persisted. It was gradually size, but the girl did not complain of pain or tenderness at any time. Then again mother took the child to her family doctor. This time he was referred for evaluation at the hospital.

The mother also said that there was a history of fever which was mild to moderate degree. This was not associated with chills and rigor. Fever used to be more in the evening. The mother also gave a history of loss of appetite and loss of weight. The girl also complained of early fatiguability.

CASE AT A GLANCE

Basic Findings
Height	:	118 cm (50th centile)
Weight	:	18 kg (25th centile)
Temperature	:	37°C
Pulse rate	:	100 beats/min
Respiratory rate	:	22 breaths/min
Blood pressure	:	70/60 mm Hg

Positive Findings

History:
- Swelling in the neck
- Anorexia
- Fever
- Weight loss

Examination:
- Poorly built
- Nontender swelling
- Pallor
- Splenomegaly

Investigation:
- *Hb:* Anemia
- *Excision biopsy:* Presence of Reed–Sternberg cells
- *ESR:* Raised

(ESR: erythrocyte sedimentation rate; Hb: hemoglobin)

Past History of the Patient

She was the first child of a consanguineous marriage. She was born at term with normal vaginal delivery. She cried immediately after delivery. She started taking feeds, i.e., breastfeeds immediately, weaning started by the age of 4 months and completed by 1 year. Her developmental milestones were normal. Her performance at school was above average.

EXAMINATION

The girl was moderately built and poorly nourished. She was sitting comfortably on the examination table. There was an anxious look in her eyes. Her anthropometric measurements included, the height was 118 cm (50th centile), and the weight was 18 kg (25th centile).

She was afebrile, the heart rate was 100 beats/min, and the respiratory rate was 22 breaths/min. The blood pressure recorded was 70/60 mm Hg.

She was pale, the swelling was present on the left part of the neck measuring about 3 × 4 cm. The swelling was nontender, rubbery in consistency there was matting. There was no change in the skin. The lymph nodes were discrete and mobile. There was no icterus and no cyanosis.

The per abdomen examination revealed the presence of splenomegaly measuring about 3 cm below the costal margin. There was no hepatomegaly. The cardiovascular and respiratory systems were normal.

INVESTIGATION

- *Hemoglobin:* 9 g/dL
- *TLC:* 8,600 cells/mm^3
- *DLC:* $P_{62}L_{30}E_8$
- *ESR:* 56 mm in the first hour
- *AEC:* 506 cells/cumm
- *Mantoux test:* Negative
- *X-ray chest:* No abnormality detected
- *Excision biopsy:* Presence of Reed-Sternberg (RS) cells

DISCUSSION

A child with a history of painless swelling at the neck, loss of appetite, loss of weight, and presence of splenomegaly along with excision biopsy findings suggests lymphoma.

Hodgkin's disease (HD) is a malignant disorder of the lymphoreticular system. The RS cell represents the malignant cell in HD. It is characterized by progressive enlargement of lymph nodes. The disease is usually considered unicentric in origin. It has a predictable pattern of spread by extension to contiguous nodes. This is one of the lymphoreticular malignancies. It is associated with impaired cellular immunity in the host.

The incidence is highest in late childhood and early adulthood (15–35 years). It is very uncommon to be under 5 years of age and almost never seen under 2 years of age. The sex ratio progresses from one of male preponderance of 10:1 under the age of 7 years falling to 1.1:1 after the age of 12 years.

Infectious agents may be involved, such as human herpesvirus 6, *Cytomegalovirus* (*CMV*), and Epstein–Barr virus (EBV). The role of EBV is supported by prospective serologic studies. Infection with EBV confers a fourfold higher risk of developing Hodgkin's lymphoma (HL) and may precede the diagnosis by years. EBV antigens have been demonstrated in HL tissues, particularly type II latent membrane proteins (LMPs) 1 and 2, although EBV status is not thought to be prognostic of outcome.

Some studies have suggested that elevated copies of EBV by PCR correspond to a worse prognosis. The EBV antigens LMP 1 and 2 have been used as targets for cytotoxic T-lymphocyte (CTL) therapy in patients with relapsed/refractory HL.

Reactive infiltration of eosinophils and a cluster of differentiation 68 (CD68) macrophages and increased concentrations of cytokines, such as interleukin 1 (IL-1) and IL-6 and tumor necrosis factor (TNF), are all associated with an unfavorable prognosis. Other factors associated with a worse prognosis include the advanced stage, the presence of B symptoms, decreased response to therapy, and slow response to therapy.

A genetic predisposition to HL is suggested by the variation in incidence among racial and ethnic groups, familial aggregation of the disease, and association with specific human leukocyte antigens (HLAs). Many investigators have observed concordance of HL in first-degree relatives, including sibling and parent-child pairs. Standardized incidence ratios range from threefold for parent-child pairs to over 50-fold for monozygotic twins. HL also develops more frequently in individuals with congenital or acquired immunodeficiency, leading to the speculation that an inherited subtle immune abnormality may predispose to the development of HL by increasing the risk of malignant transformation induced by environmental factors. Genome-wide association studies have identified HLA and non-HLA susceptibility loci.

Classical HL has a bimodal incidence, with a first peak among adolescents and young adults and another among adults in the seventh to eighth decade of life. The young adult form (ages 15–34 years) shows a predominance of the nodular sclerosing histologic subtype in white adolescents and young adults in developed countries. HL is uncommon among preadolescent children, where it is associated with poorer socioeconomic environments, male sex, EBV infection, and the mixed cellularity (MC) histologic subtype.

Hodgkin's lymphoma is more common in males than in females in all parts of the world. The male predominance is most marked in patients younger than age 10 years. In adolescents, the gender difference in incidence is less conspicuous, particularly for the nodular sclerosing histologic subtype.

■ PATHOLOGY

The normal architecture of the lymph nodes is distorted. Architecture is pleomorphic with a varying number of lymphocytes. Giant cells with a mirror image called RS cells are found. RS can be seen in reactive lymphoid hyperplasia, NHL, and in nonlymphoid malignancies. The lesions are classified histologically as:
- Lymphocyte—predominant (10–20%)
- Nodular sclerosis (NS) (most common type) (40–60%)
- MC (20–40%)
- Lymphocyte—depleted (5–10%)

■ PATHOGENESIS

The RS cell, a pathognomonic feature of HL, is a large cell (15–45 μm in diameter) with multiple or multilobulated nuclei. This cell type is considered the hallmark of HL, although similar cells are seen in infectious mononucleosis, NHL, and other conditions. The RS cell is clonal in origin and arises from the germinal center B cells but typically has lost most B-cell gene expression and function, i.e., malignant transformation. EBV has been linked to HD and suggests EBV activation may contribute to HD.

This typically leads to cell regulation defects such as constitutive activation of the nuclear factor-kB pathway and abnormal regulation of the B-cell leukemia/lymphoma 2 protein (Bcl-2) family of proteins. HL is characterized by a variable number of RS cells surrounded by an inflammatory infiltrate of lymphocytes, plasma cells, and eosinophils in different proportions, depending on the HL histologic subtype. The interaction between the RS cell and these background inflammatory cells with their associated cytokine release is important in the development and progression of HL.

Reactive infiltration of eosinophils and CD68+ macrophages, arid increased concentrations of cytokines, such as IL-1 and 6, and TNF, are all associated with an unfavorable prognosis, including advanced stage, the presence of "B" symptoms (constitutional)—decreased response to therapy, and reduced survival.

■ CLINICAL FEATURES (FIG. 1)

Hodgkin's disease has an insidious onset. The most common presentation (80%) of patients is painless cervical lymphadenopathy, of whom 60% have symptomatic involvement of the mediastinum.

Patients commonly present with painless, nontender, firm, rubbery, cervical or supraclavicular lymphadenopathy and usually some degree of mediastinal involvement. They may be discrete or matted together and are fixed surrounding tissue.

There is a painless enlargement of the lymph node which occurs usually on one side. This progressively involves adjacent nodes. Posterior cervical lymph nodes are easily affected. Initially, auxiliary and anterior mediastinal lymph nodes are involved. The deeper lymph nodes may cause pressure on surrounding structures and produce related symptoms.

Mediastinal compression may cause dysphagia, dyspnea, or brassy cough. Engorgement of the neck veins and hoarseness are due to pressure on the neck veins and recurrent laryngeal nerve. Depending on the extent and location of nodal and extranodal disease, patients may present with symptoms and signs of airway obstruction (dyspnea, hypoxia, and cough), pleural or pericardial effusion, hepatocellular dysfunction, or bone marrow infiltration (anemia, neutropenia, or thrombocytopenia). Uncommon extranodal sites are CNS, bone, gastrointestinal tract (GIT), and skin. A reduced cell-mediated immunity results in an increased susceptibility to infections.

Lymph node biopsy **(Table 1)** indicates a lack of identifiable infection in the region drained by an enlarged node, anode >2 cm in size, supraclavicular adenopathy, or abnormal chest X-ray lymphadenopathy increasing in size after 2 weeks or failing to resolve within 4–8 weeks.

Retroperitoneal lymph nodes may cause abdominal pain, lymph nodes are discrete, mobile, and nontender. Fever, anemia, anorexia, and weight loss develop within a few months after enlargement of lymph nodes.

Hematogenous spread involves the liver, spleen, bone, and bone marrow **(Table 2)**. This will lead to systemic symptoms. Constitutional or class "B" symptoms are more common with advanced disease (stage I: 5%, stage IV: 81%) and are associated with

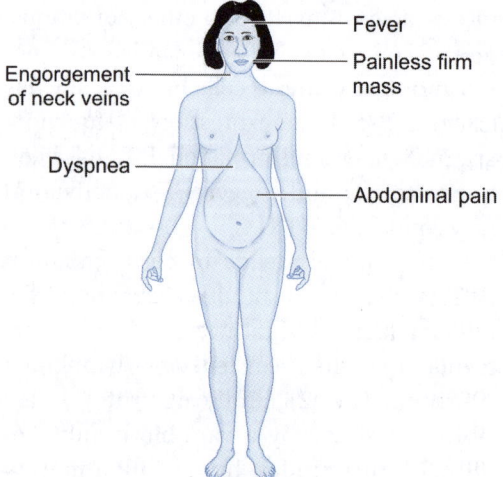

Fig. 1: Clinical features.

TABLE 1: Histopathologic classification of Hodgkin's disease.

Rye	Distinctive features
LP	Benign lymphocytes appearing with or without histiocytes. Few RS cells. No fibrosis
NS	Thickened capsule with proliferation of orderly collagenous bands, that divide lymphoid tissue in nodules: Lacunar variant of RS cells
MC	5–15 RS cells per high power field. Fine fibrosis in the interstitium. Focal necrosis may be present
LD	Abnormal cells with relative paucity of lymphocytes. Fibrosis and necrosis were common but diffuse

(MC: mixed cellularity; NS: nodular sclerosis; LD: lymphocyte depletion; LP: lymphocyte predominant; RS: Reed–Sternberg)

TABLE 2: Modified Ann Arbor classification of Hodgkin's disease.

Stage	Description
I	Involvement of a single lymph node region (I) or of a single extralymphatic or site (IE) by direct extension
II	Involvement of two or more lymph node regions on the same side of the diaphragm or localized involvement of an extralymphatic organ or site and of one or more lymph node regions on the same side of the diaphragm (IIE)
III	• Involvement of lymph node regions on both sides of the diaphragm • Abdominal disease is limited to the upper abdomen (i.e., spleen, splenic hilar nodes, celiac nodes, and portahepatic nodes)
III$_2$	• Involvement of lymph node regions on both sides of the diaphragm • Abdominal disease includes para-aortic, mesenteric, and iliac involvement with or without disease in the upper abdomen
IV	Disseminated involvement of one or more extralymphatic organs or tissues with or without associated lymph node disease
A	No symptoms
B	Fever, night sweats, or weight loss of >10% of body weight in the previous 6 months
X	Bulky disease (>10 cm in maximum dimension; >⅓ of the internal transverse diameter of the thorax at the level T5/T6)
E	Limited involvement of a single extranodal site
CS	*Clinical stage:* When based solely on physical examination and imaging technique
PS	*Pathologic stage:* When based on biopsies

a poorer outcome. Systemic symptoms, (constitutional) classified as "B" symptoms that are considered important in staging, are unexplained fever (100.4°F), weight loss >10% total body weight over 6 months, and drenching night sweats. The type of fever noted in HD is Pel–Ebstein type. There will be regular alteration of recurrent bouts of fever and afebrile state.

Active autoimmune conditions are occasionally coexistent at the time of diagnosis with HL. The most common among these are autoimmune cytopenias: Coombs-positive hemolytic anemia and immune thrombocytopenic purpura (ITP). Both tend to resolve with the initiation of HL-directed therapy. Other abnormalities of the immune system can either predate or present concurrently with a diagnosis of HL, including enhanced sensitivity to suppressor T-lymphocytes and reduction of natural killer cell cytotoxicity, leading to deficient cell-mediated immunity.

Clinical Staging of Hodgkin's Disease

Currently, the clinical staging can be done by CT scan or gallium scan.
- *Stage I:* Lymph nodes in a single anatomic zone are affected.
- *Stage II:* Lymph nodes of two or more contiguous or adjacent regions are involved. All of them are on the same side of the diaphragm.
- *Stage III:* Lymphatic tissues are enlarged on both sides of the diaphragm but are limited to lymph nodes, Waldeyer's ring, and spleen.
- *Stage IV:* Involvement of the visceral organs
- *Stages II and III* are subdivided. Those without constitutional symptoms are denoted by (a), and those associated with constitutional symptoms by (b).

ESSENTIAL DIAGNOSTIC POINTS
- Painless cervical, or supraclavicular adenopathy
- Mediastinal mass in 50%
- Fatigue, anorexia, and weight loss
- Fever, night sweats, pruritus, and cough

GENERAL FEATURES
- Anemia
- Anorexia
- Dysphagia
- Brassy cough
- Nephrotic syndrome

DIAGNOSIS

Evaluation includes history, physical examination, and imaging studies, including chest radiograph; CT scans of the neck, chest, abdomen, and pelvis; and PET scan.

Laboratory abnormalities in HL are nonspecific, usually indicating an inflammatory state, with activation of the reticuloendothelial system and subsequent acute phase reactants. Frequent findings include elevation of the ESR, ferritin, and C-reactive protein, as well as a normocytic anemia of chronic inflammation. Elevations of serum lactate dehydrogenase (LDH) or alkaline phosphatase are less common.

A chest radiograph is particularly important for measuring the size of the mediastinal mass in relation to the maximal diameter of the thorax, the extent of a mediastinal mass if present and identities hilar nodes and pulmonary parenchymal involvement, which may not be evident a chest radiographs.

Computed tomography scan of the chest provides information about pulmonary parenchyma, chest wall, pleura and pericardium that may not be apparent on chest X-ray. CT scan of the abdomen and pelvis is done to examine for involvement of the viscera and lymph nodes. Although lymphangiography is a reliable method for retroperitoneal lymph nodes, it is rarely performed in children. Bone marrow biopsy should be performed in all children with systemic symptoms and in advanced stage (III and IV) disease. A staging laparotomy is not performed because of concerns related to operative morbidity and splenectomy.

Formal excisional biopsy is preferred over needle biopsy to ensure that adequate tissue is obtained, both for light microscopy and for appropriate immunohistochemical and molecular studies. Once the diagnosis of HL is established, the extent of the disease (stage) should be determined to allow the selection of appropriate therapy.

Bone marrow aspiration and biopsy should be performed in patients with advanced disease (stage III/IV), B-symptoms, and bony involvement or abnormal count. Bone scans are performed in patients with bone pain and/or elevation of alkaline phosphatase.

Bone scans are performed in patients with bone pain and/or elevation of alkaline phosphatase. Gallium scan can be particularly helpful in identifying areas of increased uptake, which can then be reevaluated at the end of treatment, fluorodeoxyglucose PET imaging has advantages over gallium scanning, as it is a 1-day procedure with higher resolution, better dosimetry, loss of intestinal activity, and the potential to quantify disease. PET scans are being evaluated as a prognostic tool in HL, enabling therapy to be reduced in those predicted to have a good outcome and identifying those at risk of relapse.

Positron emission tomography scan of the whole body: PET scanning may identify more sites of initial disease than conventional imaging and is more accurate in detecting viable HL in post-therapy residual masses. Rapid early response documented by a significant reduction in disease volume and PET negativity at an early stage (after one or two cycles of chemotherapy) is associated with a favorable outcome. PET scanning should be performed at baseline and a minimum of 3 weeks postchemotherapy completion and 8–12 weeks postradiation.

A definitive diagnosis of HL can be made only by histologic confirmation. Most frequently this is achieved with an excisional lymph node biopsy. Noninvasive needle biopsies are typically insufficient, as they do not provide material adequate to view the malignant cells, the Hodgkin and Reed–Sternberg (HRS) cells, within the context of surrounding stromal cells and nodal architecture.

Hodgkin and Reed–Sternberg cells are thought to derive from germinal center B cells that have lost their mature B-cell features, including expression of the mature B-cell marker cluster of differentiate 20 (CD20). Instead, a cluster of differentiate 30 (CD30), a TNF family member and transmembrane receptor, is present. One of the more frequent genetic changes in classical Hodgkin lymphoma (CHL) is an amplification of the 9p24.1 locus, leading to over-expression of the tyrosine kinase Janus kinase 2 (JAK2).

> **LABORATORY SALIENT FINDINGS**
> - ESR and acute phase reactants are elevated
> - *Autoantibody phenomena:* Hemolytic anemia and idiopathic thrombocytopenic purpura
> - Histological examination of lymph node
> - Bone marrow examination
> - Radiograph of chest
> - Lymphangiography and ultrasound scanning
> - CT scan of chest, abdomen, and pelvis
>
> (CT: computed tomography; ESR: erythrocyte sedimentation rate)

■ DIFFERENTIAL DIAGNOSIS

- Non-Hodgkin disease
- Lymphoblastic leukemia
- Tuberculosis

■ MANAGEMENT (TABLE 3)

Treatment is determined largely by disease stage, presence or absence of B symptoms, and the presence of bulky nodal disease. To achieve long-term disease-free survival while minimizing treatment toxicity, HD is increasingly treated by chemotherapy alone- and less often by radiation therapy.

TABLE 3: Treatment modalities and results in Hodgkin's disease.

Stage	Treatment modality	Survival deficits%
I, II	Involved field RT + MOPP or COPP/ABVD three to four cycles	96–98
III, IV	Involved field RT+MOPP or COPP/ABVD six cycles	70–75

(ABVD: adriamycin, bleomycin, vinblastine, dacarbazine; COPP: cyclophosphamide, vincristine, procarbazine and prednisolone; MOPP: mechlorethamine, vincristine, procarbazine, and prednisolone; RT: radiotherapy)

Most children are treated with combination chemotherapy alone or in combination with RT.

Radiation therapy alone, once given at higher doses, initially resulted in prolonged remission and cure rates in patients with low-stage HL. However, this treatment also caused significant long-term morbidity in pediatric patients, including growth retardation, thyroid dysfunction, and cardiac and pulmonary toxicity.

The development of effective multiagent combination chemotherapy was a major milestone in the treatment of HL resulting in a complete response rate of 70–80% and a cure rate of 40–50% in patients with advanced-stage disease.

Agents such as those that disrupt the nuclear factor kappa B (NF-κB) pathway and monoclonal antibodies (mAbs) that target RS tumor cells, as well as the benign reactive cells that surround them, are currently being investigated. Ongoing clinical trials report encouraging results with anti-CD20 antibody (rituximab), particularly in nodular lymphocyte-predominant HL, for which trials in relapsed disease have shown an overall response rate of 94%. In addition, anti-CD30 agents are being used that are targeted to the RS cells themselves, where CD30 is abundantly expressed. Brentuximab vedotin is an antibody-drug conjugate approved to treat HL.

Both brentuximab and rituximab have been combined with combination chemotherapy either alone or together in newly diagnosed patients, allowing for the elimination of toxic alkylator agents, topoisomerase inhibitors, bleomycin, and radiation in these patients. EBV-specific CTLs can also be generated from allogeneic donors for patients with advanced HL.

Management is largely determined by disease stage, patient's age, and presence of bulky nodal disease. The RT includes 3,500–4,500 cGy. The adverse reaction may be growth retardation, thyroid failure, and cardiac and pulmonary dysfunction.

Treatment in the pediatric population is different in certain respects from adults. As HD is treated with curative intention, growth, and development are important issues in pediatric protocols.

Principles of Radiotherapy

Radiotherapy has historically been an essential component of HL therapy. Whereas RT is routinely incorporated into the treatment plan for adults with early-stage disease who are treated with ABVD (adriamycin, bleomycin, vinblastine, dacarbazine) chemotherapy. Pediatric regimens omit RT for rapid or complete responders or utilize reduced RT dose and or volume strategies. The risk of radiation-induced secondary cancers, cardiovascular disease, and thyroid dysfunction throughout life is the primary driver of the different approaches for pediatric HL.

- Low dose involved field radiation with combination chemotherapy in growing children.

- For adolescents and fully grown patients with localized disease, high-dose extended-field RT alone remains the standard treatment.
- Transposition of ovaries to midline and midline pelvic block to protect ovarian function. Testicular shield or sperm banking in male children.
- High-dose radiation therapy should be avoided in young children because of late complications such as diminished growth of soft tissue and bone, hypothyroidism, gonadal dysfunction, and secondary malignancies.
- The RT includes 15–25 Gy. The adverse reaction may be growth retardation, thyroid failure, cardiac and pulmonary dysfunction.

Chemotherapy

Chemotherapy agents commonly used to treat children and adolescents with HL include cyclophosphamide, procarbazine, vincristine or vinblastine, prednisone or dexamethasone, doxorubicin, bleomycin, dacarbazine, etoposide, methotrexate (MTX), and cytosine arabinoside.

Superior efficacy and absence of significant toxicity have made ABVD the preferred regimen for HL.

The recommended chemotherapy includes:
- MOPP (nitrogen mustard, vincristine, prednisolone, and procarbazine)
- ABVD
- High doses of anthracyclines and bleomycin should be avoided to reduce cardiopulmonary toxicity and alkalizing agents because of gonadal toxicity.

Early response to chemotherapy is currently being studied as a means of further refining therapy planning: Directing those with an inadequate response toward more intensive therapy and reducing therapy for those with a rapid early response. Clinical trials by the Children's Oncology Group, for example, have demonstrated that RT can be safely omitted for those with an adequate response to chemotherapy. Fluorodeoxyglucose PET has become an established technique for assessing response to treatment by detecting metabolic activity and distinguishing between residual disease and necrosis or fibrosis. It is important to emphasize that interim PET CT has not been validated as a predictive endpoint and its use in this setting remains investigational. Reduction in tumor mass as measured by 2-dimensional area or volume on CT, or in total metabolic volume on PET may add predictive value over PET alone.

In Stage I, II, and IIIA

Four cycles of MOPP or ABVD are given every 28 days. Again, the patient should be clinically staged, if the patient has responded then two more cycles of ABVD should be given with the standard dose of radiation therapy to the area involved, i.e., 4,000 rds.

Stages IIB, IIIB, and IV

Six to eight total courses of MOPP alternating with ABVD are given every 28 days. 6 weeks after the completion of chemotherapy all patients should be given radiation therapy to bulk disease.

Relapse

Most relapses occur within the first 3 years after diagnosis, but relapses as late as 10 years have been reported. Relapse cannot be predicted accurately with this disease. Poor prognostic features include tumor bulk, stage at diagnosis, extralymphatic disease, and presence of B symptoms Patients who achieve an initial chemosensitive response but relapse or progress <12 months from diagnosis are candidates for myeloablative chemotherapy and autologous stem cell transplantation with or without the addition of radiation therapy.

Most recurrences of HL occur within 3 years after initial diagnosis, although some patients may relapse as long as 10 years after initial diagnosis. Treatment and ultimate prognosis depend on initial staging and treatment, time to relapse, extent of disease at relapse, and presence of B symptoms at relapse.

Patients with lower-risk relapses (e.g., those with late relapse of low-stage disease) may be cured with salvage chemotherapy, with or without consolidative RT. Those with primary refractory disease or very early progression (<3 months from the end of primary therapy) tend not to respond to conventional salvage therapy and have a poor prognosis for long-term disease-free survival (30–55%). For those with higher-risk relapses or primary refractory disease who can achieve complete remission with chemotherapy, a consolidation with myeloablative therapy followed by autologous stem cell rescue improves disease-free survival over chemotherapy alone.

Multiple salvage regimens have been used in this context, including ICE (ifosfamide, carboplatin, and etoposide), IV (ifosfamide and vinorelbine), MIED (high dose MTX, ifosfamide, etoposide, and dexamethasone), and GV (gemcitabine and vinorelbine). Although these regimens have never been compared head-to-head, all have similar overall response rates. As with initial therapy, clinicians must weigh treatment intensity against toxicity, often choosing to start with the least toxic regimen and advancing to more aggressive regimens if the initial response is inadequate.

Reduced intensity or nonmyeloablative allogeneic hematopoietic stem cell transplantation (HSCT) is under evaluation as a retrieval therapy for children with recurrent/refractory disease after autologous HSCT. Nonmyeloablative conditioning regimens most often use a nontoxic. immunosuppression with the goal of establishing a graft versus-lymphoma effect that provides a platform for adoptive cellulitis.

Treatment of relapse includes stem cell transplantation. Other novel approaches include iodine-131 (^{131}I) labeled antibody directed against ferritin and radionucleotide yttrium.

- *Cyclophosphamide:* 400 mg/m^2 orally from day 1 to day 5
- *Procarbazine:* 100 mg/m^2 orally from day 1 to day 14
- *Vincristine:* 1.4 mg/m^2 intravenously daily on day 1 and day 8
- *Vinblastine:* 0.1–0.15 mg/kg from daily on day 1 and day 8
- *Prednisolone:* 40 mg/m^2 orally from day 1 to day 14
- *Nitrogen mustard:* 0.4 mg/kg for 5 days
- *Adriamycin:* 25 mg/m^2 IV daily 1 and 15

PROGNOSTIC FACTORS

Poor prognostic features include tumor bulk, stage at diagnosis, extralymphatic disease, and the presence of B symptoms.
- Stage of the disease
- *Histopathological subtype:* Risk increase from lymphocyte predominant (LP) to NS, MC to lymphocyte depletion (LD)

- Presence of "B" symptoms
- Bulky mediastinal disease
- Extensive splenic involvement
- >5 nodal sites in stage III

LATE EFFECTS

- Hypothyroidism following RT to the neck
- Subfertility in males with alkylating agents
- Premature ovarian dysfunction with the use of alkylating agents
- Adverse cardiac events following anthracycline-based regimens with/without mediastinal RT.
- Pulmonary dysfunction with bleomycin
- Second malignant neoplasm

BIBLIOGRAPHY

1. Freed J, Kelly KM. Current approaches to the management of pediatric Hodgkin lymphoma. Paediatr Drugs. 2010;12(2):85-98.
2. Friedman DL, Chen L, Wolden S, Buxton A, McCarten K, FitzGerald TJ, et al. Dose-intensive response-based chemotherapy and radiation therapy for children and adolescents with newly diagnosed intermediate-risk hodgkin lymphoma: a report from the Children's Oncology Group Study AHOD0031. J Clin Oncol. 2014;32(32):3561-8.
3. Jachimowic RD, Engert A. The challenging aspects of managing adolescents and young adults with Hodgkin's lymphoma. Act Haematol. 2014;132(3-4):274-8.

CASE 95

Leukemia

■ PRESENTING COMPLAINTS

An 8-year-old girl was brought with the complaint of:
- Tiredness since 2 months
- Not taking food properly since 2 months
- Loss of weight since 1 month

History of Presenting Complaints

A girl aged about 8 years was brought to the hospital with a history of not doing well with health and tiredness. Her mother noted that her daughter was not taking food properly. She noticed her daughter used to be lethargic and irritable. She also found that there should be loss of weight since the last 2 months. She used to sit in one place and never used to play along with her friends.

Past History of the Patient

The girl was the first sibling of a nonconsanguineous marriage. She was born at full term by normal vaginal delivery. The birth weight of the child was 3 kg. There was no significant postnatal event. The child was on breast milk exclusively for 6 months. Weaning started later and the child was on family food by 1 year. Her developmental milestones were normal. Her performance at school was average.

CASE AT A GLANCE

Basic Findings
Height	: 124 cm (50th centile)
Weight	: 16 kg (below 10th centile)
Temperature	: 37°C
Pulse rate	: 110 beats/min
Respiratory rate	: 22 breaths/min
Blood pressure	: 100/70 mm Hg

Positive Findings

History:
- Tiredness
- Loss of weight
- Lethargy

Examination:
- Pallor
- Splenomegaly
- Sternal tenderness
- Endothelial cell specific molecule (ESM)
- Retinal hemorrhage

Investigation:
- Anemia
- *Peripheral blood smear:* Presence of blast cells
- *Bone marrow:* Blast cells
- *X-ray of hand:* Osteolytic lesions

■ EXAMINATION

She was moderately built and moderately nourished. She was looking very much pale. She was not interested in her surroundings. Her anthropometric measurements included, the height was 124 cm (50th centile), and the weight was 16 kg (below 10th centile).

CASE 95: Leukemia

The girl was afebrile, the pulse rate was 110 beats/min, and the respiratory rate was 22 breaths/min. The blood pressure recorded was 100/70 mm Hg. There was pallor, no edema, and no lymphadenopathy.

Bony tenderness was present on the left hand and sternal tenderness was present. Per abdomen examination revealed the presence of splenomegaly. The spleen was palpable about 2 cm below the costal margin. It was nontender and a splenic notch was felt. There was no hepatomegaly.

■ INVESTIGATION

- *Hemoglobin:* 6.2 g/dL
- *TLC:* 100,000 cells/mm^3
- *Differential leukocyte count (DLC):* $P_{68}L_{25}E_2M_1$
- *ESR:* 30 mm in the first hour
- *Platelet count:* 200,000 cells/mm^3
- *Peripheral blood smear:* Revealed pressure of blast cells
- *Bone marrow examination:* Showed the presence of blast cells
- *X-ray of the hand:* Osteolytic lesion in the humerus

■ DISCUSSION

An 8-year-old girl with a history of tiredness, generalized weakness, bony tenderness, pallor, and splenomegaly was investigated. The investigation revealed leukemia. The diagnosis is supported by bony tenderness, presence of blast cells in the peripheral blood smear. Bone marrow examination revealed blast cells in the marrow.

Leukemia is the most common form of childhood malignancy. 95% of leukemia cases are of acute variety. Acute lymphatic leukemia (ALL) appears to be a heterogeneous disorder. There is uninhibited proliferation of lymphoblasts in bone marrow which invade blood and viscera. Acute myeloid leukemia (AML) accounts for about 10–15% of childhood leukemias. The remaining subset consists of uncommon childhood leukemias viz., chronic myeloid leukemia (CML) and juvenile myelomonocytic leukemia (JMML).

Leukemias may be defined as a group of malignant diseases in which genetic abnormalities in a hematopoietic cell give rise to an unregulated clonal proliferation of cells. The progeny of these cells has a growth advantage over normal cellular elements, because of their increased rate of proliferation and a decreased rate of spontaneous apoptosis. The result is a disruption of normal marrow function and ultimately, marrow failure. The clinical features, laboratory findings, and responses to therapy vary depending on the type of leukemia.

The diagnosis of ALL is often initially suspected by the presence of circulating blasts in the peripheral blood that often occur in the setting of concomitant anemia and thrombocytopenia. Leukemia cells may also infiltrate extramedullary sites (e.g., CNS, testes, lymphatic system, and solid organs). Patients with extramedullary lymphoid masses, but <25% blasts in the bone marrow, are considered to have lymphoblastic lymphoma. ALL may arise from precursor B cells (B-ALL) or T cells (T-ALL).

The incidence of childhood ALL peaks between 2 and 3 years of age and is slightly more common in males than females. The incidence of leukemia is substantially higher in white children compared to black children, with the highest rates in children of Hispanic ethnicity. With the exception of Down syndrome and rare familial leukemia predisposition syndromes, causal factors of childhood ALL remain largely unknown. Various environmental factors (e.g., viral infections, parental smoking living near power lines) are potentially associated with increased risk of childhood ALL, although definitive associations have not been proven.

Exposure to very high doses of ionizing radiation, chemicals such as benzene, and certain chemotherapies have been associated with an increased risk of AML, but not ALL.

In clinical practice, the course and prognosis of ALL are related to the type of cells involved in the leukemia process.

In virtually all cases, the etiology of ALL is unknown, although several genetic and environmental factors are associated with childhood leukemia. Most cases of ALL are thought to be caused by postconception somatic mutations in lymphoid cells. However, the identification of the leukemia-specific fusion-gene sequences in archived neonatal blood spots of some children who develop ALL at a later date indicates the importance of in utero events in the initiation of the malignant process in some cases.

Although the etiology of acute leukemia is unknown, several genetic conditions and environmental agents are known to be associated with childhood leukemia. Certain inherited conditions such as Down syndrome (trisomy 21), Fanconi's syndrome, Bloom syndrome, Schwachman syndrome, Klinefelter syndrome, Turner's syndrome (45,XO), neurofibromatosis, ataxia telangiectasia, severe combined immunodeficiency, and Li–Fraumeni syndrome (p53 deletion) are known to predispose to leukemia. Ionizing radiation, exposure to benzene, and certain drugs such as alkylating agents and epipodophyllotoxins have been incriminated in the pathogenesis of acute leukemias.

Congenital leukemia **(Fig. 1)** is very rare. It is diagnosed at birth or within one of life. At birth they have respiratory distress, fever, hepatomegaly, loose motion and petiche.

It is characterized by malignant, clonal proliferation of cell precursors, i.e. blast cells. These cells will occupy and inhibit the function of bone marrow. They may circulate in blood forming leukemia deposits in any tissue.

In ALL blast cell morphology resembles precursor and lymphoid cells. In AML, the malignant cells resemble myeloid precursors.

Morphology

Morphology is usually adequate alone to establish a diagnosis, but the other studies are essential for disease classification, which can have a major influence on the prognosis and the choice of appropriate therapy. The rare leukemia of mature B cells is termed Burkitt leukemia and is one of the most rapidly growing cancers in humans, requiring a different therapeutic approach than other subtypes of ALL.

The PCR and FISH techniques offer the ability to pinpoint molecular genetic abnormalities and can be used to detect small numbers of malignant cells at diagnosis as well as during follow-up [minimal residual disease (MRD)].

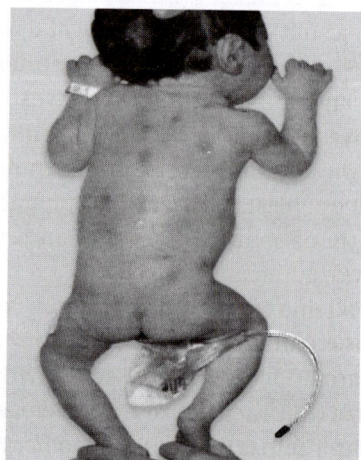

Fig. 1: Congenital leukemia.
(For color version, see Plate 11)

Typing of leukemia requires an adequate number of blast cell samples for cytogenetic studies. It should be done urgently when there are no symptoms and signs of raised intracranial tension. The diagnostic cerebrospinal fluid (CSF) is collected and if the pleocytosis is present, it indicates CNS involvement. If there are signs of raised intracranial tension, then a CT scan is advised.

Other rare sites of extramedullary involvement include the heart, lungs, kidneys, ovaries, skin, eye, or GIT.

Acute Lymphoblastic Leukemia

Factors predisposed to childhood leukemia are discussed further.

Genetic Conditions

- Down syndrome
- Fanconi anemia
- Bloom syndrome
- Diamond–Blackfan anemia
- Shwachman–Diamond syndrome
- Neurofibromatosis type 1
- Ataxia telangiectasia
- Severe combined immune deficiency
- Paroxysmal nocturnal hemoglobinuria

Environmental Factors

- Ionizing radiation
- Drugs
- Alkylating agents
- Epipodophyllotoxin
- Benzene exposure

In certain developing countries, there is an association between B-cell ALL (B-ALL) and Epstein–Barr viral infections.

The classification of ALL has evolved from one, which was based predominantly on morphology to one, which is based on immunophenotyping, karyotyping, and molecular biology techniques. For ALL, the results of immunophenotyping are used to classify leukemia as either B-cell derived, or T-cell derived. The morphologic classification (the French-American-British (FAB) classification) is still used by many centers, due to its ease and familiarity. It classifies the blasts as L1, L2, and L3 depending on the cell size, amount of cytoplasm, and the presence of nucleoli and vacuoles.

Progenitor B-cell-derived ALL constitutes 80–85% of childhood ALL. 15% are derived from T-cells and 1–2% from mature B-cells. Certain chromosomal abnormalities are associated with a favorable prognosis viz., t(12;21) and simultaneous presence of trisomy 4 and 10. Others such as t(4;11) and the Philadelphia chromosome (9;22) and t(8;14) cannot have a poor prognosis. In general, patients with hyperdiploidy (DNA index >1.16) fare better than those with hypodiploidy.

For AML, the FAB classification is widely used. However, the new classification is now gaining acceptance. According to this classification, the presence of >20% blasts in the bone marrow is diagnostic of acute leukemia.

The presence of t(8;21), trisomy 8, and t(15;17) is associated with favorable prognosis whereas del (7) and t(4;11) are poor prognostic chromosomal abnormalities.

■ CLINICAL FEATURES (FIG. 2)

Most of the clinical features are related to the proliferation of lymphoblasts, and displacement of erythrocytes, granulocytes, and thrombocytes from the marrow, causing anemia, neutropenia, and thrombocytopenia. This explains most of the clinical features of leukemia. Leukemia cells invade tissues. Immunological functions are impaired and hence these children are prone to infections.

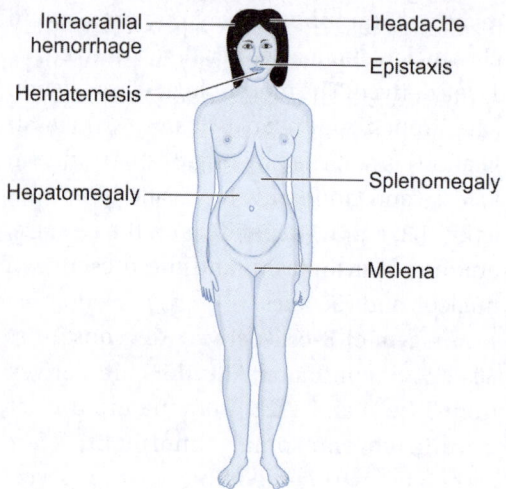

Fig. 2: Clinical features.

Clinical features of acute leukemia are related to the decrease in the normal cells in the bone marrow viz., red blood cells (RBCs), WBCs, and platelets, as well as the leukemic cell infiltration of various organs (extramedullary outside bone marrow) sites. The average duration of symptoms before diagnosis varies from 1 to 2 weeks to 1 to 2 months.

Initial symptoms may be vague, such as anorexia, fatigability, and low-grade fever. Intermittent fever occurs as a result of cytokine induced by leukemia itself or infections secondary leukopenia. Bone pain is severe and can wake the patient at night. Bone pain is seen especially in the pelvis, vertebral, and legs. As the disease progresses, signs and symptoms of bone marrow failure become more obvious with the occurrence of pallor, fatigue, exercise intolerance, bruising, or epistaxis, as well as fever, which may be caused by infection or the disease.

In many cases of childhood ALL, production of the various types of blood cells other than lymphocytes is seriously impaired. Children may present with decreased hemoglobin and hematocrit (anemia), manifesting as pallor or fatigue. Decreased platelets (thrombocytopenia) can lead to bruising and spontaneous bleeding. Low white blood cell (WBC) counts can lead to serious bacterial, fungal, or viral infections manifesting with fever, particularly in the context of prolonged neutropenia or lymphopenia.

The triad of fever, pallor, and bruising is a common presentation of ALL, particularly in younger children. Some children also initially present with bone pain or refusal to walk due to leukemic infiltration of the bone marrow. Many patients with ALL presents with palpable lymphadenopathy, hepatomegaly, or splenomegaly due to infiltration of organs by leukemic blasts.

Children and adolescents with ALL less commonly present with respiratory compromise due to the presence of a large anterior mediastinal mass, which is more common in patients with T-ALL. Large mediastinal masses causing respiratory distress are considered a medical emergency and often require immediate intervention. The presence of lytic bone lesions diagnosed by radiography or MRI is another rare presentation of ALL. Prior to performing a biopsy of a lytic bone lesion, a complete blood count and a careful review of the peripheral blood smear should be performed.

Organ infiltration can cause lymphadenopathy, hepatosplenomegaly, testicular enlargement, or CNS involvement (cranial neuropathies, headaches, and seizures). Respiratory distress may be due to severe anemia or mediastinal node compression of the airways.

On physical examination, patients are usually pale with evidence of petechiae, purpura, or ecchymosis.

Generalized lymphadenopathy is common either localized or generalized to cervical, axillary, and inguinal regions and hepatosplenomegaly is present in 60% of patients with high tumor burden. Findings of pallor, listlessness, purpuric and petechial skin lesions, or mucous membrane hemorrhage can reflect bone marrow failure. The proliferative nature of the disease may be manifested as lymphadenopathy, splenomegaly, or, less commonly, hepatomegaly.

In patients with bone or joint pain, there may be exquisite tenderness over the bone or objective evidence of joint swelling and effusion. Nonetheless, with marrow involvement, deep bone pain may be present, but tenderness will not be elicited.

Chloroma **(Figs. 3A and B)** is extramedullary myeloblastoma and is associated with myeloblastic leukemia.

Rarely, patients show signs of increased intracranial pressure that indicates leukemic involvement of the CNS. These include papilledema, retinal hemorrhages, and cranial nerve palsies.

Respiratory distress usually is related to anemia but can occur in patients with an obstructive airway problem (wheezing) as the result of a large anterior mediastinal mass (e.g., in the thymus or nodes). Tachypnea and respiratory distress may be present secondary to severe anemia leading to congestive cardiac failure or secondary to the presence of a mediastinal mass leading to tracheal compression. A large mediastinal mass may also cause superior vena cava syndrome with facial edema and plethora, throbbing headache, conjunctival congestion, and dilated neck veins. This problem is most typically seen in adolescent boys with T-cell ALL (T-ALL), T-ALL also usually has a higher leukocyte count.

B-lymphoblastic leukemia is the most common immunophenotype, with onset at 1–10 years of age. Testicular involvement is rarely evident at diagnosis, but prior studies indicate occult involvement in 25% of boys. There is no indication for testicular biopsy.

Bleeding tendencies such as easy bruising, gum bleeding, epistaxis or petechiae, and ecchymosis are common. Fever may be due to an infection such as otitis media, pneumonitis, and an abscess, or due to leukemia itself. Oral ulcers or thrush may be present at diagnosis. Bone and joint pains and occasionally joint swelling are common symptoms.

The course of illness is rapid. Early symptoms are nonspecific, such as anorexia,

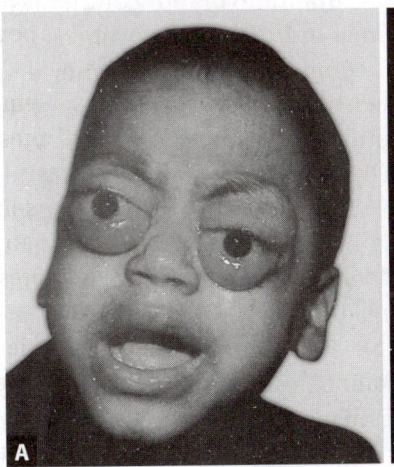 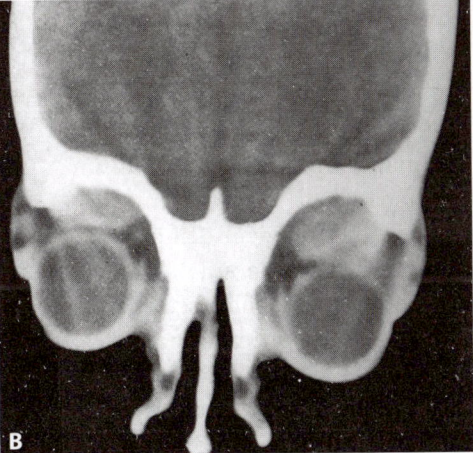

Figs. 3A and B: Chloroma. *(For color version, see Plate 11)*

irritability, and lethargy. The child becomes markedly pale and cardiac dilatation produces a hemic murmur. Hemorrhage manifestation includes epistaxis, hematemesis, melena, and intracranial bleeds. Sternal tenderness and bony pain are present. The spleen is moderately enlarged. Hepatosplenomegaly and lymphadenopathy are less marked. Because of neutropenia, phagocytosis is diminished and hence patients become more vulnerable to infection and fever. Invasion of the meninges and CNS produces symptoms of headache, vomiting, and neck rigidity. Papilledema is also encountered.

At the time of diagnosis, a child with acute leukemia is often ill. This may be because of bone marrow failure, anemia, infection, or bleeding. Leukemia may present as an acute emergency with life-threatening complications such as infection, hemorrhage, organ dysfunction secondary to leukocytes, and signs and symptoms of superior vena cava syndrome caused by mediastinal adenopathy compressing superior vena cava.

Patients with high tumor burden can occasionally present in tumor lysis syndrome with decreased urine output and azotemia secondary to uric acid nephropathy. They may have metabolic disturbances due to tumor lysis syndrome. Deposition of leukemia cells in organs or body cavities can lead to disturbances of organ functions such as superior vena cava obstruction, pleural effusion, cardiac tamponade, ascitic effusion, and renal, hepatic, or splenic infiltration. They may have neurological disturbances, secondary to either intracranial bleeding, tumor deposition, or metabolic disturbances.

About 5–10% of patients have CNS involvement at diagnosis and present with headaches or cranial nerve palsies and nuchal rigidity. It may be associated with papilledema and other signs of raised intracranial pressure. Testes may either unilaterally or bilaterally enlarge secondary leukemic infiltration. Testicular involvement at diagnosis is extremely rare but can be present, usually with painless testicular enlargement.

Patients with AML are more likely to present with bleeding manifestations. Acute promyelocytic leukemia (APML, i.e., AML-M3) case presents with disseminated intravascular coagulation (DIC) due to the release of thromboplastin from the promyelocytic granules. Gum hypertrophy and skin deposits (leukemia cutis) are characteristic of AML M4/M5. Rarely patients may present with a soft tissue mass (an extramedullary myeloid cell tumor) and this may precede leukemia in the bone marrow by several weeks.

GENERAL FEATURES
• Anorexia • Irritability • Lethargy • Pallor • Neutropenia

DIAGNOSIS

The complete blood count may reveal anemia and/or thrombocytopenia. The white cell count may be increased or decreased; in either case, it is characterized by neutropenia. Hyperleukocytosis (WBC count >100,000/mm^3]) is more commonly seen in ALL than AML. The peripheral blood smear may or may not reveal blasts. Often, they may be reported as atypical lymphocytes or immature cells. Coagulopathy may be present with elevated prothrombin time (PT), partial thromboplastin time (PTT), and fibrinogen degradation products (FDPs).

The diagnosis of leukemia is established by bone marrow aspiration. The presence of 25% blasts confirms the diagnosis of ALL (20% in the case of AML). Rarely in the case of dry tap, bone marrow biopsy may be needed.

In patients with high WBC, there may be elevation of uric acid and LDH. Tumor lysis syndrome is characterized by elevated potassium, phosphorus, uric acid, and depressed calcium. In severe cases, renal function may be compromised with elevation of blood urea nitrogen and creatinine. Elevated transaminases and hyperbilirubinemia may occasionally be present in cases of extensive liver involvement.

Indications for Bone Marrow Examination

- Presentation suggestive of leukemia/aplastic anemia
- Sick child
- Persistent thrombocytopenia beyond 6 months
- Presence of generalized lymphadenopathy or bony tenderness
- Anemia disproportionate to the severity of bleeding
- Presence of weight loss
- Before starting corticosteroids.

The diagnosis of ALL is strongly suggested by peripheral blood findings that indicate bone marrow failure. Anemia and thrombocytopenia are seen in most patients. The WBC count may be elevated or depressed, in either case, it is characterized by neutropenia. Blasts may or may not be present in the peripheral blood as may be reported as atypical lymphocytes. Leukemic cells might not be reported in the peripheral blood in routine laboratory examinations. Many patients with ALL presents with TLCs of <10,000/μL. In such cases, the leukemic cells often are reported initially to be atypical lymphocytes, and it is only on further evaluation that the cells are found to be part of a malignant clone.

When the results of an analysis of peripheral blood suggest the possibility of leukemia, the bone marrow should be examined promptly to establish the diagnosis. It is important that all studies necessary to confirm a diagnosis and adequately classify the type of leukemia be performed, including bone marrow aspiration and biopsy, flow cytometry, cytogenetics, and molecular studies.

ALL is diagnosed by a bone marrow evaluation that demonstrates >25% of the bone marrow cells as a homogeneous population of lymphoblasts. Bone marrow aspiration smears confirm the diagnosis when >30% blasts are present [>20% for AML by the World Health Organization (WHO) classification).

Initial evaluation also includes CSF analysis, including cytology is necessary for staging. If lymphoblasts are found and the CSF leukocyte count is elevated, overt CNS or meningeal leukemia is present. This finding reflects a worse stage and indicates the need for additional CNS and systemic therapies.

Morphology along with cytochemistry can accurately diagnose about 80% of acute leukemias. Immunophenotyping is useful for further subtyping according to the lineage and for tailoring treatment and for prognostication. Rarely a bone marrow biopsy is necessary for adequate tissue to rule out other causes.

Biochemical evaluation including liver and renal function tests, serum LDH, uric acid, electrolytes, and calcium, phosphorus, and magnesium levels should be performed to establish baseline organ function and to rule out tumor lysis syndrome.

Serology for human immunodeficiency virus (HIV), hepatitis B and C, and EBV and

CMV should be performed at diagnosis. Coagulation profile with PT, PTT, fibrinogen level, and FDP should be done to rule out DIC.

Chest X-ray may reveal a mediastinal mass, more often, in T-cell ALL, hepatosplenomegaly, and occasionally nephromegaly may be documented by sonography.

> **LABORATORY SALIENT FINDINGS**
>
> - Anemia, neutropenia, and thrombocytopenia
> - *Peripheral blood smear:* Elevated lymphoblasts, tear drop RBCs, decreased platelet counts
> - Decreased hemoglobin
> - Uric acid and LDH are elevated
> - *Bone marrow examination:* Leukemic blast cells
> - Chest X-ray
> - Abdominal ultrasonography
> - Plain X-ray of long bones
>
> (LDH: lactate dehydrogenase; RBCs: red blood cells)

The staging lumbar puncture (LP) may be performed in conjunction with the first dose of intrathecal chemotherapy if the diagnosis of leukemia was previously established from bone marrow evaluation. An experienced proceduralist should perform the initial LP because a traumatic LP is associated with an increased risk of CNS relapse.

■ DIFFERENTIAL DIAGNOSIS

- Idiopathic thrombocytopenic purpura
- Scurvy
- Rheumatoid arthritis
- Lymphoma
- Histiocytosis

The differential diagnosis of ALL several benign and malignant conditions, Viral infection-induced cytopenias are the most common conditions, which mimic leukemia, Infectious mononucleosis, CMV infection and a host of other viral infections may present with fever and lymphadenopathy along with anemia, thrombocytopenia, and/or neutropenia with atypical lymphocytosis.

Immune thrombocytopenia presents with sudden onset of thrombocytopenia with petechiae, purpura, and ecchymosis, in an otherwise well child. The presence of atypical features such as fever, lymphadenopathy, and anemia may warrant a bone marrow examination to rule out leukemia.

Drug-induced cytopenias can be suspected by a detailed history, and withdrawal of the offending drug usually leads to recovery of the concerned cell lines. Bone marrow failure syndromes, myelodysplastic syndromes, and hypoplastic/aplastic anemia usually have a long-standing history and need a bone marrow biopsy for confirmation. Some collagen vascular disorders such as rheumatoid arthritis and systemic lupus erythematosus can present with symptoms of leukemia, Langerhans cell histiocytosis with or without marrow involvement is another common differential.

Malignant conditions that mimic acute leukemia include metastases from solid tumors such as neuroblastoma and rhabdomyosarcoma and marrow involvement in NHL.

The differential diagnosis of acute leukemia includes other hematologic malignancies such as CML, JMML, CML in blast crisis, and lymphoma evolving to the leukemic phase. Bone marrow failure is secondary to marrow infiltration by metastatic deposits in neuroblastoma, rhabdomyosarcoma, and EWS can occasionally mimic acute leukemia.

■ PROGNOSTIC FACTORS

The combination of age and WBC is currently used for initial risk group allocation in patients with B-ALL. Standard risk B-ALL is defined as age >1 and <10 years and a WBC of <50,000/µL, while high-risk B-ALL is defined as age 2–10 years and/or initial WBC 50,000/µL. Children with CNS positivity

(CNS-3) are also generally considered high risk. Hepatosplenomegaly and other extramedullary involvement at diagnosis have no independent prognostic significance. CNS involvement of leukemia is a less favorable prognostic factor, and testicular involvement with leukemia in males is also considered high risk.

■ TREATMENT

Modern treatment for childhood ALL consists of multiagent chemotherapy administered in several phases: induction, consolidation, intensification, and maintenance phases of therapy. The induction phase of treatment generally lasts 1 month, and over 95% of children achieve a remission at the end of this phase. The next phases of treatment (consolidation and intensification) are designed to intensify systemic and CNS-directed therapy to eradicate any residual disease. The final and longest phase of treatment (maintenance) is designed to prevent disease recurrence. In general, treatment is 2-3 years in duration. Some earlier ALL studies treated boys for longer than girls because the male gender was associated with inferior outcomes.

The management of acute leukemia is intense and prolonged. It needs the combined efforts of the pediatric oncologist, the radiotherapist, the dietician, the psychologist, and the medical social workers to treat these children.

Treatment of Acute Lymphatic Leukemia

Chemotherapy

It consists of induction of remission and consolidation to attain disease control. Maintenance treatment is to avoid the recurrence of leukemia in the bone marrow and CNS prophylaxis.

Induction of Remission

Initial therapy, termed *remission induction*, is designed to eradicate leukemic cells from the bone marrow. During this phase, therapy is given for 4 weeks and consists of vincristine weekly a corticosteroid such as dexamethasone and prednisone, and usually a single dose of a long-acting, pegylated asparaginase preparation. Patients at higher risk also receive daunomycin at weekly intervals. With the tins approach, 98% of patients are in *remission*, as defined by <5% blasts in the marrow and a return of neutrophil and platelet counts to near normal levels after 4-5 weeks of treatment and at least once more during induction. Intrathecal chemotherapy is always given at the start of treatment and at least once more during induction.

The drugs used are vincristine 15 mg/m^2, prednisolone 60 mg/m^2, and Adriamycin 20 mg/m^2/week, for 4-5 weeks. L-asparaginase 10,000 units/m^2/three times/week for 2 weeks. The total induction treatment is 4-6 weeks. If normal bone marrow is not achieved, treatment can be carried out for two additional weeks.

Central Nervous System Prophylaxis

Central nervous system prophylaxis is carried out weekly by intrathecal injection of MTX for 5-6 weeks followed by every 8 weeks of intrathecal injection for the maintenance therapy period. Patients with CNS involvement may sometimes require cranial radiation of 1,800-2,000 rads and intrathecal MTX. This is combined with hydrocortisone (12 mg/m^2) given as triple intrathecal therapy. This is followed by CNS therapy.

Consolidation Chemotherapy

The second phase of treatment, consolidation, focuses on intensive *CNS therapy* in combination with continued intensive systemic therapy in an effort to prevent later CNS relapses. CNS therapy consists of cranial irradiation and intrathecal chemotherapy. The concept of CNS preventive therapy is based on the assumption that undetectable CNS leukemia is present at diagnosis.

Cranial irradiation with intrathecal MTX has been in use as CNS preventive therapy. This causes significant adverse effects on neurocognitive function in some survivors. Hence most western protocols reserve cranial irradiation for patients with CNS disease at presentation and those who are at high risk for CNS relapse. Children younger than 3 years of age are given high-dose chemotherapy using cytosine arabinoside, in an attempt to prevent radiation to the developing brain.

Intrathecal chemotherapy is given repeatedly by lumbar puncture. The likelihood of later CNS relapse is thereby reduced to <5%, from historical incidence as high as 60%. A small percentage of patients with features that predict a high risk of CNS relapse may receive irradiation to the brain in later phases of therapy. This includes patients who, at the time of diagnosis, have lymphoblasts in the CSF and either an elevated CSF leukocyte count or physical signs of CNS leukemia, such as cranial nerve palsy.

Consolidation chemotherapy follows CNS therapy and is aimed at decreasing the leukemic burden further. Drugs used include vincristine, cyclophosphamide, daunorubicin, and cytosine arabinoside.

Consolidation therapy is carried out by cyclophosphamide, L-asparaginase, or multiple drug combinations. These include newer agents, such as VP-16, VM-26, and high-dose cytosine arabinoside, i.e., 1–2 g/m².

Subsequently, many regimens provide 14–25 weeks of therapy, with the drugs and schedules used vary depending on the risk group of the patient. This period of treatment is often termed and includes phases of aggressive treatment (delayed *intensification*) as well as relatively nontoxic phases of treatment (interim maintenance), multiagent chemotherapy, including such medications as cytarabine, MTX, asparaginase, and vincristine, is used airily, these phases to eradicate residual disease.

Maintenance Chemotherapy

Finally, patients enter the maintenance phase of therapy, which lasts for 2–3 years, depending on the protocol used. Patients are given daily mercaptopurine and weekly oral MTX, usually with intermittent doses of vincristine and corticosteroid.

Maintenance chemotherapy using mercaptopurine and MTX is continued for 2 years in order to eradicate dormant leukemia cells. Maintenance therapy is done with 6-mercaptopurine at a dose of 50–75 mg/m²/day and MTX at a dose of 20 mg/m²/week. The period of maintenance therapy is 130 weeks of continuous remission. Absolute neutrophil count should be maintained between 750 and 1,500 cells/mm³. Prophylactic treatment with cotrimoxazole helps to reduce infection.

Complete response can be achieved in 92% of the patients at the end of induction. Relapse of disease occurs in 25–30% of patients treated with this protocol at various centers. Most relapses occur during maintenance and within the first 6 months of completion of therapy.

A small number of patients with particularly poor prognostic features, such as those with induction failure and extreme hypodiploidy, may undergo bone marrow transplantation during the first remission.

Adolescents and young adults with ALL have an inferior prognosis compared to children younger than 15 years old. They often have adverse prognostic factors and require more intensive therapy. Patients in this age group have a superior outcome when treated with pediatric treatment as opposed to adult treatment protocols. Although the explanation for these findings may be multifactorial, it is important that these patients be treated with pediatric treatment protocols, ideally in a pediatric cancer center.

Treatment of Acute Myeloid Leukemia

Induction chemotherapy for AML consists of aggressive multiagent protocols **(Table 1)**. An anthracycline (daunorubicin or idarubicin) is used in combination with cytosine arabinoside, given over 7–10 days. The resultant myelosuppression takes about 3–4 weeks to recover. About 70% of patients achieve remission at the end of induction chemotherapy. Postremission treatment consists of two courses of high-dose chemotherapy using cytosine arabinoside. 3–4 months of maintenance chemotherapy is recommended in children.

TABLE 1: Protocol for ALL.

Cycle	Chemotherapy	Dose and schedule
Induction 1 (I$_1$)	Prednisone	40 mg/m^2 PO days 1–28
	Vincristine	1.4 mg/m^2 IV days 1, 8, 15, and 22
	Methotrexate	12 mg/m^2 IT, days 1, 8, 15, and 22
	L-asparaginase	6,000 μ/m^2 IM QOD × 10 doses, days 2, 20
	Daunorubicin	30 mg/m^2 IV days 8, 15, and 29
Induction 2 (I$_2$)	Mercaptopurine	75 mg/m^2 PO daily, days 1–7 and days 15–21
	Cyclophosphamide	750 mg/m^2 IV days 1–15
	Methotrexate	12 mg/m^2 IT days 1, 8, 15, and 22
	Cranial radiation	180 cGy daily × 10 days (total 1,800 cGy)
Repeat induction (RI$_1$)	Same as I$_1$	Doses and schedules as per I$_1$
Consolidation (C)	Cyclophosphamide	750 mg/m^2 IV day 1
	Vincristine	1.4 mg/m^2 IV days 1 and day 15
	Mercaptopurine	75 mg/m^2 PO daily days 1–7 and days 15–21
	Cytarabine	100 mg/m^2 SC every 12 hours × six doses on days 1–3 and days 15–17
	Daunorubicin	30 mg/m^2 IV days 15
Maintenance (M, six cycles)	Prednisone	40 mg/m^2 PO days 1–7
	Vincristine	1.4 mg/m^2 IV on day 1
	Daunorubicin	30 mg/m^2 IV on day 1
	L-asparaginase	6,000 μ/m^2 IM days 1, 3, 5, and 7
	Methotrexate	15 mg/m^2 PO once a week. Missing every fourth for a total of 12 weeks. Begin on day 15
	Mercaptopurine	75 mg/m^2 PO daily, 3 weeks out of every 4 for a total of 12 weeks. Begin on day 15

(ALL: acute lymphatic leukemia; IM: intramuscular; IT: intrathecally; IV: intravenous; PO: per os; SC: subcutaneous)

> **BOX 1:** IOSG protocol for AML.
>
> - *Induction:*
>   - Daunorubicin (60 mg/m^2/day × 3 days) or idarubicin (12 mg/m^2/day × 3 days)
>   - Cytosine arabinoside (100 mg/m^2/day as 24-hour continuous infusion × 7 days)
> - *Consolidation I:*
>   - High dose cytosine arabinoside (1.5 g/m^2/dose every 12 hourly × 5 days)
> - *Consolidation II:*
>   - Same as consolidation I
> - *Maintenance × four cycles:*
>   - Daunorubicin (45 mg/m^2/day × 1 day)
>   - Cytosine arabinoside (100 mg/m^2/every 12 hourly SC × 5 days)
>
> (AML: acute myeloid leukemia; IOSG: Indian Oncology Study Group; SC: subcutaneous)

The Indian Oncology Study Group (IOSG) protocol **(Box 1)** has given good results in children with AML. Acute promyelocytic (APML) is characterized by the t(15;17) involving the retinoic acid receptor A (RAR-α). The use of all transretinoic acid (ATRA) causes the differentiation of the promyelocytes leading to their maturation with resolution of the coagulopathy. Its use in combination with chemotherapy like anthracycline leads to complete remission. Maintenance therapy with ATRA improves long-term disease-free survival. Arsenic trioxide, alone or in combination with ATRA has also produced excellent response rates in APML patient.

Supportive Care

Supportive care is extremely important in the treatment of acute leukemias. This includes blood component therapy and aggressive management of infectious complications. Packed RBC transfusions are indicated to maintain hemoglobin over 8 g/dL in good children and over 10 g/dL in patients with fever and infection. Platelet transfusions are indicated if the platelet count is <10,000/mm^3 or in the case of overt bleeding, especially in patients with fever and infection. Every episode of febrile neutropenia should be treated aggressively with broad-spectrum antibiotics after drawing blood cultures.

All patients should receive prophylaxis for pneumocystis carinii pneumonia with cotrimoxazole and for fungal infections with clotrimazole. Maintenance of oral and perianal hygiene reduces the risk of infections to a significant extent. The use of hematopoietic growth factors [granulocyte colony-stimulating factor (G-CSF) and granulocyte-macrophage colony-stimulating factor (GM-CSF)] reduces the period of neutropenia but are expensive and do not improve the overall outcome of the patients. The use of long-term indwelling venous access devices, which allows for easy blood collection and for the administration of intravenous medication and blood products makes and treatment of acute leukemias less painful and more patient-friendly.

The successful therapy of ALL is a direct result of intensive and often toxic treatment. However, such intensive therapy can incur substantial academic, developmental, and psychosocial costs for children with considerable financial costs and stress for their families. Both long-term and acute toxicity effects can occur. An array of cancer care professionals with training and experience in addressing the myriads of problems that can arise is essential to minimize the complications and achieve an optimal outcome.

Infants with AML often present with CNS or skin involvement and have a subtype known as acute myelomonocytic leukemia. The treatment may be the same as that for older children with AML, with similar outcomes. Meticulous supportive care is necessary because of the young age and aggressive therapy needed in these patients.

Several new biological agents, including tyrosine kinase inhibitors and immunotoxins, are currently in various stages of research.

Bone Marrow Transplantation

Bone marrow transplantation or stem cell transplantation is indicated in patients with acute leukemia in the first remission only if associated with very high-risk factors, viz., ALL with t(9;22) or t(4;11) or in AML with monosomy 5 or 7, t(9;22) or t(6;9).

Patients whose blasts contain certain chromosomal abnormalities, hypodiploidy (<44 chromosomes), and patients with very slow response to therapy may have a better cure rate with early HSCT from a HLA-DR-matched sibling donor, or a matched unrelated donor, than with the intensive chemotherapy alone. HSCT cures about 50% of the patients who relapse, provided that a second remission is achieved with chemotherapy before transplant.

Any patient with acute leukemia, who relapses needs a transplant while in second remission in an attempt to achieve a cure.

Treatment of Relapse

Despite numerous advances in the treatment and supportive care for children with ALL, 2–3% will die of infectious or other toxic complications, 1% will develop a second malignant neoplasm, and 10–15% will relapse. Recurrent or relapsed ALL remains a significant challenge, as fewer than 50% of patients will survive long-term. Relapse can occur in the bone marrow or extramedullary sites, with CNS and testes being most common or in both locations. The most important prognostic factors for recurrent ALL are the site and timing of the recurrence relative to the initial diagnosis. In general, isolated bone marrow relapse carries a worse prognosis compared to extramedullary or combined relapse. Early relapse (<36 months from initial diagnosis) has a worse outcome than late relapse. Relapses of T-ALL are particularly challenging to treat and have very few long-term survivors.

The major impediment to a successful outcome is a relapse of the disease. Outcomes remain poor among those that relapse, with the most important prognostic indicators being lime from diagnosis of the site of relapsed disease, in addition, other factors, such as immunophenotype (T-ALL worse than All) and age at initial diagnosis, have prognostic significance.

Relapse occurs in the bone marrow in 15–20% of patients with ALL and carries the most serious implications, especially if it occurs during or shortly after completion of therapy, Intensive chemotherapy with agents not previously used in the patient followed by allogeneic Stem cell transplantation can result in long-term survival for some patients with bone marrow relapse.

The incidence of CNS relapse has decreased to <5% since the introduction of preventive CNS therapy. CNS relapse may be discovered at the time of a routine lumbar puncture in the asymptomatic patient, symptomatic patients with relapse in the CNS usually present with signs and symptoms of increased intracranial pressure and call present with isolated cranial nerve palsies. The diagnosis is confirmed by demonstrating the presence of leukemic cells in the CSF. The treatment includes intrathecal medication and cranial or craniospinal irradiation. Systemic chemotherapy also must be used, because these patients are at high risk for subsequent bone marrow relapse. Most patients with leukemic relapse confined to the CNS do well, especially those in whom the CNS relapse occurs longer than 18 months after initiation of chemotherapy.

Testicular relapse occurs in <2% of boys with ALL, usually after completion of therapy. Such relapse occurs as a painless swelling of 1 or both testes. The diagnosis is confirmed by a biopsy of the affected testis. Treatment includes systemic chemotherapy and possibly local irradiation. A high proportion of boys with a testicular relapse can be successfully retreated and the survival rate of these patients is good.

PROGNOSIS

The two most important prognostic factors are age at diagnosis and initial WBC count. The prognosis is unfavorable in children with age below 2 years and above 8 years. Significant hepatosplenomegaly, lymphadenopathy, mediastinal enlargement, CNS, and testicular involvement carry a poor prognosis. The prognosis is poor if the WBC count is >50,000 cell/mm^3 hypogammaglobulinemia, hypodiploidy.

Acute lymphatic leukemia is a heterogeneous disease and prognosis depends on the subtype, the tumor burden at presentation, the associated cytogenetic abnormality, the ploidy, and most importantly, the response to treatment. Early clearance of blasts from the peripheral blood (day 7 absolute blast counts) after initiation of treatment and evidence of bone marrow remission on day 14 of induction therapy has been associated with a very good prognosis.

BIBLIOGRAPHY

1. Advani AS, Hunger SP, Burnett AK. Acute leukemia in adolescents and young adults. Semin Oncol. 2009;36(3)213-26.
2. Gaynon PS, Angiolillo AL, Carroll WL, Nachman JB, Trigg ME, Sather HN, et al. Long-term results of the children's cancer group studies for childhood acute lymphoblastic leukemia 1983-2002: a Children's Oncology Group Report. Leukemia. 2010;24(2):285-97.
3. Martin A, Morgan E, Hijaya N. Relapsed or refractory pediatric acute lymphoblastic leukemia: current and emerging treatments. Paeditric Drugs. 1012;14(6):377-87.
4. Nguen K, Devidas M, Cheng SC, La M, Raetz EA, Carroll WL, et al. Factors influencing survival after relapse from acute lymphoblastic leukemia: a Children's Oncology Group study. Leukemia. 2008;22(12):2142-50.
5. Vrooman LM, Silverman LB. Childhood acute lymphoblastic leukemia: update on prognostic factors. Curr Opin Pediatr. 2009;21(1):1-8.

CASE 96

Neuroblastoma

■ PRESENTING COMPLAINTS

An 18-month-old boy was brought with the complaints of:
- Swelling in abdomen since 2 months
- Loose motion since 15 days
- Vomiting since 3 days

History of Presenting Complaints

An 18-month-old boy was referred by a general practitioner for evaluation of swelling in the abdomen. According to the mother, his son was taken to a doctor for treatment of loose motion and vomiting. During the examination, the doctor had found a mass in the upper abdomen. Hence, he referred the boy to a hospital for evaluation of the mass. Mother also revealed the history of the presence of swelling in the child.

Past History of the Patient

The patient was the only sibling of a consanguineous marriage. He was born at full term with normal vaginal delivery. The baby cried immediately after the delivery. The birth weight of the child was 3 kg, the length of the child was 51 cm, and the head circumference was 35 cm. There was no significant postnatal history except for transient tachypnea of the newborn which settled by itself without any treatment. He was on breast milk exclusively for 4 months. Weaning started with cereals and fruits. His developmental milestones were normal. According to mother, his son was suffering mainly from loose motion and vomiting for which he was seeking treatment by his family doctor.

CASE AT A GLANCE

Basic Findings
Height	: 84 cm (90th centile)
Weight	: 10.5 kg (50th centile)
Temperature	: 37°C
Pulse rate	: 120 beats/min
Respiratory rate	: 32 breaths/min
Blood pressure	: 70/50 mm Hg

Positive Findings

History:
- Mass per abdomen
- Loose motions
- Sweating

Examination:
- Mass per abdomen
- Sign of moderate dehydration

Investigation:
- Serum electrolytes:
  - Sodium (Na): 110 mEq/L
  - Potassium (K): 3 mEq/L
  - Chlorine (Cl): 90 mEq/L
- Urinary vanillylmandelic acid (VMA): Increased
- Excretory urogram: Showed displacement of left kidney
- Biopsy: Neuroblast cells and large amount of cytoplasm

EXAMINATION

The child was moderately built and nourished. The child was irritable and signs of moderate dehydration were present. Anthropometric measurements included that the height was 84 cm (90th centile), the weight was 10.5 kg (50th centile), and the head circumference was 48 cm. Anterior fontanelle was normal. The heart rate was 120 beats per minute, the respiratory rate was 32 breaths per minute. The blood pressure recorded was 70/50 mm Hg. There was no pallor, no icterus, no lymphadenopathy, and no cyanosis.

Per abdomen examination revealed the presence of mass in the epigastric region. The mass measured about 3 cm × 2 cm. The consistency was firm. The mass was nontender. Other systemic examinations were normal.

INVESTIGATION

- *Hemoglobin:* 12 g/dL
- *TLC:* 7,600 cells/mm^3
- *Serum electrolytes:*
  - Sodium (Na): 110 mEq/L
  - Potassium (K): 3 mEq/L
  - Chlorine (Cl): 90 mEq/L
- *Urinary vanillylmandelic acid (VMA):* 20 mg/24 h (Normal range: 2–10 mg/24 h)
- *Excretory:* Showed urogram displacement of left kidney downward and slightly lateral suprarenal mass
- *Biopsy:* Showed primitive neuroblast cells, cytoplasmic process rosettes, and central fibrillar material.
- *CT scan of abdomen and chest:* Normal

DISCUSSION

Neuroblastomas are embryonal cancers of the peripheral sympathetic nervous system with heterogeneous clinical presentation and course, ranging from tumors that undergo spontaneous regression to very aggressive tumors unresponsive to very intensive multimodal therapy. Neuroblastoma and related neoplasms arise from those neural crest cells that differentiate in cells of the sympathetic ganglia and adrenal medulla. Because neuroblastoma arises from any site along the sympathetic chain, the location of primary tumor at diagnosis is varied and change with age. The most common sites are adrenal, sympathetic chain, retroperitoneal area, posterior mediastinum, and cervical area.

Increased incidence of neuroblastoma is associated with some maternal and paternal occupational chemical exposures, farming, and work related to electronics, although no single environmental exposure has been shown to directly cause neuroblastoma.

The enigmatic characteristics of neuroblastoma with paraneoplastic syndromes and spontaneous regression under some circumstances have led some researchers to suggest that neuroblastoma may originate as a neurodevelopmental disorder.

Neuroblastoma, a tumor of the sympathetic nervous system, is the most common extracranial solid tumor of childhood. Neuroblastoma is a clinically heterogeneous disease, as infants with metastatic disease may experience complete tumor regression without therapy, while other children may experience relentless disease progression despite modern multimodality therapy. Current risk classification schemes use clinical, histologic, and genomic features at diagnosis to predict tumor behavior and to assign patients to an appropriate treatment regimen based on risk of recurrence. Children with lower-risk disease are spared unnecessary therapies yet still achieve excellent outcomes. Nevertheless, outcome remains poor for patients classified as high-risk.

EPIDEMIOLOGY

Neuroblastoma is the most common extracranial solid tumor in children and the most commonly diagnosed malignancy in infants. It accounts for 7–10% of childhood cancer. The etiology is unknown. Occasionally, it is congenital with metastasis to the placenta. Neuroblastoma accounts for >15% of the mortality from cancer in children. The median age of children at diagnosis of neuroblastoma is 2 years, and 90% of cases are diagnosed by 5 years of age. The incidence is slightly higher in boys and in white children.

Neuroblastoma is unique with a high rate of spontaneous regression. Neuroblastoma in situ is related to nodular clusters of the neuroblasts. There is an association with neurofibromatosis, Hirschsprung's disease, heterochronic fetal hydantoin and fetal alcohol syndrome, and Friedreich's ataxia. Rearrangement or deletion of the short arm of chromosome number 1 has been found.

PATHOLOGY

Neuroblastoma is one of the small blue round-cell tumors of childhood (others are EWS, NHL, PNET, and rhabdomyosarcoma). The typical neuroblastoma is composed of small, uniform cells with hyperchromatic nuclei and scanty cytoplasm that may form a rosette pattern. The presence of neuritic processes (neutrophil) and Homer Wright pseudorosettes help to distinguish neuroblastoma from other round-cell tumors. The fully differentiated, benign counterpart of neuroblastoma is ganglioneuroma, which is composed of mature ganglion cells, neutrophils, and Schwann cells. Ganglioneuroblastoma has features intermediate to those of the other two.

Neuroblastoma tumors, which are derived from primordial neural crest cells, form a spectrum with variable degrees of neural differentiation, ranging from tumors with primarily undifferentiated small round cells (neuroblastoma) to tumors consisting of mature and maturing Schwannian stroma with ganglion cells (ganglioneuroblastoma or ganglioneuroma).

In gross pathology, this tumor is seen as a firm grey mass. Hemorrhage into the tumor produces variegated maroon color often with necrosis and calcification. Most tumors contain primitive neuroblastoma cells. Some tumors have large amount of cytoplasm, with the cytoplasmic process, rosettes, and central fibrillar material.

The prognosis of children with neuroblastoma varies with the histologic features of the tumor, and prognostic factors include the presence and amount of Schwannian stroma, the degree of tumor cell differentiation, and the mitosis-karyorrhexis index.

PATHOGENESIS

The etiology of neuroblastoma in most cases remains unknown. Familial neuroblastoma accounts for 1–2% of all cases, is associated with a younger age at diagnosis, and is linked to mutations in the *PHOX2B and ALK* genes. The *BARD1* gene has also been identified as a major genetic contributor to neuroblastoma risk. Neuroblastoma is associated with other neural crest disorders, including Hirschsprung disease, central hypoventilation syndrome, neurofibromatosis type I, and potentially congenital cardiovascular malformations. Children with Beckwith-Wiedemann syndrome (BWS) and Hemihypertrophy also have a higher incidence of neuroblastoma.

Genetic characteristics of neuroblastoma tumors that are of prognostic importance include amplification of the *MYCN* (N-myc) proto-oncogene and tumor cell DNA content, or ploidy. Amplification of *MYCN* is strongly associated with advanced tumor stage and poor outcomes. Hyperdiploidy confers a better prognosis if the child is younger than 1 year of age at diagnosis. Other chromosomal abnormalities, including loss of heterozygosity of 1p, 11q, and 14q, and gain of 17q, are commonly found in neuroblastoma tumors and are also associated with worse outcomes.

Neuroblastoma arises from sympathetic neuroblasts, and neuronal differentiation is often seen in histologic evaluation. Some tumors undergo spontaneous or therapy-induced differentiation, suggesting that the malignant behavior of these cells may be maintained in part by a failed differentiation program. The factors responsible for regulating differentiation or regression are not well understood but may involve neurotrophin signaling, as neurotrophin pathways play a key role in the development of the sympathetic nervous system.

CLINICAL FEATURES (FIG. 1)

Clinical features are related to the localization of the sympathetic nervous system and the site of metastasis symptoms will be different if the tumor is located in the neck or the pelvis.

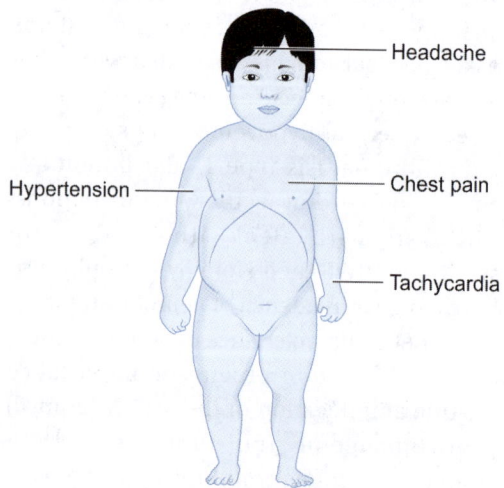

Fig. 1: Clinical features.

The most common sites of primary lesion include adrenal gland, paravertebral glands, retroperitoneum, posterior mediastinum, pelvis, and cervical area.

The primary tumor is usually in the abdomen. The mass usually is in the upper abdomen as it will be mainly in adrenal gland (40%). It presents as a firm, irregular, and nontender mass. It accounts for 25% of paraspinal ganglion. In the posterior mediastinum, the tumor is usually asymptomatic and discovered on chest X-ray accidentally. The primary tumor extends beyond midline, and margins are often poorly defined. Clinical features vary with the primary site of malignant disease and neuroendocrine functions of the tissue.

Neuroblastoma may develop at any site of sympathetic nervous system tissue. Approximately half of neuroblastoma tumors arise in the adrenal glands, and most of the remainder originate in the paraspinal sympathetic ganglia.

Metastatic spread, which is more common in children older than 1 year of age at diagnosis, occurs via local invasion or distant hematogenous or lymphatic routes. The most common sites of metastasis are the regional or distant lymph nodes, long bones and skull, bone marrow, liver, and skin. Lung and brain metastases are rare, occurring in >3% of cases. Metastatic disease can cause a variety of signs and symptoms, including fever, irritability, failure to thrive, bone pain, cytopenias, bluish subcutaneous nodules, orbital proptosis, and periorbital ecchymosis. Localized disease can manifest as an asymptomatic mass or can cause symptoms because of the mass itself, including spinal cord compression, bowel obstruction, and superior vena cava syndrome. It has a predilection for metastasis to the skull, especially to sphenoid bone and retrobulbar tissue causing periorbital ecchymosis and proptosis.

Neuroblastoma has polymorphic symptoms. This is because of numerous sites of primary tumor and the patterns in widespread metastasis. There are tumor-associated metabolic disturbances.

The signs and symptoms of neuroblastoma depend on the tumor site and extent of disease, and the symptoms of neuroblastoma can mimic many other disorders, a fact that can result in a delayed diagnosis (Fig. 1).

Hemorrhage in the enlarging tumor is common and may even produce pallor and hypotension. Hepatic enlargement and ascites will occur with hepatic involvement.

Children with neuroblastoma can also present with neurologic signs and symptoms. Neuroblastoma originating in the superior cervical ganglion can result in *Horner syndrome (unilateral ptosis, myosis, and anhidrosis)*. Paraspinal neuroblastoma tumors can invade the neural foramina, causing spinal cord and nerve root compression. It can develop either intraspinally or extraspinally. It can extend on dumbbell fashion in intervertebral foramen. This causes cord compression, back pain, sphincter dysfunction, paraplegic or quadriplegic and gait disturbances.

Neuroblastoma can also be associated with a paraneoplastic syndrome of autoimmune origin, termed *opsoclonus–myoclonus–ataxia syndrome*, in which patients experience rapid, uncontrollable jerking eye and body movements, poor coordination, and cognitive dysfunction. Some tumors produce catecholamines that can cause increased sweating and hypertension and some release vasoactive intestinal peptide, causing profound secretory diarrhea. Children with extensive tumors can also experience tumor-lysis syndrome and DIC. Child may present with paresis, paralysis and bowel and bladder dysfunction.

Encephalopathy involving the cerebellum produces a syndrome called opsomyoclonus. It is characterized by progressive ataxia, titubation of head, myoclonic jerks, and chaotic conjugate jerking movements of the eyes. With progression, secretary diarrhea occurs due to vasointestinal peptide secretion by tumor. This will be associated with atonic bladder.

There will be extreme loss of potassium. It may occur as a result of overproduction of vasoactive intestinal peptide. Hypertension is very rare with neuroblasts. It is common with pheochromocytoma. Episodes of unexplained sweating and flushing have been reported due to catecholamine release.

It may extend to surrounding tissues by local invasion or to the regional lymph nodes by lymphatics. Hematogenous spread most frequently involves liver, bone marrow, and skeleton. Metastasis to the brain is rare.

Subcutaneous nodules are bluish in color and associated with erythematous flush followed by blanching when compressed, secondary to catecholamine release.

> **ESSENTIAL DIAGNOSTIC POINTS**
> - Abdominal pain, bone pain, and irritability
> - Anorexia, weight loss, fatigue, and fever
> - Abdominal mass adenopathy and hepatomegaly
> - Periorbital ecchymosis, and proptosis
> - Skull masses, subcutaneous nodules, and spinal cord compression

> **GENERAL FEATURES**
> - Anorexia
> - Listlessness
> - Anemia
> - Loss of weight
> - Cough

DIAGNOSIS

Neuroblastoma is usually discovered as a mass or multiple masses on plain radiography, CT, or MRI. The mass often contains calcification and hemorrhage that can be appreciated on plain radiography or CT. Prenatal diagnosis of neuroblastoma on maternal ultrasound scans is sometimes possible. Tumor markers, including catecholamine metabolites, homovanillic acid (HVA), and VMA, are elevated in the urine of approximately 95% of cases and help to confirm the diagnosis. A pathologic diagnosis is established from tumor tissue obtained by biopsy.

Evaluation of Patient

Evaluations for metastatic disease should include CT or MRI of the chest and abdomen, bone scan to detect cortical bone involvement, and at least two independent bone marrow aspirations and biopsies to evaluate for marrow disease.

Iodine-123 metaiodobenzylguanidine (^{123}*I-MIBG*) studies should be used when available to better define the extent of the disease.

- *Primary site:*
  - X-ray, ultrasonography (USG), CT scan/MRI
  - 24-hour-urinary VMA
- *Metastatic disease:*
  - Bone marrow aspiration and trephine biopsy
  - Technetium bone scan

A standard evaluation to determine the extent of disease is performed at diagnosis. CT or MRI scans of the neck, chest, abdomen, and pelvis are used to evaluate the primary tumor and to detect regional or distant disease. MRI is superior to CT in evaluating paraspinal mass lesions for intraforaminal extension and spinal cord compression.

For the abdominal tumor CT scan will be helpful. Radiography of abdomen and excretory urography are done. Helpful findings include calcification or displacement of renal collecting system or the ureter.

Computed tomography scan shows mixed tissue density including both solid and cystic components. The cystic area is either hemorrhagic or necrotic in the tumor. Metrizamide myelography along with CT may be required to define the extent of intraspinal extension of the disease.

Bone scan shows periosteal lytic lesion in skull. It is helpful in defining the extent of metastatic disease. Bone marrow aspiration or biopsy should be performed for staging in all patients.

Bone marrow disease is assessed via bilateral bone marrow aspirates and trephine biopsies. Immunohistochemistry is now widely used to confirm the presence of tumor in the marrow. Molecular assays that detect neuroblastoma cells in bone marrow are highly sensitive. However, the use of these assays has not been incorporated into routine clinical practice at this time.

The specific diagnostic feature is the elevated levels of catecholamines in the urine. Increased levels of dihydroxyphenylalanine (DOPA), dopamine, norepinephrine, normetanephrine, HVA, or VMA are present. This provides an ancillary diagnostic test, as well as a means to follow disease activity.

The two enzymes primarily responsible for the catabolism of catecholamines are catechol-O-methyltransferase and monoamine oxidase. DOPA and dopamine are converted primarily to HVA, whereas norepinephrine and epinephrine are converted primarily to VMA. Both urinary VMA and HVA should be normalized for age and for urinary creatinine.

Imaging

Conventional radiography often reveals mediastinal widening in stippled calcification in an abdominal tumor. A complete body bone scan is useful in detecting bone metastasis and is necessary for staging. Metastatic to bone appears irregular and lytic periosteal reaction and pathological fracture.

Ultrasound scan, CT, and MRI all help to delineate the primary tumor and detect metastasis. CT scan helps to know extension of primary lesion and presence of metastasis in lymph node and liver. MRI is helpful to detect the presence of spinal cord involvement and that appears to involve neural foramina.

The methylidobenzylguanidine (MIBG) scintigraphy scan is a radiolabeled, specific, and very sensitive method for the evaluation and follow-up of primary and metastatic disease. Recent reports also suggest its very useful therapeutic role in the treatment of advanced and relapsed disease.

Myelography is very important in the evaluation of primary or metastatic spinal disease and if performed early can diagnose the exact location and site of lesions causing impending motor weakness of the limbs. However, safer modes of investigations (e.g., MRI) are preferred.

LABORATORY SALIENT FINDINGS
• *Elevated urinary catecholamine:* HVA, and VMA • Plain X-ray, CT scan of primary tumor • *Bone scan:* Periosteal lytic lesion of the skull • Histopathological examination
CT: computed tomography; HVA: homovanillic acid; VMA: vanillylmandelic acid

■ DIAGNOSTIC CRITERIA

The gold standard for the diagnosis of neuroblastoma is the examination of tumor tissue by histopathology and immunohistochemistry.

The criteria is:
- An unequivocal pathological diagnosis made from tumor tissue by light microscopy, with or without immunohistochemistry and electron microscopy and/or increased urine catecholamines or metabolites [>3 standard deviations (SD) above the mean for age]

  Or
- Bone marrow aspirate or biopsy containing unequivocal tumor cells and increased urine catecholamines or metabolites (>3 SD above the mean for age)

Other investigations include blood counts, urinary catecholamine excretion, bone marrow aspiration and biopsy, liver function tests, abdominal ultrasound, and X-ray and bone scan for metastasis. Nuclear scanning with I-123 or ^{131}I-MIBG detects tumors and metastasis accurately. CT scan of chest, abdomen, and pelvis is indicated to assess the extent of disease. MRI is preferred for paraspinal tumors to assess spinal cord compression.

■ STAGING OF NEUROBLASTOMA

Clinical staging as per Evans (CCSG) staging system is done if surgery is not done upfront. International Neuroblastoma Staging System (INSS) is used when surgical details are available and is one of the most important prognostic factors **(Table 1)**.

■ RISK STRATIFICATION

Risk stratification depends upon many factors as follows:
- Age
- Stage
- *Pathology (prechemotherapy biopsy or specimen):* The Shimada classification appears to have prognostic significance. It is based on histological features such as the presence or absence of stroma, degree of differentiation, and mitosis-karyorrhexis index.
- *Biological factors:* Chromosome 1p deletion and DNA index.

TABLE 1: International neuroblastoma staging system and evans staging system.

International neuroblastoma staging system	Evans staging system
Stage 1: Localized tumor confined to the area of origin; complete gross excision with or without microscopic residual disease, ipsilateral and contralateral lymph nodes negative microscopically	*Stage I:* Tumor-limited organ or structure of origin
Stage 2A: Unilateral tumor with incomplete gross excision; identifiable ipsilateral and contralateral lymph nodes negative microscopically	*Stage II:* Tumor with regional spread that does not cross the midline; ipsilateral lymph node may be involved
Stage 2B: Unilateral tumor with complete or incomplete gross excision; positive ipsilateral lymph nodes identifiable contralateral negative microscopically	
Stage 3: Tumor with spread to midline with or without the involvement of regional lymph node or unilateral tumor with contralateral regional lymph node involvement or midline tumor with bilateral regional lymph node involvement	*Stage III:* Regional tumor crossing the midline; bilateral lymph nodes may be involved
Stage 4: Dissemination of tumor to distant lymph nodes, bone, bone marrow, liver, and/or other organs	*Stage IV:* Tumor with metastases to distant sites
Stage 4-S: Localized primary tumor as defined for stage I or II with dissemination limited to liver, skin, and/or bone marrow	*Stage IV-S:* Localized primary tumor and disseminated disease limited to liver, skin and/or bone marrow

DIFFERENTIAL DIAGNOSIS

Differential diagnosis includes the following.
- Multicystic kidney
- Wilms tumor (WT)
- Pheochromocytoma
- Lymphosarcoma
- Hydronephrosis
- Brucellosis
- Teratoma

TREATMENT

The mainstay of therapy is surgical resection coupled with chemotherapy. Massive size of the tumor often makes primary resection impossible. Under these circumstances, only biopsy is performed. Following the chemotherapy, a surgical correction may allow the resection of primary tumor. Radiation therapy is also sometimes necessary.

Treatment depends upon the staging and severity.

Stages	INSS
Stage I:	Confined to the area of origin with complete gross excision
Stage IIA:	Unilateral tumor with incomplete gross excision
Stage IIB:	Unilateral tumor with positive ipsilateral regional lymph nodes
Stage III:	Tumor infiltrating across the midline with or without regional lymph nodes
Stage IV:	Dissemination of tumor to distant lymph nodes, bone, bone marrow, liver, or other organs
Stage IVS:	Localized primary tumor as defined with dissemination limited to liver, skin, or bone marrow

Stage I: Surgery alone

Stage IIA or 3 (<12 months): Surgery followed by cyclophosphamide and Adriamycin for 5 cycles

Stage IIB (>12 months): Cyclophosphamide and Adriamycin for 5 cycles with radiation therapy beginning at 3 weeks. If complete response obtained, patients should be treated with 2 more cycles of chemotherapy followed by 2 cycles of VM-26 and cisplatinum.

Stage III (>12 months): Surgical removal of primary tumor plus alternate cycles of chemotherapy with oncovin, cyclophosphamide, etoposide, and cisplatinum (OPEC) and oncovin, cyclophosphamide, etoposide, and carboplatin (OJEC)

Stage IV (<12 months): Initial surgery followed by 9–12 months of chemotherapy with the following:

- *CADO:* Vincristine, cyclophosphamide, doxorubicin
- *PECADO:* Vincristine, cyclophosphamide, doxorubicin, cisplatin, teniposide

Treatment strategies **(Table 2)** vary according to the risk groups. For identical age, stage, and presence of unfavorable histology, upgrade the patient to the next risk category.

The patients' age and tumor stage are combined with cytogenetic and molecular features of the tumor to determine the treatment risk group and estimated prognosis for each patient.

The usual treatment for children with low-risk neuroblastoma is surgery for stages 1 and 2 and observation for stage 4S with cure rates generally >90% without further therapy. Treatment with chemotherapy or radiation for the rare child with local recurrence can still be curative. Children with spinal cord compression at diagnosis also may require urgent treatment with chemotherapy, surgery, or radiation to avoid neurologic damage. Stage 4S neuroblastomas have a very favorable prognosis, and many regress spontaneously without therapy.

TABLE 2: Treatment strategy based on risk categories of the patients.

Risk	Stage	Age (years)	Treatment	Survival
Low	1	Any	Surgery	90%
	2A/2B	Any	Surgery followed by low-dose chemotherapy (cyclophosphamide and doxorubicin)	85–90%
	4S	<1	Observation if asymptomatic, chemotherapy/RT if symptomatic	
Intermediate	3	Any	Multiagent chemotherapy (cyclophosphamide, cisplatin, etoposide, and doxorubicin) + 2nd look surgery ± RT to tumor bed ± lymph node ± maintenance chemotherapy	75%
	4	<1		
	4S	<1		
High	2A/2B	>1	Multiagent chemotherapy as induction, additional treatment such as MIBG therapy, high-dose chemotherapy with autologous BMT as consolidation, and biological therapy (13-cis-retinoic acid) as treatment of minimal residual disease	40–50%
	3	Any		
	4 and 4S	>1		
	4	>1		

BMT: bone marrow transplant; MIBG: metaiodobenzylguanidine; RT: radiotherapy

Chemotherapy or resection of the primary tumor does not improve survival rates, but for infants with massive liver involvement and respiratory compromise, small doses of cyclophosphamide or low-dose hepatic irradiation may alleviate symptoms. For children with stage 4S neuroblastoma, who require treatment for symptoms, the survival rate is 81%.

Treatment of intermediate-risk neuroblastoma includes surgery, chemotherapy, and in some cases, radiation therapy. The chemotherapy usually includes moderate doses of cisplatin or carboplatin, cyclophosphamide, etoposide, and doxorubicin given for several months. Radiation therapy is used for tumors with incomplete response to chemotherapy. Children with intermediate-risk neuroblastoma, including children with stage 3 disease and infants with stage 4 disease and favorable characteristics, have an excellent prognosis and >90% survival with this moderate treatment.

Children with high-risk neuroblastoma have long-term survival rates between 25% and 35% with current treatment that consists of intensive chemotherapy, high-dose chemotherapy with autologous stem cell rescue, surgery, radiation, and l3-cis-retinoic acid (isotretinoin). Induction chemotherapy for children with high-risk neuroblastoma includes combinations of cyclophosphamide, topotecan, doxorubicin, vincristine, cisplatin, and etoposide. After completion of induction chemotherapy, resection of the residual primary tumor is followed by high-dose chemotherapy with autologous stem cell rescue and focal radiation therapy to tumor sites.

The further addition of 13-cis-retinoic acid after autologous stem cell transplantation resulted in further improvements in survival rates. In addition, a national clinical trial has demonstrated an increase in short-term survival rates with the addition of the monoclonal antibody ch14.18, IL-2, and granulocyte-macrophage stimulating factor to 13-cis-retinoic acid therapy.

Cases of high-risk neuroblastoma are associated with frequent relapses, and children with recurrent neuroblastoma have a <50% response rate to alternative chemotherapy regimens. New treatment strategies and agents are needed for children with both high-risk and recurrent neuroblastoma. Therapies currently under investigation include new chemotherapeutic agents and other novel therapies directed against critical intracellular signaling pathways, radiolabeled targeted agents (such as 131 I-MIBG), immunotherapy, and antitumor vaccines.

Radiotherapy

Indications

- *Low-risk patients:* For symptomatic life- or organ-threatening tumor
- *Intermediate-risk patients:* Whose tumor has responded incompletely to both chemotherapy and attempted resection and also has unfavorable biologic characteristics
- *High-risk patients:* Even in cases of complete resection
- *Bone marrow transplant:* As a part of preparatory regimen
- *Metastatic disease:* Palliative radiation therapy.

■ CONCLUSION

Neuroblastoma represents one of the most challenging malignancies for treatment decisions because of its unusual biological behavior which includes spontaneous regression at one end to maturation to ganglioneuroma and treatment-resistant progression at other end of the spectrum. The main achievements in the management of neuroblastoma during the last two decades have been the reduction of chemotherapy in patients with low-risk disease and the increased efficacy of chemotherapy in high-risk disease.

■ BIBLIOGRAPHY

1. London WB, Castleberry RP, Matthay KK, Look AT, Seeger RC, Shimada H, et al. Evidence for an age cutoff greater than 365 days for neuroblastoma risk group stratification in children oncology group. J Clin Oncol. 2005;23(27):6459-65.
2. Mattay KK, Reynolds CP, Seeger RC, Shimada H, Adkins ES, Haas-Kogan D, et al. Long-term results for children with high-risk neuroblastoma treated on a randomized trial of myeloablative therapy followed by 13-cis retinoic acid: A children's oncology group study. 2009;27(7):1007-13.
3. National Cancer Institute. (2024). Neuroblastoma—patient version. [online] Available from http/www. cancer.gov/cancertopics/types/neuroblastoma [Last accessed June 2024].
4. Schmidt ML, Lal A, Seeger RC, Maris JM, Shimada H, O'Leary M, et al. Favorable prognosis for patients 12 to 18 months of age with stage 4 nonamplified MYCN neuroblastoma: A Children's Cancer Group Study. J Clin Oncol. 2005;23(27):6474-80.
5. Yu AL, Gilman AL, Ozkaynak MF, London WB, Kreissman SG, Chen HX, et al. Anti GD2 antibody with GM-CSF, interleukin-2, and isotretinoin for neuroblastoma. N Eng J Med. 2010;363(14)1324-34.

CASE 97

Osteosarcoma

■ PRESENTING COMPLAINTS

A 10-year-old boy was brought with the complaints of:
- Pain in the leg since 15 days
- Decreased movements since 15 days
- Swelling in the leg since 5 days

History of Presenting Complaints

A 10-year-old boy came to pediatric outpatient department (OPD) with a history of pain in the lower end of thigh. Mother complains that his son was apparently normal 15 days back. To begin with, he developed pain in lower part of thigh and was shown to a general practitioner. He was diagnosed with myalgia and analgesics were given. Pain used to come down for some time. After about 1 week, pain in the thigh limited his movements. The child started to limp. His mother had noticed a small swelling at the site of pain. She then noted the swelling was tender and hard, and brought the child to the hospital for specialist consultancy.

Past History of the Patient

The patient was the second sibling of a nonconsanguineous marriage. He was born at full term by normal vaginal delivery. There was no significant postnatal event. All the developmental milestones were normal. He had been completely immunized. His performance at school was satisfactory. He was a good athlete. He used to have minor usual ailments and for those, he was getting treatment from a general practitioner. His elder sister maintained apparently good health.

■ EXAMINATION

On examination, the boy was moderately built and moderately nourished. He looked

CASE AT A GLANCE

Basic Findings
Height	: 130 cm (25th centile)
Weight	: 27 kg (50th centile)
Temperature	: 38°C
Pulse rate	: 106 beats/min
Respiratory rate	: 24 breaths/min
Blood pressure	: 90/70 mm Hg

Positive Findings

History:
- Pain
- Limping
- Swelling

Examination:
- Swelling
- Limping
- Tenderness
- Erythema

Investigation:
- Alkaline phosphatase: Increased
- X-ray of femur: Sclerosis
- Fine-needle aspiration cytology (FNAC): Showed highly malignant pleomorphic spindle cells

very much sick because of the pain. He came to the OPD limping.

Anthropometric measurements included a height of 130 cm (25th centile) and a weight of 27 kg (50th centile). He was febrile, i.e., 38°C. The heart rate was 106 beats per minute, the respiratory rate was 24 breaths per minute. The blood pressure recorded was 90/70 mm Hg.

Pallor was present. Localized edema was present at the lower end of the femur. There was inguinal lymphadenitis on the right side.

Local examination showed that there was a palpable mass at the lower end of the femur. There was limitation of the movement and limping. There was tenderness and local erythema.

■ INVESTIGATION

- *Hemoglobin:* 9 g/dL
- *TLC:* 7,600 cells/mm^3
- *DLC:* $P_{80} L_{18} E_2$
- *Serum alkaline phosphatase:* 200 U/L (*Normal range:* 30–120 U/L)
- *X-ray chest:* No abnormality detected
- *X-ray of the femur:*
  - Sclerosis and periosteal new bone formation
  - Showed well-defined soft-tissue mass, sclerosis, and lysis in the medullary cavity
- *FNAC:* Malignant and pleomorphic spindle cells

■ DISCUSSION

Osteosarcoma is the most common malignant tumor of bone constituting nearly 20% of the malignant tumors of the bone. It occurs in the young population between the ages of 10 and 20 years. It is more common in males. The common sites of occurrence are the distal end of femur (40%), the proximal end of tibia, and the proximal end of humerus in the metaphysis.

The peak incidence occurs in the second decade of life when the most longitudinal growth occurs. The adolescent peak occurs at age 13 years in girls and between ages 15 and 17 years in boys, corresponding with the age of greatest growth velocity in each gender. The peak occurrence during the adolescent growth spurt suggests a casual relationship between rapid bone growth and malignant transformation.

Osteosarcoma is slightly more common in males. Other evidence supporting the relationship with growth includes its skeletal distribution with the majority occurring in regions that undergo the most extensive longitudinal growth. In addition, osteosarcoma typically occurs in the metaphyses of bones, which is the site where new bone arises from the growth plates. Osteosarcoma is rare in children under the age of 5 years.

The highest risk period for the development of osteosarcoma is during the adolescent growth spurt, suggesting an association between rapid bone growth and malignant transformation.

The sites of osteosarcoma in these patients were initially thought to be only in previously irradiated areas, but later, studies show them to arise in sites far from the original retinoblastoma radiation field.

There are some predisposing diseases to osteosarcoma. These include osteochondromatosis, multiple hereditary exostosis, osteogenesis imperfecta, and Paget's disease.

Kindreds with Li–Fraumeni syndrome have a spectrum of malignancies in first-degree relatives, including carcinoma of the breast, soft-tissue sarcomas, brain tumors, leukemia, adrenocortical carcinoma, and other malignancies. Rothmund–Thomson syndrome is a rare condition associated with short stature, skin telangiectasia, small hands and feet, hypoplasticity or absence of the thumbs, and a high risk of osteosarcoma. Osteosarcoma also can be induced by irradiation for EWS, craniospinal irradiation for brain tumors, or high-dose irradiation for other malignancies. Other benign conditions that can be associated with malignant transformation to osteosarcoma include Paget's disease, enchondromatosis, multiple hereditary exostoses, and fibrous dysplasia.

One well-known etiologic factor is ionizing radiation, although there is typically a long interval between irradiation and the development of osteosarcoma, making it less relevant to most pediatric patients. However, it should be noted that the incidence of osteosarcoma is markedly increased among survivors of hereditary retinoblastoma, who harbor germline mutations of the retinoblastoma gene. This risk is further increased in those who received RT as a component of their treatment. Similarly, germline mutations in the *p53* gene (the basis of Li–Fraumeni syndrome) can lead to a high risk of developing multiple malignancies including osteosarcoma. It is a highly malignant spindle cell neoplasm-producing osteosarcoma.

Osteosarcoma is a primary malignant tumor of the bone. It arises from the multipotent mesenchymal tissue of bone. Neoplastic cells will produce osteoid. They arise within medullary canal of the shaft and may break through the cortex of the bone of origin. This will form shaft tissue mass. This can attain a considerable size. The tumor may extend along the medullary cavity.

■ PATHOLOGY

The tumor is located in the metaphyseal region and reaches the subperiosteal area through the cortex. It is grayish white, the consistency may be hard and fleshy with streaks of tumor bone or it may be soft and vascular with areas of hemorrhage. The tumor edge stops at the epiphyseal cartilage and does not break through it. The tumor also extends into the medullary canal. In advanced cases, the tumor breaks through the periosteum, invades the soft tissues, and even fungates through the skin.

The most characteristic features are the anaplastic sarcomatous stroma with newly formed woven bone and the presence of malignant osteoid. It may also show areas of malignant cartilage and fibrous tissue. The stromal cells are spindle-shaped osteoblasts showing excessive mitosis, pleomorphism, and hyperchromatism. There may be areas of hemorrhage and necrosis.

■ PATHOGENESIS

Although the cause of osteosarcoma is unknown, certain genetic or acquired conditions predispose patients to the development of osteosarcoma. Patients with hereditary retinoblastoma have a significantly increased risk for development of osteosarcoma. Predisposition to development of osteosarcoma in these patients may be related to loss of heterozygosity of the *RB* gene. Osteosarcoma also occurs in the Li-Fraumeni syndrome, which is a familial cancer syndrome associated with germline mutations of the *P53* gene.

The pathologic diagnosis of osteosarcoma is made by demonstration of a highly malignant, pleomorphic, spindle cell neoplasm associated with the formation of malignant osteoid and bone. There are four pathologic subtypes of conventional high-grade osteosarcoma: Osteoblastic, fibroblastic, chondroblastic, and telangiectatic.

Osteosarcoma has some important classifications: Two variants of osteosarcoma, parosteal and periosteal, should be distinguished from conventional osteosarcoma because of their characteristic clinical features.

- *Parosteal osteogenic sarcoma (also called juxtacortical osteosarcoma):* It is a well-differentiated extramedullary tumor. This has got a low metastatic potential. This tumor is found exclusively in long bones, for example, femur and shows extensive central ossification. Parosteal osteosarcoma is low-grade, well-differentiated tumor that does not invade the medullary cavity and most commonly is found in the posterior aspect of the distal femur. Surgical resection alone often is curative in this lesion, which has a low propensity for metastatic spread.
- *Periosteal osteogenic sarcoma:* It is a histologically pleomorphic lesion. It clinically behaves more aggressively. Periosteal osteosarcoma is a rare variant that arises on the surface of the bone but has a higher rate of metastatic spread than the parosteal type and an intermediate prognosis.
- *Telangiectatic osteosarcoma:* It is a bloody cystic lesion. It is confused with aneurysmal bone cyst because of its lytic appearance on radiography. High-grade osteosarcoma typically arises in the diaphyseal region of long bones and invades the medullary cavity. It also may be associated with a soft-tissue mass. Surgical resection alone often is curative in this lesion, which has a low propensity for metastatic spread.

CLASSIFICATION

Osteosarcomas are broadly classified as:
- *Central (intramedullary) type:*
  - Primary
    - Conventional
    - Telangiectatic
    - Small cell
    - Multicentric
  - Secondary
    - Paget's disease
    - Radiation-induced
    - Arising from other benign conditions like fibrous dysplasia and osteochondroma
- *Juxtacortical (surface) type:*
  - Parosteal
  - Periosteal
  - Differentiated

CLINICAL FEATURES (FIG. 1)

The onset of the disease is more common among the adolescent period. The mean age of the onset is 15 years. It occurs more frequently within long bones at metaphyseal ends. These are places of most active growth and reconstruction. The most common primary sites are distal femur, proximal humerus, and proximal tibia. The children with bilateral retinoblastoma have an increased incidence of osteosarcoma. The gene associated with retinoblastoma may predispose the patient to osteosarcoma as well.

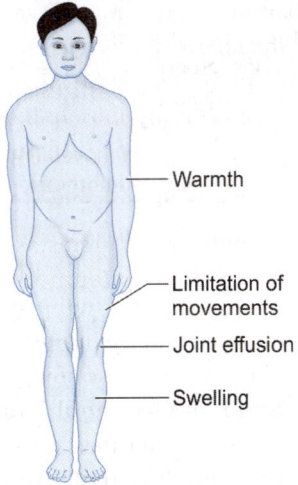

Fig. 1: Clinical features.

The highest risk period for the development of osteosarcoma is during the adolescent growth spurt, suggesting an association between rapid bone growth and malignant transformation. Patients with osteosarcoma are taller than their peers of similar age.

The most common initial finding is pain at the site of the tumor. Later, there is a limitation of movements. Palpable or visible tumor may develop. There may be limping or alteration in gait with involvement of the legs and pelvis. There will be tenderness and local erythema and hyperthermia may occur (Fig. 1).

On examination, the swelling is fusiform and the skin is stretched, shiny, and vascular with prominent veins. The swelling is warm to touch and may also show pulsation if the tumor is very vascular. It is firm to hard in consistency with areas of softening where the tumor has invaded the soft tissues. In the later stages, the tumor fungates. The patient's general health deteriorates with anemia, loss of weight, and cachexia. The patient develops pulmonary symptoms due to secondaries.

> **ESSENTIAL DIAGNOSTIC POINTS**
> - Occurs in long tubular bones, arises from metaphysis
> - Pain is the initial symptom
> - Bone swelling, progressively increasing in size
> - Radiography; trabecular pattern with indistinct margin
> - Limping and limitation of movements
> - Pleural effusion and pneumothorax

The common site of metastasis is lung. Pleural effusion and pneumothorax can occur. Other sites of metastasis include other bones, hilar lymph node, and CNS.

> **GENERAL FEATURES**
> - Pain
> - Tenderness
> - Fever

DIAGNOSIS

Persistent unexplained bone pain, associated with a palpable mass, requires radiography. In radiograph, sclerosis of the bone and periosteal new bone formation are common. It shows permeative destruction of normal bony trabecular pattern with indistinct margin.

The tumor arises at the metaphyseal region of the bone, either centrally or over the cortex. There are mottled areas of rarefaction with areas of osteosclerosis. When it extends beyond the cortex, the periosteum is raised and there is new bone formation in lines at right angles to the cortex. This causes the "sun-ray" appearance on the radiograph. There is also reactive new bone formation subperiosteally to the junction of the lifted periosteum and the normal bone. This is called Codman triangle. The radiographs may also show a pathological fracture.

Radiograph of the chest must be taken. It may show round shadows caused by secondary deposits (cannon-ball appearance).

Results of routine laboratory tests, such as a complete blood cell count and chemistry panel, are usually normal, although alkaline phosphatase or LDH values may be elevated.

The recommended imaging studies for osteosarcoma at the time of diagnosis are a plain radiograph and MRI. As with other musculoskeletal conditions, such as slipped capital femoral epiphysis (SCFE), symptom localization in osteosarcoma may not be precise. Consequently, if symptoms persist and imaging is negative, obtaining imaging of adjacent bones or joints should be considered.

A plain radiograph is often the most appropriate initial test to order if the presence of a malignant bone tumor is suspected. A plain radiograph often identifies the anatomic region of abnormality and shows features of the bone and tumor that help narrow the differential diagnosis.

On plain radiographs, osteosarcoma usually has a mixed pattern of bone lysis and sclerosis, the boundary between tumor and normal bone is usually irregular, and the bone cortex is often disrupted by tumor growth into the surrounding soft tissue. Osteoid formation within the tumor results in areas of calcification visible in the bony and soft-tissue components of the tumor. Periosteal new bone formation in osteosarcoma can be irregular or can occur in a sunburst pattern.

Magnetic resonance imaging should be performed with contrast, and the entire bone from which the tumor arises as well as the closest adjacent joint should be imaged.

Before the biopsy, MRI of the primary lesion and the entire bone should be performed to evaluate the tumor for its proximity to nerves and blood vessels, soft tissue, joint extension, and skip lesions. The metastatic workup, which should be performed before biopsy, includes CT of the chest and radionuclide bone scanning to evaluate for lung and bone metastases, respectively. The differential diagnosis of a lytic bone lesion includes histiocytosis, EWS, lymphoma, and bone cyst.

Cranial irradiation with intrathecal MTX has been in use as CNS preventive therapy. This causes significant adverse effect on neurocognitive function in some survivors. Hence, most Western protocols reserve cranial irradiation for patients with CNS disease at presentation and those who are at high-risk for CNS relapse. Children younger than 3 years of age are given high-dose chemotherapy using cytosine arabinoside, in an attempt to prevent radiation to the developing brain.

The tumor is pleomorphic, spindle cell tumor that forms an extracellular matrix of osteoid. Metastatic bony lesions and lung involvement must be looked at. It includes CT scan of the chest. MRI provides the best assessment of tumor extent to plan surgery.

In all cases, the diagnosis should be established by a biopsy. This should be done at the growing periphery of the tumor, which gives the typical microscopic appearance.

PET-CT may be considered in monitoring the response to treatment.

> **LABORATORY SALIENT FINDINGS**
> - *Radiographic findings:* Mottled areas of rarefaction, periosteum is raised, new bone formation in lines at right angles to cortex—sun-ray appearance
> - CT scan and MRI of chest and bone scan
> - Biopsy
> - Histopathological examination
>
> CT: computed tomography, MRI: magnetic resonance imaging

DIFFERENTIAL DIAGNOSIS

Differential diagnosis of osteosarcoma includes:
- EWS
- Osteomyelitis
- Septic arthritis

TREATMENT

Broadly speaking, the treatment of osteosarcoma is usually a combination of surgery, RT, and chemotherapy. Osteosarcomas are fully radioresistant lesions.

Surgery

Complete surgical resection of the tumor is important for cure. The current approach is to treat patients with preoperative chemotherapy in an attempt to facilitate limb-salvage operations and to treat micrometastatic disease immediately. Up to 80% of patients are able to undergo limb salvage operations after initial chemotherapy. It is important to resume chemotherapy as soon as possible after surgery. Lung metastases present at diagnosis should be resected by thoracotomies at some time during the course of treatment. Active agents currently in use for multidrug chemotherapy regimens for conventional osteosarcoma include doxorubicin, cisplatin, MTX, and ifosfamide.

A limb-saving surgery may be possible if the case is diagnosed early and the lesion is small. In such a situation, after neoadjuvant chemotherapy, the lesion is excised widely, including a margin of normal tissue all around and the gap thus created may be bridged by bone grafts or artificial prosthesis whatever is feasible.

Amputation remains the mainstay of treatment if limb salvage is not feasible. The amputation can be a palliative amputation if the disease is advanced. In this situation, the goal of the operation is either pain relief or to prevent complications in a fungating tumor. A definitive amputation removes the tumor completely. The level of amputation and the length of the remaining stump of the limb, etc., can be better planned.

For patients who require amputation, early prosthetic fitting and gait training are essential to enable patients to resume normal activities as soon as possible. Before definitive surgery, patients with tumors of weight-bearing bones should be instructed to use crutches to avoid stressing the weakened bones and causing pathologic fractures. The role of chemotherapy in parosteal and periosteal osteosarcomas is not well defined, and chemotherapy is generally reserved for use in patients with tumors that have a high-grade microscopic appearance.

Contraindications for limb-saving surgery include major involvement of neurovascular bundle by tumor, immature skeletal age, inappropriate biopsy site, and extensive muscle involvement.

Radiotherapy

Radiotherapy is indicated for local control of the disease after incomplete surgical removal of the tumor and also for tumors situated at surgically inaccessible sites.

Chemotherapy

Chemotherapy is often administered prior to the definitive surgery—neoadjuvant therapy. This permits an early attack on micrometastatic disease and may also shrink the tumor, facilitating limb-salvage procedure. Preoperative chemotherapy makes detailed histologic evaluation of tumor response to chemotherapy agents possible. If the histological response is poor, postoperative chemotherapy can be changed accordingly. Chemotherapy can be given intra-arterially or intravenously.

It consists of drugs—MTX, bleomycin, cyclophosphamide, adriamycin, doxorubicin, ifosfamide, and cisplatinum—given pre and/or postoperatively to control the micrometastasis. A regular follow-up every 3 months is mandatory to detect any recurrence or spread of the tumor in time. Postsurgical chemotherapy is generally continued until the patient has received 1 year of treatment.

■ PROGNOSIS

The prognosis is best with low-grade tumor such as parosteal osteosarcoma or juxtacortical osteosarcoma. More than two-thirds of patients presenting without metastasis have long-term survival and are cured. The cure rate in metastatic disease is <25%.

One of the most important prognostic factors in osteosarcoma is the histologic response to chemotherapy. An international cooperative group is performing a randomized trial of the postoperative addition of high-dose ifosfamide with etoposide to standard three-drug therapy with cisplatin, doxorubicin, and MTX to improve the patients with poor histologic response. After limb salvage surgery, intensive rehabilitation and physical therapy are necessary to ensure maximal functional outcome.

The most important prognostic factor in the treatment of osteosarcoma is the presence of grossly visible metastatic disease at the time of diagnosis, which confers a much worse prognosis. That said, the general principles of treatment for these patients remain the same, including chemotherapy and resection of all sites of bulk disease, including pulmonary metastases.

Other adverse prognostic factors include older age and an unresectable primary tumor, which can be related to tumor site or tumor size. Approximately 80% of patients with osteosarcoma are diagnosed with localized disease and with current therapy 60–70% of those patients will be long-term survivors.

Patients with the localized disease having 90% or greater turnout necrosis have 70–75% long-term disease survival rate. Favorable prognostic factors include distal skeletal lesion, longer duration of symptoms, age older than 20 years, female gender, and near diploid tumor DNA index.

■ BIBLIOGRAPHY

1. Geller DS, Gorlik R. Osteosarcoma: A review of diagnosis, management and treatment strategies. Clin Adv Hematol Oncol. 2010; 8(10):705-18.
2. Grimer RJ. Surgical options for children with osteosarcoma. Lancet Oncol. 2005;6(2): 85-92.

CASE 98

Retinoblastoma

PRESENTING COMPLAINTS

A 20-month-old boy was brought with the complaint of:
- Asymmetric movements of eyeball since 2 months
- Doubtful vision in the left eye since 1 month

History of Presenting Complaints

A 20-month-old boy was brought to the pediatric outpatient department with history of squint in left eye. His mother complained that he was apparently normal till 2 months back. Later she noticed the asymmetric movement of the eyeball. It was more on the left side. She even developed the doubt whether the child could see with left eye. Hence, she brought him to the hospital. There was no history of pain or trauma to eye.

Past History of the Patient

The boy was the only sibling of a consanguineous marriage. He was born at full term by normal vaginal delivery. The baby cried immediately after the delivery. There was no significant postnatal event. The mother and child were discharged on third day. The child was on breast milk exclusively for the first 3 months. Weaning started later, and child was on normal family food from 15 months. All the developmental milestones are normal. He had been completely immunized.

CASE AT A GLANCE

Basic Findings
Height	: 83 cm (50th centile)
Weight	: 11 kg (75th centile)
Temperature	: 38°C
Pulse rate	: 116 beats/min
Respiratory rate	: 26 breaths/min
Blood pressure	: 60/46 mm Hg

Positive Findings

History:
- Squint
- Doubtful of vision

Examination:
- Loss of vision
- Squint

Investigation:
- *Fundoscopy:* Presence of white reflex
- *Plain X-ray skull:* Calcification

EXAMINATION

Child was moderately built and nourished. He was playing with toys on examination table. On careful observation, it was found that he was moving his whole body for toys on left side to play with them.

There was conjugate gaze on left eye. Eye examination revealed presence of loss of vision on left eye with squint. Anthropometric measurements included the height 83 cm (50th centile) and the weight 11 kg (75th centile). The head circumference was 46 cm.

He was febrile, the heart rate was 116 beats/min, and the respiratory rate was

26 breaths/min. The blood pressure recorded was 60/46 mm Hg. There was no pallor and no lymphadenopathy. There was no cyanosis and clubbing. Fundus examination showed presence of white reflex. Other systemic examinations were normal.

■ INVESTIGATION

- *Hemoglobin:* 13 g/dL
- *TLC:* 7,600 cells/cumm
- *ESR:* 32 mm in the first hour
- *AEC:* 340 cells/dL
- *Plain X-ray skull:* Calcification is seen within the globe
- *Fundoscopy:* Presence of white reflex is evident

■ DISCUSSION

Retinoblastoma is the most common primary malignant intraocular tumor of childhood. It occurs in approximately 1 in 20,000 infants.

Retinoblastoma is an embryonal malignancy of the retina and the most common intraocular tumor in children. Retinoblastoma progresses to metastatic disease and death in over 50% of children worldwide.

In heritable cases, the first mutation arises during gametogenesis, either spontaneously (90%), or through transmission from parents (10%). This mutation is present in every retinal cell and in all other somatic and germ cells. 90% of persons, who carry this germline mutation will develop retinoblastoma.

For tumor formation loss of second RB1 allele within the cell must occur. Loss only is insufficient for tumor formation. The second mutation occurs in somatic (retinal) cell. In inheritable cases (60%) both mutation arise in somatic cell after gametogenesis has taken place.

Hereditary and nonhereditary patterns of transmission occur; there is no sex or race predilection. The average age at diagnosis for bilateral tumor is 12 months and for unilateral tumors it is 21 months.

In trilateral retinoblastoma syndrome, pineal tumors develop in approximately 1 in 100 patients with bilateral ocular disease. Characteristically, the diagnosis is made by ophthalmoscopic, radiographic, and ultrasonographic appearance, without pathologic confirmation. The locus is present on chromosome 13. It is associated with osteosarcoma, pineal tumor, and lung and breast cancer.

Genetics and Molecular Biology

Different causative mutations have been identified, including translocations, deletions, insertions, point mutations, and epigenetic modifications such as gene methylation. The nature of the predisposing mutation can affect the penetrance and expressivity of retinoblastoma development.

According to Knudson's "2-hit" model of oncogenesis, two mutational events are required for retinoblastoma tumor development. In the hereditary form of retinoblastoma, the first mutation in RB1 is inherited through germinal cells, and a second mutation occurs subsequently in somatic retinal cells. Second mutations that lead to retinoblastoma often result in the loss of the normal allele and concomitant loss of heterozygosity. Heterozygous carriers of oncogenic RB1 mutations demonstrate variable phenotypic expression.

It occurs either spontaneously or as an inherited disorder. Retinoblastoma shows an autosomal dominant inheritance pattern with high penetrance. Approximately 55% of tumor occur as nonhereditary, unifocal, unilateral tumor.

An additional 15% are unilateral, but are hereditary with a family history. 30% occur as heritable bilateral unifocal or multifocal tumors. Hereditary cases usually are diagnosed at a younger age and are multifocal and bilateral, whereas sporadic cases are usually diagnosed in older children who tend to have unilateral, unifocal involvement.

The retinoblastoma gene is a tumor suppressor gene and retinoblastoma tumors are homozygous for chromosome 13q14 abnormalities with either deletions or alterations of genetic material at that locus. The hereditary form is associated with loss of function of the retinoblastoma gene (RB1) via gene mutation or deletion. The RB1 gene is located on chromosome 13q14 and encodes the retinoblastoma protein, a tumor-suppressor protein that controls cell-cycle phase transition and has roles in apoptosis and cell differentiation. Hereditary cases show a germline abnormality in one gene at this locus. Some affected children have other systemic features of the 13q deletion syndrome.

Genetic counseling for patients with retinoblastoma and their families is complex, but a few generalizations can be made. Patients with the hereditary form are at risk for other cancers later in life, including soft tissue and bone sarcomas and melanoma. This risk is increased in patients treated with RT. It is estimated that 10% of individuals who carry an abnormal RB1 gene do not develop retinoblastoma, because the second event did not occur in any cell; however, they are still at risk of developing other cancers during their lifetime.

Screening: Children with a positive family history of retinoblastoma should undergo a dilated eye examination under general anesthesia early in life and at regular intervals until genetic testing is performed and results are available. Infants with a negative genetic test require no further screening; infants with a positive genetic test require regular screening ophthalmologic examinations until age of 5 years.

PATHOLOGY

This tumor, which usually arises from the posterior portion of the retina, consists of small sound closely packed malignant cells with scanty cytoplasm. Tumor may grossly appear crumbly and friable with gelatinous areas of degradation and patches of calcification or pigmented hemorrhage. It may appear as a single tumor in the retina, but typically has multiple foci.

Tumors can also be both endophytic and exophytic. The growth may be endophytic (forward into the vitreous cavity) or exophytic (into the subretinal space with detachment of retina). Endophytic tumors arise from the inner surface *of* the retina and grow into the vitreous, and can also grow as tumors suspended within the vitreous itself, known as vitreous seeding. Exophytic tumors grow from the outer retinal layer and can cause retinal detachment. Diffuse infiltrating tumors grow intraretinally and remain flat. These are less common and can cause iris neovascularization. The tumor fragments may break off and float free in the vitreous to seed other parts of retina. The most frequent extraocular sites of involvement are the optic nerve, orbit and periorbital tissues, cranial tissue, and bone and bone marrow.

Histologically, retinoblastoma appears as a small, round, blue cell tumor with rosette formation (Flexner–Wintersteiner rosettes). It may arise in any of the nucleated layers of the retina and exhibit various degrees of differentiation. Retinoblastoma tumors tend to outgrow their blood supply, resulting in necrosis and calcification.

These tumors can also spread by direct extension to the choroid or along the optic nerve beyond the lamina cribrosa to the CNS, or by hematogenous or lymphatic spread to distant sites, including bones, bone marrow, and lungs.

■ CLINICAL FEATURES (FIG. 1)

It is the most common primary ocular tumor of childhood arising from embryonic retina. This occurs between 3 and 5 years. There is no sex predilection.

The most common presenting sign of retinoblastoma is leukocoria. When a tumor is small and at the macula, the initial sign may be sensory strabismus. When disease is very advanced, presenting symptoms may include pain due to secondary glaucoma, buphthalmos, proptosis, hyphema, or orbital cellulitis.

The differential diagnosis of retinoblastoma includes persistent hyperplastic primary vitreous (PHPV), retinal detachment, Coats disease, glial hamartoma, retinal hemangioma, myelinated nerve fibers, congenital cataract, chorioretinal coloboma, uveitis, larval granulomatosis, congenital retinal folds, retinal dysplasia, and retinopathy of prematurity.

The tumor usually presents with leukokoria **(Figs. 2A and B)**, i.e., yellow white reflex in the pupil. Other presenting complaints may be loss of vision reflected as a squint in the affected eye. The other symptoms may be pain, pupillary irregularity, and hyphema. Proptosis may present with advanced tumor. There may be signs of increased intracranial pressure. There may be bone pain associated with metastatic disease.

The common presenting sign is strabismus followed by painful glaucoma, redness of eye, diminished vision.

Tumor spreads locally—bones, CSF, bone marrow, liver, and spleen. Extension of retinoblastoma into choroid usually occurs with massive tumors. This may indicate hematogenous metastasis. Extensions of tumor through lamina cribrosa and optic nerve will lead to involvement of CNS.

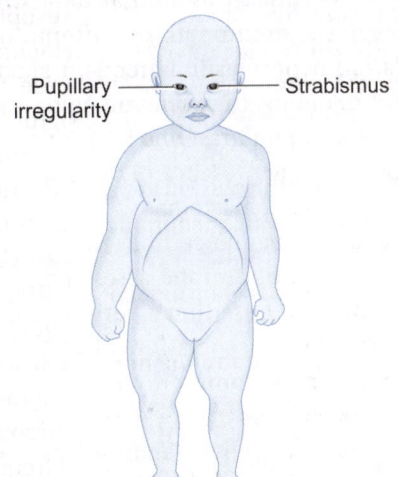

Fig. 1: General features.

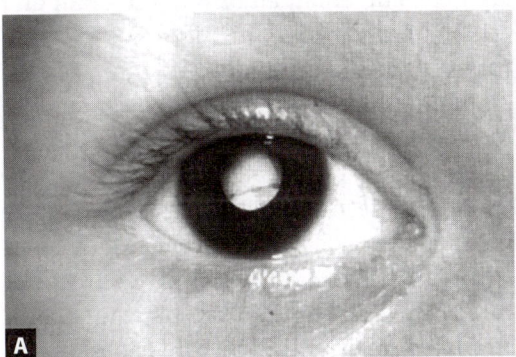
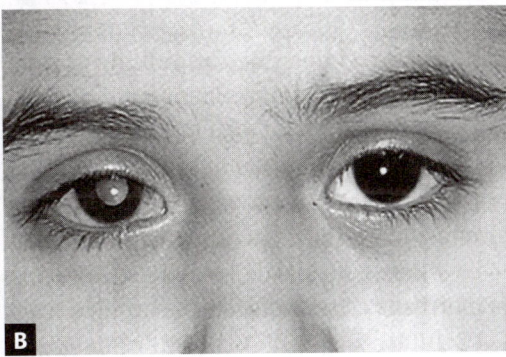

Figs. 2A and B: Leukocorea.

For proper staging children should have CT scan of the orbit and skull assessment of local orbital and intracranial extension, bone marrow biopsy, and CSF examination for cytology. Rarely, a painful eye with glaucoma, hyphema, or proptosis are the initial manifestation. Bilateral involvement is seen in 20–30% of children.

GENERAL FEATURES
- White pupillary reflex
- Orbital inflammation
- Hyphemia
- Glaucoma
- Retinal detachment

ESSENTIAL DIAGNOSTIC POINTS
- It is the neuroectodermal malignancy
- Arises from embryonic retinal cells
- Leukocoria, unusual appearance asymmetry of eyes
- Strabismus is present

■ DIAGNOSIS

Diagnosis is by finding of the leukokoria. Other causes of white reflex include retinal detachment, hyperplasia of primary vitreous, visceral larva migrans, cataract, coloboma of choroid, and retinopathy of prematurity. The findings of leukokoria must be followed by careful fundoscopic examination under anesthesia.

Indirect ophthalmoscopy with slit-lamp evaluation can detect retinoblastoma tumors, but a complete evaluation requires an examination under general anesthesia by unexperienced ophthalmologist to obtain complete visualization of both eyes, which also facilitates photographing and mapping of the tumors. Retinal detachment or vitreous hemorrhage can complicate the evaluation.

Orbital USG, CT, or MRI is used to evaluate the extent of intraocular disease and extraocular spread. Occasionally (60%), a pineal area (primitive neuroectodermal) tumor is detected in a child rise in with hereditary and bilateral retinoblastoma, a phenomenon known as trilateral retinoblastoma. MRI allows for better evaluation of optic nerve involvement.

Computed tomography scan of the orbit should be performed to evaluate extent of tumor and to assess whether optic nerve, bony structures or pineal gland are involved. Most intraocular retinoblastoma show evidence of intratumoral calcification.

Ultrasound may aid in the differential diagnosis, which includes other causes of leukokoria such as retinal detachment or dysplasia, retinopathy of prematurity, persistent hyperplastic vitreous, nematode endophthalmitis, cataract, and coloboma of the choroids. An ultrasound of the globe can demonstrate the presence of calcium, which is typical of retinoblastoma.

Magnetic resonance image of the brain is an essential part of the assessment of all children with hereditary retinoblastoma because of the association of a PNET in the brain, most commonly located in the pineal region. This trilateral retinoblastoma syndrome is usually diagnosed at a very young age, and screening and early detection may improve survival. If metastatic disease is a consideration, an MRI of the brain and spine, bone scan, bone marrow aspiration and biopsy, and a lumbar puncture to examine the CSF for tumor cells should be performed. These are not routinely indicated if the history, examination, blood count, and MRI indicate intraocular disease only.

Radionuclide bone scan and examination of bone marrow and CSF for tumor cells are necessary only if there is evidence of transscleral extension or extension beyond the cut end of optic nerve. Metastatic disease of the bone marrow and meninges can be ruled out with bilateral bone marrow aspiration and biopsies plus CSF cytology.

> **LABORATORY SALIENT FINDINGS**
> - Fundus examination: White or creamy pink mass protruding into the vitreous
> - CT scan of the orbit
> - Bone marrow aspirate and biopsy
> - CSF cytology
> - Bone scan, CT scan of liver
>
> (CSF: cerebrospinal fluid; CT: computed tomography)

■ DIFFERENTIAL DIAGNOSIS

- Retinal detachment
- Vitreous hemorrhage
- Cataract
- Choroidal coloboma
- Retinopathy of prematurity

The differential diagnosis of retinoblastoma includes other causes of leukocoria, including PHPV, Coats disease, vitreous hemorrhage, cataract, endophthalmitis from *Toxocara canis*, choroidal coloboma, retinopathy of prematurity, and familial exudative vitreoretinopathy.

■ TREATMENT

The primary goal of treatment is always cure; the secondary goals include preserving vision and the eye itself and decreasing the risk of late side effects, mainly secondary malignancies.

The modalities of treatment include photocoagulation, localized radioactive plaque, and systemic chemotherapy.

Cryotherapy, photocoagulation, and radioactive plaques can be used for local tumor control.

It is highly curable when the disease is intraocular. Local therapy includes cryotherapy, photo (laser) coagulation, brachytherapy (plaque) radiation, and/or external beam RT. It enhances the risk of secondary malignancy.

Local ophthalmic measures include laser photocoagulation, thermotherapy, and/or cryotherapy.

Laser therapy includes argon or diode laser is the primary treatment for smaller tumors, but is also sometimes used after chemoreduction.

Cryotherapy: A special probe is applied through the sclera to produce low temperature ($-60°$ to $-80°C$) is suitable for tumors smaller than 4 disc diameters close to retina.

Chemotherapy: It enables salvaging the affected eye, avoiding enucleation or external beam RT and risk of secondary malignancies. Systemic chemotherapy includes combination of vincristine, carboplatin, and etoposide. Chemotherapy may also be used for chemoreduction, as an adjunct modality or for therapy of metastasis. Newer routes of drug (melphalan, carboplatin) administration by periocular, intravitreal, and intraophthalmic artery injection have improved outcomes in intraocular retinoblastoma.

Radiotherapy: External beam RT is considered, if chemotherapy and focal therapy fail. Although this approach may result in significant orbital deformity and increased incidence of second malignancies in patients with germline RB1 mutations. RT may lead to orbital deformity, sicca syndrome, cataract, radiation retinopathy, neovascular glaucoma, and risk of a second malignancy.

Hematopoietic stem cell transplantation: Patients with extraocular disease have poor prognosis with respect to the survival. Those with regional extraocular disease (involving orbit, optic nerve, or periauricular region) may be treated with a combination of conventional chemotherapy and external beam RT. Patients with distant metastasis require high-dose chemotherapy, external beam RT, and HSCT.

Photocoagulation is generally used for small tumors confined to the retina. Peripheral tumors too large to be treated effectively with photocoagulation may be treated more appropriately with cryotherapy. This combined approach of chemoreduction followed by local therapy has been shown to improve visual outcome and delay or avoid external beam radiation and enucleation. More recently, promising alternate routes of chemotherapy delivery such as intra-arterial (ophthalmic artery) or intravitreal injections have been employed in an attempt to preserve the affected eyes in both unilateral and bilateral retinoblastoma.

Most unilateral disease presents with a solitary, large tumor. Enucleation is performed if there is no potential for the salvage of useful vision. With bilateral disease, chemoreduction in combination with focal therapy (laser photocoagulation or cryotherapy) has replaced the traditional approach of enucleation of the more severely affected eye and irradiation of the remaining eye. The dose of the irradiation is 4,000–4,500 rads if there is painful glaucoma eye should be enucleated. Irradiation is preferred if tumor is very small.

Absolute indications for enucleation are no vision, glaucoma, inability to examine the treated eye, and inability to control tumor growth conservative treatment.

If feasible, small tumors can be treated with focal therapy with careful follow-up for recurrence or new tumor growth; larger tumors often respond to multiagent chemotherapy, including carboplatin, vincristine, and etoposide. If this approach fails, external-beam irradiation should be considered, although this approach may result in significant orbital deformity and increased incidence of second malignancies in patients with germline RB1 mutations. Brachytherapy, or episcleral plaque RT, is an alternative with less morbidity. Enucleation may be required for unresponsive or recurrent tumors.

When enucleation is planned an attempt should be made to resect as much optic nerves as possible, i.e., 10 mm or more. Radiation therapy should be considered if there is regional extraocular extension of tumor found at the time of enucleation.

Chemotherapy is also used as an adjunct to primary surgery in those cases that are high risk for metastases, such as eyes with optic nerve, massive choroidal or scleral invasion. Children with metastatic retinoblastoma require more intensive therapy. Modalities include systemic chemotherapy, external beam RT, and high-dose chemotherapy followed by autologous hematopoietic stem cell rescue.

Patients with extraocular and metastatic disease or those considered to be a great risk for metastatic disease because of significant involvement of choroid, sclera, or ciliary body or because of extension of tumor beyond lamina cribrosa should be treated with combination chemotherapy probably including carboplatin, etoposide, and vincristine.

Local therapy such as laser therapy, cryotherapy, RT, or enucleation should be considered depending upon the response to chemotherapy. Bone marrow transplantation has been advocated for metastatic retinoblastoma.

Alternative treatment options currently under investigation include other systemic chemotherapy agents, such as topotecan, and intense multiagent chemotherapy with autologous stem cell rescue for patients with metastatic disease.

■ PROGNOSIS

The overall survival rate is >90%, although survival into the third and fourth decades of life may be decreased considerably, by the high incidence of second malignancies. The prognosis is directly related to the size and extension of the tumor. Most tumors that are confined to the eye can be cured. Cures are infrequent when extensive orbital or optic nerve extension has occurred or patient has CNS or distal metastasis.

Children with retinoblastoma confined to the retina (whether unilateral or bilateral) have excellent prognosis with 5-year survival rate >90%. Mortality is directly correlated with optic nerve involvement, orbital extension of tumor, and choroid invasion. Patient's disease in optic nerve beyond the lamina cribrosa have 5-year survival rate of 40%. Meningeal and metastatic spread will rarely survive.

■ BIBLIOGRAPHY

1. Abramson DH, Schefler AC. Update on retinoblastoma. Retina. 2004;24:828-48.
2. Canty CA. Retinoblastoma: an overview for advanced practice nurses. J Am Acad Nurse Pract. 2009;21(3)149-55.
3. Kiss S, Mukai S. Diagnosis, classification, and treatment of retinoblastoma. Int Ophthalmol Clin. 2008;48(2):135-47.
4. Rodriguez-Galindo C et al.; Treatment of intraocular retiblastoma with vincristine and caroplatin.
5. Shields CL, Meadows AT, Leahey AM, Shields JA. Continuing challenges in the management of retinoblastoma with chemotherapy. Retina. 2004;24:849-62.

CASE 99

Wilms' Tumor

■ PRESENTING COMPLAINTS

A 6-year-old girl was brought with the complaint of:
- Abdominal pain since 3 days
- Fever since 2 days
- Breathlessness since 1 day

History of Presenting Complaints

A 6-year-old girl presented with history of abdominal pain for 3 days. The pain was present in right side. There was radiation of pain down to medial aspects of thigh. Her mother also gave history of fever which was of moderate to high degree. It used to be intermittent and more so in evening. It was associated with chills and rigors. There was no history of vomiting and bowel disturbances. Later child becomes much toxic, restless, and also breathless. Then the child was brought to the hospital.

Past History of the Patient

The child was the second sibling of consanguineous marriage. She was delivered at term by normal vaginal delivery. She cried immediately after the delivery. There was no significant postnatal event. The child was on breast milk exclusively for the first 4 months. Later weaning was started, and child was on family food by 15 months of age. She never had any urinary and bowel disturbances. She had been completely immunized. Her developmental milestones were normal. Her performance at school was above average.

■ EXAMINATION

The child was moderately built and nourished. She was looking much anxious. She was pale. Anthropometric measurements included her

CASE AT A GLANCE

Basic Findings
Height	: 116 cm (75th centile)
Weight	: 15 kg (25th centile)
Temperature	: 38°C
Pulse rate	: 120 beats/min
Respiratory rate	: 40 breaths/min
Blood pressure	: 90/60 mm Hg

Positive Findings

History:
- Abdominal pain
- Fever

Examination:
- Abdominal mass
- Tenderness
- Abdominal distension
- PSM of grade 3/6

Investigation:
- Urine: RBCs ++, protein ++
- Ultrasound abdomen: Large mass, displaced aorta, IVC not visible
- Excretory urogram: Displacement of pelvis and calyces

(IVC: inferior vena cava; PSM: pan systolic murmur; RBC: red blood cell)

height 116 cm (75th centile) and weight 15 kg (25th centile).

She was febrile, the pulse rate was 120 beats/min, and the respiratory rate was 40 breaths/min. The blood pressure recorded was 90/60 mm Hg. There was pallor, no clubbing, no cyanosis, and no lymphadenopathy.

Per abdomen examination revealed presence of abdominal distension. A large mass was palpable. It was present on right loin and was tender. Bowel sounds were normal. Cardiac examination revealed presence of grade 3/6 pansystolic murmur in left sternal edge.

■ INVESTIGATION

- *Hemoglobin:* 6 g/dL
- *TLC:* 9,660 cells/mm^3
- *ESR:* 36 mm in first hour
- *Urine examination:* Protein ++ RBCs ++
- *Ultrasound abdomen:* Normal organs could not be visualized because of large right-sided mass; aorta is displaced to left kidney and IVC cannot be visualized
- *Excretory urogram:* It showed tumor originating from lower pole of kidney displacing pelvis and calyces upward

■ DISCUSSION

Large right-sided abdominal mass with hematuria suggests nephroblastoma. The child started developing signs of tricuspid regurgitation possibly because of disruption of tricuspid valve due to tumor thrombus impinging on valve. Congestive cardiac failure should be treated first.

Wilms' tumor develops as a result of abnormalities in the development of metanephric blastoma. It is the second most common malignant tumor of abdomen in childhood. It is the most common malignant tumor of kidney. Bilateral disease is more common among familial type.

It is congenital in origin. The usual age of onset is 4 months to 6 years. It is mainly unilateral. About 5–10% may have bilateral disease. 1.5% cases of WT are familial. It constitutes 6% of all childhood cancers.

Tumor appears as a large well-defined capsulated mass that replaces the kidney tissue. It is soft and pliable. It may grow into the surrounding tissues. Metastasis occurs in liver and lungs. Prognosis is better in tumors with the dominance of epithelial components.

It can arise in one or both kidneys; the incidence of bilateral WT is 7%. In 8–10% of patients, WT is observed in the context of hemihypertrophy, aniridia, genitourinary anomalies, and a variety of rare syndromes, including BWS and Denys–Drash syndrome. An earlier age at diagnosis and an increased incidence of bilateral disease are generally observed in syndromic and familial cases.

Germline truncating mutations are usually associated with WT in the context of genitourinary anomalies or the WAGR syndrome (WT, aniridia, genitourinary anomalies, mental retardation). Missense germline mutations are usually observed in children with Denys–Drash syndrome, resulting in early-onset renal failure. In instances of germline mutation, the wild-type allele present in the germline is mutated or lost in the tumor, resulting in loss of WT1 function.

The *Wnt signaling pathway* plays a critical role in regulating the differentiation of the fetal kidney. CTNNB1 encodes β-catenin, which has a major regulatory point in this pathway, and CTNNBI mutations are observed in approximately 15% of WTs, very often those that have sustained WTI mutations. WTX, a gene located on the X chromosome that encodes a protein that also plays a role in Wnt pathway regulation, is mutated in approximately 20% of tumors. CTNNBI and WTX mutations are somatic.

One class of genes encodes proteins essential for the biogenesis of mature miRNAs and are mutated in one-fifth to one-third of WT. DROSHA missense mutations in the catalytic domains critical or the processing of pre-miRNA occur in approximately 10% of tumors. These are invariably heterozygous, and in vitro studies have supported a dominant-negative mechanism of action by which they impair miRNA biogenesis. Additionally, mutations genes encoding other components of the miRNA biogenesis pathway (DICER, DGCR8, XPO5, and TARBP2) are observed in WT. DICER1 mutations are usually missense mutations and can be somatic or germline. Germline DICER1 mutations are observed, albeit infrequently, in WT families and, more frequently, in families with pleuropulmonary blastoma.

Germline mutations have been identified in a minority of families, and each of those genes identified (e.g., *WT1*, *DICER1*, *MYCN*, *REST*, *BRCA2*) is altered in <5% of WT families.

■ EPIDEMIOLOGY

The median age at diagnosis of WT is approximately 3.5 years, with some variation based on gender and ethnic group. The majority of WT cases occur prior to 5 years of age, and WT is very rare in children over 10 years of age. Renal cell carcinoma (RCC) is the second most common renal neoplasm in pediatric and adolescent patients, accounting for 2–6% of renal malignancies in this age-group. While WT is more common in younger children, RCC is most common in ages 15–19 years old.

Wilms' tumor cases that have been reported are WAGR, Denys-Drash (WT diffuse mesangial sclerosis leading to early-onset renal failure, and intersex disorders that can range from ambiguous to normal-appearing female genitalia in both XY and XX individuals), and BWS (embryonal tumors, macrosomia, macroglossia, hemihyperplasia, visceromegaly; omphalocele, neonatal hypoglycemia, and ear creases/pits).

Wilms' tumor has been reported to be associated with hemihypertrophy, aniridia, genitourinary anomalies, and various anomalies. Genitourinary anomalies are the most common and account for incidence of 4–8%. The anomalies include fused kidney, renal dysplasia, cryptorchidism, hypospadias, duplication of the collecting system, WAGR syndrome. WT is also featured in many disorders of overgrowth including BWS, Perlman syndrome, and isolated hemihypertrophy.

Although most patients with WT are karyotypically normal, genomic studies have led to the localization and subsequent cloning of WT genes in two regions—11p13 and 11p15. The former is *WT1* gene and is associated with WAGR syndrome and the latter is *WT2* gene, which is associated with BWS.

The important deletion that is found in patients with WT is the deletion in the region of 11p13 with large deletion malformation such as mental retardation, aniridia, abnormal genitalia are found.

■ PATHOLOGY

While the classic description of WT is of triphasic morphology, including blastemal, stromal, and epithelial elements, remarkable histologic diversity can be seen among these tumors. The variety of cellular types and patterns that are normally seen in the developing kidney can be found in WT. Further, tissues that are not usually noted within the kidney, such as skeletal muscle, cartilage, and squamous epithelium, also can be present. It is postulated that a variety of cell types arise due to the pluripotent potential of the primitive metanephric blastemal cells.

On gross examination, areas of tumor within the kidney are well-circumscribed, lobular masses, and are usually gray or pink in color. Multiple nodules of differing sizes can be found, and cystic changes, necrosis, and hemorrhage are often seen. These tumors are frequently friable.

The classic triphasic WT [favorable histology (FH)] is made up of varying proportions of three cells types—blastema stromal and epithelial cells, recapitulating stages of normal renal development. Unfavorable histology is characterized by qualitative variation from the classical type. Presence of focal or diffuse anaplasia, clear cell sarcoma, and rhabdoid tumor is considered to be unfavorable histologic features. Most WT are unicentric, 11% are multicentric but unilateral and 7% are bilateral.

> **ESSENTIAL DIAGNOSTIC POINTS**
> - Asymptomatic abdominal mass, or swelling
> - Hematuria, fever
> - Hypertension
> - Genitourinary malformations
> - Aniridia, hemihypertrophy

■ CLINICAL FEATURES (FIG. 1)

The most common initial clinical presentation is the mass, which can be quite large, because retroperitoneal masses can grow unhampered by strict anatomic boundaries. The child may present with mass in abdomen. Pain in the abdomen or hematuria are rarely seen. Aniridia and hemihypertrophy may be associated.

Cataract, genitourinary abnormalities, and mental retardation are present. A nontender mass is palpable in the renal area. It generally does not cross the midline. At time mass is pushed. Hypertension is present in approximately 25% is of tumors at presentation and has been attributed to increased renin activity. Palpation should be gentle and minimum to obviate the spread of metastasis.

Abdominal pain, gross painless hematuria, and fever are other frequent findings at diagnosis. Occasionally, rapid abdominal enlargement and anemia occur as a result of bleeding into the renal parenchyma or pelvis.

Wilms' tumor thrombus extends into the inferior vena cava (IVC) in 4–10% of patients and rarely into the right atrium; dislodgment of the intravascular tumor may produce a fatal pulmonary embolism. Patients might also have microcytic anemia from iron deficiency or anemia of chronic disease, polycythemia, elevated platelet count, and acquired deficiency of von Willebrand factor or factor VII deficiency.

Wilms' tumor lesions are metabolically active and concentrate fluorodeoxyglucose (FDG). Regional spread and metastatic lesions can be visualized on PET/CT scanning. The diagnosis is usually made by imaging studies and confirmed by histology at the time of nephrectomy. Although biopsy is a reliable diagnostic tool, it is discouraged since it results in disease upstaging. A core needle biopsy obtained through a posterior approach (to limit contamination of the peritoneal cavity) should be performed in cases of unusual presentation (10 years old, signs of infection, inflammation) or unusual imaging findings (significant adenopathy, no renal parenchyma seen, intratumoral calcification).

The classic presentation of a child with WT is the discovery of an abdominal mass by a parent bathing or dressing the child or by the pediatrician on a routine well-child visit. Symptoms can include constipation, abdominal pain and/or

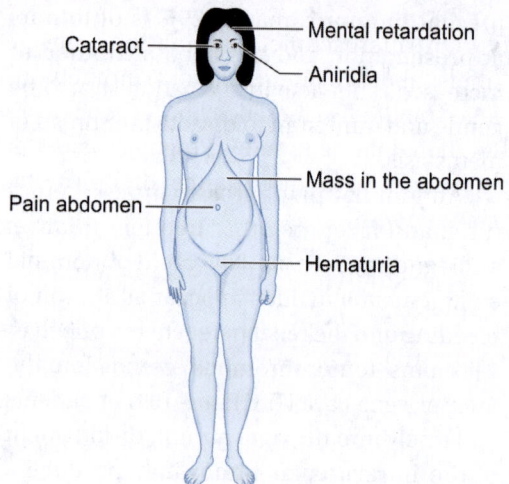

Fig. 1: Clinical features.

distension, and hematuria, but the patient can also be asymptomatic. Clinical signs can include hypertension and anemia. Rarely, spontaneous rupture of a WT can occur, leading to sudden pain and anemia due to bleeding within and surrounding the tumor. The majority of WT cases are unilateral, affecting only one kidney. Bilateral WT comprises 7% of total cases and is more common in individuals with genetic predisposition syndromes.

GENERAL FEATURES
• Hemihypertrophy • Genitourinary abnormalities

◼ DIAGNOSIS (TABLE 1)

Patients with a suspected renal mass should have a complete blood count and differential, a full electrolyte panel, blood urea nitrogen and creatinine (to evaluate kidney function), and liver function tests. Coagulation studies should be done prior to surgical intervention, since WT has been associated with acquired von Willebrand disease, a bleeding disorder that affects primary hemostasis. Urinalysis may reveal hematuria, and urine

TABLE 1: Investigations and purpose.

Investigation	Purpose
Abdominal USG	• Organ of origin • Identify contralateral kidney • Presence/absence of tumor thrombus in IVC
CT scan	• Further evaluation of extent of tumor • Extension into adjoining structures • Such as liver spleen and colon • Visualization and function of contralateral kidney
Chest X-ray	Pulmonary metastasis
Bone scan and skeletal survey	Bone mets in clear cell sarcoma of kidney
Brain imaging (MRI/CT scan)	Intracranial mets in rhabdoid tumor
Fine-needle aspiration cytology of mass	Cytological confirmation of diagnosis prior to prenephrectomy chemotherapy

(CT: computed tomography; IVC: inferior vena cava; MRI: magnetic resonance imaging; USG: ultrasonography)

catecholamine levels will be negative in WT and positive in most cases of neuroblastoma. These findings can help distinguish these two abdominal tumors, which occur in similar age groups.

It should be considered as an emergency. Intravenous pyelography (IVP) shows distortion of renal pelvis with or without minimum displacement. Plain radiograph shows unilinear calcifications. Resection is undertaken as soon as possible.

Regional lymph nodes with slightest suspicion should be removed. Preoperative irradiation is not recommended, because it induces fibrosis and makes resection difficult.

Although USG is helpful in diagnosing the presence of a renal tumor, subsequent cross-sectional imaging with MRI or CT is necessary to define better the anatomy of the tumor and to aid in surgical planning. The classic finding consistent with WT on cross-sectional imaging is the "claw sign" in which the tumor displaces normal kidney tissue, giving the appearance of tumor surrounded by a "claw of normal kidney tissue. Computed tomography is the most commonly used imaging modality for initial staging of pediatric renal tumors because of its easy accessibility and short duration; however, some institutions have been using MRI to spare the patients exposure to ionizing radiation.

Ultrasonography with Doppler imaging of renal veins and the inferior vena cava is a useful first study that not only can look for WT but also can evaluate the collecting system and demonstrate tumor thrombi in the renal veins and IVC.

Computed tomography is useful to define the extent of the disease, integrity of the contralateral kidney, and metastasis. MRI in may be helpful in defining an extensive tumor thrombus that extends up to the level of the hepatic veins or even into the right atrium, and to distinguish WT from nephrogenic rests.

Chest CT is more sensitive than chest radiography to screen for pulmonary metastasis, and is preferably performed before surgery, because effusions and atelectasis can interpretation of postoperative imaging studies. Liver scan is done to look for hepatic metastasis.

A bone scan is performed if the histologic diagnosis confirms clear cell sarcoma of the kidney to look for bone metastasis. Brain imaging with CT or MRI is obtained in cases of clear cell sarcoma of the kidney or rhabdoid tumor of the kidney as these tumors can spread to the brain.

On microscopic examination, muscle fibers, abortive glomeruli, and undifferentiated spindle-like mesenchymal cells encloses epithelial lining tubules. Prognosis is better in tumor with dominance of epithelial components.

NATIONAL WILMS' TUMOR STUDY STAGING

This is a clinicopathologic staging system.
- *Stage I*: Tumor confined to the kidney and completely excised
- *Stage II*: Tumor extending beyond the kidney but is completely excised local tumor spillage during surgery lymph nodes negative
- *Stage III*: Residual nonhematogenous disease confined to the abdomen perioperative rupture of renal capsule diffuse tumor spillage during surgery peritoneal implants positive lymph nodes
- *Stage IV*: Hematogenous metastases to lungs, liver, bones, or brain
- *Stage V*: Bilateral WT

The differential diagnosis of WT includes benign processes such as renal cysts, dysplastic kidneys, a renal abscess, or other renal malignancies. Neuroblastoma should also be considered because WT and neuroblastoma occur in the same age-group and affect adjacent organs of the abdomen: WT arises from the kidney and neuroblastoma arises from the adrenal gland. Lymphoma involving the kidneys can masquerade as a renal tumor. Finally, benign renal tumors such as cystic nephroma, metanephric tumors, and cystic partially differentiated nephroblastoma should be included in the differential diagnosis. Age of presentation, clinical and laboratory features, and imaging appearance may provide clues to the diagnosis, but histologic assessment remains the gold standard for diagnosis.

DIFFERENTIAL DIAGNOSIS
- Neuroblastoma
- Leukemia
- Hydronephrosis
- Pyelonephritis
- Multicystic disease of kidney

TREATMENT

The three modalities of treatment include surgery, chemotherapy, and radiotherapy (RT). The immediate treatment for unilateral disease is removal of affected kidney. Many prefer preoperative chemotherapy, because it diminishes the size of the tumor and makes it possible to come to better tumor staging. Actinomycin D and vincristine are used for 4 weeks. Commonly used drugs are vincristine, actinomycin D, and adriamycin.

Surgical removal of the primary tumor is a cornerstone of WT treatment. Regardless of surgical timing (prior to or after chemotherapy), radical nephrectomy is recommended for unilateral WT. A transverse abdominal incision is generally used as it is important to avoid tumor rupture, which has been associated with increased risk of local recurrence. Regional lymph node sampling is also performed to ensure optimal staging. Partial nephrectomy is recommended for patients with bilateral WT to spare as much normal renal parenchyma as possible.

After nephrectomy and lymph node sampling, chemotherapy and RT depend upon the stages:
- Stage I and II (FH) and stage I (focal or diffuse anaplasia); nephrectomy and 18 weeks of chemotherapy with vincristine and pulse intensive dactinomycin
- Stage II–IV (focal anaplasia); nephrectomy, abdominal irradiation (10 Gy) and 24 weeks of chemotherapy with vincristine, doxorubicin, and pulse-intensive dactinomycin
- Stage I–IV (clear cell) and stage II–IV (diffuse anaplasia); nephrectomy, RT (10 Gy) for abdomen (12 Gy) for lungs 24 weeks of chemotherapy with vincristine, doxorubicin, cyclophosphamide, and VP-16
- Stage I–IV (rhabdoid); nephrectomy, RT, carboplatin, VP-16 and cyclophosphamide

Actinomycin D in the dose of 15 µg/kg is given intravenously for 5 consecutive days from day 1. The course is repeated after 6, 12, 25, 38, 51, and 64 weeks.

Vincristine is given in a dose of 1.5 mg/m^2, or a maximum of 2 mg, intravenously once a week for 8–12 weeks. Cyclophosphamide in high doses for tumor regression is recommended. Adriamycin also gives good results.

Doxorubicin and abdominal radiation are additional therapies for stage III illness. Cyclophosphamide, carboplatin, and etoposide are used for anaplasia and metastatic disease. Pulmonary radiation is used for pulmonary metastasis.

Bilateral tumors and tumors considered inoperable at first surgery should receive 4–6 weeks of chemotherapy followed by second-look surgery. In case of bilateral tumors, effort should be made to preserve as much of each kidney as possible. In such cases, chemotherapy may have to be given for a longer period to enable partial nephrectomy to be done.

Prenephrectomy Chemotherapy

Prenephrectomy chemotherapy helps to decrease the need for postoperative abdominal radiation therapy in the event of tumor rupture during nephrectomy. Risks of prenephrectomy chemotherapy include modification of tumor histology and loss of staging information.

Absolute indications for prenephrectomy chemotherapy:
- Large tumor technically difficult to deliver at surgery
- Presence of major tumor thrombus in the IVC
- Bilateral WT
- WT in a solitary kidney or horse shoe kidney

Radiotherapy for Wilms' Tumor

Indications
- Stage II unfavorable histology
- Stage III favorable and unfavorable histology
- Stage IV lung bath for pulmonary metastases; need for RT to tumor bed is determined by local stage
- Local recurrence
- Palliative RT for metastatic disease

Principles of Radiation Therapy

Radiotherapy is very effective in the treatment of WT; however, its use is reserved for higher-stage FH WT or anaplastic histology (AH) WT due to the risk of acute and long-term toxicities. Patients with local stage II WT receive either flank or whole abdominal radiation, depending on the local extent of spread.

Radiotherapy should be planned starting within 10 days of surgery, without change of RT dose for favorable and unfavorable histology.

Target Volume

Volume should encompass tumor bed and site of excised kidney with 2–3 cm margin. Entire vertebral body to be encompassed to avoid disproportionate growth.

Special Considerations

In patients with stage V, or bilateral disease, an initial 6–12 weeks of chemotherapy precedes surgery in order to optimize tumor shrinkage prior to nephron-sparing surgery or partial nephrectomy. This is done in order to preserve as much renal function as possible.

Treatment of recurrent WT has improved over time with the introduction of new active chemotherapy drugs. The most important prognostic factor at the time of recurrence is the therapy that was administered for the original WT treatment. Patients treated initially with just vincristine and dactinomycin have an 80% survival rate after recurrence, whereas patients treated initially with three or more agents have a 50% survival rate after recurrence. The role of high-dose therapy with autologous stem cell rescue has been the subject of considerable debate. Although a randomized clinical trial to assess the benefit of high-dose therapy has not been conducted, a meta-analysis of the available literature suggested that the benefit of high-dose therapy is restricted to patients who received >4 agents as part of their initial treatment.

■ PROGNOSIS

Prognostic factors for risk-adapted therapy include age, stage, tumor weight, and loss of heterozygosity at chromosomes 1p and 16q. Histology plays a major role in risk stratification of WT. Absence of anaplasia is considered a favorable histologic finding. Presence of anaplasia is further classified as focal or diffuse, both of which are unfavorable histologic findings.

Prognostic factors are determined by staging. Another factor is pathology. Tumor with favorable pathology have better prognosis and require only surgical excision. Tumor with unfavorable histology, i.e., bone metastasis, pleomorphic, and ruptured have poor prognosis. They require intensive therapy. Tumor with standard histology, treatment has to be adjusted to staging. Ploidy is another prognostic sign, diploid tumors have a better prognosis than hyperdiploid tumor.

Anaplastic histology (focal and diffuse) accounts for approximately 11% of WT cases. Patients with diffuse anaplasia, in particular have a poor outcome. They are treated with intensive chemotherapy regimens (fiat includes vincristine, cyclophosphamide, doxorubicin, etoposide, lobaplatin, and ifosfamide, in addition to radiation therapy).

■ RECURRENT DISEASE

Approximately 15% of FH and 50% of AH WT relapse; most relapses occur early (within 2 years of diagnosis). Factors associated with a favorable outcome after relapse include low stage (I/II) at diagnosis, treatment with vincristine and actinomycin D only, no prior RT, FH, relapse to lung only, and interval from nephrectomy to relapse >12 months. Other agents used to treat recurrent WT include doxorubicin, carboplatin, cyclophosphamide, ifosfamide, etoposide, and topotecan. Metachronous WT may not represent tumor relapse, but may lead to development of a new tumor in the opposite kidney.

■ CONCLUSION

Since WT is one of the most curable malignancies of childhood, special emphasis needs to be laid on the need for surveillance for late effects of development, fertility, and second malignant neoplasm.

■ BIBLIOGRAPHY

1. Buckley KS. Pediatric genitourinary tumors. Curr Opin Oncol. 2011;23(3):297-302.
2. Davidoff AM. Wilms' tumor. Curr Opin Pediatr. 2009;21(3):357-64.
3. Davidoff AM, Giel DW, Jones DP, Jenkins JJ, Krasin MJ, Hoffer FA, et al. The feasibility and outcome of nephron-sparing surgery for children with bilateral Wilms tumor. The St Jude Children's Research Hospital experience: 1999-2006. Cancer. 2008;112(9):2060-70.
4. National Cancer Institute. Cancer Types. [online] Available from https://www.cancer.gov/types [Last accessed June, 2024].
5. Wright KD, Green DM, Daw NC. Late effects of treatment of Wilms tumor. Pediatr Hematol Oncol. 2009;26(6):407-13.

SECTION 13

Rheumatic Diseases

- Case 100 Acute Rheumatic Fever
- Case 101 Hurler's Syndrome
- Case 102 Dermatomyositis
- Case 103 Juvenile Rheumatoid Arthritis

CASE 100

Acute Rheumatic Fever

■ PRESENTING COMPLAINTS

A 7-year-old girl was brought with the complaint of:
- Sore throat since 15 days
- Pain in the joint since 10 days
- Palpitation since 7 days
- Fever since 5 days

History of Presenting Complaints

A 7-year-old girl came with history of pain in left knee joint. Her mother noted that there was swelling of the joint. The swelling was very painful and the child was not allowing to move her leg. She also complained of similar type of pain in the left shoulder. She also told that the pain in the left shoulder joint has disappeared by the time she noticed pain in left knee joint. There was also associated history of fever. Fever used to be of moderate to high degree. There was no history of chills and rigors. Fever used to be more in the evening and night. She also complained of abnormal awareness of the heartbeat. She used to feel much tired even for the routine work.

Past History of the Patient

She was the only sibling of nonconsanguineous marriage. She was born at full term by normal vaginal delivery. Her birth weight was 3 kg. She cried immediately after the delivery. There was no significant postnatal event. She was exclusively on the breastfeeds for the first 3 months. Later weaning was started as per the advice of the family doctor and the

CASE AT A GLANCE	
Basic Findings	
Height	: 117 cm (50th centile)
Weight	: 19 kg (50th centile)
Temperature	: 38°C
Pulse rate	: 116 beats/min
Respiratory rate	: 24 breaths/min
Blood pressure	: 90/60 mm Hg
Positive Findings	
History:	
• Fleeting type of joint pain	
• Fever	
• Sore throat	
• Palpitation	
Examination:	
• Febrile	
• Arthritis	
• Diastolic murmur	
• Loud first heart sound	
Investigation:	
• Hemoglobin: 9 g/dL	
• ESR: Raised	
• Chest X-ray: Cardiomegaly	
• ASLO: Raised	
• CRP: Raised	
• ECG: Prolonged PR interval	
(ASLO: antistreptolysin O; CRP: C-reactive protein; ECG: electrocardiogram; ESR: erythrocyte sedimentation rate)	

child was on family food by 18 months. Her developmental milestones were normal. She had been completely immunized. Her performance at the school was good.

Her mother complained that her daughter used to develop repeated attacks of throat pain, for which she was seeking medical treatment. She had pain in the joints occasionally.

■ EXAMINATION

On examination, the girl was moderately built and moderately nourished. She was in agony with pain in the joint. Her anthropometric measurement included her height 117 cm (50th centile) and the weight 19 kg (50th centile).

She was febrile, i.e., 38°C, the pulse rate was 116 beats/min, and the respiratory rate was 24 breaths/min. Blood pressure recorded was 90/60 mm Hg.

There was pallor, no lymphadenopathy, and no cyanosis. There was pain and swelling in the left knee joint. There were limitations of the movements.

Cardiovascular system revealed the presence of diastolic thrill at the apex associated with the mid-diastolic murmur at the apex. The first heart sound was loud. Second heart sound was normal. Respiratory system revealed presence of crepitation at the base. Per abdomen examination revealed no significant abnormality.

■ INVESTIGATION

- *Hemoglobin:* 9 g/dL
- *Total leukocyte count (TLC):* 7,600 cells/cumm
- *Differential leukocyte count (DLC):* $P_{72} L_{18} M_2 E_6 B_2$
- *Erythrocyte sedimentation rate (ESR):* 28 mm in the first hour
- *X-ray chest:* Cardiomegaly
- *Antistreptolysin O (ASLO):* 400 Todd units
- *C-reactive protein (CRP):* 1,100 µg/dL (normal range: 67–1,000 µg/dL)
- *Throat culture and sensitivity:* Sterile
- *Blood culture and sensitivity:* Sterile
- *Electrocardiogram (ECG):* PR interval is prolonged, right ventricular hypertrophy seen

■ DISCUSSION

Rheumatic fever is a multisystem disease, triggered by group A beta-hemolytic *Streptococcus*. Its acute manifestations include arthritis, carditis, chorea, subcutaneous nodules, and erythema marginatum. It is recurrent in nature and results in chronic heart disease. Hence it is said, rheumatic fever licks the joints and bites the heart.

Acute rheumatic fever (ARF) is a non-suppurative sequela of pharyngeal infection with group A *Streptococcus* (GAS). Target organs of the resultant autoimmune process include the heart, joints, central nervous system, and subcutaneous tissues. Permanent cardiac damage is the most important consequence of this disease.

Acute rheumatic fever is an immunological disorder. This is initiated by group A beta-hemolytic streptococci. Antibodies produced against the streptococcal protein and sugar react against the connective tissue of the body as well as heart. This results in rheumatic fever.

Predisposing factors include poor socio-economic condition leading to unhygienic living conditions and overcrowded households. Under and poor nutrition will alter the immune system.

The most common age involved is 5–15 years. Mitral valve disease and chorea are common in female. Aortic valve involvement is common in males. Rheumatic fever occurs during winter season.

As many as two-thirds of patients with an acute episode of rheumatic fever a have history of an upper respiratory tract infection several weeks before, and the peak age and seasonal incidence of ARF closely parallel that of GAS pharyngitis. Patients with ARF almost always have serologic evidence of a recent GAS infection. Their antibody titers are usually considerably higher than those seen in patients with uncomplicated GAS infections.

Rheumatic fever follows an attack of streptococcal infection of upper respiratory tract and usually there will be laboratory evidence of recent streptococcal infection. The latent period of rheumatic fever is 1–3 weeks and that of chorea is 2–6 months. The major epidemiological risk factor for the development of ARF is group A β-hemolytic streptococcal infection of the upper respiratory tract. Almost all serotypes of streptococci are involved.

Not all serotypes of GAS can cause rheumatic fever. When some GAS strains (e.g., M type 4) cause acute pharyngitis in a very susceptible rheumatic population. Certain serotypes of GAS (M types 1, 3, 5, 6, 18, 19, 24, 27, and 29) are more frequently isolated from patients with ARF than are other serotypes.

The concept of rheumatogenicity is further supported by the observation that although serotypes of GAS frequently associated with skin infection can be isolated also from the upper respiratory tract, they rarely cause recurrences of rheumatoid factor (RF) in individuals with a previous history of RF or first episodes of RF.

Certain populations with increased genetic susceptibility such as polymorphisms of interferon gamma (IFN-γ), angiotensin-converting enzyme (ACE), FCN, FcgRIIA, toll-like receptor 2 (TLR-2), and human leukocyte antigen (HLA) can explain why rheumatic fever occurs specifically in certain individuals.

PATHOGENESIS

The cytotoxicity theory suggests that a GAS toxin is involved in the pathogenesis of ARF and rheumatic heart disease. However, a major problem with the cytotoxicity hypothesis is its inability to explain the substantial latent period (usually 10–21 days) between GAS pharyngitis and onset of acute RF.

In addition to the specific characteristics of the infecting strain of GAS, the risk of developing ARF is also dependent on various host factors. The incidence of both initial attacks and recurrences of ARF peaks in children aged 5–15 years, which is the age-group greatest at risk for GAS pharyngitis. Patients who have had an attack of ARF tend to have recurrences, and the clinical features of the recurrences tend to mimic those of the initial attack. In addition, there appears to be a genetic predisposition to ARF.

The streptococcal cell wall proteins as well as carbohydrates have the capacity to produce antibodies capable of reacting with human connective tissue resulting in rheumatic fever. It appears to be the result of host's unusual response at both the cellular and humoral level to the *Streptococcus*. Antibodies against the heart muscle, antiheart antibodies and the nervous system, antineuronal antibodies are found in high titers with carditis and chorea.

An immune-mediated pathogenesis for ARF and rheumatic heart disease has been suggested by its clinical similarity to other illnesses with an immunopathogenesis and by the latent period between the GAS infection and ARF. The antigenicity of several GAS cellular and extracellular epitopes and their immunologic cross-reactivity with cardiac antigenic epitopes also lends support to the hypothesis of molecular mimicry.

Common epitopes are shared between certain GAS components (e.g., M protein, cell membrane, group A cell wall carbohydrate, capsular hyaluronate) and specific mammalian tissues (e.g., heart valve, sarcomere, brain, joint). Additionally, the involvement of GAS superantigens such as pyrogenic exotoxins in the pathogenesis of ARF has been proposed.

A more recently proposed pathogenetic hypothesis is that the binding of an M protein N-terminus domain to a region of collagen type IV leads to an antibody response to the collagen, resulting in ground substance inflammation especially in subendothelial areas like cardiac valves and myocardium.

■ PATHOLOGY

Acute rheumatic fever occurs most often in the winter and spring seasons and in children ages 5–15 years. Much less commonly, it has been reported in the preschool age-group. Patients with ARF have a high likelihood of recurrence when reinfected with GAS; this tendency declines with age and age increased time since the last episode. Environmental factors such as nutrition, wading, and age all appear to influence the incidence of ARF, probably because the same factors influence the incidence of streptococcal pharyngitis.

Antigenic differences among GAS serotypes are related to the bacterial M protein, found within its cell wall. Recent data demonstrated a shift in prevalence from "rheumatogenic" to "nonrheumatogenic" M types over the past 40 years that parallels, the decrease in the incidence of ARF over this period. The period of 10 days to 3 weeks between streptococcal pharyngitis and ARF is consistent with a cellular and humoral immune response. Cross-reactivity or streptococcal antigens and human cardiac, synovial, and brain antigens also support an immune mechanism of ARF.

Pathologic changes are found throughout the body in connective tissue and around small blood vessels. The pathognomonic, lesson of rheumatic fever is the Aschoff body, a painless nodular connective tissue lesion consisting of fibrinoid changes and a collection of lymphocytes, plasma cells, and histiocytes. Within the heart, the endocardium and myocardium are most often affected; the pericardium involved by extension or as serositis. Active valvulitis results in variable degrees of valve insufficiency, with chronic changes possibly leading to valvar stenosis. The mitral and aortic valves are affected most commonly, the tricuspid less frequently, and the pulmonary valve rarely.

Pathologic changes in the joints consist of joint effusion, exudation with edema of synovial membranes, focal necrosis in the joint capsule, and edema and inflammation in periarticular tissue. These changes are completely reversible. Subcutaneous nodules seen during the acute phase of the disease histologically resemble Aschoff bodies.

The pathological process is described in two stages:
1. Exudative stage
2. Proliferative stage

Exudative stage: In this acute phase, there is fibrinoid necrosis of connective tissues with edema of collagen fibers, resulting in two major clinical signs.
1. *Arthritis:* Without residuals
2. *Pancarditis:* It is a life-threatening condition

Proliferative stage: It is a more prolonged process, resulting in scarring of myocardium and endocardium. During acute RF, Aschoff bodies involve all the layers to produce pancarditis. The hallmark of the proliferative phase is the formation of Aschoff bodies. These are granulomas due to injury to collagen. Other important event is deposition of gamma globulins in heart. Lesion in pericardium is a fibrinous inflammation and macroscopically shows a "bread and butter" appearance. Endocarditis affects the valvular or mural endocardium. When the valvular endocardium heals, it results in scarring and deformity of valves. The valves damaged usually are mitral, aortic, tricuspid, and pulmonary.

CLINICAL FEATURES (FIG. 1)

The classical clinical picture of rheumatic fever includes streptococcal sore throat with fever. Rheumatic fever is diagnosed depending upon presence of criteria, which may be major or minor. Major criteria include carditis, subcutaneous nodules, chorea, and erythema marginatum. The minor criteria include fever, arthralgia, ASLO titer value, positive throat culture, acute phase reactions, and prolonged PR interval.

Diagnosis requires that an individual have either two major criteria or one major criterion plus two minor criteria along with evidence of streptococcal infection. Exceptions are chorea or indolent carditis, which each may by itself indicate rheumatic fever.

The essential criteria include evidence of recent streptococcal infections such as raised ASLO titer and positive throat culture.

> **ESSENTIAL DIAGNOSTIC POINTS**
> - Migratory polyarthritis
> - Carditis
> - Sydenham's chorea
> - Evidence streptococcal infection such as scarlet fever, positive throat culture, ASLO titer
> - Acute phase reactants are elevated
> - EEG changes
>
> (ASLO: antistreptolysin O; EEG: electroencephalogram)

CLINICAL MANIFESTATIONS AND DIAGNOSIS

There is no single specific clinical manifestation or specific laboratory test that establishes the diagnosis. There are a number of selective clinical findings (Jones criteria) that make diagnosis of RF highly probable. The revised Jones criteria are described in **Table 1**.

TABLE 1: Revised Jones criteria.

Major criteria	Minor criteria
• Carditis • Polyarthritis migratory • Erythema marginatum • Chorea	• Fever • Arthralgia • Previous history of rheumatic fever • Elevated acute phase • Phase reactants (ESR, CRP) • Prolonged PR interval on an ECG
Subcutaneous nodules	
Plus (essential criteria)	
Evidence of a preceding group A streptococcal infection (culture, rapid rise in antigen–antibody titer)	

(CRP: C-reactive protein; ECG: electrocardiogram; ESR: erythrocyte sedimentation rate)

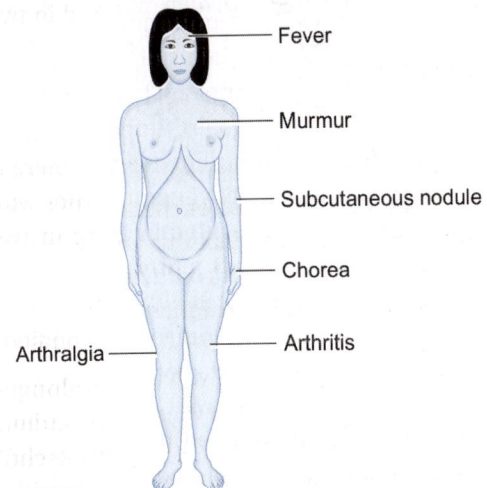

Fig. 1: Clinical features.

(Labels: Fever, Murmur, Subcutaneous nodule, Chorea, Arthritis, Arthralgia)

The presence of two major criteria or one major and two minor criteria indicates a high probability of the presence of rheumatic fever. Evidence of preceding streptococcal infection greatly strengthens the possibility of ARF. Its absence should make the diagnosis doubtful, except of Sydenham's chorea or long-standing carditis.

The *Jones criteria*, as revised in 2015, is now intended for diagnosis of the initial attack of ARF and recurrent attacks. There are five major and four minor criteria and a requirement of evidence of recent GAS infection.

Diagnosis of a first attack or recurrent attack of ARF can be established when a patient fulfills two major or one major and two minor criteria and has evidence of preceding GAS infection. Diagnosis of recurrent ARF can also be made only in the moderate/high-risk population by presence of five minor criteria with evidence of preceding GAS infection. In the 2015 Jones criteria revision, a major change from previous versions expands the definition of the major criterion carditis to include subclinical evidence [e.g., in the absence of a murmur, echocardiographic evidence of mitral regurgitation (MR) meeting specific criteria to distinguish physiologic from pathologic MR].

Migratory Polyarthritis

In rheumatic fever, 60–70% suffer from acute arthritis. Arthritis, the early manifestation of rheumatic fever lasts for 3–7 days and leaves no residual damage. It is polyarthritis involving the large joints such as knee, ankles, and elbows. Acute arthritis affecting the major joints is the characteristic involvement. The joints show signs of acute inflammation grade-IV tenderness and limitation of movements. The arthritis is migratory and fleeting and leaves behind no residual changes.

Arthritis occurs in approximately 75% of patients with ARF and typically involves larger joints, particularly the knees, ankles, wrists, and elbows. Involvement of the spine, small joints of the hands and feet, or hips is uncommon. Rheumatic joints are classically hot, red, swollen, and exquisitely tender, with even the friction of bed clothes being uncomfortable. The pain can precede and can appear to be disproportionate to the objective findings. The joint involvement is characteristically migratory in nature, i.e., a severely inflamed joint can become normal within 1–3 days without treatment, even as one or more other large joints become involved. Severe arthritis can persist for several weeks in untreated patients. Polyarthritis is the most common of the major criteria and lasts <4–6 weeks when untreated. Characteristic is a dramatic response to salicylates and nonsteroidal anti-inflammatory drugs (NSAIDs); early use in febrile children may confound diagnosis.

Carditis

Carditis occurs in approximately 50–60% of all cases of ARF. Recurrent attacks of ARF in patients who had carditis with their initial attack are associated with high rates of carditis with increasing severity of cardiac disease. The major consequence of acute rheumatic carditis is chronic, progressive valvular disease, particularly valvular stenosis, which can require valve replacement. In developing countries, 60–80% cases of rheumatic fever have clinical features of carditis and in 40% is seen during the first attack of rheumatic fever.

A major change in the Jones criteria is the acceptance of subclinical carditis (defined as without a murmur of valvulitis but with echocardiographic evidence of valvulitis) or clinical carditis (with a valvulitis murmur) as fulfilling the major criterion of carditis in all populations.

Echocardiography is an important tool to confirm cardiac involvement in ARF.

The following are the echocardiographic criteria developed in 2012:
- *Doppler criteria:*
  - Pathological mitral regurgitation—four criteria (all must be met)
  - Visible at least in two projections
  - Regurgitation jet length ≥2 cm at least in one projection
  - Regurgitation peak velocity >3 m/s; regurgitation pansystolic
  - Pathological aortic regurgitation—four criteria (all must be met)
  - Visible at least in two projections:
    - Regurgitation jet length ≥1 cm at least in one projection
    - Regurgitation peak velocity >3 m/s
    - Regurgitation pandiastolic
- *Morphological criteria:*
  - In acute mitral valve involvement:
    - Dilatation of mitral annulus
    - Elongation of chordae tendinae
    - Rupture of chordae tendinae with acute mitral regurgitation
    - Prolapse of anterior (less often posterior) leaflet
    - Nodular lesions on leaflets
  - In chronic mitral valve involvement (invisible in acute involvement):
    - Thickening of leaflets
    - Thickening of chordae tendinae with their fusion
    - Limited mobility of leaflets
- *Calcifications:*
  - Lesions in acute and chronic aortic valve involvement:
  - Symmetrical or focal thickening of leaflets
  - Disturbed leaflet coaptation (leaflet closing during systole)
  - Limited mobility of leaflets
  - Prolapse of leaflets

Acute rheumatic carditis usually presents as tachycardia and cardiac murmurs, with or without evidence of myocardial or pericardial involvement. Moderate-to-severe rheumatic carditis can result in cardiomegaly and heart failure with hepatomegaly and peripheral and pulmonary edema. Echocardiographic findings are not diagnostic but include pericardial effusion, decreased ventricular contractility, and aortic and/or mitral regurgitation.

Mitral regurgitation is characterized typically by a high-pitched apical holosystolic murmur radiating to the axilla. In patients with significant Initial regurgitation, this may be associated with an apical mid-diastolic murmur of relative mitral stenosis. Aortic insufficiency is characterized by a high-pitched decrescendo diastolic murmur at the left sternal border.

It is pancarditis involving pericardium, myocardium, and endocardium. Carditis occurs within 2 weeks of the onset of the fever. It is an early manifestation of the rheumatic fever so that by the time a patient seeks help, he/she had already had carditis.

Pericarditis may appear suddenly and may be associated with precordial pain and a friction rub. More often, however, patients with pericarditis are asymptomatic. Pericarditis seldom appears without endocarditis and myocarditis, the combination being termed pancarditis. Death may occur during the acute phase of carditis; permanent cardiac damage may result in long-term disability, usually because of mitral or aortic valvar insufficiency and/or stenosis. Pericarditis results in pericardial pain. The pain may be quite severe. Friction rub may be heard on auscultation. ECG shows ST and T wave changes. A patient of rheumatic pericarditis always has additional mitral or mitral and aortic regurgitation murmur.

Myocarditis presents with cardiac enlargement, soft heart sound, and congestive cardiac failure (CCF). Carey Coombs murmur is a delayed diastolic mitral murmur heard during the course of ARF. S_3 gallop may be present. Gallop rhythm is an abnormal array of heart sounds in which third and fourth heart sounds may also be present, and usually indicates active disease of the heart. Arrhythmias are present.

Endocarditis (valvulitis) is represented by pansystolic murmur of mitral regurgitation. Tricuspid valvulitis results in tricuspid regurgitation. The severity of the valvular endocarditis causes acute or later chronic hemodynamic overload. Acute hemodynamic overload is the main reason of morbidity and mortality of the rheumatic fever. The most frequent murmur is an apical regurgitant systolic murmur of mitral regurgitation. With severe mitral regurgitation, the third heart sound may be followed or replaced by a low-pitched mid-diastolic rumble. The early diastolic murmur of aortic regurgitation is the second most common murmur in ARF and generally occurs only in patients who also have mitral regurgitation.

Cardiomegaly may be evident on radiograph. Severe myocarditis may result in congestive heart failure with signs including jugular venous distention, hepatomegaly, and pulmonary edema with rales. Prolongation of the PR demonstrated on an electrocardiogram interval is common but does not indicate carditis.

Clinical Features of Carditis

- Murmurs:
  - Significant apical systolic murmurs (musical quality of grade III)
  - Apical mid-diastolic murmur due to edema of valve (Carey Coombs murmur)
  - Basal diastolic murmur
- Enlarged heart
- Congestive heart failure
- Presence of pericardial rub

Others include:
- Tachycardia (sleeping)
- Heart sounds (decreased or muffled)
- Gallop, arrhythmias, changing murmurs
- Subcutaneous nodules
- Persistent dry cough, ECG changes, laboratory findings, raised ESR, and presence of CRP
- Valves affected in frequency of occurrence are mitral 70%, mitral and aortic (7%), and tricuspid and pulmonary valves are rarely affected

Subcutaneous Nodules

They appear as early as 6 weeks after the onset of fever. These lesions are very infrequent and are present in 1–10% of patients with rheumatic fever. Nodules are better seen than felt. They are firm, nontender, pea-sized nodules seen over the extensor aspects of forearm, elbows, wrist, knees, ankles, spine, scalp, and along tendons. The presence of rheumatic nodules indicates presence of activity in 100% of cases and underlying carditis in 70% of cases. Subcutaneous nodules are a rare finding (<1% of patients with ARF) and consist of firm nodules approximately 1 cm in diameter along the extensor surfaces of tendons near bony prominences. There is a correlation between the presence of these nodules and significant rheumatic heart disease.

Chorea

Chorea occasionally is unilateral (hemichorea). The latent period from acute GAS infection to chorea is usually substantially longer than for arthritis or carditis and can be months. Onset can be insidious, with symptoms being present for several months before recognition. Sydenham chorea occurs in approximately 10-15% of patients with ARF and usually presents as an isolated, frequently subtle, movement disorder, emotional lability, incoordination, poor school performance, uncontrollable movements, and facial grimacing, all exacerbated by stress and disappearing with sleep are characteristic.

Sydenham chorea is characterized by sudden, aimless, irregular movements of the extremities, frequently associated with emotional instability and muscle weakness. Whereas carditis and arthritis develop within weeks after an inciting streptococcal infection; chorea presents after several months and is not often associated with other futures of ARF except perhaps mild carditis. The onset may be gradual complaints that the child is nervous. The child may become clumsy and stumble, fall, or drop objects. Often there are complaints of poor attention and deteriorating handwriting and school performance. Facial grimacing and various speech disorders occur. As chorea becomes more severe, irregular jerking movements can be sufficiently violent to cause injuries. Muscle weakness may be profound.

The choreiform movements subside during sleep and are exaggerated by emotion. Characteristically, when the patient is asked to extend the arms, hands, and lingers, flexion of the wrists and hyperextension of the metacarpophalangeal joints ("silver forking") are observed. The pronator sign may be elicited; after the arms are raised above the head, there is gradual pronation of the hands (apposition of the dorsal aspects of the hands). Other signs are an inability to hold the tongue still when it is protruded and spasmodic contractions of the hands when the patient intentionally grips objects or the examiner's hand (milkmaid's grip). Chorea can also be caused by diseases other than ARF, such as systemic lupus erythematosus (SLE) or Wilson disease, and patients who present with chorea as the only manifestation of ARF should undergo a full evaluation.

Chorea develops much later than other manifestation of rheumatic fever and 25% of these cases develop carditis after 10 years. This appears 3 months after onset of the fever. It consists of purposeless jerky movements, resulting in deranged speech, muscular incoordination, awkward gait, and weakness. It is more common among females. It is a self-limiting disease. The duration of illness is 2–6 weeks.

Erythema Marginatum

These are erythematous nonpruritic annular lesions with serpiginous borders, usually seen over the anterior aspects of chest, abdomen, and thigh. It is more specific. The rash is more faintly reddish, not raised above the skin. Erythema marginatum occurs in <10% of *ARF* patients; it may be seen *more frequently in children* <5 years old. The characteristic rash consists of an evanescent, pink, erythematous macule, with a clear center and serpiginous outline. The rash is transient, migratory, and not pruritic; it blanches with pressure and is exacerbated by warmth. It occurs primarily on the trunk and extremities, but not on the face, and it can be accentuated by warming the skin.

Minor Criteria

- *Clinical:*
  - Fever
  - Arthralgia
- *Laboratory evidence:*
  - Acute phase reactants:
    - Polymorphonuclear reactants
    - ESR raised

- CRP is raised
- Prolonged PR interval

The two laboratory minor criteria are: (1) Elevated acute phase reactants [defined as ESR at least 60 mm/h and/or CRP at least 3.0 mg/dL (30 mg/L) in low-risk populations, and ESR at least 30 mm/h and/or CRP at least 3.0 mg/dL (30 mg/L) in moderate-/high-risk populations] and (2) prolonged PR interval on ECG (unless carditis is a major criterion). However, a prolonged PR interval alone does not constitute evidence of carditis or predict long-term cardiac sequelae.

Recent Group A *Streptococcus* Infection

An absolute requirement for the diagnosis of ARF is supporting evidence of a recent GAS infection. ARF typically develops 2–4 weeks after an acute episode of GAS pharyngitis at a time when clinical findings of pharyngitis are no longer present. One-third of patients with ARF have no history of an antecedent pharyngitis. Therefore, evidence of an antecedent GAS infection is usually based on elevated or rising serum antistreptococcal antibody titers.

If only single antibody is measured (usually ASLO), only 80–85% of patients with ARF have an elevated titer; however, 95–100% have an elevation if three different antibodies (ASLO, anti-DNase B, antihyaluronidase) are measured. Therefore, when ARF is suspected clinically, multiple antibody tests should be performed. Except for chorea, the clinical findings of ARF generally coincide with peak antistreptococcal antibody responses. Most patients with chorea have elevation of antibodies to at least GAS antigen. The diagnosis of ARF should not be made in those patients with elevated or increasing streptococcal antibody titers who do not fulfill the Jones criteria.

GENERAL FEATURES
• MCarditis
• Fever
• Erythema marginatum
• Antistreptolysin O (AsLo) titer

The diagnosis of acute RF can be made without strict adherence to the Jones criteria in three circumstances: (1) When chorea occurs as the only major manifestation of acute RF, (2) when indolent carditis is the only manifestation in patients who first come to medical attention only months after the apparent onset of acute RE, and (3) in a limited number of patients with recurrence of acute RF in particularly high-risk populations.

Laboratory Diagnosis of Rheumatic Fever

Proof of previous streptococcal infection is required in addition to combinations of major and minor criteria. Paired, increasing serum antistreptococcal antibody titers are probably the most specific and reliable proof of previous streptococcal infection. A rising antibody titer to specific streptococcal antigens is more specific than a single elevated value. However, if the patient presents with chorea >3 months after the acute streptococcal infection, then antibody titers may be declining or low. The most widely used serologic test is antibody formation against streptolysin O. Titers of at least 333 U in children and 250 U in adults are usually considered elevated.

Acute phase reactants like erythrocyte sedimentation rate (ESR) and C-reactive protein (CRP) are always elevated at the onset of rheumatic fever. There may be neutrophilic leukocytosis and anemia.

- Serial chest X-rays are required to assess the progressive cardiac enlargement
- ECG shows conduction defects and signs of carditis and pericarditis

Preceding streptococcal infections are confirmed by following tests:
- *Throat culture:* This remains the gold standard for confirmation of presence of group A streptococci and 25–40% of the individuals have positive throat culture.
- *Serodiagnosis:* Antistreptolysin O titer has been the widely accepted diagnostic test for rheumatic fever. A titer of 333 Todd units and above is suggestive of ARF.

Other streptococcal antigens tested are:
- Antistreptokinase
- Antihyaluronidase
- Anti-DNAse B

LABORATORY SALIENT FINDINGS

- *Elevated acute phase reactants:* Raised ESR, C-reactive protein, leukocytosis
- Rise in ASLO titer
- Chest X-ray
- ECG changes

(ASLO: antistreptolysin O; ECG: electrocardiogram; ESR: erythrocyte sedimentation rate)

■ DIFFERENTIAL DIAGNOSIS

- Juvenile rheumatoid arthritis (JRA)
- Lyme disease
- Osteomyelitis
- Pharyngitis
- Viral fever

■ TREATMENT

Rheumatic fever treatment may be divided into three stages:
1. Management of acute stage
2. Eradication of streptococcal infection
3. Prevention of recurrence

Management of Acute Stage

Arthritis, carditis, and Sydenham's chorea are the three acute systemic manifestation of ARF. So, the acute therapy is planned, at the management of these three conditions.

Strict bed rest is advised for all three conditions.

Mainstay of the treatment is strict bed rest especially when there is evidence of carditis is present. Bed rest is advised till the evidence of the activity subsides. Salt restriction is advised in CCF associated with carditis. Throat culture and sensitivity test should be done. Procaine penicillin 4 units can be given for 10 days. This may be followed by prophylactic penicillin.

If a child with ARF is free of clinical carditis, normal activity can be resumed once the pain and fever resolve. There is mild carditis, and a period of 1–2 weeks resting at home is reasonable. The murmur may persist indefinitely, and its disappearance is not a requisite for return to activity. The ESR may remain high for weeks, showing gradual decline. All patients with ARF should be placed on bed rest and monitored closely for evidence of carditis. However, patients with carditis require longer periods of bed rest.

Anti-inflammatory Therapy

Anti-inflammatory agents (e.g., salicylates, corticosteroids) should be withheld if arthralgia or atypical arthritis is the only clinical manifestation of presumed ARF. Acetaminophen can be used to control pain and fever while the patient is being observed for more definite signs of ARF or for evidence of another disease.

Patients with typical migratory polyarthritis and those with carditis without cardiomegaly or congestive heart failure should be treated with oral salicylates. The usual dose of aspirin is 50–70 mg/kg/day in four divided doses PO for 3–5 days, followed by 50 mg/kg/day in four divided doses PO for 3 weeks and half that dose for another 2–4 weeks. If rebound of rheumatic activity occurs, full therapy may have to be reinstituted for an additional 4-6 weeks.

Patients with carditis and more than minimal cardiomegaly and/or congestive heart failure should receive corticosteroids. The usual dose of prednisone is 2 mg/kg/day in four divided doses for 2-3 weeks followed by half the dose for 2-3 weeks and then tapering of the dose by 5 mg/24 h *every* 2-3 days. When prednisone is being tapered, aspirin should be started at 50 mg/kg/day in four divided doses for 6 weeks to prevent rebound of inflammation. Supportive therapies for patients with moderate-to-severe carditis include digoxin, fluid and salt restriction, diuretics, and oxygen. The cardiac toxicity of digoxin is enhanced with myocarditis.

In patients with moderate-to-severe carditis, neither salicylates nor steroids demonstrate superiority over the other drug in modifying the duration of acute disease or lessening the residual heart damage. However, steroids are indicated in patients who develop congestive heart failure. Current understanding suggests unlikely benefit from digoxin, with the exception of associated arrhythmias. Occasionally, severe incompetence of aortic and/or mitral valves leads to refractory heart failure, which requires surgical implantation of a prosthetic valve.

Sydenham Chorea

Because chorea often occurs as an isolated manifestation after the resolution of the acute phase of the disease, anti-inflammatory agents are usually not indicated. Sedatives may be helpful early in the course of chorea phenobarbital (16-32 mg every 6-8 hours PO) is the drug of choice. If phenobarbital is ineffective, then haloperidol (0.01-0.03 mg/kg/24 h divided bid PO) or chlorpromazine (0.5 mg/kg every 4-6 h PO) should be initiated. Some patients may benefit from a few-week course of corticosteroids.

Specific treatment for chorea is not available. Physical and mental stress should be minimized, and protective measures to prevent injury during severe episodes should be instituted. In very severe cases, steroids, phenobarbital, and valproic acid have been helpful.

Eradication of *Streptococcal* Infection

Antibiotic Therapy

A full course of oral or intramuscular penicillin as given for GAS pharyngitis should be administered to all patients with ARF even if testing tor GAS is negative. An oral cephalosporin is an acceptable alternative; macrolide antibiotics, such as erythromycin, clarithromycin, or azithromycin, should be limited to penicillin-allergic patients.

Once the diagnosis of ARF has been established and regardless of the throat culture results, or a single intramuscular injection of benzathine penicillin to ensure eradication of GAS from the upper respiratory tract. Long-acting benzathine penicillin depending on age and weight of child, a single intramuscular injection of 0.6-1.2 million IU, 250-500 mg orally 2-3 times a day for 10 days or amoxicillin 50 mg/kg (maximum 1 g) once daily for 10 days. If patient is penicillin-allergic, 10 days of erythromycin, azithromycin (5 days) or clindamycin is indicated. After this initial course of antibiotic therapy, lung-term antibiotic prophylaxis should be instituted.

Primary Prevention

The following preventive regimens are in use:
- Penicillin G Benzathine 6,00,000 units for <27 kg, 1.2 million units for more 27 kg

intramuscularly every 4 weeks is the drug of choice.
- Penicillin V-250 mg orally twice daily is much less effective than intramuscular Benzathine penicillin.
- Sulfadiazine 500 mg for <27 kg 1 g >27 kg once daily; this is recommended regimen for penicillin patients.
- Erythromycin 250 mg orally twice a day may be given to the patients allergic to both penicillin and sulfonamides. Azithromycin or clarithromycin may also be used.

Prophylaxis against recurrent ARF should be instituted immediately following acute therapy. The most effective prophylaxis consists of benzathine penicillin G intramuscular injections every 4 weeks; the injection can be painful and may lead to reactions. Alternative therapy consists of either oral penicillin V twice daily or oral sulfisoxazole once daily. Patients without rheumatic heart disease are at lower risk of recurrence than patients with carditis or valvar disease. In pediatric ARF patients without carditis, prophylaxis should continue for at least 5 years or until age of 21 years, whichever is longer.

Most acute pharyngitis is caused by virus and less commonly, other bacteria. The epidemiologic peak of GAS pharyngitis and the risk for developing ARF are between 5 and 15 years of age. Protocols testing for acute GAS pharyngitis in adults account for the lower GAS prevalence and risk for ARF beyond 15 years of age and are not to be used in children.

Preferred regimens include oral penicillin V 2-3 times daily or a single daily dose of amoxicillin for 10 days. Parenteral benzathine penicillin is generally reserved for patients with poor compliance. Penicillin-allergic patients should receive a first-generation cephalosporin, clindamycin, or a macrolide. Macrolide resistance by GAS varies geographically. Testing for cure is not generally indicated.

Appropriate antibiotic therapy instituted before the 9th day of symptoms of acute GAS pharyngitis is highly effective in preventing the first attacks of ARF. Long-term (possibly lifelong) prophylaxis is recommended for patients with residual rheumatic heart disease.

Antibiotic prophylaxis should continue in these patients until the patient reaches 21 years of age or until 5 years have elapsed since the last rheumatic fever attack, whichever is longer. The decision to discontinue prophylactic antibiotics should be made only after careful consideration of potential risks and benefits and of epidemiologic factors such as the risk for exposure to GAS infections.

Secondary Prevention

The chemoprophylaxis for recurrences of acute rheumatic fever (secondary prophylaxis) is given in **Table 2**.

Secondary prevention is directed at preventing acute GAS pharyngitis in patients at substantial risk of recurrent ARF. The regimen of choice for secondary prevention is a single intramuscular injection of benzathine penicillin G (600,000 IU for children weighing <27 kg and 1.2 million IU for those weighing >27 kg) every 4 weeks. In certain high-risk patients, and in certain areas of the world where the incidence of rheumatic fever is particularly high, use of benzathine penicillin G every 3 weeks may be necessary, because serum concentrations of penicillin may decrease to marginally effective levels after 3 weeks.

Secondary prevention requires continuous antibiotic prophylaxis, which should begin as soon as the diagnosis of ARF has been made and immediately after a full course

TABLE 2: Chemoprophylaxis for recurrences of acute rheumatic fever (secondary prophylaxis).

Drug	Dose	Route
Penicillin G Benzathine	600,000 IU for children weighing ≤60 lb and 1.2 million IU for children >60 lb, every 4 weeks	Intramuscular
Or Penicillin V	250 mg, twice daily	
Or Sulfadiazine or Sulfisoxazole	0.5 g, once daily for patients weighing >60 lb	Oral
	1.0 g, once daily for patients weighing >60 lb	Oral
For people who are allergic to penicillin and sulfonamide drugs		
Macrolide or azalide	Variable	Oral

TABLE 3: Duration of prophylaxis for people who have had acute rheumatic fever.

Category	Duration
• Rheumatic fever without carditis	• 5 years or until 21 years of age, whichever is longer
• Rheumatic fever with carditis but without residual heart disease (no valvular disease)	• 10 years or until 21 years of age, whichever is longer
• Rheumatic fever with carditis and residual heart disease (persistent valvular disease)	• 10 years or until 40 years of age, whichever is longer; sometimes lifelong prophylaxis

of antibiotic therapy has been completed. Because patients who have had carditis with their initial episode of ARF are at higher risk for having carditis with recurrences and for sustaining additional cardiac damage, they should receive long-term antibiotic prophylaxis well into adulthood and perhaps for life.

Table 3 gives the duration of prophylaxis for people who have had acute rheumatic fever.

■ BIBLIOGRAPHY

1. Cilliers A, Manyemba J, Adler AJ, Saloojee H. Anti-inflammatory treatment for carditis in acute rheumatic fever. Cochrane Database Syst Rev. 2012;6:CD003176.
2. Gerber MA, Baltimore RS, Eaton CB, Gewitz M, Rowley AH, Shulman ST, et al. Prevention of rheumatic fever and diagnosis and treatment of acute post Streptococcal pharyngitis: a scientific statement from the American Heart Association Rheumatic Fever, Endocarditis, and Kawasaki Disease Committee of the Council on Cardiovascular Disease in the Young, the Interdisciplinary Council on Functional Genomics and Translational Biology, and the Interdisciplinary Council on Quality of Care and Outcomes Research: endorsed by the American Academy of Pediatrics. Circulation. 2009;119:1541-51.

CASE 101

Hurler's Syndrome

■ PRESENTING COMPLAINTS

A 9-year-old girl was brought with the complaint of:
- Delay in developmental milestones since birth
- Deafness since 6 years
- Behavioral problems since 4–5 years

History of Presenting Complaints

A 9-year-old girl was brought by the parents with a history of behavioral problems to pediatric psychiatry outpatient department. The behavioral problems include both aggressive and depressive moods. She was fighting with her brothers in the house. Sometimes she was banging her own head on the table or against the wall. The child was admitted in the ward for the control of the behavioral problems.

Past History of the Patient

The child was the elder sibling of the consanguineous marriage. Her parents were cousins. She was born at term with the normal delivery. There was no history suggestive of the birth asphyxia. The newborn was breastfed soon after delivery. At the time of birth, the weight was 3.5 kg, the length was 45 cm, and head circumference was 35 cm.

The weaning of the child started at 4 months and the girl was eating family food by 18 months onward. The child used to have feeding problems such as vomiting and sometimes choking. Motor development was slightly delayed. Speech development

CASE AT A GLANCE	
Basic Findings	
Height	: 130 cm (40th centile)
Weight	: 36 kg (90th centile)
Temperature	: 37°C
Pulse rate	: 100 beats/min
Respiratory rate	: 26 breaths/min
Blood pressure	: 100/80 mm Hg

Positive Findings

History:
- Mental retardation
- Deafness
- Consanguineous marriage
- Behavioral problems
- Delay in motor milestones

Examination:
- Upward slanting of eyeball
- Short stature
- Short thick neck
- Hirsute features
- Hepatomegaly

Investigation:
- Upward slanting of eyeball
- Urinary excretion of keratin and dermatan phosphate
- *X-ray hand:* Wide metacarpals
- *X-ray skull:* Long vertical diameter, shallow pituitary fossa, deep serration of the coronal suture

was impaired probably because of deafness. She was mentally retarded and partially deaf. The child was immunized as per schedule.

■ EXAMINATION

The girl was moderately built and nourished. She was plotted on the 90th centile for weight, i.e., 36 kg and 40th centile for the height, i.e., 130 cm. She had coarse and hirsute features. She was short and had a thick neck. She was sitting quietly.

She was afebrile. The pulse rate was 100 beats/min and the respiratory rate was 26 breaths/min. The blood pressure recorded was 100/80 mm Hg.

There was no pallor, no lymphadenopathy, and no clubbing. She was partially deaf. Eye examination was normal. Per abdomen examination revealed the presence of hepatomegaly measuring about 4 cm below the costal margin. It was nontender and firm in consistency. Cardiovascular system revealed no murmurs. Respiratory system was normal. Skull and spine were normal.

■ INVESTIGATION

- *Hemoglobin:* 12 g/dL
- *TLC:* 6,800 cells/cumm
- *ESR:* 32 mm in the first hour
- *Absolute eosinophil count:* 426 cell/dL
- *Urine routine:* Normal
- *Urine:* Keratin level is increased, dermatan phosphate level also increased
- *X-ray of hand:* Showed wide metacarpal
- *X-ray of skull:* Showed long vertical diameter, shallow pituitary fossa, deep serration of coronal suture

■ DISCUSSION

Family history of the consanguineous marriage, mentally retarded child with behavioral problems, and associated deafness give the clue to hereditary disease, Hurler's disease. Along with the physical examination findings such as short stature, thick neck, hirsute features, and hepatomegaly, the diagnosis of the mucopolysaccharidosis is made. Urinary excretion of the keratin and dermatan phosphate and radiograph of hand revealing the wide metacarpal will consolidate the diagnosis.

Hurler's disease is a severe progressive disorder. This involves the multiple organs and tissues such as cornea, heart, brain, and skeletal leading to premature death. Usually before the age of 10 years.

The basic defect is the deficiency of alpha-L-iduronidase. This results in the accumulation of the dermatan sulfate and heparin sulfate in the tissues. These are also excreted in urine. Almost all the tissues in the body are involved. There will be progressive mental and physical deterioration.

In the brain, the lipid storage occurs with the mucopolysaccharide accumulation. There is unusual hyalinization of collagen bundles. This leads to joint deformities and stiffness, thickened meninges, hydrocephalus, peripheral nerve compression, and tendency to develop hernia.

There will be narrowing of the coronary arteries, thickening of the cardiac valve and endocardium. Stiffening of the myocardium leads to CCF. Acute cardiomyopathy may be a feature of some infants. The constricted thorax contributes to the clinical deterioration of the patient.

ESSENTIAL DIAGNOSTIC POINTS
• Autosomal recessive
• Mental retardation
• Hepatosplenomegaly
• Umbilical hernia
• Coarse facies
• Corneal clouding
• Dorsolumbar gibbus
• Severe heart disease
• Heparin sulfate and dermatan sulfate are found in urine

CASE 101: Hurler's Syndrome

■ CLINICAL FEATURES (FIG. 1)

The infant with Hurler's disease appear normal at birth. Hepatosplenomegaly, skeletal deformity, corneal clouding, coarse facial features, large tongue, prominent forehead, short stature, and stiffness in the joint occur in between the ages of 6 and 24 months. There will be delay in language development as a result of chronic hearing loss and large tongue. There will be both conductive and sensorineural hearing loss.

The facial features appear progressively coarser. There will be frontal bossing, prominent sagittal and metopic sutures. There is a depressed nasal bridge. Nose is broad and flat. The child will deteriorate rapidly at second and third years of life. These children become immobile. Joints become progressively stiff and contracted **(Fig. 2)**.

Communicating hydrocephalus can occur as a result of progressive ventricular enlargement. The head will be large—dolichocephalic **(Fig. 3)**. Recurrent respiratory tract infection, ear infection, noisy breathing, persistent nasal discharge are present. Clouding of the cornea **(Fig. 4)**, umbilical, and inguinal

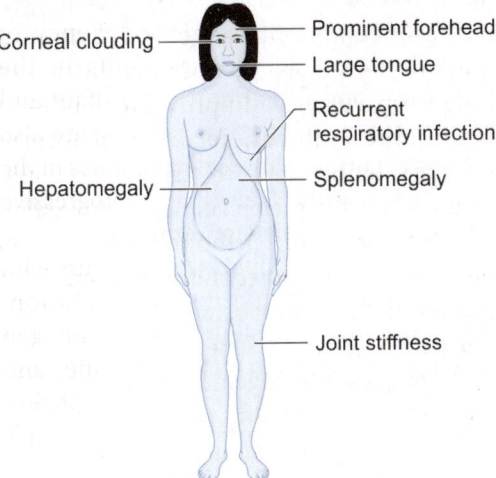

Fig. 1: Clinical features.

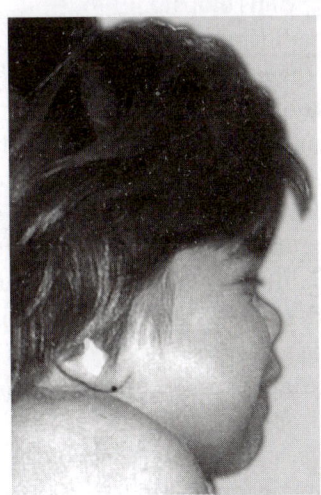

Fig. 3: Dolichocephalic.

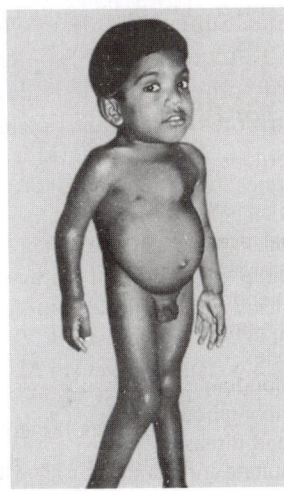

Fig. 2: Hurler syndrome. *(For color version, see Plate 11)*

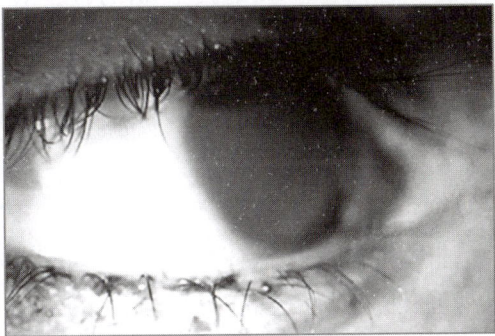

Fig. 4: Corneal clouding. *(For color version, see Plate 12)*

hernia are common. Mental retardation is obvious. Glaucomas and retinal detachment are common.

DIAGNOSIS

The initial diagnostic test is the urinary excretion of glycosaminoglycans. Any individual who is suspected of clinical features, radiographic reports, urinary screening definitive diagnosis should be done by enzyme assay. Serum, leukocytes, or cultured fibroblasts are used as a tissue source for measuring lysosomal enzymes. Prenatal diagnosis is routinely carried out on cultured cells from the amniotic fluid or chorionic villus biopsy.

The radiograph of the patient in Hurler's disease reveals dysostosis multiplex. This includes dolichocephalic head and thickened calvarium. The medial third of the clavicle is thickened. There will be a beak-like projection on the lower anterior margin. There will be premature closure of the lambdoid and sagittal sutures. There will be enlarged J-shaped sella, shallow orbits, abnormal spacing of teeth with the dentigerous cyst.

The diaphyses of the long bones are enlarged and irregular appearance of the metaphyses. The pelvis is poorly formed with a small femoral head. Coxa valga is present. The clavicles are short, thickened, and irregular. The ribs are narrowed at the vertebral end and flat and broad at sternal end. The phalanges are short.

GENERAL FEATURES
- Skeletal deformity
- Coarse facial features
- Glaucoma
- Hearing problem
- Retinal degeneration
- Kyphosis

DIFFERENTIAL DIAGNOSIS

Differential diagnosis includes Hurler–Scheie syndrome, Scheie syndrome, Hunter's syndrome, Sanfilippo syndrome, and Morquio's syndrome.

TREATMENT

These is no definitive treatment. The corrective factors are the missing lysosomal enzymes. Replacement of these enzymes by the administration of plasma or leukocytes are not satisfactory. Bone marrow transplantation has resulted in significant clinical improvement of the somatic disease and increased long-term survival. Improvement is seen with joint stiffness, facial appearance, hepatosplenomegaly, heart disease, and hearing loss. But skeletal or ocular anomalies are not corrected. Orthopedic correction includes femoral osteotomies, acetabular reconstruction, and posterior spinal fusion. The neurological outcomes are varied.

Supportive management with particular attention to respiratory, cardiac complications, hearing loss, carpal tunnel syndrome, spinal cord compression, and hydrocephalus improves the quality of life. These patients require evaluation of their clinical status on a regular basis.

BIBLIOGRAPHY

1. Landau YE, Lichter-Konecki U, Levy HL. Genomics in newborn screening. J Pediatr. 2014;164(1):14-9.
2. Matern D, Oglesbee D, Tortorelli S. Newborn screening for lysosomal storage disorders and other neuropathic conditions. Dev Disabil Rev. 2013;17(3):247.
3. Tomatsu S, Fujii T, Fukushi M, Oguma T, Shimada T, Maeda M, et al. Newborn screening and diagnosis of mucopolysaccharidoses. Mol Genet Metab. 2013;110(1-2):42-53.

CASE 102

Dermatomyositis

■ PRESENTING COMPLAINTS

A 5-year-old boy was brought with the complaints of:
- On-and-off fever since 3 months
- Rashes since 2 months
- Ulcerative wound since 15 days
- Pain in leg since 1 week

History of Presenting Complaints

A 5-year-old boy came to the hospital with a history of tiredness, listlessness, and intermittent pain in the legs. There was history of recurrent attacks of fever since 3 months. The mother had also noted presence of rashes over exposed parts of the body since last 2 months. Rashes are more common on the face and hands. After few days, the mother noticed a painful ulcer over the third knuckle on the left hand. The pain in the leg was not allowing him to stand. He was not able to stand up from the bending posture.

Past History of the Patient

The child was the second sibling of a non-consanguineous marriage. He was born at full term with normal vaginal delivery. He was breastfed exclusively for 3 months.

Later, weaning started, and he was on family food by 18 months. The child had been completely vaccinated. There was no significant delay in developmental milestones.

CASE AT A GLANCE	
Basic Findings	
Height	: 110 cm (90th centile)
Weight	: 15 kg (25th centile)
Temperature	: 37.9°C
Pulse rate	: 96 beats/min
Respiratory rate	: 20 breaths/min
Blood pressure	: 80/60 mm Hg
Positive Findings	

History:
- Recurrent flu-like illness for last 3 months
- Rashes over the exposed area of body
- Ulcer over the hand
- Pain in legs

Examination:
- Facial erythema
- Moderate cervical and lymphadenopathy enlargement
- Nodule scar, perforating calcific masses over legs
- Diminished power in quadriceps

Investigation:
- CPK: Elevated
- LDH: Increased X-ray chest: Normal
- Muscle biopsy: Inflammatory cell infiltrate and perifascicular degeneration

(CPK: creatine phosphokinase; LDH: lactate dehydrogenase)

He had two siblings, one was elder by 2 years and the other was younger by 3 years.

■ EXAMINATION

The boy was thin, average built, and moderately nourished. Rashes were present on the face. Erythema was present on the back of the hands and knee. The anthropometric measurements included the height 110 cm (90th centile) and the weight 15 kg (25th centile).

He was afebrile. The pulse rate was 96 beats/min and respiratory rate was 20 breaths/min. The blood pressure recorded was 80/60 mm Hg.

There was no pallor. There was cervical and inguinal lymphadenopathy. There was no clubbing or cyanosis. Subcutaneous nodules, scars, and perforating calcific masses were present over the legs (**Fig. 1**). There was some wasting in quadriceps muscles. The power was decreased in these muscles. This was more on right side. Other systemic examinations were normal.

■ INVESTIGATION

- *Hemoglobin:* 10.2 g/dL
- *TLC:* 12,400 cells/cumm
- *Platelets count:* 4,00,000 cells/cumm
- *ESR:* 20 mm at the first hour
- *Creatine phosphokinase (CPK):* 500 U/L
- *Lactate dehydrogenase (LDH):* 400 U/L
- *ECG:* Normal
- *X-ray chest:* Normal
- *Muscle biopsy:* Showed inflammatory cell infiltrate and perifascicular degeneration

■ DISCUSSION

The boy has photosensitive rashes on the exposed body parts, generalized weakness, tiredness, and pain in legs. Along with these, there were cervical and inguinal lymphadenopathies. All these make diagnosis of dermatomyositis.

The etiology of juvenile dermatomyositis (JDM) is multifactorial, based on genetic predisposition and an unknown environmental trigger. HLA alleles such as B8, DRB1*0301, DQA10501, and DQAl*0301 are associated with increased susceptibility to JDM in selected populations. Maternal microchimerism may play a part in the etiology of JDM by causing graft-versus-host disease (GVHD) or autoimmune phenomena. Persistent maternal cells have been found in blood and tissue samples of children with JDM. An increased number of these maternal cells are positive for HLA-DQA1*0501, which may assist with transfer or persistence of chimeric cells.

Specific cytokine polymorphisms in tumor necrosis factor-alpha (TNF-α) promoter and variable-number tandem repeats of the interleukin 1 (IL-1) receptor antagonist may increase genetic susceptibility. These polymorphisms are common in the general population. A history of infection in the 3 months before disease onset is usually reported, multiple studies have failed to produce a causative organism.

The characteristic heliotropic rash on the face is because of vasculitis. This produces erythema over the joint surface of the knuckles and knee. The inflammatory process may be associated with local area of tenderness, edema, and ulceration. Myositis may result in profound stiffness and weakness. Hence, a child may be unable to stand from the sitting position.

■ PATHOGENESIS

Interferon upregulates genes critical in immunoregulation and major histocompatibility complex (MHC) class I expression, activates natural killer (NK) cells, and supports dendritic cell (DC) maturation.

Upregulation of gene products controlled by type 1 IFNs occurs in patients with dermatomyositis, potentially correlating with disease activity and holding promise as clinical biomarkers.

It appears that children with genetic susceptibility to JDM (HLA DQAI0501, HLA-DRB-0301) may have prolonged exposure to maternal chimeric cells and/or an unknown environmental trigger. Once triggered, an inflammatory cascade with type I IFN response leads to upregulation of MHC class I expression and maturation of DCs. Overexpression of MHC class I upregulates adhesion molecules, which influence migration of lymphocytes, leading to inflammatory infiltration of muscle.

In an autoregulatory feedback loop, muscle inflammation increases the type 1 IFN response, regenerating the cycle of inflammation. Cells involved in the inflammatory cascade include NK cells (CD56), T-cell subsets (CD4, CD8, Th17), monocytes/macrophages (CD14), and plasmacytoid DCs. Neopterin, IFN-inducible protein 10, monocyte chemoattractant protein, myxovirus resistance protein, and von Willebrand factor products, as well as other markers of vascular inflammation, may be elevated in patients with JDM who have active inflammation.

It is an autoimmune angiopathy affecting the muscle and skin predominantly. The skin rash takes the form of violaceous discoloration in upper eyelid. The erythematous eruption on the upper cheeks and telangiectasia on knuckles and nail-folds are seen. Investigations are not always helpful, and the diagnosis is essentially a clinical one. It is not associated with underlying malignancies in childhood.

It is a multisystem disease associated with nonsuppurative inflammation of the striated muscle. The cause is unknown. Cellular immune system may play a basic role in pathogenesis. Immunoglobulin and complement deposition occur in blood vessels of the affected muscle.

The prominent lesion in children is an occlusive vasculitis involving arterioles, venules, and capillaries in connective tissue in skin, and subcutaneous tissue and muscle. In muscles, there is a patchy degeneration and regeneration of muscle fibers and interstitial edema. Myopathies, polymyositis, Guillain-Barré syndrome, and myasthenia gravis are casually associated with skin manifestation. The inflammatory process may involve eyes, joints, lungs, and gastrointestinal (GI) tract.

CLINICAL FEATURES (FIG. 1)

Constitutional signs and upper respiratory symptoms predominate, but one-third of patients report preceding GI symptoms. GAS, upper respiratory infections, GI infections, coxsackievirus B, toxoplasma, enteroviruses, parvovirus B19, and multiple other organisms have been postulated as possible pathogens in the etiology of JDM.

Onset is usually insidious with general development in proximal muscle group and trunk muscles. The child may develop an awkward gait. There will be nonpitting and thickening of the skin and subcutaneous

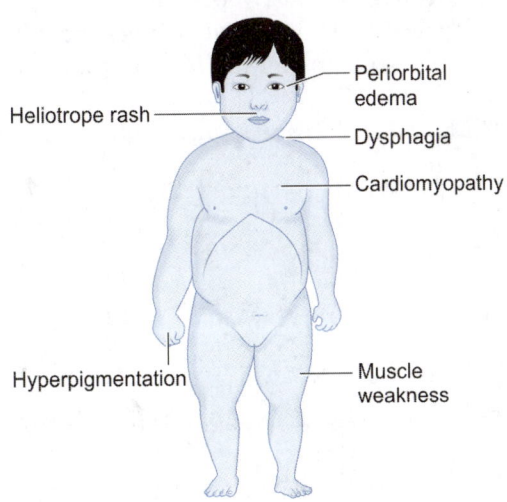

Fig. 1: Clinical features.

tissue. Palatorespiratory muscles may lead to respiratory difficulty, aspiration, and death.

The upper eyelid assumes a pathognomonic violaceous discoloration—heliotrope eyelid. A butterfly rash similar to that of SLE is present. The capillaries of nail-bed may become tortuous or occluded. A dusty erythema may cover the upper trunk and proximal extremities.

In long-standing disease, there may be cutaneous atrophy with binding of skin. In underlying structure calcium may be deposited in affected subcutaneous tissue, muscle, and fascia. Low-grade fever is often present. Systemic involvement is represented by lymphadenopathy, hepatosplenomegaly, and GI manifestation.

Some of the clinical features are as follows:
- Insidious
- Fatigue
- Low-grade fever
- Weight loss
- Irritability
- Heliotropic rash
- Periorbital or facial edema
- Hyperpigmentation at knuckles **(Fig. 2)**
- Proximal muscle weakness
- Dysphagia cardiomyopathy

Typical dermatological changes include goitrous papules over the dorsal aspects of metacarpophalangeal and interphalangeal joint, edema over the eyelids, photosensitivity, a truncal rash, and calcinosis.

CRITERIA FOR THE DIAGNOSIS
- Characteristic heliotrope discoloration over the upper eyelid
- Symmetrical proximal muscle weakness
- Elevate levels of muscle enzymes
- Electromyographic evidence of myopathy
- Muscle biopsy findings, myonecrosis, myophagocytosis, perifascicular atrophy

Magnetic resonance imaging shows muscle edema and inflammation, fibrosis, atrophy, and fatty infiltration.

Methotrexate is a steroid-sparing agent. It allows the rapid reduction total corticosteroid dose. Additional immunomodulatory agents include cytosine. Intravenous (IV) immunoglobulin may be used. Newer biological agents include etanercept.

LABORATORY SALIENT FINDINGS
- Muscle enzyme levels—aspartate aminotransferase, alanine aminotransferase, lactate dehydrogenase
- Magnetic resonance imaging (MRI)—suggestive of myositis
- Electromyography
- Muscle biopsy suggestive of myositis

DIAGNOSIS

Tests for RFs and antinuclear antibodies (ANAs) are generally negative. Radiograph shows calcium deposits in soft tissue.

Elevated serum levels of muscle-derived enzymes [creatine kinase (CK), aldolase, aspartate transaminase, alanine transaminase (ALT), LDH] reflect muscle inflammation. Not all enzyme levels rise with inflammation in a specific individual; ALT is usually elevated on initial presentation, whereas CK level may be normal.

Serologic testing results are divided into two groups: Myositis-associated

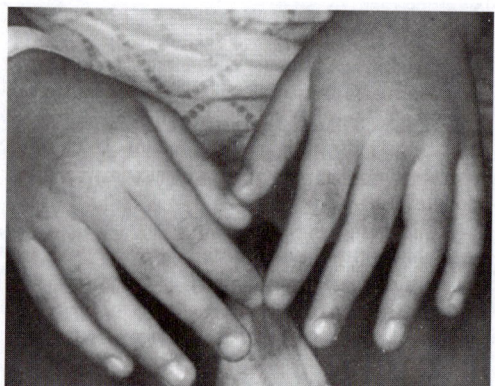

Fig. 2: Hyperpigmentation of knuckle.

antibodies (MAAs) and myositis-specific antibodies (MSAs). MAAs are associated with JDM but are not specific and can be seen in both overlap conditions and other rheumatic diseases. MSAs are specific for myositis. Presence of MAAs such as SSA, SSB, Sm, ribonucleoprotein (RNP), and double-stranded (ds) DNA may increase the likelihood of overlap disease or connective tissue myositis.

Anti-p155/140 antibodies also known as transcriptional intermediary factor 1-gamma (TIF-1-γ) are reported in 23–30% of children with JDM and are associated with photosensitive rashes, ulceration, and lipodystrophy. Unlike in adults, this antibody is not associated with malignancy in children with JDM. Anti-MJ antibodies, also known as NXP2, are reported in children with JDM and are associated with cramps, muscle atrophy, contractures, and dysphonia. Anti-MDA5 antibodies have been recently reported in children with JDM, and are concerning for development of interstitial lung disease.

Radiographic studies aid both diagnosis and medical management. MRI using T2-weighted images and fat suppression identifies active sites of disease, reducing sampling error and increasing the sensitivity of muscle biopsy and EMG, results of which are nondiagnostic in 20% of cases if the procedures are not directed by MRI.

Electromyogram (EMG) shows myopathic pattern with areas of fibrillation and indicating necrosis. It shows mixture of myopathic small, short polyphasic units, and denervation changes, i.e., fibrillation and positive sharp waves at rest. Blood immunoglobulin levels are elevated in some cases.

Muscle biopsy typically shows fiber degeneration and regeneration of inflammatory round cell infiltration and perifascicular atrophy. These changes are often focal and patchy. This may explain why muscle biopsy can occasionally be negative. Muscle ultrasound shows patchy, high-signal changes and may be used as a guide for the best site for muscle biopsy.

DIFFERENTIAL DIAGNOSIS

Differential diagnosis includes hematological malignancies and infectious diseases such as human immunodeficiency virus (HIV) and toxoplasmosis.

TREATMENT

Nursing care is mandatory. Corticosteroids will suppress the symptoms effectively. Prednisolone (1–2 mg/kg/24 hours) reduces the enzyme levels toward the normal value within 1–2 weeks. Clinical improvement with decreased pain and swelling in muscles and increased muscle strength usually follows. A low dose of steroid is sufficient to suppress clinical symptoms, and serum enzyme levels should be maintained for 1 month. Physiotherapy is also important.

Weekly oral, IV, or subcutaneous methotrexate (the lesser of 1 mg/kg or 15 mg/m^2, maximum 40 mg) is often used as a steroid-sparing agent in JDM. The concomitant use of methotrexate halves the cumulative age of steroids needed for disease control.

Risks of methotrexate include immunosuppression, blood count dyscrasias, chemical hepatitis pulmonary toxicity, nausea/vomiting, and teratogenicity. Folic acid is typically given with methotrexate starting at a dose of 1 mg daily to reduce toxicity and side effects of folate inhibition (oral ulcers, nausea, anemia). Children who are taking immunosuppressive medications such as methotrexate should avoid live-virus vaccination, although inactivated influenza vaccination is recommended yearly.

An international trial found the combination of methotrexate plus corticosteroids to perform better than corticosteroids alone and with fewer side effects than corticosteroids plus cyclosporine A.

Hydroxychloroquine has little toxicity risk and is used as a secondary disease-modifying agent to reduce rash and maintain remission. Typically, it is administered at doses of 4–6 mg/kg/day orally in either tablet or liquid form. Ophthalmologic follow-up 1–2 times per year to monitor for rare retinal toxicity is recommended. Other side effects include hemolysis in patients with glucose-6-phosphate deficiency, GI intolerance, and skin/hair discoloration.

The use of rituximab in a trial of steroid-dependent patients with resistant inflammatory myopathies, including JDM, did not meet the primary study endpoint showing a difference in time to improvement between individuals given rituximab at baseline or at 8 weeks, but overall, 80% of all patients met the definition of improvement in the trial. Reports of the use of other biologic agents are based on case reports with mixed results.

■ BIBLIOGRAPHY

1. Ernste FC, Reed AM. Recent advances in juvenile idiopathic inflammatory myopathies. Curr Opin Rheumatol. 2014; 26(6):671-9.
2. Rider LG, Katz JD, Jones OY. Developments in the classification and treatment of the juvenile idiopathic inflammatory myopathies. Rheum Dis Clin North Am. 2015;39(4):877-904.

CASE 103

Juvenile Rheumatoid Arthritis

■ PRESENTING COMPLAINTS

A 6-year-old girl was brought with the complaint of:
- Pain in the finger since 1 week
- Swelling of the small joint since 1 week
- Fever since 3 days

History of Presenting Complaints

A 6-year-old girl was brought to the outpatient department with history of pain in fingers of the hand and swelling of the small joints. Her mother told that her daughter developed these complaints since 1 week. In the beginning, she developed pain in the joints of the fingers of the hands. Pain became severe restricting the movements. The presence of the swelling at the joint was also noted. It was associated with history of fever. Fever was of moderate to high degree continuous type. There was no history of rigors and chills.

Past History of the Patient

The child was the only sibling of nonconsanguineous marriage. She was born at term by normal vaginal delivery. There was no significant postnatal event. Her birth weight was 3 kg. She started taking breast milk on the first day itself. She was exclusively on breast milk for 4 months, weaning of the feeds started later with cereals, and she was on family food by 15 months. Her developmental milestones were normal. She had been completely immunized. Her performance at school was above average. There was no family history of similar complaints.

■ EXAMINATION

The girl was moderately built and moderately nourished. She was looking toxic and was crying in agony. She was not allowing anybody to touch her fingers. Her anthropometric

---

CASE AT A GLANCE

Basic Findings
Height	: 114 cm (50th centile)
Weight	: 18 kg (50th centile)
Temperature	: 38°C
Pulse rate	: 124 beats/min
Respiratory rate	: 26 breaths/min
Blood pressure	: 80/60 mm Hg

Positive Findings

History:
- Joint pain
- Joint swelling
- Fever

Examination:
- Febrile
- Toxic
- Lymphadenopathy
- Splenomegaly

Investigation:
- *Hb:* 9 g/dL
- *ESR:* Raised
- *X-ray of joint:* Soft tissue swelling and increased joint space

(ESR: erythrocyte sedimentation rate; Hb: hemoglobin)

measurements included the height 114 cm (50th centile) and the weight 18 kg (50th centile). She was febrile, i.e., 38°C. The heart rate was 124 beats/min and the respiratory rate was 26 breaths/min. The blood pressure recorded was 80/60 mm Hg.

The child was pale. There was no cyanosis and no clubbing. There was cervical lymphadenopathy and no icterus. Per abdomen examination revealed presence of splenomegaly. Spleen was palpable about 3 cm below the costal margin. Respiratory cardiovascular system were normal.

INVESTIGATION

- *Hemoglobin:* 9 g/dL
- *TLC:* 9,800 cells/cumm
- *DLC:* $P_{72}\ L_{26}\ E_2\ M_0$
- *ESR:* 56 mm in the first hour
- *Serum immunoglobulin M (IgM):* Increased
- *X-ray of the joints:* Soft tissue swelling and increase in joint space

DISCUSSION

A girl presented with history of pain in the finger of the hand and associated with the swelling in joint. These symptoms along with the raised ESR and radiographic finding help in diagnosis of Juvenile idiopathic arthritis (JRA).

Juvenile idiopathic arthritis (JIA) is the most common rheumatic disease in children and one of the more common chronic illnesses of childhood. JIA represents a heterogeneous group of disorders all sharing the clinical manifestation of arthritis. The etiology and pathogenesis of JIA are largely unknown, and the genetic component is complex, making clear distinction among various subtypes difficult.

Juvenile rheumatoid arthritis is a clinical syndrome in which one or more joints show inflammatory changes lasting for >3 months. It may occur at any time after infancy. The peak age of the onset is children 2.5 years. Girls are more prone than boys.

It is an autoimmune disease with major histocompatibility complex (MHC) associated with genetic predisposition. Environmental triggering factors include, e.g., infection with rubella virus, parvovirus 19, mycobacterium, trauma, and psychological stress are linked to the onset of JRA.

There is nonspecific inflammation of the synovial membrane. Synovial tissue is edematous, hyperemic, and infiltrated with lymphocytes and plasma cells. Joint spaces are filled with inflammatory fluid.

Complement activation and consumption probably play an important role in the inhibition and perpetuation of the inflammatory response. These are believed to secrete inflammatory cytokine. A number of autoantibodies, i.e., ANAs and antismooth muscle antibodies are seen. The immunoglobulin M (IgM) rheumatoid factor (RF) is usually negative.

ETIOLOGY

The etiology and pathogenesis of JIA are not completely understood though both immunogenetic susceptibility and an external trigger are considered necessary. JIA is a complex genetic trait in which multiple genes may affect disease susceptibility. There is evidence that the interleukin-6 (IL-6) gene, confers susceptibility to systemic JIA (sJIA), with increased transmission of the -174G allele in patients older than 5 years. Possible nongenetic triggers include bacterial and viral infections, enhanced immune responses to bacterial or mycobacterial heat shock proteins, abnormal reproductive hormone levels, and joint trauma.

PATHOGENESIS

Juvenile rheumatoid arthritis is an autoimmune disease associated with alterations in both humoral and cell-mediated immunity. T-lymphocytes have a central role, releasing proinflammatory cytokines favoring a type 1 helper T-lymphocyte response. Studies of T-cell receptor expression confirm recruitment of T-lymphocytes specific for synovial non-self-antigens. B-cell activation, immune complex formation, and complement activation also promote inflammation. Inheritance of specific cytokine alleles may predispose to upregulation of inflammatory networks, resulting in systemic disease or more severe articular disease.

Systemic JIA is characterized by dysregulation of the innate immune system with a lack of autoreactive T-cells and autoantibodies. It is therefore may be more accurately classified as an autoinflammatory disorder.

As disease of persistent inflammation of the synovium, JIA has long been considered a manifestation of autoimmunity; however, intense investigation has failed to identify autoantibodies or target antigens. It is postulated that persistence of microbial antigens initiates synovial inflammation through the action of antibodies against microbial antigens that cross-react with self (molecular mimicry). Another line of investigation presents evidence that an infection promotes the presentation of self-human leukocyte antigen (HLA) peptides to T-cells.

Evidence for an infectious initiation of synovial inflammation includes the persistent arthritis seen after a variety of infections, including rubella and parvovirus. The clinical features (abrupt onset, high-spiking fever, rash, hepatosplenomegaly, lymphadenopathy, and serositis) and a clustering of cases in the autumn also suggest infection as an inflammatory trigger. Further, polymerase chain reaction has allowed identification of microbes and their antigens in synovial tissue in some arthritides not previously thought to be due to infection.

The immunologic cascade involved in JIA appears to be initiated by presentation of antigen(s) to T-lymphocytes by antigen-presenting cells (macrophages, B-cells, DC, fibroblasts, and endothelial cells). Cytokines then trigger polyclonal T-cell expansion and production of a variety of additional inflammatory mediators including prostaglandins, complement proteins, kinins, proteases, matrix metalloproteases, and lysosomal enzymes. The result is migration of additional inflammatory cells into the synovial tissue and fluid, increased vascular permeability, and damage to cartilage and bone.

The histology of the inflamed synovium in all categories of JIA is identical to that of adult rheumatoid arthritis, with characteristic lymphocytic and plasma cell infiltration, and later villous hypertrophy and hyperplasia of the synovial lining. This process is accompanied by prominent vascular endothelial cell hyperplasia and angiogenesis, resulting in the secretion of large amounts of protein-rich synovial fluid and the migration of neutrophils, lymphocytes, and macrophages into the joint. Synovial-fluid white cell counts usually range from 2,000 to 30,000/mL. However, even counts exceeding 100,000/mL may be seen in patients with sJIA.

An exuberant inflammatory process leads to aggressive expansion of the synovium onto the articular cartilage, resulting in the so-called pannus formation. Lysosomal hydrolyses that break down proteoglycans and collagen facilitate invasion of the avascular cartilage by the pannus. Prolonged synovial inflammation causes irreparable damage to the cartilage, as well as erosion and destruction of subchondral bone. Formation of synovial-lined bony cysts can occur. New investigations have documented migration of activated macrophages into subchondral bone, with activation of osteoclasts, further contributing to chronic erosive changes.

Small areas of bone at the margins of articular cartilage (bare areas) are exposed directly to the inflamed synovium; erosions at these sites provide an early radiographic clue to bony destruction in inflammatory arthritis.

All these immunologic abnormalities cause inflammatory synovitis characterized pathologically by villous hypertrophy and hyperplasia with hyperemia and edema of the synovial tissue. Vascular endothelial hyperplasia is prominent and is characterized by infiltration of mononuclear and plasma cells with a predominance of T-lymphocytes. Advanced and uncontrolled disease leads to pannus formation and progressive erosion of articular cartilage and contiguous bone.

■ CLINICAL FEATURES (FIG. 1)

Arthritis must be present to make a diagnosis of any JIA subtype. Arthritis is defined by intra-articular swelling or the presence of two or more of the following signs: limitation in range of motion, tenderness or pain on motion, and warmth. Initial symptoms may be subtle or acute and often include morning stiffness with a limp or gelling after inactivity. Easy fatigability and poor sleep quality may be associated. Involved joints are often swollen, warm to touch, and painful on movement or palpation with reduced range of motion, but usually are not erythematous.

Arthritis in large joints, especially knees, initially accelerates linear growth and causes the affected limb to be longer, resulting in a discrepancy in limb lengths. Continued inflammation stimulates rapid and premature

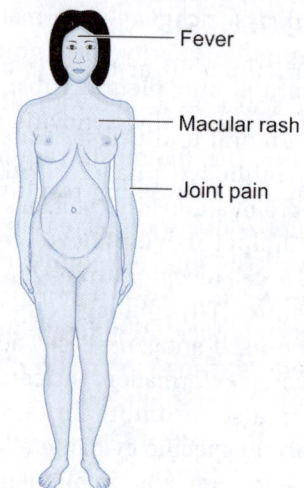

Fig. 1: Clinical features.

closure of the growth plate, resulting in shortened bones.

The patient's history and physical examination assume critical importance in establishing the diagnosis of JIA. A cardinal feature of inflammatory synovitis is morning stiffness of at least 30 minutes, with improvement over time or following movement and warming of the joint. Parents and other caregivers may observe changes in walking, running climbing stairs, or eagerness to play. Children may need help with dressing, eating, bathing, toileting, and other activities that were previously performed independently. Enuresis may recur in a recently toilet-trained child, and developmental milestones may be lost. Children not old enough to describe stiffness or pain may be cranky or irritable in the morning or after a nap or have generally decreased activity.

On physical examination, all joints must be thoroughly assessed for swelling, tenderness, pain, motion, and bony enlargement. Muscles should be examined for strength and possible atrophy. In addition, extra-articular signs of juvenile arthritis, including abnormal pupils, rash, lymphadenopathy, organomegaly, and pericardial and pleural rubs, should be sought. Occasionally, synovitis may be painless, but the diagnosis requires the physical finding of swelling resulting from inflammation. Loss of or decreased motion with pain of the affected joints indicates chronicity of the joint inflammation and is indirect evidence of synovitis in those joints where swelling cannot be visualized (i.e., spine, hip, and shoulder).

Oligoarticular Juvenile Idiopathic Arthritis

Oligoarticular type is most common type. It constitutes about 30–40% of patients. It is often asymmetrical. Children may develop leg-length discrepancy, in which involved leg grows longer due to increased blood and growth factor.

Oligoarticular JIA, defined as arthritis in four or fewer joints over the first 6 months of symptoms. The ratio of males to females is 1:6.5; the usual age of onset is 1–3 years. Typically, the arthritis has an insidious onset and is minimally symptomatic. Many of these children will report no pain and come to medical attention after joint swelling is found incidentally. The knee is most frequently involved, followed by the ankle and then the small joints of the hand or the wrist; almost any joint, however, may be affected. Children with oligoarticular JIA are systemically well otherwise.

Type I: It is more common among females. Knees, ankles, and elbows are commonly involved. There will be low-grade fever and easy fatigability. Iridocyclitis is observed in 25% patients. These require slit-lamp examination. Secondary glaucoma and cataract may develop. ANAs are positive. RF is negative.

Type II: It is less common. Hip and girdle joints are involved. Sacroiliitis will develop. ANA antibodies and RFs are negative. Family history of psoriasis, Reiter's disease, and low back pain will be present.

Asymptomatic uveitis (inflammation of the uveal tract—iris, ciliary body, and choroid) develops in approximately 20% of children with oligoarticular JIA, and 80% of these children will have a positive ANA test. Prompt diagnosis and treatment of uveitis are critical to prevent later cataracts and glaucoma and potential loss of vision. Consequently, ophthalmologic screening by slit-lamp examination every 3–4 months is essential for these high-risk children. Persistent or difficult-to-treat uveitis becomes the most prominent chronic feature in a subset of children with JIA.

Over time, approximately 80% of children with oligoarthritis will continue to have episodes of arthritis with four or fewer joints involved (persistent oligoarthritis), whereas 20% will have extension of synovitis into additional joints, which will be labeled as having extended oligoarthritis.

Enthesitis refers to inflammation at the site where ligaments, tendons, fascia, or capsules attach to bone. This group includes children most likely be from the International League of Associations for Rheumatology (ILAR) categories of enthesitis-related arthritis, psoriatic arthritis, and undifferentiated arthritis, but may include patients from any of the ILAR JIA categories. Active enthesitis is tenderness and/or swelling of the entheses.

Enthesitis is most common in males, older 10 years of age. It is typically associate with lower extremity and large arthritis. The hallmark of this form is inflammation of tendinous insertion (enthesopathy), such as tibial tubercle or the heel. Carriage of HLA-B27 antigen is associated with increased risk of developing enthesitis-associated arthritis.

Psoriatic arthritis have typical psoriasis present and subtle changes such as nail pitting are present. They may also present with dactylitis or "sausage digit", which is painful swelling of entire finger or toe.

The presence of a positive ANA confers 20% increased risk for asymptomatic anterior uveitis, requiring periodic slit-lamp examination. ANA positivity may also be correlated with younger age at disease onset, female sex, asymmetric arthritis, and lower number of involved joints over time. Slit-lamp examination must performed at 3 months' interval if ANA positive and at 6 months' interval if ANA negative for at least 4 years after onset of arthritis as this the period of highest risk.

Anemia is mild-to-moderate, normocytic, or microcytic hypochromic type. Total leukocyte count is increased. Serum protein shows increase alpha 2 and gamma globulin fractions.

Lupus erythematosus may be demonstrated in few cases. IgM levels are elevated, radiograph of joints show soft tissue swelling and increased joint space. With destruction of articular cartilages, bone ends approximate and joint space is reduced.

Synovial fluid aspiration for microscopy and culture are indicated. Fluid predominantly shows polymorphonuclear response with low sugar and decreased complement.

Polyarticular Juvenile Idiopathic Arthritis

Polyarticular JIA is defined as involvement of at least five joints during the first 6 months of illness; it is found in approximately 25% of children with JIA. This group is further subclassified into the categories of RF-negative and RF-positive disease. Those children who are considered to be RF-positive must have this test confirmed with repeat testing at least 3 months from the initial test. Females predominate, with two peak ages of onset: 1–3 years, and again during early adolescence.

Both large and small joints may be affected; presentations vary from scattered joint involvement to symmetric synovitis of nearly all joints in the body. Involvement of the cervical spine, hips, shoulders, and temporomandibular joints (TMJ) is common finding. Micrognathia reflects chronic TMJ disease. Cervical spine involvement, manifesting as decreased neck extension, occurs with a risk of atlantoaxial subluxation and neurologic sequelae. Hip disease may be subtle, with findings of decreased or painful range of motion on examination. Flexion deformities of the knees, wrists, and hips may develop. Proximal interphalangeal joints are involved.

In most patients, the onset is insidious and accompanied by fatigue. Additionally, some patients have low-grade fever, weight loss, hepatosplenomegaly, lymphadenopathy, pleuritis pericarditis, and pneumonitis. These patients are more likely to have elevated acute-phase reactants, including ESR, C-reactive protein (CRP), and platelet counts, and often may have mild anemia of chronic disease. White blood cell counts typically are normal.

The disease of children with a positive RF closely resembles adult rheumatoid arthritis, including occasional development of rheumatoid nodules, vasculitis, and Felty syndrome (splenomegaly and leukopenia). Antibodies to cyclic citrullinated peptide (anti-CCP) are found in many of the same patients, although they may develop earlier than the RF and may be a more sensitive marker of severe disease. Other serologic markers generally are negative; approximately 30% of patients with polyarticular JIA have positive ANA test results.

Systemic Juvenile Idiopathic Arthritis

In acute febrile, or systemic disease, i.e., Still's disease (sJIA). It accounts for 5–10%. The systemic manifestation includes fever, and rashes. Fever is intermittent. There is nonpruritic evanescent maculopapular rash in 90% of the patients. sJIA is characterized by arthritis, fever, rash, and prominent visceral involvement, including hepatosplenomegaly, lymphadenopathy, and serositis (pericarditis). The characteristic fever, defined as spiking temperatures to ≤39°C (102.2°F), occurs on a daily or twice-daily basis for at least 2 weeks, with a rapid return to normal or subnormal temperatures. The fever is often present in the evening and is frequently accompanied by a characteristic faint, erythematous, macular rash. The peak of the fever curve is often in the evening and may be accompanied by intense arthralgia and myalgia. When the temperature is normal, the child may feel quite well only to appear ill again when the fever spikes. Often the fever and other systemic features will precede the development of arthritis, so in general, systemic-onset JIA is a diagnosis of exclusion. Such patients must have an extensive or most reasonable evaluation to rule out other sources of fever, especially infections and malignancies.

Patients with sJIA may have a wide variety of systemic manifestations. Among them is a. macular, evanescent, salmon-colored rash. It typically exhibits discrete borders with or without central clearing and is often best seen during the fever. The rash may be raised, is usually, nonpruritic, and is migratory, appearing anywhere, but most commonly over the trunk, thighs, and axillae. It may be induced by mild trauma (Koebner phenomenon). Other common systemic manifestations include pericarditis, myocarditis, pleuritis, lymphadenopathy, hepatosplenomegaly, abdominal pain, fatigue, anorexia, weight loss, and, rarely, asymptomatic iritis. With time, few or many inflamed joints will appear. They tend to be markedly swollen and more painful than the arthritis of other subgroups. Nighttime pain and awakening are not unusual, but they nonetheless should prompt investigation for underlying malignancy or infection.

Neutrophilic leukocytosis (20,000–30,000 cells/cumm) mild anemia, elevated sedimentation rate, and elevated acute phase reactants are present. ANAs are present, but RFs are negative.

Variants in MHC class I and class II regions have indisputably been associated with different JIA subtypes. Non-HLA candidate loci are also associated with JIA, including polymorphisms in the genes encoding protein tyrosine phosphatase nonreceptor 22 (PTPN22), TNF-0, macrophage inhibitory factor, IL-6 and its receptor, and IL-1a. Possible nongenetic triggers include bacterial and viral infections, enhanced immune responses to bacterial or mycobacterial heat shock proteins, abnormal reproductive hormone levels, and joint trauma.

The fever is often present in the evening and is frequently accompanied by a characteristic faint, erythematous, macular rash. The evanescent salmon-colored lesions, classic for sJIA, are linear or circular and are usually distributed over the trunk and proximal extremities. The classic rash is nonpruritic and migratory with lesions lasting <1 hour. Koebner phenomenon, a cutaneous hypersensitivity in which classic lesions are brought on by superficial trauma, is often present. Heat can also evoke rash. Fever, rash, hepatosplenomegaly, and lymphadenopathy are present in >70% of affected children.

Macrophage activation syndrome (MAS) is a rare but potentially fatal complication of sJIA that can occur at any time (onset, medication change, active or remission) during the disease course. It is also referred to as secondary hemophagocytic syndrome or hemophagocytic lymphohistiocytosis (HLH). MAS classically manifests as acute onset of high-spiking fevers, lymphadenopathy, hepatosplenomegaly, and encephalopathy. Laboratory evaluation shows thrombocytopenia and leukopenia with elevated liver enzymes, LDH, ferritin, and triglycerides.

Patients may have purpura and mucosal bleeding, as well as elevated fibrin split product values and prolonged prothrombin and partial prothromboplastin times. The ESR falls because of hypofibrinogenemia and hepatic dysfunction, a feature useful in distinguishing MAS from a flare of systemic disease.

An international consensus panel developed a set of classification criteria for sJIA-associated MAS, including hyperferritinemia (>684 ng/mL) and any two of the following: thrombocytopenia <1.5 lakh, elevated liver enzymes (aspartate transaminase >48 U/L), hypertriglyceridemia (>156 mg/dL), and hypofibrinogenemia <360 mg/dL.

These criteria apply to a febrile patient suspected of sJIA and in the absence of disorders such as immune-mediated thrombocytopenia, infectious hepatitis, familial hypertriglyceridemia, or visceral leishmaniasis. A relative change in laboratory values is likely more relevant in making an early diagnosis than are absolute normal values.

A bone marrow aspiration and biopsy may be helpful in diagnosis, but evidence of hemophagocytosis is not always evident. Emergency treatment with high-dose intravenous (IV) methylprednisolone, cyclosporine, or anakinra may be effective.

Laboratory features:
- Cytopenias
- Abnormal liver function tests
- Coagulopathy (hypofibrinogenemia)
- Decreased erythrocyte sedimentation rate
- Hypertriglyceridemia
- Hyponatremia
- Hypoalbuminemia
- Hyperferritinemia
- Elevated sCD25 and sCD163

Clinical features:
- Nonremitting fever
- Hepatomegaly
- Splenomegaly
- Lymphadenopathy
- Hemorrhages
- Central nervous system dysfunction (headache, seizures, lethargy coma, disorientation)

Histopathological features:
- Macrophage hemophagocytosis in the bone marrow aspirate
- Increased CD163 staining of the bone marrow
- Proposed criteria for MAS in sJIA
- Serum ferritin >684 ng/mL and any two of the following:
- Thrombocytopenia <1.5 lakh
- Elevated liver enzymes (aspartate transaminase >48 U/L)
- Hypertriglyceridemia (156 mg/dL)
- Hypofibrinogenemia <360 mg/dL

The child with typical fever and rash but without arthritis may be treated empirically for probable sJIA after other diagnoses are exhaustively excluded. The diagnosis is not firm until synovitis appears and other potential causes of the child's symptoms have been duly considered. Many of these children will require bone marrow aspiration and/

or lymph node biopsy to exclude malignant diseases. However, severe sequelae largely may be avoided with prompt recognition and treatment with pulse IV methylprednisolone and further immunosuppression (e.g., with interleukin blockade with anakinra, or IV cyclosporine).

> **ESSENTIAL DIAGNOSTIC POINTS**
> - Nonarticular, monoarticular, or polyarticular arthropathy
> - Proximal interphalangeal joints and large joints are involved
> - Duration will lasts for >3 months
> - Fever erythematous rashes, nodules leukocytosis
> - Iridocyclitis, pleuritis pericarditis
> - Anemia, fatigue, and growth failure

■ DIAGNOSIS

As described for each category of JIA, there is no test or combination of tests that can differentiate JIA from other diseases. JIA remains a clinical diagnosis dependent on the finding of unexplained synovitis. The major role of laboratory tests is to exclude other potential diagnoses, particularly infection and/or malignancy, and to stratify patients' risk of developing disease sequelae. In cases of systemic arthritis, laboratory tests additionally help define severity of systemic inflammation.

Investigations in oligoarticular JIA:
- Primarily to exclude alternate diagnosis such as infections and malignancy
- Complete blood count (CBC) with peripheral smear
- C-reactive protein, ESR
- Consider LDH levels if suspicion of malignancy is high
- Koch's screen if history suggestive
- ANA by immunofluorescence (IF)
- RF is usually negative
- Imaging to be considered on case-to-case basis

- Ultrasound scan or MRI of affected joint in select cases
- Eye screening for uveitis

Investigations in polyarticular course of JIA:
- Complete blood count with peripheral smear
- CRP and ESR
- RF
- HLA-B27
- X-ray pelvis/magnetic resonance imaging (MRI)/computed tomography (CT)
- Tuberculosis (TB) screening before starting DMARDs

Investigations in systemic arthritis:
- Complete blood count with peripheral smear
- C-reactive protein, ESR
- Liver function test
- Ferritin levels
- LDH, bone marrow aspiration to exclude malignancy
- Triglycerides, fibrinogen levels if suspicion of MAS is high
- ANA-F and RF usually negative
- Infection screen as deemed suitable by treating physician
- Imaging to be considered on a case-to-case basis: Ultrasound/plain radiograph/MRI
- Intra-articular corticosteroid injection
- Adjunct NSAIDs

Radiographic Changes

The earliest changes are soft tissue swelling and periarticular osteopenia, although this latter finding is only visible on plain radiographs when 50% of the bone mineral content has been lost because of inflammation. The intense inflammation of the tendon sheath, joint, and tendon attachments can stimulate periosteal new bone formation in the tubular bones of the phalanges, metacarpals and metatarsals, and, occasionally, long bones.

A characteristic radiographic finding in children with JIA involving a finger is widening of the midportion of a phalange from periosteal new bone formation. Plain radiographs are also useful for monitoring chronic joint changes and effectiveness of treatment, but ultrasound, CT, and MRI evaluations are more sensitive.

In young children, joint space widening can initially be seen because of increased intra-articular fluid or synovial hypertrophy. The hypervascularity of involved joints may stimulate adjacent growth plates and result in bony enlargement (e.g., knee or ankle) or epiphyseal advancement or closure (often seen in the wrist or hip).

Ultrasonography can identify synovial expansion, increased synovial fluid, and bony erosions. Ultrasound provides an inexpensive, easily available imaging technique that can assist clinicians in demonstrating subclinical synovitis and enthesitis as an adjunct to clinical examination and assessment, especially on the hips, shoulders, wrists, and ankles. MRI with IV gadolinium contrast provides the most complete imaging analysis, can assess the extent of synovitis and bone marrow edema, and can reliably show early erosive changes. CT is most useful for identifying bony abnormalities and erosions.

Joint space narrowing on plain radiographs and CT scanning is detectable only after a significant amount of cartilage has been destroyed. This detection typically takes longer in children than in adults because of the relative thickness of cartilage during growth and may first become manifest in the TMJ. The TMJ is at particular risk for destruction, because the epiphysis is as immediately adjacent to a thin fibrocartilage, which is not as robust as is true articular cartilage. When the epiphysis is destroyed, micrognathia due to lack of mandibular growth becomes evident. Coronal CT of the TMJ currently provides the best images for evaluation of joint damage in the TMJ. Whereas MRI with IV gadolinium can detect active synovitis.

Children with JIA involving the neck should be followed with flexion and extension lateral radiographs of the cervical spine to assess the stability of C1 and C2 movement. Repeat films should be obtained before general anesthesia and if children are involved in gymnastics and contact sports.

Laboratory abnormalities of sJIA are often dramatic, including significant leukocytosis (>40,000), thrombocytosis (>1 million), and elevated inflammatory markers (e.g., CRP >20 mg/dL and ESR 100 mm/h). Elevated transaminases, anemia, and low serum albumin levels are found frequently, but urinalysis is normal.

During the acute phase of disease, some children become severely ill, with development of leukopenia, thrombocytopenia, profound anemia, and hypofibrinogenemia, and an acute decrease in the sedimentation rate. In addition, D-dimer and ferritin levels may rise dramatically, and prothrombin time and partial thromboplastin time become prolonged, consistent with disseminated intravascular coagulation. This crisis is called macrophage activation syndrome (MAS), and it appears to be related to hereditary lymphohistiocytosis. As it progresses, serum transaminases may abruptly increase to greater than 1,000 U/L, the bone marrow may exhibit hemophagocytosis, and further sequelae of disseminated intravascular coagulation and cytokine storm may develop.

Elevated ANA titers are present in 40–85% of children with oligoarticular or polyarticular JIA, but are rare with sJIA. ANA seropositivity is associated with increased risk of chronic uveitis in JIA.

Children with sJIA usually have striking elevations in inflammatory markers and white blood cell and platelet counts. Hemoglobin levels are low, typically in the range of 7–10 g/dL, with indices consistent with anemia of chronic disease. The ESR is usually high.

The main indication for joint aspiration and synovial analysis is to rule infection. A positive Gram stain and culture is definitive test for infection. A leukocyte count >2,000/μL suggests inflammation. A very low glucose concentration (<40/mg/dL) or very leukocyte count >60,000/μL is suggestive of bacterial arthritis.

Laboratory Criteria

- Cytopenias
- Abnormal liver function tests
- Coagulopathy (hypofibrinogenemia)
- Decreased ESR
- Hypertriglyceridemia
- Hyponatremia
- Hypoalbuminemia
- Hyperferritinemia
- Elevated sCD25 and sCD163

Clinical Criteria

- Nonremitting fever
- Hepatomegaly
- Splenomegaly
- Lymphadenopathy
- Hemorrhages
- CNS dysfunction (headache, seizures, lethargy, coma, disorientation)

Histopathological Criteria

- Macrophage hemophagocytosis in the bone marrow aspirate
- Increased CD163 staining of the bone marrow.

GENERAL FEATURES

- Morning stiffness
- Fatigue
- Oligoarthritis
- Polyarthritis

LABORATORY SALIENT FINDINGS

- Rheumatoid factor is positive
- Antinuclear antibodies (ANA) is present in pauciarticular disease
- Joint fluid analysis
- Anemia—normocytic or microcytic hypochromic, leukocytosis
- Increased alpha 2 and gamma globulin in serum.
- Immunoglobulin M (IgM) levels are elevated
- *Radiograph of joint:* Increased joint space soft-tissue swelling
- Synovial fluid aspiration for microscopy and culture

■ DIFFERENTIAL DIAGNOSIS

- Systemic lupus erythematosus (SLE)
- Dermatomyositis
- Vasculitis syndrome
- Scleroderma
- Lyme disease
- Reactive arthritis
- Rheumatic fever

■ COMPLICATIONS

- Chronic anterior uveitis
- Joint contractions
- Growth disturbances
- Amyloidosis

■ TREATMENT

Treatment includes: (1) Medical therapy, (2) physiotherapy, and (3) psychotherapy.

Medical Therapy

The goals of treatment are to achieve disease remission, prevent or halt joint damage, and foster normal growth and development. All children with JIA need individualized treatment plans, and management is tailored according to disease subtype and severity, presence of poor prognostic indicators, and response to medications.

Early diagnosis of JIA is the cornerstone of most effective therapy. The goals of treatment are to minimize or resolve symptoms, prevent joint destruction, maintain normal growth and development, and achieve inactive disease. Inactive disease is defined as no joints with active arthritis; no systemic features such as fever, rash, serositis, splenomegaly, or generalized lymphadenopathy attributable to JIA; no uveitis; normalization of inflammatory markers such as ESR or CRP; and normal physician's global evaluation.

Medications (Table 1)

Timely use and correct choice of currently available medications to achieve sustained remission with as few side or adverse effects as possible remain the most challenging issues in the treatment of JIA.

Nonsteroidal anti-inflammatory drugs (NSAIDs) are no longer the mainstay of treatment for arthritis, but they continue to be useful in the initial treatment for reduction of pain and as mild anti-inflammatory agents.

Intra-articular injections of triamcinolone acetonide or triamcinolone hexacetonide, in place of or in addition to systemic therapies, can be particularly effective in quickly suppressing inflammation in a limited number of joints. Depending on the age of the child and the number and location of joints to be injected, brief general anesthesia may be necessary for the injections. Repeat injections (up to three per joint) can be an important treatment strategy.

The administration (orally or intravenously) of systemic corticosteroids is mainly restricted to the management of the extra-articular features of sJIA (e.g., fever, anemia, pericarditis). A short course of low-dose prednisone may be considered for severe polyarthritis refractory to other therapies or while awaiting the effect of the recently initiated second-line or biologic therapy.

Corticosteroids are used for severe unremitting arthritis, systemic manifestation, i.e., pericarditis, myocarditis, and vasculitis.

Dose of prednisolone is 1–2/kg/ mg/day; occasionally methylprednisolone (10–30 mg/kg) are necessary for severe unremitting arthritis, systemic manifestations such as pericarditis, myocarditis, and vasculitis. Local steroid joint injection may be helpful.

TABLE 1: Drugs and doses.

Drugs	Doses
Naproxen	10–20
Indomethacin	1.5–3
Ibuprofen	30–40
Conventional disease-modifying antirheumatic drugs (DMARDs)	
Methotrexate	10–15 mg/m^2, once weekly, oral (preferably on empty stomach) or subcutaneous; administer with folic acid or folinic acid
Sulfasalazine	30–50 mg/kg/day in two divided doses (maximum 2 g/day)
Leflunomide	<20 kg: 10 mg every other day 20–40 kg: 10 mg daily >40 kg: 20 mg daily, oral

Triamcinolone hexacetonide is long-acting steroid that can be used injection.

Methotrexate remains the most widely used initial disease-modifying therapy in JIA because of its efficacy at achieving disease control and acceptable adverse effects. Methotrexate can be given either orally or as a subcutaneous injection, with the latter having greater bioavailability at higher doses. For patients with polyarthritis or persistent or extended oligoarthritis, methotrexate should be started as early as possible.

Folic or folinic acid supplementation may help prevent some or the adverse effects of methotrexate, in particular oral sores and ulcerations, nausea, and hematologic and liver enzyme abnormalities. Hydroxychloroquine is a useful adjunct and used along with methotrexate. Leflunomide may have efficacy and safety similar to those of methotrexate and is a reasonable alternative in a child with intolerance to methotrexate.

Nonsteroidal anti-inflammatory drugs alone rarely induce remission in children with polyarthritis or sJIA. Methotrexate is the oldest and least toxic of the DMARDs available for adjunctive therapy. It may take 6–12 weeks to see the effects of methotrexate. A low dose of methotrexate (5–10 mg/m^2/week or up to 1 mg/kg/weeks as a single dose) is generally well tolerated. A complete blood count and liver function tests should be obtained every 2–3 months.

Some NSAIDs are given as follows:
- *Naproxen:* 15–20 mg/kg/day; maximum dose per day is 750 mg/day given twice daily.
- *Ibuprofen:* 20–40/mg/day; maximum dose per day is 2,400 mg/day given four times daily.
- *Aspirin:* 50–75mg/kg/day; maximum dose per day is 2,000 mg/day given four times daily.
- *Indomethacin:* 1–2.5 mg/kg/day; maximum dose per day is 150 mg/day given three times daily.
- *Diclofenac:* 2–3 mg/kg/day; maximum dose per day is 150 mg/day given four times daily.
- *Piroxicam:* 0.3–0.6 mg/kg/day; maximum dose per day is 20 mg/day given once daily.

Failure of methotrexate monotherapy warrants the addition of a biologic DMARD (disease-modifying antirheumatic drug).

Some of the DMARDs are given as follows:
- Gold salts—0.25 mg/kg/week increased gradually to 1 mg/kg/week
- d-penicillamine
- Hydroxychloroquine.

With the advent of newer DMARDs, the use of systemic corticosteroids can often be avoided or minimized. Systemic steroids are recommended only for management of severe systemic illness, for bridge therapy during the wait for therapeutic response to a DMARD, and for control of uveitis. Steroids impose risks of severe toxicities, including Cushing syndrome, growth retardation, and osteopenia, and they do not prevent joint destruction.

Intra-articular injections of glucocorticoids —triamcinolone are preferred therapy for children with oligoarthritis who do not respond to an initial trail of NSAIDs. Systemic glucocorticoids usually prednisolone 1–2 mg/kg/day. Occasionally methylprednisolone (10–30 mg/kg) are necessary for severe unremitting arthritis, systemic manifestations such as pericarditis, myocarditis, vasculitis.

Cytotoxic agents: These are cyclophosphamide and azathioprine and very rarely required. Cyclosporine A is used in difficult cases.

Uveitis treatment is initiated with corticosteroid eye drops and dilating agents to prevent scarring between iris and lens.

In patients who fail to topical treatment, methotrexate, cyclosporine, and/tumor necrosis inhibitor such as infliximab or adalimumab may be used.

Newer modalities include biological: NSAIDs alone rarely induce remission in children with polyarthritis or sJIA. Methotrexate is the oldest and least toxic of the DMARDs available for adjunctive therapy. It may take 6–12 weeks to see the effects of methotrexate. Failure of methotrexate monotherapy warrants the addition of a biologic DMARD. Biologic medications that inhibit pro-inflammatory cytokines, such as TNF-a, IL-1, and IL-6, demonstrated excellent disease control.

During the past decade and a half, there has been quite a remarkable evolution in biologic therapy for adult and childhood arthritis. More focused anticytokine agents have been introduced and, to date, have been shown to be effective in better controlling arthritis and preventing joint damage, especially when administered earlier in the disease process.

In children with persistent enthesitis despite treatment with NSAIDs, TNF inhibitor (TNFi) is considered over methotrexate or sulfasalazine. However, in our settings DMARDs can be considered if TNFi is not feasible due to cost constraints.

A short course of bridge steroids may also considered for significant symptoms. Short course (3 months) and the lowest dose needed to control symptoms. The usual starting dose for this is 0.5–1 mg/kg/day in divided doses, which is gradually tapered and stopped over 3 months. This may be considered during initiation or escalation of therapy in children with moderate or high disease activity.

Intra-articular glucocorticoid injections (triamcinolone acetonide) can be used for ameliorating the symptoms in limited number of joints in any of the JIA subtype.

These include anakinra (IL-1 receptor antagonist); canakinumab (monoclonal antibody to IL-1); tocilizumab (monoclonal antibody to IL-6 receptor); infliximab, golimumab, and adalimumab (monoclonal antibodies to TNF alpha); etanercept (recombinant soluble TNF receptor p75 fusion protein); and abatacept (inhibitor of T-cell activation).

Tumor necrosis factor-alpha antagonists (e.g., etanercept, adalimumab) are used to treat children with an inadequate response to methotrexate, with poor prognostic factors, or with severes disease onset, aggressive therapy with a combination or methotrexate and a TNF-a antagonist may result in earlier achievement of clinically inactive disease. Abatacept, a selective inhibitor of T-cell activation, and tocilizumab, an IL-6 receptor antagonist, have demonstrated efficacy in and are approved for treatment of polyarticular JIA.

Etanercept was the first anti-TNF therapy that was approved in the treatment of JIA; others with similar pharmacologic activity include infliximab, adalimumab, and golimumab. Co-stimulatory blocking agents (abatacept) provided another therapeutic option for those without good control with an anti-TNF agent. Anti-IL-1 (anakinra, rilonacept, canakinumab) and anti-L-6 (tocilizumab) agents have shown efficacy and tolerability for the treatment of sJIA.

Tumor necrosis factor inhibition is not as effective for the systemic symptoms found in sJIA. When systemic symptoms dominate, systemic corticosteroids are started followed by the initiation of IL-I or IL-6 antagonist therapy, which often induces a dramatic and rapid response. Patients with severe disease activity may go directly to anakinra. Canakinumab, an IL-1 inhibitor, and tocilizumab are Food and Drug Administration (FDA)-approved treatments for sJIA in children older than 2 years. Standardized consensus treatment plans to guide therapy for sJA, outline for treatment plans based on glucocorticoids, methotrexate, anakinra, or tocilizumab, with optional glucocorticoid use in the latter three plans as clinically indicated.

All of the medications mentioned here (including NSAIDs) have potential side effects and require ongoing laboratory monitoring. Cytopenias and liver function abnormalities are seen most commonly for patients on methotrexate, complete blood count (CBC), aspartate aminotransferase (AST), blood urea nitrogen (BUN), and creatinine are recommended after 1 month of treatment and then every 2–4 months. For NSAID use, the same monitoring (with a urinalysis) should be done 1 month after starting the medication and then every 4 months thereafter. Similar monitoring is recommended for most biologic agents.

Oral Janus kinase (JAK) inhibitors (tofacitinib, ruxolitinib) inhibit JAK signaling pathways involved in immune activation and inflammation. Tofacitinib is approved by FDA for adults with rheumatoid arthritis.

Management of JIA must include periodic slit-lamp ophthalmologic examinations to monitor for asymptomatic uveitis. Optimal treatment of uveitis requires collaboration between the ophthalmologist and rheumatologist. Initial management of uveitis may include mydriatics and corticosteroids used topically, systemically, or through periocular injection. DMARDs allow for a decrease in exposure to steroids, methotrexate and antibodies to TNF-alpha. (adalimumab and infliximab) are effective in treating severe uveitis.

Dietary evaluation and counseling to ensure appropriate calcium, vitamin D, protein, and caloric intake are important for children with JIA. Physical therapy and occupational therapy are invaluable adjuncts to any treatment program. A social worker and nurse clinician can be important resources for families to recognize stresses imposed by a chronic illness, identify appropriate community resources, and aid compliance with the treatment protocol.

■ PROGNOSIS

Children with persistent oligoarthritis JIA have high rate of clinical remissions. Children with RF factor-positive disease are at higher risk for chronic erosive arthritis, which may continue in adulthood. Prognosis in systemic disease is worse in patients with persistent systemic disease after 6 months, thrombocytosis, and more extensive arthritis.

Tuberculosis screening should be done prior to initiation of any biologic treatment and repeat surveillance should be performed annually while on anti-TNF agents.

Clinical follow-up of children with active JIA should occur every 1–3 months to allow for thorough evaluations and medication adjustments, with the goal of achieving disease remission. Meticulous surveillance for medication-related adverse effects is of prime importance, especially with the use of biologic agents. After inactive disease is achieved, medications are kept stable for 6 months to several years before they are gradually tapered and discontinued.

■ PHYSIOTHERAPY

Physical and occupational therapies are important components of the care and treatment of children with JIA. Its goals include improving range of motion, strength, and function, and preventing further deterioration. Because loss of age-appropriate developmental skills can occur, functional skills should be monitored by a therapist experienced in working with children with arthritis. Frequency of therapy visits varies considerably, but all therapy is based on a daily home program done by the child and parent. With severe ongoing disease, long-term cooperation with physical and occupational therapy can be difficult but is enhanced if the therapist tailors the home program to take into account age, extent and severity of disease, school activities, sports, hobbies, and family dynamics. An active lifestyle is important for maintaining bone and joint health; low-impact exercises, like swimming, are preferable when disease is active.

Night time splinting of the wrist, hand, knee, elbow, or ankle may decrease morning stiffness and help to prevent flexion contractures during active disease. Loss of extension can often be improved after corticosteroid injection followed by serial casting of a knee, ankle, wrist, finger, or elbow. Ice, heat ultrasound, or a combination of these modalities may help restore motion and decrease pain caused by muscle spasm. When a difference in leg length is present, a shoe lift for the shorter limb will help to prevent contralateral knee or hip flexion contractures. Children with arthritis of the tarsal and metatarsal joints may ambulate more easily with shoe splints (soft orthotics).

BIBLIOGRAPHY

1. Beukelman T, Patkar NM, Saag KG, Tolleson-Rinehart S, Cron RQ, DeWitt EM, et al. 2011 American College of Rheumatology recommendations for the treatment of juvenile idiopathic arthritis: initiation and safety monitoring of therapeutic agents for the treatment of arthritis and systemic features. Arthritis Care Res (Hoboken). 2011; 63:465-82.
2. Cassidy JT, Levison JE, Bass JC, et al. Arthritis Rheum. 29:174-181, 1996.
3. Kahn PJ. Juvenile idiopathic arthritis—what the clinician needs to know. Bull Hosp Jt Dis (2013). 2013;71(3):194-9.
4. Ringold S, Weiss PF, Beukelman T, Dewitt EM, Ilowite NT, Kimura Y, et al.; American College of Rheumatology. 2013 update of the 2011 American College of Rheumatology recommendations for the treatment of juvenile idiopathic arthritis: recommendations for the medical therapy of children with systemic juvenile idiopathic arthritis and tuberculosis screening among children receiving biologic medications. Arthritis Care Res (Hoboken). 2013;65(10): 1551-63.
5. Stoll ML, Cron RQ. Treatment of juvenile idiopathic arthritis: a revolution in care. Pediatr Rheumatol Online J. 2014;12:13.

SECTION 14

Miscellaneous

- Case 104 **Congenital Dislocation of Hip**
- Case 105 **Leprosy**
- Case 106 **Marfan's Syndrome**
- Case 107 **Osteogenesis Imperfecta**
- Case 108 **Talipes**

CASE 104: Congenital Dislocation of Hip

■ PRESENTING COMPLAINTS

A newborn baby girl was brought with the complaint of:
- Deformity in hip joint since birth.

History of Presenting Complaints

A newborn baby girl was brought to the orthopedic department as the resident doctor of the pediatric department found some deformity in the hip joint.

The baby was born by cesarean section at the term. The indication for the cesarean section was breech presentation. The baby cried immediately after the delivery. The cry of the baby was normal. The birth weight of the child was 3 kg. Activity of the child was normal. The pediatric resident who attended the delivery found hip of the child was abnormal. All movements at the hip joint were possible. Hence the child was sent to the orthopedic department to rule out congenital dislocation of the hip.

■ EXAMINATION

The baby was lying on the bed. She was alert and active. She appeared normal. The anthropometric measurements included, the length of the child was 51 cm (50th centile), the weight of the child was 3 kg (50th centile), and the head circumference was 35 cm. There was no pallor, no cyanosis, no lymphadenopathy, and there was no icterus. The pulse rate was 120 beats/min, and the respiratory rate was 22 breaths/min. The blood pressure recorded was 50/40 mm Hg.

Both the hips can be put through a full range of movements. Conventional clinical examination of the hip reveals no abnormality. Ortolani's maneuver was positive. Other systemic examinations were normal.

■ INVESTIGATION

- *Hemoglobin:* 14 g/dL
- *Total leukocyte count (TLC):* 8,600 cells/cumm

CASE AT A GLANCE

Basic Findings

Length	: 51 cm (50th centile)
Weight	: 3 kg (50th centile)
Temperature	: 37°C
Pulse rate	: 120 beats/min
Respiratory rate	: 22 breaths/min
Blood pressure	: 50/40 mm Hg

Positive Findings

History:
- Breech presentation
- Lower segment cesarean section (LSCS)
- Deformities in the hip

Examination:
- Active and normal child
- Ortolani's test positive

Investigation:
- Normal

- Differential leukocyte count (DLC): $P_{67}L_{26}E_4M_3$
- X-ray hip: Normal

DISCUSSION

The hip may be either dislocated or dislocatable at birth. The ligaments of the hips are unduly lax so that the femoral head can be dislocated from the acetabulum. The infant may lie on the hip in a dislocated position. The hip may be in a reduced position but easily dislocatable. If the femoral head is allowed to remain out to the acetabulum, the shortening of ligaments reduces the dislocation and increases difficulty. If a hip is allowed to remain dislocated until the child crawls and walks, the acetabulum fails to develop normally.

Developmental dysplasia of the hip (DDH) refers to a spectrum pathology in the development of the immature hip joint form called *congenital dislocation of the hip*, DDH is more accurately described as the variable presentation of the disorder, encompassing mild dysplasia (as well as frank dislocations).

The etiology of DDH is multifactorial, but numerous predisposing factors have been identified. The classic risk factors for DDH include breech positioning, family history of DDH, firstborn, female sex, and a history of oligohydramnios. Breech positioning is considered a packaging issue (intrauterine crowding) predisposing to DDH. Torticollis, metatarsus adductus, and oligohydramnios are other packaging-related conditions strongly associated with DDH.

Developmental dysplasia of the hip is a condition in which the femoral head has an abnormal relationship to the acetabulum, specifically, the acetabulum does not completely cover the femoral head. It can result in hip joint instability. Dislocation is defined as the complete displacement of a joint, with no contact between the original articular surfaces. Subluxation is defined as the displacement of a joint with some contact remaining between the articular surfaces. Dysplasia refers to the abnormal or deficient development of the acetabulum. A teratologic dislocation is a distinct condition that occurs before birth, is generally nonreducible on physical examination, and causes the hip to be stiff. Teratologic dislocations often are associated with other syndromes and conditions, particularly arthrogryposis and myelodysplasia, and treatment depends on the underlying condition.

It commonly affects the left hip. At birth both the acetabulum and femur are underdeveloped. Although the etiology remains unknown, the final common pathway in the development of DDH is increased laxity of the joint, which fails to maintain a stable femoroacetabular articulation. This increased laxity is probably the result of a combination of hormonal, mechanical, and genetic factors.

Any condition that leads to a tighter intrauterine space and, consequently, less room for normal fetal motion may be associated with DDH. These conditions include oligohydramnios, large birth weight, and first pregnancy.

Although most newborn screening studies suggest that some degree of hip instability can be detected in 1 in 100 to 1 in 250 babies, actual dislocated or dislocatable hips are much less common, being found in 1–1.5 of 1,000 live births.

PATHOANATOMY

Developmental dysplasia of the hip, several secondary anatomic changes can develop that can prevent reduction. Both the fatty tissue in the depths of the socket, known as the pulvinar and the ligamentum teres can hypertrophy, blocking the reduction of the femoral head. The transverse acetabular ligament usually thickens as well, which effectively narrows the opening of the acetabulum. In addition, the shortened iliopsoas tendon becomes taut across the front of the hip, creating an hourglass shape to the hip capsule, which limits access to the acetabulum. Over time, the dislocated femoral head places pressure on the acetabular rim and labrum, causing the labrum to infold and become thick. The shape of a normal femoral head and acetabulum depends on a concentric reduction between the two. The more time that a hip spends dislocated, the more likely that the acetabulum will develop abnormally. Without a femoral head to provide a template, the acetabulum will become progressively shallow, with an oblique acetabular roof and a thickened medial wall.

■ CLASSIFICATION

Developmental dysplasia of the hip is classified into two major groups: (1) Typical and (2) teratologic.

The condition may be unilateral or bilateral. It is related to a predisposition to joint laxity. This condition is predominant in females and in breech malposition of the fetus.

Congenital dislocation of the hip is classified into two major groups:
1. *Typical:* Occurs in neurologically normal infants.
2. *Teratologic:* Associated with underlying neuromuscular disorders, such as myelodysplasia and arthrogryposis multiplex. The cause is multifactorial, physiological, mechanical and postural and occur before birth.

■ CLINICAL FEATURES (FIG. 1)

At birth, the hips are not dislocated except the hip capsule and ligamentum teres are normal. If dislocation is allowed to occur acetabular dysplasia occurs. Maldirection and excessive femoral and hip muscle contractures occur.

At birth the appearance of an infant is normal, and the hips can be put through the full range of movements. Conventional clinical examination reveals no abnormality. Radiologically the epiphyses of the femoral head do not appear until the first year of life. The acetabulum is largely cartilaginous so that even if the hip is dislocated, there is no obvious radiological abnormality. Relaxing is the hormone attributed to the condition (Fig. 2).

The Neonate

Developmental dysplasia of the hip in the neonate is asymptomatic and must be screened for by specific maneuvers. Physical examination must be carried out with the infant unclothed and placed supine in a warm, comfortable setting on a flat examination table.

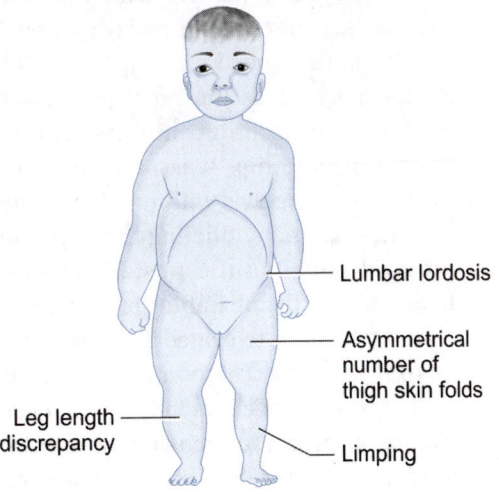

Fig. 1: Clinical features.

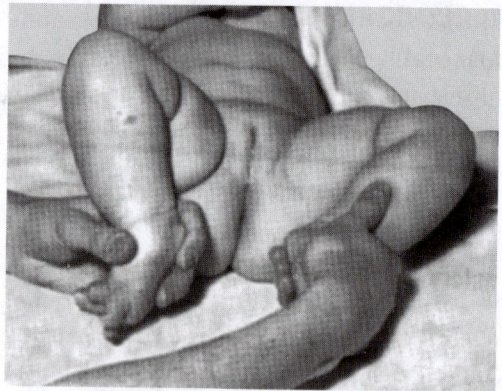

Fig. 2: Congenital dislocation of the hip.

- *Ortolani's test:* The demonstration includes eliciting the click from the hip. The hip is flexed at 90° and adducted. While the adduction is taking place, gentle pressure is exerted by examining the hand in a proximal direction along the axis of the femoral shafts. The femoral head rolls over the posterior hip of the acetabulum if the hip is dislocatable. The femoral head slips out of the acetabulum if the hip is dislocated. In unilateral congenital dislocation of the hip, skin creases in the groin and buttocks are seen asymmetrically. The affected hip will have a full range of movements and telescoping may be demonstrated.
- *Barlow's test:* It is the most important maneuver to examine hip dislocation of an unstable hip. It is performed by stabilizing the pelvis with one hand and then flexing and adducting the opposite hip and applying the posterior force. If the hip is dislocatable, it is usually readily felt. It gets relocated if the posterior force is released. The common concern is the presence of clicks in infants. These will be secondary to breaking the surface tension across the hip joint, the snapping of the gluteal tendons, and femorotibial rotation, or patellofemoral rotation.

In older children, limping, waddling, increased lumbar lordosis, toe walking, and leg length discrepancy indicate undiagnosed congenital dislocation of the hip.

- A *hip click* is the high-pitched sensation (or sound) felt at the very end of abduction during testing for DDH with Barlow and Ortolani maneuvers. Classically, a hip click is differentiated from a *hip clunk*, which is felt as the hip goes in and out of the joint. Hip clicks usually originate in the ligamentum teres or occasionally in the fascia lata or psoas tendon and do not indicate a significant hip abnormality.

The Infant

As the baby enters the second and third months of life, the soft tissues begin to tighten and the Ortolani and Barlow tests are no longer reliable. In this age group, the examiner must look for other specific physical findings, including limited hip abduction, apparent shortening of the thigh, proximal location of the greater trochanter, asymmetry of the gluteal or thigh folds, and positioning of the hip. Limitation of abduction is the most reliable sign of a dislocated hip in this age group.

Shortening of the thigh, the Galeazzi sign, is best appreciated by placing both hips in 90° of flexion and comparing the height of the knees, looking for asymmetry of thigh and gluteal skin folds may be present in 10% of normal infants but suggests DDH.

Another helpful test is the Klisic test, in which the examiner places the third finger over the greater trochanter and the index finger of the same hand on the anterior superior iliac spine. In a normal hip, an imaginary line drawn between the two fingers points to the umbilicus. In the dislocated hip, the trochanter is elevated, and the line projects halfway between the umbilicus and the pubis.

The Walking Child

The walking child often presents to the physician after the family has noticed a limp, a waddling gait, or a leg-length discrepancy. The affected side appears shorter than the normal extremity, and the child toe-walks on the affected side. The Trendelenburg sign is positive in these children, and an abductor lurch is usually observed when the child walks. As in the younger child, there is limited hip abduction on the affected side and the knees are at different levels when the hips are flexed (the Galeazzi sign). Excessive lordosis, which develops secondary to altered hip mechanics, is common and is often the presenting complaint.

GENERAL FEATURES

- Positive Barlow's test
- Positive Ortolani's test
- Palpable click
- Hip adduction
- Waddling

ESSENTIAL DIAGNOSTIC POINTS

- Positive Barlow's test
- Positive Ortolani's test
- Palpable click
- Hip adduction
- Asymmetrical number of thigh skinfolds
- Limping
- Waddling
- Increased lumbar lordosis
- Leg length discrepancy

■ DIAGNOSIS

Ultrasonography

The ultrasound examination can be used to monitor acetabular development, particularly of infants in Pavlik harness treatment; this method can minimize the number of radiographs taken and might allow the clinician to detect failure of treatment earlier.

Because it is superior to radiographs for evaluating cartilaginous structures, ultrasonography is the diagnostic modality of choice for DDH before the appearance of the femoral head ossific nucleus (4–6 months). During the early newborn period (0–4 weeks), however, physical examination is preferred over ultrasonography because there is a high incidence of false-positive sonograms in this age group. Therefore, waiting to obtain an ultrasound until the infant is at least 1 month of age is preferred unless the child has a strongly positive physical exam. In addition to elucidating the static relationship of the femur to the acetabulum, ultrasonography provides dynamic information about the stability of the hip joint. The ultrasound examination can be used to monitor acetabular development, particularly of infants in Pavlik harness treatment; this method can minimize the number of radiographs taken and might allow the clinician to detect treatment failure earlier.

In the Graf technique, the transducer is placed over the greater trochanter, which allows visualization of the ilium, the bony acetabulum, the labrum, and the femoral epiphysis. The angle formed by the line of the ilium and a line tangential to the bony roof of the acetabulum is termed the *alpha angle* and represents the depth of the acetabulum. Values >60° are considered normal, and those <60° imply acetabular dysplasia. The *beta angle* is formed by a line drawn tangential to the labrum and the line of the ilium; this represents the cartilaginous roof of the acetabulum. A normal beta angle is <55°; as the femoral head subluxates, the beta angle increases.

Another useful test is to evaluate the position of the center of the head compared to the vertical line of the ilium. If the line of the ilium falls lateral to the center of the head, the epiphysis is considered reduced. If the line falls medial to the center of the head, the epiphysis is uncovered and is either subluxated or dislocated.

Radiography

Radiographs are recommended for an infant once the proximal femoral epiphysis ossifies, usually by 4–6 months. In infants of this age, radiographs have proved to be more effective, less costly, and less operator-dependent than an ultrasound examination. An anteroposterior (AP) view of the pelvis can be interpreted with the aid of several classic lines drawn on it.

- *Hilgenreiner's line* is a horizontal line drawn through the top of both triradiate cartilages (the clear area in the depth of the acetabulum).
- *Perkins line* is a vertical line through the most lateral ossified margin of the roof of the acetabulum, drawn perpendicular to Hilgenreiner's line. The ossific nucleus of the femoral head should be located in the medial lower quadrant of the intersection of these two lines.
- *Shenton's line* is a curved line drawn from the medial aspect of the femoral neck to the lower border of the superior pubic ramus. In a child with normal hips, this line is a continuous contour. In a child with hip subluxation or dislocation, this line consists of two separate arcs and is described as "broken."

The *acetabular index* is the angle formed between Hilgenreiner's line and a line drawn from the depth of the acetabular socket to the most lateral ossified margin of the roof of the acetabulum. This angle measures the development of the osseous roof of the acetabulum. In the newborn, the acetabular index can be up to 40°; by 4 months in the normal infant, it should be no >30°. In the older child, the *center-edge angle* is a useful measure of femoral head coverage. This angle is formed at the juncture of the Perkins line and a line connecting the lateral margin of the acetabulum to the center of the femoral head. In children 6–13 years old, an angle >19° is normal, whereas in children 14 years and older, an angle >25° is considered normal.

Radiological Evaluation

Dynamic ultrasonography may be helpful in assessing acetabular development and hip stability. In the lateral radiograph of the pelvis, the ossific nucleus of the femoral head does not appear until 3–7 months of age. It may be further delayed in congenital heart disease (CHD).

> **LABORATORY SALIENT FINDINGS**
> - Dynamic ultrasonography to assess acetabular development and hip stability
> - Arthrography
> - CT or MRI
>
> (CT: computed tomography; MRI: magnetic resonance imaging)

■ DIFFERENTIAL DIAGNOSIS

- Septic arthritis
- Osteomyelitis
- Perthes disease
- Tuberculosis

■ COMPLICATIONS

- Avascular necrosis of femoral head
- Redislocation
- Residual subluxation
- Acetabular dysplasia
- Wound infection

■ TREATMENT

The goals in the management of DDH are to obtain and maintain a concentric reduction of the femoral head within the acetabulum in order to provide the optimal environment for the normal development of both the femoral head and the acetabulum.

Treatment is directed toward the reduction of the femoral head into the acetabulum. Pavlik harness in the treatment of choice. This attempts to place the hip in a human position by flexing them >90° (160-110°) and maintaining relatively full. But gentle abduction redirects the femoral head to the acetabulum. Spontaneous relocation occurs within 3-4 weeks. If it does not occur surgical closed reduction is advised:

- Preliminary skin traction for 1-3 weeks to bring the femoral head opposite to the acetabulum
- Percutaneous adductor tenotomy
- Closed reduction
- Arthrography to assess correction of reduction

Newborns and Infants Younger Than 6 Months

Newborns hips that are Barlow-positive (reduced but dislocatable) or Ortolani-positive (dislocated but reducible) should generally be treated with a Pavlik harness as soon as the diagnosis is made. The management of newborns with dysplasia who are younger than 4 weeks of age is less clear. A significant proportion of these hips normalize within 3-4 weeks; consequently, many physicians prefer to reexamine these newborns after a few weeks before making treatment decisions.

The Pavlik harness remains the most commonly used device worldwide. By maintaining the Ortolani-positive hip in a Pavlik harness on a full-time basis for 6 weeks, hip instability resolves in 95% of cases. After 6 months of age, the failure rate for the Pavlik harness is >50% because it is difficult to maintain the increasingly active and crawling child in the harness. Frequent examinations and readjustments are necessary to ensure that the harness is fitting correctly. The anterior straps of the harness should be set to maintain the hips in flexion (usually 90-100°); excessive flexion is discouraged because of the risk of femoral nerve palsy. The posterior straps are designed to encourage abduction. These are generally set to allow adduction just to neutral, as forced abduction by the harness can lead to avascular necrosis of the femoral epiphysis.

Children 6 Months to 2 Years of Age

The principal goals in the treatment of late-diagnosed dysplasia are to obtain and maintain reduction of the hip without damaging the femoral head. Closed reductions are performed in the operating room under general anesthesia. The hip is moved to determine the range of motion in which it remains reduced.

The reduction is maintained in a well-molded spica cast, with the "human position" of moderate flexion and abduction being the preferred position, After the procedure, single-cut computed tomography (CT) or magnetic resonance (MR) may be used to confirm the reduction. 12 weeks after closed reduction, the plaster cast is removed; an abduction orthosis is often used at this point to encourage further remodeling of the acetabulum. Failure to obtain a stable hip with a closed reduction indicates the need for an *open reduction*. In patients younger than 2 years of age, a secondary acetabular or femoral procedure is rarely required. The potential for acetabular lar development after closed or open reduction is excellent and continues for 4-8 years after the procedure.

Children Older Than 2 Years

Children 2–6 years of age with a hip dislocation usually require an open reduction. In this age group, a concomitant femoral shortening osteotomy is often performed to reduce the pressure on the proximal femur and minimize the risk of osteonecrosis. Because the potential for acetabular development is markedly diminished in these older children, a pelvic osteotomy is usually performed in conjunction with the open reduction. Postoperatively, patients are immobilized in a spica cast for 6–12 weeks.

BIBLIOGRAPHY

1. American Academy of Pediatrics. Clinical practice guideline: Early detection of developmental dysplasia of the hip. Pediatrics. 2000;105(4):896-905.
2. Bialik V, Blazer S, Blazer S, Sujov P, Wiener F, Berant M. Developmental dysplasia of the hip: a new approach to incidence. Pediatrics. 1999;103(1):93-9.
3. Holman J, Crroll KL, Murray KA, Macleod LM, Roach JW. Long-term follow-up of open reduction surgery for developmental dislocation of the hip. J Pediatr Orthop. 2012;32(2):121-6.
4. Wang TM, Wn KW, Shih SF, Huang SC. Outcomes of open reduction for developmental dysplasia of the hip: does bilateral dysplasia have a poorer outcome? J Bone Joint Surg Am. 2013;95(12):1081-6.
5. Weinstein SL. Natural history of congenital hip dislocation (CDH) and hip dysplasia. Clin Orthop Relat Res. 1987;225:62-76.

CASE 105

Leprosy

■ PRESENTING COMPLAINTS

A 7-year-old boy was brought with the complaint of:
- Hypopigmented patch since 2–3 months.

History of the Presenting Complaints

A 7-year-old boy was brought by the mother to the pediatric outpatient with a history of hypopigmented patches over the buttocks and on the inner side of the right thigh. Mother had noticed the development of the white patch in the last 2–3 months. It was increasing in size. That worried her and made her take the son to the hospital.

Past History of the Patient

He was the first sibling of a nonconsanguineous marriage. He was born at full term with normal delivery. He cried immediately after the delivery. There was no significant postnatal event. He was discharged on the third day. He was on breast milk exclusively for 4 months. Weaning started at 4 months and completed at 18 months. There was no delay in developmental milestones.

■ EXAMINATION

The boy was moderately built and nourished. The boy was sitting comfortably on the examination table. Anthropometric measurements included a height of 122 cm (75th centile), and a weight was 21 kg (50th centile).

He was afebrile, the pulse rate was 120 beats/min and the respiratory rate was 20 breaths/min. The blood pressure recorded was 100/70 mm Hg. There was no pallor, no lymphadenopathy, and no edema.

There were hypopigmented patches present over the buttocks and on the medial side of the thigh. There was a loss of feeling to light toner, temperature, and pain. Other systemic examinations were normal.

■ INVESTIGATION

- *Hemoglobin:* 10 g/dL
- *TLC:* 8,000 cells/mm^3

CASE AT A GLANCE

Basic Findings

Height	: 122 cm (75th centile)
Weight	: 21 kg (50th centile)
Temperature	: 37.2°C
Pulse rate	: 120 beats/min
Respiratory rate	: 20 breaths/min
Blood pressure	: 100/70 mm Hg

Positive Findings

History:
- White patches over the buttocks

Examination:
- Hypopigmented patch
- Anesthetic patch

Investigation:
- Buttock skin smear test

- DLC: $P_{75}L_{20}E_3M_2$
- *Platelet count:* 600,000 cells/mm^3
- *Erythrocyte sedimentation rate (ESR):* 32 mm in the first hour
- *Urine routine:* No abnormalities detected (NAD)
- *Buttock skin smear test:* Lepra bacilli found

■ DISCUSSION

Leprosy is a heterogeneous, chronic mycobacterial infection that primarily affects the upper airway, skin, and peripheral nerves. Disease manifestations are determined by the host's immunopathologic response to infection, resulting in a wide clinical spectrum.

■ ETIOLOGY

Mycobacterium leprae, the etiologic agent of leprosy, is an obligate intracellular acid-fast gram-positive bacillus of the family Mycobacteriaceae measuring 1–8 μm in length. The bacillus multiplies slowly, with a doubling time of 11–13 days. It is the only bacterium known to infect Schwann cells of peripheral nerves. Identification of acid-fast bacilli (AFB) in peripheral nerves is pathognomonic of leprosy.

Identification depends on criteria other than those used routinely for cultivable mycobacteria. Current criteria for *M. leprae* are the following: (1) It does not grow on routine laboratory media, (2) it characteristically infects the footpads of mice, (3) acid fastness is abolished by exposure to pyridine, (4) the organism invades nerves of the host, (5) suspensions of dead bacilli produce a characteristic pattern of reactions when injected into the skin of patients (lepromin reaction) in accordance with the various clinical forms of leprosy, (6) it produces the species-specific antigen phenolic glycolipid-1 (PGL-1), and (7) it exhibits species-specific deoxyribonucleic acid (DNA) sequences.

The incubation period between natural infection and overt clinical disease in humans ranges from 3 months to 20 years, with a mean of 4 years for tuberculoid (TT) leprosy and 10 years for lepromatous leprosy (LL). The infectiousness of patients with leprosy becomes negligible within 24 hours of the first administration of effective multidrug therapy (MDT).

■ PATHOGENESIS

Mycobacterium leprae causes disease by its ability to survive and multiply in macrophages. If macrophages of the host digest the bacilli early, the disease is not detectable, or the patient has only minimal lesions. If the macrophages are totally incapable of destroying the organisms, widely disseminated LL will follow. Apoptosis of host cells occurs but is not as important in the pathogenesis of leprosy as in some other mycobacterial infections. Survival of *M. leprae* in macrophages depends on the immune response of the patient.

The role of immunologic processes in damage to nerves in leprosy is poorly understood. Some observations suggest that antineural antibodies in the sera of many patients, especially those with lepromatous disease, are related to such damage. Tumor necrosis factor (TNF) is associated with macrophage infiltration of peripheral nerves in reversal reactions. Infected Schwann cells present antigens to T cells, making them targets for immune attack.

Mycobacterium leprae is the only bacterium known to infect nerves. *M. leprae* has been shown to colonize perineural space and gain entry into the endoneural space. The organism then binds to the laminin-2 glycoprotein present in the basal lamina of

Schwann cells in peripheral nerves. It is then taken up inside the Schwann cell, where it replicates slowly intracellularly over several years.

Specific T cells recognize the mycobacterial antigens within the nerve and initiate a chronic inflammatory response. In addition to the direct nerve invasion by *M. leprae*, the immune response to infection also contributes to nerve damage. Schwann cells express human leukocyte antigen class 2 molecules and play an important role in the immunologic reaction by presenting mycobacterial peptides to the human leukocyte antigen class 2—restricted clusters of differentiation 4 (CD4)-positive T cells. This likely explains the nerve damage seen in paucibacillary disease and in reversal reactions. Swelling within the perineurium leads to ischemia, further nerve damage, and eventually to fibrosis and axonal death.

■ METHODS OF TRANSMISSION

The infected patient is the only reservoir of the infection. Only those who are capable of discharging bacilli from their bodies transmit the infection (infectious or open cases). All active lepromatous or near lepromatous cases are open. During periods of reaction (acute exacerbation) closed or noninfectious cases may also become temporarily open or infectious.

The exact mechanism of transmission is not fully understood but is thought to occur primarily via the respiratory route. Up to 10^7 viable bacilli per day can be shed in the respiratory secretions of patients with multibacillary leprosy. The upper respiratory tract is considered the most probable site of entry of the organism into the human body. However, it is currently accepted that nasorespiratory transmission is most common. The nasal mucosa of lepromatous patients harbors massive numbers of *M. leprae*, known since Hansen's original discovery. *M. leprae* appears to bind to nasal mucosal cells by first binding to fibronectin and then attaching to fibronectin receptors on mucosal cells. *M. leprae* organisms ejected during sneezing remain viable under ambient conditions for as long as 1 week, and disseminated leprosy develops in immunosuppressed mice after the inhalation of aerosol that contains *M. leprae*. Breast tissue and milk from lepromatous patients contain *M. leprae*, and infants may acquire infection from this source.

For many years, skin-to-skin contact between the patient and healthy subjects was considered the most important means of transmission, and this concept cannot be abandoned readily. Intact skin of heavily infected patients discharges small numbers of *M. leprae*, but ulcers in the skin may be a source of large numbers of bacilli. Thus, skin-to-skin contact and fomites containing *M. leprae* could be sources of infection.

Entry of the bacillus into the bodies of the infected persons produces widely different results because of differences in the sensitivity of the host. On one end of the spectrum, in persons with high specific resistance, the bacilli are killed on entry into the body, and no disease is produced. In persons with fairly high specific resistance, the bacilli can multiply only to a limited extent resulting in the production of mild, localized, self-limiting disease with scanty bacilli, viz., the TT type. In persons with little or no specific immunity, the bacilli can multiply rapidly and spread widely in the body, resulting in generalized progressive disease with a large number of bacilli, viz., the lepromatous type.

Type of disease (multibacillary) and proximity to contact cases are important determinants of human-to-human transmission.

The relative risk for developing disease in household contacts is 8–10 for lepromatous disease and 2–4 for the TT form.

Discharge from ulcers in the nose and skin are the usual sources of organisms. Infants may acquire bacilli through breast milk. Discharges from the neuropathic ulcers in feet and hands do not contain bacilli.

■ CLINICAL FEATURES (FIG. 1)

Disease classification is important to determine potentially infectious cases and prognosis. Based on the cellular immune response and disease dissemination, two classification schemes for leprosy are frequently used: The Ridley–Jopling scale and the World Health Organization (WHO) classification:

- The *Ridley–Jopling scale* is used and describes the five types of leprosy, according to the clinical spectrum of disease, bacillary load, and findings on histopathology.
  - *TT form:* Patients usually have a vigorous and specific cellular immune response to *M. leprae* antigens and have a small number of skin lesions, generally, one to three well-demarcated macules or plaques with elevated borders and reduced or absent sensation. The lesions are infiltrated by T-helper 1 (Th1) cells producing abundant interferon gamma (IFN-γ) and TNF-α, forming well-demarcated granulomas, with few, if any bacilli found within the lesions.
  - Borderline tuberculoid (BT) form
  - Borderline form
  - Borderline lepromatous (BL)
  - *Lepromatous form:* Patients have an absence of specific cellular immunity to *M. leprae* (but intact immunity to *Mycobacterium tuberculosis*) and present the most severe form of the disease. They manifest clinically apparent infiltration of peripheral nerves and skin lesions (usually many lesions and not all hypoesthetic or anesthetic), with a high load of bacilli in the absence of an effective cell-mediated immune response. Skin biopsies reveal extensive infiltration of the skin and nerves, containing messenger RNA for Th2 cytokines such as interleukin (IL)-4 and IL-10, poorly formed granulomas, and uncontrolled proliferation of bacilli within foamy macrophages. A large amount of circulating antibody to *M. leprae* is present but does not confer protective immunity. Over time, patients with the lepromatous form develop a systemic disease with symmetric peripheral nerve involvement and a diffuse infiltrative dermopathy that includes thickening of the facial skin and hair loss of the eyelashes and eyebrows (madarosis), leading to the classic presentation of the leonine

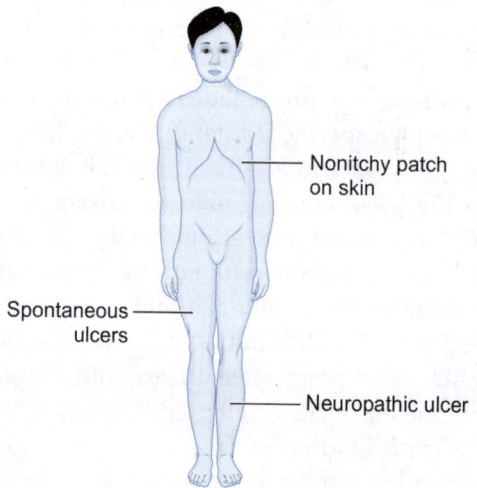

Fig. 1: Clinical features.

facies. They also have involvement of the nasal mucosa causing nasal congestion and epistaxis.
- The WHO classification can be used when histologic evaluation and confirmatory diagnosis are unavailable, a common scenario in the field. This simplified scheme is based on the number of skin lesions:
  - Paucibacillary (one to five patches)
  - Multibacillary (more than five patches).

The disease is classified as lepromatous, borderline, indeterminate, maculoanesthetic, TT, and polyneuritic. While lepromatous and TT represent the LL and TT types of immunological classification; the maculoanesthetic group may comprise the BT and TT variants. The borderline group represents BT, borderline borderline (BB), and BL variants.

Classic manifestations of leprosy include hypopigmented, erythematous, or infiltrative skin lesions with or without neurologic symptoms, such as hypoesthesia or anesthesia, weakness, autonomic dysfunction, and peripheral nerve thickening.

The period from infection to clinical disease varies (usually, 2–5 years but up to 15 years reported), and no prodromal manifestations are well established. After an incubation period, lesions of varying description appear. The nature of the lesions depends on the immune response of the patient to *M. leprae*. Classification is important because it aids in establishing the treatment program and prognosis of the patient.

The cardinal signs of leprosy are hypoesthetic lesions of the skin, enlarged peripheral nerve or nerves, and AFB in skin smears. In the absence of another clear explanation, any one of these signs strongly suggests leprosy.

Virtually all patients with leprosy have peripheral neuropathy if cutaneous sensory changes are included, and approximately 25% have significant deformity, depending on the intensity of leprosy case finding and the inherent delays in detection. In experimental studies, the pathogenesis of peripheral neuritis in leprosy involves the uptake of bacilli by the endothelial cells of epineural and perineural blood vessels and lymphatics. Surface proteins of *M. leprae* may bind the bacillus to Schwann cells via laminin.

Ocular complications in leprosy are well known. All patients with leprosy should be evaluated by an ophthalmologist at diagnosis and periodically thereafter, especially during any reactional episodes.

Indeterminate Leprosy

An indeterminate lesion is the first manifestation of leprosy in most patients and may heal spontaneously, remain unchanged for months or years, or gradually progress toward TT or LL disease. Patients with indeterminate leprosy have a single or a few macules in the skin. The macule is poorly defined and mildly hypopigmented in deeper-pigmented skin and slightly erythematous in lighter skin. Skin texture, sensation, and sweating within early macules are normal or only slightly altered. Peripheral nerves are not affected, and skin smears from lesions rarely contain bacilli.

Tuberculoid Leprosy

Patients with TT have a single or several asymmetrically distributed hypopigmented skin lesions. TT lesions arise de novo or evolve from indeterminate macules. The lesion may be macular or infiltrated, but the borders are always sharply demarcated from the surrounding normal skin and are frequently finely papulated. Lesions range from <1 cm to those that cover entire regions, such as the thigh or buttock. Many TT lesions heal spontaneously. In large, active lesions, the centers are often healed and repigmented, although somewhat atrophic.

In TT lesions, there is sensory loss with impaired sweating and eventually loss of hair. On the face, because of its rich innervation, the detection of hypoesthesia in early lesions requires discriminating tests. Conversely, clinicians may mistakenly diagnose leprosy in areas of the body that normally have reduced sensory acuity (e.g., over the elbows or knees).

Involvement of peripheral nerves commonly develops in TT leprosy and cutaneous nerves can often be palpated adjacent to or within lesions. The regional nerve trunks most commonly enlarged are the ulnar nerve from the olecranon groove to midarm, the lateral popliteal nerve just distal to the head of the fibula, and the posterior tibial nerve in the medial aspect of the ankle. Enlarged or tender nerves anywhere should alert the clinician to the possibility of leprosy. Any readily palpable cutaneous nerve is probably enlarged, but evaluating the size of nerve trunks requires experience because of the wide range in normal size.

Borderline Leprosy

Borderline leprosy, sometimes called dimorphous or intermediate leprosy, has features of both the LL and the TT forms and represents a continuous spectrum of disease ranging from near-TT to near-lepromatous. It is an unstable form of leprosy and may evolve gradually toward TT leprosy by undergoing reversal reactions or be downgraded toward LL leprosy. The three major subgroups of BL: are BT, BB, and BL.

In BT leprosy, the number of lesions is usually greater than in TT leprosy, and the borders of each lesion, macule, or plaque are defined less sharply than in TT leprosy. There may be central clearing within lesions or small satellite lesions. may develop around larger macules or plaques. BL leprosy often presents with widespread nodular infiltrations or plaques of varying sizes.

Damage to nerves and the resulting deformity develop early and are often widespread. Pain in nerves or neuropathic changes (e.g., sensory changes that lead to damaged hands or feet or muscular weakness such as footdrop) frequently bring the patient to the physician. Severe damage to nerves is infrequent in early childhood but can be disastrous. Prevention of this complication is an important goal of leprosy detection programs and to treatment of every leprosy patient.

Lepromatous Leprosy

In LL leprosy, the bacilli multiply freely and the disease disseminates widely, often before striking cutaneous manifestations develop, in contrast to the strict localization of lesions in TT leprosy. LL leprosy may evolve from indeterminate or BB leprosy or may be the first recognizable form.

In its earliest form, LL leprosy manifests as "juvenile leprosy," a clinical entity delineated from observations on large numbers of children in homes for children of patients with leprosy in India. This form, also called pre-LL, is difficult to detect and frequently goes unrecognized until a more advanced stage develops skin texture may be altered slightly, but the vague macules with indistinct borders are detected only under appropriate lighting, preferably daylight. There are no changes in sensation or sweating in the macules, and frequently AFB is not detectable in smears from the skin. Histopathologic sections may reveal a few bacilli to confirm the diagnosis.

If leprosy is suspected, the patient should be monitored until an explanation for the mild skin changes is found. If leprosy is present but not detected and treated, advanced forms of LL leprosy will develop in many of these patients.

The hypopigmented or slightly erythematous macules of early LL leprosy, like those of juvenile leprosy, are missed easily because they are vague and have slight if any, sensory changes. These macules are usually small but gradually may coalesce and cover large areas of skin, even nearly the entire body. A clinical diagnosis then is often missed, and over the course of a few years, advanced LL leprosy develops. If skin smears or biopsy specimens are taken in the macular stage, diagnosis is almost assured. If the disease is not diagnosed and treated in the macular stage, infiltration of the skin will increase gradually, and nodules may develop. The skin is infiltrated most heavily in the cooler portions of the body, notably the ears (pinnae) and face. By this time, nerves are usually enlarged, with early signs of sensory loss in the hands and feet. Eyebrows are thinned and eventually lost, beginning at the lateral edges. These advanced changes of LL leprosy are not common findings in young children but are well known.

Neuritic Leprosy

Rarely, leprosy involves one or more major nerve trunks unaccompanied by cutaneous lesions. These patients have anesthesia, paresis, or wasting of muscles in the affected area. Nerve trunks are frequently painful, enlarged, and tender. Leprosy must be suspected in patients with any peripheral neuritis that has these features. Chronic neuritis with pain, enlargement, and tenderness of peripheral nerves often persists for years after the patient has completed chemotherapy for leprosy. Large leprotic nerve abscesses are rare but are exquisitely painful and may require surgical intervention for drainage. However, most clinicians prefer to treat such lesions with corticosteroids.

GENERAL FEATURES
• Loss of feeling to touch, temperature, and pain • Loss of sensation • Numbness • Pins and needles

Skin Involvement

Examination of the skin should ideally be performed in natural sunlight and be tested for hypoesthesia to light touch, pinprick, temperature, and anhidrosis. The most common skin lesions are macules or plaques. Diffuse infiltrative lesions and subcutaneous nodules are less common. Initial lesions are insidious hypopigmented macules, although they may appear erythematous on pale skin.

Cutaneous lesions (**Fig. 2**) range from apparently innocuous-looking and probably self-healing solitary lesions to extensive involvement of skin and mucous membranes with lesions of divergent nature. Skin is thick, red, and shiny, especially on the face and hands.

Lesions may involve any area of the body, are more pronounced in cooler areas

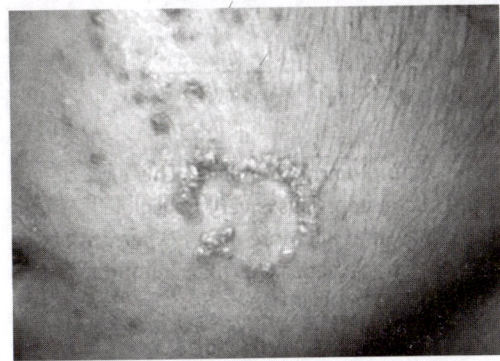

Fig. 2: Cutaneous lesions.
(For color version, see Plate 12)

(e.g., the earlobes and nose), and occur less frequently on the scalp, axillae, or perineum. Approximately 70% of skin lesions have reduced sensation; the degree of hypoesthesia depends on the location and size of the lesion. Patients with tuberculous leprosy generally have one to three well-demarcated macules or plaques with elevated borders and reduced or absent sensation. In the lepromatous form, multiple lesions are present but are not all hypoesthetic or anesthetic.

Nerve Involvement

The skin lesions overlying a nerve trunk distribution predict the involvement of nerves in the vicinity. Peripheral nerves are most commonly affected early in the disease course and should be palpated for thickness and tenderness and evaluated for both motor and sensory function (particularly temperature and light touch).

The posterior tibial nerve (medial malleolus) is the most common nerve affected, followed by the ulnar (elbow), median (wrist), lateral popliteal (fibular neck), and facial nerves. A nerve biopsy (usually of the sural nerve) is required to demonstrate granulomatous histopathology, thereby confirming the diagnosis.

Reactions

The course of leprosy, treated or untreated, is often interrupted by acute immunologically based episodes called reactions, which fall into two general categories: Reversal reactions (or type 1) and erythema nodosum leprosum (ENL) or type 2 reactions.

Reversal Reactions

Patients may also present with leprosy reactions. Leprosy reactions are acute clinical exacerbations reflecting disturbances of the immunologic balance to *M. leprae* infection occurring in 30–50% of all leprosy patients. These sudden changes occur most commonly during the initial years after infection and in patients with borderline and multibacillary leprosy, but can occur before, during, or after completion of treatment. Three types of leprosy reactions have been described and require immediate treatment so as to prevent complications.

1. *Type 1 reactions* (also known as reversal reactions) occur in one-third of patients with borderline disease and are caused by a spontaneous increase in T-cell-mediated reactivity to mycobacterial antigens. Reversal reactions are characterized by acute edema and increased erythema, warmth, and painful inflammation of preexisting cutaneous plaques or nodules with acute swelling and tenderness of peripheral nerves that can quickly progress to cause nerve abscesses and necrosis. There may be peripheral lymphocytosis and an increased cytokine response, but systemic symptoms are uncommon. Rapid and sustained reversal of the inflammatory process using corticosteroids is essential to prevent continued nerve damage.

   Patients who are lepromin positive and have immunoglobulin M (IgM) antibodies to PGL-I are most at risk for reversal reactions. The proliferation of sensitized T lymphocytes initiates reversal reactions, releasing lymphokines that amplify the inflammatory response, calling in and activating macrophages. Immunohistopathologic evidence has shown that effective chemotherapy for both paucibacillary and multibacillary patients may activate cell-mediated immunity (CMI) and provoke clinical or subclinical reversal reactions.

Differentiating reversal reactions from relapsing lesions is frequently difficult and requires careful correlation of clinical and histopathologic findings.

2. *Type 2 reactions* (ENL) occur in LL and lepromatous forms, as these patients have the highest levels of *M. leprae* antigens and antibodies, most commonly in the first 2 years after starting chemotherapy. ENL is distinguished from reversal reactions by the development of new painful, erythematous subcutaneous nodules with an accompanying systemic inflammatory response. ENL is accompanied by high circulating concentrations of TNF-alpha. Patients develop high fever and signs of systemic toxicity, and in severe cases, ENL can be life-threatening, presenting with features similar to septic shock.

   Patients are present with either a single, acute episode, a relapsing form comprised of multiple acute episodes, or a chronic, continuous form. Deposition of extravascular immune complexes leads to neutrophil infiltration and activation of complement in the skin and other organs. Tender, erythematous dermal papules or nodules (resembling erythema nodosum) occur in clusters, typically on extensor surfaces of the lower extremities and face. Immune complex deposition also contributes to migrating polyarthralgias, painful swelling of lymph nodes and spleen, iridocyclitis, vasculitis, orchitis, and, rarely, and nephritis.

3. *Type 3 reaction:* Lucio's phenomenon (erythema necroticans) is an uncommon but potentially fatal reaction distinct from type 1 or 2 reactions that occur in patients with untreated LL. It is a necrotizing vasculitis caused by *M. leprae* directly invading the endothelium. Clinically, patients develop violaceous or hemorrhagic plaques, followed by ulcerations in the absence of systemic complaints. Secondary bacterial infections are common.

■ DIAGNOSIS

A case of leprosy is defined as a person having one/more of the following features, and who has yet to complete a full course of treatment:
- Hypopigmented or reddish skin lesions with definite loss of sensation
- Involvement of peripheral nerves, demonstrated by definite thickening with loss of sensation
- Skin smear positive for AFB.

The disease should not be diagnosed if only nerve thickening is present, without any accompanying symptoms or signs. Diagnostic evaluation includes physical examination plus examination of skin smears. The examination should include evaluation of skin lesions, palpation of peripheral nerves such as the ulnar at the elbows, median and superficial cutaneous at the wrists, greater auricular in the neck, and the common peroneal at the popliteal fossa, for enlargement and/or tenderness together with sensory (skin lesions and distal extremities) and motor evaluation.

ESSENTIAL DIAGNOSTIC POINTS
• Hypopigmented or reddish skin lesions
• Definite loss of sensation
• Involvement of peripheral nerves
• Definite thickening with loss of sensation
• Skin smear positive for acid-fast bacilli

Bacteriological Examination

If no definite patches of thickened skin are visible, a smear should be taken from the ear lobes and buttocks. The small material thus obtained should be uniformly spread on a clean glass slide, dried over the flame, stained with the Ziehl–Neelsen method, and examined under the microscope. At least 100 fields should be examined before recording a negative result.

> **LABORATORY SALIENT FINDINGS**
> - *Skin smear:* Earlobes and buttocks
> - Stained with Ziehl–Neelsen method
> - Lepromin test
> - Tests for humeral response
> - Serology

Obtaining and examining smears for AFB is an important diagnostic procedure and should be controlled carefully by experienced laboratories. Briefly, smears are made from the edge of discrete macules or plaques, nodules, ear lobes, and nasal mucosa. Skin smears are made by squeezing and holding a fold of skin between the thumb and forefinger to avoid getting blood in the smear, and by making a short, shallow slit in the skin with a sterile razor blade or scalpel. The instrument is then turned at a right angle to the slit, and the edges of the incision are scraped. The cells and fluid thus obtained are spread on a slide, heat-fixed, and stained by the Ziehl–Neelsen method. Evaluation of smears should not be done by researchers unfamiliar with their interpretation.

Lepromin test: The lepromin test is carried out by injecting 0.1 mL of Mitsuda lepromin intradermally into the forearm and noting the reaction later at 21 days. It is of little use in diagnosis, though it is of value in classification and prognosis. The test is graded as follows:

As a routine, the reaction is read at 48 hours and 21 days. Two types of positive reactions have been described.

Early reaction: It is also known as the Fernandez reaction. As inflammatory reaction, i.e., response develops within 24–48 hours and this tends to disappear after 3–44 days. It is evidenced by redness and induration at the site of inoculation. If the diameter of the red area is >10 mm at the end of 48 hours, the test is considered as positive.

The early reaction indicates whether or not a person has been previously sensitized by exposure and infection by leprosy bacilli.

Negative: Nothing to see or feel
- ±: Papule 3 mm in diameter
- +: Erythematous papule 4–7 mm diameter, no ulcer
- ++: Erythematous papule 7–10 mm diameter, no ulcer
- +++: >10 mm erythematous nodule or less with ulceration.

Bacillus Calmette–Guérin (BCG) vaccination is capable of converting lepra reaction from negative to positive in a large number of patients.

It has been generally accepted as a useful tool in evaluating the immune status—CMI. It is of value in confirming the results of the classification of cases of leprosy on clinical and bacteriological grounds. It helps in the classification of the type of disease.

It is useful in estimating the prognosis in case of leprosy of all types. It is strongly positive in typical TT cases. Positivity gets weaker through the spectrum of the lepromatous end. Typical lepromatous patient being lepromin negative indicating failure of CMI.

Tests for Humeral Response
- *Florescent leprosy antibody absorption (FLA-ABS) test:* It is used for the identification of subclinical infections. It is 92.3% sensitive, and 100% specific in detecting *M. leprae*.
- *Monoclonal antibodies:* These antibodies recognize specific and nonspecific epitopes of *M. leprae* antigens. If antibodies against specific antigens are found, they

will become the reagents of choice for identifying *M. leprae*. SACT is based on this approach and has been found to be quite sensitive for the detection of *M. leprae* antibody. An enzyme-linked immunosorbent assay (ELISA) based on a particular PGL, derived from *M. leprae* is also in use.

A full-thickness skin biopsy should be taken from the most active skin lesion, entirely within the lesion and including the active margin to confirm the diagnosis. *M. leprae* is best identified in tissue using the Fite stain. Lesions from patients with the lepromatous form reveal numerous AFB in clumps (globi), whereas patients with the TT form of the disease rarely have mycobacteria identified but demonstrate well-formed noncaseating granulomas and nerve involvement.

Biopsy specimens from well-defined lesions of leprosy should be taken from the active border and fixed in buffered 10% formalin or other suitable fixative unless molecular studies are requested, in which case formalin should be avoided. The Fite-Faraco staining method is used because the Ziehl-Neelsen stain does not demonstrate *M. leprae* optimally in tissue sections. A histopathologic diagnosis of leprosy must not be made unless the evidence is convincing. DNA probes specific for *M. leprae* are available and are useful in identifying leprosy bacilli in tissue or nasal secretions. Specimens for DNA evaluation or polymerase chain reaction (PCR) amplification should be preserved in 70% ethyl alcohol.

The presence of neural inflammation differentiates leprosy from other granulomatous disorders. Hematoxylin and eosin staining, and immunohistochemistry may also contribute to the diagnosis. Mycobacterial culture of lesions is performed to exclude *M. tuberculosis* and nontuberculous cutaneous infections. Antibodies to *M. leprae* are present in 90% of patients with untreated lepromatous disease, 40–50% with paucibacillary disease, and 1–5% of healthy controls. Serologic testing is insensitive, however, and is not used for diagnosis.

■ DIFFERENTIAL DIAGNOSIS

Vitiligo, nutritional dyschromia especially of the face, tinea versicolor, nevus anemicus (hypopigmented birthmarks), hypopigmented scars left by pyogenic infections, etc., are considered in the differential diagnosis of macular patches.

■ TREATMENT

Once a diagnosis of leprosy is established, chemotherapy must be initiated. Because of drug-resistant *M. leprae*, combined MDT regimens, such as WHO-MDT, are mandatory for the treatment of all forms of leprosy. Currently, drugs used in WHO-MDT and US-HT are a combination of rifampicin, clofazimine, and dapsone for multibacillary leprosy, and rifampicin and dapsone for paucibacillary leprosy. Rifampicin, the most important antileprosy drug, is used in both types of leprosy.

Appropriate measures are also begun for preventing or correcting deformity in patients with neuropathic changes. Neuropathic changes involve primarily nerves and other structures in the cooler parts of the body and are most profound in the eyes, face, hands, and feet. Damage to the hand, for example, is related to loss of normal autonomic, sensory, and motor function. Early appropriate surgical intervention can often restore motor function, and physiotherapy will maintain useful hands.

Patients of leprosy are classified into three groups based on a clinical assumption: (1) Paucibacillary single lesion (one skin lesion),

(2) paucibacillary leprosy (two to five skin lesions), and (3) multibacillary leprosy (more than five skin lesions).

The primary goal of treatment is early antimicrobial therapy to prevent permanent neuropathy. Effective treatment of leprosy requires MDT with dapsone, clofazimine, and rifampicin.

Combination therapy is employed to prevent antimicrobial resistance.

Before starting combination MDT, patients should be tested for glucose-6-phosphate dehydrogenase deficiency, have a baseline complete blood cell count and liver function testing, and be evaluated for evidence of concomitant tuberculosis infection. The latter is imperative so as to avoid giving rifampicin monotherapy to someone with active tuberculosis.

Darkening of the skin is a common adverse reaction to clofazimine; this generally resolves 6–12 months after completing therapy. Bone marrow suppression and hepatotoxicity have been reported and should be monitored every 3 months during therapy. Yearly, a screening urinalysis should be performed.

Minocycline, clarithromycin, rifapentine, diarylquinoline, and some fluoroquinolones (ofloxacin and moxifloxacin) have been shown to be bactericidal against *M. leprae*.

The commonly used drugs for the treatment of leprosy are dapsone, clofazimine (both bacteriostatic), and rifampicin (bactericidal); others are minocycline, ofloxacin, and clarithromycin. Monotherapy with any drug should not be used for fear of early drug resistance.

Single lesion paucibacillary disease: Single lesions account for almost 20–80% of cases in various parts of India and are mainly detected during school surveys and may be cured by a limited amount of chemotherapy. The current regime used for these lesions is termed ROM (rifampin, ofloxacin, and minocycline). ROM consists of a single dose of 600 mg of rifampicin, 400 mg ofloxacin, and 100 mg of minocycline administered orally.

Paucibacillary cases: The treatment regimen for paucibacillary cases consists of 6 monthly pulses of MDT to be completed within 9 months. Each pulse is given over a period of one month as per the following guidelines:

	Age group	
	6–14 years	0–5 years
Rifampicin once a month (supervised)	450 mg	300 mg
Dapsone daily dose (domiciliary)	50 mg	25 mg

Multibacillary cases: The treatment regimen for multibacillary cases consists of 12 monthly pulses of MDT to be completed within 18 months. Each pulse is given over a period of 1 month as per the following guidelines.

	Age group	
	10–14 years	6–9 years
Rifampicin once a month (supervised)	450 mg	300 mg
Clofazimine once a month (supervised)	150 mg	100 mg
Clofazimine (self-administered)	50 mg (alternate days)	50 mg (twice a week)
Dapsone once a month (supervised)	50 mg	50 mg
Dapsone daily dose	50 mg	25 mg

Side effects of MDT include flu-like syndrome, acute renal failure, cutaneous reactions, toxic hepatitis, gastrointestinal complaints, hemolytic anemia, methemoglobinemia, thrombocytopenic purpura, disseminated intravascular coagulation, and hypotension.

Treatment of Reactions in Leprosy

Patients undergoing a reversal (type 1) reaction or ENL (type 2) reaction should be observed daily in the early stages and hospitalized if the symptoms are severe so that sensory loss and deformities are minimized. By repeated reversal reactions, BL, and even cases close to LL disease, may be gradually upgraded to TT leprosy, often with disastrous peripheral neuropathy.

Formerly, specific antileprosy therapy was stopped or the dosage reduced during reactions, but these measures are no longer recommended. Damage to the eyes and neuropathic changes may ensue rapidly without immediate attention. Nerve tenderness and function must be assessed frequently during reactions. Acute inflammation of isolated lesions without damage to nerves is likely to be of little consequence except for cosmetic considerations.

Without chemotherapy, the prognosis in all patients except those with limited and self-healing disease is potentially poor. Patients with borderline or advanced TT leprosy frequently become mutilated because of damage to nerves. Borderline patients can downgrade toward LL leprosy. In patients with LL leprosy, the disease is progressive and can cause death from laryngeal obstruction.

Reversal Reactions

For reversal reactions, analgesics are given, and the affected area is put at rest. Large daily doses of corticosteroids are started and tapered to a minimal effective dose until the reaction subsides. Conversion to alternate-day steroid regimens may be attempted when long-term treatment is necessary. Some clinicians use clofazimine for chronic reversal reactions, but it is not recommended for the initial treatment of reactions with acute neuritis. For reactions, clofazimine is probably consistently efficacious only for ENL.

Erythema Nodosum Leprosum

Mild ENL reactions are treated with analgesics; more severe ENL is treated with thalidomide or corticosteroids. Pediatric doses of thalidomide in ENL have not been established, but the initial adult dose is 100 mg four times daily followed by a minimally effective dose, usually 100 mg daily. The teratogenic action of thalidomide demands that appropriate measures be taken in the treatment of fertile females. For the rare patient who does not respond to thalidomide or in fertile females, corticosteroids, or clofazimine are used. Corticosteroids, if used, are administered in the usual dosage schedules, beginning with large doses, and tapering to a minimal effective level. Some clinicians use an alternate-day regimen when long-term steroid therapy is necessary, thus minimizing the well-known side effects. A few studies suggest that pentoxifylline or pentoxifylline plus clofazimine may be effective for ENL.

Clofazimine is effective in most patients with ENL and does not have the disadvantages of thalidomide or corticosteroids. The anti-inflammatory action of clofazimine is not manifested until after 4–6 weeks of continuous use. The dosage must be adjusted to the minimal effective level.

- *Type 1 reaction:*
  - *Mild:* Nonsteroidal anti-inflammatory drug (NSAID)
  - *Moderate:* NSAIDs and oral corticosteroids
  - *Severe:* NSAIDs and oral corticosteroids
- *Type 2 reaction:*
  - *Mild:* NSAIDs

- *Moderate:* NSAIDS, thalidomide, chloroquine, and clofazimine
- *Severe:* Thalidomide and corticosteroids.

For type 1 lepra reactions addition of prednisone 1 mg/kg/day orally (40–60 mg) with a slow taper (decreasing by 5 mg every 2–4 weeks after evidence of improvement over 3–6 months) is recommended in addition to standard MDT. If there is evidence of peripheral nerve deterioration, higher doses and longer tapers may be needed. Nerve function improves after corticosteroid treatment in 60–70% of patients who did not have preexisting neuritis.

For type 2 reactions in patients older than 12 years of age with systemic symptoms, thalidomide (100 mg/day for 4 days) is the drug of choice. In younger patients or pregnant females in whom thalidomide is contraindicated or in older patients with thalidomide-refractory ENL, corticosteroids may be used in daily doses of 1 mg/kg for 12 weeks. Clofazimine (300 mg/day tapering to <100 mg/day for 12 months) has been useful in managing patients with chronic ENL as well. Lucio's phenomenon is managed with corticosteroids and treatment of underlying infections.

In endemic countries, close monitoring of household contacts of Hansen's disease (HD) patients, particularly those with multibacillary disease, and either chemoprophylaxis or early treatment to contacts with evidence of early HD are effective control strategies. A single dose of BCG vaccine gives variable protective efficacy against leprosy ranging from 28 to 80%; an additional dose demonstrated increased protection. A heat-killed leprosy vaccine, given as an immunotherapeutic adjuvant along with combination MDT, is approved for use in India.

LONG-TERM COMPLICATIONS

The major chronic complications and deformities of leprosy are caused by segmental demyelination and permanent nerve injury. The prognosis for arresting progression of tissue and nerve damage is good if therapy is started early, but recovery of lost sensory and motor function is variable and frequently incomplete. Nerve impairment may be purely sensory, motor, or autonomic, or maybe a combination. Sensory deficits lead to undetected trauma, ulceration, and osteomyelitis. Motor deficits result in muscle paralysis, atrophy, and limb deformities, especially of small muscles of the hand and foot (claw hand or foot, foot drop).

Nerve function impairment can occur before diagnosis, during MDT, or after MDT and can develop without overt signs of skin or nerve inflammation (silent neuropathy). Patients at highest risk of nerve impairment are those with multibacillary leprosy and preexisting nerve damage. These patients should undergo regular monthly surveillance during therapy and for at least 2 years from the time of diagnosis. In children, deformities can occur in 3–10% of cases and mainly in those with nerve enlargement. Other factors contributing to the risk of deformities include increasing age in children, delay in accessing medical care, multiple skin lesions, multibacillary disease, smear positivity, multiple nerve involvement, and leprosy reaction at presentation.

BIBLIOGRAPHY

1. Duthie MS, Raychaudhuri R, Tutterrow YL, Misquith A, Bowman J, Casey A, et al. A rapid ELISA for the diagnosis of MB leprosy based on complementary detection of antibodies against a novel protein-glycolipid conjugate. Diagn Microbiol Infect Dis. 2014;79(2):233-9.

2. Oliveira MB, Dniz LM. Leprosy among children under 15 years of age: literature review. An Bras Dermatol. 2016;91(2):196-203.
3. Richardus JH, Oskam L. Protecting people against leprosy: chemoprophylaxis and immunoprophylaxis. Clin Dermatol. 2015;33(1):19-25.
4. Smith CS, Noordeen SK, Richardus JH, Sansarricq H, Cole ST, Soares RC, et al. A strategy to halt leprosy transmission. Lancet Infect Dis. 2014;14(2):96-8.

CASE 106

Marfan's Syndrome

■ PRESENTING COMPLAINTS

A 9-year-old boy was brought with the complaints of:
- Palpitation since 6 months
- Chest pain since 1 month

History of Presenting Complaints

A tall slender boy aged about 9 years was brought to hospital with a history of palpitation. He was complaining of abnormal awareness of the heartbeat. He had noticed that it used to be more on exertion, stress, and strain. He also complained of occasional chest pain on the left side. Chest pain used to be aggravated by exertion.

Past History of the Patient

The patient was the second sibling of a consanguineous marriage. He was born at term by normal vaginal delivery. His birth weight was 2.75 kg, length was 52 cm, and head circumference was 35 cm. He started to take the breast milk as soon as possible. His developmental milestones were normal. He had been completely immunized. His performance at school was good. He was suffering from repeated respiratory tract infections. He was the tallest boy in the school. He had a sore eye problem associated with vision which was corrected by the spectacles.

CASE AT A GLANCE	
Basic Findings	
Height	: 136 cm (>90th centile)
Weight	: 25 kg (50th centile)
Temperature	: 37°C
Pulse rate	: 100 beats/min
Respiratory rate	: 20 breaths/min
Blood pressure	: 110/60 mm Hg
Positive Findings	
History:	
• Palpitation	
• Chest pain	
Examination:	
• Tall and thin	
• Long extremities	
• Displaced apex beat	
• Diastolic thrill	
• Diastolic murmur	
Investigation:	
• *Electrocardiography (ECG):* Deep S waves in V_1 and tall R waves in V_6	
• *X-ray chest:* Showed cardiac enlargement of left ventricular type	

■ EXAMINATION

The boy was moderately built and nourished. He was tall and slender. The extremities were long. The fingers were long and tapered. Anthropometric measurements included the height of 136 cm (>90th centile) and the weight of 25 kg (50th centile). The arm span was 140 cm.

He was afebrile, the pulse rate was 100 beats per minute and collapsing type. The respiratory rate was 20 breaths per minute. The blood pressure recorded was 110/60 mm Hg. There was no pallor, no lymphadenopathy, no cyanosis, and no clubbing.

Apex beat was displaced downward and outward. It was forcible and heaving in character. Diastolic thrill was palpable at the right sternal border. High-pitched decreased diastolic murmur was present starting with aortic component of the second sound. Other systemic examinations were normal.

INVESTIGATION

- *Hemoglobin:* 12 g/dL
- *TLC:* 7,600 cells/mm^3
- *ESR:* 20 mm in the 1st hour
- *Electrocardiography (ECG):* Deep S waves in V_1 and tall R waves in V_6
- *X-ray chest:* Showed cardiac enlargement of left ventricular type

DISCUSSION

A tall slender boy with a history of palpitation, chest pain, and presence of features of cardiac disease puts the diagnosis of Marfan's syndrome (MFS).

Marfan syndrome is autosomal dominantly inherited, systemic, connective tissue disorder caused by mutations in the gene encoding the extracellular matrix (ECM) protein fibrillin-1. The abnormalities are found in elastin and collagen.

It is primarily associated with skeletal, cardiovascular, and ocular pathology. The diagnosis is based on clinical findings, some of which are age-dependent.

The disorder shows with high penetrance but variable expression; both interfamilial and intrafamilial clinical variations are common. There is no racial or gender preference.

The clinical findings of aortic root aneurysm and ectopia lentis (displacement of the lens from the center of the pupil) are particularly important diagnostic criteria because of their specificity and clinical significance.

PATHOGENESIS

Marfan's syndrome is associated with abnormal production, matrix deposition, and/or stability of fibrillin-1, a 350-kDa ECM protein that is the major constituent of microfibrils, with prominent disruption of microfibrils and elastic fibers in diseased tissues. The *fibrillin-1 (FBN1)* locus resides on the long arm of chromosome 15 (15q21), and the gene is composed of 65 exons.

There have been greater than 1,300 pathogenic variants identified in this gene, which are highly penetrant; however, there is a great degree of phenotypic variability with this disorder. A majority of affected individuals (75%) have an affected parent, whereas the rest (25%) are de novo.

Marfan's syndrome was traditionally considered to result from a structural deficiency of connective tissues. Reduced fibrillin-1 was thought to lead to a primary derangement of elastic fiber deposition, because both skin and aorta from affected patients show decreased elastin, along with elastic fiber fragmentation. In response to stress (such as hemodynamic forces in the proximal aorta), affected organs were thought to manifest this structural insufficiency with accelerated degeneration.

ESSENTIAL DIAGNOSTIC POINTS

- Disproportionate growth
- Skeletal abnormalities
- Arachnodactyly and tall stature
- Joint hyperextensibility
- Lens dislocation and aortic insufficiency
- Mitral valve prolapse
- Dural ectasia

> **GENERAL FEATURES**
> - Tall stature
> - Failure to thrive
> - Arachnodactyly
> - Mitral valve prolapse
> - Aortic regurgitation

■ CLINICAL FEATURES (FIG. 1)

The patient is generally tall and slender. Subcutaneous tissue is lacking. Tall stature may be present at birth and persist postnatally. Diminished subcutaneous tissue may suggest failure to thrive. Hypotonia and ligamentous laxity may suggest developmental delay, but cognitive performance is normal. In newborns, this present with hypotonia, arachnodactyly, joint laxity, and dislocation.

Marfan's syndrome is a multisystem disorder, with cardinal manifestations in skeletal, cardiovascular, and ocular systems.

Skeletal System

Excessive bone growth is typically noted in MFS, particularly in the long, tubular bones of the extremities, leading to disproportionally long extremities compared to the trunk (known as dolichostenomelia). This alters the arm span-to-height and upper-to-lower segment ratios. The lower segment is measured from the pubic symphysis to the floor, and the upper segment is calculated by subtracting the lower segment from the height. An increased arm span-to-height ratio (>1.05) and a reduced upper-to-lower segment ratio (<0.85) are considered positive findings.

The extremities are long. The lower segment measurement is greater than the upper segment measurement. The arm span exceeds the height. The fingers are long and tapered. The wrist sign, i.e., the thumb and the fifth finger when clasped around the wrist is overlapping.

Anterior chest deformity is likely the result of excessive rib growth, pushing the sternum either outward (pectus carinatum) or inward (pectus excavatum). Abnormal curvatures of the spine (most commonly thoracolumbar scoliosis) may also partly result from increased vertebral growth. Other skeletal features include an inward bulging of the acetabulum into the pelvic cavity (protrusio acetabuli), flatfeet (pes planus), and joint hypermobility or joint contracture.

Contracture of the fingers (camptodactyly) and elbows are commonly observed. A selection of craniofacial manifestations may be present including a long narrow skull (dolichocephaly), deep-set eyes (enophthalmos), recessed lower mandible (retrognathia), or small chin (micrognathia), flattening of the midface (malar hypoplasia), a high-arching palate, and downward-slanting palpebral fissures. The recurrent dislocation of the patella is observed. The thumb may be adducted, i.e., Sternberg sign.

Other skeletal features include progressive scoliosis or thoracic kyphosis and abnormally deep acetabulum of the hip

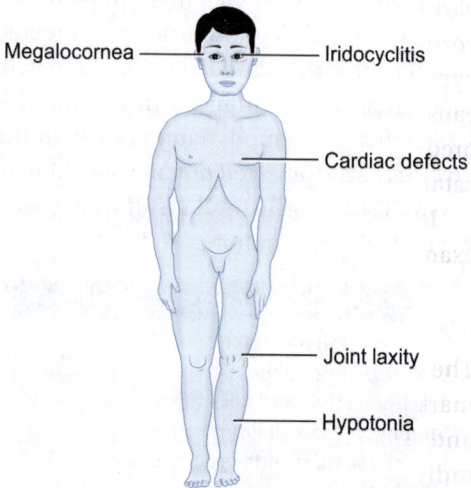

Fig. 1: Clinical features.

known as protrusio acetabuli (which can be associated with pelvic or upper leg pain). Flat feet (pes planus) as well as a hindfoot deformity defined as medial rotation of the medial malleolus may also be observed in individuals with MFS.

Cardiovascular System

The major sources of morbidity and mortality from this disorder are the complications noted in the cardiovascular system namely dilation of the aorta, aortic valve insufficiency, aortic aneurysm and dissection, mitral valve prolapse, tricuspid prolapse, and enlargement of the proximal pulmonary artery.

Within the heart, thickening of the atrioventricular valves is common and often associated with valvular prolapse. Variable degrees of regurgitation may be present. In children with early onset and severe MFS, insufficiency of the mitral valve can lead to congestive heart failure, pulmonary hypertension, and death in infancy; this manifestation is the leading cause of morbidity and mortality in young children with the disorder. Supraventricular arrhythmias and ventricular dysrhythmias may be seen in association with mitral valve dysfunction. Dilated cardiomyopathy occurs with increased prevalence in patients. Aortic valve dysfunction is generally a late occurrence and is attributed to stretching of the aortic annulus by an expanding aortic root aneurysm.

The aortic dilation is seen mainly at the level of the sinuses of Valsalva but can be seen in other parts of the aorta as well. The aortic root measurements are interpreted on the basis of normal values for age and body surface area (Z-score). Aortic dilatation is progressive over time and, if left uncorrected, increases the risk for dissection in these individuals; however, the onset and rate of progression are highly variable, and hence, close surveillance is warranted by a cardiologist familiar with MFS.

Aortic aneurysm, dissection, and rupture, principally at the level of the sinuses of Valsalva (aortic root), remain the most life-threatening manifestations of MFS, promoting lifelong monitoring by ECG or other imaging modalities. The most important risk factors for aortic dissection are the maximal aortic root size and a positive family history. The characteristic histologic findings from the aortae of patients with MFS include cystic medial necrosis of the tunica media and disruption of elastic lamellae.

Stretching of the chordae tendineae may lead to mitral valvular disease such as mitral valve prolapse. Congestive cardiac failure and rupture of the aorta secondary to the dissecting aneurysm are the common causes of death.

Ocular System

Dislocation of the ocular lens (ectopia lentis) occurs in approximately 60–70% of patients, although it is not unique to the disorder. Other ocular manifestations include early and severe progressive myopia, flat cornea, increased axial length of the globe, hypoplastic iris, and ciliary muscle hypoplasia causing decreased miosis. Patients are also predisposed to retinal detachment and early cataracts or glaucoma.

It is most reliably diagnosed by slit-lamp examination with pupillary dilation.

Skin Findings

The main skin findings in MFS are stretch marks or striae across the back, shoulders, and inguinal and axillary regions. These individuals can also have widened scars. Individuals with MFS are at risk for hernias, and primary hernia repairs should use synthetic mesh to minimize the risk of recurrence. These findings are not necessarily specific to this disorder.

Central Nervous System and Dural Manifestations

The dural sac in the lumbosacral region in individuals with MFS can stretch and result in dural ectasia. A majority of patients with this finding are asymptomatic; however, some individuals have pain, weakness, and numbness. This dural abnormality is identified by MRI or CT scans. Cognitive deficits are not known to be a part of the spectrum of MFS.

Pulmonary Features

The pulmonary features of MFS include spontaneous pneumothorax from lung bullae, reduced pulmonary reserve from pectus deformity or severe scoliosis, obstructive sleep apnea, and emphysematous lung disease.

Craniofacial Features

The craniofacial features of MFS are notable for a long narrow face with deep-set eyes, enophthalmos, downward slanting palpebral fissures, malar hypoplasia, micrognathia, high arched palate, and dental crowding. The facial features are highly variable and not specific to this disorder. However, these individuals can have difficulty with anesthesia and intubation secondary to their craniofacial features.

The disease is most commonly confused with homocystinuria. This may be differentiated by the character of the lens dislocation, i.e., upper dislodgement is seen in MFS. In homocystinuria, there is malar flush, generalized osteoporosis, and moderate mental retardation. There is a positive nitroprusside test and homocysteine is present in urine.

■ DIAGNOSIS

Laboratory studies should document a negative urinary cyanide nitroprusside test or specific amino acid studies to exclude cystathionine beta-synthase deficiency (homocystinuria). Although it is estimated that most, if not all, people with classic MFS have an *FBN1* mutation.

In the absence of a conclusive family history of MFS, the diagnosis can be established in four distinct scenarios:

1. The presence of either aortic root dilatation when standardized to age and body size (an aortic root Z-score 22) or aortic dissection combined with ectopia lentis allows for the unequivocal diagnosis of MFS, irrespective of the presence or absence of any systemic features, except when these are indicative of an alternate diagnosis.
2. The presence of aortic root dilatation (Z-score 22) or aortic dissection and the identification of a bona fide *FBN1* mutation are sufficient to establish the diagnosis even if ectopia lentis is absent.
3. When aortic root dilatation (an aortic root Z-score 22) or aortic dissection is present, but ectopia lentis is absent and the *FBN1* status is either unknown or negative, the diagnosis may be confirmed by the presence of sufficient systemic findings (a systemic score 27 points). However, features suggestive of an alternate diagnosis must be excluded, and the appropriate alternative molecular testing should be performed.
4. In the presence of ectopia lentis, but the absence of aortic root dilatation or aortic dissection, an *FBN1* mutation, which has previously been associated with aortic disease, is required before the diagnosis can be made. If the *FBN1* mutation

is not unequivocally associated with cardiovascular disease in either a related or unrelated proband, the patient should be classified as "isolated ectopia lentis syndrome" (see differential diagnosis).

In an individual with a positive family history of MFS (where a family member has been independently diagnosed using the above criteria), the diagnosis can be established in the presence of:
- Ectopia lentis
- A systemic score of 27 points
- Aortic root dilatation with Z-score 22 in adults (20 years old) or Z-score 23 in individuals <20 years old.

DIFFERENTIAL DIAGNOSIS

Differential diagnosis includes:
- Rickets
- Chondrodystrophy
- Homocystinuria
- Hereditary arthro-ophthalmopathy
- Lujan syndrome
- Ehlers–Danlos syndrome

COMPLICATIONS

Complications include:
- Progressive scoliosis
- Astigmatism
- Myopia
- Mitral valve prolapse
- Aortic root dilation
- Aortic aneurysm

TREATMENT

Treatment includes mainly prevention of complications and genetic counseling. Physiotherapy may improve neuromuscular tone and strength of the affected infants. Maximum exercise should be discouraged. This is because stress increases the cardiac output.

Management of MFS requires a multidisciplinary approach with involvement of different specialists. Yearly ophthalmologic exams are recommended and should be performed by a physician who is familiar with MFS. Most eye problems are controlled with corrective lenses, but some may require surgery. In patients with pectus deformities that interfere with cardiac or pulmonary functioning, a surgical intervention is required. Yearly evaluations for scoliosis and kyphosis are recommended, and it is important to have an orthopedic surgeon involved in the care of these patients.

Current Therapies

Important advances have been made in the cardiovascular management of patients with MFS. Management recommendations include serial cardiac imaging, medications to decrease progressive aortic root dilation and prophylactic aortic root replacement. Generally, yearly cardiac imaging evaluations with echocardiograms alternating with computed tomography angiography (CTA) or magnetic resonance angiography (MRA) are preferred. Due to the fragility of the aorta, contact sports and isometric exercise are prohibited in individuals with aortic root dilation. Current medical therapies that have been approved to decrease the rate of progressive aortic root dilation include beta blockers and angiotensin II type 1 receptor blockers.

Activity Restrictions

Physical therapy can improve cardiovascular performance, neuromuscular tone, and psychosocial health, and therefore aerobic exertion in moderation is recommended.

Aortic Surgery

Surgical guidelines for aortic root repair in young children with MFS are determined by (i) the rate of increase of the aortic root diameter (>1 cm/yr), (ii) progressive and severe aortic regurgitation, and (iii) size of the maximal aortic root (if it exceeds 5 cm). If possible, a valve-sparing procedure is preferred to avoid chronic anticoagulation therapy. However, valvular dysfunction can be seen, which leads to volume overload with resultant heart failure. The leading cause of morbidity and mortality in young children with MFS is mitral valve prolapse, leading to congestive heart failure. It should be noted that children are at high risk for repeat cardiac operations.

Pregnancy

There is a higher risk of aortic dissection during pregnancy in women with MFS. Prophylactic aortic root replacement can minimize the risk of aortic dissection and death in women with MFS who wish to become pregnant.

Patients with MFS should continue to receive prophylaxis for bacterial endocarditis, in part because it remains unknown, but possible, that the myxomatous valves typical of MFS are a preferred substrate for bacterial infection.

Current Pharmacologic Approaches

Endocarditis prophylaxis should be started with beta-adrenergic blocking drugs such as propranolol, or atenolol. Beta blockers have traditionally been considered the standard of care in MFS and multiple small observational studies suggest there is a protective effect on aortic root growth, with the dose typically titrated to achieve a resting heart rate <100 beats/min during submaximal exercise. Given the putative role of hemodynamic stress in aortic dilation and aortic dissection in MFS, these effects are attributed to the negative isotropic and chronotropic effects of beta blockade.

Deficient extracellular fibrillin-1 has led to the discovery that myopathy in MFS reflects excessive signaling by transforming growth factor beta TGF-β, an inhibitor of myeloblast differentiation. Studies have suggested that aortic aneurysm can be prevented by TGF-beta antagonists including blocker of angiotensin II type/receptors.

Emerging Therapeutic Strategies

Angiotensin II Receptor 1 Blockers

There is extensive evidence linking angiotensin II signaling to TGF-beta activation and signaling. In a mouse model of MFS, the angiotensin I Type 1 receptor blocker (ARB) losartan was shown to completely prevent pathologic aortic root growth and to normalize both aortic wall thickness and architecture findings that were absent in placebo-treated and propranolol-treated mice. These data suggest the potential for productive aortic wall remodeling in MES after TGF-beta inhibition.

Angiotensin-converting Enzyme Inhibitors

It has been proposed that angiotensin-converting enzyme (ACE) inhibitors might prove as effective as, or more effective than, ARBs in the treatment of MFS through their ability to limit signaling through both the type 1 and type 2 angiotensin receptors (ATIR and AT2R, respectively).

Extracellular Signal-regulated Kinase Inhibitors

It is known that ligand-dependent TGF-beta receptor activation can also initiate noncanonical cascades, including the mitogen-activated protein kinases (MAPKs). There is an increase in ERK1/2 activation in the aortas of MFS mice, while administration of an orally bioavailable selective inhibitor of ERK1/2 activation, and RDEA119 completely prevented pathologic aortic root growth in MFS mice, suggesting that ERK1/2 is a critical mediator of disease pathophysiology and a potentially viable therapeutic target.

PROGNOSIS

The major cause of mortality is aortic root dilation, dissection, and rupture, with the majority of fatal events occurring in the 3rd and 4th decade of life. A re-evaluation of life expectancy in MFS suggests that early diagnosis and refined medical and surgical management have greatly improved the prognosis for patients with the condition.

GENETIC COUNSELING

Genetic counseling is mandatory. 15–30% of the affected individuals are the firstborn. Paternal age is a contributing factor. This leads to new dominant mutations with minimal recurrence risk to the future offspring of the normal parents. The heritable nature of MFS makes recurrence risk (genetic) counseling mandatory. Fathers of these sporadic cases are, on average, 7–10 years older than fathers in the general population. This paternal age effect suggests that these cases represent new dominant mutations with minimal recurrence risk to the future offspring of the normal parents. Each child of an affected parent, however, has a 50% risk of inheriting the MFS mutation, and thus being affected. Recurrence risk counseling is best accomplished by professionals with expertise in the issues surrounding the disorder.

BIBLIOGRAPHY

1. Kumar A, Agarwal S. Marfan syndrome: An eyesight of syndrome. Meta Gene. 2014;2: 96-105.
2. Labreiro A, Martins E, Cruz C, Almeida J, Maciel MJ, Cardoso JC, et al. Marfan syndrome: Clinical manifestations, pathophysiology and new outlook on drug therapy. Rev Port Cardiol. 2010;29(6):1021-36.

CASE 107

Osteogenesis Imperfecta

■ PRESENTING COMPLAINTS

A 7-day-old girl was brought with the complaints of:
- Excessive crying since 3 days
- Swelling in head and leg since 2 days

History of Presenting Complaints

A baby girl aged about 1 week was brought to hospital with a history of excessive crying.

CASE AT A GLANCE	
Basic Findings	
Length	: 47 cm (3rd centile)
Weight	: 1.7 kg (LBW)
Temperature	: 37°C
Pulse rate	: 126 beats/min
Respiratory rate	: 26 breaths/min
Blood pressure	: 50/35 mm Hg
Positive Findings	
History:	
• Excessive crying on handling	
• Multiple swellings on the head and the extremities	
• Low birth weight	
Examination:	
• Low birth weight	
• Excessive crying	
• Breaking of nose	
• Short limbs	
• Multiple fractures	
Investigation:	
• *Infantogram:* Multiple old and fresh fractures	
LBW: low birth weight	

Paradoxically, the child was crying a lot when she was consoled by taking her close to her mother's chest. Her mother noticed the small swellings on the head and along the long bones of both legs. The mother also told that the swellings were painful and hard in consistency. The child was taking feeds regularly. Her bowel and bladder habits were normal.

Past History of the Patient

The baby was born at term by normal vaginal delivery. She cried immediately after delivery. Cry of the baby was normal. All the neonatal reflexes were normal. The weight of the baby was 1.7 kg. The length of the baby was 46 cm and the head circumference was 33 cm. She started taking breast milk immediately.

■ EXAMINATION

The child was a low birth weight (LBW) baby. She was irritable and was lying on the bed and crying. She was crying a lot when she was taken into the hands. The features of intrauterine growth retardation (IUGR) were present. Anthropometric measurements included the height of 47 cm (3rd centile), the weight of 1.7 kg, and the head circumference of 33 cm.

The child was afebrile and her heart rate was 126 beats per minute. Respiratory rate was 26 breaths per minute. The blood pressure recorded was 50/35 mm Hg. There was no pallor, no lymphadenopathy, no cyanosis, and no edema.

The child was lying with broad thigh, fixed at right angles to the hip. There was beaking of the nose. Short and deformed limbs were present. The child had blue sclera. There were signs of multiple fractures at the swelling sites. The systemic examinations were normal.

■ INVESTIGATION

- *Hemoglobin:* 14 g/dL
- *TLC:* 7,200 cells/dL
- *ESR:* 30 mm in the 1st hour
- *Absolute eosinophil count (AEC):* 360 cells/mm^3
- *Infantogram:* Showed evidence of multiple fractures which are fresh and old

■ DISCUSSION

Osteogenesis imperfecta (OI) is a rare group of genetic disorders of collagen metabolism and connective tissue causing bone fragility, with bowing and frequent multiple fractures. The incidence is 1 in 15,000.

Osteogenesis imperfecta (brittle bone disease) is the most common genetic cause of osteoporosis. The spectrum of OI ranges from forms that are lethal in the perinatal period, i.e., OI congenita to a mild form in which the diagnosis may be equivocal in an adult.

This is the statistical chance that 1 parent has germline mosaicism. The collagen mutation in the mosaic parent is present in some germ cells and may be present in somatic tissues. If a parent is a mosaic carrier, the risk of recurrence may be as high as 50%.

The fibrillin-1 (*FBN1*) locus resides on the long arm of chromosome 15 (15q21), and the gene is composed of 65 exons. Linkage analysis has suggested an absence of locus heterogeneity and the involvement of *FBN1* is demonstrated in >90% of cases, with >1,000 disease-causing mutations identified to date (the majority of which are missense point mutations and unique to a given family).

■ ETIOLOGY

Osteogenesis imperfecta is a primary bone dysplasia. The majority of cases (90%) are caused by autosomal dominant variants of two genes that form type I collagen, *COLIA1* and *COLIA2*. Type I collagen is formed by two COLIA1 and one COLIA2 proteins to create a structurally strong triple helix. These large structural proteins contain a helical domain with glycine-X-Y repeats, where X is primarily proline and Y is primarily hydroxyproline.

Structural or quantitative defects in type I collagen cause the full clinical spectrum of OI (types I–IV). Type I collagen is the primary component of the ECM of bone and skin. These cases are caused by defects in genes whose protein products interact with type I collagen. One group of patients has overmodified collagen with similar biochemical findings, and other group with collagen structural defects has severe or lethal OI bone dysplasia.

The most recent set of genes added to the recessive OI causative panel (*SP7*, type XIII OI; *TMEM38B*, type XIV OI; *WNT1*, type XV OI; *CREB3L1*, type XVI OI, *SPARC*, type XVII OI; and *MBTPS2*, type XVIII OI) not only are involved in osteoblast differentiation but also affect collagen synthesis and cross-linking. There are very few individuals with OI whose genetic defect is not in a known causative gene.

■ PATHOLOGY

The collagen structural mutations cause OI bone to be globally abnormal. The bone matrix contains abnormal type I collagen fibrils and relatively increased levels of types

III and V collagen. Several noncollagenous proteins of bone matrix are also reduced.

Cortical thickness is reduced in the shafts of long bones and skull bones that are completely surrounded by cranial sutures—Wormian bones are present in skull. Bone cells contribute to OI pathology, with abnormal osteoblast differentiation and increased numbers of active bone-resorbing osteoclasts. The hydroxyapatite crystals deposited on this matrix are poorly aligned with the long axis of fibrils, and there is paradoxical hypermineralization of bone.

PATHOGENESIS

Collagen structural defects are predominantly of two types.

80% are point mutations causing substitutions of helical glycine residues or crucial residues in the C-propeptide by other amino acids, and 20% are single exon splicing defects.

The clinically mild OI type I has a quantitative defect, with null mutations in 1 alpha (I) allele leading to a reduced amount of normal collagen.

The glycine substitutions in the two alpha chains have distinct genotype–phenotype relationships. One-third of mutations in the alpha 1 chain are lethal, and those in alpha 2 are predominantly nonlethal. Two-third regions in alpha 1(I) align with major ligand-binding regions of the collagen helix. Lethal mutations in alpha 2(I) occur in 8 regularly spaced clusters along the chain that align with binding regions for matrix proteoglycans in the collagen fibril.

Type of collagen is a heterotrimer composed of two alpha 1(I) chains and one alpha 2(I) chain. The chains are synthesized as procollagen molecules with short globular extensions on both ends of the central helical domain. The helical domain is composed of uninterrupted repeats of the sequence Gly-X-Y, where Gly is glycine, X is often proline, and Y is often hydroxyproline. The presence of glycine at every third residue is crucial to helix formation because its small side chain can be accommodated in the interior of the helix. The chains are assembled into trimers at their carboxyl ends; helix formation then proceeds linearly in a carboxyl-to-amino direction. Concomitant with helix assembly and formation, helical proline and lysine residues are hydroxylated by prolyl-4-hydroxylase and lysyl hydroxylase, and some hydroxylysine residues are glycosylated.

CLINICAL FEATURES (FIG. 1)

Osteogenesis imperfecta is the most common osteoporotic disease of the newborn. This is characterized by fractures and skeletal deformities. In OI congenita condition, the child dies in newborn period with extreme fragility of bones and numerous fractures. It is distinguished by multiple intrauterine or perinatal fractures.

In OI tarda, the child manifests bone fragility in life and half a normal lifespan. These are genetic syndromes that account for variability.

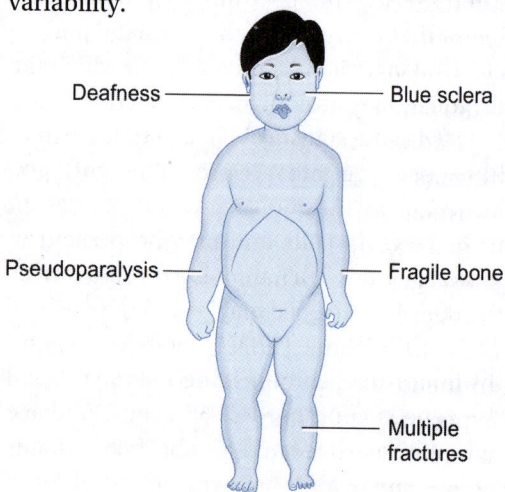

Fig. 1: Clinical features.

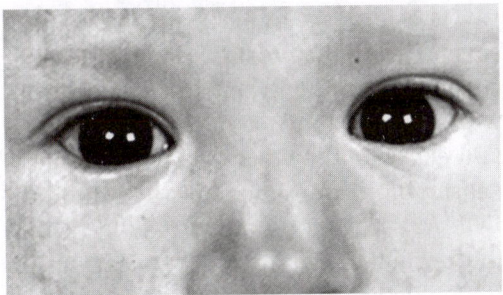

Fig. 2: Blue sclera.

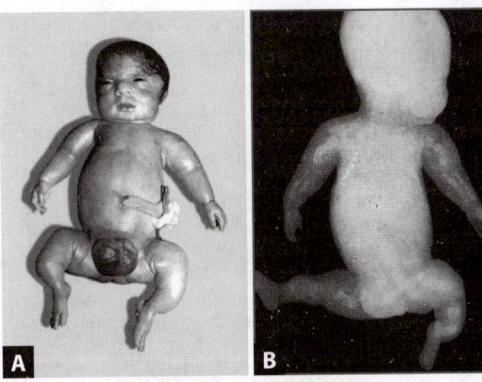

Figs. 3A and B: Osteogenesis imperfecta (type I).
(For color version, see Plate 12)

Osteogenesis Imperfecta Type I (Mild)

Osteogenesis imperfecta type I (mild) is of autosomal dominant type, with most cases being familial. Classically, it is defined as nondeforming OI with blue-gray sclera (**Fig. 2**). It is characterized by osteoporosis and excessive bone fragility. The child will have a blue sclera. There is presenile conductive deafness.

Deformities are mainly due to fractures. There are rarely fractures or limb bowing present in utero or at birth. Fractures result from mild-to-moderate trauma but decrease after puberty. The risk again increases in late adulthood, particularly in postmenopausal women. Vertebral fractures and scoliosis are a risk in childhood and may require therapeutic intervention.

Radiographic features that suggest a diagnosis of type I OI include the presence of Wormian bones in the skull and the finding of generalized osteopenia. The radiograph shows general osteopenia and evidence of a previous fracture (**Figs. 3A and B**). Bowing of the lower limb is common. Other possible connective tissue abnormalities include hyperextensible joints, easy bruising, thin skin, joint laxity, scoliosis, Wormian bones, hernia, and mild short stature compared with family members.

The diagnosis of type I OI can be made by performing sequence and deletion/duplication evaluation of COLIA1 and COLIA2 or by collagen studies on fibroblasts.

Both types I and IV are divided into A and B subtypes, depending on the absence (A) or presence (B) of dentinogenesis imperfecta.

Osteogenesis Imperfecta Type II

Osteogenesis imperfecta type II is a perinatal lethal form of OI (**Fig. 4**). It is of autosomal recessive type. Biochemically, there is a marked reduction in the type I collagen, i.e., the principal collagen of bone (**Figs. 5A and B**). It is typically caused by de novo glycine substitutions in *COLIA1* or *COLIA2*. There is severe fragility of the skeleton with consistent findings including the presence of in utero fracture, short and severely bowed extremities, enlarged fontanelles, and low birth length and weight for gestational age. There is a deep blue-grey sclera.

Radiograph shows crumpled long bones with fractures and beaded ribs. Multiple rib fractures create a beaded appearance, and the small thorax contributes to respiratory insufficiency.

There is a beaking of nose with hypotelorism. Short and deformed bowing of

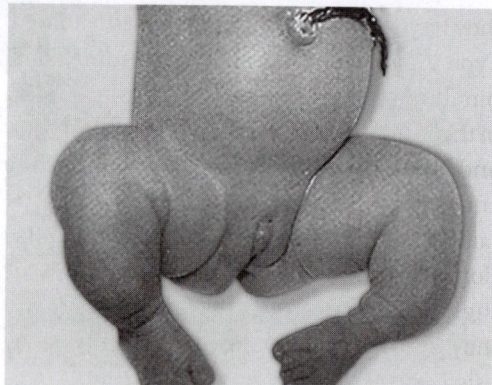

Fig. 4: Osteogenesis imperfecta type II.

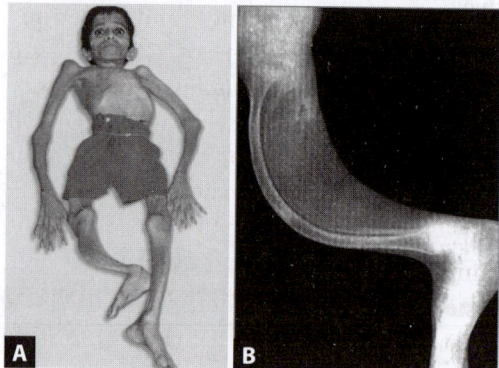

Figs. 5A and B: Osteogenesis imperfecta (type II).

Osteogenesis imperfecta type II is a severe nonlethal form, termed progressively deforming type, and can present with multiple in utero or at-birth fractures and extremity bowing. This type is usually caused by missense variants in COL1A1 or COL1A2. While the length may be within the normal range at birth, typically there is a reduction to below the normal range by 1–2 years. In infancy, fractures occur frequently from minimal trauma or manipulation. The presence of dentinogenesis imperfecta and scleral color are variable.

Radiographic findings include long bone and vertebral anomalies from infancy. Many patients with this subtype are not able to bear weight or ambulate on their own. Orthopedic management, medical management with bisphosphonates, and physical therapy/rehabilitation care are all required to manage this form of OI. Basilar invagination, caused by compression of the skull on the cervical spine, is common and may progress to brain stem compression, obstructive hydrocephalus, or syringomyelia.

limbs are present. The thighs are broad and fixed at right angles to hip. The legs are held abducted at right angles to the body in the frog leg position. The skull is large for body size, with enlarged anterior and posterior fontanelles. Sclerae are dark blue–gray. The cerebral cortex has multiple neuronal migrations and other defects (agyria, gliosis, and periventricular leukomalacia).

Death typically occurs in the 1st week and is caused by respiratory insufficiency as a result of the narrow chest, rib fractures, and potentially the presence of a flail chest. The recurrence risk has been reported to be 6% for de novo changes in OI, given the presence of paternal gonadal mosaicism.

Osteogenesis Imperfecta Type III

Osteogenesis imperfecta type III is of autosomal recessive type. OI type III is the most severe nonlethal form of OI and results in significant physical disability. Birthweight and length are often below normal. It is characterized by severe bone fragility and multiple fractures leading to progressive skeletal deformities. Fractures usually occur in utero. There are relative macrocephaly and triangular facies. Postnatally, fractures occur from inconsequential trauma and heal with deformity. The sclera may be blue at birth and become less blue with age.

A considerate proportion of patients succumb to cardiorespiratory complications in infancy or childhood. The rib cage has flaring at the base, and pectus deformity is frequent. Virtually, all type III patients have scoliosis and vertebral compression. Growth falls below the curve by the 1st year. All type III patients have extremely short stature.

Radiograph shows generalized osteopenia and multiple fractures. There is no beading of the ribs and crumpling of the long bones. The skull shows osteopenia and multiple Wormian bones. Disorganization of the bone matrix results in a "popcorn" appearance at the metaphyses. Dentinogenesis imperfecta, hearing loss, and kyphoscoliosis may be present or develop over time.

Osteogenesis Imperfecta Type IV

Osteogenesis imperfecta type IV is the most common type. It is of autosomal dominant type. It is characterized by osteoporosis. Patients with OI type IV can present at birth within utero fractures or bowing of lower long bones. They can also present with recurrent fractures after ambulation and have normal-to-moderate short stature. Most children have moderate bowing even with infrequent fractures. Patients typically have bowing of tibias and have moderate short stature. Children with OI type IV require orthopedic and rehabilitation intervention, but they are usually able to attain community ambulation skills. Fracture rates decrease after puberty. Patients with type IV have moderate short stature. Scleral hue may be blue or white. This form of OI is also typically caused by single nucleotide variants in COL1A1 and COL1A2.

Osteogenesis Imperfecta Type V (Hyperplastic Callus) and Type VI Hyperosteoidosis (Mineralization Defect)

Types V and VI OI patients clinically have OI similar in skeletal severity to type IV, but they have distinct findings on bone histology. Type V patients also usually have some combination of hyperplastic callus, calcification of the interosseous membrane of the forearm, and/or a radiodense metaphyseal band. They constitute <5% of OI populations. All type V OI patients are heterozygous for the same mutation, which generates a novel start codon for the bone protein BRIL. Ligamentous laxity may be present; blue sclera or dentinogenesis imperfect are not present. Patients with type VI OI have progressive deforming OI that does not manifest at birth. They have distinctive bone histology with broad osteoid seams and fish-scale lamellation seen under polarized light.

Osteogenesis Imperfecta Types VII, VIII, and IX (Autosomal Recessive)

Types VII and VIII patients overlap clinically with types II and III OI but have distinct features including white sclerae, rhizomelia, and small-to-normal head circumference. Surviving children have severe osteochondrodysplasia with extreme short stature.

Osteogenesis Imperfecta Type IX

Type IX OI is very rare (only 8 cases reported). The severity is quite broad, ranging from lethal to moderately severe. These children have white sclerae but do not have rhizomelia.

Osteogenesis Imperfecta X and XI

Type X OI is severe to lethal form caused by defects affecting serine type endopeptidase inhibitor domain of HSP47. Type XI OI is more prevalent recessive form with moderate to severe skeletal phenotype, including white sclera and normal teeth. Congenital contracture of the joints may occur.

Defects in Osteoblast Differentiation (Types XII–XVIII Osteogenesis Imperfecta)

The most recent functional grouping of genes causing recessive OI (types XII to XVII) affects osteoblast differentiation and is collagen-related. *SP7* (type XIII OI) regulates osteoblast differentiation and is critical for bone formation.

GENERAL FEATURES
• Low birth weight • Excessive crying • Beaking of nose • Short limbs

High Bone Mass Osteogenesis Imperfecta (Cleavage of the Procollagen C-Propeptide)

Autosomal dominant mutations in the C-propeptide cleavage site of procollagen or recessive defects in the enzyme responsible for its cleavage cause bone fragility with normal or elevated dual-energy X-ray absorptiometry bone density Z-scores. Individuals with dominant mutations have normal stature, white sclerae and teeth, and mild-to-moderate OI. Null mutations in *BMP1* lead to a more severe skeletal phenotype with short stature, scoliosis, and bone deformity because *BMP1* has other substrates in addition to type I collagen.

ESSENTIAL DIAGNOSTIC POINTS
• Dominantly inherited with multiple and recurrent fractures • Bony deformities and growth retardation • Blue sclera and thin skin • Hyperextensibility of ligaments • Otosclerosis with significant hearing loss • Hypoplastic deformed teeth • Intelligence not affected

■ DIAGNOSIS

Deoxyribonucleic acid sequencing is the first diagnostic laboratory test; several diagnostic laboratories offer panels to test for dominant and recessive OI. Mutation identification is useful to determine the type with certainty and to facilitate family screening and prenatal diagnosis. It is also possible to screen for type VI OI by determination of serum pigment epithelium-derived factor level, which is severely reduced in this type.

Severe OI can be detected prenatally by level II ultrasonography as early as 16 weeks of gestation. OI and thanatophoric dysplasia may be confused. Fetal ultrasonography might not detect OI type IV and rarely detects OI type I. For recurrent cases, chorionic villus biopsy can be used for biochemical or molecular studies. Amniocytes produce false positive biochemical studies but can be used for molecular studies in appropriate cases,

In the neonatal period, the normal-to-elevated alkaline phosphatase levels present in OI distinguish it from hypophosphatasia.

Diagnosis is confirmed by collagen biochemical studies using fibroblast cultured from the skin—percutaneous biopsy.

LABORATORY SALIENT FINDINGS
• Biochemical studies using fibroblast • Skin—percutaneous biopsy • Ultrasonographically at 16 weeks • Chorionic villus biopsy for biochemical assay.

■ COMPLICATIONS

Complications include:
- Cardiopulmonary
  - Recurrent pneumonia
  - Cardiac failure
- Neurological
  - Basilar invagination
  - Brainstem compression
  - Hydrocephalus
  - Syringohydromyelia

MANAGEMENT

For OI type I and type II, no therapeutic intervention is effective. Prompt splinting of the fractures and correction of deformities are recommended. Calcitonin therapy will increase the skeletal mass and decrease the frequency of the fractures.

There is no cure for OI. For severe nonlethal OI, active physical rehabilitation in the early years allows children to attain a higher functional level than orthopedic management alone. Children with OI type I and some with type IV are spontaneous ambulators. Individuals with OI type III are usually wheelchair dependent. With aggressive rehabilitation, they can attain transfer skills and household ambulation.

Children with types III, IV, V, VI, and XI OI benefit from gait aids and a program of swimming and conditioning. Severely affected patients require a wheelchair for community mobility but can acquire transfer and self-care skills. Teens with OI can require psychologic support with body image issues. Growth hormone improves bone histology in growth-responsive children (usually types I and IV).

Orthopedic management of OI is aimed at fracture management and correction of deformity to enable function. Fractures should be promptly splinted or cast; OI fractures heal well and cast removal should be aimed at minimizing immobilization osteoporosis. Correction of long bone deformity requires an osteotomy procedure and placement of an intramedullary rod.

Hearing Assessment and Regular Dental Checkup

Formal audiologic assessment should be completed at the time of diagnosis, and a CT or MRI scan should be considered in individuals with severe OI to evaluate for basilar invagination. Twice yearly dental evaluations should be completed starting at age of 3 years. Serum vitamin D should be measured and supplemented if low.

Bisphosphonates

Geneticists and endocrinologists use bisphosphonates to decrease the incidence of fractures. The use of bisphosphonates in OI has been demonstrated to increase bone density and decrease bone pain, although studies have not clearly shown a reduction in fracture risk (although the studies have significant limitations). Criteria for starting intravenous (IV) bisphosphonate therapy in OI include multiple fractures within a 1-year period, the presence of bowing, or the presence of vertebral compression fractures. IV bisphosphonate therapy has also shown benefit in treating bone pain. Although bisphosphonates improve bone density, it is unclear if they improve bone quality; thus, bisphosphonates should be used cautiously, and the presence of side effects should be closely monitored.

A several-year course of treatment of children with OI with bisphosphonates (IV pamidronate or oral olpadronate or risedronate) confers some benefits. Bisphosphonates decrease bone resorption by osteoclasts; OI patients have increased bone volume that still contains the defective collagen. Bisphosphonates are more beneficial for vertebrae (trabecular bone) than long bones (cortical bone). Treatment for 1-2 years results in increased is LI-LA dual-energy X-ray absorptiometry and, more importantly, improved vertebral compressions and area.

Emerging therapies include teriparatide, an anabolic agent, which was demonstrated to improve density in OI type I, and preclinical antibody therapies against TGF-beta, which has been demonstrated to be upregulated in OI, and an antisclerostin antibody.

Genetic Counseling

For autosomal dominant OI, the risk of an affected individual passing the gene to offspring is 50%. An affected child usually has about the same severity of OI as the parent; however, there is variability of expression, and the child's condition can be either more or less severe than that of the parent. The collagen mutation in the mosaic parent is present in some germ cells and may be present in somatic tissues. If a parent is a mosaic carrier, the risk of recurrence may be as high as 50%.

For recessive OI, the recurrence risk is 25% per pregnancy. No known individual with severe nonlethal recessive OI has had a child.

■ PROGNOSIS

Osteogenesis imperfecta limits both the lifespan and functional level.
- *In Type II OI:* Death within a month to year
- *In Type III OI:* Reduced lifespan with rehabilitation
- *In Type I and IV:* Compatible with full lifespan

■ BIBLIOGRAPHY

1. Harrington J, Sochett E, Howard A. Update on the evaluation and treatment of osteogenesis imperfecta. Pediatr Clin North Am. 2014;61(6):1243-57.

CASE 108

Talipes

■ PRESENTING COMPLAINTS

A 6-month-old boy was brought with the complaint of:
- Deformity of leg since 6 months.

History of Presenting Complaints

A 6-month-old boy was brought to the hospital with history of deformed legs. Her mother had noticed the deformity at birth. But the concerned doctor assured that it can be corrected by splinting. She told that the foot was bent inward. Whenever, she tried to make the child to stand, the dorsum of the foot was touching the ground. The sole was completely bent inward.

CASE AT A GLANCE	
Basic Findings	
Length	: 67 cm (>50th centile)
Weight	: 7 kg (50th centile)
Temperature	: 37°C
Pulse rate	: 106 beats/min
Respiratory rate	: 22 breaths/min
Blood pressure	: 60/40 mm Hg
Positive Findings	
History:	
• Deformed legs	
Examination:	
• Adduction deformity of foot	
Investigation:	
• Normal	

Past History of the Patient

The boy was the first child of nonconsanguineous marriage. He was born at full term by normal vaginal delivery. He cried immediately after delivery. His birth weight was 3 kg. He took breast milk on the first day itself. There was no significant postnatal event. His mother had noticed the inward bent of the foot. The doctor had advised splinting and surgery in the later part of childhood.

■ EXAMINATION

The child was moderately built and nourished. He was active and alert. He was lying on the bed and playing with the dolls given to him. Anthropometric measurements included the length 67 cm (>50th centile) the weight 7 kg (50th centile), the head circumference 40 cm.

Child was afebrile. The heart rate was 106 beats/min. The respiratory rate was 22 breaths/min. The blood pressure recorded was 60/40 mm Hg. There was no pallor, no lymphadenopathy, no cyanosis, and no icterus.

The deformities consist of adduction and rotation of the forefoot. The child's sole was resting on the medial aspect of tibia. Spine and other joints were normal.

INVESTIGATION

- *Hemoglobin:* 13 g/dL
- *TLC:* 7,600 cells/cumm
- *ESR:* 32 mm in the first hour
- *X-ray chest:* No abnormality detected
- *X-ray of the foot:* No significant bony deformities

DISCUSSION

This deformity is called as talipes. Clubfoot or congenital talipes equinovarus (CTEV) is the term used to describe a deformity involving malalignment of the caleaneotalar–navicular complex. Components of this deformity may be best understood using the mnemonic CAVE (cavus, adductus, varus, equinus).

The features of this disorder are:
- Plantar flexion of the foot at ankle joint—equinus
- Inversion deformity heel—varus
- Medial deviation of the forefoot—adductus.

It is the common foot deformity. It can be congenital, teratologic or positional. The positional (or postural) clubfoot is a normal foot that has been held in a deformed position in utero and is found to be flexible on examination in the newborn nursery. The incidence of the deformity is 1:1,000. Male to female ratio is 2:1.

It is now considered as multifactorial with single autosomal dominant gene. In majority of the patients etiology is unknown. It has been suggested that raised intrauterine pressure forces the lower limb of the fetus against the wall of the uterus. This leads to the molding of the feet.

It has been thought alternatively that the deformities are due to fiber-typed disproportion and increased neuromuscular junction in the muscles of the calf or the soft tissues of the foot. This is the primary neuromuscular cause. All the deformities are secondary to medial dislocation of the talonavicular joint. The atrophy of the calf muscle and foot are more evident in older children.

The pathoanatomy involves both abnormal tarsal morphology (plantar and medial deviation of the head and neck of the talus) and abnormal relationships between the tarsal bones in all three planes as well as associated contracture of the soft tissues on the plantar and medial aspects of the foot.

CLINICAL FEATURES (FIG. 1)

Newborn Evaluation

Examination of all joints for range of motion and stability, including the hips is important, as is examination of lower extremities for equal length and symmetry. The severity of newborn foot deformity is determined more by the foot's flexibility than by its appearance. Newborn foot deformities that can be easily manipulated into an overcorrected position are considered positional rather than true clubfoot deformities. These resolve with minimal or no treatment. Unless a limb deficiency such as fibular hemimelia, tibial

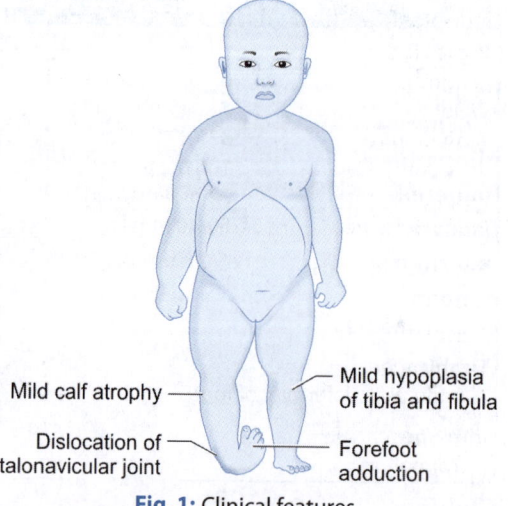

Fig. 1: Clinical features.

hemimelia, or congenital short femur is noted, radiography is not necessary.

Several syndromes are known to be associated with clubfoot, including classic arthrogryposis, multiple pterygium syndrome, distal arthrogryposis, amniotic band syndrome, and Freeman–Sheldon syndrome. Geneticists can help to evaluate when there is suspicion of a syndrome. Neurologic causes include myelomeningocele, lipomeningocele, tethered cord syndrome, diastematomyelia, and sacral agenesis. A careful examination of the spine is needed to detect the sometimes subtle findings associated with tethered cord such as sacral dimple or hair patch.

It occurs more commonly in males (2:1) and is bilateral in 50% of cases. The pathoanatomy involves both abnormal tarsal morphology (plantar and medial deviation of the head and neck of the talus) and abnormal relationships between the tarsal bones in all three planes, as well as associated contracture of the soft tissues on the plantar and medial aspects of the foot.

The congenital variety will constitute 75% of the cases. It is characterized by variable rigidity of the foot, mild calf atrophy, mild hypoplasia of tibia, fibula, and bones of the feet. Positional clubfoot is normal that had been held in deformed position in uterus.

The congenital clubfoot can either be idiopathic or syndromic. Idiopathic may be hereditary. Congenital clubfoot may be paralytic or secondary to myelodysplasia, the deformities in the arthrogryposis multiplex congenita may also include clubfoot. Sometimes this may be associated with clubbing in the hand.

Syndromic clubfoot associated with neuromuscular diagnoses or syndromes is typically rigid and more difficult to treat. Clubfoot is also extremely common in patients with myelodysplasia, arthrogryposis, Larsen syndrome, and other chromosomal syndromes such as trisomy 18 and chromosome 22q11 deletion syndrome.

There will be adduction and external rotation of the bone of the forefoot. The adduction occurs at midtarsal and tarsometatarsal joint. The external rotation is produced by torsion of the shaft of the metatarsals **(Figs. 2 and 3)**.

The extent of the deformities are variable. In the mildest cases, the deformities consist of adduction and some rotation of the forefoot. In extreme cases foot is so deformed that, the sole rests on medial aspect of the tibia.

A complete physical examination should be performed to rule out coexisting musculoskeletal

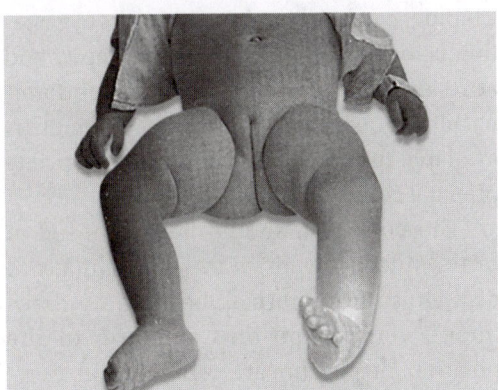

Fig. 2: Congenital talipes.

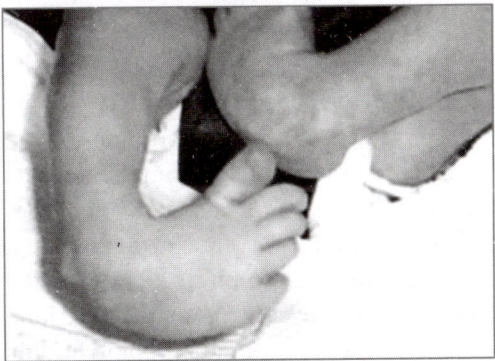

Fig. 3: Talipes equinovarus.

and neuromuscular problems. The spine should be inspected for signs of occult dysraphism. Examination of the infant clubfoot demonstrates forefoot cavus and adductus and hindfoot varus and equines. The degree of flexibility varies, and all patients will exhibit calf atrophy. Internal tibial torsion, foot-length shortening, and leg-length discrepancy (shortening of the ipsilateral extremity) will be observed in a subset of cases.

GENERAL FEATURES
• Hand–foot equinus • Midfoot varus

■ DIAGNOSIS

Clubfoot can be detected at 13 weeks of gestation using transvaginal ultrasonography and at 16 weeks of gestation using transabdominal ultrasonography. No prenatal treatment is available for clubfoot; however, appropriate prenatal counseling is important.

The condition should be diagnosed at birth. Mild deformities may be difficult to distinguish from normal, because newborn infants tend to posture the foot, in the position of equinovarus. In normal newborn, dorsiflexion occurs till the dorsum touches the anterior aspect of the skin. If this is impossible, the minor degree of talipes exists.

Radiographic Evaluation

Multiple radiographic measurements can be made to describe malalignment between the tarsal bones. The navicular bone does not ossify until 1–6 years of age, so the focus of radiographic interpretation is the relationships between segments of the foot, forefoot to hindfoot. A radiographic finding is "parallelism" between lines drawn through the axis of the talus and the calcaneus on the lateral radiograph, indicating hindfoot varus. X-ray may be particularly useful for older children with persistent or recurrent deformities that are difficult to assess.

ESSENTIAL DIAGNOSTIC POINTS
• Mild calf atrophy • Mild hypoplasia of tibia, fibula • Hand–foot equinus • Midfoot varus • Forefoot adduction • Dislocation of talonavicular joint

■ DIFFERENTIAL DIAGNOSIS

- Calcaneovalgus feet
- Congenital vertical talus
- Hypermobile pes planus
- Tarsal coalition

■ TREATMENT

Nonoperative treatment is initiated in all infants. It should be started as soon as possible following birth. Techniques include taping and strapping, manipulation and serial casting, and functional treatment. It is done between 3 and 12 months of age.

Manipulation of the foot is to stretch the contracted tissues on medial and posterior aspects followed by casting to hold correction is the preferred treatment. Serial casting are typically performed on weekly basis for 6–8 weeks.

Functional treatment, or the "French method", involves daily manipulations (supervised by a physical therapist) and splinting with elastic tape, as well as continuous passive motion (machine required) while the baby sleeps. Although many feet remain well aligned after surgical releases, a significant percentage of patients have required additional surgery for recurrent or residual deformities. Weekly cast changes are performed; 5-10 casts are typically required.

If the deformity is slight, foot can be dorsiflexed to little beyond the plantigrade position. The mother should be taught to manipulate her child's foot after every feed. Sufficient pressure should be applied and maintained for about 2 seconds. The pressure is released and reapplied over a period of about 5 minutes.

Ponseti Treatment Method

The method consists of three phases of treatment:
1. Manipulation and casting
2. Tenotomy
3. Bracing

The first phase involves manipulation and weekly serial above-knee casting performed by an individual trained in the technique. This phase typically lasts for 5-8 casts. Treatment can start anytime in the neonatal period, ideally the first 1-3 weeks. Weekly cast changes are performed; 5-10 casts are typically required.

In the second phase, after all of the elements of the deformity except equinus have been corrected, a percutaneous Achilles tenotomy is performed under local anesthesia by a surgeon in the clinic. A final cast is placed immediately after the tenotomy and worn for 3 weeks. About 90% of infants with clubfoot require a tenotomy. The most difficult deformity to correct is the hindfoot equinus, and approximately 90% of patients will require a percutaneous tenotomy of the heel cord as an outpatient. Following the tenotomy, a long leg cast with the foot in maximal abduction (up to 70°) and dorsiflexion is worn for 3-4 weeks; the patient then begins a bracing program.

The third and most important phase is the bracing phase, which starts immediately after removal of the post-tenotomy cast. The brace is a foot abduction orthosis that consists of two shoes or splints connected by a bar, which holds the feet shoulder width apart. During the first 3 months, the brace is worn 23 hours per day, allowing the brace to come off for dressing and bathing only. After the first 3 months, the brace is worn at nighttime and nap time only, with a goal of 12-14 hours of brace wear, until the child is 4-5 years old.

An abduction brace is worn full-time for 3 months and then at nighttime for 3-5 years. A small subset of patients (up to 20%) with recurrent, dynamic supination deformity will require transfer of the tibialis anterior tendon to the middle cuneiform for recurrence.

Splinting can be done by aluminous splint using zinc oxide plaster. The splint is removed and reapplied with little more correction every week. Denis Brown splint may be used throughout the day instead of maternal manipulation until child walks, and thereafter it may be used at night.

Complete correction both clinically and radiologically should be achieved by 3 months. If this happens, holding the cast is then advised for next 3-6 months followed by arthroses and correction shoes until the child is walking well.

If there is remaining equinus, surgery may be required in the form of percutaneous Achilles tenotomy in order to full correction. After the full correction is obtained, night braces is necessary for long-term maintenance of correction.

Failure of clinical and radiological correction is indication of surgery. 15-50% require surgical release. The surgical treatment is the complete soft-tissue release. This is usually performed between 6 and 12 months of age. The use of tendon transfer and bone procedure including arthrodesis (i.e., fusing), centralization of the tibialis anterior tendon have been useful in young children.

Common surgical approaches include a release of the involved joints (realignment of the tarsal bones), a lengthening of the shortened posteromedial musculotendinous units, and usually pinning of the foot in the corrected position. For older children with untreated clubfeet or those in whom a recurrence or residual deformity is observed, bony procedures (osteotomies) may be required in addition to soft-tissue surgery. Triple arthrodesis is reserved as salvage for painful, deformed feet in adolescents and adults.

Triple arthrodeses are indicated in painful deformity in adolescence.

Although most patients require some form of surgery, the procedures are minimal in comparison with extensive surgical release, which requires lengthening and/or release of muscles and tendons about the ankle and capsulotomy of the major joints to reposition the foot.

■ BIBLIOGRAPHY

1. Dobbs MB, Gurnett CA. Update on clubfoot: etiology and treatment. Clin Orthop Relat Res. 2009;467(5):1146-53.
2. Sankar WN, Weiss J, Skaggs DL. Orthopaedic conditions in the newborn. J Am Acad Orthop. 2009;17(2):112-22
3. Zionts LE, Packer DF, Cooper S, Ebramzadeh E, Sangiorgio S. Walking age of infants with idiopathic clubfoot treated using the ponseti method. J Bone Joint Surg Am. 2014; 96(19):e164.

Glossary

Achondroplasia: It is an autosomal dominant disease. It is characterized by limb dwarfism, frontal bossing, trident hand, and occasionally hydrocephalus. The limb shortening is more in proximal segments. A skeletal radiograph confirms the diagnosis. Genetic counseling is important.

Abdominal paracentesis: It is performed for diagnostic purposes to determine the etiology of peritoneal fluid and to determine whether infiltration is present, or for therapeutic reasons, i.e., to remove large volumes of abdominal fluid which impair respiratory function.

Abetalipoproteinemia: This is an autosomal recessive disorder caused by a defect in the gene for microsomal triglyceride transfer protein. Clinical features include fat malabsorption, failure to thrive, acanthocytosis severe anemia ataxia, and retinitis pigmentosa.

Absence attack: These start abruptly in children. A typical attack is not preceded by an aura. There will be a brief lapse of consciousness. Patients may show sudden discontinuation of activity with staring spells, eye fluttering, or rhythmic movements. This may last for <30 seconds.

Acne: It is a pleomorphic eruption usually seen on the face and trunk. It is observed most commonly during adolescence. It may persist for 1–5 years.

Acrocephaly: Skull appears like a turret due to the involvement of all the sutures.

Acrodermatitis enteropathica: It is an autosomal recessive disorder that usually manifests in the first year of life. The causative mechanism is the deficiency of zinc-binding ligandin. There will be depigmentation of hair and chronic diarrhea. Administration of zinc sulfate 50–100 mg per day is useful.

Acromegaly: This occurs because of the hypersecretion of the pituitary hormone after the fusion of epiphyses. The child is taller. Peripheral parts of the body like the hands and feet are large. There is a prominent jaw, broad nose, enlarged tongue, bushy eyebrows, thick skin and subcutaneous tissue, and kyphosis.

Acute flaccid paralysis: Acute onset of flaccid paralysis in a child aged <15 years. Poliomyelitis is an important cause.

Acute phase proteins: A protein, proteinase inhibitors, and coagulase proteins collectively constitute acute phase proteins. They enhance resistance to infection and promote repair of damaged tissue. These levels fluctuate in response to infection, inflammation, and tissue injury.

Acute kidney injury: It denotes acute impairment of renal function resulting in retention of nitrogenous wastes and other metabolic derangements.

Acute tubular necrosis: There will be dehydration. The oliguric phase lasts for 3–10 days.

The biochemical and clinical abnormalities gradually worsen. Subsequently, urine output increases steadily, i.e., diuretic phase. This lasts for a week.

Adenoid facies: It occurs as a result of enlarged pharyngeal tonsils. Adenoid facies are characterized by an open mouth, narrow, high-arched palate, and elongated mandible.

Adreno leukodystrophy: It usually presents between the ages of 4 and 12 years. The symptoms include behavioral changes, gait disturbances, dysarthria, dysphagia, loss of vision, seizures and decorticate posturing. One-third of the patients show evidence of adrenal insufficiency.

Albinism: It is an inherited disorder due to the deficiency of enzyme tyrosinase with diminished or absent melanin in skin, hair, and eyes. The synthesis of melanin is defective.

Algid malaria: The majority of patients with severe malaria remain well-perfused and warm. However, some may develop shock with cold extremities. This is known as algid malaria. This may result from secondary gram-negative bacteremia and hypovolemia.

Alopecia areata: It is a skin-specific auto-immune disease, due to inappropriate immune response to hair follicle-associated antigens. Children present with discoid areas of non-inflammatory, noncicatricial alopecia with exclamation mark hair at the periphery.

Alport's syndrome: It is characterized by hereditary glomerulonephritis. It is associated with hematuria and proteinuria. It is also associated with sensory neural deafness. The symptoms include high-colored urine, puffiness of the face, and generalized edema. Hypertension, urinary tract infection, and chronic renal failure are the complications.

Anemia: Reduction in the number of red blood cells, the quantity of hemoglobin, and the volume of the packed red cells per 100 mL of blood below normal level A hemoglobin level of <11 g/dL. indicates anemia in children between 6 months to 6 years old. The cut-off in children older than 6 years is 12 g/dL.

Anisocytosis: The term is used to describe an increase in variation in the size of the red cells. It may be due to an increase in the number of small or large cells or both.

Annular pancreas: This is due to the failure of complete rotation of the ventral segment during the development. Hence the collar of the pancreatic tissue surrounds the second part of the duodenum. Usually, it does not cause symptoms.

Anoxic crisis: This occurs in anemia. The anemia is complicated by leucopenia and thrombocytopenia. This occurs as a result of secondary infection due to anemia.

Anoxic spell: It is seen in the tetralogy of Fallot. It occurs predominantly after waking up or after following exertion. The child starts crying and becomes dyspneic. It becomes cyanosed. Convulsions may also occur.

Antinuclear antibodies: These antibodies are responsible for a variety of self-antigens. These cause damage to several organs and tissue systems. These produce a generalized autoimmune process.

Apgar score: It is a semiobjective measure of assessing the infant's respiratory, circulatory, and neurological status at birth. Normal babies have an Apgar score of >8 at 1 and 5 minutes. The most important cause of cardiopulmonary neurological depression is indicated by a low Apgar score.

Aplastic crisis: It is caused by sudden cessation of the marrow erythropoiesis. This leads to hemolysis and red cell mass is diminished.

Apneic spell: Cessation of respiration >20 seconds or any respiratory pause accompanied by bradycardia (heart rate <100 beats/min) and cyanosis.

Arnold–Chiari malformation: This refers to the extension and displacement of the medulla oblongata and cerebellum through the foramen magnum. This malformation may lead to the development of communicating hydrocephalus and clinically may be presented with signs of raised intracranial pressure and respiratory distress because of involvement of the lower cranial nerve. Shunting and surgery may be required to treat this condition.

Arthrogryposis multiplex: It is a symptom complex characterized by multiple joint contractures present at birth. The involved muscles are replaced partially or completely by fat and fibrous tissue. Most children who have this nonprogressive disorder survive. Some die in infancy as a result of the involvement of the respiratory muscles.

Ascites: It is a pathological accumulation of fluid within the peritoneal cavity and it can occur at any age and in utero. Sometimes a large intraabdominal cyst, i.e., cystic lymphangioma, an omental or ovarian cyst can mimic as ascites, this is known as pseudoascites.

Ataxia telangiectasia: It is an autosomal recessive disorder. It is characterized by progressive ataxia, choreoathetosis, pulmonary infection, and telangiectasia of the conjunctiva, face, and knees. These have higher chances of developing lymphoreticular tumors. Death occurs due to infection or tumor dissemination.

Athetosis: This is one of the types of involuntary movements. These are slow, rhythmic, writhing movements present more in the proximal group under the cover of the hypertonia. The patient is unable to maintain fingers and toes in one position. The lesion is in the caudate nucleus and putamen.

Autism: It is characterized by the triad of qualitative impairment of social behavior, and communication (verbal and nonverbal) skills associated with stereotypic and restrictive behavioral patterns, with onset before 3 years of age.

Azotemia: Retention in the blood of excessive amounts of nitrogenous waste products of metabolism. It is a result of the failure of the kidneys to remove the urea from the blood; also known as uremia.

Babinski's sign: This is one of the methods of eliciting plantar reflex. This is done by stroking along the lateral border of the sole. The normal response is flexion of big and all the toes. The extensor response includes dorsiflexion of the big toe, fanning of the small toes, dorsiflexion of the ankles, and contraction of the tensor fascia lata. The causes of extensor response include pyramidal lesion, coma, infancy, and postictal.

Baby mass index: This is defined as weight/height^2 (in kg^2). It correlates significantly with subcutaneous and total body fat in adolescents.

Barlow's test: This is the provocative test to find dislocation of the hip joint. This is performed by stabilizing the pelvis with one hand and then flexing and adducting the opposite hip and applying the posterior force. Dislocatable hip readily displaces. After the release of the posterior force, the hip usually relocates spontaneously.

Bartter syndrome: It occurs as a result of excessive chloride potassium and sodium wasting in the thick ascending limb of the loop of Henle. Clinical features include failure to thrive, polyuria, polydipsia, and recurrent episodes of dehydration.

Bacillus Calmette-Guérin (BCG) test: It is a more sensitive test than purified protein derivative (PPD). An induration of >6 mm after 3 days of the BCG vaccination is considered a positive reaction.

Beckwith's syndrome: It is the syndrome that consists of intractable hypoglycemia. This is seen with infants with microglossia, large size, visceromegaly, mild microcephaly, omphalocele, and facial naevus. It is associated with renal medullary dysplasia. Pancreatic hyperplasia is seen. Some infants also have polycythemia.

Beriberi: It occurs as a result of thiamine deficiency, and mainly affects the nervous system—dry beriberi, or the cardiovascular system, wet beriberi. In dry beriberi, symptoms include irritability, fatigue, emotional disturbances, headache, and polyneuritis. The wet beriberi is characterized by palpitation, tachycardia, dyspnea, and edema.

Bitemporal hemianopsia: Blindness is present in the temporal half of both fields. This occurs in the lesion of the nasal halves of both optic nerves.

Blackwater fever: This is characterized by sudden and massive intravascular Hemolysis and passage of black-colored urine due to hemoglobinuria. In some cases, renal failure occurs.

Bloom's syndrome: It is inherited as an autosomal recessive. Erythema and telangiectasia develop during infancy in a butterfly distribution on the face after exposure to sunlight. A balloonous eruption on the lips and telangiectatic erythema on the hands and forearms may develop. Intellect is normal. Patients usually have low levels of immunoglobulin A (IgA), immunoglobulin M (IgM), and immunoglobulin G (IgG). They are susceptible to infections and are sensitive to ultraviolet radiation. Affected children have an unusual tendency to develop lymphoreticular malignancies.

Bronchopleural fistula: This is one of the peculiar complications of thoracic operation involving resection of lung tissue. This may be due to poor surgical technique and malignant infiltration or tuberculous endobronchitis of the bronchial stump. Symptoms appear at the end of the first week after the operation. The symptoms may be fever and blood-stained sputum. Treatment is by early aspiration of the fluid from the pleural cavity and by nursing the patient with the affected side down. Smaller fistulas can be controlled by aspiration, larger fistula requires reopening of the chest and resuturing of the bronchus.

Brushfield's spots: It refers to a speckled or marbled rash that is found on the iris in Down syndrome.

Bullous impetigo: It appears as large fluid-filled blisters that rupture to form superficial erosions. Face, palm, and soles are involved.

Buphthalmos: It is the congenital rise of intraocular pressure. It should be suspected whenever the anteroposterior diameter and corneal curvatures are increased in size.

Burr cells: These are contracted cells which have one or more spiny projections on the surface. These are seen in chronic renal failure.

Burrow: Grayish thread-like tortuous due to travel of aitch mite in the epidermis.

Cafe-au-lait: These are uniformly hyperpigmented, sharply, and demarcated macular lesions. They are tan or light brown in color. They vary in size and may be large sometimes. Borders are smooth. The lesions are characterized by an increasing number of melanocytes and melanin in the epidermis. One to three spots are commonly found in normal individuals. They may be present at birth or may develop during childhood. These are present in neurofibromatosis, McCune–Albright syndrome, Russel–Silver syndrome, ataxia, telangiectasia, tuberous sclerosis, and Bloom's syndrome.

Canthal index: It helps in determining hypertelorism. It is calculated by:

$$\frac{\text{Inner canthal distance}}{\text{Outer canthal distance}} \times 100$$

This is normally 38 in males, and 38.5 in females. This index is increased in hypertelorism.

Capillary hemangioma: This refers to congenital abnormalities of vessels. These are of three types. There can be (1) salmon patches, (2) port-wine stain, and (3) strawberry angioma. They are present over the forehead and over the occiput. They disappear by 1 year.

Caput succedaneum: It is the edema of the scalp that follows local pressure and trauma during delivery. It is soft, and pits on pressure. It is not fluctuating. It does not have a well-defined margin.

Cardiomyopathy: It is an intrinsic of the myocardium that is not associated with structural deformity of the heart. Etiology may be unknown, and secondary if it is attributable to systemic disease.

Caries: A microbial disease resulting in demineralization of inorganic material and destruction of organic content of the hard tissues of teeth.

Carey Coombs murmur: It is the delayed diastolic murmur heard during the course of acute rheumatic fever. This occurs as a result of pancarditis.

Carpenter syndrome: Here craniosynostosis is associated with mental retardation and preaxial polysyndactyly of the feet. Soft tissue syndactyly of hands is also present. Patella is displaced.

Carrier: Presence of specific infectious agent in the absence of clinical disease. A carrier serves as a potential source for further transmission. Temporary carrier lasts <6 months. A chronic carrier state may last lifelong.

Cellulitis: It is a spreading inflammatory exudate along subcutaneous and facial planes. The most common causative organism is *Streptococcus pyogenes*. Redness, itching, or stiffness commences followed by tenderness and swelling. The skin becomes shiny in appearance. Local gangrene may occur. Appropriate antibiotics and rest are the mainstay of treatment.

Cephalohematoma: It is the subperiosteal hemorrhage that usually involves the parietal and temporal bones. It depends on obstetric maneuvers. It is more frequent with forceps delivery vacuum extraction and prolonged labor.

Chemosis: This is edema of conjunctiva, due to orbital cellulitis, nephritis, angioneurotic edema, or cavernous sinus thrombosis.

Cherry red spot: This is the round bright white area at the macula whose center is occupied by a cherry red circular spot. It is seen in Tay Sach's disease, gangliosidoses, and Niemann–Picks disease.

Cheyne-Stoke breathing: It is a periodic breathing that indicates bilateral damage to the cerebral cortex with an intact brain stem. It is attributed to an abnormally increased ventilatory response to CO_2 followed by posthyperventilation apnea.

Chloromas: These are the localized collection of leukemic cells seen almost exclusively in patients with acute myeloid leukemia. They may occur at any site including the central nervous system (CNS), bones, and skin.

Cholesteatoma: It is a sac of squamous epithelium extending from the tympanic membrane to the middle ear.

Chorea: It is a purposeless jerky movement, resulting in deranged speech and muscular incoordination. This results in an awkward gait and weakness. This involves commonly distal muscles under the cover of hypotonia. The lesion will be in the putamen and caudate nuclei. They are increased by agitation, decreased by voluntary activities, and disappear during sleep. The causes are rheumatic fever, typhoid, thyrotoxicosis, Wilson's disease, and drugs.

Choreoathetosis: It is characterized by sudden onset of unilateral or bilateral dystonic posturing of the leg or arms. It is associated with facial grimacing and dysarthria. This is precipitated by sudden movements, particularly on rising from a sitting posture. It is typically seen between 8 and 14 years. It can be managed by anticonvulsants.

Clinodactyly: This is the deviation of deflection of the fingers seen in Down's syndrome and trisomies.

Clutton's joint: This condition is due to bilateral effusion developing in the knee joint. This is usually seen in congenital syphilis and is painless.

Coeur en sabot: Here the absence of the main pulmonary artery segment makes the heart shadow resembling that of the boot. Hence it is called coeur en sabot. The right ventricle is enlarged and is prominent. This occurs in the tetralogy of Fallot.

Cold chain: A series of events undertaken to maintain the vaccines at a lower temperature, from the manufacture to the place of administration to maintain efficacy.

Complimentary feeding: It refers to the food that compliments breast milk and ensures that the child continues to have enough energy, protein, and other nutrients to grow normally.

Conduct disorder: It is characterized by aggressive and destructive activities that disrupt the child's environment.

Conn syndrome: It is characterized by episodic and reversible weakness. Proximal myopathy may become irreversible. CPK levels are elevated. Myoglobinuria occurs in acute attacks.

Coxa vara: It is a deformity of the hip joint with a decrease in the angle of inclination between the neck and shaft of the femur.

Craniotabes: This occurs because of a reduction in mineralization of the skull. This results in abnormal softness. This is evident in the parietal and occipital bones. This is seen characteristically in rickets.

Crigler–Najjar syndrome: It is inherited as an autosomal recessive. It is characterized by hyperbilirubinemia type II is autosomal dominant. It responds to treatment with phenobarbitone.

Crohn's disease: It is one of the inflammatory diseases characterized by abdominal mass, strictures, and fistulae. The lesion is characterized by skip lesions and transmural involvement. Erythema nodosum and mouth ulcers are common. The most common place of involvement is the ileum. The treatment aims to alleviate the symptoms. Oral prednisolone may be tried. Surgical therapy involves bowel resection if there is a high recurrence rate. Nutritional therapy is the effective primary treatment.

Crouzon syndrome: It is characterized by acrocephaly, hypertelorism, exophthalmos, hypoplastic maxilla, beak-shaped nose, short upper lip, and protruding lower lip. It is autosomal dominant.

Cryptorchidism: It can be due to imperfect descent of the testes. This can also be incomplete descent or ectopic. Many a times, testes will be retained within the abdomen, in the inguinal canal, or the superficial inguinal pouch. Treatment is by orchiopexy.

Cubitus valgus: It is a deformity of the hip joint with an increase in the angle of inclination between the neck and shaft of the femur.

Cysticercosis: It is the infection with the intermediate stage of, i.e., the larva of *Taenia solium*. Neurocysticercosis is the most common parasite infection of the CNS. The common target organs for cysticercosis are the brain, muscle, and subcutaneous tissue.

Cystinosis: It is the autosomal disorder present in infancy. Affected patients later show photophobia, enlarged liver, and spleen, and blonde hair. The presence of cystine crystals in the cornea and elevated levels of leucocyte cystine are useful in diagnosis.

Cystinuria: It is a metabolic disorder with autosomal recessive inheritance. There is a selective increase in the renal clearance and urinary excretion of the basic amino acids.

Dacryoadenitis: It is an acute bilateral inflammation of the lacrimal gland. It occurs with influenza, mumps, and infectious mononucleosis. Chronic dacryoadenitis is associated with syphilis, tuberculosis, and sarcoidosis.

Dandy-Walker syndrome: In this syndrome, there is a cystic dilatation of the fourth ventricle leading to congenital hydrocephalus. This causes obstruction of the foramina of Magendie and Luschka. The associated anomalies include agenesis of the posterior cerebellar vermis and corpus callosum. There will be a rapid increase in the size of the head and transillumination tests are positive. It is managed by shunting the cystic activity.

Darting tongue: Here child cannot maintain the tongue in a protruding position, i.e., darting tongue. This is seen with Sydenham's chorea.

Delinquency: Neglecting a legal obligation; failing to do so in accordance with law.

Dermatomyositis: This is a collagen disease characterized by nonsuppurative inflammation of the skin, subcutaneous tissues, and muscles. There will be necrosis of muscle fibers. Oral corticosteroids such as prednisolone and cyclophosphamide are used. Physical and occupational therapy is also important.

De Musset's sign: It is nodding of the head. May be present with each systole due to the sudden filling of the carotid vessels in severe aortic regurgitation.

Development: Increase in capability or maturation of function. It is related to the maturation and myelination of the nervous system and the acquisition of a variety of skills for a variety of functioning of the individual.

Diaper dermatitis: It is irritant dermatitis in infants due to prolonged contact with feces and ammonia (produced by the action of urea-splitting organisms in urine).

Disseminated intravascular coagulation (DIC): This is a serious disorder where the blood gets coagulated within the circulation, using up coagulation factors and platelets.

DiGeorge syndrome: This is characterized by defects in embryogenesis of the third and fourth pharyngeal pouches. It presents with unusual facies, hypocalcemia tetany, aortic arch anomalies, and an absent thymus.

Dolichocephaly: This occurs due to premature closure of the sagittal suture. The skull grows perpendicular to the open coronal suture. It appears to expand anteroposteriorly in the direction of the sagittal sutures.

Doll's eye response: If the head is suddenly turned to one side, there is conjugate deviation of the eye in the opposite direction. This response occurs if the brainstem is intact. It is not seen in normal conscious infants. It is absent when the brainstem centers for eye movements are damaged.

Double-bubble sign: It is the type of gas shadow seen on a plain abdominal radiograph. The appearance is caused by a distended and gas-filled stomach and proximal duodenum. This is seen in duodenal atresia.

Drooling: It is common in infancy but persists beyond 2–3 years in children with neuromuscular disorders and in mouth breathers.

Dubin–Johnson syndrome: It is an autosomal recessive disorder of childhood characterized by elevated levels of conjugated bilirubin. This presents as intermittent obstructive jaundice. There will be elevated levels of coproporphyrin in the urine.

Duchenne muscular dystrophy: It is the most common hereditary neuromuscular disease. It is an X-linked recessive trait. It is characterized by proximal muscle weakness. Respiratory muscle involvement is expressed by weak cough and recurrent lung infections. There will be pseudohypertrophy of calf muscles. The creatine phosphokinase (CPK) and lactate dehydrogenase (LDH) levels are consistently elevated.

Duodenal stenosis: Stenosis occurs at the point of fusion of the fore and midgut. It is frequently accompanied by other congenital anomalies. Laparotomy should be undertaken. Duodenojejunostomy is done.

Duroziez's sign: A systolic murmur may be heard if the pressure is applied to partially occlude the artery proximal to the chest piece. The diastolic murmur is heard if the pressure is applied distally. This combination of systolic and diastolic murmur is the Duroziez's sign.

Dysentery: It refers to the presence of grossly visible blood in the stools and is a consequence of infection of the colon by either bacteria or ameba.

Dysostosis multiplex: It is characterized by a dolichocephalic skull with a thickened calvarium. A medial third of the clavicle is thickened. There will be tapering of the phalanx. This is seen in mucopolysaccharidoses.

Dysphagia: It refers to a sensation of food being hindered in its passage from mouth to stomach, i.e., difficulty in swallowing.

Dysphoria: It is a disorder of the mood. It consists of major depression, dysrhythmic disorder, and bipolar disorder.

Dystonia: It is the slow intermittent twisting motion. This produces exaggerated turning and posture of the extremities and trunk. The principal causes include perinatal asphyxia, dystonia musculorum deformans, Wilson's disease, and drugs such as L-Dopa and lithium.

Ebstein anomaly: In this anomaly, the tricuspid valve is set into the right ventricle. This creates a large square-shaped heart.

There is a downward displacement of the tricuspid valve. It is associated with Wolff–Parkinson–White (WPW) syndrome and supraventricular tachycardia. Treatment is by prostaglandin infusion.

Ecchymosis: A large superficial hemorrhage, usually blue in color. These are seen in platelet count <50,000/mm^3.

Eczema: Infantile eczema manifests as a rosy erythema over the cheeks. There is brawny desquamation, small papule formation, and some crusting. Most children show a resolution by the age of 1 or 2 years. However, the illness may continue with remission and exacerbation in a few cases.

Edward syndrome: It is the second most common autosomal trisomy. The majority of the cases are postmature with low birth weight. These are hypertonia, elongated skull, lowest and malformed ear, micrognathia, and shield-shaped chest. The mean survival is about 3 months.

Ehlers–Danlos syndrome: The basic manifestations are joint hypermobility, skin hyperextensibility, dystrophic scarring of the skin, and easy bruising and connective tissue fragility. Wound healing is delayed and there are free movable subcutaneous nodules.

Eisenmenger syndrome: It is a cyanotic heart disease with pulmonary arterial hypertension. This results in a right-to-left shunt at the atrial, ventricular, or pulmonary arterial level.

Encephalocele: It is the herniation of the brain and meninges through the defect in the calvaria.

Encopresis: It is defined as the passage of stools in clothes beyond the age when bowel control should have been achieved usually by 4 years.

Endocardial fibroelastosis: This is a thickening of the endocardium. This presents with cardiac failure in infancy. Aortic stenosis, aortic atresia, and hypoplastic left heart syndrome are the causes. Dyspnea, cough, anorexia, hepatomegaly, and edema are the manifestations.

Enuresis: It is defined as normal nearly complete evacuation of the bladder at the wrong place and time at least twice a month after the fifth year of life.

Epidermolysis bullosa: It is an autosomal recessive condition. It is life-threatening. Serum morbidity and disfigurement can occur as a result of complications. Blisters appear at birth and involve the perioral, scalp, legs, and diaper area. Healing is delayed. Mild atrophy may be seen in the area of recurrent blisters. Most patients die in the first 3 years of life.

Epidermolysis hyperkeratosis: It is inherited as an autosomal trait. Onset is at birth. There is generalized erythroderma and severe hyperkeratosis. The scales are small, hard, verrucous, and distinctive. Hyperkeratosis persists throughout adult life. Recurrent blistering is present. Palms and soles are thickened. Some may have crumpled ears and ectropion. Treatment is difficult. Oral antibiotics, keratolytic agents, and oral retinoids are useful.

Epistaxis: It is bleeding from the nose is frequent in children and usually follows injury to the anterior portion of the nasal septum in Little's area, location of Kiesselbach arterial plexus.

Epstein pearl: These are epithelial inclusion cysts that appear as whitish spots on the hard palate. No treatment is required.

Erythema infectiosum: It is also called the fifth disease and the most common manifestation of the human parvovirus infection. The characteristic skin lesion occurs in three stages.

Erythema marginatum: It is a type of skin discoloration showing red areas. These are disk-shaped with elevated ridges. It is one of the major criteria of acute rheumatic fever.

Erythema multiforme: The most important characteristic is an acute target lesion. This may appear erythematous, macular, urticarial, papular, vesicular, or bullous. This is believed to be an immune-complex disease.

Erythema toxicum: On the second and third day of the newborn, these appear as discrete, erythematous papules may appear on the trunk and face. The rash disappears spontaneously in 1–3 days.

Erythropoiesis: This is the term used to describe the development of nucleated red cells. It is characterized by diminution in cell size, ripening of cytoplasm, and ripening of muscles.

Exostosis: It occurs due to failure of bone remodeling at metaphysis. A variable number of extra growth develops at the metaphyseal region. These may stop growing at the completion of the skeletal growth.

Failure to thrive: Weight for the age <2 SD or below third centile or downward change in growth that has crossed two major growth percentiles (i.e., 75th percentile to below 25th percentile) in a short time.

Fallot's tetralogy: It is associated with infundibular obstruction, overriding of the aorta, ventricular septal defect, and right ventricular hypertrophy. Cyanosis is present at birth which deepens on crying. An anoxic spell occurs. Medical management is limited to the treatment of complications and correction of anemia.

Fanconi's anemia: It is an autosomal recessive disorder. It is characterized by congenital malformation of bones of the forearm, short stature, and mental retardation. There will be hyperpigmentation, cafe-au-lait spots. The main complications are liver disorders, infection, and bleeding.

Flag sign: It is characterized by bands of pigmented and depigmented zones of hair present in malnutrition, especially kwashiorkor.

Floppy infant: It is described as an infant with marked hypotonia of all the muscles. They may be associated with frequent respiratory infections, feeding difficulties, and facial weakness. Contractures may develop in later stages.

Foster Kennedy syndrome: This is seen with intracranial spaces occupying the lesion. There may be optic atrophy in the fundus on the same side and papilledema on the opposite side.

Friedreich's ataxia: It is due to autosomal recessive inheritance. It presents usually in late childhood. There is progressive dysfunction of the cerebellum and spinal cord. Patients can have myocarditis, cardiac failure, kyphosis, scoliosis, hammer toes, and diabetes mellitus.

Froehlich syndrome: It is characterized by obesity, short stature hyperphagia, sexual infantilism, and sometimes blindness.

Furunculosis: It is an acute infection of the hair follicle which usually precedes suppuration and necrosis. A painful indurated swelling appears which gradually extends. After 2 or 3 days, the center softens and a small slough is discharged. It is common on the back of the neck.

Gallop rhythm: It is an auscultatory finding of the three of four heart sounds. The extra sound is heard in the diastole. It is related either to atrial contraction or to rapid filling of the ventricle.

Genetic counseling: It is a communication process, dealing with human problems associated with the occurrence and recurrence of genetic disorders in a family. Patients should be provided with risk figures for future offspring based on genetic facts.

Gigantism: Hypersecretion of the growth hormone in children, usually due to pituitary adenoma results in somatic overgrowth or gigantism. The child is taller than his peers. Peripheral parts of the body such as hands and feet are large. Muscle weakness, bony, and cartilaginous overgrowth, and cardiomyopathies may be present.

Gliosis: It is the excess of astroglia seen in the damaged area of the central nervous system.

Gower's sign: This is seen in Duchenne's muscular dystrophy. Here child turns to the side, lifts his trunk by supporting his weight on his arms, and then stands as if he is climbing upon his arms and is standing up.

Grasp reflex: When the baby's palm is stroked with the examiner's index finger, the baby's fingers close on it and grasp it. As the examiner lifts his index finger, the flexor muscles of the infant's forearm become tight. The grasp reflex usually disappears by the age of 12 weeks. Persistence beyond this age should arouse the suspension of brain damage.

Graves' disease: It is the toxic goiter. It occurs due to the presence of thyroid-stimulating autoantibodies. This binds to the receptor of the thyroid-stimulating hormone. Ophthalmopathy is caused by antibodies that bind to the extraocular muscles and orbital fibroblasts.

Greenstick fracture: Here one cortex may be fractured, while the other bends. The resultant angulation may be hard to correct without completing the fracture. This type of fracture is more common in children.

Grey Turner's sign: It is dark discoloration around the umbilicus seen in pancreatitis.

Growth: It is the net increase in the mass of tissues, due to the multiplication of cells and the increase in intracellular substances.

Guillain-Barré syndrome: It is a post-infection polyneuropathy. This causes demyelination in motor and sometimes in sensory nerves. The paralysis of muscles occur. Weakness begins in the lower limbs and extends upwards. CSF protein is increased. Treatment is self-limiting and symptomatic.

Guthrie's test: It is the microbiological test based on the principle that phenylalanine is necessary for the growth of the *Bacillus subtilis*.

Gynecomastia: It is an occurrence of mammary tissue in males. It is almost always a sign of the estrogen-androgen imbalance. The main causes include physiological changes, Klinefelter's syndrome, ketoconazole drugs, and Peutz–Jeghers syndrome.

Hemangioma: Vascular lesions on the skin. These can be superficial (strawberry) or deep (cavernous). These are primarily composed of capillaries. Most are situated on the head and neck.

Hemarthrosis: This is seen in hemophilia. It may occur spontaneously but usually results from minor joint strain or from a direct injury. This happens during the active phase of bleeding. The pain and disability depend upon the rapidity and duration of bleeding.

Hematuria: The presence of blood in urine imparts it a color, which includes various shades of deep red, smoky brown, cola color, and faint pink.

Hemochromatosis: It is a disorder of iron metabolism with excess deposition of iron in tissues leading to bronze skin pigmentation, hepatic cirrhosis, and diabetes mellitus.

Hemolytic uremic syndrome: It is characterized by acute renal failure (ARF), microangiopathic hemolytic anemia, and thrombocytopenia. It is the most common cause of ARF. Onset is preceded by gastroenteritis, pallor, irritability, weakness, and oliguria. The complications include acidosis, anemia, cardiac failure, hypertension, and uremia. Peritoneal dialysis and management of hematological and renal manifestations are recommended.

Hemopoiesis: It is the formation and development of blood cells. This can be either extramedullary or in the spleen, liver, and lymph nodes.

Hemoptysis: It means the presence of blood-stained sputum. Many a time it is confused with hematemesis. The causes of this are tuberculosis, bronchiectasis, whooping cough, pneumonia, mitral stenosis, and bleeding disorders.

Harrison's groove: It is a horizontal depression, seen along the lower border of the chest corresponding to the insertion of the diaphragm. This is seen in rickets.

Head banging: It involves rhythmic hitting of the head against a solid surface. It results in callus formation at the site of banging abrasion and contusion.

Hemianopsia: Here one half of the visual field is lost. It can be homonymous, bitemporal, or binasal.

Hemiparesis: It is associated with decreased arm swing on the affected side and lateral circular motion of the leg.

Hiatus hernia: It may be acquired or congenital. There are three types: (1) sliding, (2) paraesophageal, and (3) mixed. Pain, heartburn, dysphagia, and secondary anemia may be present.

Hills sign: It is the exaggeration of the systolic pressure difference between the brachial and femoral arteries, seen in aortic regurgitation.

Hirschsprung's disease: It is a congenital megacolon characterized by the absence of ganglion cells of the myenteric plexus. There will be delayed passage of meconium. Failure to pass stool leads to dilatation of proximal bowel and abdominal distension. Rectal manometry and rectal suction biopsy are the most reliable indicators. Surgery is the treatment of choice.

Histiocytosis: Here there will be prominent proliferation or accumulation of the monocyte-macrophage system of bone marrow origin. The diagnostic classification depends on histopathological findings. The clinical manifestations vary. Bone involvement, skin involvement, exophthalmos, pituitary dysfunction, and weight loss are present. Immunosuppressive therapy includes cyclosporin and antithymocyte globin.

Hodgkin's disease: This is a type of lymphoma where the normal architecture of the lymph node is distorted. The lymph nodes contain giant cells with mirror-image nuclei called Reed–Sternberg cells. These cells are associated with painless enlargement of lymph nodes and hepatosplenomegaly with fever. Treatment is by chemotherapy.

Hoarseness: Vocal nodules are the chief cause of hoarseness in children, caused by vocal abuse. The severity of hoarseness fluctuates worsening with vocal abuse and improving with rest.

Homocystinuria: It is a metabolic error with autosomal recessive inheritance. Cystathionine is not synthesized from the homocysteine and serine because of the deficiency of the enzyme cystathionine synthetase.

Horner's syndrome: There will be sinking of the eyeball, ptosis of the upper lid, slight elevation of the lower lid, miosis, narrowing of palpebral tissue, and anhidrosis and flushing of the affected side of the face. This is due to paralysis of cervical sympathetic nerves.

Hutchinson's teeth: These are also called screwdriver teeth. This is seen in children with congenital syphilis. The upper edge of the incisor is centrally notched and widely spaced.

Hypoxic ischemic encephalopathy: It refers to CNS dysfunction associated with perinatal asphyxia.

Hyphema: It is the presence of blood in the anterior chamber of the eye. It may follow either blunt or perforating injury. It appears as a bright or dark red fluid level between the cornea and iris. Treatment is by rest.

Hypospadias: It is the most common congenital anomaly of the urethra. The external meatus is situated at some point under the surface of the penis or in the perineum. The types include glandular, coronal, penile, penoscrotal, and perineal.

Hypotonia: It is characterized by flabby muscles which offer less resistance to passive movements.

Ichthyosis: It is an inherited keratinizing disorder of the skin associated with a distinct pattern of visible scaling. These are hyperproliferative and retention types.

Incontinentia pigmenti: It is an X-linked dominant multisystemic disorder. It is characterized by vesicular, hyperpigmented, and hypopigmented stages.

Imperforate anus: It occurs as a result of an imperfect fusion of the postallantoic gut with the proctodeum. These are of two types, high, and low, depending upon the termination of the bowel above and below the pelvic floor. Surgery is the treatment.

Impetigo: It is a superficial bacterial skin infection involving the upper epidermis. There are two types, i.e., (1) nonbullous and (2) bullous type.

Interferons: These are the proteins produced and secreted by blood leucocytes, fibroblasts, and epithelial cells. These influence many cell functions. These include restoration, augmentation, and/or modulation of the host immune system.

Jaw thrust: It is used for victims of neck injury and can be accomplished without extending the neck. The fingers of each hand are placed under the sides of the lower jaw to lift it up and outward.

Jitteriness: Symmetrical tremulous movements of the extremities More proximal than distal, suggests cerebral hyperexcitability or metabolic defect, such as hypoglycemia.

Juvenile delinquency: The term refers to a person under 18 years of age who is brought to the attention of the juvenile justice system for committing a criminal act or displaying other illegal behaviors.

Kangaroo mother care: It is a powerful easy-to-use method to promote the health and wellbeing of low-birth-weight babies. Its key features include early continuous prolonged skin-to-skin contact between the mother and baby.

Kartagener's syndrome: This is a hereditary syndrome associated with dextrocardia, bronchiectasis, and sinusitis. Immotile cilia are also present in this condition. It is characterized by recurrent otitis media, conductive hearing, deafness, and loose productive cough. Treatment is symptomatic.

Keratoconus: It is a conical cornea in which the cornea is thin near the center and progressively bulges forward. It is present in Down syndrome, Marfan syndrome, and osteogenesis imperfecta.

Keratomalacia: Here the cornea is softened and ulcerated. It is usually irreversible and results in sear formation or phthisis bulbi.

Kernicterus: The term is used to describe the pathological finding of bilirubin toxicity within the brain. This includes staining and necrosis of neurons.

Kernig's sign: This is usually seen in meningitis and refers to an inability to completely extend the leg when sitting or lying with the thigh flexed upon the abdomen.

K-F ring: This is seen in Wilson's disease. It occurs because of the golden-brown deposits of copper in Descemet's membrane of the cornea.

Knock-knee: It is a deformity of the thigh or leg or both knees. The knees are abnormally close together and space between the ankles is increased. This is seen in rickets.

Koilonychia: This is a dystrophy of fingernails in which they are thin and concave with raised edges. This is present in iron deficiency anemia.

Koplik's spots: These are greyish or bluish-white grain rashes seen inside the cheek opposite to the upper molar. These are seen in measles.

Kussmaul breathing: This is characterized by deep rapid respiration. This is seen in diabetic ketoacidosis.

Kyphosis: It is an abnormally increased convexity in the curvature of the thoracic spine as viewed from the side.

Larva migrans: It is caused by nematodes that are normally parasitic for other species, the larva hatch and invade the intestinal mucosa to be carried by the bloodstream to different organs.

Laurence–Moon–Biedl syndrome: It is characterized by pleomorphic pigmentary retinal degeneration with a progressive vision impairment. There will be prominent macular involvement. Obesity is one of the clinical features.

Legg–Perthes syndrome: It is an idiopathic avascular necrosis of the hip joint. It is caused by an interruption of blood supply. It is associated with protein C, protein S, thrombophilia, and hypofibrinolysis. Children with this syndrome will have delayed bone age, disproportionate growth, and mild short stature.

Lennox–Gastaut syndrome: It is characterized by mixed seizures including myoclonic, atypical absence generalized tonic-clonic, or partial seizures.

Lepromin test: It is carried out by injecting 0.1 mL of Mitsuda lepromin intradermally onto the forearm and reaction is noted later at 21 days.

Live-born: It is the product of conception irrespective of weight or gestational age that after separation from the mother, shows any evidence of life such as breathing, heart rate, pulsation of the umbilical cord, or definite movement of voluntary muscle.

Loeffler's syndrome: The pulmonary phase of migration of Ascaris larva may cause wheezing, pulmonary problems, and eosinophilia in the blood.

Lorber criteria: This is for surgical treatment for neural tube defects. Surgery is not done if there is severe paraplegia at or below the L3 level, kyphosis or scoliosis, or gross hydrocephaly.

Lordosis: It is the forward curvature of the lumbar spine.

Lowe syndrome: This is an X-linked condition that presents within the first few months of life with Fanconi syndrome, rickets, ocular defects, hypotonic, and developmental delay.

Macewen's sign: It is a hyperresonant note heard on percussion of the skull behind the junction of the frontal, temporal, and parietal bones. This is seen in *hydrocephalus*, cerebral abscess, and in raised intracranial tension.

Malrotation: It is rotational abnormalities developing during maturation of the gut that cause recurrent obstruction, occurring either in the Ladd's bands or volvulus of the gut over the narrow mesenteric pedicle.

Mantoux reaction: 0.1 mL of a suitable dilution of tuberculin is injected intradermally. A weal of 5 mm should be raised. The reaction is read after 48 hours.

Marasmus: It is characterized by gross wasting of muscle and subcutaneous tissues resulting in emaciation, marked stunting, and no edema.

Marfan's syndrome: It is an autosomal dominant disorder with mesodermal dystrophy. The patients are tall and slender. Muscles are hypotonic and joints are hyperextendable. There may be subluxation of lens, cataract, coloboma, squint, nystagmus, and megalocornea.

McBurney's point: It lies at the junction of the lateral third with the medial two-thirds of a joining anterosuperior iliac spine and the umbilicus. It is the classical site of the greatest tenderness in appendicitis.

McCune–Albright syndrome: This is also called polyostotic fibrous dysplasia. This disease is characterized by precocious puberty in females, melanotic pigmentation of the skin, hyperthyroidism, epileptic seizures, headache, and mental derangement.

Meckel's diverticulum: It is a remnant of an embryonic yolk sac. It is also referred to as the omphalomesenteric duct or vitellointestinal duct. Partial or complete failure of involution results in residual structures. Meckel's diverticulum is one such structure. It presents with brick-colored or currant jelly stool. This is painless. Sometimes it may be associated with partial or complete bowel obstruction.

Megalocornea: Here the corneal diameter is >13 mm. It is observed in Marfan syndrome and osteogenesis imperfecta.

Megaloencephaly: It is also called *hydrocephalus*. It represents a diverse group of conditions that result from impaired circulation and absorption of cerebrospinal fluid (CSF). Sometimes it can be due to choroid plexus papilloma.

Meningeal tuberculosis: This is also called tuberculous meningitis. This is characterized by meningeal signs, headache, vomiting, and convulsion. The CSF analysis should be done. The treatment is antitubercular medicine.

Meningococcemia: This occurs as a result of meningococcal infection. It will vary from fever to occult bacteremia to sepsis, shock, and death.

Mental retardation: Significant subaverage intellectual function with intellectual quotient (IQ) <2 SD below the mean. It is associated with deficits in adaptive behavior.

Metachromatic leukodystrophy: The inheritance is autosomal recessive. The characteristic metabolic defect is decreased. urinary or leukocyte aryl sulfatase. Clinically it manifests as ataxia, stiffness starting in the second year of life.

Metaphysis: It is the wider part at the end of the shaft of the long bone adjacent to the epiphyseal disk.

Methemoglobinemia: It occurs due to an imbalance between oxidation and reduction of hem iron. When the hemiron is oxidized to a ferric state, methemoglobin is formed.

Microalbuminemia: It is defined as the period of incipient nephropathy with a urinary albumin excretion rate (AER) of 20–200 µg/min or 30–300 mg/24 h. Microalbuminemia is related to the duration of diabetes and is most common in postpubertal adolescents.

Microangiopathic anemia: This is mechanical hemolytic anemia in which red cell fragmentation is due to contact between red cells and abnormal intima of partly thrombosed, narrowed, or necrotic small arteries.

Microcytic: The mean corpuscular volume is reduced, i.e., <76 fL and mean corpuscular hemoglobin concentration (MCHC) is within the normal range, i.e., 30–35 g/dL.

Miliary tuberculosis: This usually occurs within a year of primary infection. The pulmonary form presents with temperature, dyspnea, and cyanosis. In septicemia form, the child is delirious, and disturbance of the sensorium is seen.

Milkmaid sign: The child relaxes his grip off and on as if he is milking the cow. This is seen in Sydenham's chorea.

Molluscum contagiosum: It is caused by a pox virus and is characterized by well-circumscribed dome-shaped tiny pearly papules or nodules up to 1 cm in size, especially in intertriginous areas.

Mongoloid facies: It includes bossing of the skull. Prominent frontal and parietal eminence with flattened vault, straight forehead, and hypertrophy of maxilla. Prominent malar eminence, depressed nasal bridge, and puffy eyes.

Mongolian spots: These are bluish well-demarcated spots on the buttocks and trunk.

Moon face: It is characterized by a round face with prominent flushed cheeks and a double chin seen in Cushing's syndrome.

Moro's reflex: The supine infant's hands are grasped, and shoulders are lifted a few centimeters while keeping the back of the head on the bed. Then the hands are suddenly released. A positive response consists of sudden adduction of the arms at the shoulder and extension of the arm at the elbow. This is followed by adduction of the arms and flexion of the forearm.

Mulberry molar: Abnormal first molar characterized by a small surface and an excessive number of cusps. This is seen in congenital syphilis.

Mullerian inhibitory substance: It is a glycoprotein hormone secreted by the Sertoli cells of fetal testes. During sexual differentiation, it causes the involution of embryonic precursors of the cervix, uterus, and fallopian tubes.

Myelodysplasia: It describes various abnormal conditions of the vertebral column that affect spinal cord function. These include meningomyelocele and meningocele.

Nadas criteria: This criteria help in the assessment of the child for the presence or absence of heart disease. The criteria is divided into major and minor criteria. The presence of one major or two minor criteria is essential for indicating the presence of heart disease.

Neural tube defects: These are structural congenital anomalies. This implies the failure of improper closure of neural tube and covering mesoderm and ectoderm.

Neurofibromatosis: It is autosomal dominant. It is characterized by cafe u lait spots, neurofibromas, and freckling in the axillary or inguinal region.

Neutropenia: It is defined as a reduction in the number of neutrophils below the lower normal limit, i.e., 2,500 cells/mm^3.

Newborn/neonate: An infant from birth to 4 weeks (28 days) is called a neonate or a newborn. The first week (7 days) of life is called an early neonatal period. The late neonatal period extends from 7 to less 28th days.

Nikolsky's sign: The outer epidermis separates easily from the basal layer on exertion of firm sliding manual pressure. This is seen with staphylococcal skin scalded syndrome (SSSS) and pemphigus.

Nissen fundoplication: This is curative surgical treatment of hiatus hernia. Here the fundus of the stomach is wrapped around the lower 5 cm of the esophagus.

Nondisjunction: These are the most common numeric chromosomal aberration. In the metaphase of the first mitotic division, both members of the paired chromosome may move jointly during the ana phase to either of the daughter cells.

Noonan syndrome: The clinical features include a broad forehead, hypertelorism, epicanthic folds, ptosis, low-set ears, and webbing of the neck. It is associated with cardiac disease, pulmonary stenosis, and mental retardation.

Non-Hodgkin's disease: This is common among younger children. Clinical manifestations depend on the anatomical site and extent of involvement. Systemic symptoms include malaise, anorexia, and low-grade fever. Chemotherapy and radiotherapy are a mainstay of management.

Normocytes: Here mean corpuscular volume is within the normal range, i.e., 76–97 fL.

Obstructive sleep apnea: It is characterized by partial or complete upper airway obstruction during sleep. The main cause is adenotonsillar hypertrophy. Sequelae are hypoxemia, hypercapnia, and acidosis which contribute to behavioral and neurocognitive impairment.

Esophageal atresia: It is usually associated with tracheoesophageal fistula. The child may regurgitate; saliva pours, coughing, and cyanosis occur on feeding.

Olympian brow: It is associated with recurrent periostosis and thickening of bone. This includes frontal bossing resulting in bony prominence of the forehead.

Opsomyoclonus: It is a paraneoplastic syndrome. The affected children have chaotic eye movements, myoclonus, and ataxia. It is seen associated with neuroblastoma.

Optic atrophy: This is an irreversible degeneration of the optic disk in which the disk becomes pale or white with a reduction in the number of capillaries on the disk. There are two types, i.e., (1) primary and (2) secondary optic atrophy.

Optic neuritis: It is the inflammation of the optic nerve. If it is visible on the disk is called papillitis.

Osteopetrosis: It is here do familial disorder in which partly calcified cartilaginous intercellular ground substance is not regularly reabsorbed and replaced by regular osteoid tissue and bone.

Ortolani's maneuver: The knees of the babies are flexed. The examiner places his thumb over the inner aspect of the thigh and his middle finger presses the greater trochanter of the femur. Baby's thigh is then adducted in dislocation of the hip. The femoral head returns to the acetabulum with a jerk.

Otomycosis: It is fungal otitis externa. It is most common in humid weather. There is pain and pruritus in the affected ear. Examination reveals fungal spores and filaments along with cloudy discharge.

Oxytocin reflex: Oxytocin is a hormone produced by the posterior pituitary. It is responsible for the contraction of myoepithelial cells around the alveoli. This causes the ejection of milk from the gland into the lactiferous sinuses and lactiferous ducts.

Paget's disease: It is an autosomal recessive disorder where serum levels of both calcium and phosphates are normal. Urinary leucine peptidase activity and serum acid phosphatase levels are increased. Bone turnover is reduced.

Pagophagia: It refers to a desire to ingest unusual substances such as ice or dust. This occurs in iron deficiency anemia.

Panarteritis nodosa: It is a necrotizing vasculitis affecting small and medium-sized arteries. Aneurysms and nodules may form at irregular intervals throughout affected arteria.

Pancytopenia: It occurs due to either failure of production of hematopoietic progenitors, their destruction, or replacement of bone marrow by tumor or fibrosis.

Papilledema: It occurs as a result of increased intracranial tension. The optic nerve will have blurred disk margins and venous congestion. A disk is edematous and raised. Hemorrhages are evident with a disk. The causes are increased intracranial tension, hypertension, Guillain-Barré syndrome, central retinal vein thrombosis, and pseudotumor cerebri.

Patau syndrome: It is characterized by severe developmental and physical retardation, microcephaly with a sloping forehead, and holoprosencephaly type of defect with varying degrees of incomplete development of the forebrain, olfactory, and optic nerve.

Pectus excavatum: The lower part of the sternum appears depressed, or funnel-shaped. This may be a result of rickets or may follow chronic upper respiratory obstruction.

Pel-Ebstein fever: This type of fever is encountered in lymphoma. The fever is irregular and intermittent with febrile and afebrile states.

Pemphigus: It is a large flaccid bullae emerging on erythematous skin. It is commonly seen on the face, trunk, pressure points, groin, and axilla. Nikolsky's sign is positive. The disease is best treated initially with a high dose of systemic corticosteroids. Azathioprine, cyclophosphamide, methotrexate, and gold therapy have been useful.

Pendred syndrome: It is an autosomal recessive fashion. It is associated with congenital deafness and goiter. Hearing loss is usually presented at birth but goiter generally appears at puberty.

Periodic breathing: Respiration characterized by regular cycles of respiration of 10–18 seconds interrupted by a pause of at least 3 seconds. The pattern recurs for at least 3 seconds.

Pertussis: It is a highly contagious infectious disease of the respiratory tract caused by Bordetella pertussis. It is characterized by catarrhal phase, paroxysmal phase, and convalescent phase. The triad of the disease is whoop, absolute lymphocytosis, and decreased erythrocyte sedimentation rate (ESR).

Phakomatoses: These are nodular lesions, yellowish in color, refractile in nature, or observed in tuberous sclerosis.

Phimosis: Normally seen up to the age of 2 years, the prepuce cannot be fully retracted because of congenital adhesions with the glands. In children, it may predispose to recurrent urinary tract infection.

Pica: It is a habit of eating nonedible substances such as clay, paint, earth, chalk, etc. These children usually have a history of neonatal insults. There is no specific treatment.

Pierre Robin syndrome: It is a syndrome associated with micrognathia, occurring in association with cleft palate, glossoptosis, and absent gag reflex.

Pilonidal sinus: It is a dimple located in the midline intergluteal cleft at the level of the coccyx. It is seen relatively frequently in normal infants. An open sinus is a benign condition and is usually asymptomatic.

Plantar fasciitis: It is an inflammation of the supporting structure of the longitudinal arch owing to repetitive cycling. Pain increases with the first step out of bed in the morning. Treatment is by shin splints.

Platybasia: The first and second occipital segment and the first and second cervical vertebra may be fused together. In this disorder, medulla oblongata may get kinked over the odontoid process resulting in the compression of the spinal cold tract and quadriplegia.

Plumbism: Toxic effects of lead are collectively known as plumbism. It involves many body systems principally resulting in nervous, hematological, and renal manifestations in children.

Pneumatocele: It is pathognomonic of staphylococcal pneumonia. These are progressively inflated abscess. These ultimately resolve and disappear within a period of a few weeks.

Poikilocytosis: It is used to describe varied cell shapes. Alterations include oval cells, pear and tear-shaped cells, and sickle cells.

Polyhydramnios: This is a clinical condition wherein the amniotic fluid level will be >2,000 mL. The associated anomalies include anencephaly, hydrops fetalis, ectopia vesicae, high intestinal obstruction, and multiple pregnancies.

Pompe disease: Signs and symptoms of this disease result from lysosomal storage of glycogen in skeletal muscles, cardiac muscle, and central nervous system. The heart is enlarged and appears globular. Death usually occurs before the age of 1 year.

Port-wine stains: These represent progressive ectasia of the superficial vascular plexus. These do not resolve spontaneously. These stains are typically pink in infancy. The face is commonly involved. This is best treated by a 585 nm pulsed dye laser.

Portal hypertension: It is defined by elevation of portal venous pressure to values above 10–12 mm Hg.

Potter's facies: It is characterized by wildly separated eyes, epicanthic fold, low set ear, and broad nose. Chin is receding and limb abnormalities are seen. This is seen as associated with infantile polycystic kidney.

Prader-Willi syndrome: Here both hypogonadotropic hypogonadism and hypergonadotropic occur secondary to cryptorchidism.

Primary complex: It is a combination of draining lymphangitis and inflamed regional lymph nodes. This is seen in tuberculosis.

Primary focus: The inflamed area at the point of the entry of the tubercle bacilli is called primary focus.

Proptosis: Protrusion of the eye is called proptosis. It may be caused by shallowness of the orbit as in many craniofacial malformations. It may occur because of neoplastic vascular and inflammatory disorders.

Puberty: It is the period of life when the ability to reproduce sexually begins; characterized by the maturation of genital organs, development of secondary sexual characteristics, and onset of menstruation in females.

Pulsus paradoxus: Normally systolic blood pressure falls by 3-10 mm during inspiration. But in some conditions, it falls below 10 mm, then the pulse is called pulsus paradoxus. The causes include bronchial asthma, emphysema, cardiac tamponade, and congestive cardiac failure (CCF).

Rachitic rosary: These are prominent costochondral junctions seen in rickets.

Radial streak: Pyelogram reveals opacification of dilated collecting ducts. Because these ducts extend from the cortex to the medulla, they appear as radial streaks similar to the spokes of a wheel. This is seen in polycystic kidney disease.

Railroad calcification: This is the type of calcification found in Sturge-Weber syndrome. It is seen in the occipital and temporal regions on the skull radiograph.

Ramstedt's operation: This is also called pyloromyomotomy. The hypertrophied circular muscle fibers are cut longitudinally completely without damaging the mucosa.

Ranula: Ranula are the cystic lesions of the floor of the mouth. They are thought to be caused either by salivary gland obstruction or by salivary leakage from a traumatized sublingual and minor salivary gland.

Red currant jelly: It is a typical description of the stool in intussusception. This occurs as a result of inflammation of the bowel.

Red reflex: It is the red flare seen through the fundoscopy through the pupil in a normal infant.

Reed-Sternberg cells: These are giant cells with multiple or multiloculated nuclei. It is the hallmark of Hodgkin's disease.

Refsum disease: This is due to the disturbances in phytanic acid metabolism. Clinical features include ataxia, ichthyosis, and conduction defects in the heart. These patients are treated by withholding green vegetables.

Renal tubular acidosis: It encompasses a condition characterized by renal acidification. This result is hyperchloremic metabolic acidosis and inappropriately high urine pH.

Retinal detachment: This is the separation of the inner layers of the retina from its pigment epithelium. In children, it usually occurs after the injury and will lead to blindness if not detected and treated.

Retinitis pigmentosa: It is a bilateral disease resulting in blindness by middle age. Rods are mainly involved, and night blindness is present. The disease may be primary or secondary to intrauterine infection or drugs.

Reye's syndrome: It follows confirmed adenovirus infection of several serotypes. It is characterized by bronchopneumonia, hepatitis, seizures, and DIC.

Rhabdomyosarcoma: It is the most common soft tissue sarcoma. It is one of the small round cell tumors. These are present with mass. The most common primary site is the neck.

Rheumatoid factor: It is an autoantibody present in rheumatoid arthritis. It acts as an antibody Fc fragment of immunoglobin.

Rickety rosary: It is an apparent costochondral junction seen in rickets.

Riley-Day syndrome: It is an autosomal recessive disorder involving the peripheral nervous system. This is characterized pathologically by a reduced number of nerve fibers that carry pain, temperature, and taste sensations. There will be poor sucking and swallowing. Breath-holding spells are present.

Risus sardonicus: It occurs as a result of intractable spasms of the facial and buccal muscles in tetanus.

Roseola infantum: It is caused by the human herpes virus. The onset is abrupt. High-grade fever is associated with mild pharyngitis and coryza. Macular, maculopapular rashes appear and last for 24 hours.

Sabre tibia: It is the anterior bowing of the midportion of the tibia. It is seen in congenital syphilis.

Saddle nose: It is a depression of the root of the nose. It occurs as a result of syphilitic rhinitis. It destroys adjacent bone and cartilage.

Salmon patch: These are the most common vascular lesions in infancy. These are pale, pink to red macules seen over the glabella, upper eyelids, or neck. Most fade by 1–2 years of age.

Schaumann disease: It is idiopathic kyphosis. This develops during adolescence. The cause is not known. There will be increased pressure on the anterior vertebral growth plate.

Scoliosis: It is defined as lateral curvature of the spine. The lateral curvature is always complicated by rotational deformity. It can be idiopathic, congenital, paralytic, or postural.

Scorbutic rosary: This is a prominent sharp and angular costochondral junction seen in scurvy.

Sequestrum: It is a piece of dead bone separated from normal bone. This is seen in osteomyelitis.

Simian crease: This refers to a single palmar crease seen in Down's syndrome.

Spur: It is a projecting bone spike seen in the scurvy.

Stammering: It is dysfluency of speech characterized by abnormal repetition of syllables and prolonged interruptions.

Staple sign: It is subglottic narrowing seen in the lateral chest radiograph. It is seen in the croup.

Status epilepticus: It is characterized by repetitive prolonged seizures and the patient remains unconscious in between the seizures or if the duration of the attack is >1 hour.

Steatorrhea: It is an excess of fat found in the stools of people with cystic fibrosis

Stillbirth: A fetal death (a product of conception that, after separation from the mother does not show any evidence of life) at gestation age 20 weeks or more or weighing >500 g.

Still's disease: It is the systemic phase that precedes juvenile rheumatoid arthritis. It is characterized by hepatosplenomegaly and rashes.

Strabismus: It is a deviation of the eye that the patient cannot overcome. It may be of paralytic or nonparalytic type. The visual axes of the lens of the eye do not fall in a parallel plane. This results in diplopia or defective vision.

Stridor: Abnormal produced due to narrowing/obstruction of the larynx or trachea, mainly inspiratory in nature.

Sunset sign: It is a downward deviation of the eyes so that each iris appears to set beneath the lower lid. This is commonly seen in hydrocephalus. The white sclera is exposed between the sunset sign and the upper eyelid. This is indicative of raised intracranial tension.

Talipes: It is characterized by plantar flexion and inversion of the ankle. Dorsiflexion of the foot is limited. Corrective casts should be applied.

Tay-Sachs disease: It is an autosomal recessive disease. Low serum beta-hexosaminidase level is the characteristic metabolic defect. As a result, ganglioside monosialic (GM2) ganglioside accumulates in neurons. A cherry red spot is seen over the macular region or the retina. Death occurs in 2–4 years.

Temper tantrum: It is a kind of physically aggressive behavior. This happens when a child cannot express his autonomy. The aggressive behavior may be in the form of biting, crying, and throwing objects.

Thermoneutral temperature: The ideal environmental temperature for a newborn at a basal metabolic rate of the body is at minimum, oxygen utilization is least and maintains a core temperature between 36.5 and 37.5°C.

Thumb sucking: It is normal in infants and toddlers. It peaks by 18–21 months of age and usually disappears by the age of 4 years. Beyond 4 years of age, the child should be motivated to refrain from this habit. Both positive and negative reinforcement can be used.

Thrombocytopenia: It refers to a reduction in platelet count below 15,000/mm^3. The causes include decreased production and sequestration of platelets in the enlarged spleen.

Todd paralysis: It is paralysis or hemiparesis. It follows focal seizures. However, weakness and neurological signs disappear completely within 24 hours.

Tonic neck reflex: The supine infant's head is suddenly turned to one side. The arm and leg on the same side extend while the opposite limbs go into flexion. The reflex is prominent in 2–4 months. Persistence of the reflex beyond 6–9 months indicates spastic cerebral palsy.

TORCH: It is a combination of infections, such as toxoplasmosis, rubella, cytomegalovirus, and herpes simplex.

Tracheomalacia: It is a congenital anomaly associated with flabbiness of airway walls leading to collapse and airway obstruction. Tracheomalacia may be associated with bronchomalacia.

Trendelenburg gait: Here the glutei muscle on the affected side cannot keep the pelvis at a level when the affected limb bears the weight so the pelvis is tilted to the unaffected side. The level of the pelvis is checked by placing a hand on the iliac crest.

Trismus: This condition occurs as a result of motor disturbance of the trigeminal nerve. This is due to spasms of masticatory muscles which result in difficulty in opening the mouth. This is one of the characteristic early symptoms of tetanus.

Trophic feeding: This type of feeding is practiced in premature infants whose illness severity otherwise prevents the advancement of enteral feeding volume. The purpose is to stimulate the gastrointestinal (GI) tract's functional and structural integrity.

Tuberculoma: It is a common space-occupying lesion, occurring alone or with tuberculous meningitis. Symptoms include seizures, focal neurological deficits, and raised intracranial pressure.

Turner's syndrome: It is the most common monosomy. The finding is due to loss of the part or all of one of the sex chromosomes. The affected individual will have 45x. The phenotype is female and is characterized by short stature and underdeveloped gonad.

Tzanck preparation: This is useful in the diagnosis of some viral infections such as herpes simplex, varicella, herpes zoster, etc. The base of the blister is scraped with blunt-edged instruments. Staining with Giemsa stain is preferable. Balloon cells and multinucleated giant cells are characteristic of pemphigus.

Vasoocclusive crisis: It consists of sudden attacks of bone pain, usually in limbs, joints, back, and chest, or of abdominal pain. Infection is the precipitating factor.

Vesicometeric reflux: It refers to the retrograde flow of urine from the bladder to the upper urinary tract. The rest of the intravesical pressure occurring during the micturition is freely transmitted to the ureter, renal pelvis, papillary collecting ducts, and renal tubules.

Von Gierke disease: This is a glycogen storage disorder. Clinical features include hepatomegaly, failure to thrive, hypoglycemia, ketosis, and acidosis.

Von Hippel–Lindau disease: In this disorder, there are retinal, and cerebellar hemangioblastomas besides the spinal cord angiomas and cystic tumors of pancreas, kidneys, and epididymis. Patients show nystagmus, ataxia, and signs of increased intracranial pressure.

Von Willebrand disease: It is an autosomal dominant disorder, and it occurs due to the deficiency of the von Willebrand factor. A child presents with mucosal bleeding.

Wegener's granuloma: It is the vasculitis affecting the upper and lower respiratory tract and kidneys. It is characterized by necrotizing granuloma. There will be nonspecific complaints. Ophthalmic involvement includes uveitis and orbital pseudotumor.

Wheeze: Abnormal high-pitched musical sound produced due to the narrowing/obstruction of terminal airways, i.e., bronchi, mainly expiratory in nature.

White reflex: Absence of red flare when seen through the pupil with the help of a fundoscope. It is seen in retinoblastoma.

Wimberger sign: It is seen in scurvy, epiphyseal centers of ossification surrounded by a white ring is called Wimberger sign.

Wiskott–Aldrich syndrome: It is an X-linked recessive disorder characterized by eczema, thrombocytopenia, and recurrent infections. There is profound immunoglobulin M (IgM) deficiency in addition to defective T cells.

Xeroderma pigmentosum: This is an autosomal recessive (AR) condition, due to defective nucleotide excision repair of photodamaged deoxyribonucleic acid (DNA) and characterized by extreme photosensitivity with the onset of infancy. Over the next 2–3 years the child develops hyperpigmented (freckles) and hypopigmented lesions predominantly on the photoexposed skin on a background of xerosis.

Xerophthalmia: This occurs because of a deficiency of vitamin A in the diet. There is pigmentation of the cornea with the loss of normal luster and moist appearance of the palpebral conjunctiva, which appears dry and wrinkled.

Zoonosis: An infectious disease that can be transmitted from vertebrate animals to human beings. Common animals associated with zoonosis include cattle, dogs, cats, pigs, rats, and monkeys.

Index

Page numbers followed by *b* refer to box, *f* refer to figure, *fc* refer to flowchart, and *t* refer to table

A

Abdomen 861
    Distension of 121, 173, 282*f*, 290, 304, 875, 932
    mild distension of 253
    palpation of 290, 862
    ultrasound of 584, 643
    upper 311*f*
    X-ray of 237, 254, 256, 282, 311*f*
Abduction brace 1103
Abductor muscles, discomfort of 869
Abetalipoproteinemia 1105
ABO
    hemolytic disease 837
    incompatibility 362
    isoimmunization 847
Abortive poliomyelitis 745, 748
    signs of 746
Abscess 773
    cerebral 487
    fluid 300
    hepatic 295, 296
    metaphyseal 734
    multiple 104, 296
    myocardial 158
    periannular extension of 160
    periosteal 737
    peritonsillar 75
    retropharyngeal 75
    subphrenic 299
Absolute eosinophil count 37, 237, 595
Academia, respiratory 897
Acellular pertussis vaccines 786, 794
Acetabular dysplasia 1064
Acetabular index 1064
Acetabulum 1061
Acetaminophen 408
Acetazolamide 521
Achalasia 263, 318
Achondroplasia 1105
Acid–base
    balance 882
    gas analysis 821
    homeostasis 897
    status 899
Acidemia, metabolic 897
Acid-fast bacilli 121, 740
    cultures 756
Acidosis 213, 446, 827, 894
    correction of 43, 615
    metabolic 44, 221, 305, 672, 894
    mild 675
    organic 312
    respiratory 67
Acinetobacter 476
Acne 1105
Acquired immunodeficiency syndrome 688, 924
Acridine orange 559
Acrocephaly 1105
Acrodermatitis enteropathica 1105
Acromegaly 63, 1105
Actinomycin D 1012
Activated prothrombin complex concentrates 341
Acute bacterial meningitis 553, 558, 558*t*
    complications of 560
Acute diarrhea 208
    types of 209
Acute leukemia 943
    differential diagnosis of 972
    etiology of 966
Acute lymphatic leukemia 965, 975, 978
    treatment of 973
Acute myeloid leukemia 965, 976
    treatment of 975
Acute otitis media 31, 86, 89, 93*t*, 209, 311, 312
    microbiology of 87
    treatment of 92
Acute poststreptococcal glomerulonephritis 429, 437
    diagnosis of 430
Acute pyogenic meningitis
    diagnosis of 557
    falls, treatment of 560
Acute respiratory distress syndrome 312, 709
Acute rheumatic fever 180, 757, 1017, 1020, 1029, 1030*t*
    recurrent attack of 1022
Acyclovir 684, 703, 783
    intravenous 685
    oral 684, 685
Adalimumab 1055
Adenoid 27, 28
    enlargement 30
    facies 1106
    hypertrophied 28*f*
Adenoidectomy 31
Adenoma
    benign cortical 600
    pituitary 599
Adenopathy 658, 699
    supraclavicular 956, 958
Adenosine triphosphate 815
Adenovirus 88, 175
Adenylate cyclase 787
Adhesive otitis 90
Adipocytes 912

Adipose genital dysmorphy 913
Adipose tissue 911, 912
Adipsia 604
Adrenal androgen 639
    moderate hypersecretion of 595
    production 578
        disorders of 578
Adrenal enzyme defects 589*t*
Adrenal glands 633
Adrenal hyperplasia
    congenital 583, 586, 587, 588*f*, 638
    nonclassic congenital 587
Adrenal insufficiency 241, 613, 827, 828
    signs of 588
Adrenaline stimulates 48
Adrenocortical carcinoma 991
Adrenocorticotropic hormone 521, 522, 596
    prohormone precursor of 911
Adrenoleukodystrophy 1106
Adriamycin 960, 962
Aedes
    aegypti 650, 671
    africanus 650
Afebrile 4, 375, 601
    seizure 528
Aganglionic megacolon, congenital 279
Aganglionic segment 280
    irregular sawtooth contraction of 283
Agenesis 620
Aggregatibacter actinomycetemcomitans 156
Aggressive respiratory support 250
Agonal bradycardia 810
Air
    embolism 848
    swallowing 260
Air-blood barrier 888
Air-fluid level 81
Airway
    foreign body 59
    inflammation 34
    maintenance 764
    management 764
    obstruction 700
        episodic symptoms of 36
    remodeling 36
Alanine
    aminotransferase 297, 913
    transaminase 272, 1038

Albendazole 927
Albinism 1106
Albumin 810, 842, 843
    bound bilirubin 842
    serum 449
Albuterol 70
Aldolase 1038
Aldosterone 584, 589
    deficiency 613
    resistance 613
    serum 584
Algid malaria 1106
Alkalemia, respiratory 897
Alkaline phosphatase 270, 272, 297, 322, 929, 936
Alkylating agents 462, 967
Allergen immunotherapy 51
Allergic bronchopulmonary aspergillosis 55
Allergy tests 37, 95
Alloimmunization 420
Alopecia areata 1106
Alpha-amino-3-hydroxy-5-methyl-4-isoxazolepropionic acid receptors 813
Alpha-angle 1063
Alpha-antitrypsin deficiency 56
Alpha-globin chains 414, 415
Alpha-thalassemia 413, 415
    disease 419
    silent carrier 415
    syndromes 415
Alport's syndrome 1106
Alveolar air block syndrome 118
Alveolar rupture 248
Alveolar ventilation 891
Alzheimer's disease 7, 8, 13
Ambiguous genitalia 575, 576, 577*f*, 581, 582, 864
Ambulation 511
Amebiasis 299
Amebic liver abscess 297
    treatment of 300
Ameliorate early infections 793
Amenorrhea 20, 326
Amikacin 127, 129, 130, 135
Amino acid 393, 501, 881
    chromatography 821
    metabolism disorder 815
Aminoaciduria 546
Aminocaproic acid 371
Aminoglycoside 61, 135, 299, 561, 758

Aminophylline 41
    role of 44
Ammonia, serum 820
Ammonium tetrathiomolybdate 329
Amniocentesis 10, 840
Amniocytes 1096
Amoxicillin 93, 105, 135, 478, 774, 924
Ampicillin 77, 105, 127, 561, 564, 793, 924
Amplatzer Duct Occluder 171
Amylin 910
Amyloid precursor protein gene 13
Amyloidosis 1051
Anabolic agent 1097
Anabolic steroids
    endogenous excess of 388
    exogenous excess of 388
Anaerobes 281
Anakinra 1055
Anal stenosis 282
Analgesia 401
Analgesics 670, 685
Anaphylactoid purpura 292, 436
Anaplasia 1012
Anasarca 449
Anastomotic suture line 288, 289
Ancestral morbillivirus 717
Androgen
    insensitivity 578
    resistance syndrome 581
    treatment 645
Androgenic influence, evidence of 631
Anemia 159, 160, 333, 362, 622, 706, 876, 924, 942, 958, 1046, 1051, 1106
    aplastic 273
    correction of 194
    disproportionate 971
    hemolytic 361, 445, 659, 666, 876, 1078
    management of 925
    microangiopathic 1120
    mild-to-moderate 361
    onset of 379
    severe 363, 708
        malarial 708
    sideroblastic 382
Aneuploidy 15
Angelman syndrome 10, 500
Angiocardiography 191, 200

Angiodestructive disorder 700
Angioedema, acute 75
Angioma 546
Angiomatous lesion 871
Angiopathy, autoimmune 1037
Angiotensin-converting
enzyme 1019
inhibitors 437, 1088
Angular stomatitis 379
Anhidrosis 983
Aniridia 1008
Anisocytosis 1106
Ankle
broad 933f, 934f
joint 1100
widening of 929, 932f
Anopheles mosquito 707
bites 705
Anorectal malformations 282, 284
Anorectal manometry 283
Anorexia 89, 176, 231, 274, 382,
719, 720, 920, 942,
958, 968
Anoxic brain damage 792
Anoxic spell 30, 191, 192, 1106
Antacids, aluminum-
containing 930
Antenatal corticosteroid
prophylaxis 889
Anterocephaloid
malalignment 187
Anthropometric measurements
315, 333, 352, 375, 516,
541, 552, 565, 628, 640,
752, 761, 776, 813, 854,
874, 918, 947
Antiandrogen 638
Antibiotic 77, 82, 105t, 233, 904
empiric oral 478t
indications of 222
intra-articular 758
oral 163
prophylaxis 480, 480t, 481,
1029
selection 306
therapy 93, 163, 561, 564, 737,
757, 773, 927, 1028
treatment 562
Antibodies
myositis-specific 1039
nonfunctional 689
Anticholinergics 41, 42
Anticoagulant warfarin 347
Anticonvulsant 823

drugs, pediatric dosages
of 521t
phenytoin 347
therapy 823
Antidiuretic hormone, lack of 602
Antiepileptic drug 506, 522, 523,
523t
treatment 522
Antiepileptic therapy 531
Anti-Epstein–Barr virus
antibodies 701, 702
Antifibrinolytic agents 371
Antiganglioside antibodies 537
Antigen detection tests 772
Antiglobulin test 368
Antigravity gastrocnemius
muscles 497
Antihyaluronidase 1027
Anti-inflammatory therapy 1027
Anti-islet cell antibody 612
Antimicrobial agents 155
Antimicrobial prophylaxis 165
Antimicrobial susceptibility
testing 774
Antimicrobial therapy 104,
299, 739
Antineutrophil antibody 436
Antinuclear antibody 1038, 1106
testing 368
Antiperoxidase antibodies 623
Antiplatelet antibodies, removal
of 372
Antiretroviral prophylaxis 691
Antiretroviral resistance
testing 693
Antiretroviral therapy 694, 695
Anti-Rh (D) globulin 372
Antisclerostin antibody 1098
Antisecretory drug 224
Antisickling agents 411
Antismooth muscle antibodies
1042
Antispasticity drugs 506
Antistaphylococcal agent plus
third-generation
cephalosporin 738
Antistaphylococcal
antibiotics 738
Antistaphylococcal penicillin 738
Antistreptokinase 1027
Antistreptolysin O 183, 185, 429,
436, 1017, 1021, 1027
elevated levels of 355
Antithyroid antibodies 22
Antitrypsin deficiency 328

Antituberculous drug 127, 135
Antiviral drug 684, 782
Anus 863
Anxiety 34
Aorta
aneurysm of 152
coarctation of 20, 148, 150
descending 168
dissection of 152
Aortic aneurysm 1085, 1087
Aortic dissection, higher risk
of 1088
Aortic ejection systolic
murmur 151
Aortic regurgitant murmur 151
Aortic root 1086
aneurysm 1083, 1085
dilatation 1086, 1087
Aortic stenosis 155
Aortic surgery 1087
Aortic valve 172, 1020
acute 1023
chronic 1023
Aortopulmonary transposition
143
Apathy 923
Apert syndrome 237, 239
Apgar score 493, 802, 803, 810,
825, 1106
Aplastic crisis 363, 405, 1106
secondary, risk for 362
Apnea 67, 788, 791, 792, 804, 816,
819, 827, 874, 884
recurrent 67
risk of 822
Apneic spell 67, 1107
Appendectomy, laparoscopic 234
Appendicitis 226, 227, 475
acute 233
chronic 234
diagnosis of 233
gangrenous 227
perforated 235
Appendix 288
Appetite, loss of 557, 699, 706, 709
Apt test 349
Arachnodactyly 1083, 1084
Arachnoid
cyst 633
villi 542
Arachnoiditis 560
Arcuate arteries 442
Arginine vasopressin 602, 608
Arnold-Chiari malformation 1107
Arrhenoblastoma 578

Arrhythmias 146, 1024
  cardiac 35
  development 160
Artane 506
Artemether 712
Artemisinin-based combination therapies 714
Arterial blood gas 46, 69, 187, 302, 895
Arterial carbon dioxide, partial pressure of 39, 563
Arterial oxygen
  partial pressure of 901
  saturation 190
Arteries
  intra-acinar pulmonary 246
  intralobular 442
Artesunate 712
Arthralgia 355, 660
Arthritis 328, 354, 355, 660, 1020, 1022, 1027, 1044
  fungal 757
  juvenile idiopathic 176, 1042
  reactive 1051
  systemic 1049
  traumatic 757
Arthrodesis 1104
Arthrogryposis 1060
  multiplex 1101, 1107
Arthro-ophthalmopathy, hereditary 1087
Arthropod borne viruses 671
Arthrotomy 753
Arthus reactions 766
Articular cortical degradation 753
Articular surfaces 1060
Ascaris 872
Ascites 324, 1107
Ascorbic acid 943
Aspartate
  aminotransferase 297, 651, 913
  transaminase 406, 1038
Asphyxia 495, 800, 828, 887
  causes of 800
  pathophysiology of 799
  perinatal 889
  progresses 800
Aspiration 876
  percutaneous 299
  pneumonia 55
    recurrent 317
  pneumonitis 249
  syndrome 896
Aspirin 391, 408, 1053
Asplenia, functional 396

Asthenia 678
Asthma 49, 56, 105
  acute exacerbation of 39*t*
  bronchial 32, 68, 76
  classification of 48*t*
  diagnosis of 36
  severe persistent 48
  therapy, long-term 47
Astigmatism 1087
Ataxia telangiectasia 502, 1107
Ataxic cerebral palsy 499
  motor disorder 499
Atelectasis 792, 888, 894
  minimize 903
Atelectatic theory 56
Atelectrauma 888
Atenolol 437
Atherogenic plasma lipid profile 456
Athetoid cerebral palsy 499, 501
Athetosis 1107
Atopic dermatitis 684
Atovaquone 713
Atresia 316, 892
Atrial fibrillation 541
Atrial septal defect 6, 141, 142
Atrial surgery 181
Atrophic glossitis 379
Atrophy, cerebral 496, 548
Atropine 810, 818
Attack, acute 530
Attention-deficit hyperactivity disorder 8, 21
Audiology 12
Auditory abnormalities 843
Auerbach's plexuses 279
Auramine O staining 123
Autism 658, 1107
Autoantibody phenomena 959
Autoimmune
  disease 1042
  disorder 388
  hemolysis 706
    anemia 362, 368
  inflammatory 177
  process 359
Autoimmunity, manifestation of 1043
Autologous stem cell 988
Automatisms 518
Autosomal dominant 602
  aquaporin-2 defect 605
  hypophosphatemic rickets 930
Autosomal recessive 602, 1032
  aquaporin-2 defect 605

  hypophosphatemic rickets 930
Axillary regions 115
Azathioprine 372
Azithromycin 83, 105, 222, 774, 775, 793, 1028
Azoospermia 16
Azotemia 1107
Aztreonam 61

B

Babinski's sign 1107
Baby mass index 1107
Bacillus
  entry of 1069
  subtilis 1115
Bacillus–Calmette-Guérin
  adenitis 132
  diagnostic test 125
  test 118, 1108
  vaccination 1076
Back pain, severe 674
Baclofen 506
  intrathecal 506
Bacteremia 156, 160, 163, 397, 770, 781
  non-*Staphylococcus* 163
  rate of 398
Bacteria 99, 469, 753, 787
  gram-positive 300
  proliferation of 281
  rapid killing of 563
Bacterial colonization 87
Bacterial heat shock proteins 1042
Bacterium, gram-negative 768
Bacteriuria, asymptomatic 473
Bacteroides 233
  fragilis 296
Ballard score 854
Bariatric surgery 914
Barium
  enema 279, 282, 283, 287
  reduction 356
  maximum permissible height of 291
  study 231, 241
  swallow 149, 151, 258, 259, 263
Barlow's test 1062, 1063, 1107
Barotrauma 248
Barrett's esophagus 265
Bart hemoglobin 415
Bartonella 157, 159
  henselae 733

Bartter syndrome 1107
Basal ganglia 841
    appearance of 499
Basilar invagination 1096
B-cell
    activation 688
    gene expression 955
    leukemia 955
    lymphomas 698
Becker muscular dystrophy 509
Beckwith-Wiedemann syndrome 387, 828, 981, 1108
Beclomethasone 49
Bell's palsy 699, 857f
Benzathine 1030
    penicillin G 1029
Benzene exposure 967
Benzodiazepines 504, 506, 531, 532, 822, 823
Benzoic acid 822
Benzothiazide 828
Berger's disease 355
Beriberi 1108
Beta-adrenergic
    blockers 437
    drugs 70
Beta-agonists 40
Beta-blockers 1088
Beta-cell
    autoimmune destruction of 612
    damage 612
Beta-globin 414
    alleles 414
    gene production 414, 415
Beta-hemolytic streptococcus 353
Beta-lactams 135, 163, 561
    inhibitors 135
Betamethasone 905
Beta-thalassemia 359, 393, 413, 417
    intermedia 414
    major 414, 415
    syndromes 414
    trait 419
Bethanechol 268
Bile duct atresia 6
Bilevel positive airway pressure 503
Biliopancreatic diversion 915
Bilirubin 843, 845
    displacement of 843
    encephalopathy 843
    metabolism 834
    protein ratio 844
    serum 358, 393, 838, 839, 844, 846, 846t
Biochemistry 445
Biopsy 125, 264, 737, 979, 1077
    testicular 17
Bipedal edema 921
Birth
    asphyxia 797, 798, 816, 827
    injury 816
    marks, hypopigmented 1077
    multiple 800
    weight 838, 846
        low 308, 653, 873, 884, 929, 1090
Bisphosphonates 1097
Bitot spots 927
Blackwater fever 709, 1108
Bladder 571
    emptying of 477
    fleeting paralysis of 746
    incontinence 568
    paralysis 749
Blalock-Taussig shunt 155, 194
Bleeding 337, 848, 942
    diathesis 884
    disorders 340
    fundamental treatment of 338
    gastrointestinal 21, 312, 336, 675, 676
    gum 942, 942f
    intracerebral 816
    periventricular 876
    prevention of 339
    tendencies 969
    time 346, 653
    vaginal 629, 639
    variceal 324
Bleomycin 960, 961, 963
Block steroid synthesis 638
Blood 598, 790
    area, level of 435
    brain barrier 560, 840, 842
    count dyscrasias 1039
    culture 159, 160, 163, 302, 736, 755, 772, 821
    disorder 875
    examination 457
    flow
        cerebral 815
        pulmonary 188
        umbilical 799
    gas analysis 892
    glucose 821
    group 839
    intrapulmonary shunting of 894
    loss 375, 377
    pressure 148, 456, 822, 827, 873
        accurate measurement of 471
        cuff 178
        measurements of 438
        studies 529
    sugar 913
    tests 476
    transfusion 409, 410
        annual 420
        role of 409
        therapy, primary toxic effect of 410
    urea 595
        levels 457
        nitrogen 106, 429, 436, 456, 520, 675, 1010
    vessels 940, 1020
    volume 848
Bloodstream, massive seeding of 111
Bloom's syndrome 1108
Blue sclera 1093f
Blueberry muffin 656
    lesions 656
Bluish retention cyst 858
Bluish-white spots 719
Blunt trauma 296
B-lymphoblastic leukemia 969
Body weight loss 214
Bone 986
    age 637
        advanced 637
    aspiration 737
    cultures 737
    dysplasia 1091
    marrow 973, 982, 986
        aspirate 985, 1048
        disease 984
        examination 367, 368, 382, 959, 971
        failure syndrome 368
        infiltration 956
        iron staining 382
        transplantation 424, 977, 987, 988, 1004
        trilineage
            myeloproliferation 390
    metaphysis of 991
    sarcomas 1000
    scans 959
    softening of 929

Bony deformities 1096
Borderline leprosy 1072
Borderline tuberculoid 1070
Bordetella
    bronchie septicum 786
    organisms 786
    parapertussis 786
    pertussis 786, 787, 789
Borrelia burgdorferi 560
Bottle feeding 87
Botulinum toxin 506
Bounding pulses 170
Bow legs 934*f*
Bowel
    disease, inflammatory 21, 377
    loops of 245*f*
    neurogenic 571
    obstruction 982
        signs of 281
    perforation 355
    sounds 248
Bradycardia 674, 678, 803
Bradykinin 34
Brain 911, 1020
    abnormalities, congenital 604
    abscess 192, 633, 815
    capillaries 706
    dysplasia of 7
    injury, hypoxic 603
    tumor 312, 548, 991
Brainstem
    auditory pathways 841
    compression 1096
    oculomotor nuclei 841
Brassy cough 958
Breast
    bilateral enlargement of 14
    development 635, 860*f*
    enlargement 635
    milk 617
        jaundice 834, 837
    size 853
Breastfeeding 218, 470, 881
Breath
    nitric oxide 37
    periodic 67, 1122
    shortness of 389
Breathlessness 63, 97, 148, 186, 301, 894
Brilliant transillumination 545
Broad-spectrum antibiotic therapy 470
Brodie abscesses 735

Bronchial asthma 32, 68, 76
    acute attack of 41*t*
    hallmark of 35
    long-term management of 47
Bronchial diameter 60
Bronchiectasis 54-56, 59, 105, 791
    acquired 57
    congenital 55
Bronchiolar obstruction 66
Bronchiolitis 37, 63, 65, 68, 791
    obliterans 107
Bronchitis, diffuse 61
Bronchoalveolar lavage 66
Bronchodilators 40, 48, 61, 70
    effect 50
    therapy 43
Bronchography 59
Bronchopneumonia 76, 98, 720, 721, 792
Bronchopulmonary infection, recurrent 262
Bronchoscopy 59, 123
Bronchospasm, refractory 317
Bronze baby syndrome 846
Brucella 157, 733
Brucellosis 773, 986
Brudzinski sign 556
Brushfield's spots 7*f*, 8, 1108
Budesonide 49
Bulbar function 538
Bulbar muscle 538
Bulging anterior fontanelle 556, 558, 656, 658
Bullous impetigo 1108
Bullous rash 666
Bumetanide 464
Buphthalmos 1108
Burkitt's leukemia 966
Burkitt's lymphoma 700, 709
Burning micturition 471
Burr cells 1108
Burrow 1108
Buttocks 1076
Butyrate 424
Butyric acid analogs 411

C

Cafe-au-lait 1108
Calcaneovalgus feet 1102
Calcineurin inhibitors 462
Calcium 529, 813, 882, 929
    deficiency 930
    serum 418, 821, 935, 936

    therapy 820
    urinary 935
Caleaneotalar-navicular complex, malalignment of 1100
Calf muscles, pseudohypertrophy of 1112
Calves, enlargement of 510
Campylobacter 222, 441, 691
    infection 534
    jejuni 534
    serologic tests for 537
Canavan disease 546
Cancer incidence 633
Candida albicans infections 469
Canthal index 1109
Capreomycin 127, 129, 135
Capsular hyaluronate 1020
Caput succedaneum 855*f*, 1109
Carbamazepine 185, 519, 521
Carbon dioxide 66
Carbonic anhydrase inhibitors 548
Carboplatin 962, 988, 1003, 1004, 1012
Carboxyhemoglobin 834
Carcinoid tumors 228
Carcinoma, adrenal 598
Cardiac anomalies 809
Cardiac arrest 46
Cardiac catheterization 170, 190, 191, 200
Cardiac defects 656, 658
    congenital 11
Cardiac dilatation 970
Cardiac dysfunction 875
Cardiac enlargement 168, 623, 624
Cardiac failure 67, 828
    congestive 101, 150, 171, 172, 389, 411, 434, 446, 457
Cardiac flow murmur 397
Cardiac injury 179
Cardiac massage, external 808
Cardiac murmur 158
Cardiac tamponade 180
    acute 175
    causes of 175
Cardiac valve, thickening of 1032
Cardiobacterium hominis 156
Cardiomegaly 363, 1024
Cardiomyopathy 406, 511, 1109
Cardiopulmonary system 390
Cardiorespiratory monitoring 765
Cardiovascular collapse 360
Cardiovascular defects 389

Cardiovascular disease, high risk of 914
Cardiovascular system 139, 142, 187, 861, 875, 1018, 1085
   examination 154
Carditis 1022, 1023, 1027, 1030
   acute rheumatic 1023
   clinical features of 1024
   moderate-to-severe 1028
Carey Coombs murmur 1109
Carpal Tunnel syndrome 1034
Carpenter syndrome 1109
Cartilage 279, 940
   lack of 316
Catalase 375
Cataract 655, 656, 657f, 1009
   congenital 1001
   sunflower 325
Catarrhal phase 788
Catecholamine
   metabolites 984
   secretion in utero 827
Catheter tipped transducer 548
Caudate nuclei 184
Caustic injury 315
Cefazolin 738
Cefixime 478
Cefotaxime 83, 561-564, 758
Cefprozil 478
Ceftazidime 561, 562, 758
Ceftriaxone 83, 233, 561-564, 738
Cefuroxime 83, 478
   axetil 105
Celiac disease 376, 377, 931
Cell 15, 718
   ballooning degeneration of 778
   culture 747
   cytoplasm 687
   free noninvasive prenatal testing 10
   membrane 1020
   potassium leaks out of 918
   regulation defects 955
   surface proteins 787
   wall endoxin 563
Cellular damage 846
Cellular debris 66
Cellular immune system 1037
Cellulitis 1109
   deep 757
Centers for Disease Control and Prevention 721
Central diabetes insipidus 602, 603, 608

   causes of 602
   treatment of 608
Central nervous system 325, 337, 355, 390, 444, 483, 486, 495, 543, 630, 665, 690, 874, 854, 1086, 1110
   disease 118
   disorders 630
   dysfunction 819, 1048
   hemorrhage, acute 905
   infarct 396
   injury 495
   involvement 326
   lesions 245
   mass, evidence of 631
   problems 7
   prophylaxis 973
   trauma 814
   tuberculosis 118, 119
Central precocious puberty 629, 630
   causes of 630
Cephalexin 478, 480
Cephalohematoma 833, 856f, 1109
   aspiration of 848
Cephalopelvic disproportion 540, 800
Cephalosporins 163, 299, 562, 738
Cerebellar ataxia-facial neuritis 728
Cerebral dysgenesis 815
Cerebral gigantism 546
Cerebral palsy 493, 494, 496, 497f, 500, 500b, 876
   classification of 495, 496b
   dyskinetic 499
   poster criteria of 499b
   risk factors for 495b
   spastic 496
Cerebrospinal fluid 119, 490, 520, 542, 547, 549, 551, 557, 558t, 559, 656, 667, 729, 747, 781, 812, 813, 1003
   absorption 542
   analysis 490, 530
   circulation, physiology of 541
   culture 559
   examination 557, 781
   excessive accumulation of 541
   flow 541
   grain stain 559
Cerebrovascular occlusive disease 487

Ceruloplasmin, serum 322, 327
Cervic sign 241
Cervical lymph node, enlarged 27
Cervical spine X-ray 13
Cesarean section 887, 889
Cetpodoxime 478
Cheilosis 379
Chelation therapy 421
Chemical
   hepatitis pulmonary toxicity 1039
   irritants 34
Chemoprophylaxis 135, 794, 1030t
   long-term 715
   primary 135, 136fc
   short-term 714
Chemosis 1109
Chemotherapy 961, 973, 975, 988, 996, 1003, 1004, 1012
   high-dose 974, 988
   intrathecal 974
   maintenance 974
   prenephrectomy 1012
   short course 131
Cherry red spot 1109
Chest 860
   circumference 919
   compression 808
   hyperexpand 933f
   infections 147
   pain 178, 181, 679
   physiotherapy 904
   radiograph 170, 180, 191, 249, 313
   syndrome, acute 401, 402
   ultrasound of 81
   upper 893
   wall
      deformities 860
      movements 903
   X-ray of 4, 37, 81, 187, 200, 245, 552, 676, 895
Cheyne-Stoke breathing 1109
Chiari malformation 569, 570
Chickenpox, gestational 777
Chikungunya 649
   virus 651
Childhood tuberculosis 127t
   treatment of 131b
Chills 471, 473
Chlamydia 87, 98, 402, 786
Chloramphenicol 561, 758
Chloride, serum 598

Chloroma 969, 969f, 1110
Chloropropamide 609
Chloroquine 712, 713, 1080
   resistant malaria 712
Chlorpromazine 185, 353, 828
Chlorpropamide
   maternal use of 828
   oral administration of 609
Cholangiolar proliferation 323
Cholangiopancreatography,
   endoscopic
   retrograde 313
Cholecystokinin 911
Cholelithiasis 914
   risk for 915
Cholera 222
Cholestasis 272
Cholesteatoma 90, 1110
Cholesterol 449
   levels 457
   lowering medication 347
Cholinergic agonist 268
Chondrodystrophy 1087
Chordae tendinae
   elongation of 1023
   rupture of 1023
Chorea 184, 1024, 1025, 1110
Choreiform movements 1025
Choreoathetoid 501
Choreoathetosis 723, 1110
Chorionic villus sampling 10
Chorioretinal coloboma 1001
Chorioretinitis 662, 663, 666
   glaucoma 666
Choroid
   plexus papilloma 542
   tubercles 118
Choroidal coloboma 1003
Chromium 924
Chromosomal abnormalities,
   maternal age-related 4
Chromosome 261, 1091
   analysis 4, 17, 643
Chronic obstructive pulmonary
   disease 56
Chronic osteomyelitis 739, 740
   treatment of 740
Ciliary dyskinesia 105
   primary 55, 58
   pulmonary 56
Cimetidine 267
Cinchonism 713
Ciprofloxacin 130, 135, 235
Cirrhosis 122

   cryptogenic 324
   disease 718
Cisplatin 987, 988, 997
   dose of 988
Citrobacter 468
Clarithromycin 105, 135, 1078
Classical neurological signs 841
Clavicle, palpation of 860
Clavulanate 93, 478
Clavulanic acid 105, 135
Claw sign 1011
Cleft lip 858f
Clindamycin 712, 714, 738, 758
Clinicopathologic staging
   system 1011
Clinodactyly 1110
Clobazam 521
Clofazimine 1078, 1080
Clonazepam 521
Clonus 818
Closed-chest tube drainage 83
Clostridia 233
   septicemia 362
Clostridium
   difficile 222, 281
   perfringens 302
Clot retraction 346
Cloxacillin 83
Clubfoot 1100, 1101
   congenital 1101
Clutton's joint 1110
Coagulation 445
   intravascular 970
   profile 407
Coagulopathy 1048, 1051
Coarctation 248
   severity of 151
Coarse facies 1032
Coats disease 1001
Cobalamin C mutations 441
Codeine 408
Coeur en sabot 1110
Cold 690, 720
   agglutinin 104
   disease 359
   air 34
   chain 1110
Coliforms 281
Colistin 61
Collagen
   disorders 122
   structural
      defects 1092
      mutations 1091

   types of 1092
   vascular disorders 367
Colloids 677
   preparations 678
Coma 923
Combination antiretroviral
   therapy 688
Commando crawl 498
Communication disorders 500
Complement fixation 675
Complete blood count 275, 771,
   838, 1049, 1055
Complimentary feeding 1110
Computed tomography 984,
   985, 995
   angiography 1087
   detects 599
   scan 231, 232, 256, 530,
      736, 1002
   indications of 559
Concomitant femoral shortening
   osteotomy 1066
Conduct disorder 1110
Condyloma 666
   lata 664
Congenital diaphragmatic
   hernia 248
   incidence of 245
Congenital esophageal
   disorders 315
   stenosis, types of 316
Congenital heart disease 6, 142,
   153, 155, 160
   signs of 656
Congenital hypothyroidism 618,
   619, 620f, 624
   causes of 620b
Congenital neurosyphilis 662
   diagnosis of 667
Congenital rubella 653, 656, 657f
   syndrome 658
Congenital syphilis 661-665, 943
   clinical signs of 663
   diagnosis of 666
Congenital talipes 1101f
   equinovarus 1100
Congestion 437
   conjunctival 969
Conjunctivitis, phylctenular 112
Conn syndrome 1110
Connective tissue
   defective formation of 940
   disorders 176
Consciousness 708
   loss of 191

Conservative therapy 266
Consolidation chemotherapy 973, 974
Constipation 503
Contact dermatitis 684
Continuous positive airway pressure 503, 896, 900, 901
Contractures, prevention of 502
Convalescent serum specimens 721
Conventional repair surgery 194
Convulsions 528, 763, 823
Cooley's anemia 417
Coombs sera 420
Coombs test 358, 361, 368, 837, 839
   direct 368
   negative 362, 837
Cope's manure 293
Copper 323, 924
   altered incorporation of 323
   deficiency 382
   enters circulation 324
   serum 322
Cord
   clamping of 798
   compression 799, 983
   prolapses 800
Corneal clouding 1032, 1033f
Cornelia de Lange syndrome 237
Corona radiata lesions 489
Coronary artery, narrowing of 1032
Cortical sensory deficits 500
Cortical vein thrombosis 224
Corticosteroids 42, 43, 49, 112, 120, 129, 180, 372, 452, 458, 563, 600, 702, 793, 829, 1039, 1052
   high-dose 371
   oral 77
   therapy 370, 459t
   use of 77
Cortisol
   deficiency 584, 586
   levels 598
   synthesis 578
Coryza 719, 721
Cotrimaxazole 480, 774, 923
   therapy 694
Cough 54, 58, 68, 85, 97, 101, 118, 314, 690. 786, 789
   chronic productive 58
   harassing 30

illness 790
   rhinorrhea, acute-onset of 67
   whooping 785, 917
Countercurrent immuno-electrophoresis 558
Cow's milk protein 612
Coxa vara 933, 1110
Coxiella 159
   burnetii 157
Coxsackievirus 175, 228, 612
Crackled peeling patches 921
Cranial irradiation 633, 974
Cranial nerve
   deficits 560
   examination of 867
   involvement 539
   nuclei 744
   palsy 560, 666, 969
Cranial neuropathies 556
Cranial radiation 975
Craniopharyngioma 602, 630
Cranioschisis 566
Craniospinal irradiation 992
Craniotabes 932, 1110
C-reactive protein 160, 185, 231, 245, 651, 751, 812, 1017, 1021
Creatine
   kinase 1038
   phosphokinase 510, 512, 1035
Cremasteric reflex 644
Crepitations 798, 873
Cri du chat syndrome 10
Cribriform plate 553
Crigler–Najjar syndrome 839, 1110
Crisis
   abdominal 401
   anoxic 1106
   aplastic 363, 405, 1106
   hypoplastic 358
   megaloblastic 358
   vasoocclusive 400, 1127
Critical enzyme thyroperoxidase 619
Crohn's disease 21, 377, 388, 475, 1110
Cromolyn 50
   sodium 47
Cross-matched triple saline-washed packed cells 420
Croup 72, 73
   viral 74

Crouzon syndrome 1111
Crying 226
Cryoglobulin 160
Cryoprecipitate 339, 340
Cryotherapy 1003
Cryptorchid testes 642
Cryptorchidism 16, 641, 1111
   consequences of 642
Cryptosporidium 222, 223
Crystalline penicillin, aqueous 668
Crystalloid 677
Cubitus valgus 1111
Currarino triad 282, 283
Cushing's disease 595, 596, 598
Cushing's syndrome 594, 595, 597-599, 633, 912, 913, 1053
   diagnosis of 595
   signs of 597
Cyanosis 35, 70, 113, 142, 172, 187, 189, 254, 389, 709, 717, 760, 786, 827, 854, 861, 891, 893, 895, 999
   causes of 894
   central 73
Cyanotic spells 190
Cyclic adenosine monophosphate 224
   high levels of 787
Cyclophosphamide 372, 462, 463, 952, 960-962, 975, 987, 1012, 1014
Cycloserine 127
Cyclosporine 372, 462, 463, 1053
Cyproheptadine 600
Cystadenomatoid malformation 247, 896
Cystic fibrosis 35, 38, 55, 289, 931
Cystic hygroma 859f
Cysticercosis 1111
Cystinosis 937, 1111
Cystinuria 1111
Cystitis 472, 473
   acute hemorrhagic 473
   interstitial 473
Cystourethrogram, micturating 474, 476, 477
Cysts
   branchial 859f
   intestinal duplication 288, 289
Cytarabine 975
Cytochromes 375

Cytogenetics 4
Cytokine
    polymorphisms 1036
    tumor necrosis
        factor-alpha 353
Cytomegalovirus 99, 342, 353,
        612, 815
    infection 667
Cytopenia 693, 1048, 1051, 1055
    autoimmune 957
Cytosine 1038
    arabinoside 961, 976
        high-dose 976
Cytotoxic agents 1053

D

Dacarbazine 961
Dacryoadenitis 1111
Dactylitis 399f
Danazol 372
Dandy-Walker
    malformation 545
    syndrome 569, 1111
Danger sign 836, 885
Dantrolene 506
Dapsone 1078
Dark colored urine 361
Darting tongue sign 184, 1111
Daunorubicin 975, 976
De Musset's sign 1111
Deafness 655, 656, 728
Death, causes of 68
Deciduous tooth 342
Deep tendon reflexes 551
Deep venous thrombosis 915
Deferasirox 411
Deferiprone 422
Deferoxamine 410, 422
Deformity 1093, 1100
    correction of 1097
    extent of 1101
    prevention of 502
Degradation 930
Dehydration 101, 212, 214t, 217t,
        218t, 224, 242, 473, 503,
        650, 712, 757, 922
    assessment of 213, 922
    clinical signs of 214t
    mild 237
    moderate 79, 440, 687
    moderate-to-severe 70
    severe 219t, 609
    signs of 80, 270
Dehydroepiandrosterone 586,
        589, 591

Dehydrogenase, serum
    lactate 699
Deiodination 619
Delinquency 1111
    juvenile 1117
Delivery room
    management 877
    resuscitation 801
Dementia 7, 723
Demyelination, perivascular 778
Dendritic cells 717
Dengue
    diagnosis of 676
    fever 670, 671, 676, 678
    hemorrhagic fever 671, 674,
        677, 678
    infections, secondary 676
    shock syndrome 671, 673, 677
    virus 275
Dent disease 930
Dentine 940
Dentinogenesis imperfecta 1095
Deoxyribonuclease 83
Deoxyribonucleic acid 123, 246,
        667, 687, 711, 846
    deletions of 414
    methods of 512
    sequences 1068, 1096
    viral 702
Depot testosterone 645
Dermatomyositis 513, 1035,
        1051, 1111
Desferrioxamine 422
Desmin 949
Developmental dysplasia
    1060, 1061
Dexamethasone 76, 77, 961, 962
    suppression testing 598
    test, low-dose 598
Dextran sulfate sodium 677
Diabetes 612t, 613, 800, 887, 889
    insipidus 601-603
        central 602, 603, 608
        nephrogenic 602, 604,
            606, 609
        neurogenic 608
    mellitus 603, 610, 613
        diagnostic criteria for 613t
        risk of 658
Diabetic ketoacidosis 612, 614
Diamond sign 241
Diaper dermatitis 1111
Diaphragm, sac-like structure
    of 247
Diaphragmatic hernia 244, 245,
        809, 896
    types of 245

Diarrhea 67, 211, 212, 216, 221,
        224, 282, 396, 689
    acute 208
        watery 209
    bacterial 211
    chronic 921, 922
    complications of 224
    intermediate 208
    management of 925
    mild 455
    protozoal 212
    viral 211
Diarylquinoline 1078
Diastasis recti 862f
Diastolic murmur, audible
    delayed 170
Diazepam 506, 822
Diazoxide therapy 829
Diclofenac 1053
Dietary management 463, 924
Differential leukocyte count 4, 27,
        78, 226, 245, 468, 602
DiGeorge syndrome 1112
Dihydrotestosterone 576
Dihydroxyphenylalanine 501
    increased levels of 984
Diiodotyrosine 619
Dimercaptosuccinic acid 474
    scan 477
Dipalmitoylphosphatidyl-
    choline 888
Diphtheria-pertussis-tetanus,
    dose of 196
Diphtheria-toxoid-tetanus toxoid-
    acellular pertussis 766
Diphtheroids 157
Diplegia, spastic 497, 498
Diploic spaces 418
Dipstick tests 475
Direct antiglobulin test 368
Direct fluorescent antibody 68
Direct radionuclide
    cystourethrogram 477
Disseminated intravascular
    coagulation 160, 224,
    340, 672, 1078, 1111
Distal pulmonary artery
    anatomy 192
Distal renal tubular acidosis
    930, 936
Distal sensory loss 536
Disturbed sleep 63, 716
Diuretics 464
Dolichocephaly 1084, 1112
Doll's eye response 1112
Dopamine 984

Index

Dorsal root ganglia 744
Dorsolumbar gibbus 1032
Double bubble sign 256, 256*f*, 1112
Double collecting system 21
Double-outlet right ventricle 197
Down syndrome 3, 5, 6*f*, 8, 387, 500, 625
Downes score 893*t*
Doxorubicin 952, 961, 987, 988, 997, 1012, 1014
Doxycycline 712, 714
Drooling 1112
Droperidol 46
Drug-resistant tuberculosis 134
    incidence of 134
    treatment of 134
Drugs
    therapy 221
    toxicity 818
    withdrawal 819
Drumstick gram positive bacilli 764
Dry cough 720, 1024
Dry lips 27
Dry powder inhaler 52
Dubin–Johnson syndrome 1112
Duchenne muscular dystrophy 508, 509, 1112
Ductus
    arteriosus 168
    patency of 237
Duhamell's pull-through, modified 284
Duodenal atresia 11, 248, 253, 254, 257
Duodenal ileum 257
    produces stenosis, failure of recanalization of 255
Duodenal obstruction, congenital 254
Duodenal portal vein 254
Duodenal stenosis 241, 1112
Duodenoduodenostomy 257
Duodenojejunostomy 1112
Duodenum 255
    protozoal 257
Dural ectasia 1083
Duroziez's sign 1112
Dwarfism 932
Dysarthria 326, 488, 504
Dyschromia, nutritional 1077
Dyselectrolytemia 224, 242, 676
Dysentery 208, 209, 1112
Dysgenesis 620
Dyshormonogenesis 618-620

Dyskinetic syndromes 499
Dyslipidemia 465
Dysmorphic facial features 575
Dysmorphism 15
    facial 495
Dysostosis
    metaphyseal 937
    multiplex 1112
Dysphagia 263, 763, 958, 1112
    cardiomyopathy 1038
Dysphonia 52
Dysphoria 1112
Dysplasia 7, 1060
    bronchopulmonary 876
    multiple fibrous 629
    retinal 1001
Dyspnea 32, 39, 113, 118
Dystonia 326, 501, 507, 723, 1112

E

Earlobes 1076
Ears 1073
    firmness 853
Ebstein anomaly 1112
Ecchymosis 920, 969, 1113
    periorbital 982
Echinococcus granulosus 295
Echocardiography 151, 191, 200
    transesophageal 160
    transthoracic 160
    two-dimensional 146
Eclampsia 800, 873
Ectopia lentis 1083, 1086, 1087
Ectopic anus 282, 284
Ectopic pancreatic tissue 288, 289
Eculizumab 447
Eczema 1113
Edema 68, 324, 355, 434, 452, 455*f*, 456, 464, 717, 920, 921, 1036
    acute pulmonary 434
    angioneurotic 436, 457, 922
    cerebral 119
    generalized 920
    inflammatory 744
    interstitial 311
    loss of 458
    periorbital 699, 1038
    pulmonary 709, 890
Edematous malnutrition edema 921
Edward syndrome 1113
Effective feeding program 506
Ehlers-Danlos syndrome 1087, 1113

Eikenella corrodens 156
Eisenmenger syndrome 199, 200, 1113
Ejection systolic murmur 151
Electrocardiogram 55, 151, 153, 180, 185, 191, 490, 623, 764, 802, 1021
Electrocardiography 180
Electrodes 519
Electroencephalogram 185, 501, 502, 529, 530, 764, 811, 821
Electroencephalography 547
Electrographic seizure activity 820
Electrolyte 106, 879
    abnormalities 880
    disturbance 920
        management of 220
    imbalance 848, 875
        correction of 923
    panel 1010
    serum 302, 529, 584, 821
Electromyography 505, 539
Electron microscopy 323
Emboli, pulmonary 158
Embolic phenomena 158, 159
Embolism 160
Embolus, pulmonary 915
Emergency
    drug treatment 525
    lower segment cesarean section 493
    ultrasound examination 873
Emotional lability 1025
Emphysema 61, 105
    pneumomediastinum 248
    subcutaneous 791
    surgical 248
Empyema 78, 79, 781
    chronic 81
    necessitatis 80
    split pleura sign of 82
    stages 80
Encephalitis 603, 633, 659, 711, 720, 729
    optic neuritis 699
    post-varicella 778
    viral 560, 748
Encephalocele 569, 1113
Encephalomyelitis 748
Encephalopathy 560, 691, 771, 791, 814
    early signs of 833
    hepatic 328
    hypertensive 434, 815

hypoxic-ischemic 495, 818, 1117
 syndrome, reversible 400, 434
Encopresis 1113
Endocarditis 161t, 1024
 culture-negative 157
 fungal 164
 subacute bacterial 154, 432
Endocardium 1032
Endocrine 911
 disorders 913
 system 573
Endodermal cells 316
Endoluminal techniques 268
Endoscopic balloon dilation 242
Endoscopy 264
Endothelial cells 888
Endothelium 155
Endotracheal intubation 765
Endotracheal tube 76, 807, 897, 902
 size 807
Enema, saline 291
Enophthalmos 1084
Enoxacin 135
Enriched milk, composition of 926
Enteral nutrition 881
Enteritis, ischemic 444
Enterobacter 157, 233, 468
Enterococcus 476, 562
Enterocolitis 292
Enterostomy tube 288
Enteroviruses 88, 175, 743
Enthesitis 1045
Enthesopathy 1045
Enuresis 1113
Enzymatic defects 620
Enzyme 918
 deficiency 589
 immunoassay test 675, 772
 inducing antiepileptic drug 523
 proteolytic 753
Enzyme-linked immunosorbent assay 69, 123, 558, 651, 711, 721, 729, 747, 781, 790, 791, 1077
 serum 298
Enzymopathies 362
Eosinophils, reactive infiltration of 956
Ephedrine 818
Epidermal nevus syndrome 930
Epidermolysis
 bullosa 1113
 hyperkeratosis 1113
Epididymitis 729
Epilepsy 500, 515, 520, 521t, 524
 future risk of 531
 idiopathic generalized 517
 juvenile myoclonic 519
 refractory 525
 risk of 532
 surgery 523
 syndrome 520
Epinephrine 809, 829, 830
Epiphyseal advancement 1050
Epiphyseal closure 638
Epiphyseal plate 931
Epipodophyllotoxin 967
Episodic asthma, mild 47
Epistaxis 342, 676, 969, 1113
Epithelial cell 888, 890
 proliferation 431
Epithelial elements 1008
Epithelial pearls 858
Epithelium, ciliated 77
Epstein pearl 1113
Epstein-Barr nuclear antigen 701
Epstein-Barr virus 275, 353, 680, 697, 698, 702
Erb's palsy 860f
Erection 627
Erythema 755, 948
 infectiosum 1113
 marginatum 1025, 1114
 multiforme 1114
 necroticans 1075
 nodosum 112
  leprosum 1079
 toxicum 872, 1114
Erythroblastosis fetalis 828
Erythrocytapheresis 410
 automated 409
Erythrocyte 705, 706
 destruction 706
 membrane 359
 sedimentation rate 78, 120, 185, 355, 374, 429, 551, 584, 649, 731, 736, 751, 756, 916, 953, 959, 1017, 1021, 1041, 1068
 test 183
 sickle 394
Erythrocytic schizont 705
Erythrocytosis 389
Erythroid
 hyperplasia 362
 production 415
 regulator 378
Erythromycin 105, 268, 794, 1028, 1029
Erythropoiesis 378, 1114
Erythropoietic tissue, hypertrophy of 416
Escherichia coli 157, 296, 302, 440, 563, 733
Esophageal atresia 6, 314-1121
 diagnosis of 314
Esophageal manometry 264
Esophageal mucosa 265
Esophageal stenosis 315
 embryology of 316
 pathogenesis of 316
Esophageal strictures 263
Esophageal web 315, 316
Esophagitis, eosinophilic 315
Esophagus 778
 acquired disorders of 315
 biopsy of 264
 distal 319
Estradiol 913
 levels 17
 serum 636
Estrogen
 cyclic 23
 replacement
  low-dose 23
  therapy 23
 secreting adrenal neoplasms 632
Estrogenic influence, evidence of 631
Etanercept 1054
Eteplirsen 513
Ethambutol 127, 129, 130
Ethanol 603
Ethionamide 127, 130
Ethosuximide 521
Etoposide 952, 961, 962, 988, 997, 1004, 1012, 1014
Eustachian tube 65
 function 87
Evans staging system 986
Evans syndrome 368
Ewing's sarcoma 947, 949-951
Exacerbations 38, 58, 60
Excessive iron stores, primary treatment of 410
Exchange transfusion 372, 844, 846
 complications of 848

indications of 847*b*
serum bilirubin for 846*t*
Excretory urogram 476
Exercise 34, 35
Exostosis 1114
 multiple hereditary 991
External genitalia 575, 578, 579, 589
 development of 576
Extracellular signal-regulated kinase inhibitors 1088
Extracorporeal membrane oxygenation 250
Extramedullary hematopoiesis produces 416
Extramedullary myeloid cell tumor 970
Extravascular space 672
Extremities 864
 irregular movements of 1025
Extubation 905
Eye 856, 875
 checkup 12
 jerking of 816
 movements, abnormal 819
Eyeball, uprolling of 526, 812
Eyebrows 1070
Eyelids 5
 fluttering of 816
 heliotrope 1038

F

Face 856
 swelling of 148, 873
Facial
 edema 969, 1038
 grimacing 1025
 nerve 1074
  paralysis 90
 oxygen 804
 palsy 91*f*
Failure to thrive 121, 585, 662, 690, 709, 1084, 1114
Fallot tetralogy 6, 155, 186, 189, 1114
Famciclovir 685
Familial cortisol resistance syndrome 632
Famotidine 267
Fanconi's anemia 1114
Fanconi's syndrome 326, 328, 613, 930, 937
Fastidious organism 157
Fasting plasma glucose 613, 913

Fat cell
 hyperplasia 912
 size of 912
Febrile 109, 154, 270, 650, 812
 convulsion 526, 676
 disease 671
 illness 112, 528
 infections, acute 479
 seizures 532
  pathophysiology of 527
Fecal matter, incontinence of 569, 571
Fecal-oral route 272
Feeding 216, 268, 319, 499, 897
 habits 917
 intolerance 304
 problems 620, 622, 785
Feet, lymphedema of 20*f*
Felbamate 522, 523
Felty syndrome 1046
Female external phenotype 577
Femoral head 401
 avascular necrosis of 401, 1064
Femoral pulses 861
Fernandez reaction 1076
Ferric salts 383
Ferriprox 422
Ferritin, serum 380, 382
Ferroportin 378
Ferrous fumarate 383
Ferrous gluconate 383
Ferrous glycine sulfate 383
Fetal lung-to-head ratio 246
Fetal umbilical blood sampling 9
Fever 54, 97, 100, 153, 154, 159, 176, 226, 314, 397, 473, 551, 557, 768
 acute rheumatic 180, 757, 1017, 1020, 1029, 1030*t*
 control of 532
 low-grade 529, 968
 nonremitting 1048
 prolonged 158, 701
 rheumatic 122, 175, 184, 1021, 1022, 1030, 1051
 subsidence of 722
 viral 1027
Fiberoptic endoscopy 256
Fibers, parasympathetic 42
Fibrin
 degradation products 443
 purulent phase 80
 split-product values 676

Fibrinogen 346, 1049
Fibrinoid necrosis 353
Fibrinolysis, plasminogen activates inhibitor of 447
Fibrinolytic agents, instillation of 83
Fibroelastosis, endocardial 1113
Fibronectin receptors 1069
Fibroplasia, retrolental 875
Fibrosis 424
 endomyocardial 709
 idiopathic pulmonary 56
Fibula, mild hypoplasia of 1102
Fibular hemimelia 1100
Fimbrial agglutinogens 787
Fine needle aspiration cytology 115, 125, 623
Fingers
 clubbing of 57*f*, 58
 contracture of 1084
Fistula, bronchopleural 1108
Flaccid paralysis, acute 1105
Flag sign 920*f*, 1114
Flaky paint 921
Flat facies 5
Flaviviridae 672
Flexner–Wintersteiner rosettes 1000
Floppy infant 1114
Florescent leprosy antibody absorption 1076
Fluid 215, 217, 799, 879, 923
 amounts of 923
 collection 177, 313
  drainage of 233
 electrolyte
  balance 897
  equilibrium 749
 overload 446, 905
 replacement of 678
 therapy 243, 608, 615
Flu-like syndrome 1078
Fluorescent treponemal antibody absorption 667
Fluoroquinolones 129, 1078
 clinical use of 480
Fluoroscopy 249
Fluticasone 49
Focal neurological deficit 556
Folate 566
 functions 566
Folic acid 1039
 supplementation 362, 1053
Folinic acid supplementation 1053

Fontanelle 856
    anterior 856, 980
Foot
    deformities 1100
    manipulation of 1102
    plantar flexion of 1100
    segments of 1102
Foramen magnum 542
Foramen ovale 143, 894
Forced vital capacity 36, 510
Forearm, interosseous membrane of 1095
Forefoot
    adduction 1102
    medial deviation of 1100
Formoterol 49
Foscarnet 703
Fosphenytoin 822
Foster Kennedy syndrome 1114
Foul-smelling sputum 58
Fowler–Stephen procedure 645
Fracture management 1097
Frank blood 181
Frank respiratory distress 118
Frankel white line 943
Free erythrocyte protoporphyrin 380, 381
Free thyroxine 624, 913
Free triiodothyronine 624
French method 1102
Fresh frozen plasma 339, 340, 347
Fresh whole blood 340
Friction rub 181
Friedreich's ataxia 1114
Froehlich syndrome 1114
Fröhlich's syndrome 913
Frusemide 464
Fundoplication procedures 268
Fundoscope 149
Fungemia 160
Fungi 87, 157
Furunculosis 733, 1114
Fusobacterium 29, 700

G

Gabapentin 521, 522, 523
Galactosemia 827
Gallop 1024
    rhythm 1114
Gallstone 362
    formation 406
Gamma-aminobutyric acid 761
    receptor 506
Gamma-chain, synthesis of 415
Gamma-globulin 160

Gammaherpesvirus 698
Ganciclovir 703
Ganglion cells 981
Ganglioneuroblastoma 981
Ganglioneuroma 981
Ganglioside monosialic 1126
Gangliosidosis 546
Gargoylism 625
Gasping respiration 805
Gastric
    banding 915
    decompression 242
    emptying 264
    inhibitory peptide 910
    lavage 122
    peristalsis 237f, 240
    pressure-volume dynamics 260
Gastroenteritis 288, 289, 663
    acute 207
    eosinophilic 237, 239
Gastroesophageal reflux 241, 248, 258-260, 266, 315, 318
    disease 105, 252, 259, 320
Gastrointestinal system 205, 875
Gastrointestinal tract 390, 956, 1037
    anomalies 6
    full-thickness necrosis of 308
Gastroplication techniques 268
Gastrostomy 268, 319
Gaze abnormalities 843
Gemcitabine 962
Gene
    encoding extracellular matrix 1083
    manipulations 424
Generalized expiratory airflow obstruction, evidence of 67
Genetic 1, 414, 910, 999
    conditions 967
    counseling 12, 581, 1000, 1089, 1098, 1115
    defects 279
    predisposition 912
    susceptibility 87
    syndromes 913
    testing 502
Genital ambiguity 578, 644f
Genital phenotype 578
Genitalia 863, 864
    abnormal 577f
    examination 863
    external 575, 578, 579, 589
Genitoplasty, feminizing 593

Genitourinary abnormalities 855, 1009
Genitourinary anomalies 1008
    congenital 470
Genitourinary system 569
Genitourinary tract 778
Gentamicin 163, 561
Gentle oropharynx 804
Genu
    valgum 934f
    varum 935f
Germ cell malignancy 643
Germinal cells 999
Germinoma 602, 604
Germline mutations 1007, 1008
Gestational age 851
    assessment 851, 852t, 853
    estimated 807
Ghrelin 910
Gianotti–Crosti syndrome 697
Giardia 691
Giardiasis 376, 383
Giemsa stain 710
Gigantism 633, 1115
Gilbert syndrome 839
Gingival hypertrophy 942f
Gland biopsy 115
Glaucoma 658, 663, 1002
    congenital 666
Glial hamartoma 1001
Gliosis 496, 1115
Glomerular filtration barrier, major component of 452
Glomerulonephritis 160, 432
    acute 430, 436b
        poststreptococcal 429, 437
Glossitis 921f
Glossoptosis 892
Glucagon 829, 830
    like peptide-1 910
Glucocorticoids 564, 591, 599, 906
    chronic 595
    excretion products of 598
    intra-articular injections of 1053
    treatment 591
Glucose 217, 810, 882, 910
Glucose-6-phosphate dehydrogenase 359, 840
    deficiency 833, 840
Glucuronidase gene 834
Glutamate receptor 2 813
Glutamic acid decarboxylase 611
Glycine 1092

Glycogen
  granules 323
  storage disorder 827
Glycosuria 598, 613
  sudden onset of 882
Goldberg–Shprintzen syndrome 279
Gonadal dysgenesis 577
Gonadoblastomas 632
Gonadotropic stimulation, evidence of 631
Gonadotropin 17
  basal 581
  levels 636
  receptor defect 581
  serum 636
  therapy 645
Gonadotropin-releasing hormone 587, 637
  causes of 632
  stimulation tests 637
Gonococcus 753
Goodpasture syndrome 355
Gowers's sign 510, 511*f*, 1115
Graf technique 1063
Graft versus host disease 424
Gram stain 558, 559
Granulocyte colony-stimulating factor 976
Granuloma
  eosinophilic 951
  inflammatory 487
  tuberculous 127, 633
  umbilical 862*f*
Granulomatosis 107
  lymphomatoid 700
Granulomatous disease, chronic 295
Granulosa cell tumor 632, 638
Grasp reflex 869, 1115
Graves' disease 7, 619, 1115
Gravity drainage 749
Great arteries
  transportation of 155
  transposition of 894
Greenstick fractures 933, 1115
Grey Turner's sign 1115
Group A cell wall carbohydrate 1020
Growth 189, 363, 465, 925
  advanced 636
  changes 622
  disproportionate 1083
  disturbances 1051
  hormone 624
    therapy 23

  impairment 876
  physical 405, 417
  retardation 379, 622, 920, 1053
Grunt 893
Gubernaculum 641
Guillain–Barré syndrome 533-535, 699, 728, 748, 1037, 1115
  congenital 536
Gum
  bleeding 969
  hypertrophy 942, 942*f*, 970
Gut-derived peptides
  cholecystokinin 910
Guthrie's test 1115
Gynecomastia 16, 17, 1115

H

Haemophilus 176
  aphrophilus 156
  infection, treatment of 106
  influenzae 29, 99, 552, 723, 752
    infections 102
    meningitis 563
    type B 362, 397, 733
    pneumonia 102
Hair
  changes 920
  growing, length of 920
  hypoplasia 279
Halofantrine 714
Haloperidol 185
Hamartoma 288, 289
  hypothalamic 630
Hand-foot
  equinus 1102
  syndrome 401, 406
Hansen's disease 1080
Harbor malignant ovarian tumors 632
Harrison's groove 932, 935, 1116
Harrison's sulcus 933*f*
Head 855
  banging 1116
  circumference 544, 919
  drop 746, 747
  trauma 312, 633
Headache 148, 389, 533, 545, 556, 651, 706, 745, 750, 768
  throbbing 969
Healed pyogenic skin lesions 430
Healing 739
  rickets 943
Hearing 13

  assessment 12, 1097
  defects 7
  impairment 884
  loss 560, 658, 1034
    saddle nose 666
  problems 500
Heart
  block 160
  circulates blood 808
  defects, congenital 143
  disease 159, 487
    congenital 6, 60, 142, 153, 155, 160
    cyanotic 896
    rheumatic 155
    severe 1032
  enlarged 1024
  failure 147, 164
    congestive 68, 146, 160, 924, 1024
  size 151
  sounds 1024
  valve 1020
Heat-killed leprosy vaccine 1080
Heinz bodies 395
Helical proline 1092
Helicobacter
  infection 537
  pylori 366, 376, 534
Heliotropic rash 1038
Helper T-lymphocyte response 1043
Hemagglutination
  inhibition antibody titer, estimation of 659
  tests 721
Hemagglutinin 726
Hemangioma 288, 866, 1115
  capillary 1109
  retinal 1001
  subdural 892
Hemarthrosis 336*f*, 342, 1115
Hematocrit 390, 418, 676, 678
Hematogenous dissemination 111
Hematological disorders 884
Hematological system 331
Hematoma 347
  chronic subdural 548
  subcutaneous 342
Hematopoietic growth factors 976
Hematopoietic stem-cell transplantation 408, 410, 423, 1003
Hematoxylin and eosin staining 1077

Hematuria 159, 342, 456, 458, 473, 662, 942, 1115
  gross 433, 435
  microscopic 160, 454, 474
Hemianopsia 1116
  bitemporal 1108
Hemiatrophy, cerebral 492
Hemichorea 1024
Hemihyperplasia 1008
Hemihypertrophy 981, 1008
Hemimelia 1101
Hemiparesis 556, 560, 1116
Hemiplegia 192, 489
  acute 485, 487
  contralateral 489
Hemochromatosis 1116
Hemoconcentration 675, 676
Hemoglobin 4, 55, 153, 237, 245, 254, 315, 322, 346, 358, 374, 386, 387, 394, 494, 509, 595, 767, 953, 1041
  A 407
  C 393
  D 393
  fetal 394
  level of 417
  O 393
  sickle 407
  unstable 362
Hemoglobinuria 709
Hemolysis 395, 838
  acute 326
  copper-induced 328
  evidence of 359, 361
  intravascular 394
Hemolytic anemia 361, 445, 659, 666, 876, 1078
  congenital 359
  Coombs-negative 326, 327
  Coombs-positive 957
Hemolytic disease 839
  congenital 359
Hemolytic uremic syndrome 222, 368, 436, 439, 440, 1116
  pathogenesis of 442
Hemopericardium 177
Hemophilia 333, 334, 338, 342, 343
  A 335, 342, 343
  B 342, 343
  long-term complications of 343
  severity of 335
  treatment of 342
  types of 335

Hemopoiesis 1116
Hemoptysis 1116
Hemorrhage 356, 389, 983, 1048
  antepartum 495
  interventricular 874, 883
  intracranial 335, 367, 371, 487, 675, 814
  intraventricular 543
  life-threatening 342, 371
  periventricular 814
  petechial 672, 942
  postpartum 603
  primary subarachnoid 814
  retinal 708, 969
  splinter 158, 159
  subarachnoid 560, 816
  subdural 815
  vitreous 1003
Hemorrhagic
  disease 345
  disorders, congenital 346
  manifestation 673
  periventricular infarction 883
  stroke 491
    treatment of 491
  varicella lesions 782
Hemosiderosis 417
Hemuturia 457
Henoch–Schönlein purpura 288, 352, 353, 432, 757
Hepatic copper overload syndrome 328
Hepatic disease 324, 326
Hepatic dysfunction 324
Hepatic failure 326
Hepatic injury, grades of 323
Hepatitis 270, 328, 659, 690, 693, 711
  A 420
  A virus 271-275
    infection 271, 276
    vaccine 276
  autoimmune 275
  B 420
    virus 353
  C 420
    virus 420
  E virus 271
  G virus 271
  toxic 1078
  transfusion 342
  treatment of 848
  viral 676
Hepatocellular dysfunction 956
Hepatocyte 273

  damage 272
Hepatomegaly 177, 675, 707, 827, 920, 1048
Hepatosplenomegaly 389, 665, 666, 689, 701, 1032, 1047
  thrombocytopenia 658
Hepcidin 378
Hernia 247, 1093
  congenital diaphragmatic 248
  diaphragmatic 244, 245, 809, 896
  hiatal 241, 263, 318, 1116
  indirect inguinal 644, 645
  inguinal 862
  umbilical 620, 862f, 1032
Herpes simplex 667, 780f
  vesicles 680f
  virus 680
Herpes zoster 679, 680, 682, 684, 685
  incidence of 680
  rash 680f
  severe 681
Herpesviridae 698
Heterophile antibody 701, 702
Heterosexual 630, 631
Heterotaxic syndromes 60
Hiatal hernia 241, 263, 318, 1116
High-arched palate 5, 666
High-resolution computed tomography scan 60
Hilgenreiner's line 1064
Hills sign 1116
Hip 1065
  adduction 1063
  click 1062
  congenital dislocation of 1059-1061, 1062f
  developmental dysplasia of 1060
  flexion contractures 1056
  girdle weakness 510
  joint 758
  unstable 869
Hirschsprung's disease 5, 6, 248, 278-282, 306, 1116
His bundle 198
Histamine
  leukotrienes 34
  receptor antagonists 267
  sensitivity 787
Histiocytosis 972, 1116
Hoarse cry 620
Hoarseness 622, 1116

Hodgkin's disease 953, 960t, 1116
    classification of 957t
    clinical staging of 958
Hodgkin's lymphoma 452
    classical 959
Homeostasis 884
Homer Wright pseudorosettes 981
Homocystinuria 1087, 1116
Homovanillic acid 984, 985
Honeycomb appearance 54
Hookworm infestation 418
Hormone 910
    gastrointestinal 911
    levels 592
    therapy 383
Horner's syndrome 983, 1117
Horseshoe kidney 21
Human chorionic gonadotropin 637, 643
    levels, serum 637
Human herpesvirus 680, 702
Human immunodeficiency virus 56, 209, 686, 687, 694, 924, 1039
    infection 121, 688
        complications of 176
    transcription 687
    wasting syndrome 691
Human leukocyte antigen 410, 612
Human metapneumovirus 88
Human parvovirus B19 infection 405
Human tetanus immunoglobulin 764
Humid atmosphere 875
Humidified oxygen 69, 193
Huntington's chorea 185
Hurler's disease 1032
Hurler's syndrome 548, 1031, 1033f
Hutchinson's teeth 666, 1117
Hyaline membrane disease 249
    risk factors for 889
Hydration 401, 408
    maintenance of 723
Hydrocele 864
    congenital 864f
Hydrocephalus 540, 541, 544, 545, 545f, 555, 560, 569, 572, 630, 633, 883, 1034, 1096, 1119
    acute 549
    congenital obstructive 549
    diagnosis of 548
    pathogenesis of 546
    pathophysiology of 542
    severe 548
    signs of 545
    therapy for 548, 570
Hydrochlorothiazide 609
Hydrocortisone 41, 830
    challenge test 584
Hydrofluoroalkane 52
Hydronephrosis 986, 1012
Hydrops 666, 800
    fetalis 415
    severity of 836
Hydrotherapy 723
Hydroxyapatite
    crystals 1092
    form of 929
Hydroxychloroquine 1040, 1053
Hydroxyproline 1092
Hydroxyurea 409, 411, 422-424
    therapy 423
    typical starting dose of 409
Hyperalgesia, cutaneous 674
Hyperbilirubinemia 240, 360, 833, 844
    conjugated 240
    management of 844t
    pathological 832
    unconjugated 240
Hypercalcemia 605, 609
Hypercholesterolemia 662
Hypercoagulability 454
Hypercyanotic attacks, severity of 193
Hypercyanotic episodes 189, 193
Hyperesthesia, cutaneous 674
Hyperestrogenic state 629
Hyperexcitability, cerebral 818
Hyperferritinemia 1048, 1051
Hypergammaglobulinemia 689
Hyperglycemia 611, 613, 882
Hyperinflation, clinical evidence of 104
Hyperinsulinism 828
Hyperkalemia 305, 446
Hyperlipidemia 452-454, 456, 457
Hypermobile pes planus 1102
Hypernatremia 220, 815, 820
Hyperoxemia 894
Hyperperistaltic waves 240
Hyperpigmentation 921, 1038, 1038f
    mucosal 633
Hyperplasia 238, 390
    squamous 265
Hyperplastic callus, combination of 1095
Hyperpyrexia 676
Hypersensitivity
    onset of 124
    reaction 176
Hypersplenism 367
    late manifestation of 424
Hypertension 437, 446, 458, 585, 589, 662, 800, 873, 896, 913
    malignant 441
    mild 433
    mild-to-moderate 437
    portal 324, 1123
    progressive pulmonary 791
    pulmonary 147, 200, 202, 424
        arterial 171, 172
    severe pulmonary arterial 151
    transient 434
Hyperthyroidism 185
Hypertonic saline 61
Hypertriglyceridemia 1048, 1051
Hypertrophic pyloric stenosis 237, 238, 793
    congenital 236, 237
Hypertrophy, diffuse 238
Hypervolemia 678
Hyphema 1002, 1117
Hypnozoites 705
Hypoalbuminemia 456, 457, 1048, 1051
Hypocalcemia 815, 816, 818, 823, 845, 875, 876, 882, 924
Hypochromia 418
Hypocomplementemia 432, 663
Hypofibrinogenemia 1048, 1051
Hypogammaglobulinemia 454
Hypoglycemia 390, 614, 709, 815, 816, 818, 825, 826, 828, 848, 875, 876, 923, 924, 1008
    causes of 827
    clinical
        features of 826
        manifestations of 827t
    correction of 823
    development of 828
    early 882
    prevention of 828
    refractory 829

Hypogonadism 912
Hypokalemia 220, 605, 609
Hypomagnesemia 815, 924
Hyponatremia 220, 305, 672, 815, 1048, 1051
  correction of 220
Hypophosphatemia 937
Hypophysitis, lymphocytic 604
Hypopigmentation 921
Hypopituitarism, congenital 827
Hypoplasia 190, 282, 284, 618
  bilateral pulmonary 892
  pulmonary 247, 248, 809, 904
Hypoplastic deformed teeth 1096
Hypoproteinemia 281, 282, 662
Hypospadias 16, 1117
Hyposthenuria, high incidence of 408
Hypotension 898
  acute 800
  risk of 822
Hypothalamic dysfunction 580
Hypothalamus-pituitary-gonadal axis 628, 641
Hypothermia 827, 843, 918, 923
Hypothesis 453
Hypothyroidism 22, 454, 591, 617, 618, 619, 622, 623, 633, 912-914, 963
  acquired 622
  central 619, 622
  congenital 618, 619, 620f, 624
  hypopituitary 619
  neonatal 624
  primary 618, 625
    congenital 623
  severe primary 634
  subclinical 625
  transient 622
Hypotonia 5, 496, 824, 932, 1117
Hypotonic syndrome 500
Hypovolemia stimulates 456
Hypoxemia 791, 902
Hypoxemic spells 189
Hypoxia 64, 118, 800, 816, 827, 875, 876
  perinatal 815
  physiological 798

I

Ibuprofen 180, 408, 1052, 1053
Ichthyosis 1117
Icteropyloric syndrome 240
Icterus 142, 322, 836

Idarubicin 976
Idiopathic arthritis, systemic juvenile 1047
Idiopathic thrombocytopenic purpura 364, 365, 972
Ifosfamide 952, 962, 997, 1014
Ileoileal disease 291
Ileoileal intussusception 291
Ileostomy 307
Ileus 213
Illness
  acute phase of 683
  initial phase of 676
Imipenem 127
Immobility 503, 723
Immune
  deficient states 55
  serum globulin 276
  system, role of 452
  thrombocytopenia
    acute 369
    chronic 372
    diagnosis 366
Immunity 109, 684
  cell mediated 110, 698, 1043, 1074
  humoral 1043
Immunization 466, 694
  active 276, 766
Immunoadsorption 372
Immunochromatographic tests 710
Immunodeficiency
  syndrome 341, 367
  virus infection 681
Immunofluorescence examination 431
Immunoglobulin 276
  A 659
  G 659
    antibodies 368
  M 649, 651, 653, 659, 667, 721, 1074
    antibodies 650
  platelet associated 366
  prophylaxis 277
Immunologic reaction 1069
Immunomodulatory drugs 452
Immunosuppression 1039
Immunosuppressive 452
Immunotherapy 51
Imperforate anus 5, 282, 284, 855, 1117
Impetigo 433f, 733, 1117
  contagiosa 684

In utero surgical closure 569
In vivo methylation 566
Incontinentia pigmenti 1117
Indian Academy of Pediatrics classification 918
Indian Childhood Cirrhosis 328
Indian Oncology Study Group 976
Indomethacin 180, 408, 609, 898, 1052, 1053
  dose of 171
Infant stimulation program 13
Infantogram 1091
Infarctions 119, 603, 848
  cerebral 403
Infections 271, 308, 398, 465, 495, 603, 612, 617, 717, 815, 848, 875, 876, 884, 917, 923, 1049
  bacterial 222, 784, 1042
  chronic 382
  clinical signs of 884
  congenital 543, 816
  dulminant 923
  early stages of 115
  extrapulmonary 101
  fetal 666
  focus of 557
  fungal 295, 690, 691, 754
  inapparent 745
  increased risk of 272
  intercurrent 113
  intra-abdominal 296
  intracranial 819
  metastatic 160
  mycobacterial 691
  parapharyngeal 30
  perinatal 689
  peritonsillar 30
  polymicrobial 733
  primary 112, 678
  protozoal 223
  pyogenic 175
  respiratory 146, 289, 314
  retropharyngeal 30
  secondary 125, 791
    bacterial 781
  spreads 726
  streptococcal 781, 1027
  theory 56
  transplacental 662
  viral 35, 690, 1042
Infectious disease 120, 487, 647

Infectious mononucleosis 228, 696, 773, 972
    complications of 700b
Infective endocarditis 146, 153, 154, 155
    avascular vegetations of 163
    complications of 160
    prophylaxis 172
    treatment of 161t
Infertility 16, 60
Inflammation
    pancreatic 312
    perineuronal 744
    signs of 727
Inflammatory colitis, severe 444
Inflammatory disease, chronic 49
Infliximab 1055
Influenza 175, 676, 690
    virus 88, 786
Inguinal hernia 862
    bilateral 863f
Inhalation 110
    devices 51
Inhibitory gamma-aminobutyric acid, development of 813
Injury
    cerebral 878
    ischemic 888
    postinhalation 56
Insect bite 436
Insulin 611, 615, 910
    sensitizer 914
Intensive care
    management 45
    unit 45
Intercostal drainage 83
Interferons 372, 1117
    gamma release assay 125, 126
Interleukin 1042
Intermittent positive-pressure ventilation 824, 902
    weaning of 904
International League Against Epilepsy 517
International Neuroblastoma Staging System 985, 986
International Working Group Consensus Report 368
Interstitial air leaks 890
Intestinal complications 356, 444
Intestinal obstruction 263, 591
    symptoms of 281
Intestinal perforation 773

Intra-abdominal pressure 641
Intra-articular corticosteroid injection 1049
Intra-articular glucocorticoid injections 1054
Intracardiac shunts, magnitude of 199
Intracranial complications 90
Intracranial pressure monitoring 548
Intracranial space occupying lesion 487
Intragastric tube 925
Intramuscular route 384
Intratumoral calcification 1002
Intrauterine growth
    restriction 874
    babies 826
    retardation 386, 653, 1090
Intrauterine varicella 684
Intravenous anti-D therapy 370
Intravenous fluid 43
    therapy 219, 219t
Intravenous immunoglobulin 538, 846
    therapy 368, 693
Intubation 45, 806
Intussusception 286, 293
    acute 292
    chronic 290
    pediatric 288
    recurrent 288
    resection of 292
Inverted appendix stump 288, 289
Iodide
    organification 620
    transport 618
Iodine organification, defects of 619
Iodine-123 metaiodobenzylguanidine 984
Ionic changes 395
Ipratropium 42
    bromide 41
Iron 375, 378
    absorption 377
        intestinal 378
    binding capacity 380
    chelation 410
        therapy 421
    deficiency 375, 379
        anemia 374, 375, 380, 381, 385, 418
        diagnosis of 382

        mild-to-moderate 379
        risk for 377
    deficient microcytic red cells 391
    dextran, bolus injection of 384
    hemosiderin 422
    homeostasis 377
    overload 421, 424
        monitoring 421
    quantitation 421
    serum 381
    sources 376
    storage protein 380
    stores 378, 421
    supplementation 383
    therapy
        oral 383
        parenteral 384
Irrigation, arthroscopic 758
Irritability 89, 121, 176, 226, 382, 658, 916, 1038
Ischemia
    mucosal 303
    myocardial 180
Ischemic stroke 491
    prevention of 491
    treatment of 491
Islet cell antibodies 611
Isoimmune hemolytic anemia 362
Isoniazid 127, 128, 130, 134
Isosexual precocity, peripheral 633
Isospora 223
Isotretinoin 988
Isovolumetric exchange transfusion 847
Itching, history of 352

J

Janeway lesion 158, 159
Janus kinase 390
    inhibitors, oral 1055
Jaundice 270, 274, 361, 362, 471, 665, 707, 827, 828, 838, 876, 882, 885, 923
    biochemical 838
    clinical 838
    onset of 837
    pathological 831, 834f
    physiological 909
    prolonged 620, 836, 839
        physiological 236, 622
    severe 833, 836

Jaw thrust 1117
Jerking eye, uncontrollable 983
Jitteriness 818, 827, 1117
    causes of 818
Joint
    capsule, early distension of 756
    congenital contracture of 1095
    contractions 1051
    deformity 759
        prevention of 757
    fluid
        analysis 756, 1051
        cultures 757
    hyperextensibility 1083
    inflammation 1045
    laxity 1093
    pain 456, 651
    radiograph of 1051
    space narrowing 1050
    stability of 868
    subluxation of 8
    swelling of 650
    symptoms 674
    tender 650
Jones criteria 1022
    revised 1021t
Joubert syndrome 279
Jugular venous
    pressure 68, 174
    pulsations 177
Juvenile idiopathic arthritis 176, 1042
    diagnosis of 1042

K

Kala-azar 773
Kallmann syndrome 580
Kanamycin 127, 129, 135
Kangaroo mother care 1117
Kaposi sarcoma 288
Kartagener's syndrome 56, 1117
Karyotype 10, 11, 581
Kawasaki disease 355
Kawasaki syndrome 312
Kayser-Fleischer ring 322, 324, 325f, 324
Keloid 871, 871f
Kenneth Jones diagnostic criteria 126, 127t
Keratitis 665, 666
    interstitial 665, 668

Keratoconjunctivitis 683
    benign asymptomatic 721
Keratoconus 21, 1118
Keratomalacia 927, 1118
Kernicterus 495, 840, 841, 843, 1118
    clinical
        classification of 843
        features of 841
        risk factors for 843b
        symptomatic levels for 843b
Kernig's sign 556, 1118
Ketamine 46
Ketoacidosis 612, 614
Ketoconazole 638
Ketonemia 613
Ketonuria 613
Kidney 863
    disease 693
    function 935
    injury, acute 1105
    rhabdoid tumor of 1011
    severity of 433
Kingella kingae 156, 732, 754
Kinyoun stain 110
Kiss-knee sign 746, 747
Klebsiella 102, 157, 233, 296, 302, 306, 468, 472, 754
    pneumoniae 91, 298
Klinefelter's syndrome 14, 15, 580, 631, 1115
Knee
    contralateral 1056
    joint 1017
    swelling of 333
Knee-chest position 193
Knock knees 935f, 1118
Knuckle, hyperpigmentation of 1038, 1038f
Koch's screen 1049
Kocher-Debré-Sémélaigne syndrome 621
Koebner phenomenon 1047
Koilonychia 379, 1118
Koplik's spots 719, 719f, 720, 1118
Korotkoff sound 179
Kramer's criteria 833, 833t
Kupffer cells 323
    enlarged 323
    hyperplasia, diffuse 272
Kussmaul breathing 1118
Kwashiorkor 457, 919, 920
    onset of 920
Kyphosis 932, 933, 1118
Kyphotic gibbus 568

L

Labia 874
Labyrinthitis 91
Lactate dehydrogenase 81, 510, 512, 711, 972, 1035, 1112
    elevations of 406
Lactic acid concentration 757
Lactobacillus rhamnosus 222
Ladd's bands 1119
Lamivudine 695
Lamotrigine 521, 523
    blocks voltage 522
    dose 523t
Landau-Kleffner syndrome 524
Langerhans cell histiocytosis 604
Laparoscopy, diagnostic 234
Larva migrans 1118
Larval granulomatosis 1001
Laryngeal diphtheria 75
Laryngeal mask, use of 899
Laryngeal stenosis 892, 905
Laryngeal swab cultures 790
Laryngomalacia 892
Laryngoscope blade size 807
Laryngotracheobronchoscopy 265
Laryngotracheoesophageal clefts 315
L-asparaginase 975
Latex particle agglutination kits 558, 559
Laurence-Moon-Biedl syndrome 912, 1118
Lead poisoning 382
Leak urine 568
Leakiness 452
Lecithin 888, 895
Leflunomide 1052
Left ventricular outflow obstruction 143
Left-to-right shunt 105, 145, 199, 202
Legg-Perthes syndrome 1118
Legionella 353
Legs 664
    length discrepancy 1063
    long bones of 933
    swelling of 886
    ulcer, chronic 411
    valgus deformities of 930
    varus deformities of 930
Leiomyomas 288, 289
Lemierre's disease 700

Lennox-Gastaut syndrome 519, 523, 1118
Lens dislocation 1083
Lentivirus genus 687
Leprae 1068
Lepromatous leprosy 1072
Lepromin test 1076, 1118
Leprosy 1067, 1075, 1079
    cardinal signs of 1071
    classic manifestations of 1071
    indeterminate 1071
Leptin 910
Leptospirosis 275, 676, 773
Lesions 1023, 1073
    active 1072
    cutaneous 1073, 1073f
Lethargy 121, 176, 471, 496, 614, 620, 658
Leukemia 5, 125, 289, 603, 724, 964, 965, 991, 1012
    acute 943
        lymphatic 965, 975, 978
        lymphoblastic 967
        myeloid 965, 976
    chronic myeloid 965
    congenital 966f
    cutis 970
    juvenile myelomonocytic 965
    lymphoblastic 959
Leukemic cell infiltration 968
Leukocorea 1001f
Leukocyte 474, 1051
    count 598
    detection of 474
    esterase 474
    monitoring of 307
Leukocytoclastic vasculitis 273, 353
Leukocytosis 80, 159, 160, 355, 445, 790
Leukodystrophy 502, 546
    metachromatic 546, 548, 1119
Leukoencephalitis 560
Leukomalacia, periventricular 883
Leukopenia 658, 659, 720, 781, 1046
    infections secondary 968
Leukotriene modifiers 50
Leuprolide acetate 638
Levamisole 462
Levodopa 506
Levothyroxine 625, 626
    initial dose of 625t

Leydig cell 16
    agenesis 582
    hyperplasia 638
Li-Fraumeni syndrome 991, 992
Ligaments, hyperextensibility of 1096
Light spectrum 845
Limb
    deficiency 1100
    movements 819
    saving surgery 996
    splinting of 739
    tonic postures of 816
Limping 1063
Lipids 910
Lipodystrophy 693
Lipoma 866
    tufts of 546
Lips, bluish color of 186
Listeria 562
    monocytogenes 157, 552
    meningitis 563
Liver 322, 378, 863, 986
    abscess 294, 295
        solitary 298
    biopsy 421
    cell damage 273
    cryptogenic 296
    disease
        chronic 342
        develops features of 324
    enzymes 923
        mild elevation of 773
    failure 828
    function 935
        test 270, 297, 654, 659, 781, 916, 924, 971, 985, 1010, 1048, 1051
    hemosiderosis 417
    inflammation of 691
    injury 914
Lobaplatin 1014
Lobar pneumonia 98
Local anesthesia, inadvertent use of 815
Lockjaw 763
Loeffler's syndrome 1118
Lomefloxacin 135
Long-acting inhaled
    anticholinergics 51
    beta-agonists 48, 49
Long-chain polyunsaturated fatty acids 926
Lorazepam 821, 823

Lorber criteria 1118
Lordosis 1119
Louder pulmonary murmurs 145
Louder tricuspid murmurs 145
Low platelet count 659
Lowe syndrome 1119
Lower esophageal sphincter 259
Lower extremity paraparesis 570
Lower limb, scissoring of 497f
Lucey-Driscoll syndrome 837
Lucio's phenomenon 1075
Lujan syndrome 1087
Lumbar
    lordosis 935, 1063
    puncture 520, 530, 548, 820, 821
Lumboperitoneal shunts 549
Luminal obstruction leads 227
Lumirubin 845
Lung
    abscess 105, 299
    buds 247
    development 888
    disease 402, 503
        chronic 64, 411, 897
        diffuse interstitial 56
    entrapment 83
    fetal 799
    function 61, 901
        test 894t
    low compliance of 902
    malformation 894
    maturation, postnatal 891
    tissue, inflammation of 98
    ultrasound of 895
Lupus erythematosus 1046
Luschka foramina 542
Luteinizing hormone 637
    releasing hormone 637
Lyme disease 560, 1027, 1051
Lymph node 111, 132, 681, 956
    calcification 124
    distant 982, 986
    regional 986
    retroperitoneal 956
    swelling of 700
    tuberculous 791
Lymphadenitis, tuberculous 115, 131
Lymphadenopathy 121, 357, 666, 717, 786, 969, 999, 1047, 1048
    generalized 666, 689, 701, 968, 971

Lymphangiectasia, pulmonary 896
Lymphatic hypoplasia leads 55
Lymphedema, congenital 21
Lymphocyte 744, 955
    atypical 701, 702
    benign 957
    depletion 957
    infections of 698
    numbers of 689
    predominant 957
Lymphocytosis 791
Lymphohistiocytosis, hemophagocytic 700
Lymphoid tissue 718
    gut-associated 228
Lymphoma 288, 289, 368, 949, 951, 955, 972
Lymphopenia 721, 724
Lymphoproliferative disorders 700
Lymphoreticular malignancies 1108
Lymphosarcoma 986
Lysine residues 1092

M

MacEwen's sign 541, 545, 1119
Macroglossia 620, 1008
Macrolides 105, 135, 793
Macroorchidism 629
Macrophage
    activation syndrome 1048, 1050
    hemophagocytosis 1048
Macrosomia 1008
Maculopapular rashes 650, 651, 674, 697, 720 f
Madarosis 1070
Magendie foramina 542
Magnesium 529
    serum lactate 821
    sulfate 41, 44, 823
Magnetic resonance cholangiopancreatography 313
Magnetic resonance imaging 399, 490, 520, 547, 581, 607, 736, 756, 821, 943, 951, 995, 1038, 1064
Main pulmonary artery 199
Major histocompatibility complex 1036, 1042

Malabsorption syndrome 457, 922, 930
Malaise 699
Malaria 122, 676, 705, 704, 706, 707, 709, 711, 712
    cerebral 706, 706f, 708, 714
    congenital 709
    differential diagnosis of 711
    retinopathy 708
Malarial disease, acute 707
Malarial parasite, life cycle of 705
Male phenotype, development of 577
Malformations
    congenital 38, 501
    extrarenal 454
Malignancy 122, 175, 368, 700, 727, 981
    hematologic 972
    risk of 645
Malignant cells 1000
Malignant neoplasm, second 963
Malnutrition 224, 922
    acute 917
    clinical signs of 922 t
    precipitation of 224
    severe 447
        acute 921
Malpresentation 800
Malrotation 6, 248, 306, 1119
Mammalian tissues 1020
Manganese deficiency 924
Mannitol 61, 563
Manometry 264
Mantoux reaction 1119
Mantoux test 55, 120, 124, 125, 127, 457, 552, 560, 687, 786
Maple syrup urine disease 546, 821
Marasmus 919, 1119
    nutritional 919
Marfan's syndrome 1082, 1083, 1119
    diagnosis of 1083
Mask 805
Mast cell 34
    stabilizers 50
Mastoiditis, acute 91
Maternal antenatal test 9
Maturation, skeletal 623
Mature schizonts 709
Maximal cardiac impulse 861
McBurney's point 229, 1119

McCune-Albright syndrome 595, 596, 631, 930, 1109, 1119
Mean corpuscular hemoglobin 374, 418, 490
    concentration 358, 374, 418
Mean corpuscular volume 358, 374, 418, 490
Measles 716, 718, 719, 721
    croup 75
    infection, modified 720
    mumps-rubella vaccine 660
    precipitate acute malnutrition 917
    vaccine 724
    virus 717
Mechanical ventilation 900
    indications of 45
    modes of 900
Mechlorethamine 960
Meckel's diverticulum 248, 288, 289, 292, 1119
Meconium aspiration 894
    syndrome 892, 895
Meconium plug syndrome 306
Mediastinal mass 958
Mediastinum, posterior 980, 982
Medium-chain triglyceride 926
Medroxyprogesterone acetate 638
Mefloquine 713, 714
Megakaryocytic cytopenia 368
Megalencephaly 548
Megalocornea 1119
Megaloencephaly 1119
Meiotic nondisjunction 4, 15
Meissner's plexuses 279
Melanocortin-4 receptor deficiency 910
Melanocyte stimulating hormone 911
Melena 347, 942
Melphalan 1003
Membrane, prolonged rupture of 553, 889
Membranoproliferative 432
    glomerulonephritis 432
Meningeal infection 563
Meningeal irritation 556
    signs 557
Meningeal purulent 554
Meningeal signs 708
Meningism 559
Meningitis 175, 487, 551, 561-563, 711, 773, 815
    acute bacterial 553, 558, 558 t
    aseptic 559, 699, 748

bacterial 552, 553, 558, 559
basal 603
cryptococcal 560
gram-negative bacterial 561
meningococcal 563
pneumococcal 563, 564
recurrent 555
signs of 118
streptococcal 563, 564
symptoms of 118
treatment of 561t
tuberculous 119, 560, 630
Meningoceles 282, 569, 865
Meningococcemia 355, 1119
Meningococcus 562
purpuric rash of 557f
Meningoencephalomyelitis 729
Meningomyelocele 565, 566, 566f, 567f
fetal 549
Menorrhagia 383
Menstrual period 874
Mental
depression 678
retardation 5, 17, 500, 560, 666, 1032, 1119
Mercaptopurine 975
Meropenem 561
Merozoites 705
release of 707
Mesentery obstructs venous return, constriction of 289
Metabolic disorders 815, 875
evidence of 501
Metabolic dysfunction 272
Metabolism, inborn errors of 502, 820
Metaiodobenzylguanidine 987
Metalloporphyrins 846
Metallothionein 322
Metaphysis 1120
Metastatic disease 950, 984, 988
Metastatic round-cell tumors 951
Metered dose inhaler 41, 51
Metformin 914
Methemoglobinemia 418, 1120
congenital 389
Methotrexate 961, 975, 1038, 1052, 1053, 1055
effects of 1054
monotherapy, failure of 1054
risk of 1039
Methylidobenzylguanidine 985

Methylprednisolone 41, 180
Meticulous supportive care 765
Metolazone 464
Metronidazole 61, 233, 235, 765
Microalbuminemia 1120
Microangiopathy, thrombotic 440
Microcephaly 497f
Microcytic hypochromic anemia, diagnosis of 382
Microcytosis 418
Microinfarcts 396
Microorchidism normal external genitalia 16
Micropenis 579, 580
causes of 580
Microvascular injury 442
Midazolam 822, 823
Midbrain 489
Middle ear, inflammation of 89
Midfoot varus 1102
Migration inhibitory factor pathways 578
Mild calf atrophy 1102
Miliary nodules 124
Milkmaid sign 1120
Miller Fisher syndrome 534
Mineralocorticoids 592
Minimal bone tissue 949
Minimally invasive surfactant therapy 900
Minocycline 1078
Mitogen-activated protein kinase pathways, induction of 769
Mitral annulus, dilatation of 1023
Mitral atresia 143
Mitral regurgitation 164, 1023
Mitral valve 147, 1020
prolapse 155, 1083, 1084, 1087
Molecular biology 999
Molluscum contagiosum 1120
Mongolian spots 870f, 1120
Mongoloid facies 1120
Monitor arterial oxygen saturation 69
Monoclonal antibodies 1076
Monocyte chemoattractant protein 1037
Monoiodotyrosine 619
Monomorphic cells, sheets of 951
Mononucleosis 697
Monro foramen 547
Moon face 597, 1120

Moraxella catarrhalis 99
Morbillivirus genus 717
Morning stiffness 1051
Moro's reflex 812, 843, 869, 1120
Morphine 193, 408
sulfate 193
Morphology 966
Mosaicism 5, 15
Moth-eaten appearance, bilateral 664
Motilin receptor agonist 268
Motor deficits 557, 560
Motor nerve conduction velocities 537
Motor neuropathy, acute 534
Mouth 342, 858
breathing 27, 30
Movement
abnormal 504
disorder 1025
Moxifloxacin 129, 1078
Mucocutaneous lesions 664, 666
Mucolytics 61
Mucopolysaccharidoses 546
Mucosal irritation, propellant-induced 52
Mucous membrane 389, 854
Muffled heard sound 179
Mulberry molars 666, 1120
Mullerian inhibitory substance 1120
Müllerian system, regression of 580
Multiagent chemotherapy 952, 973
Multicystic kidney 986, 1012
Multifocal myoclonic movements 818
Multinucleated giant cells infiltrate 718
Multiple endocrine neoplasm 2 syndrome 279
Multiple organ defects 312
Multiple serious bacterial infections 691
Multiple sex chromosome aneuploidies 15
Multisystem disseminated disease 754
Mumps 228, 612, 725-727, 754
complications of 727
control of 729
disease 727
infection, diagnosis of 728

Neuroblastoma 279, 949, 951, 979, 982, 983, 988, 1012
 benign counterpart of 981
 cells 981
 characteristics of 980
 higher incidence of 981
 incidence of 980
 signs of 983
 staging of 985
 symptoms of 983
 tumors 982
Neurocutaneous syndrome 815
Neurodevelopmental impairment 307, 308
Neuroenteric cells, migration of 280
Neurofibroma 288, 289
Neurofibromatosis 279, 930, 1121
Neurogenic bladder, management of 571
Neurohypophysis 602
Neurologic complications 400, 699, 782
Neurologic deficits 560
Neurologic disease 325
Neurologic dysfunction 447
Neurologic examination 490, 498
Neurologic sequelae 524
Neurologic signs, interpretation of 866
Neuronal migration defects 630
Neuronal necrosis 841
Neurons 603, 910
 important sets of 910
Neuropathy 744, 1080
 peripheral 660
Neuropeptide
 numerous 911
 Y neurons 910
Neurosurgery 505
Neurosyphilis
 congenital 662
 diagnosis of 667
Neurotuberculosis 131
Neutralization test 675
Neutropenia 462, 1121
Neutrophil infiltration 353, 563
Neutrophilic leukocytosis 1047
Nevirapine 695
Niikawa-Kuroki syndrome 604
Nikolsky's sign 1121
Nissen fundoplication 268, 1121
Nitrazepam 521
Nitric oxide 251, 395
 activity of 238
Nitrites 474

Nitrofurantoin 478, 480
Nitrogen 962
Nizatidine 267
Nocardia israelli 157
Nocturia 614
Nocturnal symptoms, control of 50
Nodular sclerosis 955, 957
Nodules
 multiple 1009
 subcutaneous 1024
Noisy respiration 97
Nonbacterial thrombotic endocarditis, formation of 155
Nongastrointestinal signs 304
Non-Hodgkin's disease 959, 1121
Non-Hodgkin's lymphoma 951
Nonimmune hydrops 663
Noninvasive transcutaneous bilirubin 838
Nonnucleoside reverse transcriptase inhibitors 694
Nonspecific acute-phase reactants 160
Nonspecific tuberculous sensitivity, prevalence of 124
Nonsteroidal anti-inflammatory agents 50, 180, 182
 drugs 176, 356, 1022, 1052, 1053, 1079
Nonthrombocytopenic palpable purpura 353
Noonan syndrome 1121
Norepinephrine 984
Norfloxacin 135
Normetanephrine 984
Normocytes 1121
Norovirus 302
Nose 858
Nuchal rigidity 746, 747
Nuclear scintigraphy 264
Nucleic acid tests 126, 691
Nucleoside reverse transcriptase inhibitors 694
Nutrition 224, 504, 880, 907
Nutritional deficiencies 920

O

Obesity 465, 909, 911*f*, 912, 913
 endogenous 912
 exogenous 912

Obstruction 388
 bronchial 106, 114
 severe 189
 stimulates growth 150
 ureteral 609
Obstructive sleep apnea 8, 503, 884, 1121
Obturator internus signs 230
Occipital paroxysms 524
Occlusions, arterial 488
Occupational therapy 13
Ocular anomaly 656
Ocular disease, bilateral 999
Ocular system 1085
Ofloxacin 135, 1078
Oligoarthritis 1051, 1053
Oligoarticular juvenile idiopathic arthritis 1045
Oliguria 434, 435, 444, 456
Olpadronate, oral 1097
Olympian brow 1121
Omeprazole 267
Omphalocele 1008
Oocyte 19
Oophoritis 729
Oozing skin, development of 429
Open heart surgery 155
Open neural tube defects 566, 570
 diagnosis of 568
Ophthalmic artery 1004
Opiate antagonists 603
Opioids 401
Opisthotonus 763
Opsoclonus-myoclonus-ataxia syndrome 983
Opsomyoclonus 1121
Optic
 atrophy 1121
 glioma 602, 633
 nerve hypoplasia 602
 neuritis 1121
Oral cavity, tuberculosis of 116
Oral feeding 242
Oral glucose tolerance test 613
Oral hairy leukoplakia 700
 lesions of 702
Oral polio vaccine 196
Oral rehydration
 salt 923
  composition of 216
  limitations of 217
 solution 216, 217, 925
  dose of 218
 therapy 216

Parosteal osteogenic sarcoma 993
Parotitis 689
Parrot paralysis 664
Partial thromboplastin time 334, 337, 653
Parvovirus 175, 353, 754
   B19 infection 358, 360
Pasireotide 600
Pasteurella multocida 55
Patau syndrome 1122
Patchy atelectasis 791
Patent ductus arteriosus 6, 143, 151, 154, 158, 172, 248, 658, 875, 876
   classical triad 655
   diagnosis of 168, 169
Paterson-Kelly syndrome 379
Pathogenesis, immune mediated 1019
Pathogens, bacterial 87, 88
Patulous anal sphincter 568
Paucibacillary disease, single lesion 1078
Paucibacillary leprosy 1078
Paul-Bunnel-Davidsohn test 701
Pavlik harness 1065
Peak expiratory flow measurement 36
   rate 39
Pectus
   carinatum 933*f*
   excavatum 1122
Pedal pitting edema 174
Pediatric appendicitis score 232, 232*t*
Pefloxacin 135
Pel-Ebstein fever 1122
Pelkan spur 943
Pelvic kidney 21
Pelvic muscles, weakness of 510
Pemphigus 1122
Penciclovir 703
Pendred syndrome 618, 625, 1122
Penicillamine 328
Penicillin 61, 83, 163, 669, 738, 1028, 1029
   G 765, 1030
      benzathine 1028
Penis 912
Penoscrotal hypospadias 644*f*
Peptide hormone 378
Peptostreptococcus 29
Percutaneous drainage 299

Percutaneous umbilical blood sampling 840
Pericardial effusion 175-177, 181, 623, 956
   causes of 177
   hemodynamic effects of 177
Pericardial fluid 177
   gradual accumulation of 177
   testing of 181
Pericardial inflammation 176, 177
   manifestation of 177
Pericardial rub 1024
Pericardial sac 178
Pericardial window 181
Pericardiocentesis 181
Pericarditis 173, 175, 1047, 1052, 1053
   acute 174
   bacterial 175, 180
   causes of 180
   chest pain of 178
   infectious 176
   noninfectious 176
   purulent 175, 176, 180
   symptom of 178
   tuberculous 176
   viral etiologies of 181
Pericardium 176
   inflammation of 175
Perimembranous ventricular septal defects, nonsurgical closure of 201
Periodic acid–Schiff reaction 949
Periosteal osteogenic sarcoma 993
Periostitis 665, 667
Peripheral blood 701
   mononuclear cells 701
   parasitemia, degree of 710
   smear 358, 393, 662, 710, 917
Peripheral circulation 503
Peripheral destruction 368
Peripheral nerves 1069, 1074, 1075
   palpation of 1075
Peripheral smear 406, 709
Peritoneal dialysis 447
Peritoneal leukocyte counts 454
Peritonitis 116, 299, 456, 663
   tuberculous 116
Perkins line 1064
Perlman syndrome 1008

Permanent renal damage, risk factors for 481
Permissive hypercapnia, concept of 879
Peroxidase 375
Persistent asthma
   mild 47
   mild-to-moderate 48
   moderate 48
Pertactin 787
   deficient strains 786
Perthes disease 1064
Pertussis 786, 787, 789, 1122
   clinical 792
   diagnosis of 791
   infection 104
   toxin 787
   vaccine 794
Petechiae 872, 920, 969
Petechial rash 366*f*, 674
Peutz–Jeghers syndrome 289, 633, 634
Peyer's patches 289, 770
Phakomatoses 1123
Pharmacotherapy 914
Pharyngitis 433, 1027
   acute 1029
   exudative 701
   streptococcal 1020
Phenobarbital 347
Phenobarbitone 521, 822, 824, 846
Phenytoin 521, 603, 822
Pheochromocytoma 986
Pheumocystis jirovecii pneumonia 689
Phimosis 1123
Phlebotomy 390, 391
Phosphate 929
   ion 520
Phosphocreatinine 815
Phosphodiesterase, inhibition of 50
Phosphorus 529, 936
   deficiency 930
   homeostasis 882
Photocoagulation 1003, 1004
Photoisomerization 845
Photooxidation 845
Photophobia 651
Phototherapy 844
   contradictions of 846
   indications of 844
   intensive 844

side effects of 845
technique of 845
Physical sequelae 791
Physical therapy 13
Physiotherapy, role of 505
Pica 379, 1123
Pierre Robin syndrome 1123
Pigeon chest 932
Pilocarpine iontophoresis 60
Pilonidal sinus 1123
Pinealoma 602, 604
Piroxicam 1053
Pituitary dysfunction 580
Plantar
    fasciitis 1123
    surface 852
Plaques 1074
Plasma 678
    17-hydroxyprogesterone 627
    androgen 589
    androsterone 627
    borne infections 342
    chromatography of 502
    cortisol 584
        concentrations 598
    dehydroepiandrosterone
        sulphate 627
    glucose 525
    infusion 446
    testosterone 584
    therapy 447
    transfusion 340
Plasmapheresis 372, 446, 538
Plasmodium 376, 706
    falciparum 705
    infection 711
    malaria 432
    specific antigens 710
Platelet
    activating factor 34
    count 322, 358, 387
    function 346
Platybasia 1123
Platynychia 379
Pleocytosis 659, 666
Pleomorphic rashes 777*f*
Plethora 969
Pleural effusion 181, 676, 956
    tuberculous 114
Pleuritis 1047
Plumbism 382, 943, 1123
Plummer–Vinson syndrome 379
Pneumatocele 1123
Pneumatosis intestinalis 308

Pneumococcal conjugate
    vaccine 96
Pneumococcus 402, 453, 562, 564
Pneumocystis carinii
    pneumonia 689
Pneumomediastinum 46
Pneumonia 97, 98, 99*t*, 102, 104,
    106, 175, 663, 781, 791,
    894, 915
    acute lobar 104
    alba 665
    atypical 98
    bacterial 68, 99, 773, 791
    causes of 98
    congenital 249, 892, 896
    diagnosis of 103, 104
    eosinophilic 107
    interstitial 98, 791
    optimum antimicrobial
        management of 104
    pneumococcal 101
    recurrent 98, 1096
    right upper lobe 104
    severe 55, 102
    staphylococcal 102, 106
    upper lobe 104
    viral 99, 100
    worsening 81
Pneumonitis 98
    hypersensitivity 38, 107
    interstitial 656
    syphilitic 665
Pneumothorax 46, 248, 791,
    894, 903
Pneumovirus 65
Podocytes
    functional 452
    role of 451
Poikilocytosis 1123
Poliomyelitis 742, 743
    abortive 745, 748
    neuropathy of 744
    nonparalytic 746, 748
    paralytic 746, 748
Polioviruses 744
Polyangiitis 107
Polyarteritis nodosa 355
Polyarthritis 1051, 1053
    migratory 1022
Polyarticular juvenile idiopathic
    arthritis 1046
    treatment of 1054
Polyclonal B-cell stimulation 689
Polycystic kidney disease 605, 658

Polycythemia 386-389, 827
    acquired 388, 389
    congenital 388, 389
    familial 388
    hyperviscosity 815
    true 390
Polydactyly 865*f*
Polydipsia 614
Polyhydramnios 256, 1123
Polymerase chain reaction 64,
    159, 405, 512, 520, 559,
    651, 689, 702, 711, 791,
    951, 1077
    viral 274
Polymorphonuclear leukocyte 81,
    744, 764
    infiltration 431
    transmigration of 769
Polymorphonuclear reactants
    1025
Polymyositis 1037
Polyneuritis 513
Polyneuropathy 560
    acute inflammatory
        demyelinating 534
Polyp, intestinal 288, 289
Polyphagia 614
Polyradiculoneuropathy,
    chronic inflammatory
    demyelinating 536
Polytherapy 522
Polyuria 613, 614
    diagnosis of 613
    differential diagnosis of 613
Pompe disease 1123
Ponseti treatment method 1103
Poor feeding 70, 828
Porencephaly 496
Portal vein 296
Port-wine stains 870*f*, 1123
Positive end-expiratory
    pressure 900
Positive ventilation devices, types
    of 805*t*
Positive-pressure ventilation 877
Positron emission tomography
    519, 520, 959
Postload glucose 613
Postlung transplantation 56
Post-measles stage 720
Postpericardiotomy syndrome
    175, 176, 181
Postpolio syndrome 746

Posttransplant lymphoproliferative disease 288, 700
Potassium 217, 821, 923
    concentrations 598
Potent anti-inflammatory agents 49
Pott's shunt 194
Potter's facies 1123
Prader-Willi syndrome 10, 500, 580, 912, 913, 1123
Prechemotherapy biopsy 985
Precocious puberty 582, 591, 627, 628, 629*f*, 632
    gonadotropin-dependent 629
    gonadotropin-independent 629, 632
    idiopathic central 630
    peripheral 629, 631
    true 628*f*
Prednisolone 41, 131, 458, 459, 523, 702, 960, 962
    dose of 1052
    tapering doses of 458
Prednisone 180, 370, 961, 975
    alternate-day dosing of 459
Preeclampsia 441
Pregnancy 1088
    ectopic 60
Prematurity
    apnea of 884
    problems of 874
    retinopathy of 876, 1001, 1003
    signs of 874
Prenatal androgen excess 584
Prenephrectomy chemotherapy 1012
    absolute indications for 1013
Presacral anomaly 282
Prevotella 29
Priapism 403, 406
    acute 404
    chronic 404
Primaquine 712
Primordial neural crest cells 981
Probiotics 223
Procaine penicillin G 668
Procarbazine 960-962
Prodromal signs 346
Progesterone therapy 23
Progressive pulmonary disease 131
Proguanil 713
Prokinetic agents 268

Prominent costochondral junction 942
Promyelocytic granules 970
Proopiomelanocortin 910
Prophylactic antibiotics 480
    indications of 480
Prophylactic penicillin 408
    therapy 424
Prophylactic therapy 343
Prophylaxis 155, 531, 714
    postexposure 784
    secondary 1030*t*
Propranolol 193, 1088
Proptosis 982, 1124
Prostaglandin 34, 152
Prostate 581
Prosthetic device dysfunction 160
Protease inhibitors 694
Protein 346, 926
    acute phase 1105
    concentration 666
        serum lactate 81
    energy malnutrition 916
        classification of 918
    fibrillin 1083
    loss, heavy 454
    matrix 929
    viral nonstructural 672
Proteinuria 160, 434, 457, 662, 773
    nephrotic range 453
Proteus 468, 469, 472
    vulgaris 478
Prothrombin
    active 333
    time 337, 653
Protienuria 456
Proximal muscle weakness 1038
Prune juice 503
Pseudoaneurysm 203
Pseudocryptorchidism 644
Pseudohermaphroditism 589
    female 578, 586
    male 578, 579, 586
Pseudohypertrophy 510, 1112
Pseudohypoparathyroidism 912, 913
Pseudomonas 157, 296, 302, 469, 472, 476, 478, 479, 552, 738
    aeruginosa 60, 91, 233, 478, 553, 733
    organisms 734
Pseudoparalysis 666, 734, 755, 942

Pseudopuberty, precocious 629
Psoas 230
Psoriatic arthritis 1046
Psychiatric disorders 8
Psychogenic polydipsia 613
Psychomotor changes 920
Psychosomatic symptoms 909
Ptosis, unilateral 983
Pubertal progression 636
Pubertal status, assessment of 636
Puberty 21, 624, 1124
    central precocious 629, 630
    delayed 17, 22, 326
    precocious 582, 591, 627, 628, 629*f*, 632
    pseudoprecocious 638
Pubic hair 588, 627
Pubic tubercle 642
Pulmonary artery 190, 656
    balloon dilation of 194
    pressure 190
Pulmonary dysfunction 963
Pulmonary function tests 36, 58
Pulmonary valve 1020
    stenosis 190
Pulmonary vascular obstructive disease 198
Pulmonic valve 145
Pulse
    oximetry 69, 804
    rate 109
Pulsus paradoxus 35, 39, 178, 1124
Puncture wounds 733
Pure bulbar poliomyelitis, management of 749
Purpura 366*f*, 658
Pus 297
    anerobic culture examination of 764
Pyelography, antravenous 476
Pyelonephritis 472, 1012
    acute 471
    chronic 605
Pyloric duplication 241
Pyloric mucosa 238
Pyloric stenosis 6, 263, 591
    atypical 263
    congenital 316
    hereditary component of 238
    incidence of 237
Pyloric wall thickness 241

Pyloromyotomy, extramucosal 242
Pyoderma 732
Pyogenic arthritis 758
    source of 752
Pyogenic liver abscess 295
    development of 295
Pyrazinamide 115, 127, 128, 130
Pyridoxal dependency disorders 819
Pyridoxine 819
    dependency 815, 821, 823
Pyrogenic exotoxins 1020
Pyuria 473, 474

Q

Q fever 157
QRS complex, low-voltage 179
Quadriparesis 560
Quadriplegia 503
    spastic 498, 501
Quantitative buff coat test 710
Quinidine 353
    potential cardiac toxicity of 712
Quinine 712, 713
Quinolones 127, 135

R

Racecadotril 224
Racemic epinephrine 70, 76
Rachitic rosary 935, 1124
Radial pulses 861
Radial streak 1124
Radiation
    abdominal 1012
    ionizing 967
    therapy 960
        high-dose 961
        principles of 960, 1013
Radioactive iodine 623
Radiography, conventional 984
Radioimmunoassay testing 123
Radioiodine
    administration 619
    therapy 619
Radionuclide
    bone
        imaging 737
        scan 1002
    studies 599
Radiotherapy 988, 996, 1003, 1012, 1013

Railroad calcification 1124
Ramstedt's operation 1124
Random plasma glucose concentration 613
Ranitidine 267
Ranula 1124
Rapid antigen detection test 103
Rapid diagnostic tests 558, 710
Rashes 778f
Rasmussen's encephalitis 524
Reactive enzyme immunoassay 692
Rectal biopsy 279
Rectal examination 283
Rectal manometry 279
Rectal prolapse 863f
Red blood cell 377, 390, 429, 436, 972, 1006
    membrane 395
    transfusion 362, 409
Red cell
    distribution width 380
    indices 381
    precursor of 390
    size distribution width 381
Red reflex 1124
Reddish skin lesions 1075
Reed-Sternberg cells 959, 1116, 1124
Reflexes 813, 850, 868, 869
Reflux 261
    esophageal manifestations of 259
    esophagitis 262
Refsum disease 1124
Regurgitation 267, 876
    aortic 164, 1084
    jet length 1023
    peak velocity 1023
Rehabilitation 505, 922
    process of 505
Reifenstein syndrome 582
Relapsing malaria, treatment of 714
Renal agenesis 22
Renal anomalies 22, 248
Renal biopsy 436, 438, 445, 458, 460
    indications of 436b, 457
Renal disease 356, 395, 605
Renal disorders 613
Renal dysfunction, indicative of 445
Renal examination 863

Renal failure 160, 312, 328, 411, 709, 828
    acute 433, 434, 709, 1078
    chronic 572
Renal function 435, 476
Renal insufficiency 444
Renal losses 930
Renal parenchyma 472
    infection 469
Renal system 427
Renal tubular acidosis 328, 1124
Replacement therapy 23
Respiratory cycle 178
Respiratory disease 854
Respiratory distress 247, 248, 386, 675, 708, 886, 892, 969
    causes of 892
    grading of severity of 893t
    syndrome 886, 894, 894t, 895
        complications of 905
Respiratory insufficiency 794
Respiratory problems 6
Respiratory rate 39, 70, 893, 902
Respiratory support 878
Respiratory syncytial virus 64, 67, 99, 690
    infection 65, 66
Respiratory system 25, 73, 315, 786, 873, 874, 917
Respiratory tract infection 197
    lower 209
    recurrent 58, 932
    upper 34, 68, 288, 676, 732, 751
Respiratory viruses 68
Resuscitation 877, 922
    indications of 803
    phases of 924
    procedure: 809
Reticulocytes 445
Reticulocytosis 362, 363
Reticuloendothelial system 718, 769
    blockade of 372
Reticulosis 362
Retinal cell 999
Retinal damage 411, 846
Retinal detachment 1002, 1003, 1124
Retinal folds, congenital 1001
Retinal whitening 708
Retinitis pigmentosa 1124
Retinoblastoma 998, 999
    differential diagnosis of 1001

gene 1000
hereditary form of 999
intraocular 1002, 1003
radiation field 991
tumor development 999
Retinoic acid 988
receptor A 976
Retinopathy 395, 658
Retraction 67, 893
apnea 70
pockets 90
Retrobulbar tissue 982
Reye's syndrome 1124
Rh
blood types 837
compatibility 828
immunization 827
isoimmunization 839, 847
Rhabdomyosarcoma 949, 951, 981, 1124
Rhagades 664
Rheumatic diseases 1015
Rheumatic fever 122, 175, 184, 1021, 1022, 1030, 1051
attack of 1022
incidence of 1029
laboratory diagnosis of 1026
Rheumatoid 56
arthritis 175, 757, 972
juvenile 1027, 1041, 1043
factor 1125
nodules, occasional
development of 1046
Rhinitis 30, 86, 663
Rhizomelia 1095
Rhizotomy
procedure 503
selective dorsal 505
Rhonchi crepitation 314
Ribavirin 70, 724
Ribonucleic acid 687
paramyxovirus 718
virus, Single-stranded 271
Ribonucleotide reductase 375
Ribs, crowding of 81
Rich's foci 111
Rickets 928, 929, 933f, 1087
advanced 932
causes of 930b
hypophosphatemic 938
nonnutritional 938
pathology of 931
rosary 932f
tumor-induced 930

X-linked hypophosphatemic 930
Ridley-Jopling scale 1070
Rifabutin 135
Rifampicin 127, 128, 130, 134, 1078
derivatives 135
prophylaxis 77
susceptible 134
Rifamycin 127
Rifapentine 135, 1078
Right bundle branch block 192
Right middle lobe syndrome 55, 56
Right ventricular outflow
tract 145
Rigid bronchoscopy 318
Rigors 471, 473
Riley–day syndrome 1125
Ringer's lactate 923
Risedronate 1097
Risus sardonicus 763, 1125
Rituximab 462, 960, 1040
Robinow syndrome 580
Rolandic epilepsy 524
Rooting reflex 869
Roseola infantum 1125
Rotavirus
diarrhea 224
immunization 224
Roux-en-Y gastric bypass 915
Rovsing sign 230
Rubella 657, 667
consequences of 656
infection 655
live vaccines 754
panencephalitis, progressive 657
vaccination 660
Rubivirus 654
Rubulavirus 726
Russel-Silver syndrome 1109
Ruxolitinib 1055

S

Saber shins 666
Saber tibia 666, 1125
Saccharomyces boulardii 222, 223
Sacral bone anomalies 282, 284
Saddle nose 1125
S-adenosylmethionine, synthesis of 566
Salbutamol 41
nebulizer solution 40

Salicylates
nor steroids 1028
saturation index 844
Saline filled catheter 548
Salmeterol 48
Salmon patch 871f, 1125
Salmonella 222, 223, 228, 302, 441, 691, 733, 769, 771, 772, 775
enterica serovariant typhi 768
hirschfeldii 768
induced filament formation 769
infections 770
paratyphi 768
pathogenicity islands 769
schottmuelleri 768
septicemia, recurrent 691
typhi 768, 769
Salpingitis, tuberculous 116
Salt wasting 586
diagnosis of 590
Sandifer's syndrome 262
Sarcoid 633
Sarcoidosis 56, 603
Sarcomere 1020
Sausage-shaped mass 290
Scanty cytoplasm 981
Schaumann disease 1125
Schizogony
erythrocytic 705
pre-erythrocytic 705
stages of 705
Schwann cells 981, 1069
Schwannian stroma 981
Scintigraphy 264, 624
Sclera, hyperemia of 389
Scleral icterus 397
Scleroderma 1051
Sclerosis, multiple 718
Scoliosis 21, 81, 503, 505, 932, 933, 1093, 1125
progressive 1087
Scorbutic rosary 1125
Screening tests 9, 349, 381
Scrotum 579f, 644, 864
Scurvy 939, 941, 972
Seborrheic dermatitis 684
Secrete inflammatory
cytokine 1042
Secretion theory 56
Secundum atrial septal defect 147
Sedation 800, 904

Seizures 7, 213, 471, 516, 518, 556, 765, 791, 813-815, 817, 818, 824, 828, 883
  activity 818
  complex
    febrile 528
    partial 518
  disappearance of 524
  disorder 516
    causes of 820
  early-onset of 824
  frequency of 520
  generalized 517, 518, 522
  myoclonic 518, 818
  neonatal 518, 812, 814
  nonepileptic forms of 823
  partial 516, 517, 522
  refractory 823
  simple
    febrile 528
    partial 517
  subtle 817
  tonic-clonic 517-519
  types 817
    triad of 519
Self-human leukocyte antigen 1043
Seminoma 643
Semisolid diet 926
Sensorineural deafness 657
Sensory
  axonal neuropathy 534
  deficits 498
  examination 868
  ganglion neurons, infections of 777
  stimulation of 502
Sepsis 828
  signs of 307
  treatment of 848
Septal defect, aortopulmonary 171
Septal dropout 146
Septal perforation 663
Septic arthritis 732, 735, 751-753, 773, 1064
  sequelae of 759
Septic screen 924
Septicemia 306, 659, 711, 876
  streptococcal 896
Septooptic dysplasia 580, 602
Sequestration crisis 404
Sequestrum 1125

Serologic tests 537, 668, 669, 676, 728, 772, 773
Serology 103, 721
Serratia 298
Serum 17-hydroxyprogesterone 637
Serum adrenocorticotropic hormone concentrations 598
Serum albumin 449
  level of 452
Serum calcium 418, 821, 935, 936
  level 820
Serum glucose level 823
Serum glutamic
  oxaloacetic transaminase 270, 321, 418, 654
  pyruvic transaminase 270, 275, 321, 418, 654, 917
Serum sodium 820
  levels 457
Setting sun sign 545, 545f
Severe protein-energy malnutrition 943
  dietary management of 924
Sex development, disorders of 642
Sexual precocity, classification of 629
Shah–Waardenburg syndrome 279
Sheehan syndrome 603
Shenton's line 1064
Shigella 222, 228, 441
  dysentery 222
Shigellosis 528
Shock 471, 709, 712
  septic 603
Shone complex 149
Short neck 20f
  syndromes 892
Sibutramine 914
Sickle cell 407f
  anemia 392, 393, 418, 733
  dactylitis, acute 406
  disease 393, 487
  nephropathy 605
  pain 398
  trait 396
Sickling
  cycles of 394
  test 407
Silver forking 1025
Silverman–Anderson score 893t

Simian crease 8, 8f, 1125
Simmonds' focus 111
Simon's foci 111
Single X chromosome 509
Single-carbon transfer reactions 566
Single-photon emission computed tomography 185, 520
Sinus
  formation 131, 132
  tracts, surgical removal of 739
Sinusitis 262
Skeletal infections, optimal treatment of 737
Skeletal phenotype, severe 1095
Skeletal system 1084
Skin 852
  abnormalities 870
  biopsy, full-thickness 1077
  changes 920
  color 853
  edema of 755
  involvement 1073
  large areas of 920
  lesions 354, 776, 1074
    evaluation of 1075
    hypopigmented 1075
  prick testing 37
  redness of 735
  small vessels of 353
  soft tissue
    redness of 755
    swelling of 755
  swelling of 735
  telangiectasia 992
  testing 37
  texture 853
  tuberculosis 117
Skin-to-skin contact 1069
Skull
  bossing of 932
  X-ray of 413
Sleep-disordered breathing 503
Slit-lamp examination 325
Slit-ventricle syndrome 550
Slurred speech 488
Smear examination 122
Smith-Lemli-Opitz syndrome 237, 279
Smooth muscle
  narrow, hyperplasia of 238
  tone 280
Sneezing 68, 720
Snoring 27, 30

Snuffles 663
Soave's endorectal
pull-through 284
Social behavior, abnormal 14
Sodium 821
benzoate 822
bicarbonate 193, 810
iodide symporter 618
serum 820
valproate 185, 519, 521
Soft tissue 735, 1000
edema of 755
involvement of 950
mass 311f
sarcomas 991
surgery 1104
Solubility test 407
Somatic cell 999
Sonography
abdominal 637
pelvic 637, 639
testicular 637
Sotos syndrome 546
Sparfloxacin 135
Spasmodic croup 74
Spasms 522, 523
seizures 817
Spasticity, reduction of 502
Specific chemotherapy,
indications of 130
Speech therapy 506
Sphenoid bone 982
Spherocytes 361, 363
Spherocytic red cell 359
Spherocytosis 361, 362
hereditary 357-359
typical manifestations of 360
Sphingomyelin 895
Spina bifida occulta 569
Spinal cord 983
anterior horn cells of 744
compression 982, 1034
lesions 502
Spinal muscular atrophy,
chronic 513
Spinal rigidity 746, 747
Spine 865
tumors of 865
Spirometry 36
Spironolactone 465
Spleen 863
removal 706
Splenectomy 362, 363,
371, 372, 423

guidelines for 363
indications of 363
Splenic rupture 700
Splenomegaly 159, 160, 360, 362,
665, 827, 965, 969, 1046,
1048
Spondylodiskitis 732
Spontaneous fetal demise,
incidence of 252
Spotty paralysis 747
Spur 1125
Sputum 54
Squamous epithelium 316
Stabilization, steps of 877
Stalk, transection of 603
Standard population-based
growth charts 853
Staphylococcal
pneumonia 102
treatment of 106
skin scalded syndrome 1121
Staphylococci 102, 564
Staphylococcus 548
astrovirus 302
aureus 60, 88, 99, 100, 156,
281, 296, 553, 729, 732,
754, 757
bacteremia 398
infections 681
epidermidis 162, 549, 570
Staple sign 1125
Startle myoclonus 504
Static encephalopathy 633
Status epilepticus 524, 1125
management of 524
varies, etiology of 524
Steatorrhea 931, 1125
Steatosis, moderate-to-severe 323
Stem cell 423
Stenosis 190, 263, 284, 490
pulmonary 658
subglottic 76, 892
valvular 1022
Stensen's duct 729
Sterile pyuria 475
Sternberg sign 1084
Sternocleidomastoid muscle
tumor 859f
Steroid 135, 523, 774
beneficial effect of 564
hormone production,
enzyme of 578
resistance 460
sparing strategies 461
therapy 125

Still's disease 1047, 1125
Stillbirth 1125
Stimulation, form of 802
Stomach, dilated 240
Stool 772
cultures 537
examination 747
virus isolation 747
Storage iron depletion, first stage
of 378
Strabismus 1125
Strawberry hemangioma 870f,
871f
Streptococcal
aureus 155
cell wall proteins 1019
infection 781, 1027
eradication of 1027, 1028
organism 184
pharyngitis,
incidence of 1020
Streptococcus 296, 681, 733,
758, 1019
agalactiae 733
infection 1026
mitis group 156
mutans 156
pneumoniae 60, 99, 100, 362,
397, 440, 552, 723, 733
pyogenes 175, 754, 1109
infection 702
sanguis 156
viridans 155
Streptomyces pilosus 422
Streptomycin 127, 129, 130
Stress 183
Stridor 1125
Stroke 403, 486, 489, 490
acute ischemic 492
childhood 488
hemorrhagic 491
ischemic 491
neonatal nontraumatic
hemorrhagic 486
Sturge-Weber syndrome 524
Subdural effusion 560, 563
development of 556
Subzero temperature 718
Sucralfate 267
Sudden infant death
syndrome 266
Sugar salt solution 215
Sulfadiazine 1029, 1030

Sulfamethoxazole 222, 478, 793, 924
Sulfasalazine 1052
Sulfisoxazole 478, 1029, 1030
Sulfur-rich copper-binding protein, concentration of 322
Sunset sign 1126
Supine plain abdominal radiograph 291
Supportive care 765, 976
Supportive therapy 563
Supportive treatment 106, 848, 897
Suprapubic aspiration 475
Surfactant deficiency 888, 894, 898
Surfactant delivery, modes of 898, 899
Surfactant replacement therapy 898
   benefits of 899
   timing of 898
Surgery
   contraindications of 61
   high risk of 266
   indications of 136b, 307
Surgical therapy 758
Surgical treatment 202, 307, 593, 644
Surgical wound excision 764
Suture line 288
Sweating 709
Swelling 661, 949, 950, 979, 1069
   erythema 735
   generalized 449, 456, 916
   scrotal 356
Swollen
   knee 333, 929
   tissues 727
   wrist 929
Swyer-James-Macleod syndrome 56
Sydenham's chorea 183, 1025, 1027, 1028, 1120
Sympathetic nervous system 982
Synchronized intermittent mechanical ventilation 900
Syndactyly 865f
Syndrome of inappropriate antidiuretic hormone secretion 555, 604, 811
Synovial fluid
   aspiration 1051
   glucose 757

Synovial joint 753
Synovitis, toxic 757
Synthesis, cutaneous 930
Syphilis 815
   early congenital 663
   late congenital 665
   serologic tests for 669
Syphilitic hepatitis, manifestation of 665
Syringohydromyelia 1096
Systemic beta-2 agonists 41
Systemic inflammatory diseases 176
   response syndrome 312
Systemic lupus erythematosus 175, 355, 432, 441, 718, 1025, 1051

T

T4-binding globulin deficiency 622
Tachycardia 32, 68, 386, 760, 827, 1024
Tachypnea 32, 67, 100, 101, 177, 314, 386, 760, 791, 827, 861
   transient 249, 508, 894-896
Talipes 1099, 1100, 1126
   equinovarus 1101f
Tall stature 16, 1083, 1084
Talonavicular joint, dislocation of 1102
Tandler's theory 255
Target sign 241
Tarsal bones, realignment of 1104
Tarsal coalition 1102
Tay-Sachs disease 546, 548, 1126
T-cell subsets 1037
Technetium bone scan 984
Temper tantrum 1126
Temporomandibular joints 1046
Tender hepatomegaly 270, 386
Tenderness 226, 948
   abdominal 304
   local area of 1036
Tendon reflexes 866
Teniposide 987
Tenotomy 1103
Tension pneumothorax 809
Teratogenicity 1039
Teratoma 865, 986
Terbutaline 41
   intravenous 44
Teriparatide 1097

Testes
   abdominal 643
   ascending 642
   ectopic 641, 642
   intra-abdominal 644
   retractile 642-644
Testicular
   adrenal rest tumors 585
   dysfunction 580
   failure, idiopathic 577
   masses 663
   relapse 978
Testosterone 17, 577, 578, 913
   serum 636
   synthesis 577
Testotoxicosis 632
Tetanus 761, 762, 762f, 766
   diphtheria-pertussis 766
   management of 764
   neonatorum 760
   toxin 764
      phenomenal potency of 762
Tetrabenazine 507
Tetracycline 712
Thalassemia 382, 412, 414, 419, 423
   intermedia 417
   major 417
   minor 417, 418
   syndrome 413, 415
   trait 418
Thalidomide 1080
Thanatophoric dysplasia 1096
Thelarche 635f
   premature 635f
Theophylline 50, 815
Therapeutic diet 926
Thermal injury 362
Thermoneutral temperature 1126
Thiacetazone 130
Thiazides 464
   diuretics 353
Thomsen-Friedenreich antigen 442
Thoracic lymphadenopathy, course of 114
Thoracocentesis, diagnostic 81
Throat culture 1027
Thrombin generation 346
Thrombocytopenia 160, 368, 444, 445, 658, 675, 676, 706,

722, 773, 848, 876, 971, 1048, 1126
immune mediated 659
transient 660
Thrombocytopenic purpura 656, 722, 1078
acute infectious 671
Thrombocytosis, moderate 355
Thromboembolism 465
Thrombogenesis 155
Thrombopoietin levels 368
Thrombosis 389, 848
Thrombotic thrombocytopenic purpura 440
Thrush, oral 921f
Thumb
  printing 354
  sucking 1126
Thymolphthalein monophosphate 935
Thyroglobulin
  antibodies 22
  synthesis, defects of 619
Thyroglossal cyst 860f
Thyroid
  antibody studies 623
  aplasia 622
  areas 859
  cancer 619
  disease 367
  dysgenesis 618, 622
  dyshormonogenesis 622
  ectopy 622
  function tests 7, 12, 13
  gland 619
  hormone 623
    action 622
    amounts of 622
    concentration 622
    replacement therapy 633
    studies 637
    synthesis 618, 619
    transport 619, 622
  hypoplasia 622
  peroxidase 22
  problems 7
  stimulating hormone 7, 617, 618, 624, 913
    tests 914
  tissue, rudiments of 618
Thyroiditis 729
Thyrotoxicosis 633
  congenital 818
Thyrotropin
  deficiency 619

receptor-blocking antibodies 619
releasing hormone 622
Thyroxine 7, 617
  binding globulin
    deficiency 625
Tiagabine 522
Tibia, mild hypoplasia of 1102
Tibial nerve, posterior 1074
Ticarcillin 135
Tick-borne spirochete 560
Tiredness 148, 153, 173, 610
Tissue
  hypoxia 672
  perfusion 622
  testicular 578
Tizanidine 506
T-lymphocytes 1043
Tobramycin 61
Tocilizumab 1054
Todd's paralysis 528, 1126
Tofacitinib 1055
Togaviridae 654
Tone, active 868
Tongue 336, 617
  geographic 858f
  large 621
  thick 622
Tonic neck reflex 1126
Tonic-clonic seizures, generalized 517-519
Tonsillectomy 31
Tonsillitis, chronic 30
Tonsils, enlarged 27
Tooth extraction 342
Topiramate 523
Topotecan 988, 1004
TORCH infection 836
Total iron-binding capacity 381
Total leukocyte count 4, 27, 78, 153, 226, 245, 387, 653, 731, 751, 767, 812, 948
Toxacara
  canis 872
  catis 872
Toxic shock syndrome 781
Toxicity, acute 522
Toxin 761
Toxocara canis 1003
Toxoplasma 432
  gondii 702
Toxoplasmosis 667, 815
T-piece resuscitator 805
Trachea 68

Tracheal cytotoxin 787
Tracheitis 791
  bacterial 75
Tracheoesophageal fistula 6, 314, 317, 318f, 892
Tracheomalacia 73
  degree of 316
Traction theory 56
Tranexamic acid 371
Transcatheter device 147
Transcriptase polymerase chain reaction, reverse 728
Transcutaneous bilirubin 838
Transferrin saturation 378
Transfusion therapy 419
  chronic 410, 416
  guidelines for 420
  risk for 420
Transfusional iron overload leads 421
Transfusions 419, 420, 678
  complications of 410
Transient lower esophageal sphincter relaxation 260
Transient macular generalized rash 674
Transillumination test 856
Transsphenoidal pituitary microsurgery 600
Trauma 603
  setting of 177
Traumatic postintubation 318
Traveler's diarrhea 223
Tremors 827
Trendelenburg gait 1126
Treponema pallidum 662
Triamcinolone
  acetonide 1054
    intra-articular injections of 1052
  hexacetonide 1052
Trichuris trichiura 376
Tricuspid regurgitation 146
Trientine 329
Triethylene tetramine dihydrochloride 329
Triglycerides 449, 1049
Trihexyphenidyl 507
Triiodothyronine 7, 617
Trilateral retinoblastoma syndrome 999
Trimethoprim 222, 478, 562, 793
Tripod sign 746, 747

Trismus 1126
Trisomy 64
Tropheryma whipplei 157
Trophic feeding 1126
Trophozoites 705
Trümmerfeld zone 943
Trypsin 311
Tuber cinereum, hamartoma of 633
Tubercle 118
    bacilli, lymphohematogenous seeding of 117
Tuberculin
    syringe 124
    test 60, 115, 124
Tuberculoid leprosy 1071
Tuberculoma 1126
    paradoxical development of 120
Tuberculosis 55, 108, 109, 120, 121, 132, 134, 136*b*, 917, 959, 1064
    abdominal 116
    cardiac 120
    childhood 127*t*
    clinical features of 113*f*
    congenital 120
    cryptic miliary 124
    drug-resistant 134
    drugs for 128, 130*t*
    endobronchial 131
    flaring of 791
    genitourinary 131
    intestinal 116
    meningeal 1119
    mesenteric 116
    miliary 117, 131, 1120
    mycobacterium 87, 99, 109, 120, 175, 733, 1070
    primary 112
    pulmonary 112
    renal 117
    screening 1049
    skeletal 117
    trauma 175
Tuberculous meningitis 119, 560, 630
    clinical progression of 119
Tuberculous pleurisy, clinical onset of 115
Tubex test 772
Tubular damage, ischemic 706
Tubular necrosis,
    acute 220, 605, 1105

Tumors 288, 600, 700
    bilateral 1012
    dissemination of 986
    embryonal 1008
    formation loss 999
    hypothalamic 603
    intraocular 999
    metastatic 603
    necrosis factor 110, 1068
        alpha 1036, 1054
    primary 982
    virilizing 591, 638
Tunica vaginalis, hydrocele of 864
Turner's syndrome 18-20, 149, 581, 625, 1127
Twins, monozygotic 387
Twin-to-twin transfusion 800
Tympanic membrane 89
    inflammation of 89
    perforation 89, 90
Tympanitic sound 545
Tympanocentesis 90, 95
Tympanometry 13, 89
Tympanosclerosis 90
Typhidot test 772, 773
Typhoid 122, 711, 767
    diagnosis of 768
    fever 275, 768, 770
Tyrosine kinase Janus kinase 2 959
Tzanck preparation 679, 680, 1127
Tzanck test 684

U

Ulceration 1036
Ulcerative colitis 21, 56
Ultrasonography 179, 180, 249, 256, 476, 547, 756, 1010, 1063
    abdominal 676, 985
Ultrasound 231
    pelvic 581
    scan 985
Ultraviolet light
    examination 820
    source 710
Umbilical artery, single 855
Umbilical cord 862
Underweight 17, 382, 406
Undescended testes 248, 640, 642
    true 642
Upper gastrointestinal contrast study 256

fluoroscopy 238
radiography 263
tract 672
Upper limbs, muscles of 920
Upper respiratory tract
    epithelium of 726
    infection 34, 68, 288, 676, 732, 751
    viral 87
Urea cycle disorder arginase deficiency 501
Uremia 175
Uremic state,
    manifestation of 447
Ureteropelvic junction obstruction 21
Urethral catheterization 475
Urinalysis 456
Urinary 17-hydroxycorticosteroid excretion 598
Urinary 17-hydroxyprogesterone 584
Urinary 17-ketosteroid 589, 598
Urinary antigen 103
    tests 104
Urinary copper levels 327
Urinary intestinal fatty acid-binding protein 309
Urinary retention 536
Urinary tract
    abnormalities 256
    catheterization of 477
    infection 122, 209, 467, 472, 474*fc*, 480, 711
        diagnosis of 475*t*
        recurrent 472
        risk factors for 470
    malformation of 20
Urinary trypsin activation peptide, measurement of 313
Urine 160, 598, 772
    albumin 449
    chromatography of 502
    culture 154, 475, 839
    examination 473
    free cortisol 913
        excretion 598
    microscopy 474
    osmolality 601, 604
    output 437, 891
    routine 584, 601
    specific gravity 601
Urogenital sinus 578
Uropathy, obstructive 473, 605

Uveitis 683
    chronic anterior 1051
    treatment 1053

V

Vacuole, intracellular 768
Vaginal delivery 725, 751
Vaginal discharge 812
Vaginal mucosa, examination
    of 636
Valacyclovir 684, 685, 703
Valproic acid 531
Valsalva ruptured sinus 171
Valvar dysfunction 164
Valvular dehiscence 160
Valvular disease 656
Valvulitis 1024
    murmurs of 1022
Van Wyk-Grumbach
    syndrome 633
Vancomycin 83, 163, 564, 758
Vanillylmandelic acid 985
    urinary 979
Varicella 682, 684, 776, 777, 782
    pneumonia 781
    syndrome, congenital 780
    virus 777
    zoster
        immunoglobin 681
        virus 353, 680, 779, 780
Varicelliform rashes 779
Vascular arteriolar aneurysm 55
Vascular disease, severe
    pulmonary 202
Vascular infiltration,
    inflammatory 665
Vascular intimal proliferation 395
Vascular lesion 633
Vascular rings 315
Vasculature, pulmonary 246
Vasculitis 119, 1046, 1053
    acute leukocytoclastic 353
    syndrome 1051
    systemic 432
Vasodilator 194
    therapy 251
Vasopressin 602-604
    analogs 608
    aqueous 608
    deficiency 602
        causes of 603
    gene 603
    insensitivity 602
    response test 607
    secretion of 604

Vasopressors 193
Vater ampulla 255
Vein of Galen
    malformation 543, 569
Vena cava
    inferior 1006, 1010
    superior 142, 969, 982
Venereal Disease Research
    Laboratory 661, 667
Ventilation 749, 806
    rates 806
    strategies 250
Ventilator support 403
Ventricular septal defect 6, 143,
    153, 154, 196, 197, 200,
    248, 658
Ventriculitis 560
Ventriculoperitoneal
    shunt 548, 549
Ventriculostomy, endoscopic
    third 570
Venturi effect 156
Vernix caseosa 854, 871
Vertebral fractures 1093
Vertex vaginal delivery 855
Vertical sleeve gastrectomy 915
Vesicometeric reflux 1127
Vesicular lesion 679
Vesicular rash 680f
Vessel changes 708
Vibrios 222
Vigabatrin 521-523
Vinblastine 960-962
Vince alkaloids 372
Vincristine 372, 462, 952, 960-962,
    975, 987, 988, 1004,
    1012, 1014
Viral capsid antigen 701
Viral infection 35, 690, 1042
    evidence of 175
Viral pathogens 88
Viremia 681
Viridians streptococci 156
Virologic tests 692
Virus 99
    fecal excretion of 273
    infection 722
    isolation 651, 676
Visceral larva 872f
    migrans 872
Visceromegaly 1008
Vision, dimness of 750
Visual assessment 833t
Visual problems 500

Vitamin 924
    A 724, 924
        dose of 927
    B 920, 921
        complex factors,
            deficiencies of 921
    C 422, 940
        deficiency 941, 943
        role of 422
        supplements 943
    D
        dependent rickets 938
        disorders 930
        levels 937
        restores, supplementation
            of 931
        synthesis 930
    D3, dose of 938
    D deficiency 929, 930, 934
        congenital 930
        diagnosis of 936
        nutritional 930, 937
        secondary 930
        severe maternal 930
    dependent factors,
        concentration of 348
    E 904
    fat-soluble 915, 936
    K 348
        absorption 347
        antagonists 347
        deficiency 346, 936
        high levels of 351
        therapy 351
        transient deficiency of 347
Vitiligo 1077
Vitreoretinopathy, familial
    exudative 1003
Voiding cystourethrogram 581
Volkmann canals 734
Volutrauma 888
Vomiting 101, 211, 212, 226, 253,
    396, 473, 533, 979
    post-tussive 786
    risk of 76
von Gierke disease 1127
von Hippel-Lindau
    disease 1127
    gene 389
von Willebrand's disease 335,
    1127
von Willebrand's
    factor 333, 334, 1037

W

Waldeyer ring 29
Warm saline mouthwash 729
Warning signs 346
Warthin-Finkeledy cells 718
Water deprivation test 607
Waterston's shunt 194
Weak cry 812
Weakness 614
    first sign of 510
    relentless progression of 511
Weaning 649
Webbed neck edema 20
Wegener's granuloma 1127
Wegner sign 667
Weight
    bearing bones 117
    deficit 923
    loss 274, 610, 614, 949, 950, 1038
Welcome trust classification 918
West syndrome 506, 522
Western blot 692, 756
Wet-to-dry soaks 685
Wharton's duct 727
Wheezing 35, 67, 113, 1127
    audible 314
    recurrent 33
White blood cells 469, 736, 756, 771
White reflex 1002, 1127
White sclera 1095
Whole cow's milk protein 385
Whole-body positron emission tomography 950
Widal test 772, 773
Williams syndrome 10
Wilms' tumor 577, 986, 1006, 1008
    develops 1007
    lesions 1009
    radiotherapy of 1013
    thrombus 1009
Wilson's disease 185, 275, 321-323, 326, 328, 330, 362, 1025, 1110
    diagnosis of 327
    hallmark of 325
    hepatic manifestations of 325
    manifestation of 324
Wilson's trait 324
Wilsonian hepatic disease, forms of 324
Wimberger sign 943, 1127
Wiskott-Aldrich syndrome 1127
Wolff-Parkinson-White syndrome 1113
Wolfram syndrome 602, 604
Wormian bones 1092, 1093
Worms, treatment of 383
Wound 341, 732
    contaminated 733
    infection 915, 1064
Wrists
    broad 934*f*
    widening of 929, 932*f*, 934*f*

X

X chromosome 15, 19, 20, 602
X polysomies 580
Xerophthalmia 924, 927, 1127
Xiphoid retractions 893
X-linked lymphoproliferative disease 700
X-linked recessive
    disorder 625
    inheritance 509
    trait 509, 1112

Y

Y chromosome 577
Yeast 157
Yellow fever 676
Yellow nail syndrome 56
Yersinia 222, 228, 353, 421
Young syndrome 56

Z

Zellweger syndrome 237, 239
Zidovudine 692, 695
Ziehl-Neelsen method 1076
Ziehl-Neelsen stain 110, 122, 123, 1077
Zika virus 534
Zinc 329
    administration 223
    deficiency 924
    elemental 329
    oxide plaster 1103
    supplementation 223, 925
        role of 924
    therapy 223
Zoonosis 1127
Z-score 1086, 1087
Zygote 705